# The American Psychiatric Publishing
# Board Review Guide for Psychiatry

# The American Psychiatric Publishing
# Board Review Guide
# for Psychiatry

Edited by

**James A. Bourgeois, O.D., M.D.**
**Robert E. Hales, M.D., M.B.A.**
**Julie S. Young, M.D.**
**Stuart C. Yudofsky, M.D.**

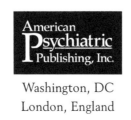

American
Psychiatric
Publishing, Inc.

Washington, DC
London, England

Copyright © 2009 American Psychiatric Publishing, Inc.
ALL RIGHTS RESERVED

Manufactured in the United States of America on acid-free paper
13  12  11  10  09      5  4  3  2  1
First Edition

Typeset in Adobe's Frutiger and Janson.

American Psychiatric Publishing, Inc.
1000 Wilson Boulevard
Arlington, VA 22209-3901
www.appi.org

**Library of Congress Cataloging-in-Publication Data**
The American Psychiatric Publishing board review guide for psychiatry / edited by James A. Bourgeois...
[et al.]. — 1st ed.
     p. ; cm.
   Includes bibliographical references and index.
   ISBN 978-1-58562-297-9 (alk. paper)
   1. Psychiatry—Examinations—Study guides. 2. Neurology—Examinations—Study guides. 3. American Board of Psychiatry and Neurology. I. Bourgeois, James. II. Title: Board review guide for psychiatry.
   [DNLM: 1. Psychiatry—Examination Questions. WM 18.2 A5121 2009]
   RC343.5.A44 2009
   616.890076—dc22

                                                                                      2009008172

**British Library Cataloguing in Publication Data**
A CIP record is available from the British Library.

# Contents

## Section I
## Basic Clinical Science

# Section II
# Psychiatric Disorders

# Section III
# Treatments and Special Topics

# Section IV
# Exams and Answer Guides

# Contributors

**Berry Anderson, B.S.N., R.N.**
Clinical Research Manager, Central Study Coordinator for National Institute of Mental Health Optimization of Transcranial Magnetic Stimulation for the Treatment of Depression (OPT-TMS Depression) Study, Brain Stimulation Laboratory, Institute of Psychiatry, Medical University of South Carolina, Charleston, South Carolina

**Linda B. Andrews, M.D.**
Associate Dean for Graduate Medical Education, Associate Professor, Menninger Department of Psychiatry and Behavioral Sciences, Baylor College of Medicine, Houston, Texas

**L. Jarrett Barnhill, M.D.**
Professor of Psychiatry and Director of the Developmental Neuropharmacology Clinic, Department of Psychiatry, Division of Child and Adolescent Psychiatry, University of North Carolina, Chapel Hill, North Carolina

**Aaron T. Beck, M.D.**
Professor of Psychiatry, University of Pennsylvania School of Medicine, Philadelphia, Pennsylvania

**Judith V. Becker, Ph.D.**
Professor of Psychology and Psychiatry, Department of Psychology, The University of Arizona, Tucson, Arizona

**Heather A. Berlin, Ph.D., M.P.H.**
Assistant Professor, Department of Psychiatry, Mount Sinai School of Medicine, New York, New York

**Jed E. Black, M.D.**
Associate Professor, Sleep Medicine Division, Stanford University; Medical Director, Stanford Sleep Medicine Clinic, Stanford, California

**Jeffrey J. Borckardt, Ph.D.**
Assistant Professor, Departments of Psychiatry and Anesthesiology, Medical University of South Carolina, Charleston, South Carolina

**James A. Bourgeois, O.D., M.D., F.A.P.M.**
Alan Stoudemire Professor of Psychosomatic Medicine, Department of Psychiatry and Behavioral Sciences, University of California, Davis Medical Center, Sacramento, California

**Daniel J. Buysse, M.D.**
Professor of Psychiatry and Clinical and Translational Science; Director, Clinical Neuroscience Research Center, University of Pittsburgh School of Medicine, Pittsburgh, Pennsylvania

**Cameron S. Carter, M.D.**
Professor of Psychiatry and Psychology; and Director, Imaging Research Center, University of California, Davis, School of Medicine, Sacramento, California

**Prabhakara V. Choudary, Ph.D., F.R.S.C.**
Professor of Psychiatry and Behavioral Sciences, Center for Neuroscience, University of California, Davis, California

**John F. Clarkin, Ph.D.**
Clinical Professor of Psychology-Psychiatry, Weill Cornell Medical College, The New York Presbyterian Hospital, White Plains, New York

**Cheryl M. Corcoran, M.D., M.S.P.H.**
Florence Irving Assistant Professor of Psychiatry, Department of Psychiatry, Columbia University at New York State Psychiatric Institute, New York, New York

**Laura B. Dunn, M.D.**
Associate Professor of Psychiatry, University of California, San Francisco, California

**Marc D. Feldman, M.D.**
Clinical Professor of Psychiatry and Behavioral Sciences, Department of Psychiatry and Behavioral Medicine, University of Alabama, Tuscaloosa, Alabama

**Ronald E. Fisher, M.D., Ph.D.**
Assistant Professor, Departments of Radiology and Neuroscience, Baylor College of Medicine, Houston, Texas; Director of Nuclear Medicine, The Methodist Hospital, Houston, Texas

**Milton J. Foust Jr., M.D.**
Assistant Professor of Psychiatry, Director, Electroconvulsive Therapy Program, Medical University of South Carolina, Charleston, South Carolina

**Albert C. Gaw, M.D.**
Clinical Professor, Department of Psychiatry, University of California San Francisco, California

**Ralph J. Gemelli, M.D.**
Clinical Associate Professor of Psychiatry, George Washington University School of Medicine, Washington, DC; Adjunct Professor of Psychiatry, Uniformed Services University of the Health Sciences, F. Edward Hébert School of Medicine, Bethesda, Maryland

**Mark S. George, M.D.**
Distinguished Professor of Psychiatry, Radiology, and Neurosciences; Director, Medical University of South Carolina (MUSC) Center for Advanced Imaging Research; Director, Brain Stimulation Laboratory; MUSC Director, South Carolina Brain Imaging Center of Excellence; Chairman, National Institute of Mental Health Optimization of Transcranial Magnetic Stimulation for the Treatment of Depression (OPT-TMS Depression) Study

**John G. Gunderson, M.D.**
Professor of Psychiatry, Harvard Medical School, Boston; and Director, Psychosocial and Personality Research, McLean Hospital, Belmont, Massachusetts

**Robert E. Hales, M.D., M.B.A.**
Joe P. Tupin Endowed Chair, and Professor and Chair, Department of Psychiatry and Behavioral Sciences, University of California-Davis School of Medicine, Sacramento, California

**Katherine A. Halmi, M.D.**
Professor of Psychiatry, Weill Cornell Medical College, White Plains, New York

**Steven P. Hamilton, M.D., Ph.D.**
Associate Professor, Department of Psychiatry, University of California–San Francisco, San Francisco, California

**Brian T. Harel, Ph.D.**
Postdoctoral Fellow, Department of Neurology, University of Iowa Hospitals and Clinics, Iowa City, Iowa

**Eric Hollander, M.D.**
Professor of Psychiatry; Director, Seaver and NY Autism Center of Excellence; Director of Clinical Psychopharmacology; Director, Compulsive, Impulsive, and Anxiety Disorders Program; Mount Sinai School of Medicine, New York, New York

**Jinger G. Hoop, M.D.**
Assistant Professor, Department of Psychiatry and Behavioral Medicine, Medical College of Wisconsin, Milwaukee, Wisconsin

**Diane B. Howieson, Ph.D.**
Associate Professor of Neurology and Psychiatry, Oregon Health and Science University, Portland, Oregon

**Robin A. Hurley, M.D., F.A.N.P.A.**
Associate Chief of Staff, Mental Health, W.G. "Bill" Hefner VAMC, Salisbury, North Carolina; Director, Education, VISN 6 Mental Illness Research, Education and Clinical Center, and Associate Professor, Departments of Psychiatry and Radiology, Wake Forest University School of Medicine; Clinical Associate Professor, Baylor College of Medicine, Salisbury, North Carolina

**Bradley R. Johnson, M.D.**
Assistant Professor of Psychiatry, University of Medicine College of Medicine, Tucson, Arizona; and Chief of Psychiatry, Arizona Community Protection and Treatment Center, Arizona State Hospital, Phoenix, Arizona

**John A. Joska, M.D., M.Med.(Psych.), F.C.Psych.(S.A.)**
Senior Specialist and Lecturer, Department of Psychiatry and Mental Health, University of Cape Town, South Africa

**Paul H. Kartheiser, M.D.**
Attending Physician, Child and Adolescent Psychiatry, Central Regional Hospital-Raleigh Campus, Raleigh, North Carolina; Assistant Professor of Psychiatry, Division of Child and Adolescent Psychiatry, Department of Psychiatry, University of North Carolina, Chapel Hill, North Carolina

**H. Florence Kim, M.D.**
Assistant Professor, Menninger Department of Psychiatry and Behavioral Sciences, Baylor College of Medicine, Houston, Texas

**Kimberly G. Klipstein, M.D.**
Director, Behavioral Medicine and Consultation Psychiatry, Department of Psychiatry, and Assistant Professor of Psychiatry, Mount Sinai School of Medicine, New York, New York

**James A. Knowles, M.D., Ph.D.**
Professor of Psychiatry, Zilkha Neurogenetic Institute, Menninger Department of Psychiatry, Baylor College of Medicine, South Central MIRECC, Department of Veterans Affairs, Houston, Texas

**Susan G. Lazar, M.D.**
Adjunct Professor, Department of Psychiatry, George Washington University School of Medicine, Washington, D.C.; Adjunct Professor, Department of Psychiatry, Uniformed Services University of the Health Sciences, F. Edward Hébert School of Medicine, Bethesda, Maryland; Training and Supervising Analyst, Washington Psychoanalytic Institute, Washington, D.C.

**Martin H. Leamon, M.D.**
Associate Professor of Clinical Psychiatry, Department of Psychiatry and Behavioral Sciences, University of California, Davis; Medical Director, Sacramento County Mental Health Treatment Center, Sacramento, California

**Raphael J. Leo, M.D.**
Associate Professor, Department of Psychiatry, State University of New York at Buffalo, School of Medicine and Biomedical Sciences; Buffalo, New York

**Muriel D. Lezak, Ph.D.**
Professor Emerita, Neurology, Oregon Health and Science University, Portland, Oregon

**Dolores Malaspina, M.D., M.S.P.H.**
Anita and Joseph Steckler Professor of Psychiatry, New York University and Adjunct Professor of Clinical Psychiatry, Columbia University, New York, New York

**José R. Maldonado, M.D., F.A.P.M., F.A.C.F.E.**
Associate Professor of Psychiatry and Behavioral Sciences; Chief, Medical and Forensic Psychiatry Section; Director, Medical Psychotherapy Clinic, Department of Psychiatry and Behavioral Sciences, Stanford University School of Medicine; Medical Director, Consultation/Liaison Service, Stanford University Medical Center, Stanford, California

**Lauren B. Marangell, M.D.**
Distinguished Scholar, Eli Lilly and Company Indianapolis, Indiana

**James M. Martinez, M.D.**
Clinical Research Physician, Eli Lilly and Company, Indianapolis, Indiana; Assistant Professor of Psychiatry, and Associate Director, Mood Disorders Center, Menninger Department of Psychiatry, Baylor College of Medicine, South Central MIRECC, Department of Veterans Affairs, Houston, Texas

**Melissa Martinez, M.D.**
Assistant Professor of Psychiatry; Interim Director, Mood Disorders Center, Menninger Department of Psychiatry, Baylor College of Medicine, Houston, Texas

**A. Kimberley McAllister, Ph.D.**
Associate Professor of Neuroscience, Center for Neuroscience, University of California–Davis, Davis, California

**Joel McClough, Ph.D.**
Independent Practice, Reston, Virginia

**Barbara E. McDermott, Ph.D.**
Associate Professor of Clinical Psychiatry, University of California, Davis School of Medicine, Department of Psychiatry and Behavioral Sciences, Division of Psychiatry and the Law, Sacramento; Research Director, Clinical Demonstration/Research Unit, Napa State Hospital, Napa, California

**Andrew H. Miller, M.D.**
William P. Timmie Professor of Psychiatry and Behavioral Sciences, Emory University School of Medicine, Atlanta, Georgia

**Michael J. Minzenberg, M.D.**
Assistant Professor, Imaging Research Center, University of California, Davis, School of Medicine, Sacramento, California

**Hugh Myrick, M.D.**
Associate Professor of Psychiatry, Medical University of South Carolina, Ralph H. Johnson VAMC, Charleston, South Carolina

**Ziad H. Nahas, M.D., M.S.C.R.**
Associate Professor; Director, Mood Disorders Program; Medical Director, Brain Stimulation Laboratory, Medical University of South Carolina, Charleston, South Carolina

**Jeffrey H. Newcorn, M.D.**
Associate Professor of Psychiatry and Pediatrics and Director, Division of Child and Adolescent Psychiatry, Mount Sinai Medical Center, New York, New York

**Stephen C. Noctor, Ph.D.**
Assistant Professor, Department of Psychiatry and Behavioral Sciences, M.I.N.D. Institute, University of California, Davis School of Medicine, Sacramento, California

**Fred Ovsiew, M.D., F.A.N.P.A.**
Professor of Clinical Psychiatry and Behavioral Sciences, Feinberg School of Medicine, Northwestern University, Chicago, Illinois

**Brooke S. Parish, M.D.**
Assistant Professor of Psychiatry, Department of Psychiatry, University of New Mexico, Albuquerque, New Mexico

**Cameron D. Quanbeck, M.D.**
Assistant Clinical Professor of Psychiatry, University of California Davis Medical Center, Sacramento, California

**Stephen Rayport, M.D., Ph.D.**
Associate Professor of Clinical Neuroscience, Department of Psychiatry, Columbia University College of Physicians and Surgeons; Research Psychiatrist, Department of Molecular Therapeutics, New York State Psychiatric Institute, New York, New York

**Phillip J. Resnick, M.D.**
Professor of Psychiatry and Director, Division of Forensic Psychiatry, Case Western Reserve University School of Medicine, Cleveland, Ohio

**Robert G. Robinson, M.D.**
Paul W. Penningroth Chair, Professor and Head, Department of Psychiatry, University of Iowa College of Medicine, Iowa City, Iowa

**Scott Schobel, M.D.**
Postdoctoral Clinical Fellow, Department of Psychiatry, Columbia University College of Physicians and Surgeons, New York, New York

**Paul E. Schulz, M.D.**
Associate Professor of Neurology, Neuroscience, and Translational Biology; Vice Chair for Education; Director, Cognitive Disorders Clinics; Director, Neuropsychiatry and Behavioral Neurology Fellowship Department of Neurology, Baylor College of Medicine, Houston, Texas

**Charles L. Scott, M.D.**
Professor of Clinical Psychiatry and Chief, Division of Psychiatry and the Law, University of California, Davis School of Medicine, Department of Psychiatry and Behavioral Sciences, Division of Psychiatry and the Law, Sacramento, California

**Jeffrey S. Seaman, M.S., M.D.**
Residency Training Director, Associate Professor of Psychiatry, Department of Psychiatry and Behavioral Sciences, University of Oklahoma Health Sciences Center, Oklahoma City, Oklahoma

**Mark E. Servis, M.D.**
Roy T. Brophy Professor and Vice Chair for Education, Department of Psychiatry and Behavioral Sciences, University of California Davis, School of Medicine, Sacramento, California

**Daniel W. Shuman, J.D.**
Professor of Law, MD Anderson Foundation Endowed Professor of Health Law, Dedman School of Law, Southern Methodist University, Dallas, Texas

**Jonathan M. Silver, M.D.**
Clinical Professor of Psychiatry, New York University School of Medicine, New York, New York

**Daphne Simeon, M.D.**
Associate Professor, Co-Director, Compulsive Impulsive Disorders Program; Director, Depersonalization and Dissociation Program, Mount Sinai School of Medicine, New York, New York

**Robert I. Simon, M.D.**
Clinical Professor of Psychiatry; Director, Program in Psychiatry and Law, Georgetown University School of Medicine, Washington, D.C.; Chair, Department of Psychiatry, Suburban Hospital, Bethesda, Maryland

**Andrew E. Skodol, M.D.**
Research Professor of Psychiatry, University of Arizona College of Medicine, Tucson, Arizona

**Stephen M. Sonnenberg, M.D**
Clinical Professor, Department of Psychiatry, Baylor College of Medicine, Houston, Texas; Adjunct Professor, Department of Psychiatry, Uniformed Services University of the Health Sciences, F. Edward Hébert School of Medicine, Bethesda, Maryland; Training and Supervising Analyst, Houston–Galveston Psychoanalytic Institute, Austin, Texas

**David Spiegel, M.D.**
Willson Professor and Associate Chair of Psychiatry and Behavioral Sciences, Department of Psychiatry and Behavioral Sciences, Stanford University School of Medicine, Stanford, CA

**Sergio E. Starkstein, M.D., Ph.D.**
Professor of Psychiatry and Clinical Neurosciences, University of Western Australia, Fremantle, Australia

**Dan J. Stein, M.D., Ph.D.**
Professor and Chair, Department of Psychiatry, University of Cape Town, South Africa

**Jill D. Stinson, Ph.D.**
Licensed Psychologist, Sex Offender Treatment Coordinator, Fulton State Hospital, Fulton, Missouri

**James J. Strain, M.D.**
Professor of Psychiatry, Mount Sinai School of Medicine, New York, New York

**Katherine H. Taber, Ph.D., F.A.N.P.A.**
Assistant Director for Education, VISN 6 Mental Illness Research, Education and Clinical Center; Research Health Scientist, W.G. "Bill" Hefner VAMC, Salisbury, North Carolina; Research Professor, Division of Biomedical Sciences, Edward Via Virginia College of Osteopathic Medicine, Blacksburg, Virginia; Adjunct Associate Professor, Department of Physical Medicine and Rehabilitation; Baylor College of Medicine, Houston, Texas

**Michael E. Thase, M.D.**
Professor of Psychiatry, Department of Psychiatry, University of Pennsylvania School of Medicine, Pittsburgh, Pennsylvania

**Daniel Tranel, Ph.D.**
Professor of Neurology and Psychology, Division of Behavioral Neurology and Cognitive Neuroscience, Department of Neurology, University of Iowa College of Medicine, Iowa City, Iowa

**Amy M. Ursano, M.D.**
Assistant Professor of Psychiatry; Associate Training Director, Child and Adolescent Psychiatry, Department of Psychiatry, Division of Child and Adolescent Psychiatry, University of North Carolina, Chapel Hill, North Carolina

**Robert J. Ursano, M.D.**
Professor and Chairman, Department of Psychiatry, Uniformed Services University of the Health Sciences, F. Edward Hébert School of Medicine, Bethesda, Maryland; teaching faculty, Washington Psychoanalytic Institute

**W. Martin Usrey, Ph.D.**
Associate Professor of Neurology, Center for Neuroscience, University of California–Davis, Davis, California

**Elisabeth A. Wilde, Ph.D.**
Assistant Professor, Department of Physical Medicine and Rehabilitation, Baylor College of Medicine, Houston, Texas

**John W. Winkelman, M.D., Ph.D.**
Assistant Professor of Psychiatry, Harvard Medical School, Boston, Massachusetts; Medical Director, Sleep Health Center, Brigham and Women's Hospital, Brighton, Massachusetts

**Jesse H. Wright, M.D., Ph.D.**
Professor and Chief of Adult Clinical Psychiatry, University of Louisville, School of Medicine, Norton Psychiatric Center, Louisville, Kentucky

**Tara M. Wright, M.D.**
Assistant Professor of Psychiatry, Medical University of South Carolina, Ralph H. Johnson VAMC, Charleston, South Carolina

**Jong H. Yoon, M.D.**
Assistant Professor, Imaging Research Center, University of California, Davis, School of Medicine, Sacramento, California

**Julie S. Young, M.D.**
Fourth-Year Resident in General Psychiatry, Department of Psychiatry and Behavioral Sciences, University of California-Davis School of Medicine, Sacramento, California

**Stuart C. Yudofsky, M.D.**
D.C. and Irene Ellwood Professor and Chairman, Menninger Department of Psychiatry and Behavioral Sciences, Baylor College of Medicine; Chairman, Department of Psychiatry, The Methodist Hospital, Houston, Texas

**Sean H. Yutzy, M.D.**
Associate Professor of Psychiatry, Department of Psychiatry, University of New Mexico, Albuquerque, New Mexico

**Phyllis C. Zee, M.D., Ph.D.**
Professor of Neurology and Director, Sleep Disorders Center, Feinberg School of Medicine, Northwestern University, Chicago, Illinois

# Disclosure of Competing Interests

*The contributors have declared all forms of support received within 12 months prior to submission of the manuscript of the textbook chapter on which their chapter in the present volume is based that may represent a competing interest, as follows:*

**L. Jarrett Barnhill, M.D.**—*Consultant:* Abbott, GlaxoSmithKline; *Speakers' Bureau:* Ortho-McNeil.

**Aaron T. Beck, M.D.**—The author may receive a portion of profits from sale of software "Good Days Ahead" for computer-assisted CBT discussed in this text. The publisher of the software is Mindstreet, LLC, Louisville, KY.

**Jed E. Black, M.D.**—*Consultant/Grant Support:* Takeda, Boehringer-Ingelheim, Jazz Pharmaceuticals, GlaxoSmithKline, Cephalon.

**Jeffrey J. Borckardt, Ph.D.**—*Grant Support:* National Institute of Neurological Disorders and Stroke, Cyberonics, Neurosciences Institute.

**Daniel J. Buysse, M.D.**—*Consultant/Speakers' Bureau:* Actelion, Cephalon, Eli Lilly, GlaxoSmithKline, Merck, Neurocrine, Neurogen, Pfizer, Respironics, Sanofi-Aventis, Sepracor, Servier, Stress Eraser, Takeda.

**Mark S. George, M.D.**—*Grant Support/Speakers' Bureau:* GlaxoSmithKline, Parke-Davis; *Consultant:* Aventis, Jazz Pharmaceuticals, Argolyn Pharmaceuticals, Abbott; *Formal Research Collaborations:* Dantec (Medtronic); Clinical Research *Grant/Consultant:* Neutonus (now Neuronetics); *Grant Support/Speakers' Bureau/Advisory Board:* Cyberonics; Advisory Board: NeuroPace; *Grant Support/Advisory Board:* Cephos.

**Robert E. Hales, M.D., M.B.A.**—Chair of industry-sponsored symposia sponsored by Bristol-Myers Squibb and AstraZeneca at the 2007 and 2008 APA Annual Meetings, respectively.

**Eric Hollander, M.D.**—*Grant Support:* Pfizer, Ortho-McNeil, Abbott.

**Bradley R. Johnson, M.D.**—*Speakers' Bureau:* AstraZeneca, Forest Pharmaceuticals.

**Lauren B. Marangell, M.D.**—*Grant Support:* Bristol-Myers Squibb, Eli Lilly, Cyberonics, Neuronetics, National Institute of Mental Health, Stanley Foundation; *Consultant/Honoraria:*

Eli Lilly, GlaxoSmithKline, Cyberonics, Pfizer, Medtronic, Forest, Aspect Medical Systems, Novartis.

**James M. Martinez, M.D.**—*Research Support:* Aspect Medical Systems, AstraZeneca, Bristol-Myers Squibb, Cyberonics, Eli Lilly, Forest Pharmaceuticals, Neuronetics, Sanofi-Aventis, National Institute of Mental Health, Stanley Foundation; *Speakers' Bureau:* AstraZeneca, Bristol-Myers Squibb, Cyberonics, Eli Lilly, Forest Pharmaceuticals, GlaxoSmithKline, Janssen, Pfizer, Wyeth Ayerst; *Consultant:* Cyberonics.

**Melissa Martinez, M.D.**—*Research Support:* Cyberonics, Eli Lilly, Sanofi-Aventis, Aspect Medical Systems, Bristol-Myers Squibb, Neuronetics.

**Andrew H. Miller, M.D.**—*Grants/Research Support:* National Institute of Mental Health, National Heart, Lung and Blood Institute (NHLBI), GlaxoSmithKline, Janssen, Schering-Plough. *Consultant:* Centecor, Schering-Plough

**Michael J. Minzenberg, M.D.**—*Research Support:* Elan, Cephalon.

**Ziad H. Nahas, M.D., M.S.C.R.**—*Grant Support:* National Institute of Mental Health, Neuronetics, Cyberonics, Medtronic, Eli Lilly, Neurospace; *Consultant:* Neuronetics, Cyberonics, Avanir Pharmaceutical, Aventis Pharmaceutical, Neuropace; *Speakers' Bureau:* Cyberonics.

**Jeffrey H. Newcorn, M.D.**—*Advisory Board/Consultant:* Abbott, McNeil, Eli Lilly, Shire, Novartis, Cortex, Pfizer, Lupin; *Research Support:* McNeil, Eli Lilly, Shire, Novartis; *Speakers' Bureau:* Novartis, Shire

**Brooke S. Parish, M.D.**—*Financial Interest/Stock Ownership:* 100 shares, Merck.

**Jeffrey S. Seaman, M.S., M.D.**—*Clinical Trials:* Bristol-Myers Squibb, Cephalon.

**Paul E. Schulz, M.D.**—*Speakers' Bureau:* Pfizer, Forest Pharmaceuticals.

**Jonathan M. Silver, M.D.**—*Consultant:* Novartis. *Speaker:* Avanir.

**Dan J. Stein, M.D., Ph.D.**—*Grant Support/Consultant Honoraria:* AstraZeneca, Eli Lilly, GlaxoSmithKline, Lundbeck, Orion, Pfizer, Pharmacia, Rocher, Servier, Solvay, Sumitomo, Wyeth.

**Michael E. Thase, M.D.**—*Advisory/Consultant:* AstraZeneca, Bristol-Myers Squibb, Cephalon, Cyberonics, Eli Lilly, GlaxoSmithKline, Janssen, MedAvante, Neuronetics, Novartis, Organon, Sepracor, Shire US, Supernus, Wyeth; *Speakers' Bureau:* AstraZeneca, Bristol-Myers Squibb, Cyberonics, Eli Lilly, GlaxoSmithKline, Organon, Sanofi Aventis, Wyeth; *Expert Testimony:* Jones Day (Wyeth litigation), Phillips Lytle (GlaxoSmithKline litigation); *Equity Holdings:* MedAvante, Inc.

**Robert J. Ursano, M.D.**—*Consultant:* Abbott, GlaxoSmithKline; *Speakers' Bureau:* McNeil.

**John W. Winkelman, M.D., Ph.D.**—*Advisory Board/Speakers' Bureau:* Boehringer-Ingelheim, Cephalon, GlaxoSmithKline, Pfizer, Sanofi-Aventis, Sepracor, Schwarz-Pharma, Takeda.

**Jesse H. Wright, M.D., Ph.D.**—The author may receive a portion of profits from sale of software "Good Days Ahead" for computer-assisted CBT discussed in this text. The publisher of the software is Mindstreet, LLC, Louisville, KY.

**Stuart C. Yudofsky, M.D.**—Co-chairman for educational symposium at the 2007 American Psychiatric Association Annual Meeting sponsored by Bristol-Myers Squibb.

**Phyllis G. Zee, M.D.**—*Consultant/Advisory Board:* Boehringer-Ingelheim, GlaxoSmithKline, Jazz, Sanofi-Aventis, Takeda.

*The following contributors stated that they had no competing interests during the year preceding submission of the manuscript for the textbook chapter on which their chapter in the present volume is based:*

Berry Anderson, B.S.N., R.N.
Linda B. Andrews, M.D.
Judith V. Becker, Ph.D.
Heather A. Berlin, D.Phil., M.P.H.
James A. Bourgeois, O.D., M.D., F.A.P.M.
Cameron S. Carter, M.D.
Prabhakara V. Choudary, Ph.D., F.R.S.C.
John F. Clarkin, Ph.D.
Cheryl M. Corcoran, M.D., M.S.P.H.
Laura B. Dunn, M.D.
Marc D. Feldman, M.D.
Ronald E. Fisher, M.D., Ph.D.
Milton J. Foust Jr., M.D.
Albert C. Gaw, M.D.
Ralph J. Gemelli, M.D.
John G. Gunderson, M.D.
Katherine A. Halmi, M.D.
Steven P. Hamilton, M.D., Ph.D.
Brian T. Harel, Ph.D.
Jinger G. Hoop, M.D.
Diane B. Howieson, Ph.D.
Robin A. Hurley, M.D., F.A.N.P.A.
John A. Joska, M.D., M.Med.(Psych.), F.C.Psych.(S.A.)
Paul H. Kartheiser, M.D.
H. Florence Kim, M.D.
Kimberly G. Klipstein, M.D.
James A. Knowles, M.D., Ph.D.
Susan G. Lazar, M.D.
Martin H. Leamon, M.D.
Raphael J. Leo, M.D.
Muriel D. Lezak, Ph.D.
Dolores Malaspina, M.D., M.S.P.H.

José R. Maldonado, M.D., F.A.P.M., F.A.C.F.E.
A. Kimberley McAllister, Ph.D.
Joel McClough, Ph.D.
Barbara E. McDermott, Ph.D.
Hugh Myrick, M.D.
Stephen C. Noctor, Ph.D.
Fred Ovsiew, M.D., F.A.N.P.A.
Cameron D. Quanbeck, M.D.
Stephen Rayport, M.D., Ph.D.
Phillip J. Resnick, M.D.
Robert G. Robinson, M.D.
Scott Schobel, M.D.
Charles L. Scott, M.D.
Mark E. Servis, M.D.
Daniel W. Shuman, J.D.
Daphne Simeon, M.D.
Robert I. Simon, M.D.
Andrew E. Skodol, M.D.
Stephen M. Sonnenberg, M.D.
David Spiegel, M.D.
Sergio E. Starkstein, M.D., Ph.D.
Jill D. Stinson, Ph.D.
James J. Strain, M.D.
Katherine H. Taber, Ph.D., F.A.N.P.A.
Daniel Tranel, Ph.D.
Amy M. Ursano, M.D.
W. Martin Usrey, Ph.D.
Elizabeth A. Wilde, Ph.D.
Tara M. Wright, M.D.
Jong H. Yoon, M.D., Ph.D.
Julie S. Young, M.D.
Sean H. Yutzy, M.D.

# Preface

Like its predecessor, *The American Psychiatric Publishing Board Prep and Review Guide for Psychiatry*, this volume, *The American Psychiatric Publishing Board Review Guide for Psychiatry* is intended to assist psychiatrists and residents in psychiatry in preparation for Part I of the American Board of Psychiatry and Neurology (ABPN) Examination in Psychiatry and similar specialty-specific examinations in other nations. It is also intended to assist psychiatrists in preparing for their maintenance of certification examination in psychiatry. Candidates are reminded that, although the Part I Examination covers both psychiatry and neurology, this volume focuses on psychiatry topics primarily. Several chapters address illnesses best conceptualized as being in the "psychiatry-neurology interface." Nonetheless, candidates are advised to seek out similar review texts and other source material for more detailed preparation for the neurology section of the examination.

Compared with the previous work, this volume, at 966 pages, is significantly expanded (the previous volume was 478 pages). Section I (Chapters 1–13) covers background basic science/neuroimaging, child development, psychometric measures, cultural and legal aspects of psychiatric illness, psychiatric interviewing, use of the clinical laboratory, and neuroimaging. There has been an effort by the volume editors to increase the detail and make greater use of tables and images throughout these background chapters.

Section II (Chapters 14–29) comprises syndrome-specific chapters that parallel the DSM-IV-TR psychiatric illness categories and, as with the scientific background chapters (Chapters 1–13), address the phenomenology and treatment of these illnesses in greater depth than our previous review book.

Section III (Chapters 30–39) includes chapters on psychopharmacology, other somatic treatments, psychotherapy, pain, suicide, violence, and ethics. All of these topics are, as in the basic science and clinical syndromes chapters, covered in greater depth and with updates reflecting the current state of the literature. Two additional chapters illustrating neuropsychiatric illness—traumatic brain injury and cerebrovascular disease—have been added for several reasons: a) these illnesses serve as illustrative models of neuropsychiatric conditions; b) with the aging of the population, these illnesses are more frequently encountered the general clinical practice of psychiatry; and c) with the current military actions in Iraq and Afghanistan, and

with their aftermaths that will persist for decades, these disorders will be prominent among psychiatrists practicing in the Department of Defense and Veterans Affairs systems, and for many other psychiatrists who care for patients in other clinical venues.

The other major structural difference between this volume and the previous work is the addition of, in Section IV, two practice examinations (each with at least 200 questions) and accompanying answer guides, following the chapters. The editors have eliminated the review questions at the end of each chapter in favor of a more realistic format in which the questions are commingled in a manner similar to the structure of the actual board examinations. The majority of these questions have been adapted from several APPI review texts. The editors emphasize that not all questions will have answers that are necessarily found within the chapters of this text; however, all questions are fully referenced in other materials. Candidates seeking additional questions and annotated answers to enhance their preparation are referred to referenced publications or to the corresponding online self-assessments (available at www.cme.psychiatryonline.org).

While it is not possible to cover all material in psychiatry required for clinical mastery, or to navigate, successfully, the Part I Examination in Psychiatry, the editors have endeavored to provide, in a single volume, a sufficiently detailed overview that may serve as a primary source for psychiatry candidates. The material herein was originally published as part of two APPI texts: *The American Psychiatric Publishing Textbook of Psychiatry* (Fifth Edition); and *The American Psychiatric Publishing Textbook of Neuropsychiatry and Behavioral Neurosciences* (Fifth Edition).

The chapters in these volumes are intended to correspond (as much as was practical in the editing process) to topics specifically mentioned in the Psychiatry Section content of the American Board of Psychiatry and Neurology (www.abpn.com) *2009 Description of Part I Examination in Psychiatry.* Chapter authors in the original source textbooks are, in most cases, carried forth in the chapters in this volume. In the chapters that are derived from more than one of the original texts, all original chapter authors are cited in a combined fashion. Authors who participate in the actual board examination process (either Part I or Part II) have had their names deleted so that they may continue to participate in such examinations.

The outline of this volume begins with background material needed to provide an overview of the clinical syndromes and clinical management covered later. There is an inherent tension between efficiency and comprehensiveness in preparing a volume of this sort. It is likely that specific material likely to be encountered on the Part I Examination is not covered here at a level of detail sufficient to please (or at least to allay the examination-related anxiety of) every candidate. On the other hand, a volume that seeks to be "completely" comprehensive runs the risk of excessive length, and impracticality by not providing sufficient emphasis on the more critical topics for study. For optimal benefit from this volume, the editors suggest that the reader use this book as a primary source for board preparation, with the candidate availing himself or herself of the textbooks upon which this book is based.

There is no substitute for excellent medical school training followed by a well-developed and executed psychiatry residency program in preparing psychiatrists for the Part I Examination. It is assumed by the editors that candidates are already well-versed in the most important clinical literature of the field and familiar with key data from several major texts in psychiatry. In addition, comprehensive clinical experience is necessary to answer Part I Examination questions based upon clinical presentations of psychiatric syndromes. Candidates often view the ABPN examinations as a daunting challenge. Indeed, with increasing emphasis on successful board certification as a "rite of passage" in the academic psychiatric community, as well as a desirable qualification for inclusion in insurance reimbursement programs, board certification is probably more important now than ever before. As such, focus on successful passing of this examination (not to mention later success on the Part 2 Examination) should ideally begin early in training and continue throughout residency, and beyond.

Patterns of lifelong learning and active maintenance of clinical knowledge is the current stock in trade in the profession. Indeed, psychiatry has been at the forefront of requiring periodic recertification and commitment to lifelong learning. Psychiatric lifelong learning CME activities such as the American Psychiatric Publishing, Inc.'s journal *FOCUS* exemplify this commitment. The editors have long experience in educating medical students and resident physicians, and it is our experience that residents who have internalized lifelong learning habits are more likely to be successful on the APBN Part 1 Examination.

Ideally, this book provides an organized and cogent review of material that is already mastered to some degree by psychiatrists who are primarily in need of active review in advance of board examinations. The editors share particular concern and empathy for otherwise well-qualified psychiatrists who, nonetheless, have had previous difficulty in passing the Part I Examination. Such candidates, perhaps, are especially in need of a single text to serve as a main study guide, to be supplemented by original source material in more comprehensive textbooks. In addition, this volume may be of utility to psychiatry residents who wish to prepare for the Psychiatry Residency in Training Examination (PRITE), which, by virtue of its similar content areas, may serve as a proxy for the later ABPN Part 1 Examination. We are also hopeful that the book will be helpful in the identification of strengths and weaknesses in categorical areas of psychiatric knowledge.

Correspondingly, neurologists who are candidates for the Neurology Examination of ABPN are likely to find this volume use in their preparation for the Psychiatry Section content of their examination. We also hope that our international colleagues in psychiatry and neurology find this book to be of assistance in preparing for their nations' specialty examinations. Finally, the editors believe this volume will prove to be helpful to mid-career psychiatrists and neurologists in their navigation of periodic recertification specialty examinations.

The editors wish to thank the thoughtful and dedicated chapter authors of the APPI books and study guides from which the material in this book was derived. Without their efforts and efficiency, we could not have compiled such a current, concise, and clinically-validated volume. These chapter authors' work represents the best of psychiatric scholarship, and we have been honored to combine their work in a volume that we hope is a vital instrument for the preparation for board examinations for the next generation of our colleagues who follow us in service to the specialty of psychiatry, the profession of medicine, and, most important, the patients and their families whom we serve.

*James A. Bourgeois, O.D., M.D.*
*Robert E. Hales, M.D., M.B.A.*
*Julie S. Young, M.D.*
*Stuart C. Yudofsky, M.D.*

# Section I

# Basic Clinical Science

1

# Normal Child and Adolescent Development

## RALPH J. GEMELLI, M.D.

Developmental tasks have been defined (Erikson 1959) for each phase of the life cycle from infancy through adulthood (Table 1–1).

## Infancy Phase of Mental Development (Birth to Age 18 Months)

### Major Developmental Tasks of Infancy

1. Infants develop the awareness that they are separate from and are valued and loved by their parents.
2. Infants develop the awareness that their parents can be trusted to feed, shelter, protect, and stimulate them in more emotionally pleasurable than emotionally displeasurable ways. (needs)
3. Infants develop the awareness that they are engaged in relationships with their parents in which both act and react to each other. ( ⇌ )

### Functions of the Social Environment

Throughout all phases of the life cycle, five functions support parents as they engage to provide a dynamically changing, developmentally enhancing, transactional goodness of fit with their children.

### *Providing Truthful Information About the Infant's Body and Surrounding World*

One major developmental task of infancy for infants is to become aware that they can trust their parents (Erikson 1959). Parents instill such a sense of trust in their infants by becoming consistently reliable conveyors of truthful information about the world the infant has entered (Magnusson and Allen 1983).

### *Providing Stimulus Modulation and Protection*

Parents also provide the social function of modulating the quality of the stimulation to which their infant is exposed so that they can keep the overall stimulation within the infant's optimal range. For example, they must protect their infant from the following:

1. Receiving too much stimulation.
2. Receiving insufficient stimulation.
3. Receiving overly repetitive and potentially monotonous stimulation.
4. Receiving stimulation in a sensory modality that the infant will process into perceptions that are overstimulating.

### *Providing Encouragement, Support, and Admiration*

Infants will turn to their parents for behavioral and emotional feedback when they are in the midst of or have

| TABLE 1–1. Developmental phases and key tasks | | |
|---|---|---|
| **Developmental phase** | **Key task** | **Associated normogenic belief** |
| Infancy (birth–18 months) | Basic trust | "I trust my parents and others." |
| Toddlerhood (18 months–3 years) | Autonomy | "I like to explore, but sometimes I get afraid when I can't see my mom or dad." |
| Early childhood (3–6 years) | Curiosity | "I am very curious, and my parents like that." |
| Late childhood (6–12 years) | Industry | "I like to show my friends what I can do." |
| Adolescence (12–19 years) | Identity | "I know who I am, and I'm not exactly like my parents." |

recently completed a behavior stimulated by one of their innate needs, new maturational advances, or new developmental achievements. Parents must respond to these infant behaviors with encouragement and admiration.

### Providing Truthful Information About Achieving Gratification of Innate Needs

Although infants are preprogrammed to gratify their own innate needs, they do not know what knowledge they must acquire and what behaviors they must master in order to become a productive member of society; nor do they know how they must adapt the expression of their innate needs and maturationally emerging capabilities to society's rules and guidelines.

### Providing Adaptive Solutions to Emotionally Displeasurable Life Events

Parents try to protect their children from traumatic experiences. However, children gradually discover that benignly emotionally displeasurable experiences are a part of life and that their parents are not omnipotent in being able to spare them from these experiences.

## The Organizational Mental Structures of the Id, Ego, Superego, and Self

Freud (1923/1963) conceptualized the mind as developing into three major structures: the id, ego, and superego.

### Id

The id, as the "container" of the infant's innate needs, has the goal of generating psychological stimuli (defined as sensory stimuli emanating from within the infant's mind).

### Ego

The ego is the collection of the individual infant's emotions, temperamental characteristics, and cognitive, verbal, and physical capabilities. The ego receives biopsychosocial stimuli and engages these stimuli in a transactional and transformational process with the mind's prior representations and conceptions and then generates mental and behavioral "products" or information.

### Superego

The superego—or its synonym, the conscience—is another "container" of specific mental functions. The superego's functions, however, are organized under the goal of providing the developing child with an inner source of familial and societal rules and standards, as well as an inner source of self-esteem. Unlike the id and ego, which are viewed as existing from birth, the superego does not begin to function fully as an effective internal authority over the id and ego until about age 5 years.

### Self

Viewed as present from birth, the fourth complex organizational structure is the *self*. The self is defined as the supraordinate organizational structure of the mind; according to this view, it exerts overriding control of the id, ego, and superego. The self not only occupies the conscious mental domain but also occupies, or has ongoing access to, the preconscious and unconscious mental domains. As such, the self, not the ego, becomes the *source of agency* of the child's developing mind.

## Maturation and Development of Innate Needs: The Oral Phase

### Satisfying Innate Needs

From birth to age 18 months, infants seek oral sensual stimulation and gratification (Brenner 1965). The sensual pleasure achieved through oral stimulation motivates infants to use their mouths to acquire new knowledge about biological stimuli (e.g., the oral mucosa and the tongue) and social stimuli (e.g., the mother's breast nipple). Freud (1923/1963) called this period of development the *oral phase* and labeled infants' sensual pleasure as *oral eroticism*.

### Signaling When Innate Needs Are Not Met

Crying—an innate behavior that triggers socializing transactions between an infant and parents or caregivers—has been proposed by several developmentalists (Ainsworth et al. 1978; Bowlby 1969; Lamb 1981) to be an innate capability that generates an innate or preprogrammed response in other humans (both children and adults), especially the infant's parents, who are biologically ready to enter into an emotional state of mind in reference to their infant that is very similar to the innate and emotional reactions to the initial stage of falling in love (Mayes 2006). When adult caregivers respond appropriately and consistently to infants' crying signals, infants learn to perceive their caregivers as predictable and reliable soothers of their distress.

### Human Motivation: The Central Role of Emotions

The pleasurable emotions (joy, excitement, pleasurable anxiety) that infants begin to experience in activating certain transactions with their parents and being allowed by their parents to assert themselves are the major motivators in infants' continued assertiveness in seeking new stimuli. Being assertively active and reactive within a transactional relationship with each parent whom an infant is learning to trust is one of the major developmental tasks of infancy.

## Maturation and Development of Physical Capabilities

### Reflexive Abilities

Two tactile reflexes are especially important in early infant–parent transactions: 1) the sucking reflex, stimulated by stroking the infant's lips, which causes the infant to produce a sucking movement of the lips and mouth; and 2) the rooting reflex, produced by stroking the infant's cheek or lips, which causes the infant to turn his or her head toward the stimulus and initiate a snapping movement with the mouth.

### Perceptual Abilities

**Visual.**  Shortly after birth, infants show a preference for disks with facial patterns painted on them over disks with

| TABLE 1–2. | Piaget's phases of cognitive maturation and development |
| --- | --- |
| Sensorimotor phase (birth to age 2 years) | |
| Preoperational phase (ages 2–7 years) | |
| Concrete operational phase (ages 7–12 years) | |
| Formal operational phase (age 12 years and onward) | |

nonfacial patterns (Fantz 1963; Kagan 1984). Also, by this age, infants are more attracted to a moving rather than a stationary face (Girton 1979).

**Auditory.**  Fantz (1961) and Hutt et al. (1968) showed that within the first days of life, infants preferentially respond to sounds that demonstrate auditory patterns similar to human speech over other types of sounds.

**Olfactory.**  Infants' innate abilities to form olfactory perceptions also show an early preferential bias for, and a discrimination of, human tastes.

## Maturation and Development of Cognitive Capabilities

According to Piaget, there are four major phases of cognitive maturation and development, each of which is qualitatively and quantitatively different from the preceding phase (Table 1–2). This phasic theory has been labeled *epigenetic* because Piaget fostered a theory of genetic epistemology, which is the "study of the manner in which a subject comes to attain objective knowledge of the world" (Case 1992).

### Acquiring Knowledge in the Sensorimotor Phase

1.  Infants' innately endowed reflexive apparatuses are not only exquisitely reactive to any available sensory stimulation but also active in seeking out more and more complex stimuli with which to interact.
2.  Newborns' and growing infants' perceptions trigger innate reflexive surface behaviors.
3.  Once an inborn reflex has been activated, an infant's maturing mind seeks to repeat the reflex.
4.  Infants continue to acquire knowledge and learn by acting on and reacting to their environment; in this way, motor actions become the initial basic triggers for acquiring new knowledge. The repetition of these behaviors makes up a set of experiences that eventually become an internal mental representation called a

*nipple schema*. This schema then becomes a new unit of knowledge for the infant.

5. Infants are motivated to initiate action when existing schemata cannot be used to integrate and comprehend new perceptions. This process of acquiring new knowledge by changing a preexisting schema into a new schema involves the following mental processes:

   a. *Habituation*—According to the *habituation principle*, when infants become selectively focused on a stimulus that appears novel in some way, their response to that stimulus will decrease over time as the stimulus is repeated without producing noxious effects.
   b. *Assimilation*—In effect, assimilation helps the infant achieve a sense of pleasure in knowing and mastering an external experience by making it equal to an existing inner experience.
   c. *Accommodation*—An infant's or child's accommodations are always limited by the cognitive phase he or she has reached developmentally.
   d. *Circular reaction*—In this mental process, which can sometimes be observed behaviorally, an infant continues trying to assimilate a new object into an old schema, and then eventually accommodates the new perception into a new schema.

## Maturation and Development of Temperamental Characteristics

*Temperament* can be defined as the style in which infants express the following temperamental characteristics (Goldsmith et al. 1987):

1. *Activity*, in stimulating the environment.
2. *Reactivity*, in responding to environmental stimulation.
3. *Emotionality*, in terms of the thresholds of stimulation that generate each emotion, the behavioral style in which each emotion is expressed, the intensity of each emotion, and the time it takes to return levels of stimulation to the infant's optimal stimulation range and thereby achieve emotional self-regulation.
4. *Sociability*, in terms of initiating social responses from others and responding to social communications.

## Maturation and Development of Emotions

### Role of Emotions

Infants at birth are capable of generating several distinct emotions in response to sensory stimuli. Their primary emotions are joy, fear, anger, sadness, disgust, and surprise. These emotions are characterized both by their early appearance and by their attendant prototypic and universal facial expressions (Lewis and Brooks-Gunn 1979).

### Parents' Interpretations of Infants' Emotions

Infants' emotions are open to interpretation by their parents and are strongly influenced by the parents' aspirations, beliefs, and projections of their own feelings, given that pre-self-aware infants do not possess an objective sense of being separate selves in a world of parents and others.

### Infants' Ability to Perceive Others' Emotions

Emde (1983) noted that pre-self-aware infants are able to perceive emotional information emanating from their parents and to use this information for emotional referencing. This ability to engage in emotional referencing propels infants to spontaneously seek and actively scan their parents' faces for emotional information as they assertively seek a novel stimulus, demonstrating infants' ever-present need to use their parents' emotions to help them regulate their own levels of stimulation so that they remain within their optimal stimulation range.

## Development of the Self and Object Relationships

### Developing Self-Value While Engaging in Transactional Relationships With Others

Kohut and Wolf (1978) defined *selfobject* as an object that is experienced as part of oneself and that one expects to control in the same manner that one controls one's own body and mind. Pre-self-aware infants perceive their parents as being both separate objects and a part of their own self-absorbed experience—that is, as selfobjects.

Normally developing infants and children are thought to need their parents to function as both *idealizing* and *mirroring selfobjects* (Kohut 1971, 1977; Kohut and Wolf 1978). Eventually, children learn to perform these mirroring and idealizing social functions for themselves. However, when parents fail to provide these functions in early life, children can grow up with serious deficits in their ability to provide these functions for themselves.

As idealizing selfobjects, parents fulfill the infants' need to idealize and otherwise view the parents as all-powerful and perfect. As mirroring selfobjects, parents fulfill the infant's need to be given and to receive acceptance and admiration for his or her performances, something that pre-self-aware infants cannot provide for themselves because they are unable to recognize their own competencies. Infants then incorporate this parental acceptance and admiration into their gradually developing self-representation. If infants do not receive this acceptance and admiration, they will not begin to establish a sense of self-value and will fail to develop self-esteem.

## Developing a Sense of Separateness

**Transactions related to infants' innate needs.** Infants discover their true selves when they begin to construct representations of their innate needs, emotions, temperamental characteristics, and cognitive abilities as belonging to themselves and come to believe (through experiences with their parents) that they will be respected and gratified.

**Low-stimulation, everyday caretaking activities with parents.** Other experiences that lead to infants' development of a sense of separateness while engaged in relationships with their parents are those that take place when infants are relatively quiet and unstimulated.

**Bodily contact.** Infants experience a sense of separateness when they are engaged in transactional relationships with their parents that involve the infants' body wholeness. *Body wholeness* is a term used to describe each individual's "sense of being a nonfragmented, physical whole with boundaries and locus of integrated action" (Stern 1985, p. 71).

**Parental responses to infants' gender.** As infants develop their self-representations, giving rise to an objective self (at about age 18 months), they will construct an early gender representation. This early gender identity is the mental conceptual representation of how infants define themselves as being a member of the category male or female.

## The Attachment Relationship

An *attachment relationship* is the specific relationship that forms between infants and their parents in a particular context (Bowlby 1988). The *attachment context* is one in which infants are completely dependent on the specific behaviors of their parents for survival. In this mutually activating and stimulating relationship, socializing transactions occur between infants and their parents (Oppenheim and Goldsmith 2007).

## The Triadic Attachment Relationship

The older *dyadic model* of attachment has been gradually replaced by a newer *triadic model* that addresses the attachment relationship as taking place among the mother, the father, and the infant (Herzog 1982; Lamb 1981).

During the first 6 months of an infant's life, the father's attachment is both similar to and different from that of the mother. A father provides more physical, spontaneous interactions as well as more novel and complex behavioral interactions (Parke and Tinsley 1981). Greenberg and Morris (1974), however, found that fathers develop unique bonds to their infant within the first 3 days of the infant's life. They labeled this strong, emotionally positive bonding experienced by fathers as *engrossment*. An engrossed father experiences feelings of elation, preoccupation, absorption, and interest in his infant. Greenberg and Morris noted that engrossed fathers also reported a strong desire to look at, touch, and stimulate their infants.

Recent findings concerning shared father–mother attachment to the infant can be summarized as follows:

1. Infants can form multiple attachments; the strength of the attachment to each parent is a function of the quantity and quality of transactions with that parent.
2. A lower quantity of high-quality care provided by a parent is more important for attachment to the mother or father than a higher quantity of poor-quality care.
3. Fathers can fulfill traditional mother-only attachment roles. Data now exist that demonstrate a stronger attachment between the infant and the father when the mother spends less time with her infant.
4. In two-career families, when the husband has supported his wife's pursuit of a career, daughters often grow up believing that the female role presents an opportunity to develop both career and motherly ambitions.

**Maternal bonding.** *Maternal bonding* is defined as "the establishment of a long-lasting, affectionate attachment of a mother toward her infant as the result of the mother's skin-to-skin contact with her newborn during a hormonally sensitive period lasting for a few hours after birth" (Campos et al. 1983, p. 820).

**Maternal attunement.** Maternal attunement (Emde 1983; Stern 1985) is similar to father engrossment in that its etiology is thought to be a genetically induced, preprogrammed capacity in the mother that is released through the nurturing experience. *Attunement* is defined as the ability in the mother to "tune in" to her infant in a form of behavior that is more similar to matching than to imitation (Stern 1985).

### Phases in the Attachment Relationship

**Phase 1: emergent social responsiveness (birth–2 months).**  Much of the actual surface behaviors that transpire between infants and parents in this phase have to do with infants' achieving homeostasis. Thus, it appears that infants, even in their first 2 months of life, are transactional social beings.

**Phase 2: discriminating social responsiveness (ages 2–6 months): the social smile.**  At age 2 or 3 months, infants develop the ability to raise their heads, which allows them to further control and direct their visual gazing. Stern (1985) observed that "by controlling their own direction of gaze, [infants] self-regulate the level and amount of social stimulation to which they are subject" (p. 21).

A major maturational advance signifying the development of infants' perceptual discrimination associated with a growing internal mental representation of their parents is the appearance of the *selective social smile*. This smile is given preferentially to the parents or to other significant caregivers, including siblings, with whom the infant has been involved since birth. The selective smile can emerge anywhere between ages 4 weeks and 12 weeks, and it also indicates that the infant is capable of recognition memory.

**Phase 3: active seeking of proximity to primary caregivers (age 6 months and onward): psychological birth.**  In Mahler's (1975) theory, at about age 6 months, the infant's *psychological birth* occurs. Mahler noted that 6-month-old infants appear more alert and are more goal-directed in their assertive pursuits than before. These new behaviors, which for Mahler usher in the separation–individuation process, appeared to Mahler as indicating the infant's psychological birth, a sort of infant "hatching." Mahler divided the separation–individuation process into three subphases: 1) differentiation, 2) early practicing and practicing proper, and 3) rapprochement.

Another behavior that emerges at ages 5–6 months is wariness of strangers. Traditionally this has been designated as *stranger anxiety* or *stranger distress* (Emde et al. 1979). At this age, infants experience a displeasurable emotional state, manifested by their reaching out and seeking proximity to the mother or father, whenever a strange face appears in front of them.

A month or so after the emergence of stranger anxiety, at about age 8 months, infants manifest a new anxiety—

*separation anxiety*—or, as it is called by Kagan (1979), *separation distress*. At this stage, infants show fretfulness, reach out toward or seek proximity to a parent, and cry when a parent leaves them.

Bowlby (1988) phenomenologically described three principal patterns of attachment:

1. *Secure attachment*—The child is confident that his or her parents (or parent figures) will be available, responsive, and helpful should he or she encounter adverse or frightening situations; the pattern of attachment consistent with healthy development.
2. *Anxious resistant attachment*—The child is uncertain whether his or her parents will be available or responsive or helpful when called on.
3. *Anxious avoidant attachment*—The child has no confidence that when he or she seeks care, he or she will be responded to, but, on the contrary, expects to be rebuffed.

## Toddlerhood Phase of Mental Development (Ages 18 Months–3 Years)

### Major Developmental Tasks of Toddlerhood

By the end of toddlerhood, children will have constructed the following:

1. An autonomous identity, in that they believe that they are separate individuals who can be autonomous, despite their wish at times to be dependent on their parents or significant others.
2. A gender identity, in that they believe that they are either boys or girls.

### Functions of the Social Environment

In nurturing their toddler to develop autonomous and gender identities, parents must be attuned to and fulfill the following functions:

- Protect the toddler in his or her *assertive explorations* from experiencing too many episodes of distressful over- or understimulation.
- Teach the toddler how to gratify his or her *needs and wishes* within the family and social environment while keeping within the limits and rules set by the parents' society.

- Provide empathically attuned encouragement, support, and admiration for the toddler's growing *autonomy* while at the same time teaching the toddler that his or her autonomy has limits and restrictions.

## Maturation and Development of Innate Needs: The Anal Phase

In the toddlerhood phase—Freud's *anal and urethral phase*—the toddler's anal and urethral mucosa become the erogenous zones.

## Maturation and Development of Physical Capabilities

Between 18 months and 3 years, toddlers walk fairly well, experiment with running, and learn more each day about how their hands can manipulate new objects and parts of their own bodies.

## Maturation and Development of Cognitive Capabilities

### Emergence of Objective Self-Awareness

Kagan (1981, 1989) described the following behaviors that emerge between ages 17 and 24 months:

1. An appreciation of right and wrong, good and bad, valued and not valued.
2. The recognition, through inferential thinking, that results have causes.
3. The use of early forerunners of empathy to motivate and guide behaviors.
4. The beginning of construction of standards.
5. The use of verbal language to identify actions.
6. The ability to visually recognize one's separateness as a person.

### Continued Development of Conceptual Thinking

**Ability to symbolize.**   The ability to form symbols emerges with toddlers' maturation of conceptual thinking (Klein 1930/1975; Werner and Kaplan 1963).

**Ability to understand concepts expressed in verbal language.**   By age 2 years, toddlers' ability to form symbolic conceptions and learn words enables them to begin to store explicit memories—information encoded in verbal form; in visual, auditory, tactile, and olfactory perceptions and conceptions; or in a combination of these forms.

**Ability to form fantasies.**   Fantasies are constructed from the same ingredients as beliefs: current sensations, perceptions, thoughts, emotions, and wishes, as well as the memories of any or all of these, including earlier fantasies and beliefs that are associated with the current experience.

**Ability to form beliefs.**   A *belief* is a conception that establishes the relation between two or more inanimate objects, aspects of nature's laws, or people (Meissner 1992).

**Ability to form categories.**   A *category* can be defined as "the symbolic representation of the qualities shared by a set of events" (Kagan 1989, p. 230).

**Development of self-reflection.**   Toddlers develop the ability to revise old conceptions through a process called *self-reflection*.

**Use of primary process and secondary process thinking.**   The further development and differentiation of toddlers' *primary process* (magical, absence of logical connections) thinking from their *secondary process* (reality based, logical) thinking is enhanced by the development of their ability to 1) use self-reflective, intuitive, and logical thinking; 2) use verbal language; and 3) create and use symbols.

**Deferred imitation.**   During the period from 18 months to 3 years, toddlers begin to demonstrate what Piaget called *deferred imitation* (Piaget 1954/1981). In deferred imitation, instead of needing to imitate an observed behavior immediately, toddlers may spontaneously attempt to imitate and repeat the behavior at a later time, often hours and sometimes days later.

**Inability to understand conservation.**   Children are unable to understand the concepts of conservation of mass and number until about age 3 years.

**Psychic equivalence mode of viewing external reality.**   The inability to understand conservation of both mass and number points to a more general cognitive inability in toddlers: the inability to perceive two physical dimensions of an object and to understand that both dimensions are properties of the same object.

## Play

The function of play for toddlers is threefold:

1. To act out, in playful fantasy, a pleasurable life experience using toys, other adults, and children as symbols for the real experience, acquiring new knowledge in the process.
2. To practice delaying the behavioral or verbal expression of wishes and feelings that are causing developmental conflicts with parents.
3. To unconsciously attempt to reconstruct a pathogenic belief, especially one resulting from a traumatic experience.

## Maturation and Development of Temperamental Characteristics

Infants and toddlers undergo changes in temperament as a result of maturation of temperamental characteristics (Baldwin and Baldwin 1978). One such maturational change involves modifications in the child's optimal stimulation range and the point at which the child signals distress when he or she is over- or understimulated.

## Maturation and Development of Emotions

When a toddler achieves self-awareness and begins to recognize himself or herself as 1) a separate agent of assertive behaviors who expresses innate needs and interests in the environment, 2) a constructor of memories, 3) a possessor of an intact and whole body, and 4) a possessor of emotions in response to sensations and perceptions (Izard 1971, 1972), the toddler begins to construct emotional conceptions about his or her emotionally tinged experiences within the environment.

## Maturation and Development of Verbal Language Abilities

### Development of Verbal Language

Two components of toddlers' earliest language are syntax (the structure and rules of language) and semantics (the meaning of language).

### Speech as Facilitator of an Autonomous Identity

**An enhancer of self-esteem.**  A parent's image of his or her toddler is mirrored in how that parent speaks to the toddler. Parents' words communicate their esteem for their child. In time, toddlers learn that their words are valued and responded to by parents with love and support.

**A means of exhibiting self-assertion and autonomy.** Speech emerges at the same time that toddlers are furthering their locomotive skills, developing their ability to defer imitation and to symbolize, and discovering that they are separate people in a world of others. Also in the midst of these advances, toddlers are becoming more autonomous, and they revel in being able to assert their autonomy through use of the word "no."

**A means of expressing self and object (other) interdependence.**  In acquiring speech, toddlers discover that they can share so much more of what they perceive externally and internally.

**A vehicle to achieve self-inhibition and to demonstrate mechanisms of defense.**  Shortly after speech acquisition begins to accelerate (i.e., around age 2½ years), toddlers are observed to generate inner speech (i.e., speech not spoken before an audience) (Berk 1994). Toddlers typically repeat aloud the shoulds and should nots they have been taught by their parents, learned about from siblings and playmates, and arrived at through their own empathic and inferential thinking.

## Maturation and Development of the Preexisting Representational World

As toddlers begin to construct, store, and retrieve explicit memories, these become differentiated into two types: semantic memories and episodic memories (Nelson 1990). *Semantic memories* store information about abstract concepts or events in time (Siegel 1993). *Episodic memories* involve the retention of information about a child's life experiences.

## Development of the Self and Object Relationships

### Formation of a Gender Identity

In becoming aware of being a separate person who possesses a particular gender, toddlers, by age 2 years, are engaged in a process of *gender categorization*, forming early categories of what it means to be a boy or a girl (Meyer 1980).

Toddlers are propelled to identify with their same-gender parent; boys wonder about being a man just like their father, and girls wonder about being a woman just like their mother (Erikson 1963).

## *Mastery Over Bodily Functions: Toilet Training*

Toilet-trained toddlers possess within their self-representation a new awareness of their self-competency, self-agency, and self-responsibility.

## *Advances and Regressions in Achievement of Autonomy*

For every advance in a toddler's capabilities, parents can describe an episode in which their toddler gave up that advance and returned to an earlier behavior. This return is called *regression*.

## *The Rapprochement Subphase of Separation–Individuation*

As toddlers experience the joy of being autonomous explorers and experimenters, they struggle with the gradual realization that their growing autonomy from their parents does not protect them from experiencing stranger and separation anxiety. In addition, parents do not always positively mirror and admire their toddler's explorations and new experiments.

This period, which occurs approximately between ages 18 and 24 months, was labeled the *rapprochement subphase* by Mahler (1975) in her separation–individuation developmental theory. The use of the term *rapprochement* (or its synonym, *reconciliation*) points to the need for toddlers to get through this relative "breakup" with their parents.

In addition, because toddlers want to view their parents as all-powerful protectors, they are slowly constructing an *ideal object representation* of each parent. This representation is an internal view of the parents the way toddlers wish their parents could be. In conjunction with constructing ideal object representations—which exist concurrently with toddlers' more general object representations of loving, admiring, and supportive parents—toddlers also construct an *ideal self-representation* that exists concurrently in their representational world with their more general self-representation. Toddlers' ideal self-representation is an internal view of themselves the way they wish they could be.

If, by about age 3 years, toddlers have had more loving than angry transactions with each parent, they will mentally integrate their good and bad representations of each parent and construct an *emotionally constant positive object representation* of each (Fraiberg 1969) (hereafter referred to as *positive object constancy*). In achieving this integration, they will possess an object representation of their mother and father as loving, admiring, and supportive even when that parent is angry with or absent from them.

## Development of the Superego

Through play, toddlers practice how to be social and construct beliefs about which behaviors are good versus which are bad. These beliefs can be called *standards* (Kagan 1984).

## Development of Adaptational Capabilities: New Defense Mechanisms

The defense mechanisms that emerge during toddlerhood are as follows:

- *Repression*—The unconscious automatic barring from consciousness of wishes, feelings, and memories that are associated with a highly displeasurable emotional state. When repression is fully effective, the repressed mental event is relegated to a toddler's unconscious but may be revived in the future by a sensation or perception that relates to the repressed mental content.
- *Projective identification*—An unconscious automatic process that is a primitive forerunner of the future capacity for empathy. In this process, a toddler unconsciously projects onto a parent or another person an intolerable mental possession and then, in inferring that the other person wishes, feels, or believes in accordance with the projected content, attempts to manipulate that person to show the projected wish, feeling, or belief (Kernberg 1976; Meissner 1980).
- *Projection*—The unconscious and automatic barring from one's consciousness of a wish, feeling, or belief while consciously being convinced that the wish, feeling, or belief is possessed by a parent or another.
- *Introjection*—The unconscious taking in of another's wish or feeling while consciously believing it is one's own.
- *Turning against the self*—Unconsciously and automatically barring from one's consciousness a wish, feeling, belief, or fantasy and then turning that mental content against oneself.
- *Identification*—According to Tyson and Tyson (1991, p. 329), *identification* is "changing the shape of one's self-representation to become more like the perception of an admired person or of some aspect of an admired person."

When used as a defense mechanism, identification allows toddlers to unconsciously affiliate themselves with parental behaviors that are causing them to experience repeated episodes of intensely displeasurable emotions, often at a traumatic level.

# Early Childhood Phase of Mental Development (Ages 3–6 Years)

By age 3 years, when children's representational worlds have begun to be "occupied" by representational composite images of both parents, memories of life experiences, and beliefs concerning emotions and rules of behavior, their minds will refer to and will be influenced by this inner world in processing more complex transactions involving biopsychosocial stimuli. Mental processing of biopsychosocial stimuli is thought to involve six steps:

1. Reception of biopsychosocial stimuli.
2. Generation of initial emotional responses and cognitive and emotional processing of transactions among biopsychosocial stimuli that evoke children's representational perceptions, conceptions, emotions, and memories.
3. Processing of mental contents into internal motivators that trigger generation of one or more of the following *initial output responses:*

   a. Initiating an action or surface behavior.
   b. Initiating speaking.
   c. Delaying acting or speaking while consciously and privately contemplating one's thoughts and emotions as internal "mental actions."
   d. Delaying acting or speaking while unconsciously activating a mental mechanism of defense, which usually involves behaving or talking in a certain way.
   e. Delaying acting or speaking while unconsciously activating the defense mechanism of somatization.

4. Activation of the capacity for self-in-relation-to-other observation.
5. Activation of the capacity for self-reflection.
6. Construction of a new representation involving final output responses and the responses or lack of responses from others in their social environment.

## Major Developmental Tasks of Early Childhood

If their first 3 years of life have gone reasonably well, children will continue to develop the following representations, which are part of their positive self-constancy and object constancy:

1. An *autonomous and valued identity.*
2. A *gender identity* as male or female.

Children's autonomous identity and gender identity are developed in the context of their belief that their parents can be trusted to continue to support, admire, protect, and love them. In addition, by age 3 years, young children begin to have experiences that enable them to construct the following additions to their self-representations, resulting in new pieces of their overall identity:

1. A *sexual identity*—A collection of beliefs, fantasies, and emotions that defines children's awareness of being able to seek sensual–sexual gratification from other individuals and that prohibits such gratification based on the rules of the family and society.
2. A *peer identity*—A collection of beliefs, fantasies, and emotions that defines children's awareness of being able to interact, cooperatively play, and negotiate conflicts with other children as a member of a peer group.
3. A *superego* or *conscience*—Children's dawning awareness that they can control their behaviors by choosing between right and wrong behaviors relatively independently of the presence of their parents.

## Functions of the Social Environment

### Fostering of Children's Healthy Narcissism in Conjunction With Their Developing Reciprocal Relationships With Others

In a mutually satisfying goodness-of-fit process, parents help their children to learn gradually that there are times that they can achieve a certain degree of gratification of their needs in a manner that is emotionally pleasurable and there are other times that the gratification of their needs must be delayed because such gratification places them in conflict with the wishes of their parents or others.

### Development of a True Self

Sensitively aware parents assist in their children's struggle to develop a true self vis-à-vis their periodically resurrected wishes to be perfect or to idealize their parents as being perfect in the following two ways:

1. Remaining aware of their child's aspirations, both conscious and unconscious, to be perfect.
2. Allowing their child both to periodically view him- or herself as perfect and to periodically view the parents as perfect.

### Healthy and Unhealthy Narcissism

*Narcissism* is generally defined as self-love (Tyson and Tyson 1984). *Healthy narcissism* is synonymous with toddlers' first objective awareness of being valued and loved by their parents. It leads to healthy self-esteem but also to children's development of esteem and love for their parents.

According to Kohut (1971), the central mechanisms "I am perfect" and "You are perfect, and I am a part of you" are the two basic narcissistic configurations used to preserve a part of the original experience of narcissistic perfection. Later, in the rapprochement phase, toddlers must face the developmental crisis of confronting limitations. They resolve this crisis by taking the "road" of emotional self-constancy and object constancy while still keeping within their minds a potential "detour," which is their "I am perfect" representation—their ideal self-representation—and their "You are perfect, and I am a part of you" representation—their ideal object representation. They use this "detour" to lead them to a periodic refuge from particularly tough days when they must face a limitation or a disappointment.

However, young children involved in a poorness of fit may develop a false self by staying permanently on the "I am perfect" or "You are perfect, and I am a part of you" road as they journey through childhood, adolescence, and adult life. Or, in the case of severe and sustained emotional and/or physical abuse, one or both parents may "inject" into the child's mind an "alien self." In response, the child will invariably generate a belief in his or her own omnipotence and will then continually attempt to control others, taking pleasure in their irritation, anger, or sadness in resisting or succumbing to his or her controlling and demeaning behaviors.

## Maturation and Development of Innate Needs: The Early Genital Phase

Freud (1923/1963) documented a progressive maturation of what he called children's *sexual drive*. This progression began with seeking sensual pleasure through oral mucosal stimulation (*oral phase*) and extended to seeking sensual pleasure through anal and urethral stimulation (*anal phase*), and then to seeking sensual and truly sexual pleasure through stimulation of the sexual organs (*phallic phase*).

## Maturation and Development of Physical Capabilities

From age 3 to age 5 years, there is a significant increase in children's body weight, size, and motor coordination—that is, walking and running abilities, hand–eye coordination, and leg–eye coordination (Ames and Ilg 1976a, 1976b, 1976c, 1979).

## Maturation and Development of Cognitive Capabilities: Maturing of the Mind's Executive Functions

In recent years, developmentalists have identified many of the cognitive functions that mature during the first 4 years of life and continue to be used by children. These functions, named *executive ego functions*, are used by the child's self, which I discussed earlier as the mind's superordinate or executive organizational structure.

## Maturation and Development of Temperamental Characteristics

Longitudinal studies of infant and child temperament (Chess and Thomas 1986; Kagan 1989) have found that some children will show continuity or temporal stability in certain temperamental characteristics they exhibited in infancy into their sixth year of life, whereas other children will show discontinuity or temporal instability between their infant temperamental characteristics and the temperamental characteristics they manifest by age 6 years.

## Maturation and Development of Emotions

### Construction of Rules for Emotional Display

In early childhood, children's emotions undergo significant maturation and development. As I described earlier, these maturational and developmental changes can be conceptualized within the framework of how emotions continue to be children's main organizers for 1) energy mobilization, 2) self-regulation, and 3) social adaptation, as well as for enhancing developmental change (Emde 1999).

### Emotions as Energy Mobilizers

As young children use both their unconscious implicit memories and their unconsciously repressed dynamic explicit memories as energy mobilizers in deciding to act or not act, they begin to learn more about what specific behavioral strategies they can use to express or withhold their emotions.

### Traumatic Emotional Memories as Unconscious Energy Mobilizers

Explicit emotional autobiographical memories of a traumatic experience will be relegated to a child's unconscious. The resulting *unconscious dynamic memory* does not lose its explicit content but instead becomes incorporated into the primary process thinking mode of the unconscious (Person 1995; Terr 1994).

### Emotions as Self-Regulators

In early childhood, children also use their emotions as organizers for developing their capacity for self-regulation. In this respect, they are assisted by a maturational advance occurring at about age 3 or 4 years, when they become able to consciously experience not only a wider range of emotions but also different *shades* of emotions (Lane and Schwartz 1987). Children now begin to become more proficient at using their own emotions as *internal signals of distress* and using the displeasurable emotions of their parents as their possible *external signals of distress*.

### Emotions as Facilitators of Social Adaptation

In the period from ages 3 to 5 years, children use their emotions as they continue to improve their social adaptation.

## Maturation and Development of Verbal Language Abilities

Starting around age 3 years, children begin to use thought, speech, and behaviors to achieve a belief in their own ability to anticipate and predict what will happen in the future. Also, they begin to remember their past—known as *reproductive memory*—and to ask questions of themselves and their parents about why things happened.

## Maturation and Development of the Preexisting Representational World

Between ages 4 and 5 years, children's mentalizing or self-reflective functions continue to develop. By age 4½ years, children have begun to engage in what will be a lifelong conscious and unconscious mental activity—the ordering of their own motivations from highest to lowest priority in terms of importance. Motives are hierarchically organized primarily on the basis of wished-for emotional states and feared emotional states (Westen 1997).

## Development of the Self and Object Relationships

### Development of a Sexual Identity: Emergence of the Early Genital Phase

In addition to continuing to learn what it means to be a boy or a girl in their society through continuing to de-

velop their gender identity, 3-year-old children begin to construct a *sexual identity*.

**Exhibitionism of genitals.**   In the initial unfoldings of the early genital phase, children are quite intensely exhibitionistic. In admiring their own clothed and nude body in the mirror, they are intensely joyous in receiving mirroring smiles of admiration from both parents.

**Curiosity about genitals.**   Parents begin to teach their children about the limits on their sexual curiosity; in the process, they teach them about a developmental task associated with constructing a sexual identity: the necessity of learning about body privacy.

**Body damage anxiety.**   Body damage anxiety is another of the developmental anxieties that Freud (1923/1963) defined as inevitable. It results from children fearing the possibility of a new developmental calamity in which their body is damaged, particularly their genitals or genital area.

**Choice of sexual object.**   Between ages 3 and 4 years, children begin to make a sexual object choice. This occurs as they begin to expand on their earlier masturbatory fantasies, which contained their early attractions to either the same gender or the opposite gender for sexual gratification.

**Emergence of the triangular phase.**   Young children's sexual object choice becomes the main organizer for their developing sexual identity, as well as a basic aspect of 4- to 5-year-old children's progression into the *triangular phase* (Mayer 1995; Tyson 1982). This was called the *oedipal phase* in the past.

The triangular phase is the phase during which the heterosexual child fantasizes about replacing his or her same-gender parent and engaging in an exclusive, sexually tinged relationship with his or her opposite-gender parent. It comprises a mixture of behaviors based on what children have learned—and carry within their object representations of their parents and others—about what constitutes being a man and a woman.

**Relative relinquishment of triangular wishes.**   Triangular wishes in heterosexual children decrease when children begin to put aside (but do not completely give up) their wishes to have what the same-gender parent has and do what the same-gender parent does.

A healthy resolution of the triangular phase in heterosexual children will enhance the identification process with the same-gender parent and other same-gender individuals in their lives.

### Development of a Peer Identity

It is during early childhood (ages 3–6 years) that the need for peer interaction becomes a crucial ingredient in fostering children's confidence in performing outside of their individual families and in taking the initiative in solving problems and resolving interpersonal conflicts.

## Development of the Superego

At about age 3 years, conventional morality begins (Kohlberg 1981). If the establishment of positive self-constancy and object constancy has led to children's construction of primarily loving object representations of their parents, children will be motivated to obey their parents' rules to keep receiving the love they have learned to expect. As the superego begins to come into being, children experience guilt when 1) they know what is a right and what is a wrong behavior, 2) they believe they have a choice between the two behaviors, and 3) they have made the bad choice. Children do not like guilt; it makes them feel they are bad and potentially unloved. In their first experiences of feeling guilty, they will try to blame someone else for their own wrong statement or behavior.

Children also begin to experience *superego anxiety*—that is, the anxiety they feel when they think about doing or saying something that is forbidden by their conscience. This superego anxiety is another internal distress signal that warns the child that guilt will ensue if a forbidden action or verbalization being considered by the child occurs.

## Development of Adaptational Capabilities

Repression is defined as an automatic unconscious mental process, viewed as an activity of children's ego under the direction of the self, that bars from their conscious awareness 1) wishes and feelings that, if gratified, would produce either parental (external) disapproval or superego (internal) disapproval (once the superego becomes an internal structure), and 2) memories of experiences that are associated with an intensely displeasurable emotional state. Repression begins to emerge at around age 18 months, but it does not become a predominant defense mechanism until children reach about the age of 3 years.

# Late Childhood Phase of Mental Development (Ages 6–12 Years)

## Major Developmental Tasks of Late Childhood

The major developmental tasks of late childhood are as follows:

1. To continue to add to and reconstruct a *peer identity*, particularly in being able to begin to relate cooperatively and competitively to peers in the formal grade-school setting
2. To construct a beginning *social identity* (the beginning belief that one is a member of various categories within one's society as a whole)

By ages 5½–7 years, children have developed the following components of their overall identity:

1. Autonomous identity.
2. Gender identity.
3. Sexual identity.
4. Peer identity.

Erikson (1963, 1968) proposed that from ages 6 to 11 years, children's developmental task is to develop a belief in their ability to be *industrious* and perform in front of peers instead of a belief of being *inferior* in front of peers and others.

## Development of a Social Identity

By age 5½ years, children are motivated to relate to their family group, playgroup, or class group, and they learn that they must follow rules and that they will be judged by the other members of the group. Group rules, standards, ethics, and principles become ingredients to be added to the child's developing superego. Once children (at ages 6–7 years) begin to use their superego anxiety signals as the "voice" of their parents when their parents are not around, they are truly becoming autonomously social.

## Functions of the Social Environment

The dominant triggering social variable in the biopsychosocial model of mental development from ages 6 to 11 years is the social requirement (in most countries, it is a law) for all children to attend school. In essence, going to school is the "job" of late childhood (Table 1–3).

**TABLE 1–3. Preparations for beginning first grade (ages 5½–6½ years)**

From infancy: "I trust my teachers."

From toddlerhood: "I feel good about being autonomous from my parents."

From early childhood: "I like being curious and assertively inquisitive."

Now: "I can be industrious and present my work to others, and I'll do well and be liked."

## Maturation and Development of Innate Needs

### Need for Fulfillment of Physiological Needs Related to Bodily Regulation and Physical Survival

One requirement for attending first grade is that children be able to take over the proper fulfillment of their physiological needs.

### Need to Assertively Explore the Social Environment

At about age 6 or 7 years, normally developing children appear to undergo what Shapiro and Hertzig (1988) called a *biodevelopmental shift*. This refers to children's maturation of physical, cognitive, language, emotional, and defense mechanisms that appear to fuel children's activation of the innate need to exhibit their autonomous identity in the social world.

### Need for Human Attachment in Emotionally Pleasurable Interactions

Children ages 5½–6½ years have developed positive self-constancy and positive object constancy, providing them with an inner representational world, or world of mind, that is a source of comfort during physical separations from the family. These self- and object-constant representations also lead them to generate *positive transference reactions* to new peers and teachers at school.

### Need for Emotionally Pleasurable Sensory–Sexual Stimulation and Gratification

Freud (1905/1963) labeled the period between ages 6 and 11 years as the period of *latency*—specifically, sexual latency. He believed that this was a period of relative "quietness" of sexual instinctual wishes in children, in which the children's oedipal (now renamed the *early trian-*

*gular*) wishes are beginning to be mastered and recede in prominence until puberty (ages 11–13 years), when some triangular wishes return and must be relinquished once again.

### Need to Signal Distress When Experiencing Emotionally Displeasurable Over- or Understimulation and to Initiate Other Fight-or-Flight Behavioral and Mental Responses

In late childhood, children become more able to organize how they activate distress signals and how they can tolerate more of a delay before activating a fight-or-flight response. New defense mechanisms maturationally emerge between ages 5½ and 11 years—namely, isolation of emotion, sublimation, reaction formation, and displacement. Fantasy formation also becomes a standard mechanism of defense. In addition, 5½- to 11-year-old children's ability to use both conscious thinking and unconscious defense mechanisms to delay action and ponder responses makes their representational world of stored knowledge more available to them than ever before.

## Maturation and Development of Physical Capabilities

Brain frontal lobe maturation mediates neuronal systems that contribute to children's self-regulatory and self-soothing capabilities. Frontal lobe maturation is associated with an increased ability to recall and to use executive control structures and emotional display rules to accomplish tasks and to use speech in the service of self-regulation and self-soothing.

## Maturation and Development of Cognitive Capabilities

### Emergence of More Complex Mental Operations

Piaget labeled the period between ages 6 and 11 years the *concrete operational phase* of cognitive development, referring to children's ability to carry out complex thinking processes about concrete events but not about abstract phenomena.

The cognitive capabilities that mature and develop between ages 6 and 11 years are as follows:

1. Ability to understand others' perspectives.
2. Ability to develop more complex categories.
3. Ability to reason logically and to understand relational rules.

4. Increased ability to use secondary process thinking.
5. Ability to understand concept of reversibility.
6. Ability to compare past and present.
7. Ability to understand conservation of mass and number.

### *Differentiation of Primary and Secondary Process Thinking: Development of Masking and Latent Symbols*

In late childhood, there is a gradual masking of primary process magical thinking within children's symbolic representations, whether through speech, play, fantasies, written stories, drawings, paintings, or models. Before age 5½ years, children could not distinguish between their symbols and what they symbolized. They now are becoming much more aware of how their symbols may reveal wishes and feelings that they 1) do not wish to acknowledge to themselves and/or 2) do not wish to reveal to their parents or others.

## Maturation and Development of Temperamental Characteristics

As noted earlier, temperament is now accepted as part of infants' innately endowed characteristics (Thomas and Chess 1977). Behavioral inhibition to the unfamiliar, for example, is a characteristic that shows temporal stability from infancy through age 7 years (Kagan 1989). However, Kagan found that some infants' inhibition to the unfamiliar could be gradually modified by their attachment relationship with their parents (Kagan 1989).

## Maturation and Development of Emotions

Between ages 6 and 11 years, children increasingly become aware of "blends" of feelings and of how new emotions can block out old remembered ones (Lane and Schwartz 1987). Children also become more consciously aware of their ambivalent feelings toward their parents and others. Finally, they begin to use their intuition and empathy more fully in appreciating the emotional states of others based on their own similar wishes and experiences.

Beginning at ages 6–7 years and continuing throughout late childhood, children are also becoming more aware of their anxious emotions or developmental anxiety. They learn to use developmental anxiety as an internal signal that warns them to become vigilant about an external threat (e.g., a physically dangerous person) or an internal threat (e.g., their own building rage toward a lit-

tle sister who has just destroyed their new video game but whom they are forbidden to physically strike).

## Maturation and Development of Verbal Language Abilities

Children now begin to think more before they speak and in the process develop their ability to delay the gratification of a feeling and to experience the feeling and think about why they are feeling this way. This form of regulating one's feelings has been called *mentalized affectivity* by Fonagy (1999).

## Maturation and Development of the Preexisting Representational World

By the time children reach the first grade (age 6 or 7 years), their representational world has become a crucial source of information that they use to strike a balance between their internal adaptation to their innate needs, wants, and wishes and their external adaptation to the demands, guidelines, and developmental taskings of their parents, peers, teachers, and others. In this process, children will call on their preexisting representational world (psychological stimuli) of beliefs, fantasies, emotional control procedures, and other mental contents in an attempt to achieve the following:

1. Use their memories to generate transference predictions about their daily experiences with people.
2. Discover which of their transference predictions about people seem to be true, thus reinforcing their prior experiences with people.
3. Discover which of their transference predictions do not seem to be true, thus challenging their prior experiences with people.

## Development of the Self and Object Relationships

Children's attainment of an autonomous and valued identity enables them to approach grade school with a sense of taking pleasure in being curious and taking the initiative in approaching the learning process (Erikson 1963). Between ages 5½ and 11 years, children begin to show "in miniature" an early picture of the personality they will have as an adult. Longitudinal data indicate that the highest correlation of childhood behavior predicting future adult behavior exists for this age period, especially for children between ages 8 and 11 years (Roff and Wirt 1984).

Throughout late childhood (ages 5½ to 11 years), children often undergo periods of being quite discouraged about their limitations. The child now perceives that he or she does not always get an A on every test or that he or she is not the best in gymnastics class. Once again, psychologically attuned parents—and teachers and coaches—must tolerate children's discouragement while being firm in not allowing them to avoid activities that might bring them face to face with their limitations and imperfections. As children reach age 10 or 11 years, compensatory fantasies and their abject discouragement about not being perfect begin to give way to the development of more realistically attainable ambitions and ideals.

## Continued Development of Gender and Sexual Identities

### Development of Gender Identity

One motivating force that propels 6- to 7-year-old children to identify with their same-gender parent is their need to feel more competent as a boy or girl and to feel a sense of power. Between ages 6 and 11 years, children learn that there are three types of mechanisms through which power or prestige may be gained in society: first, there is *intrinsic power*, which comes from being loved and valued unconditionally by their parents; second, there is *attributed power*, which is based on their performance in mastering stimuli presented to them during their first 6 years of life; and third, there is *formal or bestowed power*, which is power given by some social organization (Horner 1989).

### Development of Sexual Identity

Sexual identity development in late childhood comes under the sway of society's message that no direct sexual activity between children is permitted. Indirect activity does take place, however. The school classroom and playground become the places where children covertly and overtly develop their sexual identities concurrently with their peer and social identities.

## Development of the Superego

Normally developing 6- to 7-year-old children will experience their superego as an ally—residing within their heart or brain (labeled by Stillwell et al. [1991] as a *brain or heart conscience*)—that begins to perform two basic functions: 1) regulates and controls their behavior relatively independently of external restraints and 2) becomes a source of self-esteem that is relatively independent of external feedback.

## Development of Adaptational Capabilities: Evolution of New Defense Mechanisms

The predominant defense mechanisms used by children in late childhood are fantasy formation, isolation of emotion, sublimation, reaction formation, displacement, and suppression.

- *Fantasy formation* is used more than ever before as an adaptive defense by children in this age period. Instead of verbally or behaviorally expressing an anxiety-provoking wish or feeling that is associated with a developmental anxiety, children construct an unconscious latent fantasy that expresses the wish or feeling in a way that brings gratification.
- *Isolation of emotion* is an automatic barring from consciousness of an emotion that, if expressed, would produce an intolerable level of developmental anxiety.
- *Sublimation* is an automatic unconscious process in which gratification of a wish is achieved by changing the object or aim of the wish.
- *Reaction formation* is an automatic unconscious process that bars from consciousness an unacceptable wish or feeling and produces in consciousness the opposite wish or feeling.
- *Displacement* is an automatic unconscious mental mechanism that displaces the expression of a wish or feeling from the original person or object that is causing high levels of developmental anxiety to another, less anxiety-provoking person or object.
- *Suppression* is the conscious and willful attempt to put mental contents out of one's conscious awareness.

# Adolescence Phase of Mental Development (Ages 12–19 Years)

## Major Developmental Tasks of Adolescence

1. Construction of an emancipated identity
2. Construction of realistic ambitions and reasonable ideals
3. Further development of a sexual identity
4. Further development of a social identity

## Maturation and Development of Physical Capabilities

The "surgent" maturation at puberty of 11- to 13-year-old boys' innate need for sensual–sexual pleasurable gratification causes them to experience genital body sensations that physically are quite compelling. Boys awaken most mornings and notice that they have an erection. Likewise, 11- to 13-year-old girls have their first episode of menstruation. They wake up many mornings with obvious genital sensations that coincide with the fact that their breasts are developing and their pubic hair is beginning to show. They may avoid processing these new body perceptions or even fail to notice some of the subtle bodily changes that accompany these sexual sensations.

## Maturation and Development of Cognitive Capabilities

What Piaget termed the *formal cognitive phase*, during which formal thinking emerges, begins at about age 11 or 12 years, and it is not fully completed until about age 16 years. Some adolescents and adults, however, may never fully achieve the formal phase of cognitive maturation and development (Blackburn and Papalia 1992).

### Emergence of Hypothetical Thinking

1. The ability to be able to reason regarding a hypothesis based on verbal propositions.
2. The ability to combine propositions and isolate variables to test a hypothesis.
3. The ability to use thoughts and increasingly believe in the power of thoughts in planning for the future (Overton et al. 1992).
4. The ability to classify objects and people based on propositional or hypothetical reasoning.
5. The ability to be increasingly creative in thinking and more sophisticated in the use of symbolic thinking.
6. The ability to form personal opinions and to construct individual standards and moral values, along with an increase in the capability to separate what is theoretically possible from what is realistically possible.

### Construction of the Concept of an Unconscious Mental Domain

Adolescents' eventual discovery that they possess an unconscious mental domain is a slowly evolving process that begins during adolescence and is achieved in most adolescents by age 16 or 17 years.

## Maturation and Development of Emotions: Development of Emotional Self-Awareness

### Emotions as Energy Mobilizers

Adolescents experience a new emotion in adolescence—cognitive dissonance—as they reexamine and reflect on their beliefs and standards. As an emotion, this cognitive dissonance might be named *cognitive confusion* or even *cognitively generated ambivalent feelings*. Cognitive dissonance acts as an energy mobilizer in motivating adolescents to reflect on the logical inconsistency between a belief or standard they possess and information being obtained through new experiences. The advances in their formal thinking operations enable adolescents to become aware of much more *complex emotions* within themselves and others.

### Emotions as a Means of Self-Regulation

By the time they reach age 12 years, adolescents have already been using their emotions as internal signals to assist them in guiding their actions in order to remain within their optimal stimulation range. The new awareness of emotional blends upsets adolescents' ability to use their emotions as signals of distress.

### Emotions as an Aid in Achieving Social Adaptation

More than ever before in their lives, adolescents are able to use the emotional communications of others to guide their actions. This is attributed to their growing ability to manifest true empathy in relation to other persons.

## Maturation and Development of Verbal Language Abilities

In the psychologically aware family, the parents begin to allow their young adolescents a new "language space" in which they permit them to verbalize their thoughts and emotions within the family without always encouraging them to think before they speak.

## Development of the Self-Representation and of Object Representations

### Constructing an Emancipated Identity While Maintaining Transactional Relationships With Important Others

Young teenagers embark on this process of establishing an emancipated identity (Table 1–4) when they begin to

---

**TABLE 1–4.  Components of an emancipated identity**

1. Being separate and autonomous from one's parents and significant figures—especially the parents—while maintaining supportive transactional relationships with the parents and important others.
2. Believing in one's self-value while possessing individual points of view, ideals, and values different from those of respected parents, teachers, coaches, and similar significant figures.
3. Possessing sex-role behaviors congruent with one's sexual object choice in demonstrating heterosexuality or homosexuality.
4. Possessing social behaviors and beliefs that enable one to be comfortable in adopting a social role.
5. Attaining an appreciation of the progressive continuity in life between one's past, one's present, and one's fantasies and ambitions for the future.

---

question many of the beliefs, standards, and values that they had previously internalized as long-term memory structures within their representational world.

### *Object Relations Conflicts*

Young adolescents, in the process of reevaluating and reassessing their representational world and their current relationships with their parents and siblings, inevitably experience internal object relations conflicts.

### *Generational Conflicts*

Generational conflicts inevitably are expressed through a certain degree of normal rebellion. Rebellion in adolescents has been romanticized by some adults and overemphasized by some psychiatrists and psychologists who see only a selected population of emotionally disturbed adolescents (Offer and Schonert-Reichl 1992).

### *Adoption of a False Identity*

Erikson (1959) delineated the overall psychosocial conflict that is inevitable during adolescence as one of establishing an *emancipated identity* versus succumbing to role or self, or *identity confusion*. Significant identity confusion leads adolescents to adopt a false identity that has been attained through some combination of internal rebellion—against unloving and critically harsh parental representations contained within their superegos—and external rebellion—against unloving and critically harsh voices currently emanating from others (e.g., parents, siblings, teachers).

### *Parents' Role in Facilitating Formation of Emancipated Identity*

**Parents must empathize with the adolescent's need to confront parental values, standards, and beliefs in order to support their adolescent's verbalization and resolution of conflict.**  When parents are able to express their own views, they encourage their teenager to do the same. When there is disagreement, parents need to model for their teenager an important socially adaptive behavior: constructive arguing and conflict resolution. Collins and Laursen (1992) made the following points:

1. Conflicts tend to emerge in interpersonal relationships that are closer rather than more distant or superficial.
2. The interdependencies between adolescents and their parents—developed before the onset of adolescence—inevitably lead to generational conflict.
3. Verbalization of conflicts can be developmentally enhancing or developmentally inhibiting in relation to adolescents' construction and development of an emancipated identity.

**Parents need to be consistent in expressing their values and standards.**  Parents must be relatively consistent in expressing their values, attitudes, ideals, and points of view to provide their adolescent with a frame of reference to test out his or her own views, ideals, and beliefs by entering into verbal conflict with his or her parents.

**Parents need to encourage their adolescent's continued involvement with a peer group and not be overly competitive with that peer group.**  Parents who appreciate the crucial role of the peer group in facilitating the adolescent's development of an emancipated identity do not set up a competition between themselves and the peer group's attitudes, values, and so on.

## Further Development of Sexual and Social Identities

The first and perhaps most significant catalyst that sets into operation the process of establishing an emancipated self is puberty. This is the first step in adolescents' construction of a sexual identity. Having attained a solid gender identity (i.e., a basic sense of maleness or femaleness and associated identifications with gender-role behaviors) and sexual identity (in which they make their sexual object choice), adolescents begin to discover and consider embarking on new behaviors as they enter the world of sexual activity.

Young adolescents experience a new variant of the developmental anxiety discussed earlier as *disintegration anxiety*. Throughout development, the body has been an important source of positive or negative self-esteem, and this is no less true in adolescence. Young adolescents feel anxious that their bodily changes will not be accepted by their parents, teachers, and peers.

### Reemergence of the Early Triangular Phase

At around age 12 years, the physical and sexual changes that boys experience propel them to a new realization that they are becoming men. This brings their attention to the developmental task of putting more energy into developing their sexual identity. More often than not in contemporary American society, the heterosexual boy in his early teens learns that the male who is assertive in seeking and winning the girl is demonstrating a healthy heterosexual sexual identity (a derivative of his positive oedipal complex), and the boy who wants his father or another man to take care of him or find him a girlfriend is demonstrating a diminished or even "wimpy" heterosexual sexual identity. But the heterosexual teenage boy's negative triangular conflict is between his love and passive surrender to his father's potent caring and his fear that such passive dependency will cause him to lose his potency or even to become homosexual. Teenage heterosexual and homosexual boys fight hard to establish their assertive potency, whereas they fear passivity and impotency.

The normally developing pubertal boy will tend to avoid his mother and to spend more time with his father and other men. As his relationship with his father becomes stronger, he begins to relinquish his positive triangular wishes for the second time in his life, and as he becomes more aware of his emotional closeness with his father, he begins to deal with the issue of asserting his heterosexuality and his position in the category of "heterosexual men." When the pubertal boy is physically close to his father and other men and male peers, he may become a bit anxious: too much physical and emotional closeness makes him worry that he may be drifting toward homosexuality. His negative triangular wishes toward his father will, throughout his adolescence, cause him some measure of anxiety.

As girls between ages 12 and 15 years turn away from their fathers, there is a general reaction against their regressing to a more emotionally close and dependent relationship with their mothers. The young adolescent girl becomes anxious about wanting and needing her mother to help her develop her sexual identity. This anxiety is related to the girl's worry that she will become too dependent on her mother, thereby losing her "hard-won activity" (Dahl 1995) and burgeoning self-emancipation. As a result, girls in early adolescence undergo a period in which they turn away from involvement with their mothers, often developing a close relationship with a particular same-age peer.

As dating begins, teenagers want their parents, particularly the opposite-gender parent, to acknowledge them as a sexually attractive person because the adolescents' internalization of a belief in having a competent and attractive heterosexual identity continues to develop under the admiring gaze of the opposite-gender parent.

### Initiation of Sexual Activity

For adolescents who so choose, the first experience with sexual activity can be quite self-centered. They are initially focused on their own sexual performance rather than on caring and concern for their partner's feelings. They seek admiring feedback about how they have performed. And some adolescents may masturbate to completely avoid heterosexual or homosexual activity because of their concern about loss of virginity, pregnancy, or HIV or other sexually transmitted diseases.

## Development of the Superego

### Construction of Realistic Ambitions and Reasonable Ideals

Throughout adolescence, the conscience grows more and more internalized, gradually becoming better able to achieve its main two functions:

1. To regulate and control behavior relatively independently of external restraints.
2. To become a source of self-esteem that is relatively independent of others' evaluations of one's worth and value.

### A "Confused Conscience"

The process of idealizing and de-idealizing parents goes on for much of middle to late adolescence. The process becomes most prominent in 16- to 19-year-old adolescents when their positive triangular wishes begin to wane and their relationship and identification with the same-gender parent become stronger. A process of de-idealization of both parents now begins in which adolescents ultimately give up any residual wishes to have perfect and all-powerful parents to protect them from life's challenges.

Once again, the peer group rescues teenagers from feeling too disappointed and anxious about becoming emancipated, and they can eventually relinquish their view of their parents as all-protecting and all-admiring. In so doing, teenagers feel, for a while, a sense of loss in losing their parents as a source of admiration and positive self-esteem.

### Attainment of an Integrated Conscience

The older teenager's more highly developed superego now enables him or her to experience true structural conflicts. The superego becomes a more realistic and friendlier internal guide for behavioral choice and an internal source of admiration when older adolescents attain more realistic ambitions. Stillwell et al. (1991) labeled this more developed superego in late adolescence as the *integrated conscience*, in which good dominates evil.

## Development of Adaptational Capabilities: Emergence of More Socially Mature Mechanisms of Defense

Specific defense mechanisms have been shown to be associated with healthy adult functioning (Vaillant 1971, 1974), particularly in adults who have a good capacity to adapt to different social, educational, and professional situations. These mechanisms include the following:

- Intellectualization
- Humor
- Anticipation

## Transitioning From Adolescence to Young Adulthood: Criteria for Adulthood

### Establishment of Autonomy From Parents (Self-Autonomy)

Toward the end of adolescence, the individual begins to assert control over his or her own life, believing in his or her ability to function apart from parents or other adults. However, this emancipated or fully autonomous identity is not that of a person who is an island unto him- or herself. Self-autonomy occurs in the context of being comfortable with needing to be in emotionally intimate relationships with others (Jordan et al. 1991).

### Establishment of Realistic Goals (Realistic Self-Image)

Through a progressive relinquishment of wishes for perfection, signified by the ability to set reasonable goals and to tolerate the realization that every goal will not be achieved, the adolescent begins to manifest more self-responsibility, in that imperfections, setbacks, or faults do not generate blaming of others.

### Establishment of a Stable Sexual Identity

Establishing a stable sexual identity is often delayed because of the older adolescent's decision to avoid sexual activity in order to pursue higher education or vocational goals. In 18- to 19-year-olds who have become sexually active, this criterion addresses their growing capacity to make a mutually caring choice of a heterosexual or a homosexual partner and to treat that partner's body with kindness and respect rather than as a vehicle for demonstrating their sexual potency.

### Establishment of a Sense of Continuity Between Past Life Experiences and Current Motivations and Beliefs

Individuals in late adolescence can gain a new understanding of the relative influence of past experiences on current wishes, motivational goals, and beliefs. This understanding often entails seeking out the life histories of other family members to help one understand current problems.

# Key Points: Normal Child and Adolescent Development

The following terms and concepts are key to an understanding of normal child and adolescent development:

- **Accommodation–transformation principle**—The principle that becomes activated when stimuli create perceptions or conceptions that cannot be assimilated into prior representations. When this occurs, the infant will either change a preexisting representation to include the new perception or conception or add a new representation to his or her mental world.

- **Attachment relationship**—The specific relationship that develops between infants and their parents.

- **Belief**—A type of conception that, as a representational mental structure, establishes the relationship between two or more inanimate objects, aspects of nature's laws, or people (e.g., the child and his or her mother).

- **Child protective factor**—A characteristic within the child, the parents, the child–parent relationship, and/or the society in which the child is living that helps the child and the parents achieve developmental adaptations and maintain their goodness-of-fit transactions.

- **Developmental continuity**—The term used to address the fact that a great part, but not all, of psychological development is dependent on what took place in the past.

- **Developmental discontinuity**—An event in a person's life that is unexpected and not predictable from what has occurred in the person's past.

- **Developmentally enhancing adaptation**—An adaptation by the child that enhances the child's sense of competency, pleasure in mastering a task, and feelings of joyful pride.

- **Disintegration anxiety**—The internally generated fear that if anyone knew how imperfect or impotent the child believes himself or herself to be, others would totally reject him or her.

- **Experiential mental structures**—The emotions (e.g., shame, guilt), thoughts (perceptions and conceptions), and memories (short- and long-term) that are the result of the mind's processing of transactions between biopsychosocial stimuli.

- **Hierarchical restructuring principle**—The principle that states that as a child's cognitive abilities continue to mature and his or her mind continues to reconstruct prior representations to reflect a more advanced level of cognitive integration and comprehension, the child's mind will reorganize its representations into a hierarchy that reflects the child's unique preferences.

- **Inner mental world or representational world**—The inner world we refer to as an individual's mind, which is in contrast to the outer world of people and things.

- **Mentalizing function**—The capacity to use self-reflection to become aware of possessing a mind and to gradually understand one's own mind and the minds of others as being complex, with different emotions, beliefs, and conflicts.

- **Normal developmental external conflict**—An aspect of normal development that occurs when there is a disparity between the child's current need, wish, and/or impulse and the desires of the parents or others with whom the child is relating.

- **Normal developmental internal conflict**—An aspect of normal development that occurs when there is a disparity between what the child desires to do, fantasizes about, or believes and an inner voice that prohibits or warns the child that a developmental calamity will occur if the child acts upon his or her impulse, desire, and/or fantasy.

- **Normogenic belief**—A belief, developed by the child, that enhances the child's psychological development. Such a belief enables the child to generate positive expectancies about new life events and people.

- **Pathogenic belief**—A belief, developed by the child, that interferes with the child's psychological development. Such a belief functions as an internal inhibiting factor in that it causes the child to generate negative expectancies about new life events and people.

# References

Ainsworth MD, Belehar M, Waters E, et al: Patterns of Attachment: A Psychological Study of the Strange Situation. Hillsdale, NJ, Lawrence Erlbaum, 1978

Ames LB, Ilg FL: Your Three-Year-Old. New York, Dell, 1976a

Ames LB, Ilg FL: Your Four-Year-Old. New York, Dell, 1976b

Ames LB, Ilg FL: Your Five-Year-Old. New York, Dell, 1976c

Ames LB, Ilg FL: Your Six-Year-Old. New York, Dell Publishing, 1979

Baldwin JD, Baldwin JI: Open peer commentary: the stage question in cognitive-developmental theory. Behav Brain Sci 2:182–183, 1978

Berk LE: Why children talk to themselves. Sci Am 271:78–83, 1994

Blackburn JA, Papalia DE: The study of adult cognition from the Piagetian perspective, in Intellectual Development. Edited by Sternberg R, Berg C. New York, Cambridge University Press, 1992, pp 141–160

Bowlby J: Attachment and Loss, Vol 1: Attachment. New York, Basic Books, 1969

Bowlby J: Developmental psychiatry comes of age. Am J Psychiatry 145:1–10, 1988

Brenner C: An Elementary Textbook of Psychoanalysis. New York, International Universities Press, 1965

Campos J, Barrett KC, Lamb ME, et al: Socio-emotional development, in Handbook of Child Psychology, 4th Edition, Vol 2: Infant Development. Edited by Haith M, Campos J. New York, Wiley, 1983, pp 785–915

Case R: Neo-Piagetian theories of child development, in Intellectual Development. Edited by Sternberg RJ, Berg CA. New York, Cambridge University Press, 1992, pp 161–197

Chess S, Thomas A: Temperament in Clinical Practice. New York, Guilford, 1986

Collins W, Laursen B: Conflicts and relationships during adolescence, in Conflict in Child and Adolescent Development. Edited by Shantz CU, Hartup WW. New York, Cambridge University Press, 1992, pp 216–242

Dahl EK: Daughters and mothers. Psychoanal Study Child 50:187–204, 1995

Emde RN: The prerepresentational self and its affective core. Psychoanal Study Child 38:165–192, 1983

Emde RN: Moving ahead: integrating influences of affective processes for development and for psychoanalysis. Int J Psychoanal 80 (Pt 2):317–339, 1999

Emde RN, Gaensbauer TJ, Harmon RJ: Emotional Expression in Infancy. New York, International Universities Press, 1979

Erikson E: Identity and the Life Cycle. New York, Norton, 1959

Erikson E: Childhood and Society, Revised Edition. New York, Norton, 1963

Erikson E: Identity, Youth and Crisis. New York, Norton, 1968

Fantz RL: The origin of form perception. Sci Am 204:66–72, 1961

Fantz R: Pattern vision in newborn infants. Science 140:296–297, 1963

Fonagy P: The Process of Change and the Change of Processes: What Can Change in a "Good" Analysis. Keynote Address to the Spring Meeting of Division 39 of the American Psychological Association, New York, 16th April 1999. Available at: http://www.dspp.com/papers/fonagy.htm. Accessed September 2007.

Fraiberg S: Object constancy and mental representation. Psychoanal Study Child 24:9–47, 1969

Freud S: Three essays on the theory of sexuality (1905), in The Standard Edition of the Complete Psychological Works of Sigmund Freud, Vol 7. Translated and edited by Strachey J. London, Hogarth Press, 1963, pp 135–243

Freud S: The ego and the id (1923), in The Standard Edition of the Complete Psychological Works of Sigmund Freud, Vol 19. Translated and edited by Strachey J. London, Hogarth Press, 1963, pp 12–66

Girton M: Infants' attention to intrastimulus motion. J Exp Child Psychol 28:416–423, 1979

Goldsmith H, Buss A, Plomin R, et al: Roundtable: what is temperament? Four approaches. Child Dev 58:505–529, 1987

Greenberg M, Morris N: Engrossment: the newborn's impact upon the father. Am J Orthopsychiatry 44:520–531, 1974

Herzog JM: On father hunger: the father's role in the modulation of aggressive drive and fantasy, in Father and Child. Edited by Cath SW, Gurwitt AR, Ross JM. Boston, MA, Little, Brown, 1982, pp 163–174

Horner AJ: The Wish for Power and the Fear of Having It. Northvale, NJ, Jason Aronson, 1989

Hutt SJ, Hutt C, Lenard H, et al: Auditory responsivity in the human neonate. Nature 218:888–890, 1968

Izard CE: The Face of Emotion. New York, Appleton-Century-Crofts, 1971

Izard CE: Patterns of Emotions. New York, Academic Press, 1972

Jordan JV, Kaplan AG, Miller JB, et al: Woman's Growth in Connection: Writings From the Stone Center. New York, Guilford, 1991

Kagan J: The form of early development. Arch Gen Psychiatry 36:1047–1054, 1979

Kagan J: The Second Year: The Emergence of Self-Awareness. Cambridge, MA, Harvard University Press, 1981

Kagan J: The Nature of the Child. New York, Basic Books, 1984

Kagan J: Unstable Ideas: Temperament, Cognition and Self. Cambridge, MA, Harvard University Press, 1989

Kernberg OF: Object Relations Theory and Clinical Psychoanalysis. New York, Jason Aronson, 1976

Klein M: The importance of symbol-formation in the development of the ego (1930), in The Writings of Melanie Klein, Vol 1. London, Hogarth Press, 1975, pp 219–232

Kohlberg LA: The Philosophy of Moral Development, Moral Stages, and the Ideal of Justice: Essays on Moral Development, Vol 1. San Francisco, CA, Harper & Row, 1981

Kohut H: The Analysis of the Self: A Systematic Approach to the Psychoanalytic Treatment of Narcissistic Personality Disorders. New York, International Universities Press, 1971

Kohut H: Restoration of the Self. New Haven, CT, International Universities Press, 1977

Kohut H, Wolf E: The disorders of the self and their treatment: an outline. Int J Psychoanal 59:413–425, 1978

Lamb ME (ed): The Role of the Father in Child Development, 2nd Edition. New York, Wiley, 1981

Lane RD, Schwartz GE: Levels of emotional awareness: a cognitive-developmental theory and its application to psychopathology. Am J Psychiatry 144:133–143, 1987

Lewis M, Brooks-Gunn J: Social Cognition and the Acquisition of Self. New York, Plenum, 1979

Magnusson D, Allen V: Human Development: An Interactional Approach. New York, Academic Press, 1983

Mahler MS: On human symbiosis and the vicissitudes of individualization. J Am Psychoanal Assoc 23:740–763, 1975

Mayer LM: Towards female gender identity. J Am Psychoanal Assoc 43:17–39, 1995

Mayes LC: Arousal regulation, emotional flexibility, medial amygdala function, and the impact of early experience: comments on the paper of Lewis et al. Ann N Y Acad Sci 1094:178–192, 2006

Meissner W: A note on projective identification. J Am Psychoanal Assoc 28:43–67, 1980

Meissner WW: The pathology of belief systems. Psychoanalysis and Contemporary Thought 15:99–129, 1992

Meyer JK: Body ego, selfness, and gender sense: the development of gender identity. Psychiatr Clin North Am 3:21–36, 1980

Nelson K: Event knowledge and the development of language functions, in Research in Child Language Disorders. Edited by Miller J. New York, Little, Brown, 1990, pp 125–141

Offer D, Schonert-Reichl K: Debunking the myths of adolescence: findings from recent research. J Am Acad Child Adolesc Psychiatry 31:1003–1014, 1992

Oppenheim D, Goldsmith DF (eds): Attachment Theory in Clinical Work With Children. New York, Guilford, 2007

Overton WF, Steidl JH, Rosenstein D, et al: Formal operations as regulatory context in adolescence, in Adolescent Psychiatry, Vol 18. Edited by Feinstein SC. Chicago, IL, University of Chicago Press, 1992, pp 502–513

Parke R, Tinsley B: The father's role in infancy: determinants of involvement in caregiving and play, in The Role of the Father in Child Development. Edited by Lamb M. New York, Wiley, 1981, pp 45–76

Person ES: By Force of Fantasy. New York, Basic Books, 1995

Piaget J: Intelligence and Affectivity: Their Relationship During Child Development, Revised (1954). Palo Alto, CA, Annual Reviews, 1981

Roff JD, Wirt RD: Childhood social adjustment, adolescent status, and young adult mental health. Am J Orthopsychiatry 54:595–602, 1984

Shapiro T, Hertzig ME: Normal growth and development, in The American Psychiatric Press Textbook of Psychiatry. Edited by Talbott JA, Hales RE, Yudofsky SC. Washington, DC, American Psychiatric Press, 1988, pp 91–122

Siegel DJ: Childhood memory. Paper presented at the annual meeting of the American Academy of Child and Adolescent Psychiatry, San Antonio, TX, October 1993

Stern D: The Interpersonal World of the Infant. New York, Basic Books, 1985

Stillwell BM, Galvin M, Kopta SM: Conceptualization of conscience in normal children and adolescents, ages 5 to 17. J Am Acad Child Adolesc Psychiatry 30:16–21, 1991

Terr L: Unchained Memories: True Stories of Traumatic Memories, Lost and Found. New York, Basic Books, 1994

Thomas A, Chess S: Temperament and Development. New York, Brunner/Mazel, 1977

Tyson P: A developmental line of gender identity, gender role and choice of love object. J Am Psychoanal Assoc 30:59–84, 1982

Tyson P, Tyson RL: Narcissism and superego development. J Am Psychoanal Assoc 32:75–98, 1984

Tyson P, Tyson R: Psychoanalytic Theories of Development. New Haven, CT, Yale University Press, 1991

Vaillant GE: Theoretical hierarchy of adaptive ego mechanisms. Arch Gen Psychiatry 24:107–118, 1971

Vaillant GE: The natural history of male psychological health, II: some antecedents of healthy adult adjustment. Arch Gen Psychiatry 31:15–22, 1974

Werner H, Kaplan B: Symbol Formation: An Orgasmic-Developmental Approach to Language and the Expression of Thought. New York, Wiley, 1963

Westen D: Towards a clinically and empirically sound theory of motivation. Int J Psychoanal 78 (Pt 3):521–548, 1997

# 2

# Functional Neuroanatomy

BRIAN T. HAREL, Ph.D.

DANIEL TRANEL, Ph.D.

## Brain-Behavior Relations

### Lateral Specialization: Left Versus Right

In the vast majority of adults, the left side of the brain is specialized for language and for processing verbally coded information. This specialization is true of nearly all (about 88%) right-handed individuals, the majority (about 75%) of left-handed persons, and 43% of mixed-handed persons (Khedr et al. 2002). Moreover, compelling evidence now indicates that this applies not only to languages that are auditory based but also to languages that are based on visuogestural signals (see, e.g., American Sign Language) (Bellugi et al. 1989; Hickok et al. 1996; Poizner et al. 1987).

The right hemisphere has a very different type of specialization. It processes nonverbal information such as complex visual patterns (e.g., faces) or auditory signals (e.g., music) that are not coded in verbal form. Structures in the right temporal and occipital regions are critical for learning and navigating geographic routes (Barrash et al. 2000a). The right side of the brain is also dedicated to the mapping of "feeling states," that is, patterns of bodily sensations linked to emotions such as anger and fear. A related right hemisphere capacity concerns the perception of our bodies in space, in both intrapersonal and extrap-

ersonal terms. Table 2–1 summarizes some of the functional dichotomies of left and right hemispheric dominance.

### Longitudinal Specialization: Anterior Versus Posterior

Another useful organizational principle for understanding brain-behavior relations is an anterior-posterior distinction. The major demarcation points are the rolandic sulcus, the major fissure separating the frontal lobes from the parietal lobes, and the sylvian fissure, the boundary between the temporal lobes and the frontal and parietal lobes.

In general, the posterior regions of the brain are dedicated to sensation and perception. The primary sensory cortices for vision, audition, and somatosensory perception are located in the posterior sectors of the brain in occipital, temporal, and parietal regions, respectively. Thus, apprehension of sensory data from the world outside is mediated by posterior brain structures. Note that the "world outside" is actually two distinct domains: 1) the world that is outside the body and brain and 2) the world that is outside the brain but inside the body. Anterior brain regions, by contrast, generally comprise effector systems, specialized for the execution of behavior.

Supported by National Institute of Neurological Disorders and Stroke Grant P01 NS19632.

**TABLE 2–1.    Functional dichotomies of left and right hemispheric dominance**

| Left | Right |
| --- | --- |
| Verbal | Nonverbal |
| Serial | Parallel |
| Analytic | Holistic |
| Controlled | Creative |
| Logical | Pictorial |
| Propositional | Appositional |
| Rational | Intuitive |
| Social | Physical |

*Source.*    Adapted from Benton 1991.

## The Temporal Lobes

Several major subdivisions can be designated within the temporal lobe: 1) the mesial temporal lobe, including the hippocampus, amygdala, entorhinal and perirhinal cortices, and an additional portion of the anterior parahippocampal gyrus; 2) the remaining nonmesial portion of the temporal lobe, which includes the temporal pole (TP), the inferotemporal (IT) region, and, for purposes of the current discussion, the region of transition between the posterior temporal lobe and the inferior occipital lobe (the occipitotemporal junction); and 3) the posterior portion of the superior temporal gyrus (area 22), which, on the left side, forms the heart of what is traditionally known as Wernicke's area (Figure 2–1).

### Mesial Temporal Region

The mesial temporal lobe comprises the hippocampus, amygdala, entorhinal and perirhinal cortices, and the anterior portion of parahippocampal gyrus not occupied by the entorhinal cortex (see Figure 2–1).

#### *Hippocampal Complex*

The hippocampus and the adjacent entorhinal and perirhinal cortices can together be referred to as the *hippocampal complex*.

In a general sense, it is reasonable to describe the principal function of the hippocampal complex as the acquisition of new factual knowledge (*declarative memory*). The system is essential for acquiring records of interactions between the organism and the world outside, as well as thought processes such as those engaged in planning. It

has been posited that the hippocampal complex is primarily involved in encoding memories in terms of the relations among objects and events, even when there are no intrinsic qualities that relate them (e.g., names with faces, names with telephone numbers). This allows for multiple means of accessing information, as well as the ability for information to be used in novel situations. This is accomplished through extensive connections with many higher-order cortical processing areas. These networks, because of their interconnectedness throughout the cortex, are by their nature relational. The types of relational information range from basic sensory (e.g., relative size or shape) to higher-order relationships (e.g., Cohen and Eichenbaum 1993; Eichenbaum and Cohen 2001).

With respect to the nature of the amnesia associated with hippocampal damage, several relations have been firmly established. First, neuropsychological findings have identified selective impairments in relational memory (e.g., Ryan et al. 2000). Second, a consistent relation is found between the side of the lesion and the type of learning impairment. Specifically, damage to the left hippocampal system produces an amnesic syndrome that affects verbal material but spares nonverbal material; conversely, damage to the right hippocampal system affects nonverbal material (e.g., complex visual and auditory patterns) but spares verbal material (e.g., Frisk and Milner 1990; Milner 1968, 1972; O'Connor and Verfaellie 2002; M.L. Smith and Milner 1989).

A third point is that the hippocampal system does not appear to play a role in the learning of perceptuomotor skills and other knowledge that has been referred to as *nondeclarative memory* (e.g., Squire 1992). A patient, for example, can learn skills such as mirror drawing and mirror reading (Corkin 1965, 1968; Gabrieli et al. 1993), even though he or she has no recall of the situation in which the learning of those skills took place.

#### *Amygdala*

The role of the amygdala in memory has been a source of controversy. Studies in nonhuman primates have yielded conflicting results, with some laboratories reporting that the amygdala is critical for normal learning (e.g., Mishkin 1978; Murray 1990; Murray and Mishkin 1985, 1986) and others maintaining that the amygdala does not play a crucial role (e.g., Zola-Morgan et al. 1989). Results in the few human cases available are also equivocal (Lee et al. 1988; Nahm et al. 1993; Tranel and Hyman 1990).

However, studies have begun to clarify this issue, and it now appears that the amygdala is important for the acquisition and expression of emotional memory, but per-

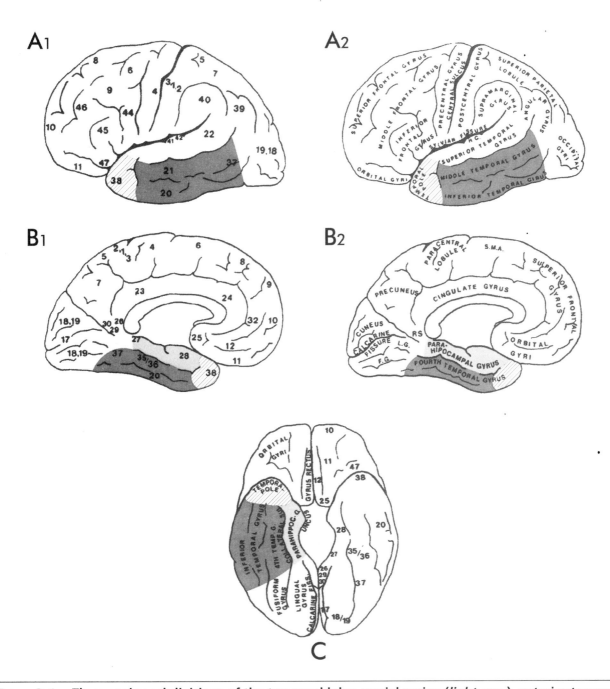

**FIGURE 2–1.** **Three major subdivisions of the temporal lobe: mesial region (*light gray*), anterior temporal pole region (*hatched*), and inferotemporal region (*dark gray*).**

Numbers corresponding to Brodmann's cytoarchitectonic areas are depicted in *Panels A1* and *B1* and the right side (left hemisphere) of *Panel C*, and standard gyrus names are shown in the corresponding *Panels A2* and *B2* and the left side (right hemisphere) of *Panel C*. Lateral (*A1* and *A2*), mesial (*B1* and *B2*), and inferior (*C*) views are represented.

haps not for neutral memory. Specifically, the amygdala contributes critically to the potentiation of memory traces for emotional stimuli during their acquisition and consolidation into long-term declarative memory (Adolphs et al. 2000, 2005; Cahill et al. 1995; Phelps et al. 1998). These findings are in accord with other evidence indicating that the amygdala is important for the recognition of emotion, especially fear, in facial expressions (Adolphs 2003; Adolphs et al. 2005; Young et al. 1995) and in the processing of other information that has emotional significance

(Markowitsch et al. 1994). Also, it has been shown that the amygdala is important for classical conditioning of autonomic responses. These findings have led to the idea that the amygdala is important for processing stimuli that communicate emotional significance in social situations; specifically, the amygdala may orchestrate patterns of neural activation in disparate sectors of the brain that would encode both the intrinsic physical features of stimuli (e.g., shape, position in space) and the value that certain stimuli have to the organism, especially emotional significance (Adolphs 2003; Adolphs and Tranel 2000).

## Anterior, Lateral, and Inferior Temporal Regions

### Retrograde Memory

The anterior and nonmesial sectors of the temporal lobes play important roles in retrograde memory—specifically, the retrieval of knowledge that was acquired before the onset of a brain injury (e.g., Hunkin et al. 1995).

### Lexical Retrieval

Structures in the anterior and inferolateral left temporal lobe play a key role in lexical retrieval, or what is commonly known as *naming*. Recent evidence has shown that neural structures in different parts of the left temporal lobe are important for the naming of objects from different conceptual categories. The neural regions under consideration here include the TP and the IT region (Figure 2–2). These regions are mostly outside the classic language areas in the left hemisphere. Structures in the right anterolateral temporal region appear to play an important role in the recognition of unique entities.

### Visual Recognition

Disorders of visual recognition are associated with damage to the posterior part of the IT region, along with the inferior portion of Brodmann areas 18 and 19 in the occipital region, a transition area known as the *occipitotemporal junction*. Lesions to the occipitotemporal junction, especially when they are bilateral, produce unimodal, visually based disorders of recognition. Patients lose the ability to recognize visual stimuli at the level of unique identity. The disturbance can affect any number of visual stimuli that normally require recognition at a unique level (e.g., faces, buildings, landmarks), but the best-studied manifestation is agnosia for faces, known as *prosopagnosia* (for review, see Barton 2003; Kanwisher and Moscovitch 2000).

## The Occipital Lobes

The neuroanatomical arrangement of structures in and near the occipital lobes is depicted in Figure 2–3. On the lateral aspect of the hemispheres, the occipital lobes comprise the visual association cortices in Brodmann areas 18 and 19. These areas continue in the mesial aspect. The mesial sector also includes the primary visual cortices (area 17), which are formed by the cortex immediately above and below the calcarine fissure. For purposes of establishing neuropsychological correlates of the occipital lobes, the region can be subdivided in the vertical plane at the level of the calcarine fissure, so that dorsal (superior) and ventral (inferior) components can be designated (Figure 2–3).

### Dorsal Component

The dorsal component of the occipital lobes comprises the primary visual cortex superior to the calcarine fissure (area 17) and the superior portion of the visual association cortices (areas 18 and 19). When situated in the primary visual cortex of area 17 and/or its connections, lesions to the dorsal sector of the occipital region lead to a loss of form vision (i.e., blindness) in the inferior visual field contralateral to the lesion, and bilateral lesions of this type will produce an inferior altitudinal hemianopia. An intriguing presentation occurs when the lesions spare the primary visual cortex and involve the association cortices of areas 18 and 19. When such lesions encroach into the adjacent parietal region comprising areas 39 and 7, patients commonly develop a constellation of defects known as *Balint's syndrome* (Figure 2–4). Balint's syndrome is based on the presence of three components: 1) visual disorientation (also known as *simultanagnosia*), 2) ocular apraxia (also known as *psychic gaze paralysis*), and 3) optic ataxia.

### Visual Disorientation

Visual disorientation (simultanagnosia) can be conceptualized as an inability to attend to more than a very limited sector of the visual field at any given moment. Patients report that they can see clearly in only a small part of the field, the rest being "out of focus" and in a sort of "fog."

### Ocular Apraxia

Ocular apraxia (psychic gaze paralysis) is a deficit of visual scanning. It consists of an inability to direct the gaze voluntarily toward a stimulus located in the peripheral vision to bring it into central vision.

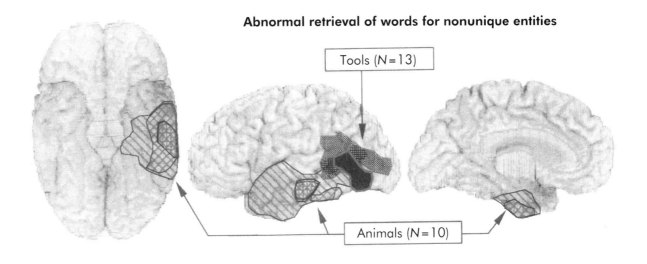

Abnormal retrieval of words for nonunique entities

Tools (N = 13)

Animals (N = 10)

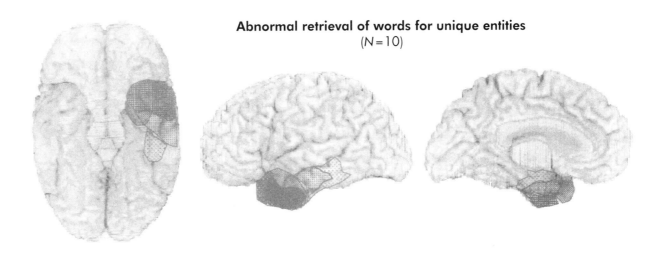

Abnormal retrieval of words for unique entities
(N = 10)

FIGURE 2–2.   **Regions in the left temporal lobe that are important for lexical retrieval, including the left temporal pole (TP) and the inferotemporal (IT) region.**

Results of analysis based on magnetic resonance (or computed tomographic) scans processed for three-dimensional reconstruction in each subject with Brainvox (H. Damasio and Frank 1992). The top section depicts defective retrieval of words for animals or tools; the bottom section depicts defective retrieval of words for persons. Abnormal retrieval of words for persons correlated with damage clustered in the left TP. Abnormal retrieval of words for animals correlated with damage in the left IT region; maximal overlap occurred in lateral and inferior IT regions. Abnormal retrieval of words for tools correlated with damage in the posterolateral IT region, along with the junction of lateral temporo-occipitoparietal cortices (posterior IT+).

## Optic Ataxia

Optic ataxia is a disturbance of visually guided reaching behavior. Patients are not able to point accurately at a target, under visual guidance. They cannot point precisely to the examiner's fingertip or to items such as a cup or coin. Optic ataxia can occur in isolation, particularly when lesions are at the border of the occipital and parietal regions or in the parietal region exclusively.

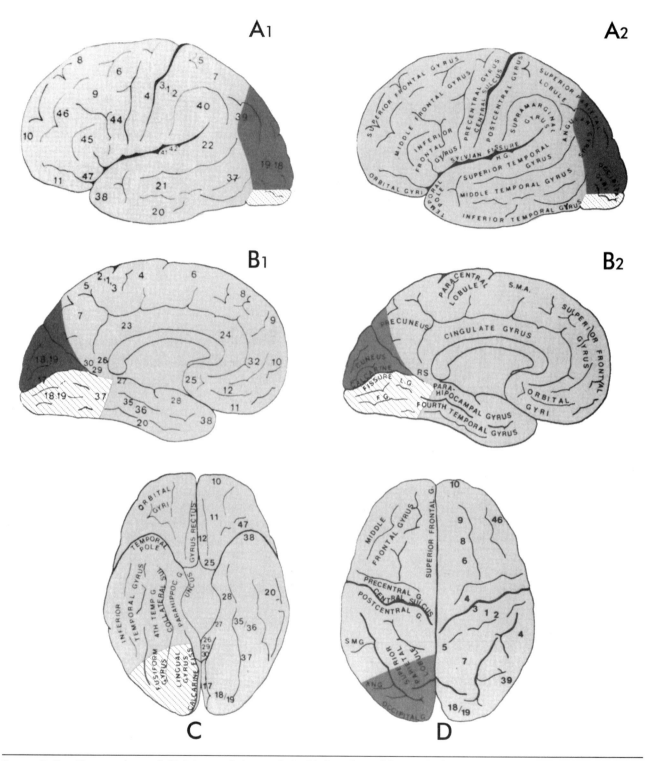

**FIGURE 2–3.  Two major subdivisions of the occipital lobe: dorsal (superior) component (*dark gray*) and ventral (inferior) component (*hatched*).**

Numbers corresponding to Brodmann's cytoarchitectonic areas are depicted in *Panels A1* and *B1* and the right side (left hemisphere) of *Panels C* and *D;* standard gyrus names are shown on corresponding *Panels A2* and *B2* and the left side (right hemisphere) of *Panels C* and *D.* Lateral (*A1* and *A2*), mesial (*B1* and *B2*), inferior (*C*), and superior (*D*) views are represented.

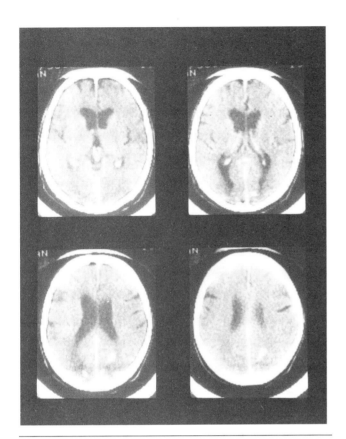

**FIGURE 2–4.** **Contrast-enhanced computed tomographic scan of a 74-year-old right-handed man, showing bilateral lesions (areas of increased density) in the superior occipital region corresponding to the supracalcarine visual association cortices.**
The man developed a complex visual disturbance (Balint's syndrome) in connection with these lesions.

## Ventral Component

The ventral component of the occipital lobes comprises the primary visual cortex immediately below the calcarine fissure (area 17) and the inferior portion of the visual association cortices (areas 18 and 19). The latter component corresponds to the lingual and fusiform gyri (see Figure 2–3C). Damage to primary visual cortex and/or its connections in the inferior bank of the calcarine fissure will produce a form vision defect (blindness) in the contralateral superior visual field. Damage to nearby structures may spare vision for form, either partially or entirely, while producing some other higher-order visual impairments. Several examples are elaborated in the following subsections.

### Acquired (Central) Achromatopsia

Acquired (central) achromatopsia is a disorder of color perception involving all or part of the visual field, with preservation of form vision, caused by damage to the inferior visual association cortex and/or its subjacent white matter (A.R. Damasio et al. 1980, 2000; Meadows 1974; Paulson et al. 1994; Rizzo et al. 1993; for review, see Heywood and Kentridge 2003; Tranel 2001).

### Apperceptive Visual Agnosia

A common form of apperceptive agnosia occurs in the visual modality in connection with right-sided lesions involving both the inferior and the superior sectors of the posterior visual association cortices. Such a lesion in a patient of this type is illustrated in Figure 2–5. Patients with apperceptive visual agnosia have difficulty in perceiving all parts of a visual array simultaneously and in generating the image of a whole entity when given a part.

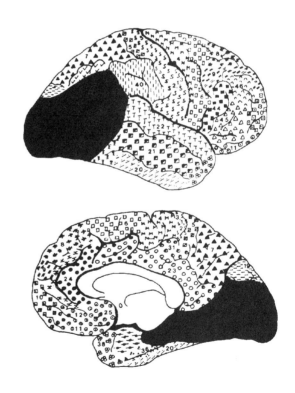

**FIGURE 2–5.** **Depiction of lesion of a 68-year-old right-handed man who had an infarction that destroyed the right posterior parietal and occipital cortices.**
Note that the lesion (marked in *black*) includes visual association cortices both above and below the calcarine fissure. The man had apperceptive prosopagnosia.

### Acquired (Pure) Alexia

Lesions that disconnect both right- and left-sided visual association cortices from the dominant, language-related temporoparietal cortices can produce a complete or partial impairment in reading, a condition known as *acquired (pure) alexia.*

# The Parietal Lobes

On the lateral aspect of the cerebral hemispheres, the parietal lobes consist of a large expanse of cortex bounded by the central sulcus anteriorly, the sylvian fissure inferiorly, and the occipital cortices posteriorly (Figure 2–6). It is important to maintain a clear distinction between the right and the left hemispheres because many cognitive and behavioral correlates of the parietal region are highly lateralized. The parietal lobes are considered together with several anatomically and functionally related neighboring regions.

## Temporoparietal Junction

In the left hemisphere, an area of cortex formed by the posterior part of the superior temporal gyrus (posterior area 22) constitutes the core of a region known as *Wernicke's area.* This region subserves a set of core speech and language functions whose disruption constitutes the syndrome known as *Wernicke's aphasia* (Caplan 2003; H. Damasio 1998; Tranel and Anderson 1999). Wernicke's aphasia is characterized by fluent, paraphasic speech, impaired repetition, and defective aural comprehension. Patients produce speech without hesitation, and the phrase length and melodic contour of utterances are normal; however, patients make frequent errors in the choice of individual words used to express an idea (paraphasias). Phonemic (also known as *literal*) (e.g., substituting *sephalot* for *elephant*) and semantic (also known as *verbal*) (e.g., substituting *superintendent* for *president*) paraphasias are common. Repetition of sentences is impaired and may be limited to single words. Repetition of digits is usually impaired as well. The comprehension defect can be quite severe and frequently involves both aural and written forms of language. The typical lesion associated with Wernicke's aphasia is depicted in Figure 2–7.

In the right hemisphere, lesions in the region of the temporoparietal junction do not cause disturbances of propositional speech but instead may impair the processing of music and spectral auditory information.

## Inferior Parietal Lobule

The inferior parietal lobule comprises the supramarginal and angular gyri. On the left side, lesions to the supramarginal gyrus and the neighboring parietal operculum (the area of cortex formed by the inferior-most portion of the postcentral gyrus) or the underlying white matter, or both, cause a speech and language disturbance known as *conduction aphasia* (e.g., Caplan 2003). An example of a computed tomographic (CT) scan from such a patient is shown in Figure 2–8. The core feature of this aphasia is a marked defect in verbatim repetition, which is disproportionately severe compared with other speech and language defects. Speech production is fluent but is dominated by phonemic paraphasias. Comprehension is only mildly compromised. Naming is defective and is dominated by phonemic errors, such as substitution of incorrect phonemes into target naming responses. Reading aloud is impaired, but reading comprehension may be normal. Another distinctive feature of conduction aphasia is that patients cannot write to dictation; however, they can write normally or nearly normally when writing spontaneously or when copying a written example.

Left-sided lesions to the parietal region, especially in the inferior parietal lobule, also have been associated with an acquired disturbance in mathematical abilities, a condition known as *acalculia.*

On the right side, the most consistent and striking neuropsychological correlates of lesions to the inferior parietal lobule are neglect and anosognosia. *Neglect* refers to a condition whereby the patient fails to attend to stimuli in the contralateral hemispace (spatial neglect). In the visual modality, for example, the patient will not attend to the left hemifield and will fail to report stimuli from that side even when it can be shown that form vision is not impaired (hemianopia). Figure 2–9 shows a typical example of a patient with a large right hemisphere lesion that includes the inferior parietal lobule. The patient had severe neglect, anosognosia, and visuospatial impairments.

Neglect also can involve intrapersonal space. For example, patients may fail to use, or even deny the existence of, the contralateral arm and leg, even when they have no motor impairment (e.g., Tranel 1995b). Representations conjured up in recall also can be affected. When asked to imagine or draw an object, the patient may omit the left half as though it did not exist.

*Anosognosia* is another frequent correlate of damage to the right inferior parietal lobule. However, there is some debate regarding the anatomical localization and lateralization of this phenomenon. The term was originally

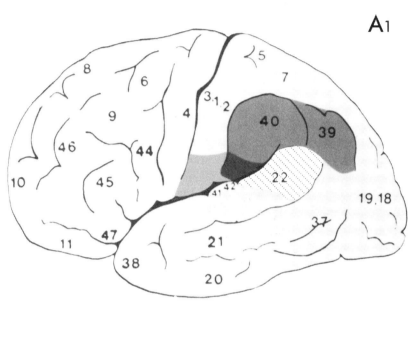

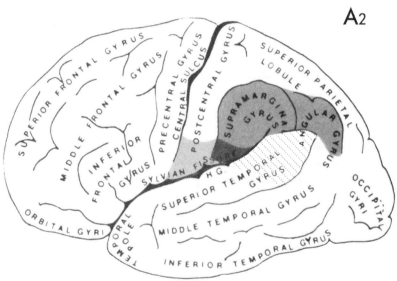

FIGURE 2–6.  **Subdivisions of the parietal lobe and nearby regions.**

The temporoparietal junction, formed by the posterior part of the superior temporal gyrus (area 22), is shown in *hatching*. The inferior parietal lobule, depicted in *medium gray*, is formed by the angular (area 39) and supramarginal (area 40) gyri. The parietal operculum is formed by the inferior aspect of the postcentral gyrus (shown in *light gray*) and a bit of the anteroinferior aspect of the supramarginal gyrus (the overlapping area shown in *dark gray*). Numbers corresponding to Brodmann's cytoarchitectonic areas are depicted in *Panel A1*, and standard gyrus names are shown on the corresponding *Panel A2*. The panels depict a lateral view.

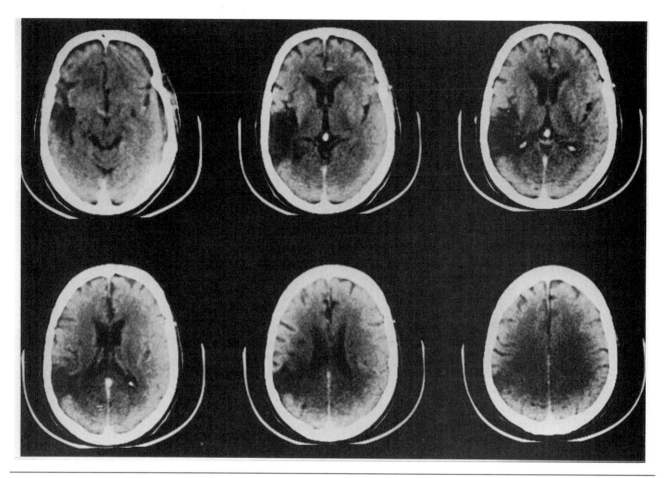

**FIGURE 2–7.   Computed tomographic scan of a 56-year-old right-handed man who developed Wernicke's aphasia after sustaining a left middle cerebral artery infarction.**
The lesion (area of low density) is centered squarely in Wernicke's area, including the posterior superior temporal gyrus (*top row*) and part of the inferior parietal lobule (*bottom row*).

applied to patients who denied that a paretic limb was in fact paretic or that it even belonged to them (Babinski 1914). Denial of sensory loss (e.g., a visual field defect) and cognitive disturbance (e.g., amnesia, dementia, aphasia) also have been included under the concept of anosognosia (see Adair et al. 2003; Anderson and Tranel 1989).

## The Frontal Lobes

The frontal lobes constitute about half of the entire cerebral mantle, and this portion of the brain has numerous functional correlates. To consider cognitive and behavioral correlates, it is helpful to divide the frontal lobes into several distinct anatomical sectors (Figure 2–10).

## Frontal Operculum

The frontal operculum is formed by areas 44, 45, and 47 (see Figure 2–10). On the left side, the heart of this region (areas 44 and 45) is known as *Broca's area*. The region is dedicated to a set of speech and language functions whose disruption produces a distinctive pattern of aphasia termed *Broca's aphasia*. Patients with Broca's aphasia have nonfluent speech, characterized by short utterances, long response latencies, and flat melodic contour. There is a marked decrease in the density of words per unit time, and the speech production has long gaps in which the patient is struggling unsuccessfully to produce sounds. A severe disturbance of grammar is also characteristic of Broca's aphasia. Paraphasias are common, usually involving omission of phonemes or addition of incorrect phonemes (phonemic paraphasias). In severe cases, speech may

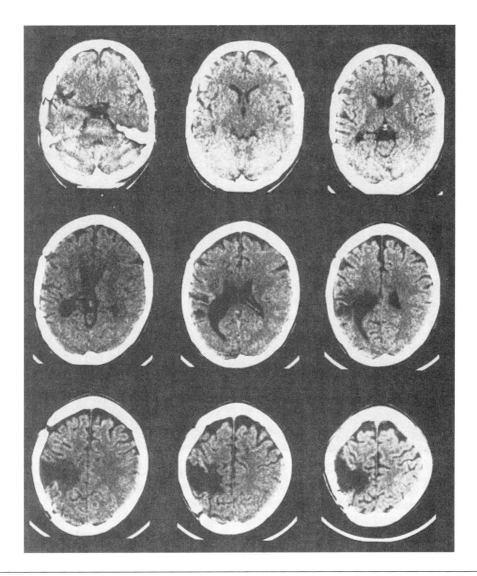

**FIGURE 2–8.** **Computed tomographic scan of a 35-year-old right-handed woman, showing a lesion (area of low density) in the left supramarginal gyrus (area 40).**
Note that the lesion spares the primary auditory cortex and the main part of Wernicke's area (posterior area 22). The woman had conduction aphasia.

be virtually unintelligible. A defect in repetition is invariably present, and most individuals with Broca's aphasia have defective naming and impaired writing. By contrast, language comprehension is relatively preserved. Persons with Broca's aphasia can comprehend simple conversations, and they generally comprehend and execute two- and even three-step commands. Reading comprehension also may be relatively preserved. An example of a CT scan from a typical patient with Broca's aphasia is shown in Figure 2–11.

In the right hemisphere, lesions to the frontal operculum have been linked to defects in paralinguistic communi-

nication, but propositional speech and language are not affected (Ross 1981). Specifically, patients may lose the ability to implement normal patterns of prosody and gesturing. Communication is characterized by flat, monotone speech; loss of spontaneous gesturing; and impaired ability to repeat affective contours (e.g., to implement emotional tones in speech, such as happiness or sadness).

## Superior Mesial Region

The superior mesial aspect of the frontal lobes comprises a set of structures that are critical for the initiation

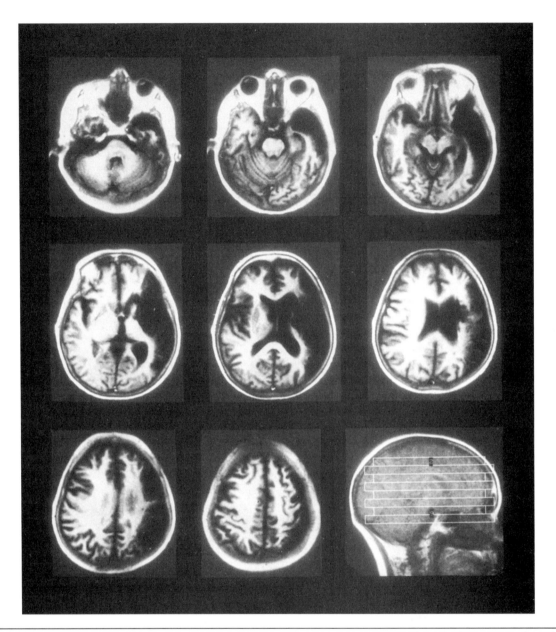

**Figure 2–9.    T1-weighted magnetic resonance images of a 34-year-old right-handed woman, showing a large right middle cerebral artery infarction.**

The lesion (shown as a *black region*) includes a significant portion of the inferior parietal lobule (areas 39 and 40). The woman had severe left-sided neglect, anosognosia, and visuospatial deficits.

of movement and emotional expression. The supplementary motor area (the mesial aspect of area 6) and the anterior cingulate gyrus (area 24) are especially important (see Figure 2–10). Lesions in this region produce a syndrome known as *akinetic mutism* (A.R. Damasio and Van Hoesen 1983; Mega and Cohenour 1997), in which the patient makes no effort to communicate, either verbally or by gesture, and maintains an empty, noncommunicative facial expression. Movements are limited to tracking of moving targets with the eyes and performing body and arm movements connected with daily necessities such as eating, pulling up bedclothing, and going to the bathroom. Otherwise, the patient does not move or speak (e.g., Tengvar et al. 2004). An example of the lesion in a patient with akinetic mutism is illustrated in Figure 2–12.

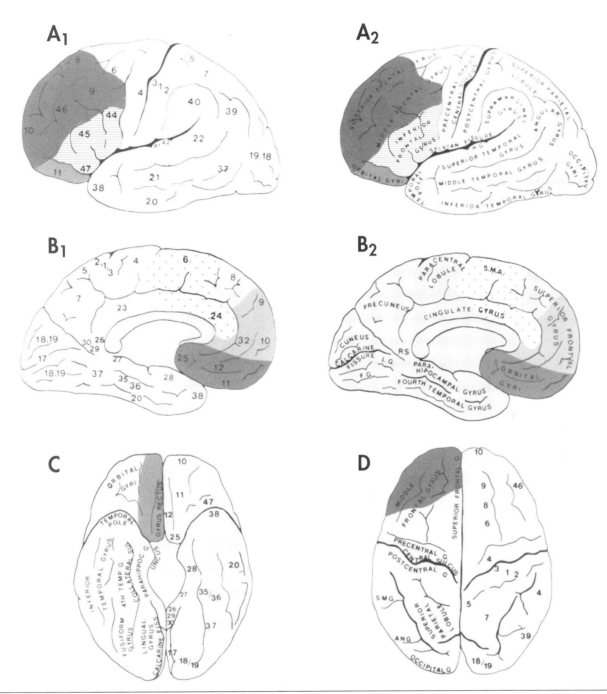

**FIGURE 2–10.** Major subdivisions of the frontal lobe: the frontal operculum, formed by areas 44, 45, and 47 (*hatched*); the superior mesial region, formed by the mesial aspect of area 6 and the anterior part of the cingulate gyrus (area 24) (*dotted pattern*); the inferior mesial region, formed by the orbital cortices (areas 11, 12, and 25) (*medium gray*) (the basal forebrain is immediately posterior to this region); and the lateral prefrontal region, formed by the lateral aspects of areas 8, 9, 46, and 10 (*dark gray*).

The ventromedial frontal lobe comprises the orbital (*medium gray*) and the lower mesial (area 32 and the mesial aspect of areas 10 and 9) cortices (*light gray*). Numbers corresponding to Brodmann's cytoarchitectonic areas are depicted in *Panels A1* and *B1* and on the right side (left hemisphere) of *Panels C* and *D*, and the standard gyrus names are shown in the corresponding *Panels A2* and *B2* and on the left side (right hemisphere) of *Panels C* and *D*. Lateral (*A1* and *A2*), mesial (*B1* and *B2*), inferior (*C*), and superior (*D*) views are represented.

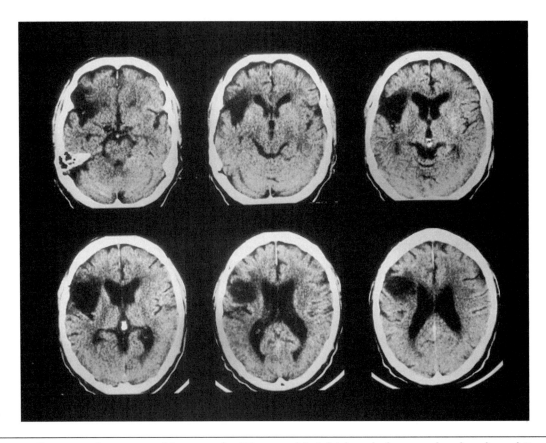

FIGURE 2–11.   **Computed tomographic scan of a 76-year-old right-handed man who developed Broca's aphasia after a left frontal infarction.**

The lesion, showing as a well-defined area of low density, is squarely in the heart of Broca's area—that is, the frontal opercular region formed by areas 44 and 45.

## Inferior Mesial Region

Inferiorly, the mesial aspect of the frontal lobes is composed of the orbital region, which includes areas 11 and 12. The basal forebrain (not part of the frontal lobes proper) is situated immediately behind the posterior-most extension of the inferior mesial region (see Figure 2–10).

### *Basal Forebrain*

The basal forebrain is composed of a set of bilateral paramidline gray nuclei that include the septal nuclei, the diagonal band of Broca, the nucleus accumbens, and the substantia innominata. Lesions to this area, commonly caused by the rupture of aneurysms located in the anterior communicating artery or in the anterior cerebral artery, cause a distinctive neuropsychological syndrome in which memory defects figure most prominently (A.R. Damasio et al. 1985, 1989; O'Connor and Verfaellie 2002; Tranel et al. 2000b; Volpe and Hirst 1983). An example

of this type of presentation is shown in Figure 2–13. Acutely, patients typically present with a confusional state and attentional problems, which resolve into an anterograde amnesia characterized by deficits in delayed free recall in the context of relatively better recognition, likely reflecting an underlying disruption of the neural mechanisms involved in strategic search processes. Evidence of temporally graded retrograde amnesia is also often seen. The amnesic profile of patients with basal forebrain lesions has several intriguing features. It is characterized by an impairment in the integration of different aspects of stimuli, wherein patients are able to learn and recall separate component features of entities and events but cannot associate those components into an integrated memory.

Another frequent manifestation in patients with basal forebrain lesions is a proclivity for confabulation. The fabrications have a dreamlike quality and occur spontaneously. They are not prompted by the need to fill gaps of

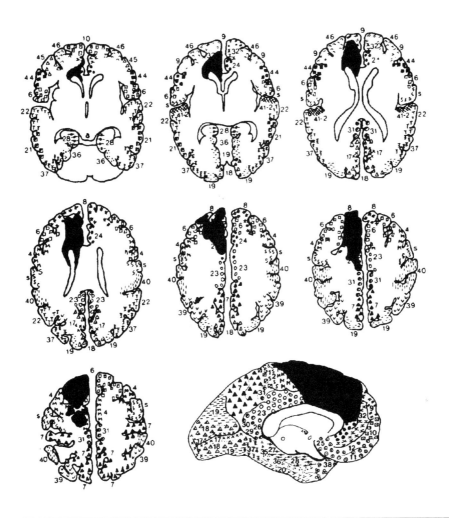

FIGURE 2–12.   **Depiction of the lesion in a 40-year-old right-handed man, marked in *black* on transverse templates and on the mesial brain.**
The lesion is in the left hemisphere and involves the mesial aspect of area 6 and the anterior part of the cingulate gyrus (area 24). Initially, the man had severe akinetic mutism, but by 3 months after onset, he had excellent recovery.

missing information in attempting to respond to an examiner's questions. In some instances, the internal experience of the patient may even include fantasies that are not recognized as such. The patient will not be capable of distinguishing reality from nonreality in his or her own recall (A.R. Damasio et al. 1985, 1989; Tranel et al. 2000b). The memory defects of patients with basal forebrain lesions can persist well into the chronic phase of recovery; even after many years, patients continue to manifest learning and recall deficits and a tendency to confabulate. In the chronic phase, however, patients usually gain some insight into their difficulties. They learn to mistrust their own recall and to cross-check their own memories against an external source.

### Ventromedial Region

The orbital and lower mesial frontal cortices (including Brodmann areas 11, 12, 25, and 32 and the mesial aspect of 10 and 9; see Figure 2–10) constitute the ventromedial frontal lobe. Patients with ventromedial frontal lobe damage develop a severe disruption of social conduct, including defects in planning, judgment, and decision making (Bechara 2004; Bechara et al. 1994, 1996; A.R. Damasio 1994; Tranel 1994; Tranel et al. 2000a), a condition that has been termed *acquired sociopathy* (Barrash et al. 2000b; A.R. Damasio et al. 1990, 1991). Preliminary evidence suggests that there may be functional asymmetries in the right and left ventromedial prefrontal sectors, with the

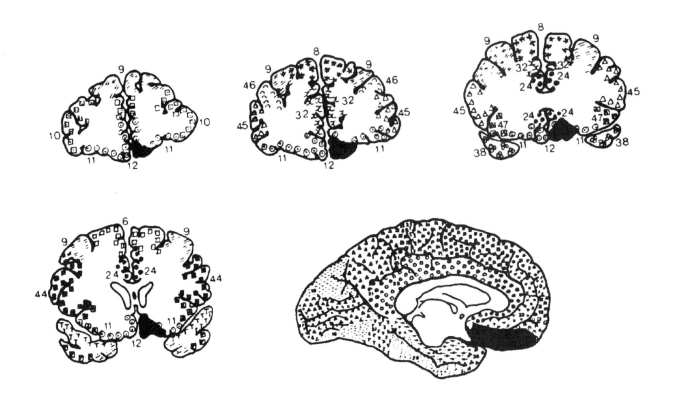

**FIGURE 2–13.** **Depiction of the lesion in a 32-year-old right-handed man who experienced rupture of an anterior communicating artery aneurysm.**
The lesion, shown in *black* on coronal sections (left hemisphere on the right) and on the mesial aspect of the hemisphere, involves the left gyrus rectus and the left basal forebrain. The man had a distinctive amnesic syndrome with confabulation and both anterograde and retrograde deficits.

right side being critical for mediating social conduct, decision making, and emotional processing and the left side playing a relatively minor role in these functions (Tranel et al. 2002). Provided that the lesion does not extend into the basal forebrain, such patients generally do not develop memory disturbances; in fact, such patients are remarkably free of conventional neuropsychological defects (A.R. Damasio and Anderson 2003; Stuss and Benson 1986; Tranel et al. 1994) (Figure 2–14).

Throughout the history of neuropsychology, investigators have called attention to the seemingly bizarre development of abnormal social behavior following frontal brain injury, especially damage to the ventromedial sector (e.g., Ackerly and Benton 1948; Brickner 1934, 1936; Harlow 1868; Hebb and Penfield 1940). The patients have a few features in common (see A.R. Damasio and Anderson 2003), including the inability to organize future activity and hold gainful employment; diminished capacity to respond to punishment; a tendency to present an

unrealistically favorable view of themselves; stereotyped but correct manners; a tendency to show inappropriate emotional reactions; and normal intelligence. It is crucial to keep in mind that in all cases, this personality and behavioral profile developed after the onset of frontal lobe damage in individuals with previously normal personalities and socialization.

Other investigators have called attention to similar characteristics in patients with ventromedial frontal lobe damage. For example, Blumer and Benson (1975) noted a personality type that characterized patients with orbital damage (which the authors termed *pseudo-psychopathic*), in which salient features were puerility, a jocular attitude, sexually disinhibited humor, inappropriate and nearly total self-indulgence, and complete lack of concern for others. Stuss and Benson (1984, 1986) emphasized that such patients have a remarkable lack of empathy and a general lack of concern about others. The patients tend to show callous unconcern, boastfulness, and unrestrained and tact-

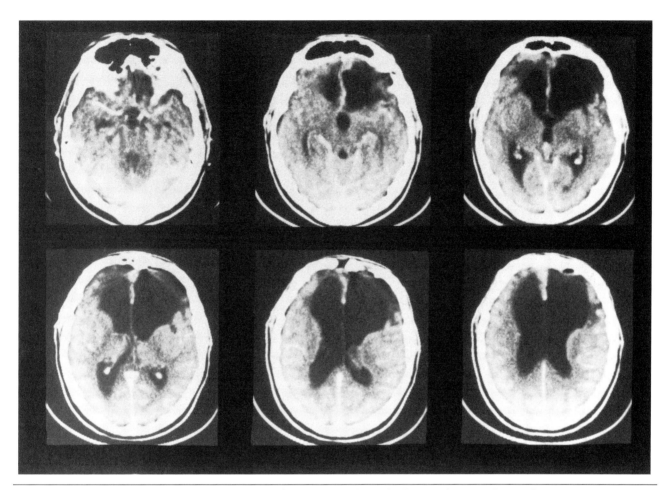

**FIGURE 2–14.** **Computed tomographic scan of a 44-year-old right-handed man who underwent resection of a large orbitofrontal meningioma.**
The lesion, showing as an area of low density, encompasses bilateral destruction of the orbital and lower mesial frontal cortices. The basal forebrain is spared. The man developed severe changes in personality but did not manifest defects in conventional neuropsychological procedures.

less behavior. Other descriptors include impulsiveness, facetiousness, and diminished anxiety and concern for the future. Mesulam (1986) emphasized the following personality features of patients with frontal lobe damage: puerile; profane; facetious; irresponsible; grandiose; irascible; erosion of foresight, judgment, and insight; loss of ability to delay gratification; loss of capacity for remorse; tendency to jump to premature conclusions; loss of capacity to grasp the context and gist of a complex situation; poor inhibition of immediate but inappropriate response tendencies; sustained shallowness; and impulsivity of thought and affect.

## Dorsolateral Prefrontal Region

The dorsolateral aspect of the frontal lobes comprises a vast expanse of cortex that occupies Brodmann areas 8, 9,

10, and 46 (see Figure 2–10). The functions of the lateral prefrontal region (exclusive of the frontal operculum and other language-related structures discussed previously) in humans are not well understood. Some of the better-established correlates are reviewed below.

One function to which the dorsolateral prefrontal region has been linked is working memory. *Working memory* refers to a relatively short (on the order of minutes) window of mental processing during which information is held "online" and operations are performed on it. For example, the demands of the Digit Span backwards test from the Wechsler Adult Intelligence Scale–III, or of the serial 7s test, are examples of working memory. The prefrontal cortex has been implicated in the mediation of working memory (Alivisatos and Milner 1989; Fuster 1989; Goldman-Rakic 1987; Jonides et al. 1993; McCarthy et al. 1994;

Milner et al. 1985; Petrides 2005; E. E. Smith et al. 1995; Wilson et al. 1993).

The dorsolateral prefrontal region also appears to be involved in higher-order integrative and executive control functions, and damage to this sector has been linked to intellectual deficits (see Stuss and Benson 1986; Stuss and Levine 2002). Patients fail to remember how often, or how recently, they have experienced a certain stimulus, but they do recognize the stimulus as familiar (Milner and Petrides 1984; Milner et al. 1985; M. L. Smith and Milner 1988).

The dorsolateral frontal cortices have been linked to the verbal regulation of behavior (Luria 1969), and verbal fluency, as measured by the ability to generate word lists under certain stimulus constraints, is notably impaired in many patients with dorsolateral lesions, especially when those lesions are bilateral or on the left (Benton 1968; Stuss et al. 1998). Finally, deficits on laboratory tests of executive function, which test the ability to form, maintain, and change cognitive sets, as well as the tendency to perseverate (the Wisconsin Card Sorting Test is a paradigmatic example), can be fairly pronounced in patients with dorsolateral lesions (Anderson et al. 1991; Milner 1963; Stuss and Levine 2002; Tranel et al. 1994).

## Subcortical Structures

Two sets of subcortical structures are considered: the basal ganglia and the thalamus.

### Basal Ganglia

The basal ganglia are a set of deep gray nuclear structures, the caudate nucleus and the lenticular nucleus, with the latter being divided into the putamen and the globus pallidus. On the left side, lesions to these structures produce a speech and language disturbance that involves a mixture of manifestations that cannot be easily classified according to standard aphasia nomenclature; hence the pattern has come to be known as *atypical aphasia* (Alexander 1989; A. R. Damasio et al. 1982; Naeser et al. 1982; for review, see Radanovic and Scaff 2003). Because damage in this region will almost invariably include the anterior limb of the internal capsule, right hemiparesis is a common accompanying manifestation. The aphasia is characterized by speech that is usually fluent but is paraphasic and dys-

arthric; (typically) poor auditory comprehension; and, in some cases, impaired repetition. An example of magnetic resonance imaging from a patient with a basal ganglia lesion and atypical aphasia is shown in Figure 2–15.

It has been noted that patients with basal ganglia lesions and atypical aphasia nearly always have lesions that involve the head of the caudate nucleus, together with the putamen and anterior limb of the internal capsule (H. Damasio 1989). Lesions confined to the putamen, or to laterally adjacent structures such as the anterior insula and subjacent white matter, do not produce an aphasic disturbance, although defects in articulation and prosody may be noted.

### Thalamus

Disturbances of speech and language have been linked to damage in the dominant thalamus (e.g., Mohr et al. 1975; for review, see Radanovic and Scaff 2003). The language disorder tends to be primarily a deficit at the semantic level, with prominent word-finding impairment, defective confrontation naming, and semantic paraphasias. This pattern has some resemblances to the transcortical aphasias, and it has been linked in particular to damage in anterior thalamic nuclei (e.g., Graff-Radford and Damasio 1984; Graff-Radford et al. 1985).

Another well-studied neuropsychological correlate of thalamic lesions is memory impairment. In the setting of chronic alcoholism and the development of Korsakoff's syndrome, such lesions typically involve the dorsomedial nucleus of the thalamus along with other diencephalic structures such as the mammillary bodies. In general, such patients develop a severe anterograde amnesia that covers all forms of declarative knowledge. However, nondeclarative learning, such as the acquisition of new perceptuomotor skills, is spared. A distinctive feature of Korsakoff's syndrome patients is their tendency to confabulate when asked direct questions about recent memory (Victor et al. 1989).

Individuals with diencephalic amnesia generally show some defect in the retrograde compartment. The impairment typically shows a temporal gradient, so that recall and recognition improve steadily with increasing distance between the present and the time of initial learning. Remote memories are retrieved more successfully (e.g., Cohen and Squire 1981).

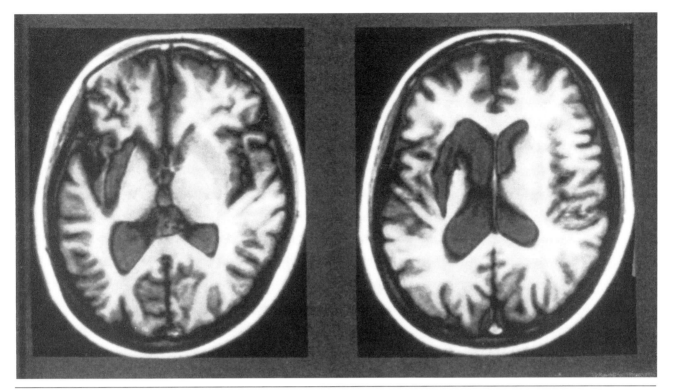

FIGURE 2–15. **T1-weighted magnetic resonance images of a 35-year-old right-handed woman who sustained a subcortical hemorrhage.**

The lesion, showing as an area of *black* on these transverse sectional images, involves the left basal ganglia, including the head and body of the caudate nucleus, and part of the putamen. The woman had a characteristic basal ganglia type of aphasia, with marked dysarthria and mixed linguistic impairments.

## Key Points: Neuropsychological Manifestations of Brain Lesions

| Structures and major subdivisions | Hemispheric side of lesion | | |
|---|---|---|---|
| | **Left** | **Right** | **Bilateral** |
| **TEMPORAL LOBES** | | | |
| Mesial | Anterograde amnesia for verbal material | Anterograde amnesia for nonverbal material | Severe anterograde amnesia for verbal and nonverbal material |
| Temporal pole | Impaired retrieval of proper nouns | Impaired retrieval of concepts for unique entities | Impaired retrieval of concepts and names for unique entities |
| | | Impaired memory for episodic and declarative knowledge | Impaired episodic memory |
| Inferotemporal | Impaired retrieval of common nouns | Impaired retrieval of concepts for some nonunique entities | Impaired retrieval of concepts and names for some nonunique entities |

| Structures and major subdivisions | Hemispheric side of lesion | | |
|---|---|---|---|
| | Left | Right | Bilateral |
| **TEMPORAL LOBES** (continued) | | | |
| Occipitotemporal junction | "Deep" prosopagnosia | Transient or mild prosopagnosia | Severe, permanent prosopagnosia |
| | Impaired retrieval of concepts for some nonunique entities | Impaired retrieval of concepts for some nonunique entities | Visual object agnosia |
| **OCCIPITAL LOBES** | | | |
| Dorsal | Partial or mild Balint's syndrome | Partial or mild Balint's syndrome | Balint's syndrome (visual disorientation, ocular apraxia, optic ataxia) |
| | | | Defective motion perception |
| | | | Astereopsis |
| Ventral | Right hemiachromatopsia | Left hemiachromatopsia | Full-field achromatopsia |
| | "Pure" alexia | Apperceptive visual agnosia | Visual object agnosia |
| | Impaired mental imagery | Defective facial imagery | Impaired mental imagery |
| | | | Prosopagnosia |
| **PARIETAL LOBES** | | | |
| Temporoparietal junction | Wernicke's aphasia | Amusia | Auditory agnosia |
| | | Defective music recognition | |
| | | "Phonagnosia" | |
| Inferior parietal lobule | Conduction aphasia | Neglect | Body schema disturbances |
| | Tactile object agnosia | Anosognosia | Anosognosia |
| | Acalculia | Anosodiaphoria | Anosodiaphoria |
| | | Tactile object agnosia | |
| **FRONTAL LOBES** | | | |
| Frontal operculum | Broca's aphasia | "Expressive" aprosody | Broca's aphasia |
| | Defective retrieval of words for actions (verbs) | | Defective retrieval of words for actions (verbs) |
| Superior mesial region | Akinetic mutism | Akinetic mutism | Severe akinetic mutism |
| Basal forebrain (inferior mesial region) | Anterograde and retrograde amnesia with confabulation (worse for verbal stimuli) | Anterograde and retrograde amnesia with confabulation (worse for nonverbal stimuli) | Anterograde and retrograde amnesia with confabulation for verbal and nonverbal stimuli |
| Orbital (inferior mesial region) | Defective social conduct | Defective social conduct | Defective social conduct |
| | "Acquired" sociopathy | "Acquired" sociopathy | "Acquired" sociopathy |
| | Prospective memory defects | Prospective memory defects | Prospective memory defects |

| | Hemispheric side of lesion | | |
|---|---|---|---|
| **Structures and major subdivisions** | **Left** | **Right** | **Bilateral** |
| **FRONTAL LOBES** *(continued)* | | | |
| Dorsolateral prefrontal region | Impaired working memory for verbal material | Impaired working memory for nonverbal spatial material | Impaired working memory for verbal and nonverbal spatial material |
| | Impaired verbal intellect | Impaired nonverbal intellect | Impaired verbal and nonverbal intellect |
| | Defective recency and frequency judgments for verbal material | Defective recency and frequency judgments for nonverbal material | Defective recency and frequency judgments for verbal and nonverbal material |
| | Defective verbal fluency | Defective design fluency | Defective verbal and design fluency |
| | Impaired "executive functions" | Impaired "executive functions" | Impaired "executive functions" |
| **SUBCORTICAL STRUCTURES** | | | |
| Basal ganglia | Atypical aphasia | —— | Atypical aphasia |
| | Dysarthria | Dysarthria | Dysarthria |
| | Aprosody | Aprosody | Aprosody |
| | Impaired nondeclarative memory | Impaired nondeclarative memory | Impaired nondeclarative memory |
| | Defective motor skill learning | Defective motor skill learning | Defective motor skill learning |
| Thalamus | Thalamic aphasia | —— | Thalamic aphasia |
| | Anterograde amnesia with confabulation | Anterograde amnesia with confabulation | Anterograde amnesia with confabulation |
| | Retrograde amnesia with temporal gradient | Retrograde amnesia with temporal gradient | Retrograde amnesia with temporal gradient |
| | Impairments in "executive functions" | Impairments in "executive functions" | Impairments in "executive functions" |
| | Attention or concentration defects | Attention or concentration defects | Attention or concentration defects |

# References

Ackerly SS, Benton AL: Report of a case of bilateral frontal lobe defect. Research Publications—Association for Research in Nervous and Mental Disease 27:479–504, 1948

Adair JC, Schwartz RL, Barrett AM: Anosognosia, in Clinical Neuropsychology, 4th Edition. Edited by Heilman KM, Valenstein E. New York, Oxford University Press, 2003, pp 185–214

Adolphs R: Is the human amygdala specialized for processing social information? Ann N Y Acad Sci 985:326–340, 2003

Adolphs R, Tranel D: The amygdala and processing of facial emotional expressions, in The Amygdala, 2nd Edition. Edited by Aggleton J. New York, Wiley-Liss, 2000, pp 587–630

Adolphs R, Tranel D, Denburg N: Impaired emotional declarative memory following unilateral amygdala damage. Learn Mem 7:180–186, 2000

Adolphs R, Tranel D, Buchanan TW: Amygdala damage impairs emotional memory for gist but not details of complex stimuli. Nat Neurosci 8:512–518, 2005

Alexander MP: Clinical-anatomical correlations of aphasia following predominantly subcortical lesions, in Handbook of Neuropsychology, Vol 2. Edited by Boller F, Grafman J. Amsterdam, Elsevier, 1989, pp 47–66

Alivisatos B, Milner B: Effects of frontal or temporal lobectomy on the use of advance information in a choice reaction time task. Neuropsychologia 27:495–503, 1989

Anderson SW, Tranel D: Awareness of disease states following cerebral infarction, dementia, and head trauma: standardized assessment. Clin Neuropsychol 3:327–339, 1989

Anderson SW, Damasio H, Jones RD, et al: Wisconsin Card Sorting Test performance as a measure of frontal lobe damage. J Clin Exp Neuropsychol 13:909–922, 1991

Babinski J: Contribution à l'étude des troubles mentaux dans l'hémiplégie organique cérébrale (anosognosie). Rev Neurol (Paris) 27:845–847, 1914

Barrash J, Damasio H, Adolphs R, et al: The neuroanatomical correlates of route learning impairment. Neuropsychologia 38:820–836, 2000a

Barrash J, Tranel D, Anderson SW: Acquired personality changes associated with bilateral damage to the ventromedial prefrontal region. Dev Neuropsychol 18:355–381, 2000b

Barton JJS: Disorders of face perception and recognition. Neurol Clin 21:521–548, 2003

Bechara A: The role of emotion in decision-making: evidence from neurological patients with orbitofrontal damage. Brain Cogn 55:30–40, 2004

Bechara A, Damasio AR, Damasio H, et al: Insensitivity to future consequences following damage to prefrontal cortex. Cognition 50:7–12, 1994

Bechara A, Tranel D, Damasio H, et al: Failure to respond autonomically to anticipated future outcomes following damage to prefrontal cortex. Cereb Cortex 6:215–225, 1996

Bellugi U, Poizner H, Klima E: Language, modality and the brain, in Brain Development and Cognition. Edited by Johnson MH. Cambridge, MA, Blackwell Publishers, 1989, pp 403–423

Benton AL: Differential behavioral effects in frontal lobe disease. Neuropsychologia 6:53–60, 1968

Benton AL: The Hécaen-Zangwill legacy: hemispheric dominance examined. Neuropsychol Rev 2:267–280, 1991

Blumer D, Benson DF: Personality changes with frontal and temporal lobe lesions, in Psychiatric Aspects of Neurologic Disease. Edited by Benson DF, Blumer D. New York, Grune & Stratton, 1975, pp 151–169

Brickner RM: An interpretation of frontal lobe function based upon the study of a case of partial bilateral frontal lobectomy. Research Publications—Association for Research in Nervous and Mental Disease 13:259–351, 1934

Brickner RM: The Intellectual Functions of the Frontal Lobes: Study Based Upon Observation of a Man After Partial Bilateral Frontal Lobectomy. New York, Macmillan, 1936

Cahill L, Babinsky R, Markowitsch HJ, et al: The amygdala and emotional memory. Nature 377:295–296, 1995

Caplan D: Aphasic syndromes, in Clinical Neuropsychology, 4th Edition. Edited by Heilman KM, Valenstein E. New York, Oxford University Press, 2003, pp 14–34

Cohen NJ, Eichenbaum H: Memory, Amnesia, and the Hippocampal System. Cambridge, MA, MIT Press, 1993

Cohen NJ, Squire LR: Retrograde amnesia and remote memory impairment. Neuropsychologia 19:337–356, 1981

Corkin S: Tactually guided maze learning in man: effects of unilateral cortical excisions and bilateral hippocampal lesions. Neuropsychologia 3:339–351, 1965

Corkin S: Acquisition of motor skill after bilateral medial temporal-lobe excision. Neuropsychologia 6:255–264, 1968

Damasio AR: Descartes' Error: Emotion, Reason, and the Human Brain. New York, Grosset/Putnam, 1994

Damasio AR, Anderson SW: The frontal lobes, in Clinical Neuropsychology, 4th Edition. Edited by Heilman KM, Valenstein E. New York, Oxford University Press, 2003, pp 404–446

Damasio AR, Van Hoesen GW: Emotional disturbances associated with focal lesions of the limbic frontal lobe, in Neuropsychology of Human Emotion. Edited by Heilman KM, Satz P. New York, Guilford, 1983, pp 85–110

Damasio AR, Yamada T, Damasio H, et al: Central achromatopsia: behavioral, anatomic and physiologic aspects. Neurology 30:1064–1071, 1980

Damasio AR, Damasio H, Rizzo M, et al: Aphasia with lesions in the basal ganglia and internal capsule. Arch Neurol 39:15–20, 1982

Damasio AR, Graff-Radford NR, Eslinger PG, et al: Amnesia following basal forebrain lesions. Arch Neurol 42:263–271, 1985

Damasio AR, Tranel D, Damasio H: Amnesia caused by herpes simplex encephalitis, infarctions in basal forebrain, Alzheimer's disease, and anoxia, in Handbook of Neuropsychology, Vol 3. Edited by Boller F, Grafman J. Amsterdam, Elsevier, 1989, pp 149–166

Damasio AR, Tranel D, Damasio H: Individuals with sociopathic behavior caused by frontal damage fail to respond autonomically to social stimuli. Behav Brain Res 41:81–94, 1990

Damasio AR, Tranel D, Damasio H: Somatic markers and the guidance of behavior: theory and preliminary testing, in Frontal Lobe Function and Dysfunction. Edited by Levin HS, Eisenberg HM, Benton AL. New York, Oxford University Press, 1991, pp 217–229

Damasio AR, Tranel D, Rizzo M: Disorders of complex visual processing, in Principles of Behavioral and Cognitive Neurology, 2nd Edition. Edited by Mesulam MM. New York, Oxford University Press, 2000, pp 332–372

Damasio H: Neuroimaging contributions to the understanding of aphasia, in Handbook of Neuropsychology, Vol 2. Edited by Boller F, Grafman J. Amsterdam, Elsevier, 1989, pp 3–46

Damasio H: Neuroanatomical correlates of the aphasias, in Acquired Aphasia, 3rd Edition. Edited by Sarno MT. New York, Academic Press, 1998, pp 43–70

Damasio H, Frank RJ: Three-dimensional in vivo mapping of brain lesions in humans. Arch Neurol 49:137–143, 1992

Eichenbaum H, Cohen NJ: From Conditioning to Conscious Recollection: Memory Systems of the Brain. New York, Oxford University Press, 2001

Frisk V, Milner B: The relationship of working memory to the immediate recall of stories following unilateral temporal or frontal lobectomy. Neuropsychologia 28:121–135, 1990

Fuster JM: The Prefrontal Cortex: Anatomy, Physiology, and Neuropsychology of the Frontal Lobes. New York, Raven, 1989

Gabrieli JDE, Corkin S, Mickel SF, et al: Intact acquisition and long-term retention of mirror-tracing skill in Alzheimer's disease and in global amnesia. Behav Neurosci 107:899–910, 1993

Goldman-Rakic PS: Circuitry of primate prefrontal cortex and regulation of behavior by representational memory, in Handbook of Physiology: The Nervous System. Edited by Plum F. Bethesda, MD, American Physiological Society, 1987, pp 373–417

Graff-Radford NR, Damasio H: Disturbances of speech and language associated with thalamic dysfunction. Semin Neurol 4:162–168, 1984

Graff-Radford NR, Damasio H, Yamada T, et al: Nonhemorrhagic thalamic infarctions: clinical, neurophysiological and electrophysiological findings in four anatomical groups defined by CT. Brain 108:485–516, 1985

Harlow JM: Recovery from the passage of an iron bar through the head. Publications of the Massachusetts Medical Society 2:327–347, 1868

Hebb DO, Penfield W: Human behavior after extensive bilateral removals from the frontal lobes. Arch Neurol Psychiatry 44:421–438, 1940

Heywood CA, Kentridge RW: Achromatopsia, color vision, and cortex. Neurol Clin 21:483–500, 2003

Hickok G, Bellugi U, Klima E: The neurobiology of sign language and its implications for the neural basis of language. Nature 381:699–702, 1996

Hunkin NM, Parkin AJ, Bradley VA, et al: Focal retrograde amnesia following closed head injury: a case study and theoretical account. Neuropsychologia 33:509–523, 1995

Jonides J, Smith EE, Koeppe RA, et al: Spatial working memory in humans as revealed by PET. Nature 363:623–625, 1993

Kanwisher N, Moscovitch M: The cognitive neuroscience of face processing: an introduction. Cogn Neuropsychol 17:1–11, 2000

Khedr EM, Hamed E, Said A, et al: Handedness and language cerebral lateralization. Eur J Appl Physiol 87:469–473, 2002

Lee GP, Meador KJ, Smith JR, et al: Preserved crossmodal association following bilateral amygdalotomy in man. Int J Neurosci 40:47–55, 1988

Luria AR: Frontal lobe syndromes, in Handbook of Clinical Neurology, Vol 2. Edited by Vinken PJ, Bruyn GW. Amsterdam, North-Holland, 1969, pp 725–757

Markowitsch HJ, Calabrese P, Wuerker M, et al: The amygdala's contribution to memory: a study on two patients with Urbach-Wiethe disease. Neuroreport 5:1349–1352, 1994

McCarthy G, Blamire AM, Puce A, et al: Functional magnetic resonance imaging of human prefrontal cortex activation during a spatial working memory task. Proc Natl Acad Sci USA 91:8690–8694, 1994

Meadows JC: Disturbed perception of colors associated with localized cerebral lesions. Brain 97:615–632, 1974

Mega MS, Cohenour RC: Akinetic mutism: disconnection of frontal-subcortical circuits. Neuropsychiatry Neuropsychol Behav Neurol 10:254–259, 1997

Mesulam MM: Frontal cortex and behavior. Ann Neurol 19:320–325, 1986

Milner B: Effects of different brain lesions on card sorting: the role of the frontal lobes. Arch Neurol 9:90–100, 1963

Milner B: Visual recognition and recall after right temporal-lobe excision in man. Neuropsychologia 6:191–209, 1968

Milner B: Disorders of learning and memory after temporal lobe lesions in man. Clin Neurosurg 19:421–446, 1972

Milner B, Petrides M: Behavioural effects of frontal-lobe lesions in man. Trends Neurosci 7:403–407, 1984

Milner B, Petrides M, Smith ML: Frontal lobes and the temporal organization of memory. Hum Neurobiol 4:137–142, 1985

Mishkin M: Memory in monkeys severely impaired by combined but not separate removal of amygdala and hippocampus. Nature 273:297–298, 1978

Mohr JP, Watters WC, Duncan GW: Thalamic hemorrhage and aphasia. Brain Lang 2:3–17, 1975

Murray EA: Representational memory in nonhuman primates, in Neurobiology of Comparative Cognition. Edited by Kesner RP, Olton DS. Hillsdale, NJ, Erlbaum, 1990, pp 127–155

Murray EA, Mishkin M: Amygdalectomy impairs crossmodal association in monkeys. Science 228:604–606, 1985

Murray EA, Mishkin M: Visual recognition in monkeys following rhinal cortical ablations combined with either amygdalectomy or hippocampectomy. J Neurosci 6:1991–2003, 1986

Naeser MA, Alexander MP, Helm-Estabrooks N, et al: Aphasia with predominantly subcortical lesion sites. Arch Neurol 39:2–14, 1982

Nahm FKD, Tranel D, Damasio H, et al: Cross-modal associations and the human amygdala. Neuropsychologia 31:727–744, 1993

O'Connor M, Verfaellie M: The amnesic syndrome: overview and subtypes, in The Handbook of Memory Disorders. Edited by Baddeley AD, Kopelman MD, Wilson BA. Chichester, UK, Wiley, 2002, pp 145–166

Paulson HL, Galetta SL, Grossman M, et al: Hemiachromatopsia of unilateral occipitotemporal infarcts. Am J Ophthalmol 118:518–523, 1994

Petrides M: Lateral prefrontal cortex: architectonic and functional organization. Philos Trans R Soc Lond B Biol Sci 360:781–795, 2005

Phelps EA, LaBar K, Anderson AK, et al: Specifying the contributions of the human amygdala to emotional memory: a case study. Neurocase 4:527–540, 1998

Poizner H, Klima ES, Bellugi U: What the Hands Reveal About the Brain. Cambridge, MA, Harvard University Press, 1987

Radanovic M, Scaff M: Speech and language disturbances due to subcortical lesions. Brain Lang 84:337–352, 2003

Rizzo M, Smith V, Pokorny J, et al: Color perception profiles in central achromatopsia. Neurology 43:995–1001, 1993

Ross ED: The aprosodias: functional-anatomic organization of the affective components of language in the right hemisphere. Arch Neurol 38:561–569, 1981

Ryan JD, Althoff RR, Whitlow S, et al: Amnesia is a deficit in relational memory. Psychol Sci 11:454–461, 2000

Smith EE, Jonides J, Koeppe RA, et al: Spatial versus object working memory: PET investigations. J Cogn Neurosci 7:337–356, 1995

Smith ML, Milner B: Estimation of frequency of occurrence of abstract designs after frontal or temporal lobectomy. Neuropsychologia 26:297–306, 1988

Smith ML, Milner B: Right hippocampal impairment in the recall of spatial location: encoding deficit or rapid forgetting? Neuropsychologia 27:71–81, 1989

Squire LR: Memory and hippocampus: a synthesis from findings with rats, monkeys, and humans. Psychol Rev 99:195–231, 1992

Stuss DT, Benson DF: Neuropsychological studies of the frontal lobes. Psychol Bull 95:3–28, 1984

Stuss DT, Benson DF: The Frontal Lobes. New York, Raven, 1986

Stuss DT, Levine B: Adult clinical neuropsychology: lessons from studies of the frontal lobes. Annu Rev Psychol 53:401–433, 2002

Stuss DT, Alexander MP, Hamer L, et al: The effects of focal anterior and posterior brain lesions on verbal fluency. J Int Neuropsychol Soc 4:265–278, 1998

Tengvar C, Johansson B, Sorensen J: Frontal lobe and cingulated cortical metabolic dysfunction in acquired akinetic mutism: a PET study of the interval form of carbon monoxide poisoning. Brain Inj 18:615–625, 2004

Tranel D: "Acquired sociopathy": the development of sociopathic behavior following focal brain damage, in Progress in Experimental Personality and Psychopathology Research, Vol 17. Edited by Fowles DC, Sutker P, Goodman SH. New York, Springer, 1994, pp 285–311

Tranel D: Higher brain function, in Neuroscience in Medicine. Edited by Conn PM. Philadelphia, PA, JB Lippincott, 1995a, pp 555–580

Tranel D: Where did my arm go? Contemporary Psychology 40:885–887, 1995b

Tranel D: Central color processing and its disorders, in Handbook of Neuropsychology, 2nd Edition, Vol 4. Edited by Boller F, Grafman J. Amsterdam, Elsevier Science, 2001, pp 1–14

Tranel D, Anderson SW: Syndromes of aphasia, in Concise Encyclopedia of Language Pathology. Edited by Fabbro F. Amsterdam, Elsevier, 1999, pp 305–319

Tranel D, Hyman BT: Neuropsychological correlates of bilateral amygdala damage. Arch Neurol 47:349–355, 1990

Tranel D, Anderson SW, Benton AL: Development of the concept of "executive function" and its relationship to the frontal lobes, in Handbook of Neuropsychology, Vol 9. Edited by Boller F, Grafman J. Amsterdam, Elsevier, 1994, pp 125–148

Tranel D, Bechara A, Damasio AR: Decision making and the somatic marker hypothesis, in The New Cognitive Neurosciences, 2nd Edition. Edited by Gazzaniga MS. Cambridge, MA, MIT Press, 2000a, pp 1047–1061

Tranel D, Damasio AR, Damasio H: Amnesia caused by herpes simplex encephalitis, infarctions in basal forebrain, and anoxia/ischemia, in Handbook of Neuropsychology, 2nd Edition, Vol 1. Edited by Boller F, Grafman J. Amsterdam, Elsevier Science, 2000b, pp 37–62

Tranel D, Bechara A, Denburg NL: Asymmetric functional roles of right and left ventromedial prefrontal cortices in social conduct, decision-making, and emotional processing. Cortex 38:589–612, 2002

Victor M, Adams RD, Collins GH: The Wernicke-Korsakoff Syndrome and Related Neurologic Disorders Due to Alcoholism and Malnutrition, 2nd Edition. Philadelphia, PA, FA Davis, 1989

Volpe BT, Hirst W: Amnesia following the rupture and repair of an anterior communicating artery aneurysm. J Neurol Neurosurg Psychiatry 46:704–709, 1983

Wilson FAW, O'Scalaidhe SP, Goldman-Rakic PS: Dissociation of object and spatial processing domains in primate prefrontal cortex. Science 260:1955–1958, 1993

Young AW, Aggleton JP, Hellawell DJ, et al: Face processing impairments after amygdalotomy. Brain 118:15–24, 1995

Zola-Morgan S, Squire LR, Amaral DG, et al: Lesions of perirhinal and parahippocampal cortex that spare the amygdala and hippocampal formation produce severe memory impairment. J Neurosci 9:4355–4370, 1989

# 3

# Cellular and Molecular Biology of the Neuron

A. KIMBERLEY McALLISTER, Ph.D.

W. MARTIN USREY, Ph.D.

STEPHEN C. NOCTOR, Ph.D.

STEPHEN RAYPORT, M.D., Ph.D.

## Cellular Composition of the Brain

Brain cells comprise two principal types: *neurons* and *glia*. Neurons are the substrate for most information processing, whereas glia are classically believed to play a supporting role. Neurons are highly differentiated cells that show considerable heterogeneity in shape and size; in fact, there are more types of neurons than types of cells in any other part of the body. The human brain contains $10^{12}$–$10^{13}$ neurons. Each neuron forms an average of $10^3$ connections, which is a minimal estimate, so the brain has on the order of $10^{15}$–$10^{16}$ synapses. During early development, neurogenesis can occur at a rate of up to 250,000 neurons per minute. In childhood, there is considerable refinement in neural circuits, associated with programmed cell death, or apoptosis, and a reduction in the number of synapses. In adulthood, neurogenesis continues, but in a very limited way. In later life, neurodegenerative disorders produce losses in the number of neurons and synapses.

Glial cells can be divided into three classes: 1) astrocytes, 2) oligodendrocytes, and 3) microglia. *Astrocytes* have three traditional functions: they provide the scaf-

folding of the brain, form the blood-brain barrier, and guide neuronal migration during development. Evidence is accumulating, however, that astroglial cells are more dynamic than previously suspected and are capable of cell-cell signaling over long distances (Dani et al. 1992; Fellin and Carmignoto 2004; Murphy et al. 1993). *Oligodendrocytes* produce the myelin sheath that speeds conduction of the action potential along axons. *Microglia* are the macrophages of the brain: quiescent until activated by brain injury.

## Neuronal Shape

Although neurons show a wide diversity of sizes and shapes, they generally have four well-defined regions: 1) dendrites, 2) cell body, 3) axon, and 4) synaptic specializations. *Dendrites* receive signals from other neurons, process and modify this information, and then convey these signals to the cell body. The *cell body* contains the genetic information resident in the nucleus that codes for the fabrication of the necessary elements of cellular function, as well as sites for their manufacture, processing, and transport. The *axon* makes highly specific connections and conveys information over long distances to its terminals. Finally, *synaptic specializations* comprise the active zone and synaptic terminal on the presynaptic axon and the postsynaptic density on the postsynaptic dendrite.

A neuron's shape is determined by the cytoskeleton. The cytoskeleton is composed primarily of three filamentous components: 1) microtubules, 2) neurofilaments, and 3) actin (Pigino et al. 2006). *Microtubules* are composed of tubulin subunits and form a scaffold that determines the shape of the neuron. *Neurofilaments* are the most abundant cytoskeletal components of the axon and are much more stable than microtubules. Finally, *actin* filaments form a dense network concentrated just under the cell membrane. In addition to its important structural role, the cytoskeleton is essential for intracellular trafficking of proteins and organelles and facilitates the selective transport of axonal and dendritic proteins (Burack et al. 2000; Kamal and Goldstein 2002).

## Neuronal Excitability

Neurons are capable of transmitting information because they are electrically and chemically excitable. This excitability is conferred by a number of classes of ion channels that are selectively permeable to specific ions and that are regulated by voltage (voltage-gated channels), by neurotransmitter binding (ligand-gated channels), or by pressure or stretch (mechanically gated channels). In general, neuronal ion channels conduct ions across the plasma membrane at extremely rapid rates—100 million ions may pass through a single channel in a second. This large flow of current causes rapid changes in membrane potential and is the basis for the action potential, the substrate for information transfer *within* neurons, and for fast synaptic responses, the substrate for information transfer *between* neurons.

Neurotransmitters released by one neuron at synapses activate receptors (ligand-gated channels) on dendrites of other neurons and induce ion flux across the membrane. The resulting electrical signals spread passively over some distance, often reaching the cell body in this way. In addition to passive conductances, localized regenerative mechanisms similar to those that give rise to the action potential (discussed later in this section) amplify dendritic input signals, boosting them so that they can reach the cell body (Eilers and Konnerth 1997; Magee and Carruth 1999; Yuste and Tank 1996). In the cell body, these synaptic inputs combine and, if sufficient, depolarize the initial segment of the axon, or axon hillock, which is the part

of the axon closest to the cell body that has the lowest threshold for activation. When a threshold level of depolarization is reached, the action potential is initiated. The action potential, or spike, is an electrical wave that propagates down the axon. In the axon terminals, this wave triggers an influx of calcium ($Ca^{2+}$), which leads to exocytosis of neurotransmitters from synaptic vesicles at specialized sites called active zones. The released neurotransmitter reaches and activates closely apposed receptors in the postsynaptic density on the postsynaptic cell's dendrites. Ultimately, this information flow reaches effector cells, principally motor fibers that mediate movement and thus generate behavior. Action potentials also back-propagate into dendrites (Johnston et al. 2003), which contributes to the crucial postsynaptic depolarization necessary for long-term potentiation.

The ability of neurons to generate an action potential derives from the presence of strong ionic gradients across the membrane; sodium ($Na^+$) and chloride ($Cl^-$) are highly concentrated outside the membrane, whereas potassium ($K^+$) is highly concentrated inside. These gradients are generated by the continuous action of membrane pumps energized by the hydrolysis of adenosine triphosphate. Also in the membrane are voltage-gated ion channels that regulate the flow of $Na^+$, $K^+$, and $Ca^{2+}$ ions across the membrane. At rest, $K^+$ and $Cl^-$ channels are open so that $K^+$ and $Cl^-$ gradients determine the membrane potential, causing the cell to be negative inside by about $-50$ mV to $-75$ mV. However, if the membrane is depolarized past the threshold potential for generating an action potential, voltage-gated $Na^+$ channels open rapidly. Because inflow of $Na^+$ depolarizes the membrane, this confers a regenerative property—once a threshold potential is reached, increased $Na^+$ influx leads to further depolarization, which opens more $Na^+$ channels, further enhancing $Na^+$ influx, and so on. Thus, once threshold is reached, the membrane potential switches to $+50$ mV very rapidly. The membrane potential stays depolarized for only about a millisecond because $Na^+$ channels then show a time-dependent inactivation. Simultaneously, voltage-dependent $K^+$ channels, which are also activated by depolarization but more slowly, increase their permeability. Because $K^+$ flows along its concentration gradient out of the cell, this, together with reduction in $Na^+$ current, leads to the repolarization of the membrane. Thus, the membrane potential peaks at a depolarized level determined by the $Na^+$ gradient and then rapidly returns to the resting potential, determined by the $K^+$ gradient. Once the membrane is repolarized, $Na^+$ inactivation wears off (the time this takes accounts for the refractory period of the neuron, a brief period when the threshold for firing an action potential is elevated), and the cell can fire again.

The regenerative property of the action potential not only serves to amplify threshold potentials (its principal function in dendrites) but also confers long-distance signaling capabilities in the axon. When the membrane potential peaks under the control of the increase in Na⁺ permeability, adjacent regions of the axon become sufficiently depolarized that they, in turn, are brought to threshold and generate an action potential. As successive axonal segments are depolarized, the action potential conducts at great speed down the axon. This is further enhanced by myelination, which increases the rate of conduction severalfold by restricting the current flow required for action potential generation to the gaps between myelin segments, the nodes of Ranvier. Because of its all-or-none characteristics and ability to conduct over long distances, the action potential provides a high-quality digital signaling mechanism in neurons.

## Signaling Between Neurons

Neurons communicate with one another at specialized sites of close membrane apposition called *synapses*. The prototypic axodendritic synapse connects a presynaptic axon terminal with a postsynaptic dendrite. This arrangement is typical for projection neurons that convey information from one region of the brain to another. In contrast, local circuit interneurons interact with neighboring neurons. Although interneurons may make axodendritic and axosomatic connections, they can also form several other kinds of synaptic contacts that greatly increase their functional sophistication. In some cases, dendrites may synapse with dendrites (*dendrodendritic* connections) or cell bodies with cell bodies (*somasomatic* connections), forming local neural circuits that convey information without action potential firing. Axons may synapse onto the axon terminals of other axons (*axoaxonic* connections) and modulate transmitter release by presynaptic inhibition or facilitation. Some neurons may function as both interneurons and projection neurons, the most prominent example being the medium spiny γ-aminobutyric acid (GABA) neurons of the striatum, which constitute about 95% of the neurons in the region (Smith and Bolam 1990).

A minority of local connections are mediated by electrical synapses that do not require chemical neurotransmitters at all. Electrical synapses are formed by multisubunit channels, called *gap junctions*, that link the cytoplasm

of adjacent cells (Bennett et al. 1991; Sohl et al. 2005), allowing both small molecules and ions carrying electrical signals to flow directly from one cell to another. Electrical synapses couple dendrites or cell bodies of adjoining cells of the same kind, typically dendrite-to-dendrite or soma-to-soma. During embryonic development, the ability to pass small molecules, including second messengers, between cells is important for the generation of morphogenic gradients (Dealy et al. 1994). During early brain development, such gradients regulate cell proliferation and establish patterns of connectivity (Kandler and Katz 1995). In the mature brain, electrical synapses act to synchronize the electrical activity of groups of neurons and mediate high-frequency transmission of signals (Bennett 1977; Brivanlou et al. 1998; Tamas et al. 2000).

Most central nervous system (CNS) synaptic connections are mediated by chemical neurotransmitters. Although chemical synapses are slower than electrical ones, they allow for signal amplification, may be inhibitory as well as excitatory, are susceptible to a wide range of modulation, and can modulate the activities of other cells through the release of transmitters activating second-messenger cascades. There are primarily two classes of neurotransmitters in the nervous system: 1) small molecule transmitters and 2) neuropeptides. In general, *small molecule transmitters* mediate fast synaptic transmission; are stored in small, clear synaptic vesicles; and include glutamate, GABA, glycine, acetylcholine, serotonin, dopamine, norepinephrine, epinephrine, and histamine. In contrast, the *neuropeptides* are a very large family of neurotransmitters that modulate synaptic transmission, are stored in large dense-core vesicles, and include somatostatin, the hypothalamic-releasing hormones, endorphins, enkephalins, and the opioids. Interestingly, small molecule transmitters and neuropeptides are often released from the same neuron and can act together on the same target (Hökfelt 1991).

Small neurotransmitter molecules are stored in small, clear, membrane-bound granules called *synaptic vesicles*. Each synaptic vesicle contains several thousand neurotransmitter molecules. When an action potential invades the presynaptic region, the depolarization activates voltage-dependent Ca²⁺ channels and triggers transmitter release. The subsequent Ca²⁺ influx raises the local Ca²⁺ concentration near the active zone, promoting synaptic vesicle fusion and neurotransmitter release via *exocytosis*. Neurotransmitter then diffuses a short distance across the synaptic cleft and binds to postsynaptic receptors. The dynamics and modulation of synaptic transmission are fundamental to alterations in synaptic connections that underlie both normal and pathological learning and memory. Synaptic vesicles undergo a six-step cycle:

1. Vesicles dock at active zones before exocytotic release.
2. Priming occurs, whereby vesicles become ready to respond to increases in intracellular $Ca^{2+}$. (The potent neurotoxins botulinum and tetanus toxin block synaptic transmission by proteolysis of key molecules involved in priming.)
3. Triggered by an influx in $Ca^{2+}$, fusion/exocytosis then occurs in less than a millisecond, releasing the neurotransmitter into the synaptic cleft.
4. Endocytosis recovers the synaptic vesicle membrane.
5. Synaptic vesicles are refilled with neurotransmitter, driven by an acidic intravesicular gradient.
6. The filled synaptic vesicles are transported back to the active zone to complete the cycle.

Neurotransmitter activity is typically limited in duration by several mechanisms that rapidly remove released neurotransmitter from the synapse. First, simple diffusion out of the synaptic cleft limits the duration of action of all neurotransmitters. Second, neurotransmitters may be enzymatically degraded; for example, acetylcholine is hydrolyzed by acetylcholinesterase bound to the postsynaptic membrane adjacent to the receptors. Finally, although the monoamine and amino acid neurotransmitters are also metabolized, they are principally removed from the synaptic cleft by rapid reuptake mechanisms, whereby they are repackaged in synaptic vesicles or metabolized (Masson et al. 1999).

## Rapid Postsynaptic Responses

The action of a neurotransmitter depends on the properties of the postsynaptic receptors to which it binds. Postsynaptic receptors activated by neurotransmitter fall into two classes: 1) ionotropic and 2) metabotropic (discussed in the "Metabotropic Receptors" subsection later in this chapter). Ionotropic receptors are directly linked to an ion channel; these receptors undergo a conformational change upon neurotransmitter binding that opens the channel. This action results in either depolarization, giving rise to an excitatory postsynaptic potential, or hyperpolarization, giving rise to an inhibitory postsynaptic potential.

The neuromuscular junction is the prototypic excitatory synapse; simultaneous binding of two acetylcholine molecules opens a channel in the receptor that is permeable to both $Na^+$ and $K^+$ (Karlin and Akabas 1995). This results in a strong depolarization of the postsynaptic membrane mediated by $Na^+$ influx (and moderated by $K^+$

efflux), leading to an action potential in the motor fiber that evokes contraction. Ligand-gated channels are found at synapses such as the neuromuscular junction, where rapid and reliable activation of the postsynaptic cell is required. At the neuromuscular junction, the postsynaptic response is sufficiently strong so that there is a one-to-one translation of motor neuron spikes into muscle fiber spikes, thus ensuring reliable muscle contraction.

Unlike the neuromuscular junction, CNS neurons function in dynamic networks (Vogels et al. 2005) so that generally no individual cell has so strong a synaptic connection with another cell that it alone brings it to threshold. Rather, groups of neurons—active in concert—converge on a postsynaptic neuron to generate multiple postsynaptic potentials. These potentials may summate within regions of the postsynaptic neuron (*spatial summation*) if they occur sufficiently close together in time to cause the postsynaptic neuron to fire. As a rule, fast ligand-gated channels mediate the flow of information representing patterns of sensory input and associations between sensory modalities, underlying central representations that ultimately give rise to motor outputs. In the CNS, glutamate receptors mediate most fast excitatory transmission; GABA and glycine are the most common inhibitory neurotransmitters.

## Glutamate Receptors

Excitatory postsynaptic potentials are mediated by two classes of ionotropic glutamate receptors: *N*-methyl-D-aspartate (NMDA) receptors and non-NMDA, or α-amino-3-hydroxy-5-methylisoxazole-4-propionic acid (AMPA), receptors (Hassel and Dingledine 2006). Ionotropic glutamate receptors are multimeric proteins, usually composed of four subunits. NMDA receptors are formed from combinations of NR1 and NR2 subunits; the NR1 subunit is universally expressed in neurons, whereas the NR2, which comes in several subtypes, is heterogeneously expressed both during development and among different neurons, giving rise to different response properties (Schoepfer et al. 1994). NMDA receptors depolarize cells by opening channels that principally allow $Ca^{2+}$ to enter the cell. The most striking property of NMDA receptors is that the ion channel is usually blocked by magnesium ($Mg^{2+}$) at membrane potentials more negative than about –40 mV (MacDermott et al. 1986; Nowak et al. 1984). As a result, at the resting potential of most neurons, the NMDA receptor channel is occluded. For current to flow through NMDA channels, glutamate must bind to the receptor and the membrane must be depolarized simultaneously to displace the $Mg^{2+}$. This dual requirement underlies the unique role of NMDA receptors in processes as varied as synaptogenesis, learning and memory, and even cell death. NMDA receptors are also likely to be critical for proper mental functioning. NMDA receptor hypofunction has been implicated as a pathogenic mechanism in schizophrenia (Coyle 2006).

## GABA Receptors

Inhibitory postsynaptic potentials in the brain are mediated primarily by GABA receptors (Olsen and Betz 2006). Several classes of GABA receptors have been identified. $GABA_A$ receptors are ionotropic receptors that form $Cl^-$-selective channels and mediate fast synaptic inhibition in the brain. $GABA_B$ receptors are metabotropic receptors that tend to be slower acting and play a modulatory role; they are often found on presynaptic terminals, where they inhibit transmitter release. $GABA_A$ receptors are members of the nicotinic acetylcholine receptor superfamily. The $GABA_A$ receptor–channel complex is composed of a mixture of five subunits from $\alpha$, $\beta$, $\gamma$, and $\rho$ families. This gives rise to receptors with varying properties, depending on the specific receptor subunit composition. Because most of the subunit families have multiple subtypes, some of which can undergo RNA splicing, there is the potential for an extraordinary diversity of $GABA_A$ receptor function. During early development, intracellular chloride levels are high, so $GABA_A$ receptors in fact mediate excitation (Lee et al. 2005).

## Metabotropic Receptors

Longer-term modulatory effects are generally mediated by metabotropic receptors (Greengard 2001). These non-channel-linked receptors regulate cell function via activation of G proteins that couple to second-messenger cascades. Although other non-channel-linked receptors also may be catalytic, in the CNS only G protein–linked receptors are found. In fact, most neurotransmitters and neuromodulators exert their effects through binding to G protein receptors. G protein–linked receptors are so named because they couple to intracellular guanosine triphosphate (GTP)–binding regulatory proteins. G proteins are formed from a complex of three membrane-bound proteins ($G_{\alpha\beta\gamma}$); when the receptor is activated, the $\alpha$ subunit ($G_\alpha$) binds GTP and dissociates from a complex of the $\beta$ and $\gamma$ subunits ($G_{\beta\gamma}$). Both $G_\alpha$ and $G_{\beta\gamma}$ may go on to trigger subsequent events. Activated G proteins have a life span of seconds to minutes; $G_\alpha$ auto-inactivates by hydrolyzing its bound GTP, after which it reaggregates with $G_{\beta\gamma}$, returning to the resting state. Continued transmitter binding to the receptor may reinitiate the cycle.

## Synapse Formation

When an axonal growth cone reaches a target cell, a complex series of interactions commences, ultimately resulting in the formation of a synapse. Although there is still much to be learned about the formation of synapses in the CNS, the basic process of synaptogenesis at the neuromuscular junction (the synapse between a motor neuron and a muscle cell) has been well described. Both the motor neuron and the muscle cell have the necessary molecular machinery prefabricated before synapse formation (Sanes and Lichtman 1999). The motor neuron growth cone functions like a protosynapse, showing activity-dependent neurotransmitter release. Noninnervated postsynaptic cells have transmitter receptors distributed over much of their surface, and within minutes of initial contact, a rudimentary form of synaptic transmission begins. Over subsequent days, connections become stronger and stabilize as the growth cone matures into a presynaptic terminal, gathering the cellular elements necessary for focused release of neurotransmitter at active zones. In parallel, the postsynaptic cell concentrates receptors at the site of contact, removing them from other regions, and over the course of days it develops postsynaptic specializations.

## Neuronal Maturation and Survival

Maturation of the postsynaptic cell requires de novo protein synthesis, as do learning-dependent, long-term changes in the adult CNS. Interactions between presynaptic and postsynaptic neurons can act to enhance and modulate their differentiation. For example, secretion of trophic factors by postsynaptic cells can determine whether innervating presynaptic neurons survive or undergo apoptosis. More subtle regulation of presynaptic cell differentiation occurs as well. In the developing sympathetic nervous system, young neurons are exclusively noradrenergic before synapse formation. Depending on the target tissue, they may be induced to become cholinergic, retaining only traces of the noradrenergic phenotype (Landis 1990). This target-dependent effect is mediated by the release of a soluble cholinergic-differentiation factor by the postsynaptic cells. Once synaptic contact is established, cholinergic activation of the postsynaptic cell by presynaptic spikes suppresses the release of cholinergic differentiation factor. Thus, synapse formation may trigger far-reaching changes, both pre- and postsynaptically, extending to the choice of neurotransmitter by a presynaptic neuron.

In many areas of the vertebrate nervous system, neurons are initially produced in excess. To survive, neurons must receive an adequate supply of one or more trophic factors produced by their target neurons. Competition for limited supplies of these factors ensures that surviving neurons will be correctly connected and that the number of neurons will be matched to the size of the target. In general, cells deprived of neurotrophic factors undergo apoptosis, a genetically programmed form of cell death characterized by cytoplasmic shrinkage, chromatin condensation, and degradation of DNA into oligonucleosomal fragments (Edwards et al. 1991). Unlike necrosis, this process does not stimulate an inflammatory response. Apoptosis is an active process that requires RNA and protein synthesis (Oppenheim et al. 1991; Scott and Davies 1990). Data are accumulating to support the remarkable hypothesis that apoptosis is the default program for most cells and that widespread cell suicide is prevented only by the continual presence of survival signals that suppress the intrinsic cell death program (Raff et al. 1993). The best-studied neuronal example is the dependence of sympathetic and sensory neurons on nerve growth factor (NGF), which is produced by the target tissue. Although approximately half of the sympathetic neurons normally undergo apoptosis, exogenously applied NGF prevents most of the cells from dying; in contrast, neutralizing antibodies to NGF produce widespread sympathetic cell death (Raff et al. 1993).

## Key Points: Cellular and Molecular Biology of the Neuron

- Neuropsychiatric disorders result from disordered functioning of neurons, and in particular their synapses.
- Individual neurons in the brain receive synaptic input from thousands of neurons and, in turn, send information to thousands of others.
- During development, neurons and glia are generated in proliferative zones lining the ventricular system and then migrate into the overlying cortical mantle.
- The determination of cell fate occurs at regional, local, and cellular levels.
- Neurons are initially produced in excess; their survival depends on trophic factors produced by their targets.
- Normal sensory experience is essential to the maturation of neural connections.
- The adult brain retains a significant degree of plasticity; changes in cortical organization can be induced by behaviorally important, temporally coincident sensory input.
- In both learning and development, the key molecular coincidence detector is the NMDA receptor, which requires both neurotransmitter binding and depolarization for activation.
- $Ca^{2+}$ influx mediated by the NMDA receptor triggers changes in the strength of synapses, in time leading to changes in synapse number.
- $Ca^{2+}$ regulates the growth or retraction of neurites, programmed cell death.

## References

Bennett MVL: Electrical transmission: a functional analysis and comparison to chemical transmission, in Handbook of Physiology, Vol I: The Nervous System. Bethesda, MD, American Physiological Society, 1977, pp 357–416

Bennett MVL, Barrio LC, Bargiello TA, et al: Gap junctions: new tools, new answers, new questions. Neuron 6:305–320, 1991

Brivanlou IH, Warland DK, Meister M: Mechanisms of concerted firing among retinal ganglion cells. Neuron 20:527–539, 1998

Burack MA, Silverman MA, Banker G: The role of selective transport in neuronal protein sorting. Neuron 26:465–472, 2000

Coyle JT: The neurochemistry of schizophrenia, in Basic Neurochemistry: Molecular, Cellular and Medical Aspects, 7th Edition. Edited by Siegel GJ, Albers RW, Brady S, et al. Burlington, MA, Elsevier Academic, 2006, pp 875–885

Dani JW, Chernjavsky A, Smith SJ: Neuronal activity triggers calcium waves in hippocampal astrocyte networks. Neuron 8:429–440, 1992

Dealy CN, Beyer EC, Kosher RA: Expression patterns of mRNAs for the gap junction proteins connexin43 and connexin42 suggest their involvement in chick limb morphogenesis and specification of the arterial vasculature. Dev Dyn 199:156–167, 1994

Edwards SN, Buckmaster AE, Tolkovsky AM: The death programme in cultured sympathetic neurones can be suppressed at the posttranslational level by nerve growth factor, cyclic AMP, and depolarization. J Neurochem 57:2140–2143, 1991

Eilers J, Konnerth A: Dendritic signal integration. Curr Opin Neurobiol 7:385–390, 1997

Fellin T, Carmignoto G: Neurone-to-astrocyte signalling in the brain represents a distinct multifunctional unit. J Physiol 559:3–15, 2004

Greengard P: The neurobiology of slow synaptic transmission. Science 294:1024–1030, 2001

Hassel B, Dingledine R: Glutamate, in Basic Neurochemistry: Molecular, Cellular and Medical Aspects, 7th Edition. Edited by Siegel GJ, Albers RW, Brady S, et al. Burlington, MA, Elsevier Academic, 2006, pp 267–290

Hökfelt T: Neuropeptides in perspective: the last ten years. Neuron 7:867–879, 1991

Johnston D, Christie BR, Frick A, et al: Active dendrites, potassium channels and synaptic plasticity. Philos Trans R Soc Lond B Biol Sci 358:667–674, 2003

Kamal A, Goldstein LS: Principles of cargo attachment to cytoplasmic motor proteins. Curr Opin Cell Biol 14:63–68, 2002

Kandler K, Katz LC: Neuronal coupling and uncoupling in the developing nervous system. Curr Opin Neurobiol 5:98–105, 1995

Karlin A, Akabas MH: Toward a structural basis for the function of nicotinic acetylcholine receptors and their cousins. Neuron 15:1231–1244, 1995

Landis SC: Target regulation of neurotransmitter phenotype. Trends Neurosci 13:344–350, 1990

Lee H, Chen CX, Liu YJ, et al: KCC2 expression in immature rat cortical neurons is sufficient to switch the polarity of GABA responses. Eur J Neurosci 21:2593–2599, 2005

MacDermott AB, Mayer ML, Westbrook GL, et al: NMDA-receptor activation increases cytoplasmic calcium concentration in cultured spinal cord neurones. Nature 321:519–522, 1986

Magee JC, Carruth M: Dendritic voltage-gated ion channels regulate the action potential firing mode of hippocampal CA1 pyramidal neurons. J Neurophysiol 82:1895–1901, 1999

Masson J, Sagné C, Hamon M, et al: Neurotransmitter transporters in the central nervous system. Pharmacol Rev 51:439–464, 1999

Murphy TH, Blatter LA, Wier WG, et al: Rapid communication between neurons and astrocytes in primary cortical cultures. J Neurosci 13:2672–2679, 1993

Nowak L, Bregestovski P, Ascher P, et al: Magnesium gates glutamate-activated channels in mouse central neurones. Nature 307:462–465, 1984

Olsen R, Betz H: GABA and glycine, in Basic Neurochemistry: Molecular, Cellular and Medical Aspects, 7th Edition. Edited by Siegel GJ, Albers RW, Brady S, et al. Burlington, MA, Elsevier Academic, 2006, pp 291–301

Oppenheim A, Altuvia S, Kornitzer D, et al: Translation control of gene expression. J Basic Clin Physiol Pharmacol 2:223–231, 1991

Pigino G, Kirkpatrick L, Brady S: The cytoskeleton of neurons and glia, in Basic Neurochemistry: Molecular, Cellular and Medical Aspects, 7th Edition. Edited by Siegel GJ, Albers RW, Brady S, et al. Burlington, MA, Elsevier Academic, 2006, pp 123–137

Raff MC, Barres BA, Burne JF, et al: Programmed cell death and the control of cell survival: lessons from the nervous system. Science 262:695–700, 1993

Sanes JR, Lichtman JW: Development of the vertebrate neuromuscular junction. Annu Rev Neurosci 22:389–442, 1999

Schoepfer R, Monyer H, Sommer B, et al: Molecular biology of glutamate receptors. Prog Neurobiol 42:353–357, 1994

Scott SA, Davies AM: Inhibition of protein synthesis prevents cell death in sensory and parasympathetic neurons deprived of neurotrophic factor in vitro. J Neurobiol 21:630–638, 1990

Smith AD, Bolam JP: The neural network of the basal ganglia as revealed by the study of synaptic connections of identified neurones. Trends Neurosci 13:259–265, 1990

Sohl G, Maxeiner S, Willecke K: Expression and functions of neuronal gap junctions. Nat Rev Neurosci 6:191–200, 2005

Tamas G, Buhl EH, Lorincz A, et al: Proximally targeted GABAergic synapses and gap junctions synchronize cortical interneurons. Nat Neurosci 3:366–371, 2000

Vogels TP, Rajan K, Abbott LF: Neural network dynamics. Annu Rev Neurosci 28:357–376, 2005

Yuste R, Tank DW: Dendritic integration in mammalian neurons, a century after Cajal. Neuron 16:701–716, 1996

# 4

# Genetics

Prabhakara V. Choudary, Ph.D., F.R.S.C.

James A. Knowles, M.D., Ph.D.

## Psychiatric Genetics: Aims and Methods

### Aims

1. To establish and specify the genetic component of the etiology of psychiatric syndromes and thus determine a) to what extent a psychiatric disorder is genetically caused, b) the DNA variation underlying each genetic contribution, c) the biopsychosocial abnormalities associated with the gene or genes involved, and d) the processes by which genetic abnormalities lead to symptoms.
2. To establish and specify the nongenetic component of the etiology of psychiatric syndromes and thus identify environmental factors that, acting independently of or interacting with vulnerable genotypes, produce or increase the likelihood of a disorder.
3. To validate the boundaries of diagnostic entities and subtypes within entities by determining a) the similarities in genetic variations between disorders, or between subtypes of a disorder, to establish groupings of genetically related disorders (e.g., a schizophrenia spectrum) or to split disorders established on clinical

phenomenology (e.g., different subtypes of schizoaffective disorder); and b) the characteristics (e.g., severity, subject's age at onset) of a disorder that increase its heritability, thereby helping to identify diagnostic boundaries that more closely correspond to biological boundaries.

4. To specify the genetic contribution to traits and psychological symptoms, independent of their role as components of defined psychiatric syndromes.
5. To develop methods of preventing or treating psychiatric disorders based on knowledge of genetic and environmental factors in their etiology.

### Methods

Research methods have evolved for each of the aims of genetic investigation. Over the past two decades, the methodologies have been especially productive in determining to what extent a psychiatric disorder is genetically caused (Table 4–1). New techniques hold the promise of determining the location, nature, and product of the genetic contribution to many disorders. Genetic investigation of a psychiatric disorder attempts to answer numerous interrelated questions, such as the following:

PVC and JAK gratefully acknowledge the support of the National Institute of Mental Health (NIMH) (RO1-MH60912, RO1-MH50214), the National Institute on Drug Abuse (RO1-DA12190, RO1-DA12853), the National Institute on Aging (RO1-AG15473), and the National Alliance for Research on Schizophrenia and Depression; and of the Pritzker Neuropsychiatric Disorders Research Fund L.L.C. and the NIMH (Silvio O. Conte Center for Mood Disorders Research #2P50-MH060398-07), respectively. The authors have no competing financial interests.

**TABLE 4–1.** Evidence in support of genetic transmission of various psychiatric disorders

| Illness | Family risk studies | Twin studies | Adoption studies | Molecular studies |
|---|---|---|---|---|
| Schizophrenia | + | + | + | + |
| Bipolar disorder | + | + | + | + |
| Major depression | + | + | (+) | + |
| Panic disorder and agoraphobia | + | + | | + |
| Generalized anxiety disorder | + | + | | |
| Simple phobia | + | + | | |
| Social phobia | + | + | | |
| Obsessive-compulsive disorder | (+) | + | | + |
| Posttraumatic stress disorder | | + | | |
| Anorexia nervosa | + | + | | + |
| Briquet's syndrome/somatization disorder and sociopathy | + | (+) | + | |
| Alcoholism | + | (+) | + | + |
| Personality disorders | | | | |
|   Antisocial | + | | | |
|   Schizotypal | + | + | | + |
|   Borderline | | + | | |
|   Avoidant | + | | | |
|   Dependent | + | | | |
| Alzheimer's disease | + | (+) | | + |

*Note.* Evidence discussed, with references, in text. +=most or all findings support genetic transmission; (+)=some findings support genetic transmission, but others do not.

- Is the illness familial?
- Is this familiality caused by genetic factors?
- What are the various clinical expressions of the abnormal gene(s)?
- What are the earliest manifestations of the predisposition to illness?
- What environmental variables increase or decrease the chances of predisposed individuals developing the disorder?
- What is the mode of transmission?
- Where is (are) the abnormal gene(s)?
- What is the biological, physiological, and psychological outcome of the genetic abnormality?

Different techniques, each with its own advantages and disadvantages as described in the following subsections, are used in attempts at answering these questions.

### Is the Illness Familial?—Family Risk Studies and Epidemiological Studies

Family risk studies are designed to determine the extent to which an illness runs in families, because genetic diseases show increased rates of illness among relatives, although not all familial traits are genetic (e.g., language skill). The current state-of-the-art family risk study

1. Samples patients (termed *probands* or *index cases*) in an unbiased way to obtain a sample that is representative of all patients with the disorder.
2. Either interviews family members directly or obtains detailed descriptions of a family member's illness through records and multiple informants.
3. Arrives at diagnoses while blind to the disease status of the index case.

4. Uses operationalized diagnostic criteria (such as those in DSM-IV-TR [American Psychiatric Association 2000]).
5. Demonstrates reliability in both the information gathering and the diagnostic processes.
6. Compares the data on familial psychopathology, using appropriate statistical analyses, with the rate of psychopathology in the family members of a matched control group investigated simultaneously with the same methodology.

When the lifetime morbid risks for first-degree relatives of ill and control probands are determined, a *relative risk* for first-degree relatives of ill probands can be calculated. As seen in Table 4–2, which is based on selected methodologically sound studies, this relative risk varies from approximately 3 to 25 for the psychiatric disorders studied, indicating significant familial aggregation for all of them. From these data, it appears that bipolar disorder, schizophrenia, panic disorder, and alcoholism are familial disorders.

### Do Genetic Factors Contribute to the Illness?— Twin and Adoption Studies

**Twin studies.**  Twin studies examine the concordance, or the coincidence, of a disorder in monozygotic (MZ), genetically identical twins and in dizygotic (DZ), fraternal twins, the latter sharing on average one-half of their genes, as do siblings. One strategy involves comparing concordance in MZ pairs and same-sex DZ pairs. If the rearing environment has predisposed an index case to illness, then the co-twin, whether MZ or DZ, also should be at risk, and the rates for both MZ and DZ twins should be equally elevated (compared with the population rate). If, on the other hand, pathogenic genes have predisposed the index twin to illness, then an MZ co-twin would be at a higher risk than a DZ co-twin. The concordance rate for MZ twins would be higher than that for DZ twins, and the concordance rate for DZ twins should be similar to that of siblings.

**Adoption studies.**  The four types of adoption studies are

1. *Adoptee study method:* the study of adopted-away children of a parent with a disorder.
2. *Cross-fostering strategy:* the study of children who were born of nondisordered parents and were adopted into a family with a disordered parent.
3. *Adoptees' family method:* the study of the adoptive and the biological relatives of disordered adoptees.

**TABLE 4–2.**  **Relative risks for psychiatric disorders**

| Disorder | Relative risk | Reference |
|---|---|---|
| Bipolar disorder | 24.5 | Weissman et al. 1984 |
| Schizophrenia | 18.5 | Kendler et al. 1985 |
| Bulimia nervosa | 9.6 | Kassett et al. 1989 |
| Panic disorder | 9.6 | Crowe et al. 1983 |
| Alcoholism | 7.4 | Merikangas 1989 |
| Generalized anxiety disorder | 5.6 | Noyes et al. 1987 |
| Anorexia nervosa | 4.6 | Strober et al. 1985 |
| Simple phobia | 3.3 | Fyer et al. 1990 |
| Social phobia | 3.2 | Fyer et al. 1993 |
| Somatization disorder | 3.1 | Cloninger et al. 1986 |
| Major depression | 3.0 | Weissman et al. 1984 |
| Agoraphobia | 2.8 | Crowe et al. 1983 |

*Note.*  Other studies may have relative risk ratios that differ considerably from those in these studies, especially if different diagnostic criteria were used. However, the methodological soundness of studies referenced here prompted our selection of them for discussion in the text and in this comparison.

4. *MZ twins reared apart:* the study of MZ twins reared apart, as discussed previously (see "Twin Studies").

Although adoption permits ideal separation of genetic factors from environmental influences, it has certain methodological drawbacks. Because few children are adopted away immediately after birth, usually some familial environmental influences of undetermined significance can exist, which are difficult to measure.

Also, "environment" does not necessarily begin at birth; and the uterine environment of an affected mother may have a significant role in the transmission of the illness, which may be examined by comparing the risk to the children of affected mothers with the risk to the children of affected fathers; or in the adoptees' family method, the risk to paternal half-siblings may be compared with the risk to maternal half-siblings.

### What Are the Various Clinical Expressions of the Abnormal Gene(s)?—Spectrum Studies

As evidence has accumulated suggesting that genetic factors account for the increased familial incidence of major psychiatric disorders, a hypothesis has been put forth that the other syndromes found to be increased among relatives are also the result of the same genetic predisposition. This concept has been expressed as the "spectrum" of disorders related to, for example, schizophrenia or bipolar disorder.

For many types of genetic studies, however, determining, for all family members, who in the family is ill and who is well is often of utmost importance. Studies attempting to determine the mode of transmission (i.e., segregation analysis) and linkage studies are most obviously affected by misclassification. Because problems are posed by both overinclusion and overexclusion, the issue of which phenotypic syndromes are manifestations of the genotype is essential.

### What Are the Early Manifestations of and Environmental Risk Factors for the Illness?— High-Risk Studies

High-risk research, or the study of children at risk, is a strategy that begins with a factor of known or putative importance for the development of psychopathology and examines, through controlled studies, the influence of that factor on exposed infants or children. Such a design has been used to delineate the effects of maternal alcohol consumption during pregnancy on birth weight. It has also been used to identify the early development of psychopathology among the offspring of parents with psychiatric disorders. This strategy entails selection of parent probands with an accurately diagnosed disorder, evaluation of psychopathology in the co-parents, and usually a longitudinal evaluation of the children with a battery of psychological and biological measures, as well as a record of environmental conditions during development. These studies can investigate 1) presymptomatic differences between the high-risk group and the control group and whether such abnormalities predict later psychopathology, 2) early manifestations of psychopathology in subjects who later develop the same disorder that their parents experienced, 3) the childhood psychopathological syndromes that may be genetically related to the adult psychiatric disorders of either or both parents, and 4) environmental variables that are associated with the development of illness in the genetically predisposed group.

### What Is the Mode of Transmission?— Segregation Analysis

When family, twin, and adoption studies show a role for genetic factors in the pathogenesis of a disorder, then *segregation analysis* can be attempted to determine the

mode of transmission of those genetic factors. The pattern of inheritance of the disorder is studied in a collection of families and compared with known patterns of inheritance. Mutations at any single gene are inherited in a dominant or recessive manner and may be autosomal or sex-linked. If the disorder is transmitted in families in one of these patterns, a single-gene mutation could be its cause.

### Where Is the Abnormal Gene?—Genetic Linkage Analysis and Association Studies

Two general approaches permit the discovery of genetic factors responsible for the pathogenesis of a disease: 1) genome scans followed by subsequent positional cloning and 2) candidate gene association studies. In the first approach, the broad chromosomal location of an abnormal gene is identified, perhaps containing hundreds of genes, without reference to the abnormal protein for which it codes, by the use of a genome scan and genetic linkage analysis.

# Genetics of Psychiatric Disorders

## Schizophrenia

### Family Studies

It would appear that schizophrenia, regardless of whether broadly or narrowly defined, is familial. Furthermore, schizoaffective disorder (as defined in DSM-III-R [American Psychiatric Association 1987]), paranoid personality disorder, atypical psychosis, and schizotypal personality disorder also aggregate in the relatives of schizophrenic probands, indicating possible boundaries of the phenotypic spectrum (Kendler et al. 1985). Additional studies have extended this boundary to other clinical conditions (qualitative phenotypes) and clinical and subclinical signs (quantitative phenotypes). It appears that even bipolar disorder may be elevated in the relatives of schizophrenic probands, at least in some families (Pope and Yurgelun-Todd 1990)—possibly those with schizophrenia "spectrum conditions" (Baron and Gruen 1991)—or when the mood disorder is associated with psychotic symptoms (Decina et al. 1991).

Elevated quantitative phenotypes that are clinically apparent in the relatives of schizophrenic probands include 1) positive symptoms measured by the Thought Disorder Index (Shenton et al. 1989); 2) negative symptoms measured by the Scale for the Assessment of Negative Symptoms (Tsuang et al. 1991); 3) neuropsychological signs such as deficits in abstraction (as measured by the Wisconsin Card Sorting Test) and in short-term verbal memory (Franke et al. 1992); and 4) neurological soft signs (Kinney et al. 1991).

## Twin Studies

If the contribution of genetic factors is crucial to the pathogenesis of schizophrenia, it is imperative that MZ and DZ co-twins of probands with schizophrenia differ in their risk for the disorder. In fact, this has been consistently observed since the initial twin studies conducted by Luxenberger almost 60 years ago. Up until 1986, 817 MZ twin pairs and 1,016 same-sex DZ twin pairs were studied, with weighted mean probandwise concordances of 59.2% and 15.2%, respectively, and therefore a broad-sense heritability of 88% (Kendler 1986). Nonetheless, estimates of probandwise concordance have varied, possibly reflecting differences in diagnostic criteria, case sampling, and zygosity assessment across studies.

The risk of schizophrenia in MZ co-twins of affected probands is at least three times that in DZ co-twins and about 40–60 times that in the general population. Just as noteworthy, however, is that only about half of MZ twin pairs are concordant for schizophrenia, despite genetic identity. Monochorionic MZ twins are more likely to be concordant than are dichorionic MZ twins, perhaps because the former share not only identical genes but also a similar in utero environment (Davis and Phelps 1995).

Although many nonschizophrenic MZ co-twins of affected probands show a variety of psychiatric disorders, including "neurotic" and character disorders and "schizoid" conditions, many (up to 43% in one series; Fischer 1971) appear to harbor no psychiatric disorder. Moreover, the offspring of nonschizophrenic MZ co-twins may be at as high a risk for schizophrenia as are the offspring of their affected siblings, implying that these co-twins carry the schizophrenic genotype despite their "normal" appearance. These findings argue against phenocopies as the sole explanation for MZ twin discordance in schizophrenia.

An additional argument against phenocopies is that discordant and concordant MZ twin pairs do not differ with respect to family risk, nor do they differ in birth order, birth weight, or condition at birth (Onstad et al. 1992). These findings also suggest a range of phenotypes compatible with the schizophrenic genotype and suggest an additive (or interactive) relation between genes and epigenetic (environmental) factors in the pathogenesis of the disorder.

## Adoption Studies

The adoptee study method was initially used by Heston (1966), who found a significantly greater risk for schizophrenia among the offspring of schizophrenic mothers separated at birth than among the adopted-away offspring of control mothers. This finding has been replicated in a Danish sample studied by Wender et al. (1974), which has withstood blind reanalysis with DSM-III (American Psychiatric Association 1980) criteria, and in a Finnish sample studied by Tienari et al. (2000), which has incorporated modern techniques such as direct blind interview of adoptees and detailed examination of adoptive families, the latter permitting an analysis of genotype–environmental interactions.

The sole cross-fostering study to date found equivalent rates of severe psychiatric illness among adoptees from biological parents without psychiatric illness, regardless of whether their adoptive parents had schizophrenia; both groups of adoptees had significantly lower rates of illness than did a group of adoptees from biological parents with schizophrenia and related disorders (Wender et al. 1974).

The adoptees' family method has been used in a series of studies conducted by Kety and colleagues in Denmark. They found that schizophrenia and related disorders were more common in the biological relatives of 34 schizophrenic adoptees (13 of 150 vs. 3 of 156, $P<0.01$), whereas the rates for these disorders, being low in both, did not differentiate the adoptive relatives of either adoptee group. The Danish adoption study has withstood reanalysis with DSM-III criteria and has since been replicated with a second cohort of 41 index and control adoptees (Kety 1988). The biological relatives of schizophrenic adoptees have shown higher rates not only of schizophrenia but also of DSM-III-diagnosed schizotypal and paranoid personality disorders, again expanding the boundaries of the schizophrenic syndrome (Kendler and Gruenberg 1984). Overall, the biological relatives of schizophrenic adoptees have shown a 10-fold increase in the risk for schizophrenia and spectrum disorders over the biological relatives of control subjects (Kety et al. 1994). Finally, two studies of MZ twins reared apart have shown high pairwise concordance for schizophrenia, providing further evidence for a genetic component in the etiology of this disorder (Gottesman and Shields 1982).

## High-Risk Studies

High-risk studies have examined both early characteristics that distinguish the offspring of schizophrenic parents from control subjects and premorbid features that predict which of those offspring will go on to develop schizophrenia. By age 1 year, high-risk infants were more likely than control infants to show "anxious" attachment behavior and sensorimotor deficits. By 2 years, they were seen to be more passive and less attentive in play. Later, they showed progressively less social competence. These findings have been taken as evidence of an inherited neurointegrative defect in schizophrenia (Fish et al. 1992). Alternatively, the findings might reflect developmental delays caused by obstetrical complications (such as low birth weight), which frequently befall schizophrenic mothers. In fact, psychopathology at age 6 years (especially among males) has been associated with low socioeconomic status, low Apgar score, and neonatal neurological abnormality (McNeil and Kaij 1987).

### Mode of Inheritance

A recessive monogenic model (with reduced penetrance) predicts that the incidence of schizophrenia among the offspring of two schizophrenic parents would be comparable to the probandwise concordance for MZ twins, and, in fact, this is what has been observed (Kringlen 1978). Similarly, a recessive model could allow for the maintenance of the abnormal gene in the population, despite reduced reproductive fitness of those individuals with the illness (Erlenmeyer-Kimling and Paradowski 1966). Normal rates of consanguinity in most families with schizophrenia, however, argue against recessive transmission of the disorder (Rosenthal 1970; but see Chaleby and Tuma 1987 regarding special populations).

Sex-linked models have been proposed by DeLisi and Crow (1989), who suggested that a schizophrenia susceptibility gene might reside on the X chromosome on the basis of sex differences in the clinical presentation of the illness, with a later onset and more benign course in women perhaps attributable to demonstration of random inactivation of X chromosomes carrying mutant alleles.

## Mood (Affective) Disorders

The major mood disorders—bipolar disorder (also known as manic-depressive illness) and major depression (also called unipolar depressive disorder)—have been found to be highly familial in several European and American studies, since the conceptualization of bipolar illness 35 years ago. First-degree relatives of bipolar probands have an elevated morbid risk for both bipolar and major depressive illnesses, whereas relatives of major depression probands have an elevated risk for major depression but not bipolar disorder (Weissman et al. 1984). In these studies, there have been inconsistent findings of increased rates of alcoholism and sociopathy among relatives. Schizoaffective disorder, especially schizoaffective disorder with manic symptoms, also has frequently been found to be associated with a high rate of bipolar disorder among relatives.

The results of a very large National Institute of Mental Health collaborative study (2,226 interviewed relatives) that used the Research Diagnostic Criteria (Spitzer et al. 1978), as reported by Andreasen et al. (1987) for interviewed relatives, are summarized in Table 4–3.

**TABLE 4–3.**    **National Institute of Mental Health Collaborative Study of the Psychobiology of Depression: rates of illness in interviewed first-degree relatives**

| Diagnoses in relatives (%) | Diagnosis of proband | | | | | |
|---|---|---|---|---|---|---|
| | **Bipolar I** | **Bipolar II** | **Unipolar** | **Schizo-affective—depressed** | **Schizo-affective—bipolar** | **Schizophrenia** |
| Bipolar I | 3.9 | 4.2 | 22.8 | 0.2 | 0.5 | 1.0 |
| Bipolar II | 1.1 | 8.2 | 26.2 | 0 | 0.4 | 0.4 |
| Unipolar | 0.6 | 2.9 | 8.4 | 20.3 | 0.2 | 0.3 |
| Schizoaffective—depressed | 0 | 3.7 | 21.0 | 0 | 0 | 2.5 |
| Schizoaffective—bipolar | 3.6 | 5.8 | 25.4 | 0 | 0.7 | 0.7 |

*Source.*    Data from Andreasen et al. 1987.

Twin studies have supported the importance of genetic factors in the transmission of the major mood disorders. Summed data from early twin studies that did not distinguish between bipolar disorder and major depression give a 65% pairwise concordance rate for MZ twin pairs and a 14% rate for DZ pairs (Nurnberger and Gershon 1982). The MZ rate for bipolar disorder was higher than that for major depression, but the study sample sizes were much smaller. One of the studies that found highest heritability of bipolar disorder, using strict criteria, observed a pairwise concordance rate of 58% for MZ pairs compared with 17% for DZ pairs, in a total of 110 pairs (broad-sense heritability of 82%) (Bertelsen et al. 1977). A meta-analysis of five twin studies of major depression, with a starting sample of more than 21,000 individuals, estimated that the additive genetic contribution to developing the disorder was 37%, and the rest of the variance was explained by individual-specific environmental effects, whereas none was attributable to shared familial environmental effects (Sullivan et al. 2000). Two twin studies of major depression suggested that heritability of major depression is higher in females than in males (Bierut et al. 1998; Kendler et al. 2001), particularly when a broad disease definition is used, but this was not observed in the above meta-analysis.

The few adoption studies of major mood disorders are confounded by differences in sampling and therefore have produced somewhat conflicting data. The lone study of adopted-away offspring found that the children of mothers with bipolar disorder or major depression had a higher rate of major mood disorder than did the adopted-away children of mothers with other psychiatric conditions (Cadoret 1978). Mendlewicz and Rainer (1977) found a significantly increased risk for affective illness in the biological parents of bipolar adoptee probands, compared with their adoptive parents or with the biological parents of control subjects. Wender et al. (1986) studied a group of adoptees with mixed mood disorder diagnoses (bipolar, unipolar, neurotic depression, "affect reaction") and found an increase in suicide and some mood disorders among their biological, but not their adoptive, relatives when each adoptee was compared with his or her corresponding control subject. In contrast, von Knorring et al. (1983), in a similar design, found no differences between the biological parent groups and noted an excess of psychiatric illness in the adoptive parents of the index cases, who were primarily adoptees with nonbipolar depression.

High-risk studies of children of parents with major mood disorders have quite consistently found high rates of social and psychiatric impairment. Controlled studies of specific diagnoses have noted an increased prevalence of major depression, conduct disorder, attention-deficit/hyperactivity disorder, anxiety disorder, substance abuse, and school problems, as well as poorer social functioning, among these children. These high-risk offspring had an earlier age at onset of depression (mean age = 12–13 years) than did depressed control subjects whose parents were not depressed (mean age at onset = 16–17 years).

## Anxiety Disorders

### Panic Disorder

Major anxiety disorders, including phobias and panic disorder, are complex traits sharing at least one susceptibility locus (e.g., 4q31–q34 at marker *D4S413* [Kaabi et al. 2006]). Another candidate is chromosome 9q31 at marker *D9S271*, which has been linked not just to panic disorder but to anxiety in general in 62 Icelandic families genotyped with 976 microsatellite markers and validated in a subset of 25 extended families (Thorgeirsson et al. 2003). Individuals with panic disorder are more sensitive to the anxiogenic effects of multiple substances, including cholecystokinin, lactate, and inhaled carbon dioxide (Caldirola et al. 1997). Family studies of carbon dioxide sensitivity have shown larger increases of anxiety symptoms in the first-degree relatives of panic disorder patients as compared with healthy control subjects (van Beek and Griez 2000), and segregation analysis suggested a single major locus for the transmission of carbon dioxide sensitivity (Cavallini et al. 1999).

### Obsessive-Compulsive Disorder

Obsessive-compulsive disorder (OCD) is a severe psychiatric illness characterized by intrusive and senseless thoughts and impulses (obsessions) and by repetitive behaviors (compulsions) (Willour et al. 2004). It is estimated to affect nearly 5 million people in the United States (Karno et al. 1988). Evidence for a strong genetic component and environmental susceptibility factors in OCD comes from twin studies, family genetics studies, and segregation analyses (for review, see Alsobrook et al. 2002). The results of family studies of OCD are largely inconsistent (Mataix-Cols 2006), except that early-onset OCD, like early-onset mood disorder, seems highly familial.

Substantial comorbidity of Gilles de la Tourette's syndrome is seen with OCD, and family studies together suggest a shared genetic diathesis (Barr and Sandor 1998; Leckman and Chittenden 1990).

### *Other Anxiety Disorders (Generalized Anxiety Disorder, Phobias, Posttraumatic Stress Disorder)*

Noyes et al. (1987) noted that increased rates of generalized anxiety disorder were specific and that they were not found among the relatives of patients with panic disorder. Fyer et al. (1990) reported a rate of 31% for simple phobia in first-degree relatives compared with 11% in control subjects (relative risk=3.3). For social phobia, two studies (Fyer et al. 1993; Reich et al. 1988) found a threefold increase in this disorder in the relatives of probands, with Fyer et al. (1993) reporting rates of 16% compared with 5% in the control group. When subtypes of social phobia were studied, an approximately 10-fold increase in the rate of generalized social phobia (and avoidant personality disorder), but not discrete and nongeneralized social phobia, was observed in the first-degree relatives of patients with social phobia of each respective subtype as compared with the relatives of control subjects (Stein et al. 1998). There is extensive comorbidity of these disorders in probands (Goldenberg et al. 1996), but the disorders "breed true" when the families of probands without comorbidity are studied (Fyer et al. 1995). Finally, no increase in posttraumatic stress disorder (PTSD) was found in the families of PTSD probands analyzed for depression using family history, but it has been reported to increase the risk to develop PTSD after rape (Davidson et al. 1998).

## Drug Dependence

Numerous studies (reviewed in Merikangas et al. 1989) show that alcoholism is highly familial and that the risk to first-degree relatives is increased approximately sevenfold. This work has been extended to other drugs of abuse, with most having an eightfold increased risk to first-degree relatives. A study of the siblings of the probands in the Collaborative Study on the Genetics of Alcoholism (COGA) found similar results (Bierut et al. 1998). Both studies found evidence of specific transmission of risk for each drug of abuse, in addition to general factors that predispose to all drugs.

Several adoption studies also provide evidence that genetic factors, as well as environmental ones, are involved in the etiology of alcoholism. Goodwin (1979) found elevated rates of alcoholism among both the adopted-away daughters of alcoholic persons and control adoptees, whereas Cadoret et al. (1985) found higher rates in the daughters of index cases compared with control subjects. Data from a large Swedish sample also support a genetic predisposition to alcoholism in women and men (Cloninger et al. 1981), as well as the possible importance of certain environmental factors, such as lower occupational status of the adoptive father. In the COGA, the risk of alcoholism in siblings of alcoholic females was observed to be slightly higher than for siblings of alcoholic males, suggesting a higher genetic predisposition in the females (Reich et al. 1998). In several studies, alcoholism in the adoptive environment was not found to increase the risk among adoptees.

## Suicide and Impulsive Behavior

Many family studies have found familial clustering of suicides and suicide attempts (Brent and Mann 2005). Such clustering has been observed in studies of completers that used either friends (Shafii et al. 1985), individuals from the community (Brent et al. 1996), or nonsuicidal diagnostically matched control subjects (Tsuang 1983). Although it is difficult to control for the psychiatric comorbidity that also runs in the families of the victims, Brent et al. (1996) found a fourfold increased risk of suicide attempts and completions in the relatives of suicide probands as compared with the relatives of control subjects from the community. In the Amish, 73% of suicides occur in 16% of the pedigrees, even though some of the nonsuicide pedigrees are just as severely affected with bipolar disorder (Egeland and Sussex 1985). This pattern of increased risk to relatives of suicide probands as compared with relatives of control subjects—even beyond the risk conferred by an Axis I disorder—is also seen for relatives of suicide attempters.

## Key Points: Genetics

- Multiple genes, each with a small effect, contribute to a psychiatric disease.

- Environmental influences, interacting with genetic factors, have a definite role in psychiatric illnesses.

- None of the psychiatric diseases has a confirmed disease gene as yet, but there are promising candidate genes for each disorder.

- *DISC1, NRG1, OLIG2, COMT, G72, APOL* cluster, and *SELENBP1* are strong candidate genes for schizophrenia.

- *SLC6A4, BDNF,* and *NMDAR* are promising candidate genes for bipolar illness.
- The fibroblast growth factor (FGF) system and GABA glutamate system appear to be involved in genetic etiology of major depressive disorder.
- Dysregulation of synaptic function, myelination, and oligodendrocyte function seem to be common to several psychiatric disorders.
- At the genetic level, bipolar disorder increasingly seems to share more common features with schizophrenia than with major depressive disorder.
- The HapMap project provides a bridge between linkage mapping and single nucleotide polymorphisms (SNPs).
- Combining data on linkage, SNP association, regulation of gene expression, and protein and RNA functions can be a powerful strategy for discovering psychiatric disease genes.
- It remains to be seen whether blood/peripheral blood leukocytes (PBLs) can serve as an alternative tissue that can be noninvasively accessed for routine diagnosis of psychiatric illnesses.
- Epigenetics likely has a greater role in the etiology of psychiatric illnesses than is now apparent.
- It pays to play by the rules of ethics.

# References

Alsobrook JP 2nd, Zohar AH, Leboyer M, et al: Association between the COMT locus and obsessive-compulsive disorder in females but not males. Am J Med Genet 114:116–120, 2002

American Psychiatric Association: Diagnostic and Statistical Manual of Mental Disorders, 3rd Edition. Washington, DC, American Psychiatric Association, 1980

American Psychiatric Association: Diagnostic and Statistical Manual of Mental Disorders, 3rd Edition, Revised. Washington, DC, American Psychiatric Association, 1987

American Psychiatric Association: Diagnostic and Statistical Manual of Mental Disorders, 4th Edition, Text Revision. Washington, DC, American Psychiatric Association, 2000

Andreasen NC, Rice J, Endicott J, et al: Familial rates of affective disorder: a report from the National Institute of Mental Health Collaborative Study. Arch Gen Psychiatry 44:461–469, 1987

Baron M, Gruen RS: Schizophrenia and affective disorder: are they genetically linked? Br J Psychiatry 159:267–270, 1991

Barr CL, Sandor P: Current status of genetic studies of Gilles de la Tourette syndrome. Can J Psychiatry 43:351–357, 1998

Bertelsen A, Harvald B, Hauge M: A Danish twin study of manic-depressive disorders. Br J Psychiatry 130:330–351, 1977

Bierut LJ, Dinwiddie SH, Begleiter H, et al: Familial transmission of substance dependence: alcohol, marijuana, cocaine, and habitual smoking: a report from the Collaborative Study on the Genetics of Alcoholism. Arch Gen Psychiatry 55:982–988, 1998

Brent DA, Mann JJ: Family genetic studies, suicide, and suicidal behavior. Am J Med Genet C Semin Med Genet 133:13–24, 2005

Brent DA, Bridge J, Johnson BA, et al: Suicidal behavior runs in families: a controlled family study of adolescent suicide victims. Arch Gen Psychiatry 53:1145–1152, 1996

Cadoret RJ: Evidence for genetic inheritance of primary affective disorder in adoptees. Am J Psychiatry 135:463–466, 1978

Cadoret RJ, O'Gorman TW, Troughton E, et al: Alcoholism and antisocial personality: interrelationships, genetic and environmental factors. Arch Gen Psychiatry 42:161–167, 1985

Caldirola D, Perna G, Arancio C, et al: The 35% $CO_2$ challenge test in patients with social phobia. Psychiatry Res 71:41–48, 1997

Cavallini MC, Perna G, Caldirola D, et al: A segregation study of panic disorder in families of panic patients responsive to the 35% $CO_2$ challenge. Biol Psychiatry 46:815–820, 1999

Chaleby K, Tuma TA: Cousin marriages and schizophrenia in Saudi Arabia. Br J Psychiatry 150:547–549, 1987

Cloninger CR, Bohman M, Sigvardsson S: Inheritance of alcohol abuse: cross-fostering analysis of adopted men. Arch Gen Psychiatry 38:861–868, 1981

Cloninger CR, Martin RL, Guze SB, et al: A prospective follow-up and family study of somatization in men and women. Am J Psychiatry 143:873–878, 1986

Crowe RR, Noyes R, Pauls DL, et al: A family study of panic disorder. Arch Gen Psychiatry 40:1065–1069, 1983

Davidson JR, Tupler LA, Wilson WH, et al: A family study of chronic post-traumatic stress disorder following rape trauma. J Psychiatr Res 32:301–309, 1998

Davis JO, Phelps JA: Twins with schizophrenia: genes or germs? Schizophr Bull 21:13–18, 1995

Decina P, Mukherjee S, Lucas L, et al: Patterns of illness in parent-child pairs both hospitalized for either schizophrenia or a major mood disorder. Psychiatry Res 39:81–87, 1991

DeLisi LE, Crow TJ: Evidence for a sex chromosome locus for schizophrenia. Schizophr Bull 15:431–440, 1989

Egeland JA, Sussex JN: Suicide and family loading for affective disorders. JAMA 254:915–918, 1985

Erlenmeyer-Kimling LE, Paradowski W: Selection and schizophrenia. Am Nat 100:651–665, 1966

Fischer M: Psychoses in the offspring of schizophrenic monozygotic twins and their normal co-twins. Br J Psychiatry 118:43–52, 1971

Fish B, Marcus J, Hans SL, et al: Infants at risk for schizophrenia: sequelae of a genetic neurointegrative defect: a review and replication analysis of pandysmaturation in the Jerusalem Infant Development Study. Arch Gen Psychiatry 49:221–235, 1992

Franke P, Maier W, Hain C, et al: Wisconsin Card Sorting Test: an indicator of vulnerability to schizophrenia? Schizophr Res 6:243–249, 1992

Fyer AJ, Mannuzza S, Gallops MS, et al: Familial transmission of simple phobias and fears: a preliminary report. Arch Gen Psychiatry 47:252–256, 1990

Fyer AJ, Mannuzza S, Chapman TF, et al: A direct interview family study of social phobia. Arch Gen Psychiatry 50:286–293, 1993

Fyer AJ, Mannuzza S, Chapman TF, et al: Specificity in familial aggregation of phobic disorders. Arch Gen Psychiatry 52:564–573, 1995

Goldenberg IM, White K, Yonkers K, et al: The infrequency of "pure culture" diagnoses among the anxiety disorders. J Clin Psychiatry 57:528–533, 1996

Goodwin DW: Alcoholism and heredity: a review and hypothesis. Arch Gen Psychiatry 36:57–61, 1979

Gottesman II, Shields J: Schizophrenia: The Epigenetic Puzzle. Cambridge, England, Cambridge University Press, 1982

Heston LL: Psychiatric disorders in foster home reared children of schizophrenic mothers. Br J Psychiatry 112:819–825, 1966

Kaabi B, Gelernter J, Woods SW, et al: Genome scan for loci predisposing to anxiety disorders using a novel multivariate approach: strong evidence for a chromosome 4 risk locus. Am J Hum Genet 78:543–553, 2006

Karno M, Golding JM, Sorenson SB, et al: The epidemiology of obsessive-compulsive disorder in five US communities. Arch Gen Psychiatry 45:1094–1099, 1988

Kassett JA, Gershon ES, Maxwell ME, et al: Psychiatric disorders in the first-degree relatives of probands with bulimia nervosa. Am J Psychiatry 146:1468–1471, 1989

Kendler KS: Genetics of schizophrenia, in Psychiatry Update: The American Psychiatric Association Annual Review, Vol 5. Edited by Frances AJ, Hales RE. Washington, DC, American Psychiatric Press, 1986, pp 25–41

Kendler KS, Gruenberg AM: An independent analysis of the Danish Adoption Study of Schizophrenia, VI: the relationship between psychiatric disorders as defined by DSM-III in the relatives and adoptees. Arch Gen Psychiatry 41:555–564, 1984

Kendler KS, Gruenberg AM, Tsuang MT: Psychiatric illness in first-degree relatives of schizophrenic and surgical control patients: a family study using DSM-III criteria. Arch Gen Psychiatry 42:770–779, 1985

Kendler KS, Gardner CO, Neale MC, et al: Genetic risk factors for major depression in men and women: similar or different heritabilities and same or partly distinct genes? Psychol Med 31:605–616, 2001

Kety SS: Schizophrenic illness in the families of schizophrenic adoptees: findings from the Danish national sample. Schizophr Bull 14:217–222, 1988

Kety SS, Wender PH, Jacobsen B, et al: Mental illness in the biological and adoptive relatives of schizophrenic adoptees: replication of the Copenhagen Study in the rest of Denmark. Arch Gen Psychiatry 51:442–455, 1994

Kinney DK, Yurgelun-Todd DA, Woods BT: Hard neurologic signs and psychopathology in relatives of schizophrenic patients. Psychiatry Res 39:45–53, 1991

Kringlen E: The status of schizophrenia research [in Norwegian]. Tidsskr Nor Laegeforen 98:65–69, 1978

Leckman JF, Chittenden EH: Gilles de la Tourette's syndrome and some forms of obsessive-compulsive disorder may share a common genetic diathesis. Encephale 16 (Spec No):321–323, 1990

Mataix-Cols D: Deconstructing obsessive-compulsive disorder: a multidimensional perspective. Curr Opin Psychiatry 19:84–89, 2006

McNeil TF, Kaij L: Swedish high-risk study: sample characteristics at age 6. Schizophr Bull 13:373–381, 1987

Mendlewicz J, Rainer JD: Adoption study supporting genetic transmission in manic-depressive illness. Nature 268:327–329, 1977

Merikangas KR: Genetics of alcoholism: a review of human studies, in Genetics of Neuropsychiatric Diseases. Edited by Wetterberg I. London, England, Macmillan, 1989, pp 269–280

Merikangas KR, Spence MA, Kupfer DJ: Linkage studies of bipolar disorder: methodologic and analytic issues. Report of MacArthur Foundation Workshop on Linkage and Clinical Features in Affective Disorders. Arch Gen Psychiatry 46:1137–1141, 1989

Noyes R Jr, Clarkson C, Crowe RR, et al: A family study of generalized anxiety disorder. Am J Psychiatry 144:1019–1024, 1987

Nurnberger JI Jr, Gershon ES: Genetics, in Handbook of Affective Disorders. Edited by Paykel ES. New York, Guilford, 1982, pp 126–145

Onstad S, Skre I, Torgersen S, et al: Birthweight and obstetric complications in schizophrenic twins. Acta Psychiatr Scand 85:70–73, 1992

Pope HG Jr, Yurgelun-Todd D: Schizophrenic individuals with bipolar first-degree relatives: analysis of two pedigrees. J Clin Psychiatry 51:97–101, 1990

Reich T, Cloninger CR, Van Eerdewegh P, et al: Secular trends in the familial transmission of alcoholism. Alcohol Clin Exp Res 12:458–464, 1988

Reich T, Edenberg HJ, Goate A, et al: Genome-wide search for genes affecting the risk for alcohol dependence. Am J Med Genet 81:207–215, 1998

Rosenthal D: Genetic Theory and Abnormal Behavior. New York, McGraw-Hill, 1970

Shafii M, Carrigan S, Whittinghill JR, et al: Psychological autopsy of completed suicide in children and adolescents. Am J Psychiatry 142:1061–1064, 1985

Shenton ME, Solovay MR, Holzman PS, et al: Thought disorder in the relatives of psychotic patients. Arch Gen Psychiatry 46:897–901, 1989

Spitzer RL, Endicott J, Robins E: Research Diagnostic Criteria: rationale and reliability. Arch Gen Psychiatry 35:773–782, 1978

Stein MB, Chartier MJ, Hazen AL, et al: A direct-interview family study of generalized social phobia. Am J Psychiatry 155:90–97, 1998

Strober M, Morell W, Burroughs J, et al: A controlled family study of anorexia nervosa. J Psychiatr Res 19:239–246, 1985

Sullivan PF, Neale MC, Kendler KS: Genetic epidemiology of major depression: review and meta-analysis. Am J Psychiatry 157:1552–1562, 2000

Thorgeirsson TE, Oskarsson H, Desnica N, et al: Anxiety with panic disorder linked to chromosome 9q in Iceland. Am J Hum Genet 72:1221–1230, 2003

Tienari P, Wynne LC, Moring J, et al: Finnish adoptive family study: sample selection and adoptee DSM-III-R diagnoses. Acta Psychiatr Scand 101:433–443, 2000

Tsuang MT: Risk of suicide in the relatives of schizophrenics, manics, depressives, and controls. J Clin Psychiatry 44:396–397, 398–400, 1983

Tsuang MT, Gilbertson MW, Faraone SV: The genetics of schizophrenia: current knowledge and future directions. Schizophr Res 4:157–171, 1991

van Beek N, Griez E: Reactivity to a 35% $CO_2$ challenge in healthy first-degree relatives of patients with panic disorder. Biol Psychiatry 47:830–835, 2000

von Knorring AL, Cloninger CR, Bohman M, et al: An adoption study of depressive disorders and substance abuse. Arch Gen Psychiatry 40:943–950, 1983

Weissman MM, Wickramaratne P, Merikangas KR, et al: Onset of major depression in early adulthood: increased familial loading and specificity. Arch Gen Psychiatry 41:1136–1143, 1984

Wender PH, Rosenthal D, Kety SS, et al: Crossfostering: a research strategy for clarifying the role of genetic and experiential factors in the etiology of schizophrenia. Arch Gen Psychiatry 30:121–128, 1974

Wender PH, Kety SS, Rosenthal D, et al: Psychiatric disorders in the biological and adoptive families of adopted individuals with affective disorders. Arch Gen Psychiatry 43:923–929, 1986

Willour VL, Yao Shugart Y, Samuels J, et al: Replication study supports evidence for linkage to 9p24 in obsessive-compulsive disorder. Am J Hum Genet 75:508–513, 2004

# 5

# Nervous, Endocrine, and Immune System Interactions in Psychiatry

ANDREW H. MILLER, M.D.

## Overview of the Immune System

The immune system is made of solid tissues and circulating cells that are distributed throughout the body. Solid tissues are organized into specific structures classified as either central lymphoid tissues (bone marrow, thymus) or peripheral lymphoid tissues (lymph nodes, spleen mucosa, associated lymphoid tissue). Areas of high exposure to external pathogens—such as the digestive tract, pulmonary tract, and skin—contain specialized lymphoid tissues, such as Peyer's patches in the gut.

All immune cells originate from hematopoietic stem cells in bone marrow. Under the influence of signaling molecules such as cytokines and hormones, these cells develop along myeloid or lymphoid paths of differentiation.

The myeloid cell line includes monocytes and granulocytes such as neutrophils, basophils, and eosinophils. Monocytes and basophils differentiate further into macrophages and mast cells, respectively, and take up residence in tissues throughout the body. The lymphoid cell line includes B cells, T cells, and natural killer (NK) cells.

After production in the bone marrow, the cells that will become B lymphocytes mature in the bone marrow, whereas T lymphocytes travel to the thymus, where they will mature (Abbas and Lichtman 2003). The bone marrow and thymus are for this reason termed *primary immune tissues*. Because immune cells are constantly being produced

with random recognition sites for an enormous variety of antigens, an important part of the maturational process for both types of lymphocytes is the elimination of cells that would react with self antigens. This essential and complex step occurs in the primary immune tissues. After maturation, cells circulate and take up residence in the secondary immune tissues (such as the spleen and lymph nodes), which provide sites for interaction with circulating pathogens.

Both the differentiation of the progenitor cell lines into either myeloid or lymphoid immune cells and the overall regulation of the immune system depend on many mediators, including immune signaling factors called cytokines. Cytokines are produced by a number of cells, including activated leukocytes, microglia, endothelial cells, fibroblasts, and adipocytes. The word *cytokine* (*cyto*, cell; *kinesis*, movement) derives from the original identification of these factors as important regulators of cell movement. However, cytokines have been found to have local and systemic effects on a wide variety of body functions not limited to the immune system.

## Immunity and Disease

Diseases of immune dysfunction help to illustrate how finely tuned the system is and how essential the immune system's role is in maintaining health. Diseases of the immune system can be subclassified into immune deficiencies, allergic diseases, and autoimmune disorders. In diseases of immune deficiency, the body is unable either to identify or to fight pathogens or malignancies. An example is the syndrome of severe combined immunodeficiency, in which both B and T cell functions are grossly impaired. Usually congenital, this disorder of both humoral and cell-mediated immunity prevents the body from fighting off infections of all sorts. Without treatment, affected individuals typically succumb rapidly to bacterial, viral, or fungal infection (or a combination of these). Other immune deficiencies are more specific. For example, certain cancer chemotherapy regimens that preferentially cause neutropenia make patients especially vulnerable to infection by extracellular bacteria. AIDS, associated with infection with HIV, demonstrates how deficiency in one component of the immune system can cause widespread pathology. The virus binds to the CD4+ protein on the surface of the helper T lymphocyte, enters the cell, and interferes with the cell's functioning in a variety of ways. Because the helper T lymphocyte plays such a pivotal role in immunity, loss of helper T cell function predisposes affected individuals to a variety of immune-related disorders. Patients are susceptible to opportunistic infections with organisms such as *Cryptococcus*, *Mycobacterium* species, and *Toxoplasma*. Reactivation or severe infection with cytomegalovirus or herpes viruses can occur. Patients with HIV infection also are at risk for cancers such as Kaposi's sarcoma and central nervous system lymphoma. The syndrome of HIV/AIDS demonstrates how dysfunction of one immune cell type reverberates throughout a number of immune processes.

Disorders of immunity also include those of excessive immunity. These diseases fall into two types: allergic diseases, in which the immune system responds excessively to nonpathogenic environmental antigens, and autoimmune diseases, in which the system fails to prevent reaction to self antigens. These processes have multiple pathological consequences. They can waste body energy resources, injure self tissues, and keep the immune system from functioning at an efficient level against external pathogens.

The main immunopathology in all allergic diseases is degranulation of mast cells, which are particularly abundant in the skin and the mucosa of the respiratory and gastrointestinal tracts. The pathophysiology of allergic reactions involves the activation of mast cells in response to antigens binding to immunoglobulin E and an overactive T helper 2 (Th2) cell response. Histamines are released by mast cells, leading to increased capillary permeability and smooth muscle contraction. The most severe form of allergy is the anaphylactic reaction, occurring when exposure to an antigen induces bronchospasm or a hypotensive reaction (Abbas and Lichtman 2003).

Autoimmune diseases occur when the system misidentifies self cells as foreign and the cascade of immune events results in damage of self tissue. These multifactorial illnesses arise from a combination of events, including individual genetic predisposition, exposure to an antigen, and hormonal patterns. Lymphocytes that should be eliminated for binding too robustly to self antigens may survive to maturity. Viral infections or other stimuli may cause surface changes of self cells, which cause immune cells to identify these cells as foreign and attack them. By these mechanisms, direct tissue damage can occur. Secondary effects also can occur, as in systemic lupus erythematosus (SLE), when circulating antigen-antibody complexes are deposited in and damage renal tissue and microvasculature. These examples of immune deficiency states and autoimmune disorders reflect the variety and severity of diseases that can occur when immune regulation is impaired.

## Stress, Depression, and Immunity: Effect on Disease

### Cancer

Regarding the effect of depression on the development of cancer, the data have been somewhat mixed (Raison and Miller 2003). In a meta-analysis of prospective studies by McGee and colleagues (1994), a small but statistically significant increased risk of cancer in patients with depression was identified. In a more recent review of more than 50 studies on mortality and depression by Wulsin and colleagues (1999), the authors concluded that although depression seems to increase the risk of death by cardiovascular disease, especially in men, depression does not seem to increase the risk of death by cancer. Both reviews commented on the lack of high-quality studies controlling for potential mediating variables. Of note are studies finding an increased incidence of cancer in depressed smokers (Linkins and Comstock 1990), an increased incidence of lung cancer in depressed men (Knekt et al. 1996), and an increased incidence of cancer in men with high levels of hopelessness (Everson et al. 1996). Taken together, the data suggest that depression may not in itself put individuals at substantially higher risk but may increase the risk of cancer in individuals with other risk factors, especially smoking.

Although the effect of stress and/or depression on the development of cancer may be relatively small, data support the notion that psychological factors may have a greater effect once cancer is diagnosed. Mounting evidence suggests that susceptibility to immune-related diseases, including cancer, is related to genetic factors. Therefore, if stress, depression, and other psychological factors are associated with altered immune function, then the effect of these factors may be the greatest on patients with immune-related disorders and genetic predisposition to immune dysfunction.

Ramirez and colleagues (1989) reported that severe life events and difficulties are associated with increased risk of breast cancer relapse. In addition, depression is relatively common in cancer patients (Evans et al. 1986), and depressive symptoms have been associated with decreased survival in patients with lung cancer (Buccheri 1998; Faller et al. 1999). Hopelessness also has been found to be associated with decreased survival in women with early-stage breast cancer (Watson et al. 1999, 2005). In a study by Walker and colleagues (1999), scores on depression and anxiety rating scales were independent predictors of therapeutic outcome in patients with newly diagnosed breast cancer.

Because stress or psychiatric symptoms may predispose cancer patients to worse outcomes, clinicians have wondered whether psychosocial interventions that address these factors might alter the disease outcome. To test these notions, Spiegel and colleagues (1989) and Fawzy and colleagues (1993) treated cancer patients with group psychotherapy under controlled conditions and found improved outcomes in the intervention group compared with those receiving standard therapy. These outcomes included lengthened survival in patients with metastatic breast cancer and decreased recurrence in patients with malignant melanoma. Not all studies have reproduced these findings. Two studies that used cognitive-behavior therapy in patients with metastatic breast cancer found no improved survival in the intervention group (Cunningham et al. 1998; Edelman et al. 1999).

## HIV Infection

Some researchers found an association between depressive symptoms and HIV disease progression without increased mortality (Burack et al. 1993; Lyketsos et al. 1993; Page-Schafer et al. 1996), and others reported both disease progression and increased mortality (Mayne et al. 1996). Other work reported no association between depression and disease progression (Lyketsos et al. 1996;

Perry et al. 1992; Rabkin et al. 1991). A meta-analysis by Zorrilla and colleagues (1996) reported an association between depressive symptoms and symptoms of HIV infection but not lymphocyte subsets. More recently, stress and depressive symptoms, particularly when they occurred jointly, were found to be associated with decreased cytotoxic (CD8+) T lymphocyte subsets as well as NK cells in men and women with HIV (Cruess et al. 2003; Evans et al. 2002; Leserman et al. 1997). Data from up to 7.5 years of a prospective study of HIV-infected men provide evidence that stress, social support, coping style, and depression can affect disease progression (Leserman et al. 1999, 2000). Interestingly, hopelessness as an individual variable was shown to affect disease progression, at least by CD4 count measures (Perry et al. 1992).

## Autoimmune Diseases

### *Multiple Sclerosis*

Some studies reported an association between stressors and the onset or exacerbation of multiple sclerosis (MS), whereas others found no such association. A particularly well-constructed study by Grant and colleagues (1989) found that patients with MS reported more life difficulties in the year preceding the onset of MS or within several months before exacerbations of the illness. Mohr and colleagues (2000) reported results of a prospective 2-year study examining the relation between life stress, conflict, or psychological distress and new MS lesions on magnetic resonance images. They found that an increase in conflict and disruption of life routine (but not psychological distress) were associated with new lesions found on magnetic resonance images 4 and 8 weeks later; however, conflict, disruption of routine, and psychological distress were not related to clinical exacerbation of symptoms. An interesting prospective study evaluated 32 patients with MS exposed to the threat of missile attacks during the Persian Gulf War (Nisipeanu and Korczyn 1993). The researchers reported a decrease in the number of relapses in these patients during this period of extremely high stress. Therefore, it is possible that very high levels of stress are associated with marked increases in cortisol that inhibit disease activity.

Further suggestion of a role for the hypothalamic-pituitary-adrenal axis in MS patients was provided by Then Bergh and colleagues (1999), who found that patients with MS showed glucocorticoid resistance, as manifested by altered results on dexamethasone/corticotropin-releasing hormone challenge.

### Systemic Lupus Erythematosus

Because SLE is approximately 10 times more common in women than in men, hormonal mechanisms are thought to play a critical role in the initiation and perpetuation of the illness. The proinflammatory effect of estrogen seems to influence the course of disease, as flares of the disease increase during pregnancy and drop off after menopause. Pregnancy is accompanied by a shift from T helper 1 (Th1) to Th2 activity that seems to exacerbate SLE.

Estrogen replacement therapy also increases the risk of development of SLE. DaCosta and colleagues (1999) found that a history of stressful life events in the 6 months before evaluation correlated with reduced functional ability 8 months after evaluation. Increasing severity of depression scores also was correlated with changes in functional ability 8 months after evaluation. Research on a large cohort of patients with SLE indicated that greater disease activity in SLE patients was associated with less social support and that increased physical disability was associated with depression in these patients (Ward et al. 1999).

### Graves' Disease

Graves' disease is an antibody-mediated autoimmune disorder in which antibody to the thyrotropin receptor stimulates the thyroid gland to produce thyroid hormone. Despite markedly increased levels of circulating thyroid hormones and accompanying decreases in thyrotropin-releasing hormone and thyrotropin, the thyroid gland continues to produce hormone. The illness is accompanied by an increased likelihood of possessing the human leukocyte antigen type DR3. Some studies have found an increase in stressful life events to be associated with the onset of the disease. Sonino and colleagues (1993) reported that an increase in multiple types of life events—positive and negative, controlled and uncontrolled—was associated with the onset of the illness. Another group found that stressful life events and smoking both were associated with the development of Graves' disease in women but not in men (Yoshiuchi et al. 1998).

## Psychiatric Illness and Immune Function

### Depression

The question of altered immunity in major depression has received the most attention with regard to the relation among the nervous, endocrine, and immune systems in psychiatric disorders. Immune changes accompanying depression include decreased lymphocyte count, increased neutrophil number, decreased mitogen responses of peripheral blood lymphocytes, and decreased NK cell activity.

Nevertheless, although the results in toto suggest immune alterations in depressed patients, important exceptions are apparent, indicating that the findings are not reproducible across studies. For example, Schleifer et al. (1989) and Andreoli et al. (1993) failed to detect differences in immune function in depressed patients who were compared with carefully matched control subjects. Although no mean differences between groups of depressed and nondepressed patients were found, particular subgroups of depressed patients in these and other studies have been shown to have immune abnormalities. When immune changes are found in depression, they typically accompany other characteristics of depressed patients. For example, although Schleifer and colleagues (1989) found no differences in mean values for immune measures between depressed and nondepressed groups, greater age and more severe depression were associated with decreases in CD4+ cell numbers and mitogen responsiveness of peripheral blood lymphocytes. A 1994 study reported that decreased NK cell activity in depressed patients was associated with sleep disturbance (Cover and Irwin 1994). Several studies have reported that male patients with depression are more likely than female patients with depression to have decreases in NK cells (Evans et al. 1992). Decreased circulating levels of NK cells also were associated with greater severity of depression (Evans et al. 1992).

More recent research has addressed the possibility that certain aspects of the immune response may become activated in depressed patients, particularly innate immunity as measured by acute phase proteins and proinflammatory cytokines (Raison et al. 2006). Moreover, a syndrome of "sickness behavior" resembling major depression occurs with the administration of cytokine therapies such as interferon-α and interleukin-2 (IL-2) (Capuron and Miller 2004; Dantzer 2004). Prominent features of this syndrome include depressed mood, anhedonia, sleep and appetite disturbances, malaise, and poor concentration. Overall patterns found in serum cytokine levels include increases in the proinflammatory cytokine IL-6, increases in soluble IL-6 receptor (sIL-6R) and sIL-2R, and a decrease in IL-2. Increases in acute phase proteins such as C-reactive protein, serum haptoglobin, the complement protein C4, α1-acid glycoprotein, and α1-antitrypsin also have been reported in several well-controlled studies. Not all studies have confirmed the findings of serum cytokine alterations, however.

## Schizophrenia

Specific measures of immune function in schizophrenic patients have presented an overall pattern of immune activation in this illness. Increased numbers of immune cells such as B cells, CD4+ lymphocytes, and monocytes have been reported in multiple studies. In at least two studies, a subset of patients have had increased numbers of CD5+ B cells, a B cell subset associated with autoimmune disease (McAllister et al. 1989; Printz et al. 1999).

Studies of immune measures, including cytokines and their receptors and acute phase proteins, in the cerebrospinal fluid (CSF) of schizophrenic patients have produced inconsistent results, but taken together they suggest the presence of immune activation. An increase in CSF IL-2 has been reported in untreated schizophrenia patients (Licinio et al. 1993), although no change has been found in other studies. An increased sIL-6R concentration in the CSF suggests immune activation because the IL-6 receptor when bound to IL-6 increases its activity. A relation has been suggested between high levels of sIL-6R in the CSF and positive symptoms of psychosis. Increased IL-10 in the CSF has been correlated to an increase in negative symptoms of psychosis. Other studied cytokines that have yielded conflicting results include IL-1 and tumor necrosis factor. An increase in the acute phase protein $\alpha$2-haptoglobin was found in the CSF of schizophrenic patients. Elevated CSF levels of soluble intercellular adhesion mol-ecules and albumin in schizophrenic patients suggest an impairment of the integrity of the blood-brain barrier in at least a subset of patients with schizophrenia. Impairment of blood-brain barrier integrity can accompany a process of immune activation. More recent studies have focused on the balance between Th1 and Th2 cytokines in schizophrenic patients, with some data indicating a higher Th1-to-Th2 ratio, which is attenuated by effective neuroleptic treatment (Kim et al. 2004).

## Bipolar Disorder

Tsai and colleagues (1999) used a case-control design to investigate several functional measures of immunity in patients with bipolar disorder during mania and after remission. Lymphocyte proliferative responses to the mitogen phytohemagglutinin were increased during the manic phase, as were plasma sIL-2R levels. These findings normalized after remission of the disease. One group reported increased levels of sIL-2R and sIL-6R in symptomatic patients with rapid-cycling bipolar disorder, with the levels normalizing after 30 days of treatment with lithium (Rapaport et al. 1999). Interestingly, levels of IL-2, sIL-2R, and sIL-6R also were increased in psychiatrically healthy volunteers who took lithium.

Other findings in manic patients have included significantly elevated levels of total immunoglobulins and complement proteins and lower levels of serum immunoglobulin D (Wadee et al. 2002). In addition, manic patients were found to have increased levels of organ-specific autoantibodies (Padmos et al. 2004).

## Key Points: Nervous, Endocrine, and Immune System Interactions in Psychiatry

- A bidirectional communication network exists between the immune system and the nervous system.

- Chronic stress and depression have been associated with altered immune responses, including decreased NK cell activity and T cell proliferation, as well as activation of innate inflammatory immune responses.

- Chronic stress and depression have been associated with a worse outcome in infectious diseases, cancer, and autoimmune disorders—as well as impaired responses to vaccination and delayed wound healing, possibly due to direct effects on the immune response.

- Cytokines released during activation of the immune system (especially during innate inflammatory immune responses) can access the brain and alter monoamine metabolism, neuroendocrine function, synaptic plasticity, and behavior.

- Through their effects on the brain, cytokines may contribute to behavioral comorbidities in medically ill individuals and may play a role in the pathophysiology of neuropsychiatric disorders, including depression and schizophrenia.

# References

Abbas AK, Lichtman AH: Cellular and Molecular Immunology, 5th Edition. Philadelphia, PA, WB Saunders, 2003

Andreoli AV, Keller SE, Rabaeus M, et al: Depression and immunity: age, severity, and clinical course. Brain Behav Immun 7:279–292, 1993

Buccheri G: Depressive reactions to lung cancer are common and often followed by a poor outcome. Eur Respir J 11:173–178, 1998

Burack JH, Barrett DC, Stall RD, et al: Depressive symptoms and CD4 lymphocyte decline among HIV-infected men. JAMA 270:2568–2573, 1993

Capuron L, Miller AH: Cytokines and psychopathology: lessons from interferon alpha. Biol Psychiatry 56:819–824, 2004

Cover H, Irwin M: Immunity and depression: insomnia, retardation, and reduction of natural killer cell activity. J Behav Med 17:217–223, 1994

Cruess DG, Douglas SD, Petitto JM, et al: Association of depression, CD8+ T lymphocytes, and natural killer cell activity: implications for morbidity and mortality in human immunodeficiency virus disease. Curr Psychiatry Rep 5:445–450, 2003

Cunningham AJ, Edmonds CV, Jenkins GP, et al: A randomized controlled trial of the effects of group psychological therapy on survival in women with metastatic breast cancer. Psychooncology 7:508–517, 1998

DaCosta D, Dobkin PL, Pinard L, et al: The role of stress in functional disability among women with systemic lupus erythematosus: a prospective study. Arthritis Care Research 12:112–119, 1999

Dantzer R: Cytokine-induced sickness behaviour: a neuroimmune response to activation of innate immunity. Eur J Pharmacol 500(1–3):399–411, 2004

Edelman S, Lemon J, Bell DR, et al: Effects of group CBT on the survival time of patients with metastatic breast cancer. Psychooncology 8:474–481, 1999

Evans DL, McCartney CF, Nemeroff CB, et al: Depression in women treated for gynecological cancer: clinical and neuroendocrine assessment. Am J Psychiatry 143:447–451, 1986

Evans DL, Folds JD, Petitto J, et al: Circulating natural killer cell phenotypes in males and females with major depression: relation to cytotoxic activity and severity of depression. Arch Gen Psychiatry 49:388–395, 1992

Evans DL, Mason K, Bauer R, et al: Neuropsychiatric manifestations of HIV-1 infection and AIDS, in Psychopharmacology: The Fifth Generation of Progress. Edited by Charney D, Coyle J, Davis K, et al. New York, Raven, 2002, pp 1281–1300

Everson SA, Goldberg DE, Kaplan GA, et al: Hopelessness and risk of mortality and incidence of myocardial infarction and cancer. Psychosom Med 58:113–121, 1996

Faller H, Bulzebruck H, Drings P, et al: Coping, distress, and survival among patients with lung cancer. Arch Gen Psychiatry 56:756–762, 1999

Fawzy FI, Fawzy NW, Hyun CS, et al: Malignant melanoma: effects of an early structured psychiatric intervention, coping, and affective state on recurrence and survival 6 years later. Arch Gen Psychiatry 50:681–689, 1993

Grant I, Brown GW, Harris T, et al: Severely threatening events and marked life difficulties preceding onset or exacerbation of multiple sclerosis. J Neurol Neurosurg Psychiatry 52:8–13, 1989

Kim YK, Myint AM, Lee BH, et al: Th1, Th2 and Th3 cytokine alteration in schizophrenia. Prog Neuropsychopharmacol Biol Psychiatry 28:1129–1134, 2004

Knekt P, Raitasalo R, Heliovaara M, et al: Elevated lung cancer risk among persons with depressed mood. Am J Epidemiol 144:1096–1103, 1996

Leserman J, Petitto JM, Perkins DO, et al: Severe stress, depressive symptoms, and changes in lymphocyte subsets in human immunodeficiency virus–infected men: a 2-year follow-up study. Arch Gen Psychiatry 54:279–285, 1997

Leserman J, Jackson ED, Petitto JM, et al: Progression to AIDS: the effects of stress, depressive symptoms, and social support. Psychosom Med 61:397–406, 1999

Leserman J, Petitto JM, Golden RN, et al: Impact of stressful life events, depression, social support, coping, and cortisol on progression to AIDS. Am J Psychiatry 157:1221–1228, 2000

Licinio J, Seibyl JP, Altemus M, et al: Elevated CSF levels of interleukin-2 in neuroleptic-free schizophrenic patients. Am J Psychiatry 150:1408–1410, 1993

Linkins RW, Comstock GW: Depressed mood and development of cancer. Am J Epidemiol 132:962–972, 1990

Lyketsos CG, Hoover DR, Guccione M, et al: Depressive symptoms as predictors of medical outcomes in HIV infection. Multicenter AIDS Cohort Study. JAMA 270:2563–2567, 1993

Lyketsos CG, Hoover DR, Guccione M: Depression and survival among HIV-infected persons. JAMA 275:35–36, 1996

Mayne TJ, Vittinghoff E, Chesney MA, et al: Depressive affect and survival among gay and bisexual men infected with HIV. Arch Intern Med 156:2233–2238, 1996

McAllister CG, Rapaport MH, Pickar D, et al: Increased numbers of CD5+ B lymphocytes in schizophrenic patients. Arch Gen Psychiatry 46:890–894, 1989

McGee R, Williams S, Elwood M: Depression and development of cancer: a meta-analysis. Soc Sci Med 38:187–192, 1994

Mohr DC, Goodkin DE, Bacchetti P, et al: Psychological stress and the subsequent appearance of new brain MRI lesions in MS. Neurology 55:55–61, 2000

Nisipeanu P, Korczyn AD: Psychological stress as risk factor for exacerbations in multiple sclerosis. Neurology 43:1311–1312, 1993

Padmos RC, Bekris L, Knijff EM, et al: A high prevalence of organ-specific autoimmunity in patients with bipolar disorder. Biol Psychiatry 56:476–482, 2004

Page-Schafer K, Delorenze GN, Satariano WA, et al: Comorbidity and survival in HIV-infected men in the San Francisco Men's Health Survey. Ann Epidemiol 6:420–430, 1996

Perry S, Fishman B, Jacobsberg L, et al: Relationships over 1 year between lymphocyte subsets and psychosocial variables among adults with infection by human immunodeficiency virus. Arch Gen Psychiatry 49:396–401, 1992

Printz DJ, Strauss DH, Goetz R, et al: Elevation of CD5+ B lymphocytes in schizophrenia. Biol Psychiatry 46:110–118, 1999

Rabkin JG, Williams JB, Remien RH, et al: Depression, distress, lymphocyte subsets, and human immunodeficiency virus symptoms on two occasions in HIV-positive homosexual men. Arch Gen Psychiatry 48:111–119, 1991

Raison CL, Miller AH: Cancer and depression: new developments regarding diagnosis and treatment. Biol Psychiatry 54:283–294, 2003

Raison CL, Capuron C, Miller AH: Cytokines sing the blues: inflammation and the pathogenesis of depression. Trends Immunol 27:24–31, 2006

Ramirez AJ, Craig TK, Watson JP, et al: Stress and relapse of breast cancer. BMJ 298:291–293, 1989

Rapaport MH, Guylai L, Whybrow P: Immune parameters in rapid cycling bipolar patients before and after lithium treatment. J Psychiatr Res 33:335–340, 1999

Schleifer SJ, Keller SE, Bond RN, et al: Major depressive disorder and immunity: role of age, sex, severity, and hospitalization. Arch Gen Psychiatry 46:81–87, 1989

Sonino N, Girelli ME, Boscaro M, et al: Life events in the pathogenesis of Graves' disease: a controlled study. Acta Endocrinol (Copenh) 128:293–296, 1993

Spiegel D, Bloom JR, Kraemer HC, et al: Effect of psychosocial treatment on survival of patients with metastatic breast cancer. Lancet 2:888–891, 1989

Then Bergh F, Kumpfel T, Trenkwalder C, et al: Dysregulation of the hypothalamo-pituitary-adrenal axis is related to the clinical course of MS. Neurology 53:772–777, 1999

Tsai SY, Chen KP, Yang YY, et al: Activation of indices of cell-mediated immunity in bipolar mania. Biol Psychiatry 45:989–994, 1999

Wadee AA, Kuschke RH, Wood LA, et al: Serological observations in patients suffering from acute manic episodes. Hum Psychopharmacol 17:175–179, 2002

Walker LG, Heys SD, Walker MB, et al: Psychological factors can predict the response to primary chemotherapy in patients with locally advanced breast cancer. Eur J Cancer 35:1783–1788, 1999

Ward MM, Lotstein DS, Bush TM, et al: Psychosocial correlates of morbidity in women with systemic lupus erythematosus. J Rheumatol 26:2153–2158, 1999

Watson M, Haviland JS, Greer S, et al: Influence of psychological response on survival in breast cancer: a population-based cohort study. Lancet 354:1331–1336, 1999

Watson M, Homewood J, Haviland J, et al: Influence of psychological response on breast cancer survival: 10-year follow-up of a population-based cohort. Eur J Cancer 41:1710–1714, 2005

Wulsin LR, Vaillant GE, Wells VE: A systematic review of the mortality of depression. Psychosom Med 61:6–17, 1999

Yoshiuchi K, Kumano H, Nomura S, et al: Stressful life events and smoking were associated with Graves' disease in women, but not in men. Psychosom Med 60:182–185, 1998

Zorrilla EP, McKay JR, Luborsky L, et al: Relation of stressors and depressive symptoms to clinical progression of viral illness. Am J Psychiatry 153:626–635, 1996

6

# Role of Psychiatric Measures in Assessment and Treatment

JOHN F. CLARKIN, Ph.D.

DIANE B. HOWIESON, Ph.D.

JOEL McCLOUGH, Ph.D.

## Definition and Development of Psychological Assessment Instruments

Three types of instruments are currently used in the assessment of patient functioning: psychological tests, rating scales, and semistructured interviews (Table 6–1).

Behavior rating scales are standardized devices that allow various informants or observers (e.g., therapist, nurse on a clinical inpatient unit, relatives, trained observers) to rate the behavior of the patient in specified areas. To aid the observer in a reliable rating of the behavior, anchor points are provided in one of several ways.

Semistructured interviews are standardized by controlling the questions, including specifying what kind of probes can be used, and standardizing the scoring of the patient's response, often by using rating scales as described earlier.

Demonstration of adequate test reliability is only the first step in test development. This step establishes that the test items are sufficiently closely related to one another to provide relatively stable measurements. However, a test's reliability does not guarantee its validity. Establishing a test's validity requires demonstration that the test measures what it is intended to measure. Three major types of validity can be assessed: content validity, crite-

**TABLE 6–1. Three types of psychological assessment instruments**

| Type | Example |
|---|---|
| Psychological tests | Wechsler Adult Intelligence Scale— Third Edition |
| | Minnesota Multiphasic Personality Inventory–2 |
| Rating scales | Brief Psychiatric Rating Scale |
| Semistructured interviews | Structured Clinical Interview for DSM-IV Axis I Disorders |
| | International Personality Disorder Examination |

rion-related validity, and construct validity (see Table 6–2). *Content validity* can be achieved only if the content of the test can be said to adequately sample the area of interest. *Criterion-related validity* refers to the test's relation to independent criteria of an individual's ability in a particular area (i.e., concurrent validity) or to the ability of the test to make predictions about future behavior (i.e., predictive validity). *Construct validity* can be achieved only by demonstrating that the test specifically measures a theoretical construct of interest and that scores on the test are unrelated to similar areas.

**TABLE 6–2.    Types of reliability and validity**

| Type | Description |
|---|---|
| **Reliability** | |
| Test–retest | Test yields comparable scores at two proximate points in time |
| Alternate form | Two forms of the same test yield comparable scores |
| Split-half | Subgroups of items yield scores comparable with those of other subgroups of items |
| **Validity** | |
| Content | Items adequately sample the content area |
| Criterion-related | Test score correlates with other measurements of the same area of activity |
| Construct | Test measures a theoretical construct and is unrelated to similar but different constructs |

## Goals of Assessment

Common assessment goals are as follows:

1. Screening for psychiatric disturbance
2. Clarification of diagnostic uncertainty following clinical interview
3. Specification of the severity of symptoms and other difficulties
4. Assessment of patient strengths
5. Informing differential treatment assignment
6. Role-inducing the patient into a therapeutic stance
7. Monitoring the effect of treatment over time
8. Assessment of barriers to learning for educational planning
9. Assessment of quality and cost-effectiveness of systems of care

## Clinical Decision Tree

At the present state of knowledge, we suggest that before referring a patient for assessment, the psychiatrist complete a semistructured interview (or methodical clinical interview) that elicits information about which DSM-IV-TR (American Psychiatric Association 2000) criteria (on

both Axis I and Axis II) the patient meets. Armed with this diagnostic information, the clinical psychologist can pursue questions about the patient along any one axis or mix of the axes that we describe in this chapter—symptoms, personality traits, cognitive functioning, psychodynamics, and environment and social adjustment—by selecting and administering tests, interviews, and rating scales, with the overall goal of informed differential therapeutics.

Psychological assessment currently takes many forms. The most common forms of assessment include screening, diagnostic/treatment planning assessment, and neurocognitive/neuropsychological assessment.

## Cultural Factors in Psychological Assessment

The results from the psychological tests described previously must be carefully considered in the context of the patient's culture, subculture, gender, age, and linguistic competence. The Multicultural Assessment Procedure (Ridley et al. 1998) is a flexible and pragmatic clinical procedure that allows clinicians to meaningfully incorporate cultural data into the assessment process. The four phases of the procedure are reviewed in Table 6–3.

## Major Areas of Assessment

### Assessment of Axis I Constellations and Related Symptoms

As psychiatric nomenclature has undergone revision, assessment tools have been developed that rely on interviews and self-reports (Table 6–4).

### Omnibus Measures of Symptoms

#### Minnesota Multiphasic Personality Inventory

The Minnesota Multiphasic Personality Inventory (MMPI; Hathaway and McKinley 1967) and its successor, the MMPI-2 (Hathaway and McKinley 1989), are probably the most widely used assessment instruments in existence. There are several reasons for the MMPI's extensive use, including its efficiency (the patient spends 1–2 hours taking the test, which can then be computer scored), the extensive data accumulated with the test, its normative base, the use of validity scales that indicate the patient's test-taking attitude, and its impressive cross-cultural valida-

TABLE 6–3. **The Multicultural Assessment Procedure**

1. *Identify cultural data during the initial interview.* Cultural variables include level of acculturation, economic issues, history of oppression, language, experience of racism and prejudice, sociopolitical issues (e.g., citizenship status, level of political activity), methods of child rearing, religious and spiritual practices, family composition, and cultural values (e.g., attitudes toward time, property, family, work, gender, sexuality, leisure).

2. *Interpret the cultural data.* Arrive at a working hypothesis regarding the effect of cultural variables on the patient's clinical presentation. The working hypothesis requires careful consideration of the relative contributions of the patient's current stressors, clinical presentation, experience with racism, psychiatric history, and reality testing.

3. *Incorporate the cultural data.* Measure the working hypothesis against additional data and criteria, such as medical evaluation, psychological tests, and DSM-IV-TR diagnostic criteria.

4. *Arrive at a sound assessment decision.* Once the working hypothesis has been tested with additional data, devise an assessment and treatment plan that meaningfully and fairly incorporates the cultural data.

tion. Although labeled as a personality test, the MMPI was constructed to assess what are now categorized as Axis I conditions and, to a lesser extent, a few dimensions of personality not represented on Axis II.

The MMPI has been revised and restandardized as the MMPI-2. The various MMPI-2 scales are summarized in Table 6–5. Revisions include the deletion of objectionable items and the rewording of other items to reflect more modern language usage, as well as the addition of several new items focusing on suicide, drug and alcohol abuse, type A behavior, interpersonal relationships, and treatment compliance.

## Personality Assessment Inventory

The Personality Assessment Inventory (PAI; Morey 1991) focuses on clinical syndromes that have been staples of psychopathological nosology and have retained their importance in contemporary diagnostic practice. Items were written with careful attention to their content validity, which was designed to reflect the phenomenology of the clinical construct across a broad range of severity.

## Millon Clinical Multiaxial Inventory

The Millon Clinical Multiaxial Inventory–III (MCMI-III; Millon et al. 1997) is a 175-item true/false self-report instrument that yields scores on 11 clinical personality patterns closely related to Millon's theory of personality and psychopathology, the personality disorder diagnoses of DSM-IV (American Psychiatric Association 1994) Axis II, and 9 clinical syndromes. It has been suggested that the MCMI-III should be best used primarily as a measure of Millon's theoretical conceptualization of personality and secondarily as a means of identifying personality disorder diagnoses according to DSM-IV criteria (Kaye and Shea 2000).

## Symptom Checklist–90—Revised

Briefer than the MMPI-2 and the PAI, the Symptom Checklist–90—Revised (SCL-90-R; Derogatis 1977, 1983) contains only 90 items and can be administered in 30 minutes and scored by computer. These items are combined into nine symptom scales: 1) somatization, 2) obsessive-compulsive behavior, 3) interpersonal sensitivity, 4) depression, 5) anxiety, 6) hostility, 7) phobic anxiety, 8) paranoid ideation, and 9) psychoticism. In addition, three global indices are compiled: 1) general severity, 2) positive symptom distress index, and 3) total positive symptoms.

The Brief Symptom Inventory (BSI; Derogatis 1993) is a 53-item self-report form of the SCL-90-R that assesses the same nine symptom dimensions and three global indices but is composed of a subset of items selected from the SCL-90-R, with the heaviest loadings on the nine primary symptoms dimensions so that the same symptom constructs can be reliably and validly measured. The psychometric properties of the BSI are comparable to those of the SCL-90-R, and the BSI has the advantage of increased ease of administration, taking only 8–10 minutes to complete.

## Brief Psychiatric Rating Scale

Another widely used rating scale for a range of psychiatric symptoms is the Brief Psychiatric Rating Scale (Overall and Gorham 1962), which was developed mainly for the assessment of symptoms with an inpatient population. Areas rated include somatic concern, anxiety, emotional withdrawal, conceptual disorganization, guilt, tension, mannerisms and posturing, grandiosity, depressive mood, hostility, suspiciousness, hallucinatory behavior, motor retardation, uncooperativeness, unusual thought content, blunted affect, excitement, and disorientation.

TABLE 6–4.    Instruments for the assessment of DSM-IV Axis I disorders and related symptom patterns

| Instrument | General classification | Description | Scoring features |
|---|---|---|---|
| **DSM-IV Axis I disorders** | | | |
| Structured Clinical Interview for DSM-IV Axis I Disorders (SCID-I); Patient Edition (SCID-I/P); Non-Patient Edition (SCID-I/NP); Clinician Version (SCID-CV) | Semistructured interview | Three-point rating scales of symptoms | Oriented to diagnosis using DSM-IV |
| **Related symptom patterns** | | | |
| Minnesota Multiphasic Personality Inventory–2 | Self-report | 567-item checklist, true/false format | $T$ scores for 13 criterion scales |
| Symptom Checklist–90—Revised | Self-report | 90-item checklist, 5-point intensity scales | $T$ scores for 9 symptom clusters |
| Brief Symptom Inventory | Self-report | 53-item checklist, 5-point intensity scales | $T$ scores for 9 symptom clusters |
| Brief Psychiatric Rating Scale | Clinical interview | 16 items, 7-point severity scales | 5 factor scores and total scores |
| Personality Assessment Inventory | Self-report | 344 items, true/false format | 4 validity scales, 10 clinical scales covering symptoms and severe personality disorders |
| Millon Clinical Multiaxial Inventory–III | Self-report | 175 items, true/false format | 3 validity scales, 22 clinical scales covering Axis I and II areas |

TABLE 6–5.    Minnesota Multiphasic Personality Inventory–2 scales

| Scale | Characteristics of high scorers |
|---|---|
| **Validity scales** | |
| Lie | Dishonest, deceptive, and/or defended |
| Infrequency | Exhibit randomness of responses or psychotic psychopathology |
| Correction/defensiveness | Defensive through presenting themselves as healthier than they are |
| **Clinical scales** | |
| Hypochondriasis | Somatizers, possible medical problems |
| Depression | Dysphoric, possibly suicidal |
| Hysteria | Highly reactive to stress, anxious, and sad at times |
| Psychopathic deviance | Antisocial, dishonest, possible drug abusers |
| Masculinity–femininity | Exhibit lack of stereotypical masculine interests, aesthetic and artistic |
| Paranoia | Exhibit disturbed thinking, ideas of persecution, possibly psychotic |
| Psychasthenia | Exhibit psychological turmoil and discomfort, extreme anxiety |
| Schizophrenia | Confused, disorganized, possible hallucinations |
| Hypomania | Manic, emotionally labile, unrealistic self-appraisal |
| Social introversion | Very insecure and uncomfortable in social situations, timid |

## Specific Areas of Symptomatology

Several instruments have been developed to measure specific symptoms. The classification, description, and scoring features of these instruments are shown in Table 6–6.

### Substance Abuse

Psychological distress and dysfunction arising from the abuse of a wide variety of substances is perhaps the chief reason for seeking psychological or psychiatric treatment. The threat to the validity of self-report screening instruments to detect substance abuse is such that these instruments should be buttressed by the assessment of biological markers (e.g., urine and blood) and reports from other informants. However, it is helpful to review the instruments that have been used for this purpose (see Table 6–6). The prominent instruments in this area are the MacAndrew Alcoholism Scale (MacAndrew 1965), the Addiction Potential Scale from the MMPI-2 (Weed et al. 1992), and Scales B (Alcohol Dependence) and T (Drug Dependence) from the MCMI-III.

The assessment of substance abuse potential is reflected in omnibus symptom rating scales such as the MMPI-2, which contains an item key—the MacAndrew Alcoholism Scale—for identifying patients who have histories of alcohol abuse or who have the potential to develop problems with alcohol (Hoffmann et al. 1974). A more thorough instrument, the Alcohol Use Inventory (Horn et al. 1986), is a self-administered test standardized on more than 1,200 admissions to an alcoholism treatment program. It contains 24 scales that measure alcohol-related problems and considers the subjects' responses in four separate domains: benefits from drinking, style of drinking, consequences of drinking, and concerns associated with drinking.

The Addiction Severity Index (McLellan et al. 1980) is a 142-item multidimensional, semistructured interview designed to be used as a guide for initial assessment and treatment planning for patients presenting with substance abuse disorders in both inpatient and outpatient settings. Information is gathered on seven problem areas frequently affected by substance abuse: medical status, employment and support, drug use, alcohol use, legal status, family or social status, and psychiatric status. Items include both objective indicators and subjective assessment of problem severity. The University of Rhode Island Change Assessment (McConnaughy et al. 1983) is a measure developed to assess a patient's readiness to change to address issues related to the use of drugs, alcohol, and nicotine. The instrument is based on Prochaska et al.'s (1992) Readiness to Change Stage model. The subscales define four stages of change: Precontemplation, Contemplation, Action, and Maintenance.

### Eating Disorders

Garner (1991) developed a multidimensional self-report measure to assess attitudes, behaviors, and traits associated with anorexia nervosa and bulimia nervosa. This inventory, the Eating Disorder Inventory–2, consists of 91 items rated on 6-point frequency scales that form 11 subscales.

### Affects

As one factor in the larger context of the total personality, anxiety can be assessed with the Sixteen Personality Factor Questionnaire (Cattell et al. 1970), the Eysenck Personality Inventory (Eysenck and Eysenck 1969), and the Taylor Manifest Anxiety Scale (Taylor-Spence and Spence 1966), a scale derived from the MMPI.

The Anxiety Status Inventory is a rating scale for anxiety developed for clinical use adhering to an interview guide, and the Self-Rating Anxiety Scale is a companion self-report instrument, both developed by Zung (1971).

The Beck Anxiety Scale (Beck et al. 1988) is a 21-item self-report questionnaire with a focus on somatic anxiety symptoms, such as heart pounding, nervousness, inability to relax, and dizziness or light-headedness. Items are rated on a 4-point scale ranging from 0 (not at all) to 3 (severe: I could barely stand it). This measure takes approximately 5 minutes to complete and was designed specifically to discriminate between anxiety and depression.

The State-Trait Anxiety Inventory (Spielberger et al. 1970) is a self-report instrument in which patients are asked to report on anxiety in general (i.e., trait) and at particular points in time (i.e., state). The S-R Inventory of Anxiousness (Endler et al. 1962) is a self-report measure of the interaction between the patient's anxiety and environmental situations such as interpersonal, physically dangerous, and ambiguous situations.

The Liebowitz Social Anxiety Scale (Liebowitz 1987) is a clinician-administered semistructured interview that assesses social phobias. A similar instrument is the Brief Social Phobia Scale (Davidson et al. 1991), an 11-item semistructured interview constructed to assess severity and treatment response of social phobias.

The measurement of the severity of obsessive-compulsive symptoms is often accomplished with the widely used Yale-Brown Obsessive Compulsive Scale; Goodman et al. 1989). There are two subscales in this clinician-administered semistructured interview, an Obsessions subscale and a Compulsions subscale.

**TABLE 6–6.    Instruments for the assessment of specific symptom areas**

| Instrument | General classification | Description | Scoring features |
|---|---|---|---|
| **Substance abuse** | | | |
| Alcohol Use Inventory | Self-report | 228 items rated on 2- to 6-point scales | 17 primary scales in 4 areas and 7 second-order factor scales |
| Addiction Severity Index | Semistructured interview | 142 items rated on 5-point subjective assessment scale and 10-point severity scale | 7 functional areas of problems with substances |
| University of Rhode Island Change Assessment | Self-report or interview | 32 items, 5-point scale | 4 scores corresponding to 4 stages of change |
| **Eating disorders** | | | |
| Eating Disorder Inventory–2 | Self-report | 91 forced-choice items rated on a 6-point frequency scale | 8 subscales and 3 provisional scales for issues and features pertinent to eating disorders |
| **Affects** | | | |
| State–Trait Anxiety Inventory | Self-report | Two 20-item scales, 4-point frequency ratings | Total scores for state and trait anxiety |
| S-R Inventory of Anxiousness | Self-report | 14-item responses on 5-point severity scales to 11 situations | Focus on intensity and quality of situations arousing anxiety |
| Fear Questionnaire | Self-report | 17 items reflecting specific phobias rated on 9-point avoidance scales | Total scores for agoraphobia, social phobia, and blood and injury phobias |
| Beck Anxiety Scale | Self-report | 21 items, 4-point scale | Total score |
| Panic Disorder Severity Scale | Clinical interview | 7 items, 5-point scale | Total score |
| Beck Depression Inventory | Self-report | 20 items, 4-point intensity scales | Total score |
| Hamilton Rating Scale for Depression | Clinical interview | 17–24 items, 3- to 5-point severity scales | Total score |
| Geriatric Depression Scale | Self-report | 30 items, yes/no, 10 negatively keyed, 20 positively keyed | Total number of depressive responses endorsed |
| Manic-State Rating Scale | Observer rating | 26 items, each scored for frequency and intensity | Total score |
| State-Trait Anger Expression Inventory | Self-report | | Total scores for state and trait anger |
| Anger, Irritability, and Assault Questionnaire | Self-report | 42 questions, 5 time frames, 210 items | 5 subscales, 3 overarching scales |
| **Suicidal behavior** | | | |
| Suicide Intent Scale | Self-report | 15 items, 3-point categorical scales | Total score |
| Index of Potential Suicide | Self-report or semistructured interview | 50 items, 5-point severity scales | Total score and 6 subscores |
| Reasons for Living Inventory | Self-report | 6 factors | Total score |
| **Thought disorder** | | | |
| Thought Disorder Index | Content rating | 22 categories at 4 levels of severity | Total score |
| Positive and Negative Syndrome Scale | Semistructured interview | 30 items, 7-point scale | 3 scale scores, option for composite score and conversion to T scores |
| Scale for the Assessment of Positive Symptoms | Observer rating | 30 items, 6-point scale | 4 global domain scores, summary score, and composite score |

A simple and brief instrument designed to assess the overall severity of DSM-IV panic disorder is the Panic Disorder Severity Scale (Shear et al. 1997). With the use of a scripted interview, the scale provides ratings of DSM-IV panic symptoms and consists of seven items: panic frequency, distress during panic, panic-focused anticipatory anxiety, phobic avoidance of situations, phobic avoidance of physical sensations, impairment in work functioning, and impairment in social functioning. A useful self-report instrument for quantifying the presence and severity of posttraumatic stress disorder (PTSD) symptoms is the Posttraumatic Stress Diagnostic Scale devised by Foa (1995).

The Beck Depression Inventory (BDI; Beck et al. 1996) is probably the most widely used self-report inventory of depression. The 21 items of the inventory were selected to represent symptoms commonly associated with a depressive disorder. This self-report instrument is frequently used in conjunction with the Hamilton Rating Scale for Depression, which allows a clinician to rate the severity of depressive symptoms during an interview with the patient. In contrast to the BDI, the Hamilton Rating Scale for Depression is more systematic in assessing neurovegetative signs.

The Geriatric Depression Scale (Yesavage and Brink 1983) is a commonly used instrument to screen for depressive illness in geriatric patients.

The Manic-State Rating Scale (Beigel et al. 1971) is a 26-item observer-rated scale that is useful for patients with bipolar depression. Eleven items reflecting elation–grandiosity and paranoid–destructive features of manic patients have produced the most consistent results and have been applied successfully in the prediction of inpatient lengths of stay (Young et al. 1978).

The Buss-Durkee Hostility Inventory (Buss and Durkee 1957) is a 75-item self-report questionnaire that measures different aspects of hostility and aggression. There are eight subscales: Assault, Indirect Hostility, Irritability, Negativism, Resentment, Suspicion, Verbal Hostility, and Guilt. Spielberger (1991) developed a State-Trait Anger Expression Inventory that takes about 15 minutes to complete. The Overt Aggression Scale—Modified (Coccaro et al. 1991) is a semistructured clinician interview that assesses aggression, irritability, and suicidality in the past week.

### Suicidal Behavior

Suicidal assessment instruments that are frequently used include the Beck Hopelessness Scale and the Suicide Intent Scale. In addition, it should be noted that the Koss–Butcher critical item set revised on the MMPI is a list of 22 items that are related specifically to depressed suicidal ideation. These critical items should not be seen as scales but rather as markers of particular item content that might be significant in assessing the individual patient (Butcher 1989).

The Suicide Intent Scale (Beck et al. 1974), the Index of Potential Suicide (Zung 1974), and the Suicide Probability Scale (Cull and Gill 1986) are three widely used instruments. A complementary approach has been taken, culminating in the development of the Reasons for Living Inventory (Linehan et al. 1983). Of practical interest is that the Fear-of-Suicide subscale in the inventory differentiates between those who have only considered suicide and those who have made previous suicide attempts.

### Thought Disorder

One approach to the reliable assessment of cognition is the use of semistructured interviews such as the Schedule for Affective Disorders and Schizophrenia (Endicott and Spitzer 1979) and the Structured Clinical Interview for DSM-IV (SCID). Although other commonly used measures of disordered thinking such as the Positive and Negative Syndrome Scale (Kay et al. 1987) and the Scale for the Assessment of Positive Symptoms (Andreasen 1984) supplement the information obtained from the clinical interview with collateral information from caregivers, review of clinical records, and direct behavioral observation prior to rating the presence or absence of a symptom, problems in the accuracy of judgments remain. The test most widely used in examinations for thought disorders has been the Rorschach inkblot test, which was developed by the Swiss psychiatrist Hermann Rorschach. In this test, a relatively ambiguous stimulus (a colored or achromatic "inkblot") is used, and, without additional instruction, individuals are asked to state what the blot looks like to them. Responses are scored for location (i.e., the area of the card that elicits a response), determinants (i.e., form, movement, color, and shading), form quality (i.e., the degree to which percepts are congruent with the area chosen), and content (e.g., human, animal, object). Exner (1974, 1978) developed a scoring system for the Rorschach test that attempts to integrate the best aspects of prior systems.

Holzman and his colleagues have published extensively on the relation of various forms of thought disorder and its severity to psychiatric diagnosis and treatment (Solovay et al. 1986). Although the scoring scheme can be applied to any record of verbal production, its most frequent application has been in the context of verbal records from the administration of tests such as the Wechsler Adult Intelligence Scale—Third Edition (Wechsler 1997) and the Rorschach. In its current version, the Thought Disorder Index (Solovay et al. 1986) considers 22 forms of thought disturbance ranging across four levels of severity as the basis for a total score. The total score has been found to distinguish psychotic from nonpsychotic patients, and more severe forms of thought disorder have been most frequently associated with schizophrenic disorders.

## Assessment of Personality Traits and Disorders

### Dimensional Assessment of Personality

The dimensional assessment of personality using psychological tests has been characterized by a nomothetic approach in which specific personality dimensions (e.g., introversion) are assessed (see Table 6–7). The dimensions chosen for assessment are typically derived from a personality theory, and individuals are expected to show quantitative differences on these various dimensions. The number of items relevant to a particular dimension that are endorsed is thought to reflect important aspects of that individual's personality style.

Within the field of personality measurement, much attention has been paid to the generalizability of such measures. Efforts to investigate the relation between self-report measures of interpersonal behavior and actual behavior in interpersonal situations continue to contribute to the refinement of this important area of psychological assessment.

### Assessment of Personality Disorders

A relatively new approach to the assessment of personality disorders is to construct instruments, either self-report or semistructured interviews, that evaluate the presence or absence of specific personality traits described in Axis II of DSM-IV-TR (see Table 6–7). The most promising instruments of this type include the Personality Diagnostic Questionnaire–4 (PDQ-4; Hyler 1994; Hyler et al. 1988); the MCMI-III (Millon et al. 1997); the Structured Clinical Interview for DSM-IV Axis II Personality Disorders (SCID-II; First et al. 1997); the International Personality Disorder Examination (IPDE; Loranger 1999); and the Structured Interview for DSM-IV Personality (SIDP-IV; Pfohl et al. 1997).

The PDQ-4 is an 85-item true/false self-report inventory of Axis II diagnostic criteria, and the test yields scores on each of the 10 personality disorder categories of DSM-IV. The instrument has a high false-positive rate, meaning that many patients who meet the PDQ-4 criteria do not actually have a personality disorder. In addition, patients typically report a number of traits and will often meet criteria for several diagnostic categories; therefore, the PDQ-4 may be more useful as a screening measure.

Several self-report questionnaires that assess personality and personality pathology have been carefully constructed with attention to psychometric properties. These include the Schedule for Nonadaptive and Adaptive Personality (Clark 1993), the Dimensional Assessment of Personality Pathology—Basic Questionnaire (Schroeder et al. 1994), and the Wisconsin Personality Disorders Inventory–IV (Klein et al. 1993). The latter is unique in that it is a self-report measure designed to provide a dimensional and categorical assessment of the DSM-IV personality disorders from the interpersonal perspective of Benjamin's Structural Analysis of Social Behavior.

Five semistructured interviews have been designed to assess, via the patient's report and the clinical judgment of the interviewer, the presence of Axis II disorders: the IPDE, the SIDP-IV, the SCID-II, the Diagnostic Interview for DSM-IV Personality Disorders (Zanarini et al. 1987), and the Personality Disorder Interview–IV (Widiger et al. 1995).

The IPDE is a semistructured interview that yields both dimensional and categorical scores for DSM-IV Axis II criteria based on 99 sets of questions. An important feature of this semistructured interview, which takes approximately 1–2 hours to administer, is that the criteria are assessed in related clusters such as self-concept, affect expression, reality testing, impulse control, interpersonal relationships, and work.

The SIDP-IV is a semistructured interview designed to assess DSM-IV Axis II disorders both categorically and dimensionally. The 101 sets of questions are thematically organized into 10 topic areas: interests and activities, work style, close relationships, social relationships, emotions, observational criteria, self-perception, perception of others, stress and anger, and social conformity.

The SCID-II is concerned with the assessment of Axis II personality disorders. The interview format is determined by the DSM-IV disorders and provides no guide for elaborating the assessment of the criteria.

The Diagnostic Interview for DSM-IV Personality Disorders is a 108-question interview developed to categorically assess DSM-IV personality disorders. The questions are organized according to personality disorder and appear in both yes/no and open-ended formats.

**TABLE 6–7.** Instruments for the assessment of personality traits and disorders

| Instrument | General classification | Description | Scoring features |
|---|---|---|---|
| Neuroticism, Extroversion, and Openness Personality Inventory—Revised | Self-report | 240 items, 5-point scale | 5 domain scales and 30 facet scales |
| Sixteen–Personality Factor Questionnaire | Self-report | 3 equivalent forms of 106–187 items each | Scaled scores for 16 personality traits |
| Eysenck Personality Inventory | Self-report | 57 yes/no items, parallel forms | Scores on extraversion and neuroticism |
| Schedule for Nonadaptive and Adaptive Personality | Self-report | 12 primary traits and 3 temperament dimensions | |
| Dimensional Assessment of Personality Pathology— Basic Questionnaire | Self-report | 18 scales | Scores on 18 scales |
| California Personality Inventory | Self-report | 468 items | Scores on 18 scales and 4 special scales |
| Millon Clinical Multiaxial Inventory–III | Self-report | 175 items, true/false format | Base rate scores on 22 clinical scales |
| Multidimensional Personality Questionnaire | Self-report | 300 items | 11 subscales and 3 higher-order scales |
| Structured Interview for DSM-IV Personality | Semistructured interview | 3-point rating scales | Yields DSM-IV Axis II diagnoses |
| International Personality Disorder Examination | Semistructured interview | Semistructured interview for patient and self-report by family member on patient | Dimensional and categorical scales on DSM-IV Axis II personality disorders |
| Structured Clinical Interview for DSM-IV Axis II Personality Disorders | Semistructured interview | 3-point rating scales | Categorical scales on DSM-IV Axis II personality disorders |
| Diagnostic Interview for DSM-IV Personality Disorders | Semistructured interview | 3-point rating scales | Categorical scales on DSM-IV Axis II personality disorders |
| Personality Disorder Interview–IV | Semistructured interview | 3-point rating scales | Dimensional and categorical scales on DSM-IV Axis II personality disorders |
| Structural Analysis of Social Behavior | Self-report | 36–72 statements of interpersonal behavior rated true/false | Internalized attitudes regarding self and significant others |
| Wisconsin Personality Disorders Inventory–IV | Self-report | 214 items, 10-point scale | Dimensional and categorical scales on DSM-IV Axis II personality disorders based on Structural Analysis of Social Behavior perspective |
| Shedler-Westen Assessment Procedure | Q-sort methodology | 200 descriptive statements, 7-point scale, sorted by fixed distribution | Yields categorical and dimensional DSM-IV diagnoses based on prototypes |

**TABLE 6–8.** Instruments for the assessment of psychodynamics and patient enabling factors

| Instrument | General classification | Description | Scoring features |
|---|---|---|---|
| Rorschach | Unstructured or projective test | 10 ambiguous inkblots, responses scored on multiple criteria | Accuracy of form, location, use of color, shading, etc., provide summary scores |
| Thematic Apperception Test | Unstructured or projective test | 30 ambiguous scenes | Affects, outcomes, and other qualities |
| Inventory of Personality Organization | Self-report | 83 items, 5-point scale | 3 primary scales and 2 supplementary scales |
| Defense Style Questionnaire | Self-report | 88 items, 9-point scale | 4 scales |
| Minnesota Multiphasic Personality Inventory–2 | Self-report | 566-item checklist, true/false format | $T$ scores for 13 criterion scales |
| Symptom Checklist–90—Revised | Self-report | 90-item checklist, 5-point intensity scales | $T$ scores for 9 symptom clusters |
| Millon Clinical Multiaxial Inventory–III | Self-report | 175 items, true/false format | Base rate scores for 22 clinical scales |

The Personality Disorder Interview–IV is similar to the SIDP-IV in that it is available in a thematic and a modular version. The thematic version is organized into nine topical areas, including attitudes toward self, attitudes toward others, security of comfort with others, friendships and relationships, conflicts and disagreements, work and leisure, social norms, mood, and appearance and perception. Few psychometric studies exist, and the measure's real strength appears to be its comprehensive and detailed manual.

## Assessment of Psychodynamics

The instruments used for the assessment of psychodynamics and patient enabling factors are shown in Table 6–8.

The most widely used assessment procedure for the examination of patients over a range of ego functions and dynamic factors is the Rorschach inkblot test, described earlier. Scoring systems have been developed by many authors, and Exner (1974, 1978) created a scoring system that attempts to integrate the best aspects of earlier systems. From these scores, inferences are drawn concerning the patient's self-image, identity, defensive structure, reality testing, affective control, amount and degree of fantasy life, degree of thought organization, and potential for impulsive acting out.

The Thematic Apperception Test is another widely used projective process for assessing the patient's self-concept in relation to others. Originally developed by Murray (1943), the test consists of a set of 30 pictures depicting one or more individuals. The patient is asked to make up a story based on each picture. The stories generated are then scored for the individual's needs as reflected in the feelings and impulses attributed to the major character in each story and the interactions with the environment leading to a resolution.

In an effort to systematically assess concepts related to psychodynamic theory in a manner amenable to the objective self-report of patients, two instruments have been developed: the Inventory of Personality Organization (IPO; Clarkin et al. 2001) and the Defense Style Questionnaire (Bond and Wesley 1996).

The IPO is an 83-item self-report measure consisting of three primary clinical scales and two secondary scales. The three primary clinical scales (57 items) are relevant to the central dimensions of Kernberg's personality organization model (i.e., identity diffusion, primitive psychological defenses, and reality testing). The two secondary scales (29 items) operationalize the supplementary diagnostic components of Kernberg's model (i.e., aggression and moral values). All IPO items have a five-point Likert-type format (1=never true to 5=always true). The Primitive Defenses subscale contains 16 items, the Identity Diffusion subscale contains 21 items, the Reality Testing subscale contains 20 items, the Moral Values subscale contains 11 items, and the Aggression subscale contains 18 items.

The Defense Style Questionnaire is designed to dimensionally assess conscious derivatives of defense mechanisms. The 88-item questionnaire provides scores on four defensive functioning styles: Maladaptive Action, Image-Distorting, Self-Sacrificing, and Adaptive. Each of the styles consists of several defense mechanisms.

## Key Points: Role of Psychiatric Measures in Assessment and Treatment

- Three types of instruments are used in the assessment of patient functioning: psychological tests, rating scales, and semistructured interviews.

- Tests should meet the standards of both reliability and validity.

- Establishing a test's reliability requires demonstration that the test items are sufficiently closely related to one another to provide relatively stable measurements. Three major types of reliability can be assessed: test–retest reliability, alternate form reliability, and split-half reliability.

- Establishing a test's validity requires demonstration that the test measures what it is intended to measure. Three major types of validity can be assessed: content validity, criterion-related validity, and construct validity.

- Assessment has the following objectives:
  1) screening for psychiatric disturbance
  2) clarification of diagnostic uncertainty following clinical interview
  3) specification of the severity of symptoms and other difficulties
  4) assessment of patient strengths
  5) informing differential treatment assignment
  6) role-inducing the patient into a therapeutic stance
  7) monitoring the impact of treatment over time
  8) assessment of barriers to learning for educational planning, and
  9) assessment of quality and cost-effectiveness of systems of care

- Cultural factors may influence subjects' response to assessment instruments.

- Major content areas of assessment include symptoms, cognitive functioning, personality disorders and traits, psychodynamics, and environmental demands and social adjustment.

- Therapeutic enabling factors are aspects of the patient that affect the acceptance, use, and absorption of the treatment.

- The major therapeutic enabling factors are problem severity, motivational distress, problem complexity, reactance, and coping style.

## References

American Psychiatric Association: Diagnostic and Statistical Manual of Mental Disorders, 4th Edition. Washington, DC, American Psychiatric Association, 1994

American Psychiatric Association: Diagnostic and Statistical Manual of Mental Disorders, 4th Edition, Text Revision. Washington, DC, American Psychiatric Association, 2000

Andreasen NC: Scale for the Assessment of Positive Symptoms (SAPS). Iowa City, University of Iowa, 1984

Beck AT, Schuyler D, Herman I: Development of suicidal intent scales, in The Prediction of Suicide. Edited by Beck AT, Resnick HLP, Lettieri DJ. Bowie, MD, Charles Press, 1974, pp 2045–2056

Beck AT, Epstein N, Brown G, et al: An inventory for measuring clinical anxiety: psychometric properties. J Consult Clin Psychol 56:893–897, 1988

Beck AT, Steer RA, Brown GK: Beck Depression Inventory Manual, 2nd Edition. San Antonio, TX, Psychological Corporation, 1996

Beigel A, Murphy DL, Bunney WE Jr: The Manic-State Rating Scale: scale construction, reliability, and validity. Arch Gen Psychiatry 25:256–262, 1971

Bond M, Wesley S: Manual for Defense Style Questionnaire. Montreal, QU, Canada, McGill University, 1996

Buss AH, Durkee A: An inventory for assessing different kinds of hostility. J Consult Psychol 21:343–349, 1957

Butcher JN: The Minnesota Report: Adult Clinical System MMPI-2. Minneapolis, University of Minnesota Press, 1989

Cattell RB, Eber HW, Tatsuoka MM: Handbook for the Sixteen Personality Factor Questionnaire (16 PF) in Clinical, Educational, Industrial, and Research Psychology, for Use With All Forms of the Test. Champaign, IL, Institute for Personality and Ability Testing, 1970

Clark LA: Manual for the Schedule for Nonadaptive and Adaptive Personality (SNAP). Minneapolis, University of Minnesota Press, 1993

Clarkin JF, Foelsch PA, Kernberg OF: The Inventory of Personality Organization. White Plains, NY, Weill Medical College of Cornell University, 2001

Coccaro EF, Harvey PD, Kupsaw-Lawrence E, et al: Development of neuropharmacologically based behavioral assessments of impulsive aggressive behavior. J Neuropsychiatry Clin Neurosci 3:S44–S51, 1991

Cull JG, Gill WS: Suicide Probability Scale (SPS) Manual. Los Angeles, CA, Western Psychological Services, 1986

Davidson JRT, Potts NLS, Richichi EA, et al: The Brief Social Phobia Scale. J Clin Psychiatry 52:48–51, 1991

Derogatis LR: The SCL-90-R. Baltimore, MD, Clinical Psychometric Research, 1977

Derogatis LR: SCL-90-R: Administration, Scoring, and Procedures Manual II. Baltimore, MD, Clinical Psychometric Research, 1983

Derogatis LR: Brief Symptom Inventory (BSI): Administration, Scoring, and Procedures Manual, 3rd Edition. Minneapolis, MN, National Computer Systems, 1993

Endicott J, Spitzer RL: Use of the Research Diagnostic Criteria and the Schedule for Affective Disorders and Schizophrenia to study affective disorders. Am J Psychiatry 136:52–56, 1979

Endler NS, Hunt J McV, Rosenstein AJ: An S-R inventory of anxiousness (monogr no 536). Psychol Monogr 76:1–31, 1962

Exner JE Jr: The Rorschach: A Comprehensive System, Vol 1. New York, Wiley, 1974

Exner JE Jr: The Rorschach: A Comprehensive System, Vol 2. New York, Wiley, 1978

Eysenck HJ, Eysenck SB: The Structure and Measurement of Personality. San Diego, CA, RR Knapp, 1969

First MB, Gibbon M, Spitzer RL, et al: User's Guide for the Structured Clinical Interview for DSM-IV Axis II Personality Disorders (SCID-II). Washington, DC, American Psychiatric Press, 1997

Foa EB: Posttraumatic Stress Diagnostic Scale: Manual. Minneapolis, MN, National Computer Systems, 1995

Garner DM: Eating Disorder Inventory–2: Professional Manual. Odessa, FL, Psychological Assessment Resources, 1991

Goodman WK, Price LH, Rasmussen SA, et al: The Yale-Brown Obsessive Compulsive Scale, I: development, use, and reliability. Arch Gen Psychiatry 46:1006–1011, 1989

Hathaway SR, McKinley JC: Minnesota Multiphasic Personality Inventory Manual, Revised Edition. New York, Psychological Corporation, 1967

Hathaway SR, McKinley JC: Minnesota Multiphasic Personality Inventory–2. Minneapolis, University of Minnesota Press, 1989

Hoffmann H, Loper RG, Kammeier ML: Identifying future alcoholics with MMPI alcoholism scales. Q J Stud Alcohol 35:490–498, 1974

Horn JL, Wanberg KW, Foster FM: Alcohol Use Inventory. Minneapolis, MN, National Computer Systems, 1986

Hyler SE: Personality Diagnostic Questionnaire–4. New York, New York State Psychiatric Institute, 1994

Hyler SE, Rieder RO, Williams JBW, et al: The Personality Diagnostic Questionnaire: development and preliminary results. J Personal Disord 2:229–237, 1988

Kay SR, Fiszbein A, Opler LA: The Positive and Negative Syndrome Scale (PANSS) for schizophrenia. Schizophr Bull 13:261–276, 1987

Kaye AL, Shea MT: Personality disorders, personality traits, and defense mechanisms measures, in Handbook of Psychiatric Measures. Washington, DC, American Psychiatric Association, 2000, pp 734–736

Klein MH, Benjamin LS, Rosenfeld R, et al: The Wisconsin Personality Disorders Inventory: development, reliability, and validity. J Personal Disord 7:285–303, 1993

Liebowitz MR: Social phobia. Mod Probl Pharmacopsychiatry 22:141–173, 1987

Linehan MM, Goodstein JL, Nielson SL, et al: Reasons for staying alive when you are thinking of killing yourself: the Reasons for Living Inventory. J Consult Clin Psychol 51:276–286, 1983

Loranger AW: International Personality Disorder Examination (IPDE) Manual. Odessa, FL, Psychological Assessment Resources, 1999

MacAndrew C: The differentiation of male alcoholic outpatients from nonalcoholic psychiatric outpatients by means of the MMPI. Q J Stud Alcohol 26:238–246, 1965

McConnaughy EA, Prochaska JO, Velicer WF: Stages of change in psychotherapy: measurement and sample profiles. Psychotherapy: Theory, Research, and Practice 20:368–375, 1983

McLellan AT, Luborsky L, Woody GE, et al: An improved diagnostic evaluation instrument for substance abuse patients: the Addiction Severity Index. J Nerv Ment Dis 168:26–33, 1980

Millon T, Davis R, Millon C: MCMI-III Manual, 2nd Edition. Minneapolis, MN, National Computer Systems, 1997

Morey LC: Personality Assessment Inventory. Odessa, FL, Psychological Assessment Resources, 1991

Murray HA: Thematic Apperception Test Manual. Cambridge, MA, Harvard University Press, 1943

Overall JE, Gorham DR: The Brief Psychiatric Rating Scale. Psychol Rep 10:799–812, 1962

Pfohl B, Blum N, Zimmerman M: Structured Interview for DSM-IV Personality (SIDP-IV). Washington, DC, American Psychiatric Press, 1997

Prochaska JO, DiClemente CC, Norcross JC: In search of how people change: applications to addictive behaviors. Am Psychol 47:1102–1114, 1992

Ridley CR, Li LC, Hill CL: Multicultural assessment: reexamination, reconceptualization and practical application. Couns Psychol 26:827–910, 1998

Schroeder ML, Wormworth JA, Livesley WJ: Dimensions of personality disorder and the five-factor model of personality, in Personality Disorders and the Five-Factor Model of Personality. Edited by Costa PT, Widiger TA. Washington, DC, American Psychological Association, 1994, pp 117–127

Shear MK, Brown TA, Barlow DH, et al: Multicenter collaborative Panic Disorder Severity Scale. Am J Psychiatry 154:1571–1575, 1997

Solovay MR, Shenton ME, Gasperetti C, et al: Scoring manual for the Thought Disorder Index. Schizophr Bull 12:483–496, 1986

Spielberger CD: State-Trait Anger Expression Inventory, Revised Research Edition. Odessa, FL, Psychological Assessment Resources, 1991

Spielberger CD, Gorsuch RR, Luchene RE: State-Trait Anxiety Inventory. Palo Alto, CA, Consulting Psychologists Press, 1970

Taylor-Spence JA, Spence KW: The motivational components of manifest anxiety: drive and drive stimuli, in Anxiety and Behavior. Edited by Spielberger CD. New York, Academic Press, 1966, pp 291–326

Wechsler D: Wechsler Adult Intelligence Scale–III Administrative and Scoring Manual. San Antonio, TX, Psychological Corporation, 1997

Weed NC, Butcher JN, McKenna T, et al: New measures for assessing alcohol and drug abuse with the MMPI-2: the APS and AAS. J Pers Assess 58:389–404, 1992

Widiger TA, Mangine S, Corbitt EM, et al: Personality Disorder Interview–IV: A Semi-Structured Interview for the Assessment of Personality Disorders. Odessa, FL, Psychological Assessment Resources, 1995

Yesavage JA, Brink TL: Development and validation of a geriatric depression screening scale: a preliminary report. J Psychiatr Res 17:37–49, 1983

Young RC, Biggs JT, Ziegler VE, et al: A rating scale for mania: reliability, validity and sensitivity. Br J Psychiatry 133:429–435, 1978

Zanarini MC, Frankenburg FR, Chauncey DL, et al: The Diagnostic Interview for Personality Disorders: interrater and test-retest reliability. Compr Psychiatry 28:467–480, 1987

Zung WWK: A rating instrument for anxiety disorders. Psychosomatics 12:371–379, 1971

Zung WWK: Index of Potential Suicide (IPS): a rating scale for suicide prevention, in The Prediction of Suicide. Edited by Beck AT, Resnick HLP, Lettieri DJ. Bowie, MD, Charles Press, 1974, pp 221–249

# 7

# The Neuropsychological Evaluation

DIANE B. HOWIESON, Ph.D.

MURIEL D. LEZAK, Ph.D.

## Indications for a Neuropsychological Evaluation

Neuropsychological signs and symptoms that are possible indicators of a pathological brain disorder are presented in Table 7–1.

## Role of the Referring Psychiatrist

The more explicit the referral question, the more likely it is that the evaluation will be conducted to provide the needed information. The referral question should include

- Identifying information about the patient.
- Reasons that the evaluation is requested.
- A description of the problem to be assessed.
- Pertinent history.

## The Nature of Neuropsychological Tests

Two types of standardized neuropsychological tests are available. Some tests involve, by design, cognitive or sensorimotor tasks that can be accomplished by all intact adults within the culture. Because all individuals are expected to be able to perform the task, failure to do so may be interpreted as impairment. Examples of this approach include many aphasia tests of basic language skills. Anyone from an English-speaking Western cultural background would be expected to name, describe, and demonstrate the use of common objects as tested by the Porch Index of Communicative Ability (Porch 1981). The Dementia Rating Scale–2 (Mattis et al. 2001) is based on the assumption that adults will be able to perform most of the cognitive tasks used in this test. The manual specifies the small number of errors considered normal. Most individuals without any cognitive impairment achieve a nearly perfect score on the Mini-Mental State Examination (MMSE; Folstein et al. 1975).

However, most tests of cognitive abilities are designed with the expectation that only very few persons will obtain a perfect score and that most scores will cluster in a middle range. For these tests, scores are conceptualized as continuous variables. The scores of many persons taking the test can be plotted as a distribution curve. Most scores on tests of complex learned behaviors fall into a characteristic bell-shaped curve called a *normal distribution curve* (Figure 7–1). The statistical descriptors of the curve are the *mean*, or average score; the degree of spread of scores about the mean, expressed as the *standard deviation*; and the *range*, or the distance from the highest to the lowest scores.

The level of competence in different cognitive functions as well as other behaviors varies from individual to individual and also within the same individual at different

**TABLE 7–1.    Neuropsychological signs and symptoms that may indicate a pathological brain process**

| Functional class | Symptoms and signs |
|---|---|
| Speech and language | Dysarthria |
| | Dysfluency |
| | Marked change in amount of speech output |
| | Paraphasias |
| | Word-finding problems |
| Academic skills | Alterations in reading, writing, calculating, and number abilities |
| | Frequent letter or number reversals |
| Thinking | Perseveration of speech |
| | Simplified or confused mental tracking, reasoning, and concept formation |
| Motor | Weakness or clumsiness, particularly if lateralized |
| | Impaired fine motor coordination (e.g., changes in handwriting) |
| | Apraxias |
| | Perseveration of action components |
| Memory[a] | Impaired recent memory for verbal or visuospatial material or both |
| | Disorientation |
| Perception | Diplopia or visual field alterations |
| | Inattention (usually left-sided) |
| | Somatosensory alterations (particularly if lateralized) |
| | Inability to recognize familiar stimuli (agnosia) |
| Visuospatial abilities | Diminished ability to perform manual skills (e.g., mechanical repairs and sewing) |
| | Spatial disorientation |
| | Left-right disorientation |
| | Impaired spatial judgment (e.g., angulation of distances) |
| Emotions[b] | Diminished emotional control with temper outburst and antisocial behavior |
| | Diminished empathy or interest in interpersonal relationships |
| | Affective changes |
| | Irritability without evident precipitating factors |
| | Personality change |
| Comportment[b] | Altered appetites and appetitive activities |
| | Altered grooming habits (excessive fastidiousness or carelessness) |
| | Hyperactivity or hypoactivity |
| | Social inappropriateness |

[a]Many emotionally disturbed persons complain of memory deficits, which most typically reflect the person's self-preoccupation, distractibility, or anxiety rather than a dysfunctional brain. Thus, memory complaints in themselves do not necessarily warrant neuropsychological evaluation.
[b]Some of these changes are most likely to be neuropsychologically relevant in the absence of depression, although they can also be mistaken for depression.

times. This variability also has the characteristics of a normal curve, as in Figure 7–1. Because of the normal variability of performance on cognitive tests, any single score can be considered only as representative of a normal performance range and must not be taken as a precise value. For this reason, many neuropsychologists are reluctant to report scores, but rather describe their findings in terms of ability levels. See Table 7–2 for interpretations of ability levels expressed as deviations from the mean of the normative sample.

An individual's score is compared with the normative data, often by calculating a standard or z score, which describes the individual's performance in terms of statistically regular distances (i.e., standard deviations). In this

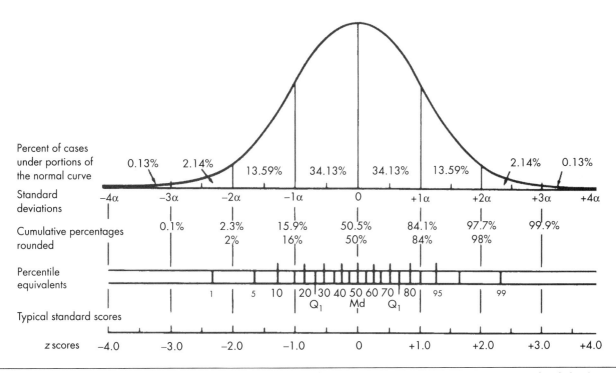

**FIGURE 7–1. A normal distribution curve, showing the percentage of cases between –4 standard deviations (–σ) and +4 standard deviations (+σ).**

The average range is defined as –0.6 to +0.6 standard deviations or the 25th to the 75th percentiles.

*Source.* Adapted from the Test Service Bulletin of The Psychological Corporation, 1955.

**TABLE 7–2. Ability test classifications expressed as deviations from the mean calculated from the normative sample**

| z Score range | Percentile | Classification |
|---|---|---|
| >+2.0 | 98–100 | Very superior |
| >+1.3 to +2.0 | 91–97 | Superior |
| +0.67 to +1.3 | 75–90 | High average |
| –0.66 to +0.66 | 26–74 | Average |
| –0.67 to –1.3 | 10–25 | Low average |
| <–1.3 to –2.0 | 3–9 | Borderline |
| <–2.0 | 0–2 | Defective |

framework, scores within ±0.66 standard deviation are considered average because 50% of a normative sample scores within this range. The z scores are used to describe the probability that a deviant response occurs by chance or because of an impairment. A performance in the below average direction that is greater than two standard deviations from the mean is usually described as falling in the impaired range because 98% of the normative sample taking the test achieve better scores. Figure 7–2 shows the performance of 34 men with schizophrenia on a set of neuropsychological tests. The z scores are calculated on the basis of the performance of a control group (the 0 line). The patient group had poorer performance than the control group on all measures.

## Major Test Categories

### Mental Ability

The most commonly used set of tests of general intellectual function of adults in the Western world is contained in the various versions and translations of the Wechsler Intelligence Scale (WIS; Wechsler 1944, 1955, 1981, 1997a). These batteries of brief tests provide scores on a variety of cognitive tasks covering a range of skills. Each version was originally developed as an "intelligence" test to predict academic and vocational performance of neurologically intact adults by giving an IQ (intelligence quotient) score, which is based on the mean performance on the tests in this battery. The entire test battery may provide the bulk of the tests included in a neuropsychological examination.

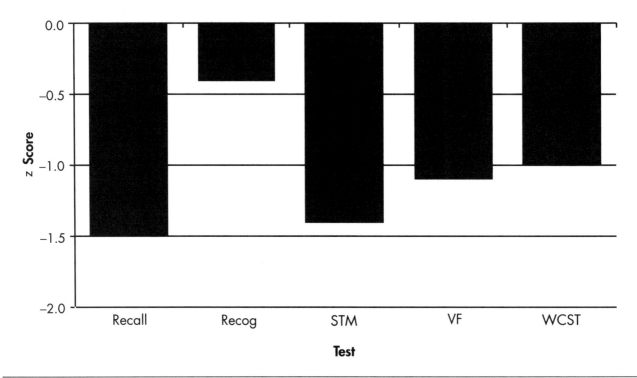

**FIGURE 7–2.** **Mean performance of patients with schizophrenia compared with control subjects on cognitive tests: delayed recall of words and stories (Recall); recognition of words when targets were mixed with distractors (Recog); short-term memory (STM) measured by the Brown-Peterson technique; verbal fluency (VF); and Wisconsin Card Sorting Test (WCST) categories achieved.**

*Source.* Adapted from Sullivan et al. 1994.

The individual tests were designed to assess relatively distinct areas of cognition, such as arithmetic, abstract thinking, and visuospatial organization, and thus are differentially sensitive to dysfunction of various areas of the brain. Therefore, these tests are often used to screen for specific areas of cognitive deficits. Many experienced neuropsychologists use and interpret these tests discretely, administering only those deemed relevant for each patient and treating the findings as they treat data obtained from individually developed tests.

When these tests are given to neuropsychologically impaired persons, summary IQ scores can be very misleading because individual test scores lowered by specific cognitive deficits, when averaged in with scores relatively unaffected by the brain dysfunction, can result in IQ scores associated with ability levels that represent neither the severity of deficits nor the patient's residual competencies (Lezak 1988).

In some cases, neuropsychologists have used discrepancies between summed scores on what Wechsler called the Verbal scale of the WIS (i.e., Verbal IQ) and summed scores on the so-called Performance scale (Performance IQ) to indicate a specific area of cognitive deficit. The pro-

cedure has developed because left hemisphere lesions tend to produce a relatively depressed Verbal IQ score, whereas both right hemisphere lesions and diffuse damage, as in dementia or any problem resulting in response slowing, produce a depressed Performance IQ score. Even this lesser amount of summation can mask important data (Bornstein 1983; Crawford 1992; Grossman 1983; Iverson et al. 2004). In the earlier example, impaired performance on one test would not be likely to produce sufficient relative lowering of the Performance IQ score to detect the cognitive deficit. Moreover, the Arithmetic and Digit Span tests of the Verbal scale are very sensitive to attentional deficits, and only three of the Performance scale measures involve motor response: one (Picture Completion) calls for a purely verbal response and loads significantly on the verbal factor in factor analytic studies.

## Language

Lesions to the hemisphere dominant for speech and language, which is the left hemisphere in 95%–97% of right-handed persons and 60%–70% of left-handed ones

(Corballis 1991; Strauss and Goldsmith 1987), can produce any of a variety of disorders of symbol formulation and use—the aphasias (Spreen and Risser 2003). Although many aphasiologists argue against attempting to classify all patients into one of the standard aphasia syndromes because of so many individual differences, persons with aphasia tend to be grouped according to whether the main disorder is in language comprehension (receptive aphasia), expression (expressive aphasia), repetition (conduction aphasia), or naming (anomic aphasia).

Many comprehensive language assessment tests are available, such as the Multilingual Aphasia Examination (Benton and Hamsher 1989). Comprehensive aphasia test batteries are best administered by speech pathologists or other clinicians with special training in this field. These batteries usually include measures of spontaneous speech, speech comprehension, repetition, naming, reading, and writing.

## Attention and Mental Tracking

A frequent consequence of brain disorders is slowed mental processing and impaired ability for focused behavior (Duncan and Mirsky 2004; Leclercq and Zimmermann 2002). Damage to the brain stem or diffuse damage involving the cerebral hemispheres, especially the white matter interconnections, can produce a variety of attentional deficits. Attentional deficits are very common in neuropsychiatric disorders. Most neuropsychological assessments will include measures of these abilities.

The Wechsler scales contain several relevant tests. Digit Span measures attention span or short-term memory for numbers in two ways: forward and backward digit repetition. Backward digit repetition is a more demanding task because it requires concentration and mental tracking plus the short-term memory component. It is not uncommon for moderately to severely brain-damaged patients to perform poorly on only the backward repetition portion of this test. Because Digits Forward and Digits Backward measure different functions, assessment data for each should be reported separately. Digit Symbol also requires concentration plus motor and mental speed for successful performance. The patient must accurately and rapidly code numbers into symbols. The Arithmetic test in the Wechsler battery is very sensitive to attentional disorders because it requires short-term auditory memory and rapid mental juggling of arithmetic problem elements. Poor performance on this test must be evaluated for the nature of the failures.

Another commonly used measure of concentration and mental tracking is the Trail Making Test (Armitage 1946). In the first part of this test (Part A), the patient is asked to draw rapidly and accurately a line connecting in sequence a random display of numbered circles on a page. The level of difficulty is increased in the second part (Part B) by having the patient again sequence a random display of circles, this time alternating numbers and letters (Figure 7–3). This test requires concentration, visual scanning, and flexibility in shifting cognitive sets (Cicerone and Azulay 2002). It shares with many attention tests vulnerability to other kinds of deficits such as motor slowing, which could be based on peripheral factors such as nerve or muscle damage, and diminished visual acuity. It is also sensitive to educational deprivation and cannot be used with persons not well versed in the alphabet common to Western languages (e.g., English, French, Dutch, Italian).

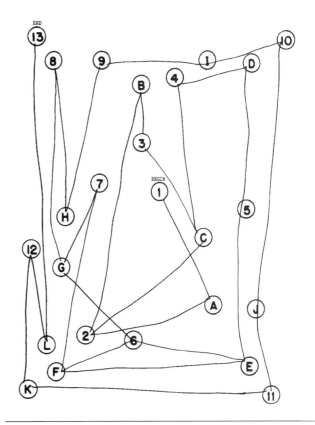

**FIGURE 7–3. Trail Making Test Part B performance by a 61-year-old man with normal pressure hydrocephalus.**

Two types of errors are shown: erroneous sequencing (1→A→2→C) and failure to alternate between numbers and letters (D→5→E→F).

## Memory

Memory is another cognitive function that is frequently impaired by brain disorders. Many diffuse brain injuries produce general impairments in abilities for new learning and retention. Many focal brain injuries also produce memory impairment; left hemisphere lesions are most likely to produce primarily verbal memory deficits, whereas visuospatial memory impairments tend to be associated with right hemisphere lesions (Abrahams et al. 1997; Ojemann and Dodrill 1985; Wagner et al. 1998), although not all visuospatial tests show a right hemisphere advantage (Raspall et al. 2005). Memory impairment often is a prominent feature of herpes encephalitis, Huntington's chorea, Korsakoff's syndrome, hypoxia, closed head injury, and a variety of neurological degenerative diseases, such as Alzheimer's disease (Baddeley et al. 2002; Bauer et al. 2003; Mayes 2000).

In most cases of brain injury, memory for information learned before the injury is relatively preserved compared with new learning. For this reason, many patients with memory impairment will perform relatively well on tests of fund of information or recall of remote events. However, amnesic disorders can produce a retrograde amnesia, with loss of memory extending weeks, months, or years before the onset of the injury. Electroconvulsive therapy also can produce retrograde amnesia (Squire et al. 1975). The retrograde amnesia of Huntington's chorea or Korsakoff's syndrome can go back for decades (Butters and Miliotis 1985; Cermak 1982). In rare cases, a patient will have retrograde amnesia without significant anterograde amnesia; that is, new learning ability remains intact (Kapur et al. 1996; Reed and Squire 1998). Isolated retrograde amnesia may include amnesia for autobiographical events (Della Sala et al. 1993; Evans et al. 1996; Kapur 1997; Levine et al. 1998). However, cases of isolated amnesia for personal identity often have a psychogenic cause (Hodges 1991).

The Wechsler Memory Scale (WMS) batteries (Wechsler 1987, 1997b) are the most commonly used set of tests of new learning and retention in the United States. These batteries are composed of a variety of tests measuring free recall or recognition of both verbal and visual material. In addition, these tests include measures of recall of personal information and attention, concentration, and mental tracking. Several of the tests provide measures of both immediate and delayed (approximately 30 minutes) recall.

## Perception

Perception in any of the sensory modalities can be affected by brain disease. Perceptional inattention (sometimes called *neglect*) is one of the major perceptual syndromes because it occurs frequently with focal brain damage (Bisiach and Vallar 1988; Heilman et al. 2000b; Lezak 1994; Rafal 2000). This phenomenon involves diminished or absent awareness of stimuli in one side of personal space by a patient with an intact sensory system. Unilateral inattention is often most prominent immediately after acute-onset brain injury such as stroke. Most commonly seen is left-sided inattention associated with right hemisphere lesions.

Several techniques can be used to detect unilateral inattention. Visual inattention can be assessed by using a Line Bisection Test (Schenkenberg et al. 1980), in which the patient is asked to bisect a series of uneven lines on a page, or by using a cancellation task requiring the patient to cross out a designated symbol distributed among other similar symbols over a page (Haeske-Dewick et al. 1996; Mesulam 2000). A commonly used test for tactile inattention is the Face–Hand Test (Berg et al. 1987; Smith 1983). With eyes closed, the patient is instructed to indicate when points on the face (cheeks) or hands or both are touched by the examiner. Each side is touched singly and then in combination with the other side, such as left cheek and right hand. The patient should have no difficulty reporting a single point of stimulation. Failure to report stimulation to one side when both sides are stimulated is referred to as *tactile inattention* or *double simultaneous extinction*.

The most commonly used forms of perceptual tests assess perceptual discrimination among similar stimuli. These visual tests may include discrimination of geometric forms, angulation, color, faces, or familiar objects (Lezak et al. 2004; McCarthy and Warrington 1990; Newcombe and Ratcliff 1989). Some perceptual tasks assess the ability to integrate isolated percepts. The Hooper Visual Organization Test (Hooper 1958) presents line drawings of familiar objects in fragmented, disarranged pieces and asks for the name of each object. Some standard cognitive tests also can be administered in a tactile version (Beauvais et al. 2004; Van Lancker et al. 1989; Varney 1986).

Frequently used tactile tests include form recognition and letter or number recognition (Reitan and Wolfson 1993).

## Praxis

Many patients with left hemisphere damage have at least one form of apraxia, and apraxia is common in progressed stages of Alzheimer's disease, Parkinson's disease, Pick's disease, and progressive supranuclear palsy (Dobigny-Roman et al. 1998; Fukui et al. 1996; Leiguarda et al. 1997). Apraxic patients' inability to perform a desired sequence of motor activities is not the result of motor weakness. Rather, the deficit is in planning and carrying out the required activities (De Renzi et al. 1983; Heilman et al. 2000a; Jason 1990) and is associated with disruption of neural representations for extrapersonal (e.g., spatial location) and intrapersonal (e.g., hand position) features of movement (Haaland et al. 1999).

Tests for apraxia assess the patient's ability to reproduce learned movements of the face or limbs. These learned movements can include the use of objects (usually pantomime use of objects) and gestures (Goodglass et al. 2000; Rothi et al. 1997; Strub and Black 2000) or sequences of movements demonstrated by the examiner (Christensen 1979; Haaland and Flaherty 1984).

## Constructional Ability

Although constructional problems were once considered a form of apraxia, more recent analysis has shown that the underlying deficits involve impaired appreciation of one or more aspects of spatial relationships. These can include distortions in perspective, angulation, size, and distance judgment. Thus, unlike apraxia, the problem is not an inability to organize a motor response for drawing lines or assembling constructions but rather misperceptions and misjudgments involving spatial relationships.

Neuropsychological assessments may include any of a number of measures of visuospatial processing. Patients may be asked to copy geometric designs, such as the Complex Figure (Mitrushina et al. 2005; Osterrieth 1944; Rey 1941; Spreen and Strauss 1998) presented in Figure 7–4 or one of the alternative forms (Lezak et al. 2004; Loring et al. 1988). The WIS battery includes constructional tasks involving copying pictured designs with blocks and assembling puzzle pieces (Wechsler 1944, 1955, 1981, 1997a).

Lesions of the posterior cerebral cortex are associated with the greatest difficulty with constructions, and right hemisphere lesions produce greater deficits than do left hemisphere lesions (Benton and Tranel 1993).

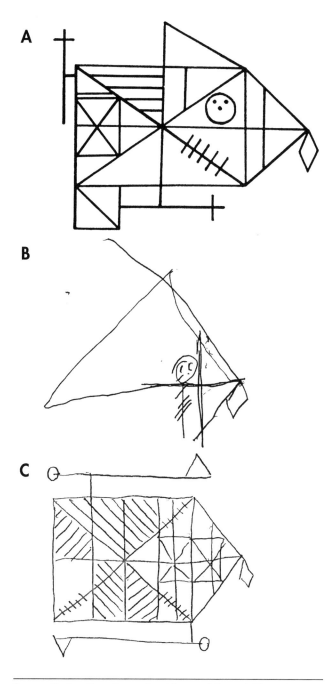

FIGURE 7–4. **Rey Complex Figure (** *Panel A***) and copy (***Panel B***) drawn by a 77-year-old man who had a right hemisphere stroke 2 days before, which produced left-sided neglect and delayed recall. Drawing in** *Panel C* **was by a 72-year-old man with strong perseverative tendencies.**

## Conceptual Functions

Tests of concept formation measure aspects of thinking including reasoning, abstraction, and problem solving. Conceptual dysfunction tends to occur with serious brain injury regardless of site. Most neuropsychological tests require that simple conceptual functioning be intact. For example, reasoning skills are required for the successful performance of most WIS tests: Comprehension assesses commonsense verbal reasoning and interpretation of proverbs; Similarities measures ability to make verbal abstractions by asking for similarities between objects or concepts; Arithmetic involves arithmetic problem solving; Picture Completion requires perceptual reasoning; Picture Arrangement examines sequential reasoning for thematic pictures; Block Design and Object Assembly test visuospatial analysis and synthesis, respectively; and Matrix Reasoning depends on pattern, spatial, and numerical relationships as well as verbal components.

## Executive Functions

Executive functions include abilities to formulate a goal, to plan, to carry out goal-directed plans effectively, and to monitor and self-correct spontaneously and reliably (Lezak 1982). Perseveration (as shown in Figure 7–4, Panel C) occurs when the response is repeated inappropriately and may involve motor acts (as shown), speech, or thoughts. Open-ended tests that permit the patient to decide how to perform the task and when it is complete are difficult tasks for many patients with frontal lobe or diffuse brain injuries (Lezak 1982; Luria 1980). Yet the abilities these tasks test are essential for fulfilling most adult responsibilities and maintaining socially appropriate conduct. An example of a class of tests that assess executive functions are tests of planning, such as mazes. The patient must plan an exit from the maze, which involves foresight to minimize trial-and-error behavior. The Tower of London (Shallice 1982) and Tower of Hanoi tests also assess planning and foresight, as disks are moved from stack to stack to reach a stated goal. Patients with frontal lobe lesions have particular difficulty with planning tests (Carlin et al. 2000; Goel and Grafman 1995). Other tasks that rely heavily on planning for successful completion are multistep tasks calling for decision-making or priority-setting abilities. Few neuropsychological tests are specifically designed to assess these aspects of behavior, yet many complex tasks depend on this analysis. An exception is a set of real-world tasks developed for this purpose called the Behavioral Assessment of the Dysexecutive Syndrome (BADS; Wilson et al. 1996), which has been shown to bring out problems with flexibility, planning, and priority setting in patients with brain injury (Norris and Tate 2000) or schizophrenia (Krabbendam et al. 1999).

# Special Assessment Tools

## Batteries

Of the commercial batteries designed for neuropsychological evaluations, by far the most popular in the United States is the Halstead-Reitan Battery. This battery was designed to assess frontal lobe disorders by Ward C. Halstead (1947) and was subsequently taken on by Ralph Reitan (1969), who added some tests and recommended this battery as a diagnostic test for all kinds of brain damage. The tests include the Category Test, which requires the patient to figure out a concept that is true for each item within the set; the Tactual Performance Test, a tactile spatial performance and memory test; the Rhythm Test, purported to be a nonverbal auditory perception test; the Speech Sounds Perception Test, purported to be a phoneme discrimination test; the Finger Tapping Test, a motor speed test; the Trail Making Test, described earlier; the Aphasia Screening Test, which was originally developed by the aphasiologist Wepman but later discarded by him for being both ineffectual and misleading; a sensory examination; and a measure of grip strength (see Lezak et al. 2004). Examiners using this battery currently administer it with one of the forms of the WIS, the WMS, and the Minnesota Multiphasic Personality Inventory–2 (Hathaway and McKinley 1989). A newer "all-purpose" battery is the Kaplan-Baycrest Neurocognitive Assessment (Leach et al. 2000). Because this is a new test battery, limited clinical data have been reported.

Examinations designed to address specific diagnostic questions are available. Several dementia examinations have been devised. The Dementia Rating Scale (Mattis et al. 2001) contains items assessing attention, initiation/perseveration, construction, conceptualization, and memory and is useful in distinguishing dementia from cognitive decline associated with aging. A brief examination for dementia by the Consortium to Establish a Registry for Alzheimer's Disease uses the MMSE and tests of category fluency, confrontational naming, verbal learning, and design copy (Welsh et al. 1992). Batteries for assessing executive deficits include the BADS (Wilson et al. 1998), the Behavioral Dyscontrol Scale (Grigsby et al. 1992), and the Executive Interview (Royall et al. 1992).

## Screening Tests

Many clinicians would like to have a brief, reliable screening examination with good sensitivity for brain damage of unknown cause or for suspected brain damage. However, there is a trade-off between the amount of information obtained in an assessment and the actual usefulness of the screening test in the detection of brain dysfunction. Brief examinations are often too restricted in range or too simple to be sensitive to subtle or circumscribed areas of dysfunction. The commonly used MMSE contains only 11 simple tasks. It is useful for examining patients with global confusion, poor memory, or dementia. However, many brain-injured patients, such as those with stroke, mild to moderate head injury, and even early dementia, perform adequately on this examination (Benedict and Brandt 1992).

The Neurobehavioral Cognitive Status Examination, also called COGNISTAT (Kiernan et al. 1987; Mysiw et al. 1989; Schwamm et al. 1987), takes about 30 minutes to administer and contains reasonably difficult items of attention, language comprehension, repetition and naming, constructional ability, memory, calculations, reasoning, and judgment, thereby increasing its sensitivity. It is a screening examination, however, and not a substitute for a thorough neuropsychological examination. It may be used to acquire information to decide whether further evaluation is warranted. As with any screening examination, intact performance does not exclude the possibility of brain dysfunction. The Repeatable Battery for the Assessment of Neuropsychological Status (Randolph et al. 1998) also takes about 30 minutes to administer and is useful in screening patients with neurological or psychiatric disease (Hobart et al. 1999; Larson et al. 2005).

# Key Points: The Neuropsychological Evaluation

- Indications for a neuropsychological evaluation
  - Assess nature and severity of known brain disorders.
  - Assess potential brain disorder in people with known risk factors.
  - Diagnose behavioral or cognitive changes of unknown etiology.
- Role of the referring clinician
  - Identify patients who might benefit from a neuropsychological evaluation.
  - Prepare the patient through education about the reasons for and nature of the examination.
  - Provide an explicit and thorough referral question.
- Assessment process
  - Interview.
  - Use standardized cognitive, behavioral, and emotional tests.
  - Interpret results on the basis of comparisons with appropriate normative data.
- Major test categories
  - Language
  - Attention and mental tracking
  - Memory
  - Perception
  - Praxis
  - Constructional ability
  - Conceptual functions
  - Executive functions
  - Motor functions
  - Personality and emotional status
- Uses of data
  - Identify patient's strengths and weaknesses.
  - Provide a diagnosis.
  - Formulate a treatment or an intervention.
  - Determine competency.

# References

Abrahams S, Pickering A, Polkey CE, et al: Spatial memory deficits in patients with unilateral damage to the right hippocampal formation. Neuropsychologia 35:11–24, 1997

Armitage SG: An analysis of certain psychological tests used for the evaluation of brain injury. Psychol Monogr (No 277) 60:1–48, 1946

Baddeley A, Kopelman M, Wilson B (eds): The Handbook of Memory Disorders, 2nd Edition. West Sussex, England, Wiley, 2002

Bauer R, Grande L, Valenstein E: Amnesic disorders, in Clinical Neuropsychology, 4th Edition. Edited by Heilman K, Valenstein E. New York, Oxford University Press, 2003, pp 495–573

Beauvais J, Woods S, Delaney R, et al: Development of a tactile Wisconsin Card Sorting Test. Rehabil Psychol 49:282–287, 2004

Benedict RH, Brandt J: Limitation of the Mini-Mental State Examination for the detection of amnesia. J Geriatr Psychiatry Neurol 5:233–237, 1992

Benton AL, Hamsher K de S: Multilingual Aphasia Examination. Iowa City, IO, AJA Associates, 1989

Benton AL, Tranel D: Visuoperceptual, visuospatial, and visuoconstructive disorders, in Clinical Neuropsychology, 3rd Edition. Edited by Heilman KM, Valenstein E. New York, Oxford University Press, 1993, pp 461–497

Berg G, Edwards DR, Danzinger WL, et al: Longitudinal change in three brief assessments of SDAT. J Am Geriatr Soc 35:205–212, 1987

Bisiach E, Vallar G: Hemineglect in humans, in Handbook of Neuropsychology, Vol 1. Edited by Boller F, Grafman J. Amsterdam, The Netherlands, Elsevier, 1988, pp 195–222

Bornstein RA: Verbal IQ–Performance IQ discrepancies on the Wechsler Adult Intelligence Scale—Revised in patients with unilateral or bilateral cerebral dysfunction. J Consult Clin Psychol 51:779–780, 1983

Butters J, Miliotis P: Amnesic disorders, in Clinical Neuropsychology, 2nd Edition. Edited by Heilman KM, Valenstein E. New York, Oxford University Press, 1985, pp 403–451

Carlin D, Bonerba J, Phipps M, et al: Planning impairments in frontal lobe dementia and frontal lobe lesion patients. Neuropsychologia 38:655–665, 2000

Cermak LS (ed): Human Memory and Amnesia. Hillsdale, NJ, Erlbaum, 1982

Christensen A-L: Luria's Neuropsychological Investigation Test, 2nd Edition. Copenhagen, Denmark, Munksgaard, 1979

Cicerone K, Azulay J: Diagnostic utility of attention measures in postconcussion syndrome. Clin Neuropsychol 16:280–289, 2002

Corballis MC: The Lopsided Ape. New York, Oxford University Press, 1991

Crawford JR: Current and premorbid intelligence measures in neuropsychological assessment, in A Handbook of Neuropsychological Assessment. Edited by Crawford JR, Parker DM, McKinlay WW. Hove, UK, Erlbaum, 1992, pp 21–49

Della Sala S, Laiacona M, Spinnler H, et al: Autobiographical recollection and frontal damage. Neuropsychologia 31:823–839, 1993

De Renzi E, Faglioni P, Lodesani M, et al: Performance of left brain–damaged patients on imitation of single movements and motor sequences. Cortex 19:333–343, 1983

Dobigny-Roman N, Dieudonne-Moinet B, Verny M, et al: Ideomotor apraxia test: a new test of imitation of gestures for elderly people. Eur J Neurol 5:571–578, 1998

Duncan C, Mirsky A: The Attention Battery for Adults: a systematic approach to assessment, in Comprehensive Handbook of Psychological Assessment, Vol 1: Intellectual and Neuropsychological Assessment. Edited by Goldstein G, Beers S, Hersen M. Hoboken, NJ, Wiley, 2004, pp 263–276

Evans JJ, Breen EK, Antoun N, et al: Focal retrograde amnesia for autobiographical events following cerebral vasculitis: a connectionist account. Neurocase 2:1–11, 1996

Folstein MF, Folstein SE, McHugh PR: "Mini-Mental State": a practical method for grading the cognitive state of patients for the clinician. J Psychiatr Res 12:189–198, 1975

Fukui T, Sugita K, Kawamura M, et al: Primary progressive apraxia in Pick's disease: a clinicopathologic study. Neurology 47:467–473, 1996

Goel V, Grafman J: Are the frontal lobes implicated in "planning" functions? Interpreting data from the Tower of Hanoi. Neuropsychologia 33:623–642, 1995

Goodglass H, Kaplan E, Barresi B: Boston Diagnostic Aphasia Examination, 3rd Edition. Philadelphia, PA, Lippincott Williams & Wilkins, 2000

Grigsby J, Kaye K, Robbins LJ: Reliabilities, norms and factor structure of the Behavioral Dyscontrol Scale. Percept Mot Skills 74:883–892, 1992

Grossman FM: Percentage of WAIS-R standardization sample obtaining verbal-performance discrepancies. J Consult Clin Psychol 51:641–642, 1983

Haaland KY, Flaherty D: The different types of limb apraxia made by patients with left vs right hemisphere damage. Brain Cogn 3:370–384, 1984

Haaland KY, Harrington DL, Knight RT: Spatial deficits in ideomotor limb apraxia: a kinematic analysis of aiming movements. Brain 122:1169–1182, 1999

Haeske-Dewick HC, Canavan AG, Hömberg V: Directional hyperattention in tactile neglect within grasping space. J Clin Exp Neuropsychol 18:724–732, 1996

Halstead WC: Brain and Intelligence. Chicago, IL, University of Chicago Press, 1947

Hathaway SR, McKinley JC: Minnesota Multiphasic Personality Inventory–2. Minneapolis, University of Minnesota Press, 1989

Heilman KM, Watson RT, Rothi LJG: Disorders of skilled movement, in Patient-Based Approaches to Cognitive Neuroscience. Edited by Farah MJ, Feinberg TE. Cambridge, MA, MIT Press, 2000a, pp 335–343

Heilman KM, Watson RT, Valenstein E: Neglect, I: clinical and anatomic issues, in Patient-Based Approaches to Cognitive Neuroscience. Edited by Farah MJ, Feinberg TE. Cambridge, MA, MIT Press, 2000b, pp 115–123

Hobart MP, Goldberg R, Bartko JJ, et al: Repeatable Battery for the Assessment of Neuropsychological Status as a screening test in schizophrenia, II: convergent/discriminant validity and diagnostic group comparisons. Am J Psychiatry 156:1951–1957, 1999

Hodges JR: Transient Amnesia: Clinical and Neuropsychological Aspects. London, WB Saunders, 1991

Hooper HE: The Hooper Visual Organization Test Manual. Los Angeles, CA, Western Psychological Services, 1958

Iverson GL, Mendrek A, Adams RL: The persistent belief that VIQ-PIQ splits suggest lateralized brain damage. Appl Neuropsychol 11:85–90, 2004

Jason GW: Disorders of motor function following cortical lesions: review and theoretical considerations, in Cerebral Control of Speech and Limb Movements. Edited by Hammond GR. Amsterdam, The Netherlands, Elsevier, 1990, pp 141–168

Kapur N: How can we best explain retrograde amnesia in human memory disorder? Memory 5:115–129, 1997

Kapur N, Scholey K, Moore E, et al: Long-term retention deficits in two cases of disproportionate retrograde amnesia. J Cogn Neurosci 8:416–434, 1996

Kiernan RJ, Mueller J, Langston JW, et al: The Neurobehavioral Cognitive Status Examination: a brief but differentiated approach to cognitive assessment. Ann Intern Med 107:481–485, 1987

Krabbendam L, de Vugt ME, Derix MM, et al: The Behavioural Assessment of the Dysexecutive Syndrome as a tool to assess executive functions in schizophrenia. Clin Neuropsychol 13:370–375, 1999

Larson E, Kirschner K, Bode R, et al: Construct and predictive validity of the Repeatable Battery for the Assessment of Neuropsychological Status in the evaluation of stroke patients. J Clin Exp Neuropsychol 27:16–32, 2005

Leach L, Kaplan E, Rewilak D, et al: Kaplan-Baycrest Neurocognitive Assessment Manual. San Antonio, TX, Psychological Corporation, 2000

Leclercq M, Zimmermann P (eds): Applied Neuropsychology of Attention: Theory, Diagnosis, and Rehabilitation. New York, Psychology Press, 2002

Leiguarda RC, Pramstaller PP, Merello M, et al: Apraxia in Parkinson's disease, progressive supranuclear palsy, multiple system atrophy and neuroleptic-induced parkinsonism. Brain 120:75–90, 1997

Levine B, Black SE, Cabeza R, et al: Episodic memory and the self in a case of isolated retrograde amnesia. Brain 121:1951–1973, 1998

Lezak MD: The problem of assessing executive functions. Int J Psychol 17:281–297, 1982

Lezak MD: IQ: R.I.P. J Clin Exp Neuropsychol 10:351–361, 1988

Lezak MD: Domains of behavior from a neuropsychological perspective: the whole story, in Integrative Views of Motivation, Cognition, and Emotion. Nebraska Symposium on Motivation. Edited by Spaulding WD. Lincoln, University of Nebraska Press, 1994, pp 23–55

Lezak M, Howieson D, Loring D: Neuropsychological Assessment, 4th Edition. New York, Oxford University Press, 2004

Loring DW, Lee GP, Meador KJ: Revising the Rey-Osterrieth: rating right hemisphere recall. Arch Clin Neuropsychol 3:239–247, 1988

Luria AR: Higher Cortical Functions in Man, 2nd Edition. New York, Basic Books, 1980

Mattis S, Jurica P, Leitten C: Dementia Rating Scale–2. Lutz, FL, Psychological Assessment Resources, 2001

Mayes AR: Selective memory disorders, in The Oxford Handbook of Memory. Edited by Tulving E, Craik FIM. Oxford, UK, Oxford University Press, 2000, pp 427–440

McCarthy RA, Warrington EK: Cognitive Neuropsychology: A Clinical Introduction. San Diego, CA, Academic Press, 1990

Mesulam M-M: Principles of Behavioral and Cognitive Neurology, 2nd Edition. New York, Oxford University Press, 2000

Mitrushina M, Boone K, Razani J, et al: Handbook of Normative Data for Neuropsychological Assessment, 2nd Edition. New York, Oxford University Press, 2005

Mysiw WJ, Beegan JG, Gatens PF: Prospective cognitive assessment of stroke patients before inpatient rehabilitation: the relationship of the Neurobehavioral Cognitive Status Examination to functional improvement. Am J Phys Med Rehabil 68:168–171, 1989

Newcombe F, Ratcliff G: Disorders of visuospatial analysis, in Handbook of Neuropsychology, Vol 2. Edited by Boller F, Grafman J. Amsterdam, The Netherlands, Elsevier, 1989, pp 333–356

Norris G, Tate RL: The Behavioural Assessment of the Dysexecutive Syndrome (BADS): ecological, concurrent and construct validity. Neuropsychol Rehabil 10:33–45, 2000

Ojemann GA, Dodrill CB: Verbal memory deficits after left temporal lobectomy for epilepsy. J Neurosurg 62:101–107, 1985

Osterrieth PA: Le test de copie d'une figure complexe. Archives de Psychologie 30:206–356, 1944

Porch BE: Porch Index of Communicative Ability: Manual. Austin, TX, Pro-Ed, 1981

Rafal RD: Neglect, II: cognitive neuropsychological issues, in Patient-Based Approaches to Cognitive Neuroscience. Edited by Farah MJ, Feinberg TE. Cambridge, MA, MIT Press, 2000, pp 115–123

Randolph C, Tierney MC, Mohr E, et al: The Repeatable Battery for the Assessment of Neuropsychological Status (RBANS): preliminary clinical validity. J Clin Exp Neuropsychol 20:310–319, 1998

Raspall T, Donate M, Boget T, et al: Neuropsychological tests with lateralizing value in patients with temporal lobe epilepsy: reconsidering material-specific theory. Seizure 14:569–576, 2005

Reed JM, Squire LR: Retrograde amnesia for facts and events: findings from four new cases. J Neurosci 18:3943–3954, 1998

Reitan RM: Manual for the Administration of Neuropsychological Test Batteries for Adults and Children. Indianapolis, IN, Author, 1969

Reitan RM, Wolfson D: The Halstead-Reitan Neuropsychological Test Battery: Theory and Clinical Interpretation, 2nd Edition. Tucson, AZ, Neuropsychology Press, 1993

Rey A: L'examen psychologique dans les cas d'encéphalopathie traumatique. Archives de Psychologie 28:286–340, 1941

Rothi LJG, Raymer AM, Heilman KM: Limb praxis assessment, in Apraxia: The Neuropsychology of Action. Edited by Rothi LJG, Heilman KM. Hove, UK, Psychology Press, 1997, pp 61–73

Royall DR, Mahurin RK, Gray KF: Bedside assessment of executive cognitive impairment: the Executive Interview. J Am Geriatr Soc 40:1221–1226, 1992

Schenkenberg T, Bradford DC, Ajax ET: Line bisection and unilateral visual neglect in patients with neurologic impairment. Neurology 30:509–517, 1980

Schwamm LH, Van Dyke C, Kiernan RJ, et al: The Neurobehavioral Cognitive Status Examination: comparison with the Cognitive Capacity Screening Examination and the Mini-Mental State Examination in a neurosurgical population. Ann Intern Med 107:486–491, 1987

Shallice T: Specific impairments of planning. Philos Trans R Soc Lond B Biol Sci 298:199–209, 1982

Smith A: Clinical psychological practice and principles of neuropsychological assessment, in Handbook of Clinical Psychology: Theory, Research and Practice. Edited by Walker CE. Homewood, IL, Dorsey Press, 1983, pp 445–500

Spreen O, Risser AH: Assessment of Aphasia. New York, Oxford University Press, 2003

Spreen O, Strauss E: A Compendium of Neuropsychological Tests, 2nd Edition. New York, Oxford University Press, 1998

Squire LR, Slater PC, Chase PM: Retrograde amnesia: temporal gradient in very long-term memory following electroconvulsive therapy. Science 187:77–79, 1975

Strauss E, Goldsmith SM: Lateral preferences and performance on non-verbal laterality tests in a normal population. Cortex 23:495–503, 1987

Strub RL, Black FW: The Mental Status Examination in Neurology. Philadelphia, PA, FA Davis, 2000

Sullivan EV, Shear PK, Zipursky RB, et al: A deficit profile of executive, memory, and motor functions in schizophrenia. Biol Psychiatry 36:641–653, 1994

Van Lancker DR, Dreiman J, Cummings J: Voice perception deficits: neuroanatomical correlates of phonagnosia. J Clin Exp Neuropsychol 11:665–674, 1989

Varney NR: Somesthesis, in Experimental Techniques in Human Neuropsychology. Edited by Hannay HJ. New York, Oxford University Press, 1986, pp 212–237

Wagner AD, Poldrack RA, Eldridge LL, et al: Material-specific lateralization of prefrontal activation during episodic encoding and retrieval. Neuroreport 9:3711–3717, 1998

Wechsler D: The Measurement of Adult Intelligence, 3rd Edition. Baltimore, MD, Williams & Wilkins, 1944

Wechsler D: WAIS Manual. New York, Psychological Corporation, 1955

Wechsler D: WAIS-R Manual. New York, Psychological Corporation, 1981

Wechsler D: Wechsler Memory Scale—Revised Manual. San Antonio, TX, Psychological Corporation, 1987

Wechsler D: WAIS-III: Administration and Scoring Manual. San Antonio, TX, Psychological Corporation, 1997a

Wechsler D: WMS-III: Administration and Scoring Manual. San Antonio, TX, Psychological Corporation, 1997b

Welsh KA, Butters N, Hughes JP, et al: Detection and staging of dementia in Alzheimer's disease: use of the neuropsychological measures developed for the Consortium to Establish a Registry for Alzheimer's Disease. Arch Neurol 49:448–452, 1992

Wilson BA, Alderman N, Burgess PW, et al: Behavioural Assessment of the Dysexecutive Syndrome. Bury St Edmunds, England, Thames Valley Test Co, 1996

Wilson BA, Evans JJ, Emslie H, et al: The development of an ecologically valid test for assessing patients with a dysexecutive syndrome. Neuropsychol Rehabil 8:213–228, 1998

# Cultural Issues

ALBERT C. GAW, M.D.

## Concepts, Components, and Essential Features of Culture

### Components of Culture

The utility of culture can be further understood by examining its components.

#### Percepts

A *percept* is "an impression in the mind of something perceived by the senses, viewed as the basic component in the formation of concepts" (Morris 1970, p. 972). Our organs for sight, smell, touch, hearing, and taste continually receive sensory impressions that are conveyed to the higher centers of the brain.

#### Concepts

*Concepts* are general ideas or understandings, especially ones derived from specific occurrences (Morris 1970). They are usually encoded in words. Many times, important concepts are embodied in and carry the force of laws, as in mandatory attendance at school or the right to vote in democratic societies.

#### Propositions

Having percepts and concepts is not enough. The mind must be able to manipulate these symbols to make sense of the relationships of things around us. The ways in which percepts and concepts are related to one another are called *propositions*. Thus, propositions allow us to use logical reasoning and inferences.

#### Beliefs

*Beliefs* are propositions considered to be *true*. When beliefs are not based on reality, cannot be dislodged by objective facts, are tenaciously held, and exert a pervasive influence on the individual's perception of the world, such false beliefs are called delusions.

#### Values

When concepts and propositions are organized into a hierarchy of preference, the result is *value*. "Do no harm" has commanded a higher order of value than blind experimentation in the ethics of patient care. Members of the medical and psychiatric professions are expected to adhere to this standard.

#### Recipes or Operational Procedures

*Recipes* are ways in which people organize their efforts to accomplish certain tasks. As such, recipes could be explicit, as in a written memorandum, or implicit, as in etiquette. We are taught to do a mental status examination, conduct a psychiatric interview, formulate a treatment plan, and prescribe medications or conduct psychotherapy. These are all operational procedures. They are part of the system of values and procedures that define who is a psychiatrist.

### Ethnicity

Closely related to culture but applied in a narrower sense is *ethnicity*. Schermerhorn (1970), a sociologist, defined *ethnicity* as "a *collectivity* within a larger society having a real or putative common ancestry, memories of a shared historical past, and a cultural focus on one or more symbolic elements defined as the epitome of their peoplehood" (p. 12; italics added).

Ethnicity is a powerful factor that binds people together. It also serves to differentiate a person or a group of individuals as a member or members of an "in- or out-group." This feeling of affiliation within an "in-group" can have a significant influence in facilitating how one learns to "trust" and identify with another person during the initial clinical encounter.

*Race*, on the other hand, is a more biologically oriented term. It refers to a number of broad divisions of the human species into groups based on a common geographic origin, certain shared physical characteristics, and a characteristic distribution of gene frequencies (Kalow 1997).

## Essential Features of Culture

1. Culture is learned.
2. *Culture* refers to systems of meanings.
3. Culture acts as a shaping template.
4. Culture is taught and reproduced.
5. Culture exists in a constant state of change.
6. Culture includes both objective and subjective patterns of human behavior.

## Summary

In summary, an understanding of culture can serve as a conceptual tool to inform psychiatry in at least the following areas:

1. Enhancing diagnosis and treatment.
2. Fostering clinicians' sensitivity toward patients.
3. Increasing psychiatric knowledge, particularly the symbolic system of healing.
4. Providing the context for differentiating "normal" from "abnormal" behavior.
5. Enhancing general understanding of human beings.

# Specific Cultural Considerations in DSM-IV-TR Diagnostic Categories

## Disorders Usually First Diagnosed in Infancy, Childhood, or Adolescence

### Mental Retardation and Learning Disorders

Because individualized testing is always required to make a diagnosis of mental retardation or a learning disorder, care should be taken that intelligence testing procedures have been validated across cultural groups.

### Language Disorder and Phonological Disorder (Formerly Developmental Articulation Disorders)

Care must be exercised when making judgments about the expressive language disorders of individuals growing up in a non-English-speaking or bilingual environment.

### Selective Mutism

Care should be exercised not to misdiagnose immigrant children with selective mutism when they are unfamiliar with or uncomfortable with the official language of their host country and refuse to speak to strangers in their new environment.

## Delirium, Dementia, and Amnestic and Other Cognitive Disorders

In the mental status examination, certain individuals may be unfamiliar with the information the test items use. Certain test items such as general fund of knowledge (e.g., names of presidents, geographic location), abstraction (e.g., proverbs), memory (e.g., date of birth, because some cultures do not celebrate birthdays), and orientation (e.g., sense of placement, because location may be conceptualized differently) are useless if the information being used is unfamiliar to the individual.

## Substance-Related Disorders

### Substance Intoxication

The acceptance of mood-altering drugs, attitudes toward drug use, exposure, and pattern of substance use vary across cultural groups.

### Alcohol-Related Disorders

Marked differences exist across different cultures in the quantity, frequency, and pattern of alcohol consumption. In most Asian cultures, the overall prevalence of alcohol-related disorders may be relatively low, and the male-to-female ratio may be high.

### Opioid-Related Disorders

In the late 1800s and early 1900s, opioid dependence was seen more often among white, middle-class individuals. Since the 1920s, in the United States, there has been an overrepresentation of opioid dependence among members of minority groups living in economically deprived areas.

## Schizophrenia and Other Psychotic Disorders

The content, course, and outcome of the symptoms of schizophrenia may vary across cultural groups. Catatonic behavior appears to be more prevalent in non-Western cultures compared with that reported in the United States. In developing countries, an acute course and a better outcome have been noted in individuals with schizophrenia.

## Mood Disorders

Depression, in some cultures, may be experienced largely in somatic terms rather than as sadness or guilt. Depressive experiences may be expressed as complaints of weakness, tiredness, "imbalance" (in Chinese and other Asian cultures), "nerves" and headaches (in Latino and Mediterranean cultures), or being "heartbroken" (in Hopi Native American culture). In some cultures, irritability as a symptom of depression may provoke greater concern than sadness or withdrawal.

## Anxiety Disorders

### Panic Disorder With or Without History of Agoraphobia

In certain cultures, panic attacks may be precipitated by intense fear of magic or witchcraft. Some culture-bound syndromes, such as *koro*, may include features of panic attack associated with fear of genital shrinkage into the body.

### Social Phobia

In Japan and Korea, instead of a marked persistent fear of social or performance situations in which embarrassment may occur (Criterion A in DSM-IV-TR [American Psychiatric Association 2000]), some individuals may develop a persistent and excessive fear of giving offense to others in social situations. In Japan, fears in social phobia in a culture-bound syndrome called *taijin kyofusho* may be in the form of extreme anxiety that blushing, eye-to-eye contact, or one's body odor will be offensive to others.

### Posttraumatic Stress Disorder

Recent immigrants from areas with considerable social unrest and war may have higher rates of posttraumatic stress disorder (PTSD). Also, these immigrants may be reluctant to divulge experiences of torture and trauma for fear of political repercussions or losing immigrant status.

## Somatoform Disorders

### Pain Disorder

There is considerable variation among ethnic and cultural groups in their reaction to painful stimuli and in the way they express their reactions to pain. In one classic study, Italian patients, compared with Irish patients, presented with significantly more pain symptoms, had symptoms in significantly more bodily locations, and noted significantly more types of bodily dysfunction (Zola 1966).

### Body Dysmorphic Disorder

Cultural factors may influence or amplify preoccupations about an imagined physical defect. *Koro*, a culture-bound syndrome reported primarily in Southeast Asia and characterized by the preoccupation of genital retraction into the abdomen and thoughts of dying, may be related to body dysmorphic disorder but differs from it by its usually brief duration, different associated symptoms of panic and fear of death, positive responses to reassurance, and occasional occurrence in epidemic proportions.

## Dissociative Disorders

### Dissociative Fugue

Culture-bound syndromes with presumed dissociative features, such as *pibloktoq* (running syndrome) among the Arctic native people, *grisi siknis* among the Miskito of Honduras and Nicaragua, *frenzy* witchcraft among the Navajo, and some form of *amok* in Western Pacific cultures, have been reported. These syndromes may meet criteria for dissociative fugue and are characterized by a sudden onset of a high level of activity, a trancelike state, potentially dangerous behavior in the form of running or fleeing (homicide in *amok*), ensuing exhaustion, sleep, and amnesia for the episode.

### Dissociative Disorder Not Otherwise Specified

Possession identity disorder, which involves a replacement of the customary sense of personal identity with a new identity attributed to the influence of a spirit, a deity, another person, an animal, or even an inanimate object, has been reported in many cultures. Possession trance with stereotypic "involuntary" movements or amnesia may be associated with *amok* (Indonesia), *bebainan* (Indonesia), *latah* (Malaysia), *pibloktoq* (Arctic), *ataque de nervios* (Latin America), and possession (India). Dissociative trance disorder should not be confused with normative induced trance states in religious or cultural practice.

## Sexual and Gender Identity Disorders

Care should be exercised in judging sexual dysfunction. An individual's ethnic, cultural, social, and religious background may influence sexual desire, expectations, and attitude about performance. In some cultures, a higher premium is placed on fertility, and sexual desire on the part of women is given less relevance.

## Eating Disorders: Anorexia Nervosa

In industrialized societies, the abundance of food and the cultural idea that attractiveness is linked to thinness for females have been suggested as reasons for the higher prevalence of anorexia nervosa. Immigrants who have assimilated the thin-body ideal may likewise be affected. Cultural expression of the motivation for food restriction may vary; instead of a disturbed perception of the body, individuals may complain of epigastric discomfort or distaste for food.

## Adjustment Disorders

The threshold for maladaptiveness varies because various cultures have different ways of experiencing and coping with stressors and interpreting the meanings of stressors. Clinicians should consider an individual's cultural setting before making a diagnosis of adjustment disorder.

## Personality Disorders

Criteria for deviancy vary across cultures. In immigrants, the factors of acculturation and the individual's customary expression of habits, customs, and political or religious values from the culture of origin should be taken into consideration when determining deviancy.

# Culture-Bound Syndromes

## Amok

*Amok* is a Malaysian term for a homicidal frenzy preceded by a state of brooding and ending with somnolence and amnesia. Afflicted individuals are usually young or middle-aged males living away from home. Precipitating factors may be a recent loss, an insult, or incidences causing such a person to "lose face."

## Ataque de Nervios

*Ataque de nervios* is characterized by sudden onset of uncontrollable shouting, trembling, heart palpitations, a sensation of heat in the chest rising to the head, fainting, and seizurelike activities in response to acute stressful experiences, such as grief during funerals, threats, being at the scene of an accident, or a family conflict. Often a person may temporarily lose consciousness. Amnesia for the episode may occur upon regaining consciousness. Considered a culturally sanctioned response to acute stresses among Puerto Ricans and Latinos, *ataque* usually afflicts socially disadvantaged women older than 45 years with less than a high school education. It is unclear how *ataque* should be classified in DSM-IV-TR.

## Brain Fag

*Brain fag* is characterized by complaints of the brain being "fatigued," with unpleasant head symptoms of burning, a crawling sensation, and a feeling of "vacancy"; visual symptoms of blurry vision, eye pain, and excessive tearing; an inability to grasp the meaning of printed symbols or spoken words; poor memory retention; and fatigue and sleepiness in spite of adequate rest. The term originated in West Africa, and the condition affects primarily male students under the stress of schooling. Brain fag has been compared with *neurasthenia* in Chinese, *hwa-byung* in Korean, and *susto* in Latino individuals. Cases of brain fag have been reported to respond to antidepressants, antianxiety medications, and relaxation therapy. Many scholars consider brain fag to be a culturally mediated anxiety, depressive, or somatoform syndrome.

## Hwa-Byung

*Hwa-byung* means "fiery illness" in Korean. Because "fire" is an Asian metaphysical expression of anger, *hwa-byung* is literally translated as an "illness of anger." Afflicted individuals complain of a feeling of oppression or pressure in the chest, a "mass" in the epigastrium or stomach, a hot sensation traveling up the chest or in the body, indigestion, dyspnea, fatigue, sighing, and headache. Emotional symptoms include fearfulness, panic, dysphoria, sad mood, nihilistic thoughts, loss of interest, suicidal ideas, and guilt. The illness affects women more than men. Kim (1993) attributes *hwa-byung* to suppression of chronic anger and indignation in Korea, where there is a long history of foreign colonization and subjugation and a culture in which open expression of feeling is not encouraged.

## Koro

*Koro* is characterized by the sudden onset of acute anxiety and panic associated with the fear of genital retraction into the abdomen and the idea of dying as a result. The condition generally affects lower-educated males, but female cases of concern about labial or breast retractions also have been reported (Bernstein and Gaw 1990). Epidemics of *koro* have been reported in Singapore, Thailand, Hainan Island of China, and India. During such epidemics, patients may be brought into the emergency department with family members, relatives, or the patient himself holding the patient's penis or using wooden clamps or strings to prevent the penis from "retracting" into the abdomen. The condition is self-limiting and can be relieved by persuasion, explanation, and education. The term *koro* is believed to derive from a Malaysian word meaning "tortoise." The symbolic association of *koro* with the phenomenon of the retraction of the head of the turtle into its body is readily apparent. Similar conditions are described as *suk-yeong* in Cantonese Chinese, *suo-yang* in Mandarin Chinese, *jinjinia bemar* in Assam, and *rok-joo* in Thailand.

## Latah

*Latah* is characterized by hypersensitivity to sudden fright or startle, often with echopraxia, echolalia, command obedience, and dissociative or trancelike behavior. Afflicted individuals typically respond to a sudden stimulus with an exaggerated startle, sometimes dropping or throwing objects held in the hand and often uttering obscene words. Such individuals are often the objects of amusement. Most cases of *latah* are in women of low socioeconomic status. *Latah* is well described among the Malays. Outside Malay, similar conditions include *amurakh, irkunii, ikota, olan, myriachit, menkeiti, bahtschi, imu, mali-mali, silok,* and *jumping.* Simons and Hughes (1985) consider *latah* to be a culture-specific elaboration of the potential of the startle reflex.

## Pibloktoq

*Pibloktoq*, also called *arctic hysteria*, is characterized by abrupt episodes of extreme excitement often followed by "seizures" and transient "coma." It is reported among the Arctic and subarctic Eskimos and affects women more than men. Afflicted individuals may show prodromes of tiredness, depressive silences, vagueness of expression, and confusion for several days. During attacks, individuals may exhibit superhuman strength and aberrant motor and ver-

bal behaviors such as tearing off clothing and becoming partially or completely nude, fleeing, rolling in snow, jumping into water, picking up or throwing things, performing mimetic acts, and engaging in choreiform movements, glossolalia, and coprophagia. Following attacks, individuals may weep, show body tremor, become feverish with bloodshot eyes, and have a high pulse rate. The exhausted individual may sleep for hours. Rational behavior is resumed after waking. Consistent with Eskimo culture, afflicted individuals, particularly women, are thought to express their sense of acute helplessness and traumatized ego with panic or anxiety in a regressive fashion.

## Possession Disorder

*Possession disorder* is characterized by the experience of one's identity being taken over by another entity that may involve a person, god, demon, spirit, animal, or even an inanimate object. Afflicted individuals may have a single or episodic disturbance of consciousness, identity, or memory associated with loss of control over their actions, loss of awareness of their surroundings, change in the tone of their voice, and loss of perceived sensitivity to pain (Gaw et al. 1998). Women are more often affected than men. Afflicted individuals usually are of lower socioeconomic and educational background. Possession disorder is found worldwide and in all cultures. Possession states are considered normal when the phenomenon occurs in the context of a broadly accepted collective cultural or religious practice.

## Shenjing Shuairuo

*Shenjing shuairuo* is characterized by feelings of physical and mental exhaustion, difficulty in concentration, memory loss, fatigue, dizziness, insomnia, loss of appetite, sexual dysfunction, irritability, and headaches. The term in Mandarin Chinese literally means "weakness of the nervous system." It is a prominent syndrome among Chinese. It is also known as *neurasthenia* in the West. Although neurasthenia currently is not an official category in DSM-IV-TR, it is officially included in the *Chinese Classification of Mental Disorders,* 2nd Edition (Chinese Society of Psychiatry 1989), and in ICD-10 (World Health Organization 1992).

## Taijin Kyofusho

*Taijin kyofusho* is characterized by an extreme concern that one's body, body parts, or bodily functions may offend, embarrass, or displease others. Symptoms include fear of embarrassment; blushing; causing discomfort by one's gaze, facial expression, or body odor; or offending others by speaking one's thoughts aloud. Considered a culture-specific social phobia among Japanese people, the condition primarily affects young people, particularly in interpersonal situations.

# Sociocultural Factors Affecting Psychopharmacotherapy and Nonadherence

Key sociocultural factors that influence noncompliance with psychotropic medications are as follows:

- Physician biases in diagnosis and prescribing
- Health beliefs
- Concomitant use of herbal and Western medicine
- Diet
- Religious beliefs
- Placebo effect
- Cost and availability of medications

## Physician Biases in Diagnosis and Prescribing

Physicians' biases in prescribing are reflected in reports of racial differences in psychiatric diagnosis and psychotropic drug responses for many diagnostic categories. For example, although the U.S. Epidemiologic Catchment Area study (Robins et al. 1991) reported no significant differences in the prevalence of affective disorders between African Americans and Caucasians, African Americans are more likely to receive a diagnosis of schizophrenia rather than affective disorder in clinical practice (Adebimpe 1994). A number of anxiety disorders, including obsessive-compulsive disorder, panic disorder, phobic disorder, and PTSD, are often underrecognized or underdiagnosed in African Americans compared with Caucasians (Lawson 1996a, 1996b). The reasons for misdiagnosis remain unclear. However, the consequences of such misdiagnosis for African American patients are serious and can include delay in the implementation of appropriate medications such as lithium therapy for bipolar disorder, the prescribing of antipsychotic medications when not indicated, the use of higher dosages of antipsychotic medications and more frequent use of as-needed medications, and a greater likelihood of receiving a depot medication.

Similarly, Hispanic patients with a confirmed diagnosis of bipolar disorder were far more likely to receive an initial diagnosis of schizophrenia (Mukherjee et al. 1983). Heterogeneity among the Hispanic subgroups and the presence of culture-bound syndromes also may confound the diagnostic picture (Mendoza et al. 1991). Some studies suggest that the dosage requirements for tricyclic agents among Hispanic women may be different from those of their Caucasian counterparts. A retrospective chart review of Hispanic female clinic patients showed a comparable treatment outcome when they were given only half the dosage of tricyclic antidepressant (Marcos and Cancro 1982). Thus, if the customary dosage of tricyclic antidepressants used for Caucasians were prescribed for this population, more complaints of side effects might occur. Indeed, more Hispanic patients in this cohort were found to complain of side effects (78% vs. 33% for Caucasian patients) and to discontinue their medication prematurely.

Among Asian patients, failure to factor in body size and potential variance due to poor metabolization of certain enzymes may lead to more reports of side effects when patients are given the usual recommended *Physicians' Desk Reference* dosages.

Thus, among ethnic patients in the United States, some studies suggest that drug dosages, patterns of drug usage, and drug nonadherence may differ from those of mainstream middle-class Caucasian patients. Clinicians who are increasingly involved in the care of ethnic patients need to be cognizant of such variations to drug reactions.

## Health Beliefs and Alternative Healing Traditions and Practices

In many non-Western cultures, long traditions of indigenous systems of healing coexist with modern Western scientific medical healing systems. Examples of indigenous healing systems include the traditional Chinese medical system and Asian Indian ayurvedic medicine. These traditional medical practices may influence patients' choices and reactions to modern treatment modalities, including drugs. For example, Chinese medical concepts such as *chi* and "energy flows" often shape the conceptions and responses of Chinese patients in the use of Western medicine (Gaw 1993). Indeed, discordance between professional and lay conceptions of causal attributions may determine the patient's satisfaction with treatment, medication adherence, and clinical outcome (Lin et al. 1993).

The study by Sing Lee (1993) in Hong Kong is instructive and illustrates that patients' reactions to side effects of medications may vary according to their health beliefs. In a biocultural study of the reports of side effects among 70 Hong Kong Chinese patients receiving chronic lithium therapy, Sing Lee found that there is "an imperfect correspondence between biomedically prescribed and culturally endorsed psychotropic side effects" (p. 301). Contrary to the usual reports of Western patients, Hong Kong patients did not usually regard the side effects of polydipsia and polyuria as bothersome symptoms or translate them into metaphors to express undesirable side effects. Although complaints of tiredness, drowsiness, and poor memory were common, their frequency was significantly lower than that in control subjects. Chinese patients had no conceptual equivalent for the complaint of "loss of creativity." Complaints of "missing of highs," loss of assertiveness, and fear of weight gain were rarely encountered.

Health beliefs are often reflected in varying ethnic expectations of Western and herbal drug actions. With the trend toward greater popularity of "alternative" or nontraditional healing methods, many individuals may simply reject the notion of introducing any "nonorganic" chemical substance into the body. Many ethnic patients regard Western medications as providing quicker action and therefore being most appropriate for treating acute illness (Lin et al. 1993). In contrast, some patients regard herbal drugs as having less tendency to induce side effects, and thus they delay or avoid taking necessary Western medications. Concerns about the addictive and toxic effects of drugs among Hispanics and African Americans in the United States may lead them to avoid taking needed medications for a longer period and may lead to premature termination of medications and psychiatric care. On the other hand, in many Asian countries where concoctions of multiple herbal drugs, as in traditional medical prac-tice, are usually prescribed, polypharmacy may come to be an accepted norm of medical practice.

## Culture and Psychotherapy: Implications for Psychotherapists and Counselors

The following points are useful to keep in mind when conducting psychotherapy across cultures:

1. *Psychotherapy is culture-bound.* Both patients and therapists are the epitome of their unique cultural heritage. It behooves both patients and therapists to understand how their respective cultural heritages affect the therapeutic encounter.
2. *Transference and countertransference phenomena may be accentuated in the cross-cultural encounter.* Conducting therapy across cultural groups is both a rewarding and a demanding experience. Variation in cultural percepts and concepts, propositions, values, beliefs, and operating procedures may accentuate transference and countertransference feelings.
3. *Therapists must be cognizant of the micro- as well as macro-sociocultural issues that may influence the structure and processes of the therapeutic relationship.* The demands of third-party payers and institutional requirements may intrude on the therapeutic relationship and undermine trust and confidentiality.
4. *There is a need for comparative research on psychotherapy across cultures.* Both the structure and the processes of symbolic healing in psychotherapy need to be examined across cultures.

## Key Points: Cultural Issues

- Culture aids psychiatric diagnosis and treatment by providing a *context* to understand a patient's distress and its symbolic meanings.
- Culture is a set of standards for behavior that a group or individual uses to orient him- or herself and that guides a person's behavior in all social circumstances, including illness behavior.
- Components of culture include percepts, concepts, propositions, beliefs, values, and operational procedures (recipes).
- Essential features of culture include the following: 1) it is learned; 2) it refers to systems of meanings; 3) it acts as a shaping template; 4) it is taught and reproduced; 5) it exists in a constant state of change; and 6) it includes patterns of both subjective and objective elements of human behavior.
- DSM-IV-TR's cultural formulation is a tool to elicit pertinent cultural data in the clinical encounter.

- Culture-bound syndromes are recurrent, locality-specific patterns of aberrant behavior and troubling experiences that are indigenously considered to be "illnesses," or at least afflictions. They are generally limited to specific societies or culture areas.

- Most culture-bound syndromes could be included in the "disorders not otherwise specified" in each of the relevant DSM-IV-TR diagnostic categories.

- Sociocultural factors that may influence drug prescribing and the taking of drugs include (but are not limited to) physician biases, patient beliefs and expectations, placebo effects, cost and availability of medications, family support, and patient adherence or nonadherence to medications.

- Sociocultural factors in psychotropic drug nonadherence are less well studied than biological factors, but they exert powerful influences on drug nonadherence.

- The phenomenon of psychotropic drug nonadherence could be understood. The contributing factors of nonadherence should be as rigorously addressed as other challenging clinical problems.

- Psychotherapy conducted across diverse cultures can be exciting, but it also is more demanding, because it requires knowledge and sensitivity to local cultural norms.

# References

Adebimpe VR: Race, racism, and epidemiologic surveys. Hosp Community Psychiatry 45:27–31, 1994

American Psychiatric Association: Diagnostic and Statistical Manual of Mental Disorders, 4th Edition, Text Revision. Washington, DC, American Psychiatric Association, 2000

Bernstein RL, Gaw AC: Koro: proposed classification for the DSM-IV. Am J Psychiatry 147:1670–1674, 1990

Chinese Society of Psychiatry: Chinese Classification of Mental Disorders, 2nd Edition [in Chinese]. Hunan, China, Hunan Medical University, 1989

Gaw AC (ed): Culture, Ethnicity and Mental Illness. Washington, DC, American Psychiatric Press, 1993

Gaw AC, Ding Q-Z, Levine RE, et al: The clinical characteristics of possession disorder among 20 Chinese patients in the Hebei province of China. Psychiatr Serv 49:360–365, 1998

Kalow W: Pharmacogenetics in biological perspective. Pharmacol Rev 49:369–379, 1997

Kim LIC: Psychiatric care of Korean Americans, in Culture, Ethnicity and Mental Illness. Edited by Gaw AC. Washington, DC, American Psychiatric Press, 1993, pp 347–375

Lawson WB: The art and science of the psychopharmacotherapy of African Americans. Mt Sinai J Med 63:301–305, 1996a

Lawson WB: Clinical issues in the pharmacotherapy of African Americans. Psychopharmacol Bull 32:275–281, 1996b

Lee S: Side effects of chronic lithium therapy in Hong Kong Chinese: an ethnopsychiatric perspective. Cult Med Psychiatry 17:301–320, 1993

Lin KM, Poland RE, Nakasaki G (eds): Psychopharmacology and Psychobiology of Ethnicity. Washington, DC, American Psychiatric Press, 1993

Marcos LR, Cancro R: Pharmacotherapy of Hispanic depressed patients: clinical observations. Am J Psychiatry 36:505–513, 1982

Mendoza R, Smith MW, Poland RE, et al: Ethnic psychopharmacology: the Hispanic and Native American perspective. Psychopharmacol Bull 27:449–461, 1991

Morris W (ed): The American Heritage Dictionary of the English Language. New York, American Heritage Publishing Company, 1970

Mukherjee S, Shukla S, Woodline J: Misdiagnosis of schizophrenia in bipolar patients: a multi-ethnic comparison. Am J Psychiatry 140:1571–1574, 1983

Robins LN, Locke B, Regier DA: An overview of psychiatric disorders in America, in Psychiatric Disorders in America: The Epidemiologic Catchment Area Study. Edited by Robins LN, Regier DA. New York, Free Press, 1991, pp 328–366

Schermerhorn RA: Comparative Ethnic Relations: A Framework for Theory and Research. Chicago, IL, University of Chicago Press, 1970

Simons RC, Hughes CC (eds): The Culture-Bound Syndromes. Dordrecht, The Netherlands, Reidel, 1985

World Health Organization: International Statistical Classification of Diseases and Related Health Problems, 10th Revision. Geneva, World Health Organization, 1992

Zola IK: Culture and symptoms: an analysis of patients' presenting complaints. Am Sociol Rev 31:615–630, 1966

# 9

# Psychiatry and the Law

ROBERT I. SIMON, M.D.

DANIEL W. SHUMAN, J.D.

The legal principles applied to the practice of psychiatry do not differ from those applied to medicine in general. Nevertheless, the diagnosis, treatment, and management of patients with psychiatric disorders present unique concerns that may pit the psychiatrist's duty to the patient against the psychiatrist's duty to the community. Issues such as informed consent, the duty of confidentiality, the right to treatment, the right to refuse treatment, substitute decision making, and advance directives are commonly confronted by clinicians when treating psychiatric patients.

The mental threshold for criminal prosecution may demand a psychiatric assessment of the defendant. To ensure fairness and accountability, we demand that regardless of whether defendants wish to accept a plea bargain and waive trial or proceed to trial, they meet minimal standards for competence. The legal standard is functional and does not confuse diagnosis with legal competence. Defendants with psychiatric impairments may not meet the competency standard. Once the issue is raised, however, they may require pretrial evaluations of their mental capacity to understand the charges brought against them and their ability to assist counsel in their own defense. Mental state or capacity is also central in deciding criminal responsibility and sentencing. The effect of a psychiatric disorder may be to reduce or avoid criminal responsibility for an act or to shape the length or the terms of confinement following conviction.

In the civil realm, psychiatrists, like all other professionals who render a service, are subject to damage claims by disgruntled clients. Specific areas of psychiatric practice are more vulnerable to psychiatric malpractice suits.

TABLE 9–1.  **Recent allegations of malpractice (approximate frequency of claims)**

| Allegation | Frequency (%) |
|---|---|
| Incorrect treatment | 33 |
| Attempted/completed suicide | 20 |
| Incorrect diagnosis | 11 |
| Improper supervision | 7 |
| Medication error/drug reaction | 7 |
| Improper commitment | 5 |
| Breach of confidentiality | 4 |
| Unnecessary hospitalization | 4 |
| Undue familiarity | 3 |
| Libel/slander | 2 |
| Other (e.g., abandonment, electroconvulsive therapy, third-party injury) | 4 |

*Source.*  Data from Benefacts 1996.

Table 9–1 describes the malpractice claims experience of the American Psychiatric Association (APA)–sponsored Professional Liability Insurance Program prior to 1996 (Benefacts 1996).

The chance of a psychiatrist being sued in the 1980s was 1 in 25 per year (Benefacts 1996). Through 1995, however, the odds increased to about 1 in 12 psychiatrists per year. The APA Professional Liability Insurance Program identifies several factors to account for the increase in malpractice suits:

1. Psychiatrists are treating "sicker" patients in managed care settings.
2. The media scrutinizes so-called recovered memories and ritual satanic abuse cases.
3. Tort reform legislation has failed.
4. Psychiatrists are specializing in new practice areas such as geriatric psychopharmacology, adolescent addiction medicine, multiple personality disorder, pain management, and adult children of alcoholic persons.
5. Psychiatrists are providing more primary care, such as in the management of patients with diabetes, hypertension, and a wide variety of acute general medical illnesses.

## Psychiatrist–Patient Relationships and the Law

### General Contours of the Relationship

#### Informed Consent

The courts typically require that a decision be knowing, intelligent, and voluntary to satisfy the requirements of informed consent (*Long v. Jaszczak* 2004):

- Competency (intelligence)
- Information (knowing)
- Voluntariness

**Competency (intelligence).** *Incompetence* refers to a court adjudication, whereas *incapacity* indicates a functional inability as determined by a clinician (Mishkin 1989). Legally, only competent persons may give informed consent. An adult patient is presumed competent unless adjudicated incompetent or temporarily incapacitated because of a medical emergency. Absent an emergency, treating an incompetent patient without substituted consent is not permitted.

Competency is not a scientifically determinable state and is situation specific. Although there are no hard-and-fast definitions, the patient's ability to do the following is legally germane to determining competency:

- Understand the particular treatment choice being proposed
- Make a treatment choice
- Communicate that choice verbally or nonverbally

A review of case law and scholarly literature reveals four standards for determining incompetency in decision making (Appelbaum et al. 1987). In order of increasing levels of mental capacity required, these standards are as follows:

1. Communication of choice
2. Understanding of relevant information provided
3. Appreciation of available options and consequences
4. Rational decision making

**Information (knowing).** In the landmark case *Canterbury v. Spence* (1972), a patient-oriented standard was applied. This standard focused on the "material" information that a *reasonable* person in the patient's position would want to know to make an informed decision.

**Voluntariness.** For consent to be considered legally voluntary, it must be given freely by the patient and without coercion, fraud, or duress.

**Exceptions and liability.** There are two basic exceptions to the requirement of obtaining informed consent. When immediate treatment is necessary to save a life or prevent serious harm and it is not possible to obtain either the patient's consent or that of someone authorized to provide consent for the patient, the law typically presumes that the consent would have been granted.

The second exception, *therapeutic privilege*, excepts informed consent if a psychiatrist determines that a complete disclosure of possible risks and alternatives might have a deleterious effect on the patient's health and welfare.

**Waivers.** A physician need not disclose risks of treatment when the patient has competently, knowingly, and voluntarily waived his or her right to be informed.

#### Confidentiality and Privilege

*Confidentiality* refers to the right of a patient, and the correlative duty of a professional, of nondisclosure of relational communications to outside parties without implied or expressed authorization. *Privilege*, or more accurately *relational privilege*, is a limitation on the power of the judge to compel disclosure of relational confidences. A psychiatrist–, psychotherapist–, or physician–patient privilege may be recognized by case law (*Jaffee v. Redmond* 1996) but is more typically a statute or rule of evidence that permits the holder of the privilege (e.g., the patient) to prevent the person to whom confidential information was given (e.g., the psychiatrist) from being compelled by a judge to disclose it in a judicial proceeding.

**Confidentiality.** The Health Insurance Portability and Accountability Act of 1996 (HIPAA) adds a layer of federal law to protect patient health care information. HIPAA limits disclosure of patient health information without patient authorization except as necessary for treatment, payment, and health care operations; however, the limitation is not absolute.

*Clinical–legal foundation.* Relational privileges require courts to compromise their search for truth by not availing themselves of relevant evidence. Thus courts have typically been reluctant to recognize a privilege and quick to find an exception applicable (Shuman and Weiner 1987). Indeed, the common law did not recognize physician–patient or psychotherapist–patient privilege. When courts have done so, it has been because they have been convinced of its necessity to further a relationship of great utility to society.

*Breaching of confidentiality.* Once the doctor–patient relationship has been created, the professional assumes a duty to safeguard a patient's disclosures. This duty is not absolute, and there are circumstances in which breaching confidentiality is both ethical and legal. Patients also waive confidentiality in a variety of situations, especially in managed care settings. Medical records may be sent to potential employers or to insurance companies when benefits are requested. Many state confidentiality statutes provide statutory exceptions to confidentiality between the psychiatrist and the patient in one or more situations (Brakel et al. 1985) (Table 9–2).

**Privilege.** Privilege statutes usually are drafted with reference to one of the following four relationships, depending on the type of practitioner:

1. Physician–patient (general)
2. Psychiatrist–patient
3. Psychologist–patient
4. Psychotherapist–patient

The last exception, known as the *patient-litigant exception*, commonly occurs in the insanity defense, will contests, workers' compensation cases, child custody disputes, personal injury actions, and medical malpractice actions.

**Liability.** An unauthorized or unwarranted breach of the duty of confidentiality can cause a patient emotional harm and result in a claim based on at least four theories:

**TABLE 9–2. Common limitations of testimonial privilege**

Valid patient consent

Civil commitment proceedings

Criminal proceedings

Child custody disputes

Court-ordered report

Patient-litigant exception

Child abuse proceedings

*Source.* Reprinted with permission from Simon RI: *Concise Guide to Psychiatry and Law for Clinicians,* 3rd Edition. Washington, DC, American Psychiatric Publishing, 2001, p. 54.

1. Malpractice (breach of professional duty of confidentiality)
2. Breach of statutory duty of confidentiality
3. Invasion of privacy
4. Breach of (implied) contract

### Right to Refuse Treatment

Buttressed by constitutionally derived rights to privacy and freedom from cruel and unusual punishment, the common law tort of battery, and the doctrine of informed consent, mentally disabled persons have been afforded protections typically available for patients of nonpsychiatric physicians—the right to refuse treatment. This right often collides with clinical judgment (i.e., to treat and protect). As a result of this conflict, the courts vary considerably regarding the parameters of this right and the procedures to be followed if it is to be overridden.

### Competency

Competency refers to a *minimal* mental, cognitive, or behavioral ability, trait, or capability required to perform a particular act or to assume a particular role. A determination of incompetency is ultimately a judicial determination. The term *incapacity*, which is often interchanged with *incompetency*, refers to an individual's functional inability to understand or to form an intention with regard to some act as determined by health care providers (Mishkin 1989).

The legal designation of "incompetent" is applied to an individual who fails one of the mental tests of capacity and is therefore considered *by law* to be not mentally capable of performing a particular act or assuming a particular role. The adjudication of incompetence by a court is now, more commonly, subject or issue specific.

Generally, the law only gives effect to decisions by a competent individual and seeks to protect incompetent individuals from the harmful effects of their acts. Adults are presumed to be competent (*Meek v. City of Loveland* 1929). This presumption, however, may be rebutted by evidence of incapacity (*Scaria v. St. Paul Fire and Marine Ins. Co.* 1975).

As a matter of law, incompetency may not be presumed from either treatment for mental illness (*Wilson v. Lehman* 1964) or institutionalization (*Rennie v. Klein* 1978). Instead, scrutiny is given to determine whether specific functional incapacities exist that render a person incapable of making a particular kind of decision or performing a particular type of task.

### Guardianship

Guardianship is a method of substitute decision making for individuals who have been judicially determined to be unable to act for themselves (Brakel et al. 1985). In some states, there are separate provisions for appointment of a "guardian of one's person" (e.g., health care decision making) and a "guardian of one's estate" (e.g., authority to make contracts to sell one's property; Sale et al. 1982). The latter type of guardian is frequently referred to as a *conservator*.

### Health Care Decision Making

Only a *competent* person is legally able to give informed consent. Health care providers work with patients who sometimes are of questionable competence because of mental illness, narcotic abuse, or alcoholism. When psychiatrists treat patients with neuropsychiatric deficits, the responsibility to obtain a valid informed consent can be clinically daunting because of the vacillating mental states associated with many central nervous system disorders.

### Right to Die

**Incompetent patients.** The U.S. Supreme Court ruled, in *Cruzan v. Director, Missouri Department of Health* (1990), that the state of Missouri could refuse to remove a food and water tube surgically implanted in the stomach of Nancy Cruzan without clear and convincing evidence of her wishes. Ms. Cruzan was in a persistent vegetative state for 7 years. Without clear and convincing evidence of a patient's decision to have life-sustaining measures withheld in a particular circumstance, the state has the right to maintain that individual's life.

**Competent patients.** A growing body of cases has emerged involving *competent* patients—with excruciating pain and terminal diseases—who seek the termination of further medical treatment. Beginning with the fundamental tenet that "no right is held more sacred...than the right of every individual to the possession and control of his own person" (*Schloendorff v. Society of New York Hospital* 1914; *Union Pacific Realty Co. v. Botsford* 1891), courts have taken this principle of autonomy seen in informed consent cases and applied it to right-to-die cases.

The right to decline life-sustaining medical intervention, even for a competent person, is not absolute. As noted in *In re Conroy* (1985), four countervailing state interests generally exist that may limit the exercise of that right: 1) preservation of life, 2) prevention of suicide, 3) safeguarding of the integrity of the medical profession, and 4) protection of innocent third parties.

### Advance Directives

The use of advance directives such as a living will, health care proxy, or durable medical power of attorney is recommended to avoid ethical and legal complications associated with requests to withhold life-sustaining treatment measures (Simon 1992a; Solnick 1985). The Patient Self-Determination Act, which took effect on December 1, 1991, requires hospitals, nursing homes, hospices, managed care organizations, and home health care agencies to advise patients or family members of their right to accept or refuse medical care and to execute an advance directive (LaPuma et al. 1991). These advance directives provide a method for individuals, while competent, to choose proxy health care decision makers in the event of future incompetency.

### Substituted Judgment

Psychiatrists often find that the time required to obtain an adjudication of incompetence is unduly burdensome and that the process frequently interferes with the provision of quality treatment. Moreover, families are often reluctant to face the formal court proceedings necessary to declare their family member incompetent, particularly when sensitive family matters are disclosed. A common solution to both of these problems is to seek the legally authorized proxy consent of a spouse or relative serving as guardian when the refusing patient is believed to be incompetent. Proxy consent, however, is becoming less available as a consent option (Simon 1992a).

The President's Commission for the Study of Ethical Problems in Medicine and Biomedical and Behavioral Research (1982) recommended that the relatives of incompetent patients be selected as proxy decision makers for the following reasons:

1. The family is generally most concerned about the good of the patient.
2. The family is usually most knowledgeable about the patient's goals, preferences, and values.
3. The family deserves recognition as an important social unit to be treated, within limits, as a single decision maker in matters that intimately affect its members.

### *Physician-Assisted Suicide*

With increasing legal recognition of physician-assisted suicide, psychiatrists are likely to be called on to become gatekeepers. Every proposal for physician-assisted suicide requires a psychiatric screening or consultation to determine the terminally ill person's competence to commit suicide. The presence of psychiatric disorders associated with suicide, particularly depression, will have to be ruled out as the driving factor behind the request.

## High-Risk Relationships

### *Psychiatric Malpractice*

Medical malpractice is a tort. Most medical malpractice claims are based in negligence rather than intentional torts (e.g., battery, false imprisonment), if for no other reason than to avoid the exclusionary language in most professional liability policies for intentional acts. *Negligence*, the fundamental concept underlying most malpractice claims, is the failure to act reasonably under the circumstances.

For a psychiatrist to be found *liable* to a patient for malpractice, the four fundamental elements of a negligence claim must be established by a preponderance of the evidence (i.e., more likely than not). Each of these four elements must be met for the claim to prevail. A psychiatrist may have rendered substandard care, but if the jury finds it caused no legally recognized harm or that any harm was caused by another actor or condition, the claim fails.

In most states, whether the psychiatrist's duty to his or her patient has been breached turns on whether the fact finder decides that the defendant acted with the degree of skill and care of the average physician in that specialty under the circumstances (*Stepakoff v. Kantar* 1985).

Nevertheless, the existence of professional treatment guidelines and procedures that are generally accepted or used by a significant number of psychiatrists should alert clinicians to consider such guidelines as practice reference sources.

Evidence that a treatment procedure is accepted by at least a respectable minority of professionals in the field can establish that a particular treatment is a reasonable profes-

**TABLE 9–3.** Required minimum standard of care for a somatic treatment of a psychiatric patient

**Pretreatment**

Complete clinical history (medical, psychiatric)

Complete physical examination as clinically indicated (performed by another physician or, if necessary, by the psychiatrist)

Administration of necessary laboratory tests and review of past test results

Disclosure of sufficient information to the patient to obtain informed consent, including information about the risks and benefits both of treatment and of no treatment

Thorough documentation of all treatment decisions, informed consent information, pertinent patient responses, and other relevant treatment data

**Posttreatment**

Careful monitoring of the patient's response to treatment, including adequate follow-up evaluations and appropriate laboratory testing

Prompt adjustments in treatment, as clinically indicated

Arrangement for additional informed consent when treatment is altered appreciably or new treatment is initiated

sional practice (Simon 1993). The standard of care associated with the use of a somatic therapy to treat a psychiatric patient, *at a minimum*, is summarized in Table 9–3.

**Theories of liability.** The potential for negligence by a psychiatrist is greatest in clinical situations involving the use of psychotropic medication. As noted earlier, claims data from the APA Professional Liability Insurance Program showed that medication error and drug reaction constituted 7% of malpractice allegations. Allegations of drug mismanagement are a significant contributor to "incorrect treatment," the most common malpractice category.

*Failure to adequately evaluate.* Sound clinical practice requires that before any form of treatment is initiated, the patient be adequately evaluated. A physical examination should be conducted or obtained, if clinically indicated. A recently performed physical examination may suffice, or patients may be referred elsewhere if the psychiatrist does not perform physical examinations. The duty to ensure that proper informed consent is obtained can be fulfilled at this time.

**TABLE 9–4.   Common negligent prescription practices**

Exceeding recommended dosages without clinical indications

Prescribing multiple drugs inappropriately

Prescribing medication for unapproved uses without a documented rationale

Prescribing unapproved medications

Failing to disclose medication risks

*Failure to monitor.*   Probably the most common act of negligence associated with pharmacotherapy is the failure to monitor the patient while he or she is taking medication. Serum drug levels are obtainable for a number of psychotropic medications. The primary indications for these laboratory tests include assessment of therapeutic and toxic levels of medication and patient compliance with treatment.

**Split treatment.**   Split-treatment situations require that the psychiatrist stay fully informed of the patient's clinical status as well as of the nature and quality of treatment the patient is receiving from the nonmedical therapist (Sederer et al. 1998). In a collaborative relationship, responsibility for the patient's care is shared according to the qualifications and limitations of each clinician. The responsibilities of each discipline do not diminish those of the other disciplines. Patients should be informed of the separate responsibilities of each discipline. Periodic evaluation by the psychiatrist and the nonmedical therapist of the patient's clinical condition and needs is necessary to determine whether the collaboration should continue. In split treatments, if negligence is claimed on the part of the nonmedical therapist, it is likely that the collaborating psychiatrist will be sued, and vice versa (Woodward et al. 1993).

**Negligent prescription practices.**   The selection of a medication, determination of initial dosage and form of administration, and other related procedures are all decisions left to the professional discretion of the treating psychiatrist. The prescribing of specific medications should be determined by the psychiatrist and the clinical needs of the patient. An appeal should be filed if a drug that is not formulary approved is denied. The law recognizes that the physician is in the best position to "know the patient" and to determine what course of treatment is best under the circumstances.

**TABLE 9–5.   Informed consent: reasonable information to be disclosed**

Although there exists no consistently accepted set of information to be disclosed for any given medical or psychiatric situation, five areas of information are generally provided:

1. Diagnosis: description of the condition or problem
2. Treatment: nature and purpose of the proposed treatment
3. Consequences: risks and benefits of the proposed treatment
4. Alternatives: viable alternatives to the proposed treatment, including risks and benefits
5. Prognosis: projected outcome with and without treatment

*Source.*   Reprinted with permission from Simon RI: *Clinical Psychiatry and the Law,* 2nd Edition. Washington, DC, American Psychiatric Press, 1992, p. 128.

A review of cases involving allegations of negligent prescription procedures reveals several common practices representing potential deviations from generally accepted treatment practice (Table 9–4).

As stated earlier, any physician who prescribes medication has a duty to first obtain the informed consent of the patient (Table 9–5). Patients lacking decision-making capacity require consent for treatment by substitute decision makers (Table 9–6).

**TABLE 9–6.   Common consent options for patients lacking the mental capacity for health care decisions**

Proxy consent of next of kin, as permitted by state law[a]

Adjudication of incompetence and appointment of a guardian

Substituted consent of the court

Advance directives (living will, durable power of attorney, health care proxy)

[a]May be excluded for treatment of mental disorders.
*Source.*   Adapted with permission from Simon RI: *Clinical Psychiatry and the Law,* 2nd Edition. Washington, DC, American Psychiatric Press, 1992, p. 109.

Other medication-related issues that have resulted in legal action include 1) failure to treat side effects after they have been recognized or should have been recognized, 2) failure to monitor a patient's compliance with prescription limits, 3) failure to prescribe medication or appropriate levels of medication according to the treatment needs of the patient, 4) failure to refer a patient for consultation or treatment by a specialist when indicated, and 5) negligent withdrawal from medication and unclear or illegible prescriptions.

### Electroconvulsive therapy (ECT).

*Pretreatment.* Although pre-ECT evaluations vary somewhat, the following procedures recommended by the APA Task Force on Electroconvulsive Therapy (American Psychiatric Association 2001a) generally should be performed:

1. Psychiatric history and examination to evaluate the indications for ECT
2. Medical examination to determine risk factors
3. Anesthesia evaluation
4. Informed consent (written)
5. Evaluation by a physician privileged to administer ECT

*Treatment.* Lawsuits involving ECT-related injuries in which the negligence is related to the actual treatment process include the following errors:

- Failure to use a muscle relaxant to reduce the chance of a bone fracture
- Negligent administration of the procedure
- Failure to conduct an adequate evaluation of the patient before continuing treatment

*Posttreatment.* The failure to attend properly to a patient for a period of time after administering ECT may result in malpractice liability. The following are examples of posttreatment circumstances that may constitute a basis for a lawsuit:

- Failure to evaluate complaints of pain or discomfort following treatment
- Failure to evaluate a patient's condition before resuming ECT treatments
- Failure to monitor a patient properly to prevent falls
- Failure to supervise properly a patient who was injured as a result of ECT

### National Practitioner Data Bank

On September 1, 1990, the National Practitioner Data Bank established by the Health Care Quality Improvement Act of 1986 went into effect. The data bank tracks disciplinary actions, malpractice judgments, and settlements against physicians, dentists, and other health care professionals (Johnson 1991).

### The Suicidal Patient

**Foreseeable suicide.** As an accepted standard of care, an evaluation of suicide risk should be done with all patients, regardless of whether they present with overt suicidal complaints. A review of case law shows that reasonable care requires that a patient who is either suspected of being or confirmed to be suicidal must be the subject of certain affirmative precautions. A failure either to reasonably assess a patient's suicide risk or to implement an appropriate precautionary plan after the suicide potential becomes foreseeable is likely to render a practitioner liable if the patient is harmed because of a suicide attempt. The law permits the fact finder to conclude that suicide is preventable if it is foreseeable. Foreseeability, however, should not be confused with preventability. In hindsight, many suicides seem preventable that were clearly not foreseeable.

*Inpatients.* Intervention in an inpatient setting usually requires the following:

- Screening evaluations
- Development of an appropriate treatment plan
- Implementation of that plan
- Ongoing case review by clinical staff

*Outpatients.* Psychiatrists are expected to reasonably assess the severity and imminence of a foreseeable suicidal act. The result of the assessment dictates the treatment and safety management options. Psychiatrists are not strictly liable whenever an outpatient commits suicide (*Speer v. United States* 1981).

**Legal defenses.** A psychiatrist's Answer to a malpractice claim arising out of a patient suicide may consist of a denial of allegations in the plaintiff's Complaint, from which the fact finder might reject the allegation that the psychiatrist breached a duty that proximately caused the patient's suicide. In addition, the defendant's Answer to the Complaint might include affirmative defenses that have the legal effect of defeating the claim even if the defendant's negligence proximately caused the patient's suicide.

The plaintiff must persuade the fact finder that the psychiatrist's negligence more likely than not caused the patient's suicide. Thus proof that the suicide was caused by an unforeseeable intervening cause negates a critical element of the claim. For example, a fact finder may find a psychiatrist not liable for the suicidal act of a borderline patient who experienced a traumatic loss of a romantic relationship between therapy sessions and then impulsively attempted suicide without trying to contact the psychiatrist.

### The Violent Patient

As a general rule, absent a special relationship, one person has no duty to control the conduct of a second person to prevent that person from harming a third person (Restatement [Second] of Torts 1965). After *Tarasoff* (*Tarasoff v. Regents of the University of California* 1976), the therapist's legal duty and potential liability significantly expanded in the outpatient setting in many, but not all, states (*Thapar v. Zezulka* 1999). In *Tarasoff*, the California Supreme Court reasoned that a duty to protect third parties was imposed when a special relationship existed between the individual whose conduct created the danger and the defendant. Finding this special relationship requirement met in this setting, the court concluded that "the single relationship of a doctor to his patient is sufficient to support the duty to exercise reasonable care to protect others [from the violent acts of patients]."

The index of suspicion for potential violence should be high in patients with a history of violence who are currently making serious threats of harm toward specific individuals. The potential for violence is further heightened if the patient is acutely psychotic, substance abusing, angry, or fearful of being harmed or is experiencing delusions of being controlled or influenced (Link and Stueve 1994).

When courts have found a duty to protect, they have required an "imminent" threat of serious harm to a foreseeable victim. The term *imminent*, however, is a problematic construct for assessing violence (Simon 2006). Just as the decisions have sought to narrow the time frame within which the violence that triggers the duty might arise, so they have sought to limit the persons who are at risk. Only a small minority of courts have held that a duty to protect exists for the population at large; most require an identifiable victim to be at risk. In some jurisdictions, courts have held that the need to safeguard the public well-being overrides all other considerations, including confidentiality.

**Release of potentially violent patients.**    Courts closely evaluate decisions made by psychiatrists treating inpa-

tients that adversely affect the patients or a third party. Liability imposed on psychiatric facilities that had custody of patients who injured others outside the institution after escape or release is clearly distinguishable from the factual situation of *Tarasoff*. In negligent-release cases, liability may arise from the allegation that the institution's affirmative act in releasing the patient caused injury to the third party. Moreover, allegations may be made that a psychiatrist or hospital personnel failed, prior to the patient's discharge, to warn individuals known to be at risk for harm from that patient. Lawsuits stemming from the release of foreseeably dangerous patients who subsequently injure or kill others are roughly five to six times more common than outpatient duty-to-warn lawsuits (Simon 1992b).

### Involuntary Hospitalization

Involuntary hospitalization of persons with mental disorders is limited to statutorily defined criteria in all states. Based on the state's decision to exercise its constitutional authority, all states have authorized civil commitment of individuals who are mentally ill and dangerous to self or others, and some states also permit commitment of individuals who are mentally ill and unable to provide for their basic needs.

Some states have enacted legislation that permits involuntary hospitalization of three other distinct groups in addition to individuals with mental illness: developmentally disabled persons, substance-addicted persons, and mentally disabled minors.

Involuntary hospitalization of psychiatric patients usually arises when violent behavior threatens to erupt toward self or others and when patients become unable to care for themselves. These patients frequently manifest mental disorders and conditions that meet the substantive criteria for involuntary hospitalization.

Courts, not clinicians, have the authority to commit patients. The psychiatrist initiates the process that brings the patient before the court, usually after a brief period of hospitalization for evaluation or after an evaluation of a prospective patient at the request of the court.

**Liability.**    Because psychiatrists are often granted conditional immunity for their good-faith participation in involuntary hospitalization proceedings, it is not surprising that most malpractice claims involving involuntary hospitalization allege an absence of good faith in the psychiatrist's behavior. Often these lawsuits are brought under the theory of false imprisonment.

TABLE 9–7.  **Indications for seclusion and restraint**

1.  To prevent harm to the patient or others
2.  To prevent disruption to treatment program or physical surroundings
3.  To assist in treatment as part of ongoing behavior therapy
4.  To decrease sensory overstimulation (seclusion only)
5.  To respond to patient's reasonable voluntary request[a]

[a]First seclusion; then, if necessary, restraints.
*Source.*   Adapted with permission from Simon RI: *Concise Guide to Psychiatry and Law for Clinicians*, 3rd Edition. Washington, DC, American Psychiatric Publishing, 2001, p. 114.

### Rights of involuntarily hospitalized patients.

Most states recognize the right of inpatients to refuse treatment. In most states, patients involuntarily hospitalized who refuse medication are entitled to a separate court hearing for an adjudication of incompetence and the provision of substituted consent by the court.

## *Seclusion and Restraint*

Seclusion and restraint have both indications and contraindications as clinical management tools (American Psychiatric Association 1985; see Tables 9–7 and 9–8).

Generally, the courts have held that seclusion and restraint are an intrusion on a patient's constitutionally protected interests and may be implemented only when a patient presents a risk of harm to self or others and no less restrictive alternative is available. Some courts have also required the following:

1.  Restraint and seclusion may be implemented only by a written order from an appropriate medical official.
2.  Orders must be confined to specific, time-limited periods.
3.  A patient's condition must be regularly reviewed and documented.
4.  Any extension of an original order must be reviewed and reauthorized.

Where they apply, federal requirements establish a floor but may be superseded by more restrictive state laws. The requirements define *seclusion* and *restraint* as follows: *Seclusion* is the involuntary confinement of a person alone in a room where the person is physically prevented from leaving, or the separation of the patient from others in a safe, contained, controlled environment. *Restraint* is the direct application of physical force to an individual, with or

TABLE 9–8.  **Contraindications to seclusion and restraint**

1.  Unstable medical and psychiatric conditions[a]
2.  Delirious patients or patients with dementia who are unable to tolerate decreased stimulation[a]
3   High-risk suicidal patients[a]
4.  Patients with severe drug reactions or overdoses or patients requiring close monitoring of drug dosages[a]
5.  For punishment of the patient or for convenience of staff

[a]Unless close supervision and direct observation are provided.
*Source.*   Adapted with permission from Simon RI: *Concise Guide to Psychiatry and Law for Clinicians*, 3rd Edition. Washington, DC, American Psychiatric Publishing, 2001, p. 117.

without the individual's permission, to restrict his or her freedom of movement. Physical force may involve human touch, mechanical devices, or a combination thereof. Under the federal rules, the use of these interventions is regarded as presenting an inherent risk to the patient's physical safety and well-being and therefore is permitted only when there is "imminent risk" that the patient may inflict harm to self or others. As do many states, federal law includes the use of drugs in the definition of restraint (Simon and Hales 2006). Federal law permits the use of seclusion and restraint only as a last resort to protect the patient's safety and dignity and never for the convenience of the staff.

## *Sexual Misconduct*

Three types of legal responses to sexual misconduct have been enacted: reporting, civil liability, and criminal prosecution. *Reporting statutes* require a therapist who learns of any past or current therapist–patient sex to disclose this information. Some states have enacted *civil statutes* that make it explicit that sexual misconduct is a violation of the standard of care and authorize a damage claim (Bisbing et al. 1995). *Criminal statutes* addressing sexual misconduct also have been enacted.

### Civil liability.

Psychiatrists who sexually exploit their patients are subject to civil and criminal sanctions as well as ethical and professional licensure disciplinary proceedings. *The Principles of Medical Ethics With Annotations Especially Applicable to Psychiatry* (American Psychiatric Association 2001b) states that sex with a current or former patient is unethical (Section 2, Annotation 1). However, a malpractice claim is probably the most common legal response.

In a medical malpractice claim for sexual misconduct, in order to prevail the plaintiff has the burden of proving, by a preponderance of the evidence, among other things, that the exploitation took place. This burden can be met by corroborating evidence such as letters, pictures, hotel receipts, and identification of incriminating body markings of the exploited, as well as the testimony of other abused (former) patients. The plaintiff is also required to demonstrate that the misconduct caused harm such as a worsened psychiatric condition, suicide attempts, or the necessity for hospitalization.

**Criminal sanctions.** Sexual exploitation of a patient may be classified as rape or sexual assault (Hoge et al. 1995). Many of the new wave of statutes criminalizing therapist–patient sexual misconduct assume, as a matter of law, that a current patient is incapable of giving consent to sexual relations with his or her therapist and treat all sexual relations between therapist and patient as a criminal act committed by the therapist (Minn. Stat. Ann. § 609.344 2005). To date, claims of psychological coercion through the manipulation of transference phenomena have not been successful in establishing the coercion necessary for a criminal case.

**Professional disciplinary action.** For the purposes of adjudicating allegations of professional misconduct, licensing boards are typically granted certain regulatory and disciplinary authority by state statutes. As a result, state licensing organizations, unlike professional associations, may discipline an offending professional by suspending or revoking his or her license to practice. A review of published reports of sexual misconduct cases adjudicated before licensing boards found that in the vast majority of cases, the evidence was reasonably sufficient to substantiate a claim of exploitation, leading to revocation of the professional's license or suspension from practice for varying lengths of time, including permanent suspension.

# Psychiatry in the Courtroom

## The Psychiatrist as a Witness

### Forensic Psychiatry

**Definition and scope.** *Forensic psychiatry* is a "a subspecialty of psychiatry in which scientific and clinical expertise is applied to legal issues in legal contexts embracing civil, criminal, correctional or legislative matters" (American Academy of Psychiatry and the Law 1989/1991, p. x).

**Forensic psychiatric evaluation.**

*Team approach.* The forensic psychiatrist who is evaluating the claimant may require the input of a neurologist, psychologist, neuropsychologist, and internist or general practitioner.

*Absence of doctor–patient relationship.* The psychiatrist should inform the claimant at the time of examination that no doctor–patient relationship will be formed—that is, the psychiatrist will not *treat* the claimant. The psychiatrist should explain that he or she has been retained by (name the specific party) to perform an independent psychiatric examination. The sole purpose of the examination is to provide information to the party retaining the psychiatrist and potentially to the court.

*Absence of confidentiality.* The claimant must be informed that confidentiality surrounding the forensic evaluation may not exist. A Protective Order issued by the court may require that the forensic psychiatrist maintain the confidentiality of specified records and documents.

*Standard diagnostic schema.* The diagnostic evaluation of claimants should be made according to the multiaxial classification system contained in DSM-IV-TR (American Psychiatric Association 2000). All five axes should be used, where applicable.

*Collateral sources of information.* The possibility of malingering should always be kept in mind (Table 9–9). Malingering is not limited to the fabrication of symptoms. More often, malingering is manifested by the *exaggeration* or even *minimization* of symptoms. Thus, the psychiatrist should consider a broad array of information.

The forensic examiner should request that the retaining lawyer provide all relevant information. Going to court with incomplete information will likely be exposed by opposing counsel, undercutting the psychiatrist's testimony and possibly damaging the claimant's case. The list of collateral sources of information in Table 9–10, although not exhaustive, indicates major areas of inquiry.

### Traumatic Brain Injury

When evaluating the mental status of a TBI claimant, the psychiatrist conducts a thorough mental status exam. Neuropsychological assessment can be a valuable adjunct to the neuropsychiatric assessment of the TBI claimant (Becker and Kay 1986). The mental status examination as described by Strub and Black (1985) provides a scored, comprehensive, reliable format for evaluation of mental status.

## TABLE 9–9. Increased index of suspicion for malingering

Litigation context (financial compensation, evasion of criminal prosecution)

Marked discrepancy between clinical findings and subjective complaints

Lack of cooperation with evaluation and treatment

Antisocial personality traits or disorder

Overdramatization of complaints

History of recurrent accidents or injuries

Evidence of self-induced injuries

Vaguely defined symptoms

Poor work history

Inability to work but retention of capacity for pleasurable activities

*Source.* Reprinted with permission from Simon RI: "Legal and Ethical Issues in Traumatic Brain Injury," in *Textbook of Traumatic Brain Injury.* Edited by Silver JM, McAllister TW, Yudofsky SC. Washington, DC, American Psychiatric Publishing, 2005, p. 598.

The role of neuropsychological testing must be critically evaluated in each case. Neuropsychological tests are not totally objective. Thus, the clinicians' motivation is critical. Low test scores may be caused by factors other than brain damage (Table 9–11).

### Posttraumatic Stress Disorder

Defendants who committed a crime while experiencing a dissociative behavioral reenactment of a prior traumatic event have successfully relied on posttraumatic stress disorder (PTSD) to support an insanity defense (Sparr 1990). The diagnosis of PTSD also has been relied on by experts for the state to bolster the credibility of the victim, by showing how other victims similarly respond or to reason backward from PTSD symptoms to establish the occurrence of a traumatic stressor. Victims of criminal acts who develop PTSD or other psychiatric disorders may institute claims under criminal injuries compensation acts.

## Psychiatry and Criminal Law: Criminal Proceedings

### Criminal Intent (Mens Rea)

Under the common law, criminal culpability for most serious crimes requires 1) the mental state or level of intent to

## TABLE 9–10. Collateral sources of information

Other physicians and health care providers (reports, direct discussions)

Hospital records

Family

Other third parties

Military records

School records

Police records

Witness information

Work records

Work products (letters, work projects)

Legal discovery (depositions, legal documents)

Prior medical and psychiatric records

Prior psychological and neuropsychological evaluations

*Source.* Reprinted with permission from Simon RI: "Legal and Ethical Issues in Traumatic Brain Injury," in *Textbook of Traumatic Brain Injury.* Edited by Silver JM, McAllister TW, Yudofsky SC. Washington, DC, American Psychiatric Publishing, 2005, p. 598.

## TABLE 9–11. Major factors influencing neuropsychological test findings

Original endowment

Environment (e.g., education, occupation, life experiences)

Motivation (effort)

Physical health

Psychological distress

Psychiatric disorders (e.g., depression, dissociative disorders)

Medications (e.g., anticonvulsants, psychotropics)

Qualifications and experience of neuropsychologist

Errors in scoring

Errors in interpretation

*Source.* Reprinted with permission from Simon RI: "Legal and Ethical Issues in Traumatic Brain Injury," in *Textbook of Traumatic Brain Injury.* Edited by Silver JM, McAllister TW, Yudofsky SC. Washington, DC, American Psychiatric Publishing, 2005, p. 599.

commit the act (known as the *mens rea*, or guilty mind), 2) the act itself or conduct associated with committing the crime (known as *actus reus*, or guilty act), and 3) a concurrence in time between the guilty act and the guilty mental state (*Bethea v. United States* 1977). To convict a person of a particular crime, the state must prove beyond a reasonable doubt that the defendant committed the criminal act with the requisite intent.

The defendant's intent determines not only the culpability for an offense but also the gravity of the offense. For instance, a person who deliberately plans to commit a crime is subject to more serious prosecution and punishment than one who does so impulsively. The difficulty, of course, is in assessing intent retrospectively (Simon and Shuman 2002).

Traditionally, legislative definitions of offenses required proof of general intent for some crimes and proof of specific intent to meet the *mens rea* requirement for others. *Specific intent* refers to the *mens rea* in crimes in which a *further intention* exists beyond the presence of a general criminal intent. For instance, the intent necessary for first-degree murder typically includes a "specific intent to kill" (Rogers and Shuman 2005). Unlike general intent, specific criminal intent may not be presumed from the unlawful criminal act alone.

Mental handicaps or impairments present a host of problems across the criminal justice system. From assessing appropriateness of diversion to the specialized mental health courts or the mental health system, the risks posed by release on bail, or competence to stand trial to face criminal charges (*Dusky v. United States* 1960); to addressing *mens rea* or an affirmative defense of insanity and the disposition of an insanity aquittee (M'Naughten's Case 1843; *United States v. Brawner* 1972); to sentencing of convicted offenders and determination of eligibility for a sentence of death (*Penry v. Lynaugh* 1989; *Tennard v. Dretke* 2004), as well as competence to be executed (*Ford v. Wainwright* 1986), the effect of mental impairment pervades the criminal justice system. The first and most common context in which mental impairment arises is competence to stand trial. However, when as the result of the defendant's conduct a question arises, the defense counsel, prosecutor, or judge may raise the issue, thus requiring the court to decide whether the defendant understands the charges brought against him or her and is capable of rationally assisting counsel with the defense.

### Competency to Stand Trial

The legal standard for assessing pretrial competency was established by the U.S. Supreme Court in *Dusky v. United States* (1960). To be competent to make decisions during the pretrial process, at trial, and during an appeal, the court succinctly and without embellishment required that the defendant have "sufficient present ability to consult with his lawyer with a reasonable degree of rational understanding" and have "a rational as well as factual understanding of the proceedings against him" (*Dusky v. United States* 1960).

Although most impairments implicated in competency examinations are functional rather than organic (Reich and Wells 1985), various forms of neuropsychiatric impairments typically raise questions about a defendant's competency to stand trial. Of the various criteria that the court established in determining the defendant's competency to stand trial, the following are directly relevant to the issue of neuropsychiatric impairment (*Wilson v. United States* 1968):

1. The extent to which the amnesia affected the defendant's ability to consult with and assist his lawyer
2. The extent to which the amnesia affected the defendant's ability to testify in his own behalf

Any disorder, whether functional or organic, that significantly impairs a defendant's cognitive and communicative abilities is likely to have an effect on competency. Nevertheless, it is the actual *functional* mental capability to meet the minimal standard of trial competency, and not the severity of the deficits, that determines whether an individual is cognitively capable to be tried. It is legal criteria, not medical or psychiatric diagnosis, that govern competency. Diagnosis is relevant only to the question of restoring the defendant's competency to stand trial with treatment.

A defendant's impairment in one particular function, however, does not automatically render him or her incompetent. For example, the fact that the defendant is manifesting certain deficits because of damage to the parietal lobe does not necessarily mean that he or she lacks the requisite cognitive ability to aid in his or her own defense at trial (Tranel 1992). The ultimate determination of incompetency is for the court to make (*United States v. David* 1975).

### *Insanity Defense*

One of the most controversial issues in American criminal jurisprudence is the insanity defense. Defendants with functional or organic mental disabilities who are found competent to stand trial may seek acquittal claiming that they were not criminally responsible for their actions because of insanity at the time the offense was committed.

Criminals may commit crimes for many reasons, but the law presumes that they do so of their own free will and that it is therefore just to impose punishment. Some offenders, however, are so mentally disturbed in their thinking and behavior that they are thought to be incapable of making a choice that could have been deterred by the criminal law and for which retribution is justified. Historically, albeit controversially, the common law has long recognized some form of limitation on the punishment of a "crazy" or insane person (Blackstone 1769; Coke 1680). Larger in legend than in life, the insanity defense is rarely used and even more rarely successful. Approximately 1% of criminal defendants plead not guilty by reason of insanity; of these, only 10%–25% are successful. The chance of exculpation is greatest when the criminal defendant was found to be psychotic at the time of the crime by the pretrial assessment (Brakel et al. 1985).

Following the acquittal by reason of insanity of John Hinckley Jr. on charges of attempting to assassinate President Reagan and murder others, an outraged public demanded changes in the insanity defense. Federal and state legislation to accomplish that result ensued. Between 1978 and 1985, approximately 75% of all states made some sort of substantive change in their insanity defense (Perlin 1989). Nevertheless, a number of states continued to adhere to the American Law Institute (ALI) insanity defense standard or some version of it. The ALI test provides that a person is not responsible for criminal conduct if at the time of such conduct, as a result of mental disease or defect, he or she lacks substantial capacity either to appreciate the criminality (wrongfulness) of his or her conduct or to conform that conduct to the requirements of law. As used in this article, the terms *mental disease* or *defect* do not include an abnormality manifested only by repeated criminal or otherwise antisocial conduct (Model Penal Code § 4.01 1962).

This standard contains both a cognitive and a volitional prong. The *cognitive prong* derives from the 1843 M'Naughten rule exculpating the defendant who does not know the nature and quality of the alleged act or does not know the act was wrong. The *volitional prong* is a vestige of the irresistible impulse test, which states that the defendant who is overcome by an irresistible impulse that leads to an alleged act is not responsible for that act.

By contrast, defendants tried in a federal court and most state courts are governed by a cognitive, pre-ALI standard. The federal standard is contained in the Comprehensive Crime Control Act of 1984 (P.L. 98–473 1984), which provides that it is an affirmative defense to all federal crimes that, at the time of the offense, "the defendant, as a result of a severe mental disease or defect, was unable to appreciate the nature and quality or the wrongfulness of his acts. Mental disease or defect does not otherwise constitute a defense." This codification eliminates the volitional or irresistible impulse portion of the insanity defense—that is, it does not allow an insanity defense based on a defendant's inability to conform his or her conduct to the requirements of the law. The defense is limited to defendants who are unable to appreciate the wrongfulness of their acts (i.e., the *cognitive portion* of the defense). The rule applicable in the federal courts requires the defendant to prove insanity by clear and convincing evidence.

### Diminished Capacity

Diminished capacity, where it is recognized, permits the accused to introduce medical and psychological evidence relating directly to the *mens rea* for the crime charged without having to assert a defense of insanity (Melton et al. 1997). When a defendant's *mens rea* for the crime charged is nullified by psychiatric evidence, the defendant is acquitted only of that charge but is likely held responsible for an offense requiring a lesser *mens rea*, such as manslaughter (Melton et al. 1997).

### Guilty But Mentally Ill

In a number of states, an alternative verdict of *guilty but mentally ill* has been established. Under these statutes, if the defendant pleads not guilty by reason of insanity, this alternative verdict is available to the jury. Under an insanity plea, the verdict may be

- Not guilty
- Not guilty by reason of insanity
- Guilty but mentally ill
- Guilty

Guilty but mentally ill is an alternative verdict that is not different in its legal effect from finding the defendant guilty. The court must still impose a sentence on the convicted person, and the length of sentence and terms of confinement are not altered.

### Exculpatory and Mitigating Disorders

**Intoxication.** Because intoxication, unlike mental illness, mental retardation, and most neuropsychiatric conditions, is usually the product of a person's own actions, the law is cautious about viewing it as a defense or mitigating factor. Most states view voluntary alcoholism as relevant to the issue of whether the defendant possessed the *mens rea* necessary for a specific intent crime. The mere fact that the defendant was voluntarily intoxicated will not justify a finding of automatism or insanity. A distinct difference arises when, because of chronic, heavy use of alcohol, the defendant has an alcohol-induced psychotic disorder, withdrawal delirium, amnestic disorder, or dementia. If competent psychiatric evidence is presented that an alcohol-related neuropsychiatric disorder caused significant cognitive or volitional impairment, a defense of insanity or diminished capacity may be considered.

**Temporal lobe seizures.** Another "mental state" defense occasionally raised by defendants charged with assault-related crimes is that the assaultive behavior was involuntarily precipitated by abnormal electrical brain patterns. This condition is frequently diagnosed as temporal lobe epilepsy (Devinsky and Bear 1984). Episodic dyscontrol syndrome (Elliott 1978, 1982) also has been advanced as a neuropsychiatric condition causing involuntary aggression.

**Metabolic disorders.** Defenses based on metabolic disorders also have been tried. In 1979, the so-called Twinkie defense was used as part of a successful diminished capacity defense of Dan White in the murders of San Francisco Mayor George Moscone and Supervisor Harvey Milk. This defense was based on the theory that the ingestion of large amounts of sugar contributed to a state of temporary insanity (*People v. White* 1981). A jury found White guilty only of voluntary manslaughter.

## Psychiatry and Civil Law: Personal Injury Litigation

### Expert Testimony

**The treating clinician.** The treating psychiatrist and the forensic psychiatric expert have different roles in litigation. Treatment and expert roles do not mix (Greenberg and Shuman 1997; Strasburger et al. 1997). The treating psychiatrist must rely heavily on the subjective reporting of the patient. In the treatment context, psychiatrists are interested primarily in the patient's perception of his or her difficulties, not necessarily the objective reality. As a consequence, treating psychiatrists usually do not speak to third parties or check pertinent records to gain additional information about a patient or to corroborate the patient's state-

ments. The law, however, is interested in truth as scrutinized by the crucible of the adversary system. Uncorroborated patient reports relied on by a treating psychiatrist are vulnerable to attack as unreliable.

Credibility issues also abound. The treating psychiatrist is, and must be, an ally of the patient. This bias *in favor of* the patient is a proper treatment stance that fosters the therapeutic alliance. The psychiatrist looks for mental disorders to treat. A treatment rather than a litigation agenda is the appropriate stance for the treating psychiatrist.

The American Academy of Psychiatry and the Law (1989/1991), in its ethics statement, advises that "a treating psychiatrist should generally avoid agreeing to be an expert witness or to perform an evaluation of his patient for legal purposes because a forensic evaluation usually requires that other people be interviewed and testimony may adversely affect the therapeutic relationship" (p. xii). The treating psychiatrist should attempt to remain solely in a treatment role. If it becomes necessary to testify on behalf of the patient, the treating psychiatrist should testify only as a fact witness rather than as an expert witness. As a fact witness, the psychiatrist will be asked to describe the number and length of visits, the diagnosis, the treatment, and the prognosis. The treatment relationship does not provide an adequate basis for going beyond these issues. Psychiatrists must remain ever mindful of the many double-agent roles that can develop when mixing psychiatry and litigation (Simon 1987, 1992a).

**The forensic expert.** The forensic expert is usually free from the encumbrances of the treating psychiatrist in litigation. No doctor–patient relationship, with its treatment biases toward the patient, is created during forensic evaluation. The forensic expert typically reviews various records and looks to multiple sources of information to verify the factual assumptions that underlie any opinions drawn (Shuman and Greenberg 2003). Furthermore, the forensic expert considers the possibility of exaggeration or malingering because of a clear appreciation of the litigation context and the absence of treatment bias. Finally, the forensic psychiatrist does not face a conflict of interest for recommending treatment from which he or she would personally (i.e., financially) benefit. However, this same absence of a traditional doctor–patient relationship may subject the expert to being labeled as a "hired gun."

## Key Points: Psychiatry and the Law

- While the risk of being sued is inherent in the practice of psychiatry, spending time and talking with patients reduces the chances of being sued when things go bad.

- Except in an emergency, a psychiatrist must obtain informed consent—intelligent, knowing, and voluntary—from a competent patient before providing treatment. If the patient is not competent, an alternative method of consent (e.g., advance directive, guardianship) must be used.

- Patient confidences are sacrosanct and may be disclosed only when authorized in writing by the patient, ordered by the court, or excepted by law (e.g., elder or child abuse).

- Although psychiatrists may be competent in many roles, they should avoid conflicting roles such as forensic expert and therapist for the same patient-litigant.

- The psychiatrist who remains informed about the legal regulation of psychiatry can more effectively manage complex clinical-legal issues that inevitably arise with patients.

## References

American Academy of Psychiatry and the Law: Ethical Guidelines for the Practice of Forensic Psychiatry. Adopted May 1987. Revised October 1989, 1991

American Psychiatric Association: The Psychiatric Uses of Seclusion and Restraint (APA Task Force Report No 22). Washington, DC, American Psychiatric Association, 1985

American Psychiatric Association: Diagnostic and Statistical Manual of Mental Disorders, 4th Edition, Text Revision. Washington, DC, American Psychiatric Association, 2000

American Psychiatric Association: The Practice of Electroconvulsive Therapy: Recommendations for Treatment, Training, and Privileging. A Task Force Report of the American Psychiatric Association, 2nd Edition. Edited by Weiner RD. Washington, DC, American Psychiatric Association, 2001a

American Psychiatric Association: The Principles of Medical Ethics With Annotations Especially Applicable to Psychiatry. Washington, DC, American Psychiatric Association, 2001b

Appelbaum PS, Lidz CW, Meisel A: Informed Consent: Legal Theory and Clinical Practice. New York, Oxford University Press, 1987, pp 84–87

Becker B, Kay GG: Neuropsychological consultation in psychiatric practice. Psychiatr Clin North Am 9:255–265, 1986

Benefacts. A message from the APA-sponsored Professional Liability Insurance Program. Psychiatric News, April 19, 1996, pp 1, 26

Bisbing SB, Jorgenson LM, Sutherland PK: Sexual Abuse by Professionals: A Legal Guide. Charlottesville, VA, Michie, 1995

Blackstone W: Commentaries, Vol 4, 1769, pp 24–25

Brakel SJ, Parry J, Weiner BA: The Mentally Disabled and the Law, 3rd Edition. Chicago, IL, American Bar Foundation, 1985

Coke E: Third Institute 6, 6th Edition, 1680

Devinsky O, Bear D: Varieties of aggressive behavior in temporal lobe epilepsy. Am J Psychiatry 141:651–656, 1984

Elliott FA: Neurological aspects of antisocial behavior, in The Psychopath: A Comprehensive Study of Antisocial Disorders and Behaviors. Edited by Reid WH. New York, Brunner/Mazel, 1978, pp 146–189

Elliott FA: Neurological findings in adult minimal brain dysfunction and the dyscontrol syndrome. J Nerv Ment Dis 170:680–687, 1982

Greenberg SA, Shuman DW: Irreconcilable conflict between therapeutic and forensic roles. Professional Psychology: Research and Practice 28:50–56, 1997

Hoge SK, Jorgenson L, Goldstein N, et al: APA resource document: legal sanctions for mental health professional–patient sexual misconduct. Bull Am Acad Psychiatry Law 23:433–448, 1995

Johnson ID: Reports to the National Practitioner Data Bank. JAMA 265:407–411, 1991

LaPuma J, Orentlicher D, Moss RJ: Advance directives on admission: clinical implications and analysis of the Patient Self-Determination Act of 1990. JAMA 266:402–405, 1991

Link BG, Stueve A: Psychotic symptoms and the violent/illegal behavior of mental patients compared to community controls, in Violence and Mental Disorder: Developments in Risk Assessment. Edited by Monahan J, Steadman H. Chicago, IL, University of Chicago Press, 1994, pp 137–159

Melton GB, Petrila J, Poythress NG, et al: Psychological Evaluations for the Courts: A Handbook for Mental Health Professionals and Lawyers, 2nd Edition. New York, Guilford, 1997

Mishkin B: Determining the capacity for making health care decisions, in Issues in Geriatric Psychiatry (Advances in Psychosomatic Medicine, Vol 19). Edited by Billig N, Rabins PV. Basel, Switzerland, S Karger, 1989, pp 151–166

Perlin ML: Mental Disability Law: Civil and Criminal, Vol 3. Charlottesville, VA, Michie, 1989

President's Commission for the Study of Ethical Problems in Medicine and Biomedical and Behavioral Research: Making Health Care Decisions, Vol 1: A Report on the Ethical and Legal Implications of Informed Consent in the Patient–Practitioner Relationship. Washington, DC, U.S. Government Printing Office, October 1982

Reich J, Wells J: Psychiatric diagnosis and competency to stand trial. Compr Psychiatry 26:421–432, 1985

Rogers R, Shuman DW: Fundamentals of Forensic Practice: Mental Health and Criminal Law. New York, Springer, 2005

Sale B, Powell DM, Van Duizend R: Disabled Persons and the Law: State Legislative Issues. New York, Plenum, 1982

Sederer LI, Ellison J, Keyes C: Guidelines for prescribing psychiatrists in consultative, collaborative, and supervisory relationships. Psychiatr Serv 49:1197–1202, 1998

Shuman DW, Greenberg SA: The expert witness, the adversary system, and the voice of reason: reconciling impartiality and advocacy. Professional Psychology: Research and Practice 34:219–224, 2003

Shuman DW, Weiner MF: The Psychotherapist–Patient Privilege: A Critical Examination. Springfield, IL, Charles C Thomas, 1987

Simon RI: The psychiatrist as a fiduciary: avoiding the double agent role. Psychiatr Ann 17:622–626, 1987

Simon RI: Clinical Psychiatry and the Law, 2nd Edition. Washington, DC, American Psychiatric Press, 1992a

Simon RI: Clinical risk management of suicidal patients: assessing the unpredictable, in American Psychiatric Press Review of Clinical Psychiatry and the Law, Vol 3. Edited by Simon RI. Washington, DC, American Psychiatric Press, 1992b, pp 3–63

Simon RI: Innovative psychiatric therapies and legal uncertainty: a survival guide for clinicians. Psychiatr Ann 23:473–479, 1993

Simon RI: The myth of "imminent" violence in psychiatry and the law. University of Cincinnati Law Review 75:631–644, 2006

Simon RI, Hales RE (eds): American Psychiatric Publishing Textbook of Suicide Assessment and Management. Washington, DC, American Psychiatric Publishing, 2006

Simon RI, Shuman DW (eds): Retrospective Assessment of Mental States in Litigation: Predicting the Past. Washington, DC, American Psychiatric Publishing, 2002

Solnick PB: Proxy consent for incompetent nonterminally ill adult patients. J Leg Med 6:1–49, 1985

Sparr LF: Legal aspects of posttraumatic stress disorder: uses and abuses, in Posttraumatic Stress Disorder: Etiology, Phenomenology, and Treatment. Edited by Wolf ME, Mosnaim AD. Washington, DC, American Psychiatric Press, 1990, pp 22–34

Strasburger LH, Gutheil TG, Brodsky A: On wearing two hats: role conflict in serving as both psychotherapist and expert witness. Am J Psychiatry 154:448–456, 1997

Strub RL, Black FW: The Mental Status Examination in Neurology, 2nd Edition. Philadelphia, PA, FA Davis, 1985

Tranel D: Functional neuroanatomy: neuropsychological correlates of cortical and subcortical damage, in The American Psychiatric Press Textbook of Neuropsychiatry, 2nd Edition. Edited by Yudofsky SC, Hales RE. Washington, DC, American Psychiatric Press, 1992, pp 70–75

Woodward B, Duckworth K, Gutheil TG: The pharmacotherapist-psychotherapist collaboration, in American Psychiatric Press Review of Psychiatry, Vol 12. Edited by Oldham JM, Riba MB, Tasman A. Washington, DC, American Psychiatric Press, 1993

## Legal Citations

Bethea v United States, 365 A.2d 64 (D.C. App. 1976), cert. denied, 433 U.S. 911 (1977)

Canterbury v Spence, 464 F.2d 772 (D.C. Cir. 1972), cert denied, Spence v. Canterbury, 409 U.S. 1064 (1972)

Cruzan v Director, Missouri Department of Health, 497 U.S. 261 (1990)

Dusky v United States, 362 U.S. 402 (1960)

Ford v Wainwright, 477 US 399 (1986)

In re Conroy, 98 N.J. 321, 486 A.2d 1209, 1222–23 (1985)

Jaffee v Redmond, 518 U.S. 1 (1996)

Long v Jaszczak, 688 N.W.2d 173 (N.D. 2004)

Meek v City of Loveland, 85 Colo. 346, 276 P. 30 (1929)

Minn. Stat. Ann. § 609.344 (West 2005)

M'Naughten's case. 10 Cl. and Fin. 200, 8 Eng. Rep 718 (HL 1843)

Model Penal Code § 4.01 (1962)

Penry v Lynaugh, 492 U.S. 302 (1989)

People v White, 117 Cal.App.3d 270, 172 Cal. Rptr. 612 (1981)

Rennie v Klein, 462 F.Supp. 1131 (D. N.J. 1978), remanded, 476 F.Supp. 1294 (D. N.J. 1979), aff'd in part, modified in part and remanded, 653 F.2d 836 (3d. Cir. 1980), vacated and remanded, 458 U.S. 1119 (1982), 720 F.2d 266 (3rd Cir. 1983)

Restatement [Second] of Torts 315(a) (1965)

Scaria v St. Paul Fire and Marine Ins. Co., 68 Wis.2d 1, 227 N.W.2d 647 (1975)

Schloendorff v Society of New York Hospital, 211 N.Y. 125, 105 N.E. 92 (1914), overruled, Bing v Thunig, 2 N.Y.2d 656, 143 N.E.2d 3, 163 N.Y.S.2d 3 (1957)

Speer v United States, 512 F.Supp. 670 (N.D. Tex. 1981), aff'd, Speer v. United States, 675 F.2d 100 (5th Cir. 1982)

Stepakoff v Kantar, 473 N.E.2d 1131 (Mass. 1985)

Tarasoff v Regents of the University of California, 17 Cal.3d 425, 551 P.2d 334; 131 Cal. Rptr. 14 (1976)

Tennard v Dretke, 542 U.S. 274 (2004)

Thapar v Zezulka, 944 S.W.2d 635 (Tex. 1999)

Union Pacific Realty Co. v Botsford, 141 U.S. 250, 251 (1891)

United States v Brawner, 471 F.2d 969 (D.C. Cir. 1972), superseded by statute, see Shannon v United States, 512 U.S. 573 (1994)

United States v David, 511 F.2d 355 (D.C. Cir. 1975)

Wilson v Lehman, 379 S.W.2d 478, 479 (Ky. 1964)

Wilson v United States, 391 F.2d 460, 463 (D.C. Cir. 1968)

# Glossary of Legal Terms

**Action**   See *civil action*.

**Adjudication**   The formal pronouncement of a judgment or decree in a cause of action.

**Assault**   Any willful attempt or threat to inflict injury.

**Battery**   An intentional and wrongful physical contact with an individual without consent that causes some injury or offensive touching.

**Beyond a reasonable doubt**   The level of proof required to convict a person in a criminal trial. This is the highest level of proof required (90%–95% range of certainty).

**Breach of contract**   A violation of or failure to perform any or all of the terms of an agreement.

**Brief**   A written statement prepared by legal counsel arguing a case.

**Burden of proof**   The legal obligation to prove affirmatively a disputed fact (or facts) related to an issue that is raised by the parties in a case.

**Capacity**   The status or attributes necessary for a person so that his or her acts may be legally and responsibly acknowledged and recognized.

**Case law**   The aggregate of reported cases as forming a body of law on a particular subject.

**Cause in fact**   The requirement of fact that without the defendant's wrongful conduct, the harm to the plaintiff would not have occurred.

**Cause of action**   The grounds of an action—that is, those facts that, if alleged and proved in a suit, would enable the plaintiff to attain a judgment.

**Civil action**   A lawsuit brought by a private individual or group to recover money or property, to enforce or protect a civil right, or to prevent or redress a civil wrong.

**Civil law**   As contrasted with criminal law, a system for enforcement of private rights arising from sources such as torts and contracts.

**Clear and convincing**   A proof that results in reasonable certainty of the truth of an ultimate fact in controversy (75% range of certainty); for example, the minimum level of evidence necessary to involuntarily hospitalize a patient.

**Common law**   A system of law based on customs, traditional usage, and prior case law rather than codified written laws (statutes).

**Compensatory damages**   Damages awarded to a person as compensation, indemnity, or restitution for harm sustained.

**Competency**   The mental capacity to understand the nature of an act.

**Consent decree**   An agreement by a defendant to cease activities asserted as illegal by the government.

**Consortium**   The right of a husband or wife to the care, affection, company, and cooperation of the other spouse in every aspect of the marital relationship.

**Contract**   A legally enforceable agreement between two or more parties to do or not do a particular thing upon sufficient consideration.

**Criminal law**   The branch of the law that defines crimes and provides for their punishment. Unlike in civil law, penalties include imprisonment.

**Damages**   A sum of money awarded to a person injured by the unlawful act or negligence of another.

**Defendant**   A person or legal entity against whom a claim or charge is brought.

**Due process (of law)**   The constitutional guarantee protecting individuals from arbitrary and unreasonable actions by the government that would deprive them of their basic rights to life, liberty, or property.

**Duress**   Compulsion or constraint, as by force or threat, exercised to make a person do or say something against his or her will.

**Duty**   The legal obligation that one person owes another. Whenever one person has a right, another person has a corresponding duty to preserve or not interfere with that right.

**False imprisonment**   The unlawful restraint or detention of one person by another.

**Fiduciary**   A person who acts for another in a capacity that involves a confidence or trust.

**Forensic psychiatry**   "A subspecialty of psychiatry in which scientific and clinical expertise is applied to legal issues in legal contexts embracing civil, criminal, correctional, or legislative matters."

**Fraud**   Any act of trickery, deceit, or misrepresentation designed to deprive someone of property or to do harm.

**Guardianship**   A legal arrangement wherein one individual (the guardian) possesses the legal right and duty to care for another individual (the ward) and his or her property.

**Hold harmless**   An agreement to protect a party from damages.

**Immunity**   The freedom from duty or penalty.

**Incompetence**    A lack of ability or fitness for some legal qualification necessary for the performance of an act (e.g., being a minor, lacking mental competence).

**Informed consent**    A competent person's voluntary agreement to allow something to happen that is based on full disclosure of facts needed to make a knowing decision.

**Intentional tort**    A tort in which the actor is expressly or implicitly judged to have possessed an intent or purpose to cause injury.

**Judgment**    The final determination or adjudication by a court of the claims of parties in an action.

**Jurisdiction**    The legal right by which courts or judicial officers exercise their authority.

**Malpractice**    Any professional misconduct or unreasonable lack of skill in professional or fiduciary duties.

**Miranda warning**    A four-part warning required to be given prior to any custodial interrogation (refers to the *Miranda v. Arizona* decision).

**Negligence**    The failure to exercise the standard of care that would be expected of a normally reasonable and prudent person in a particular set of circumstances.

**Nominal damages**    Generally, damages of a small monetary amount indicating a violation of a legal right without any important loss or damage to the plaintiff.

***Parens patriae***    The authority of the state to exercise sovereignty and guardianship of a person with legal disability so as to act on his or her behalf in protecting health, comfort, and welfare interests.

**Plaintiff**    The complaining party in an action; the person who brings a cause of action.

**Police power**    The power of government to make and enforce all laws and regulations necessary for the welfare of the state and its citizens.

**Power of attorney**    A document giving someone authority to act on behalf of the grantor.

**Preponderance of evidence**    Superiority in the weight of evidence presented by one side over that of the other (51% range of certainty); the level of certainty required in order to prevail in civil trials.

**Privileged communication**    Those statements made by certain persons within a protected relationship (e.g., doctor–patient) that the law protects from forced disclosure.

**Proximate cause**    The direct, immediate cause to which an injury or loss can be attributed and without which the injury or loss would not have occurred.

**Proxy**    A person empowered by another to represent, act, or vote for him or her.

**Punitive damages**    Damages awarded over and above those to which the plaintiff is entitled, generally given to punish or make an example of the defendant.

***Respondeat superior***    The doctrine whereby the master (i.e., employer) is strictly liable in certain cases for the wrongful acts of his or her servants (i.e., employees).

**Right**    A power, privilege, demand, or claim possessed by a particular person by virtue of law. Every legal right that one person possesses imposes corresponding legal duties on other persons.

**Sovereign immunity**    The immunity of a government from being sued in court except with its consent.

**Standard of care (negligence law)**    In the law of negligence, that degree of care that a reasonably prudent person should exercise under the same or similar circumstances.

***Stare decisis***    The duty to adhere to precedents and not to unsettle principles of law that are established.

**Statute**    An act of the legislature declaring, commanding, or prohibiting something.

**Subpoena**    A writ commanding a person to appear in court.

***Subpoena ad testificandum***    A writ commanding a person to appear in court to give testimony.

***Subpoena duces tecum***    A writ commanding a person to appear in court with particular documents or other evidence.

**Tort**    Any private or civil wrong by act or omission, not including breach of contract.

**United States Code (U.S.C.)**    The compilation of laws derived from federal legislation.

**Vicarious liability**    See *respondeat superior*.

# 10

# Epidemiological Aspects of Psychiatric Disorders

DOLORES MALASPINA, M.D., M.S.P.H.

CHERYL M. CORCORAN, M.D., M.S.P.H.

SCOTT SCHOBEL, M.D.

STEVEN P. HAMILTON, M.D., Ph.D.

## Epidemiological Studies

Epidemiological research may be viewed as a directed series of questions:

- What is the frequency of a disorder?
- Are there subgroups in which the disorder is more frequent?
- What specific risk factors are associated with the disorder?
- Are these risk factors consistently and specifically related to the disorder?
- Does exposure to these factors precede the development of disease?

A variety of epidemiological strategies have been developed to address these questions.

## Measures of Disease Frequency

The two measures of disease frequency used most often are *prevalence* and *incidence*. The former refers to the number of existing cases of a disease at a given point in time as a proportion of the total population. The latter refers to the number of new cases of a disease during a given period as a proportion of the total population at risk. The two measures are interrelated: the prevalence of a disease depends on both its incidence and its duration. One can compare two populations with and without a factor suspected of contributing to the development of disease through the calculation of the ratio of disease frequency in the two populations; this is known as the *relative risk*.

Disease incidence can be defined in several ways. *Risk* refers to the probability that an individual will develop a disease over a specified time, and thus can vary from zero (no risk) to 1 (an individual will develop the disease). A common difficulty in long-term studies is that subjects become lost to follow-up, thus distorting the risk estimate upward if the subject remains disease-free or downward if the subject develops the disease. The alternative measure of incidence, called the *rate*, is used to address this problem. The rate is the instantaneous measure of individuals newly developing the disease in relation to the number of subjects who remain at risk (i.e., new cases per person-years of follow-up). See Table 10–1 for the population prevalence, morbid risk in first-degree relatives, and relative risk of selected neuropsychiatric disorders.

TABLE 10-1.    Relative risk for neuropsychiatric disorders

| Disease | Population prevalence per 100,000 | Morbid risk in first-degree relatives (%) | Relative risk (%) |
|---|---|---|---|
| Narcolepsy | 10–100 | 30–50 | 5,000 |
| Huntington's disease | 19 | 50 | 2,630 |
| Wilson's disease | 10 | 25 | 2,500 |
| Parkinson's disease | 133 | 8.3 | 62.4 |
| Autism | 50–100 | 2–4 | 45–90 |
| Bipolar disorder | 500–1,500 | 8 | 16 |
| Schizophrenia | 900 | 12.8 | 14.2 |
| Panic disorder | 2,700 | 31 | 10 |
| Obsessive-compulsive disorder | 1,000–2,000 | 10 | 4.5 |
| Alzheimer's disease | 7,700 | 14.4 | 1.9 |
| Prion diseases | <0.1 | ? | ? |

## Descriptive Studies

Descriptive studies are conducted when little is known about the occurrence or antecedents of a disease. Hypotheses regarding risk factors then may emerge from studying several characteristics of affected individuals (e.g., sex, age, birth cohort), their place of residence, or the timing of their exposure. Descriptive studies, however, cannot be used to test etiological hypotheses.

## Analytic Studies

An analytic study commences when enough is known about a disease that specific a priori hypotheses can be examined. Such etiological hypotheses may be tested through various analytic strategies. In a prospective cohort study, information is obtained about exposure status to selected variables at the time the study begins. New cases of illness are then identified from among those who did and those who did not have the exposure to the selected variables. This contrasts with retrospective cohort studies, in which prior exposure status is established on the basis of available information, usually obtained from available documentation and/or subject interviews.

Disease incidence is determined from the time chosen by the investigator until the defined end point of the study. Case-control studies begin with the designation of disease status, and then past exposure to a risk factor is compared in those individuals who have a disease (case subjects) and in the appropriate control subjects.

## Birth Cohort Studies

Another important type of epidemiological study is the birth cohort study, in which all individuals born in a certain location at a certain time are followed up.

# Huntington's Disease

Huntington's disease (HD) is characterized by progressive dementia, chorea, and psychiatric symptoms. The mean age at onset is about 40 years, but symptoms can occur as early as age 2 and as late as age 80–90. HD usually causes death within 15–20 years of onset (Margolis and Ross 2003). In about 10% of the individuals with HD, the onset of symptoms occurs before age 20 (Gusella et al. 1993). Juvenile-onset HD or the "Westphal variant" is characterized by akinesia and rigidity instead of chorea, as well as a more rapid and severe course of illness.

Psychiatric symptoms occur in 70%–80% of the patients (Harper 1996) and can include a change in personality, paranoia, psychosis, and depression. About 40% of the patients develop a mood disorder; 25% of these have bipolar disorder (Peyser and Folstein 1990). Mood disorder may antedate other symptoms by 2–20 years (Folstein et al. 1983). In HD, the suicide rate is estimated to be as high as 12% (Harper 1996).

The overall prevalence of HD worldwide is 5–10 cases per 100,000, making it the most common neurodegenerative disorder (Landles and Bates 2004). However, the prevalence has been found to be higher (sometimes much higher) in certain places because of a large concentration of affected families; for example, the prevalence is more than 100 per 100,000 in a specific region of Venezuela (Wexler et al. 2004).

The age at onset of HD is variable and depends on the sex and the age at onset of the transmitting parent. Anticipation, which means that each successive generation tends to develop HD at an earlier age than did the previous one, occurs and is most striking with paternal inheritance.

# Parkinson's Disease

Parkinson's disease (PD) is a progressive neurological disorder that is caused by the loss of dopaminergic neurons in the substantia nigra and nigrostriatal pathway of the midbrain. The cardinal symptoms are poverty or slowness of movement (akinesia or bradykinesia), rigidity of the trunk and limb muscles, tremor or trembling that typically begins in the hands ("pill rolling"), and postural instability with impaired balance and coordination. Other common symptoms are a waxy facial expression, stooped posture, shuffling gait, and micrographia. The motor deficits arise from impairments in initiation, planning, and sequencing of voluntary movements. Some patients additionally experience difficulty in swallowing and chewing, speech impairments, and sleep disturbances. An associated dysfunction of the autonomic nervous system can cause urinary incontinence, constipation, sexual dysfunction, hypotension, and skin problems.

Many PD patients develop psychiatric syndromes, particularly depression, emotionality, and panic attacks, even in advance of the neurological signs. Treatment-emergent symptoms can include visual hallucinations, paranoid delusions, mania, and delirium. A sizable minority of patients develop cognitive slowing (bradyphrenia), and up to 40% of end-stage patients have dementia (Cedarbaum and McDowell 1987).

The onset is often subtle and gradual. Thereafter, the symptoms and their progression are quite variable, but PD frequently progresses to curtail walking, talking, and performing even simple tasks of daily living. The neuropathology includes a loss of pigmented (dopaminergic) neurons in the zona compacta of the substantia nigra and the presence of Lewy bodies in the remaining neurons. Noninvasive neuroimaging techniques can be used to examine the nigrostriatal pathophysiology (see Fischman 2005). Lewy bodies in other areas (cortex, amygdala, locus coeruleus, hypothalamus, dorsal medial nucleus of the vagus, and nucleus basalis of Meynert) may explain the nonmotor symptoms.

PD is a common condition, affecting about 1% of adults older than 60 years. The prevalence estimate is 133 in 100,000; the average age at onset is 63 years but may be increasing. The incidence of the disorder has been reported as 11 in 100,000 person-years (see Checkoway and Nelson 1999). PD may affect men at a slightly higher rate than women. Early-onset PD begins between age 21 and 40 and accounts for 5%–10% of patients. The prevalence of PD increases with age, but it is not just an acceleration of normal aging; age is associated with a decline in striatal dopamine but not with changes in the caudate and putamen (van Dyck et al. 2002).

# Alzheimer's Disease

Alzheimer's disease is the most common cause of dementia, accounting for 50%–70% of all cases. It is a neurodegenerative disease that usually begins after age 65 years, although early-onset cases also occur. Alzheimer's disease is characterized by a progressive deterioration of mental abilities, particularly memory, language, abstract thought, and judgment. Psychiatric and behavioral disturbances are among its earliest symptoms, with overt neurological signs dominating the clinical picture as the illness progresses, including rigid limbs, frontal release signs, and seizures. The course leads inevitably to the loss of independent living and death over an average course of 8–10 years. The clinical picture, history, and laboratory studies permit a probable diagnosis of Alzheimer's disease, but the definitive diagnosis depends on postmortem studies.

## Epidemiological Studies

The prevalence estimates of Alzheimer's disease depend on the population sampled (community or nursing home residents), age, and diagnostic criteria (definition of "significant impairment"). Onset before 65 distinguishes presenile (types 1, 3, 4) from senile (type 2) dementia, although the cutoff ages are indistinct. Presenile cases are more likely to be familial, to be rapidly progressive, and to show prominent temporal and parietal lobe features, including dysphasia or dyspraxia. Later-onset cases (type 2) have a more insidious course and generalized cognitive impairments.

About 3% of those ages 65–74 years and half of the population older than 85 have Alzheimer's disease. Alzheimer's disease rates approximately double every 5 years after age 40 years (Hendrie 1998); the prevalence is expected to swell as the average life span increases.

Most Alzheimer's disease cases are sporadic, particularly the senile forms, and several demographic measures, lifestyle choices, environmental exposures, and medical conditions are associated with Alzheimer's disease risk. Even in the nonfamilial cases, it is expected that genetic susceptibility plays an important role. In particular, risk is associated with alleles of *APOE* (the gene for apolipoprotein E, which is a major component of very low-density lipoproteins). The Alzheimer's disease risk for the ε4 homozygotes (*APOE\*E4*) is especially elevated, although not all patients with Alzheimer's disease have *APOE\*E4*, and many people with the ε4 allele remain free of disease. The *APOE\*E4* allele is associated with an increased number of amyloid plaques, and it may interact with other susceptibility genes and environmental factors.

Females have a greater risk for Alzheimer's disease, even after accounting for their longer life span, with males showing a higher rate of vascular dementias. It was hypothesized that the risk for women could be due to menopause, and many long-term studies suggested that women who take estrogen-based hormone replacement therapy (HRT) have a lower risk of developing Alzheimer's disease. However, because HRT use was not random among these subjects, it is possible that women who are less likely to develop Alzheimer's disease for other reasons are just more likely to use HRT. Zandi et al. (2002) found no benefit of current HRT use except for those whose use exceeded 10 years. Recently, the Women's Health Initiative Memory Study surprised investigators by showing a doubling of the risk of all-cause dementia in women randomly assigned to receive Prempro, a specific form of combination hormone therapy, after age 64 years (Shumaker et al. 2003). There is new speculation that gonadotropins, rather than estrogen and progesterone, may play the key role in determining the risk for and progression of Alzheimer's disease. As recently reviewed (see Webber et al. 2005), women with Alzheimer's disease have higher levels of luteinizing hormone (LH) than do control subjects. Both LH and its receptor are expressed in brain regions that are susceptible to Alzheimer's disease pathology.

A higher educational level is a protective factor (Launer et al. 1999), perhaps because of increased synaptic and/or dendritic complexity attendant to learning demands. A well-controlled prospective study of at-risk individuals confirmed that low educational attainment was associated with a doubling of Alzheimer's disease incidence (Stern et al. 1994). Determining whether education may directly mitigate the risk of developing Alzheimer's disease has implications for the prevention and treatment of Alzheimer's disease, such as using cognitive training to lower the risk for vulnerable individuals (Hendrie 1998).

Traumatic brain injury (TBI) has been related to Alzheimer's disease risk. A prospective study showed that TBI increased the incidence of Alzheimer's disease fourfold over the next 5 years (relative risk=4.1; 95% confidence interval=1.3–12.7), particularly in cases when *APOE\*E4* was present (Mayeux et al. 1995; Tang et al. 1996). The association between TBI and Alzheimer's disease risk may be affected by the severity of the TBI (loss of consciousness or not) and by family history (Guo et al. 2000).

Amyloid is a proinflammatory substance, and neuropathological examination shows that plaques are surrounded by signs of inflammation. Use of nonsteroidal anti-inflammatory drugs, such as ibuprofen, has shown protective effects (see Gasparini et al. 2005).

Hypertension also significantly elevates Alzheimer's disease risk, an effect that may be mediated by vascular injury and inflammation. In their review, Luchsinger and Mayeux (2004) highlighted the possible mechanisms linking cerebrovascular diseases with Alzheimer's disease. Diabetes and hyperinsulinemia are also likely to be important risk factors.

## Family and Twin Studies

Approximately a quarter of patients with Alzheimer's disease have another first-degree relative with Alzheimer's disease, and the familial nature of Alzheimer's disease has been established in case-control, family, and twin studies (reviewed in Richard and Amouyel 2001). The recurrence risks in family studies are small and variable: 0%–14.4% for parents and 3.8%–13.9% for siblings. The familial recurrences are more prominent in early-onset disease, although such cases may be just more easily ascertained, and both early- and late-onset cases frequently occur within a single family.

# Bipolar Disorder

## Epidemiological Studies

General population estimates of the prevalence of bipolar I disorder range from 1% to 1.6% in the United States and from 0.3% to 1.5% worldwide (Weissman et al. 1996). The risk for bipolar and other mood disorders has increased in successive cohorts over the course of the last century.

## Family Studies

A meta-analysis of eight family studies showed a seven-fold increase in lifetime risk for bipolar disorder in family members of bipolar probands compared with family members of control subjects (Craddock and Jones 1999). The risk for bipolar disorder appears to be especially elevated for the relatives of probands with early-onset disorder, and the risk also increases with the number of psychiatrically ill relatives (Gershon et al. 1982). Other psychiatric conditions that aggregate in the relatives of probands with bipolar disorder are bipolar II disorder, recurrent unipolar disorder, schizoaffective disorder (bipolar type), and suicide.

The age at onset of the first manic or depressive episode has been shown to be earlier, and the frequency of episodes greater, in the younger generation of two generations of affected relative pairs (McInnis et al. 1993; Nylander et al. 1994).

## Twin Studies

Ten twin studies of mood disorders that have been conducted since 1928, in which affected twins had either bipolar or unipolar disorder, have suggested higher concordance rates in monozygotic (MZ) pairs (58%–74%) than in same-sex dizygotic (DZ) pairs (17%–29%) (see Tsuang and Faraone 1990). Interestingly, as in schizophrenia, among discordant MZ twin pairs, offspring of the affected and nonaffected twin have identical risk of developing bipolar disorder; this supports the role of environmental factors in the expression of the bipolar phenotype for those who are genetically vulnerable.

## Adoption Studies

A significantly greater risk of affective disorder (unipolar, bipolar, and schizoaffective) was found in the biological parents (18%) than in the adoptive parents (7%) of adopted bipolar probands (Mendlewicz and Rainer 1977). The risk for illness in biological parents of adopted and nonadopted bipolar probands was similar. Another study of biological and adopted relatives of probands with mood disorders and control probands also showed that the biological relatives of affected probands had increased risk for the same broad spectrum of affective disorder; the biological relatives of affected probands were 8 times more likely to have unipolar depression and 15 times more likely to have completed suicide (Wender et al. 1986).

## High-Risk Studies

Structured diagnostic interviews of 60 offspring who had at least one parent with bipolar disorder yielded a 51% prevalence of psychiatric disorder, predominantly attention-deficit, unipolar, and bipolar disorders (Chang et al. 2000). The risk of bipolar disorder in offspring was associated with early age at onset of bipolar disorder in the parent. In a single extended pedigree identified by a bipolar proband, the risk of early-onset affective disorder was correlated with degree of relatedness to affected adults (Todd et al. 1994). In a series of National Institute of Mental Health (NIMH) bipolar pedigrees, children of parents with affective disorder were five times more likely to have an affective disorder than were children of healthy parents (Todd et al. 1996). Children of bipolar parents may have greater degrees of aggressiveness, obsessionality, and affective expression than do age-matched control subjects (reviewed in Goodwin and Jamison 1990).

# Panic Disorder

## Epidemiological Studies

An international epidemiological study of 40,000 persons reported a lifetime prevalence of panic disorder of 1.4%–2.9% (Weissman et al. 1997). The prevalence of panic disorder in females is about twice that in males (Eaton et al. 1994). The age at highest risk is 25–44 years (Robins et al. 1984), with a mean age at onset of 24; the hazard rates are highest at 25–34 for females and 30–44 for males (Burke et al. 1990).

## Family Studies

The first study to use DSM-III (American Psychiatric Association 1980) diagnoses showed that 31% of the first-degree relatives of panic disorder probands were affected, compared with 4% of the relatives of control subjects (R.C. Crowe et al. 1980) (relative risk=7.8). An extension of this study with twice the number of probands and relatives confirmed this finding, with a relative risk on the order of 9.9–10.7, depending on the diagnostic criteria used (R.R. Crowe et al. 1983). Among 41 families with panic disorder, 25 (61.0%) had at least one affected relative, compared with 4 of 41 control families (9.8%). The risk was double for female relatives compared with male relatives. Several subsequent studies confirmed these findings (Fyer et al. 1995; Hopper et al. 1987; Maier et al.

1993; Mendlewicz et al. 1993; Noyes et al. 1986; Weissman 1993). One group found that specific smothering symptoms increased the risk of panic disorder (Horwath et al. 1997) and that early age at onset increased the risk of panic in the first-degree relatives of panic disorder probands to 17 (Goldstein et al. 1997). On the whole, family studies of first-degree relatives of panic disorder probands suggested a relative risk of 2.6–20 (mean=7.8) (Knowles and Weissman 1995). Similar work in second-degree relatives of panic probands showed a sevenfold relative risk (Pauls et al. 1979), similar to studies in first-degree relatives. Also consistent with the first-degree relative studies, female second-degree relatives were at higher risk for panic disorder.

## Twin Studies

It was not until the 1980s that twin studies that used rigorous diagnostic criteria were published. Torgersen (1983) used DSM-III diagnostic criteria and interviewed 299 Norwegian twin pairs; in 11 twin pairs, 1 co-twin had panic disorder, and in 18 twin pairs, 1 person had panic disorder with agoraphobia. No co-twin shared the same diagnosis in this group, although in 2 MZ twin pairs, 1 twin had panic disorder, and the other twin had panic disorder with agoraphobia. A larger study that used DSM-III-R (American Psychiatric Association 1987) diagnoses identified 49 twin pairs in which 1 twin had an anxiety disorder and 32 comparison pairs without an anxiety disorder. When the co-twins were assessed, 5 of 20 (25.0%) of the MZ co-twins and 3 of 29 (10.3%) of the DZ twins were found to have panic disorder (Skre et al. 1993). The concordance rates for the comparison group were 8% and 10% in MZ and DZ twin pairs, respectively.

A much larger analysis of 1,030 female twin pairs derived from the Virginia Twin Registry was carried out by Kendler's group (Kendler et al. 1993). DSM-III-R diagnoses were made with varying levels of certainty, and 5.8% of the 2,163 interviewed twins met lifetime criteria for panic disorder. The concordance rates were 24% and 11% for MZ and DZ twins, respectively. The best-fitting model for the narrowest diagnostic scheme implied that the variance in susceptibility to panic disorder was due to individual-specific environment and additive genes, and the heritability was estimated at 46%.

## Adoption Studies

There are no known adoption studies for panic disorder.

## High-Risk Studies

Investigation of families of depressed patients showed evidence for (Weissman et al. 1984) and against (Coryell et al. 1988) the hypothesis that panic disorder would increase the risk of depression in relatives. A family study that collected patients from treatment clinics and population-based surveys showed that panic disorder itself did not increase risk for depression in relatives per se, and vice versa, whereas comorbid panic and depression increased the risk of both panic alone and depression alone, as well as comorbid panic and depression, in relatives (Weissman 1993).

Another avenue of research has identified a potential biological marker for panic disorder in high-risk individuals. Numerous groups have used inhaled carbon dioxide ($CO_2$) or infused lactate, among other compounds, to induce panic attacks in persons with panic disorder (Balon et al. 1988; Gorman et al. 1990). Subsequent work by Balon et al. (1989) has shown that when family histories of healthy subjects were taken, subjects with a high prevalence of anxiety disorders in their first-degree relatives had panic attacks after lactate infusion, whereas those who did not panic had relatives who were at lower risk. One group showed that the psychiatrically healthy first-degree relatives of panic probands had $CO_2$-induced panic attacks at significantly higher rates than did control subjects with no family history of panic disorder, although at rates lower than those in the identified probands (Perna et al. 1995). The same group studied prevalence rates of panic disorder in 895 first-degree relatives of 203 panic probands. A positive reaction to $CO_2$ inhalation in the proband conferred a morbid risk of 14.4% among first-degree relatives, whereas the rate in the families of probands with negative responses was 3.9% (Perna et al. 1996). In another study (Coryell 1997), a total of 39 persons with and without family histories of panic disorder had $CO_2$ inhalation; those with a positive family history were more likely to experience panic attacks. Bellodi et al. (1998) evaluated 20 MZ and 25 DZ twin pairs obtained from an Italian twin registry to test for concordance of the panic response to $CO_2$ inhalation and found concordance rates of 55.6% and 12.5% for MZ and DZ pairs, respectively. A segregation analysis of 165 families found that the 134 families in which a panic proband was hypersensitive to $CO_2$ fit a dominant single major locus model of inheritance (Cavallini et al. 1999). Subsequent studies showed that genetic determinants of $CO_2$ response are not necessarily enriched in panic disorder (Philibert et al. 2003) and that history of panic disorder in a parent does not predict $CO_2$ response (Pine et al. 2005).

# Obsessive-Compulsive Disorder

## Epidemiological Studies

As part of the Epidemiologic Catchment Area (ECA) study, more than 9,500 persons across three sites in the United States were interviewed for 15 DSM-III disorders, for which lifetime and 6-month prevalence data were obtained. Obsessive-compulsive disorder (OCD) was found to have a lifetime prevalence of 1.9%–3.0% among the three sites (Robins et al. 1984), whereas 6-month prevalence was estimated to be 1.3%–2.0% (Myers et al. 1984). A subsequent study extended the ECA findings to more than 18,500 persons across all five ECA sites and confirmed a lifetime prevalence of 1.9%–3.3% (Karno et al. 1988). Analysis of the temporal stability of the diagnosis of OCD with the ECA data reported that only 19.2% of those meeting diagnostic criteria for OCD continued to do so when reinterviewed 1 year later (Nelson and Rice 1997).

In a population-based study of 356 adolescents selected from an original screening set of 5,600, the DSM-III diagnosis of OCD had current and lifetime prevalences of 1.0% and 1.9%, respectively (Flament et al. 1988). Community survey data from seven countries obtained by the Cross National Collaborative Group indicated an annual prevalence rate of 1.1%–1.8% and a lifetime rate of 1.9%–2.5% (Weissman et al. 1994). Finally, a replication sample for the National Comorbidity Survey found a lifetime prevalence of 1.6% (Kessler et al. 2005).

There appears to be a slight excess of females with OCD compared with males. In a review of 11 studies performed before 1970 of treatment populations totaling 1,336 persons, 51% of the patients were women (Black 1974). Other epidemiological evidence suggests a larger female-to-male ratio, with five of the seven countries in the Cross National Collaborative Group having ratios of 1.2–1.6, with two outlying countries with proportions of 0.8 and 3.8 (Weissman et al. 1994). One striking finding has been the reversal of the sex ratio in children. In one clinic-based sample, 76.5% (13 of 17) of the patients were boys (Hollingsworth et al. 1980), and a cohort of 70 patients followed up at the NIMH showed a male-to-female ratio of 2:1 (Swedo et al. 1989b). The ratio during adolescence seems to revert to that seen with adults (Flament et al. 1988).

The mean age at onset is 20.9 years, with a significant difference between sexes (male 19.5, female 22.0; $P < 0.003$) (Rasmussen and Eisen 1992).

## Family Studies

More than a dozen family studies have been published since the 1960s and have been comprehensively reviewed (Pauls and Alsobrook 1999; Sobin et al. 2000). Nine adult studies with 686 probands and 2,427 first-degree relatives showed OCD or obsessive-compulsive symptoms at rates ranging from 0% to 20%. Two child and adolescent studies with a total of 66 probands and 186 first-degree relatives showed OCD rates of 9.5%–25%. Sobin and colleagues noted that the studies that used more direct interviews reported high morbid risk rates, although several of those also were family studies of children and adolescents, enriching for the early-onset form of the disorder (Pauls et al. 1995). Indeed, when family studies are designed to utilize children as probands, the rates of OCD in first-degree relatives are particularly elevated (Hanna et al. 2005) when compared with studies in which probands are older than 18 (Nestadt et al. 2000).

## Twin Studies

In 1936, Lewis described three sets of MZ twins with concordant obsessional traits but drew few conclusions from his data, opining, "two or three pairs tell very little: it is a pity that twins are so rare" (pp. 325–326). A later review of the largely anecdotal intervening literature calculated a concordance of 56.9% (29 of 51) among MZ pairs, with an adjusted rate of 65.0% (13 of 20) after removing 30 pairs with questionable zygosity (Rasmussen and Tsuang 1984). Unfortunately, data for direct comparison to DZ twin rates were not presented, preventing any conclusions about the contribution of genetic factors.

Three subsequent studies have been published, all including DZ twins and totaling 233 MZ and 328 DZ pairs (Andrews et al. 1990; Carey and Gottesman 1981; Torgersen 1983). In 30 twin pairs with pre-DSM-III diagnoses (15 MZ and 15 DZ), one group found MZ and DZ concordances of 87% and 47%, respectively, for obsessional symptoms but found no difference for OCD (Carey and Gottesman 1981). A twin registry–based study (446 pairs, 186 MZ and 260 DZ) and a clinically derived sample (85 pairs, 32 MZ and 53 DZ) both looked at concordance of a variety of anxiety disorders among twins (Andrews et al. 1990; Torgersen 1983). Both found no concordant DSM-III OCD, but both did note higher concordances when OCD was grouped together with other anxiety and affective disorders. For example, Torgersen observed in his clinical sample that when OCD was grouped with agoraphobia, panic disorder, and social phobia, but not with generalized anxiety disorder, respective

MZ and DZ concordances of 45.0% (9 of 20) and 15.2% (5 of 33) were seen. A sample of more than 10,000 twin pairs, all children, was analyzed for obsessive-compulsive symptoms; a prominent additive genetic influence on symptomatology was found (Hudziak et al. 2004). A smaller study of 527 adult female twin pairs suggested a smaller genetic influence on obsessive-compulsive symptoms based on the Padua Inventory (Jonnal et al. 2000).

## Adoption Studies

There are no known adoption studies for OCD.

## High-Risk Studies

The striking differences in male-to-female ratios in OCD patients with prepubertal childhood-onset (3:1) and postpubertal adolescent-onset (1:1) disorder derive from the wide differences in age at onset between males and females. Males with early-onset OCD have been reported to have persistent and severe symptoms (Flament et al. 1990) as well as a higher incidence of birth complications compared with females (Lensi et al. 1996), suggesting that males may be more vulnerable to central nervous system damage resulting in OCD than are females.

It has long been observed that OCD co-occurs with tics and Tourette's disorder (Pauls et al. 1986), particularly in males and those with early-onset OCD (Leonard et al. 1992). Early-onset OCD also predicts Tourette's disorder and tics in relatives, suggesting a distinct risk group for OCD (Pauls et al. 1995). Even after excluding Tourette's disorder from OCD probands in a family study, tics were more prevalent in OCD families (Grados et al. 2001).

Studies of children with Sydenham's chorea, a neurological manifestation of rheumatic fever, led to the discovery that many children with this poststreptococcal autoimmune syndrome showed higher rates of obsessive-compulsive symptoms (Swedo et al. 1989a). Continued investigation into this phenomenon has resulted in the definition of PANDAS (pediatric autoimmune neuropsychiatric disorder associated with streptococcal infections) (Swedo et al. 1998). Swedo's group used a monoclonal antibody (D8/17) against a B cell antigen previously found to identify probands with rheumatic fever (Khanna et al. 1989) to assay children with PANDAS, children with Sydenham's chorea, and 24 control children (Swedo et al. 1997). They found that the PANDAS and Sydenham's chorea groups were D8/17 positive significantly more often than were control subjects (85% and 89%, respectively, vs. 17%). A subsequent study appears to generalize this finding to early-onset OCD and Tourette's disorder, showing that these groups also expressed the D8/17 antigen more frequently than did control samples (Murphy et al. 1997). Khanna et al. (1989) found that 100% of the rheumatic fever probands were D8/17 positive, expressing the antigen on 33% of their B cells. Unaffected siblings and parents expressed the marker on 15% and 13% of their cells, respectively, a rate approximately twice that of control subjects.

# Schizophrenia

First-degree relatives of schizophrenic probands have an increased risk of schizophrenia, with estimated risk rates of 6% for parents, 10% for siblings, and 13% and 46% for children with, respectively, one or two affected parents (McGue and Gottesman 1991). Identical twins have a concordance rate of 53%, whereas fraternal twins have a concordance rate of 15% (Kendler and Gardner 1997); the disparity in these rates suggests that 60%–90% of the liability to schizophrenia can be attributed to genes (Cannon et al. 1998; Jones and Cannon 1998). Of interest, offspring of affected and unaffected (discordant) MZ twins have equal risk for schizophrenia (about 16%–18%), consistent with either incomplete penetrance or gene-environment interaction.

Adoption studies also support inheritance of schizophrenia liability (Heston 1966; Kety et al. 1994; Rosenthal et al. 1968) but cannot determine whether such effects are genetic or environmental (in utero) if mothers are the parent of comparison. When fathers are the parent in common (paternal half-siblings), however, the same increased risk in biological (vs. adopted) relatives holds (Kety 1988). Adoption studies also provide evidence for a gene-environment interaction because adopted-away children of biological mothers with schizophrenia are even more likely to develop schizophrenia if they are raised in an adverse environment (Tienari 1991; Wahlberg et al. 1997).

## Key Points: Paradigms of Psychiatric and Genetic Research

| Paradigm | Questions | Samples studied | Method of inquiry | Scientific goals |
|---|---|---|---|---|
| Basic genetic epidemiology | Is the disorder familial? Is it inherited? | Family, twin, and adoption studies | Statistical | To quantify the degree of familial aggregation and/or heritability |
| Advanced genetic epidemiology | What is being inherited? Are there epigenetic factors? | Family, twin, and adoption studies | Statistical | To explore the nature and mode of action of genetic risk factors |
| Gene finding | How is the disorder inherited? Where are the abnormal genes? | High-density families, trios, case–control samples | Statistical | To determine the genomic location and identity of susceptibility genes |
| Molecular genetics | What is (are) their molecular and pathological effect(s)? | Humans, animals | Biological | To identify critical DNA variants and trace the biological pathways from DNA to disorder |

*Source.* Adapted from Kendler 2005.

## References

American Psychiatric Association: Diagnostic and Statistical Manual of Mental Disorders, 3rd Edition. Washington, DC, American Psychiatric Association, 1980

American Psychiatric Association: Diagnostic and Statistical Manual of Mental Disorders, 3rd Edition, Revision. Washington, DC, American Psychiatric Association, 1987

Andrews G, Stewart G, Allen R, et al: The genetics of six neurotic disorders: a twin study. J Affect Disord 19:23–29, 1990

Balon R, Pohl R, Yeragani VK, et al: Lactate- and isoproterenol-induced panic attacks in panic disorder patients and controls. Psychiatry Res 23:153–160, 1988

Balon R, Jordan M, Pohl R, et al: Family history of anxiety disorders in control subjects with lactate-induced panic attacks. Am J Psychiatry 146:1304–1306, 1989

Bellodi L, Perna G, Caldirola D, et al: $CO_2$-induced panic attacks: a twin study. Am J Psychiatry 155:1184–1188, 1998

Black A: The natural history of obsessional neurosis, in Obsessional States. Edited by Beech HR. London, Methuen, 1974, pp 19–54

Burke KC, Burke JD Jr, Regier DA, et al: Age at onset of selected mental disorders in five community populations. Arch Gen Psychiatry 47:511–518, 1990

Cannon TD, Kaprio J, Lonnqvist J, et al: The genetic epidemiology of schizophrenia in a Finnish twin cohort: a population-based modeling study. Arch Gen Psychiatry 55:67–74, 1998

Carey G, Gottesman II: Twin and family studies of anxiety, phobic, and obsessive disorders, in Anxiety: New Research and Changing Concepts. Edited by Klein DF, Rabkin JD. New York, Raven, 1981, pp 117–136

Cavallini MC, Perna G, Caldirola D, et al: A segregation study of panic disorder in families of panic patients responsive to the 35% $CO_2$ challenge. Biol Psychiatry 46:815–820, 1999

Cedarbaum JM, McDowell FH: Sixteen-year follow-up of 100 patients begun on levodopa in 1968: emerging problems. Adv Neurol 45:469–472, 1987

Chang KD, Steiner H, Ketter TA: Psychiatric phenomenology of child and adolescent bipolar offspring. J Am Acad Child Adolesc Psychiatry 39:453–460, 2000

Checkoway H, Nelson LM: Epidemiologic approaches to the study of Parkinson's disease etiology. Epidemiology 10:327–336, 1999

Coryell W: Hypersensitivity to carbon dioxide as a disease-specific trait marker. Biol Psychiatry 41:259–263, 1997

Coryell W, Endicott J, Andreasen NC, et al: Depression and panic attacks: the significance of overlap as reflected in follow-up and family study data. Am J Psychiatry 145:293–300, 1988

Craddock N, Jones I: Genetics of bipolar disorder. J Med Genet 36:585–594, 1999

Crowe RC, Pauls DL, Slymen DJ, et al: A family study of anxiety neurosis: morbidity risk in families of patients with and without mitral valve prolapse. Arch Gen Psychiatry 37:77–79, 1980

Crowe RR, Noyes R, Pauls DL, et al: A family study of panic disorder. Arch Gen Psychiatry 40:1065–1069, 1983

Eaton WW, Kessler RC, Wittchen HU, et al: Panic and panic disorder in the United States. Am J Psychiatry 151:413–420, 1994

Fischman AJ: Role of [¹⁸F]-dopa-PET imaging in assessing movement disorders. Radiol Clin North Am 43:93–106, 2005

Flament MF, Whitaker A, Rapoport JL, et al: Obsessive compulsive disorder in adolescence: an epidemiological study. J Am Acad Child Adolesc Psychiatry 27:764–771, 1988

Flament MF, Koby E, Rapoport JL, et al: Childhood obsessive-compulsive disorder: a prospective follow-up study. J Child Psychol Psychiatry 31:363–380, 1990

Folstein SE, Abbott MH, Chase GA, et al: The association of affective disorder with Huntington's disease in a case series and in families. Psychol Med 13:537–542, 1983

Fyer AJ, Mannuzza S, Chapman TF, et al: Specificity in familial aggregation of phobic disorders. Arch Gen Psychiatry 52:564–573, 1995

Gasparini L, Ongini E, Wilcock D, et al: Activity of flurbiprofen and chemically related anti-inflammatory drugs in models of Alzheimer's disease. Brain Res Brain Res Rev 48:400–408, 2005

Gershon ES, Hamovit J, Guroff JJ, et al: A family study of schizoaffective, bipolar I, bipolar II, unipolar, and normal control probands. Arch Gen Psychiatry 39:1157–1167, 1982

Goldstein RB, Wickramaratne PJ, Horwath E, et al: Familial aggregation and phenomenology of "early"-onset (at or before age 20 years) panic disorder. Arch Gen Psychiatry 54:271–278, 1997

Goodwin FK, Jamison KR: Manic-Depressive Illness. New York, Oxford University Press, 1990

Gorman JM, Papp LA, Martinez J, et al: High-dose carbon dioxide challenge test in anxiety disorder patients. Biol Psychiatry 28:743–757, 1990

Grados MA, Riddle MA, Samuels JF, et al: The familial phenotype of obsessive-compulsive disorder in relation to tic disorders: the Hopkins OCD family study. Biol Psychiatry 50:559–565, 2001

Guo Z, Cupples LA, Kurz A, et al: Head injury and the risk of AD in the MIRAGE study. Neurology 54:1316–1323, 2000

Gusella JF, MacDonald ME, Ambrose CM, et al: Molecular genetics of Huntington's disease. Arch Neurol 50:1157–1163, 1993

Hanna GL, Himle JA, Curtis GC, et al: A family study of obsessive-compulsive disorder with pediatric probands. Am J Med Genet B Neuropsychiatr Genet 134:13–19, 2005

Harper PS: New genes for old diseases: the molecular basis of myotonic dystrophy and Huntington's disease: the Lumleian Lecture 1995. J R Coll Physicians Lond 30:221–231, 1996

Hendrie HC: Epidemiology of dementia and Alzheimer's disease. Am J Geriatr Psychiatry 6:S3–S18, 1998

Heston LL: Psychiatric disorders in foster home reared children of schizophrenic mothers. Br J Psychiatry 112:819–825, 1966

Hollingsworth CE, Tanguay PE, Grossman L, et al: Long-term outcome of obsessive-compulsive disorder in childhood. J Am Acad Child Psychiatry 19:134–144, 1980

Hopper JL, Judd FK, Derrick PL, et al: A family study of panic disorder. Genet Epidemiol 4:33–41, 1987

Horwath E, Adams P, Wickramaratne P, et al: Panic disorder with smothering symptoms: evidence for increased risk in first-degree relatives. Depress Anxiety 6:147–153, 1997

Hudziak JJ, van Beijsterveldt CEM, Althoff RR, et al: Genetic and environmental contributions to the Child Behavior Checklist Obsessive-Compulsive Scale: a cross-cultural twin study. Arch Gen Psychiatry 61:608–616, 2004

Jones P, Cannon M: The new epidemiology of schizophrenia. Psychiatr Clin North Am 21:1–25, 1998

Jonnal AH, Gardner CO, Prescott CA, et al: Obsessive and compulsive symptoms in a general population sample of female twins. Am J Med Genet 96:791–796, 2000

Karno M, Golding JM, Sorenson SB, et al: The epidemiology of obsessive-compulsive disorder in five US communities. Arch Gen Psychiatry 45:1094–1099, 1988

Kendler KS, Gardner CO: The risk for psychiatric disorders in relatives of schizophrenic and control probands: a comparison of three independent studies. Psychol Med 27:411–419, 1997

Kendler KS, Neale MC, Kessler RC, et al: Panic disorder in women: a population-based twin study. Psychol Med 23:397–406, 1993

Kessler RC, Berglund P, Demler O, et al: Lifetime prevalence and age-of-onset distributions of DSM-IV disorders in the National Comorbidity Survey Replication. Arch Gen Psychiatry 62:593–602, 2005

Kety SS: Schizophrenic illness in the families of schizophrenic adoptees: findings from the Danish national sample. Schizophr Bull 14:217–222, 1988

Kety SS, Wender PH, Jacobsen B, et al: Mental illness in the biological and adoptive relatives of schizophrenic adoptees: replication of the Copenhagen Study in the rest of Denmark. Arch Gen Psychiatry 51:442–455, 1994

Khanna AK, Buskirk DR, Williams RC Jr, et al: Presence of a non-HLA B cell antigen in rheumatic fever patients and their families as defined by a monoclonal antibody. J Clin Invest 83:1710–1716, 1989

Knowles JA, Weissman MM: Panic disorder and agoraphobia, in American Psychiatric Press Review of Psychiatry, Vol 14. Edited by Oldham JM, Riba MB. Washington, DC, American Psychiatric Press, 1995, pp 383–404

Landles C, Bates GP: Huntington and the molecular pathogenesis of Huntington's disease (Fourth in Molecular Medicine Review Series). EMBO Rep 5:958–963, 2004

Launer LJ, Andersen K, Dewey ME, et al: Rates and risk factors for dementia and Alzheimer's disease: results from EURODEM pooled analyses. EURODEM Incidence Research Group and Work Groups. European Studies of Dementia. Neurology 52:78–84, 1999

Lensi P, Cassano GB, Correddu G, et al: Obsessive-compulsive disorder: familial-developmental history, symptomatology, comorbidity and course with special reference to gender-related differences. Br J Psychiatry 169:101–107, 1996

Leonard HL, Lenane MC, Swedo SE, et al: Tics and Tourette's disorder: a 2- to 7-year follow-up of 54 obsessive-compulsive children. Am J Psychiatry 149:1244–1251, 1992

Lewis A: Problems of obsessional illness. Proc R Soc Med 29:325–336, 1936

Luchsinger JA, Mayeux R: Cardiovascular risk factors and Alzheimer's disease. Curr Atheroscler Rep 6:261–266, 2004

Maier W, Lichtermann D, Minges J, et al: A controlled family study in panic disorder. J Psychiatr Res 27 (suppl 1):79–87, 1993

Margolis RL, Ross CA: Diagnosis of Huntington disease. Clin Chem 49:1726–1732, 2003

Mayeux R, Ottman R, Maestre G, et al: Synergistic effects of traumatic head injury and apolipoprotein-epsilon 4 in patients with Alzheimer's disease [see comments]. Neurology 45:555–557, 1995

McGue M, Gottesman II: The genetic epidemiology of schizophrenia and the design of linkage studies. Eur Arch Psychiatry Clin Neurosci 240:174–181, 1991

McInnis MG, McMahon FJ, Chase GA, et al: Anticipation in bipolar affective disorder. Am J Hum Genet 53:385–390, 1993

Mendlewicz J, Rainer JD: Adoption study supporting genetic transmission in manic-depressive illness. Nature 268:327–329, 1977

Mendlewicz J, Sevy S, Mendelbaum K: Minireview: molecular genetics in affective illness. Life Sci 52:231–242, 1993

Murphy TK, Goodman WK, Fudge MW, et al: B lymphocyte antigen D8/17: a peripheral marker for childhood-onset obsessive-compulsive disorder and Tourette's syndrome? Am J Psychiatry 154:402–407, 1997

Myers JK, Weissman MM, Tischler GL, et al: Six-month prevalence of psychiatric disorders in three communities 1980 to 1982. Arch Gen Psychiatry 41:959–967, 1984

Nelson E, Rice J: Stability of diagnosis of obsessive-compulsive disorder in the Epidemiologic Catchment Area study. Am J Psychiatry 154:826–831, 1997

Nestadt G, Samuels J, Riddle M, et al: A family study of obsessive-compulsive disorder. Arch Gen Psychiatry 57:358–363, 2000

Noyes R Jr, Crowe RR, Harris EL, et al: Relationship between panic disorder and agoraphobia: a family study. Arch Gen Psychiatry 43:227–232, 1986

Nylander PO, Engstrom C, Chotai J, et al: Anticipation in Swedish families with bipolar affective disorder. J Med Genet 31:686–689, 1994

Pauls DL, Alsobrook JP 2nd: The inheritance of obsessive-compulsive disorder. Child Adolesc Psychiatr Clin N Am 8:481–496, 1999

Pauls DL, Noyes R Jr, Crowe RR: The familial prevalence in second-degree relatives of patients with anxiety neurosis (panic disorder). J Affect Disord 1:279–285, 1979

Pauls DL, Towbin KE, Leckman JF, et al: Gilles de la Tourette's syndrome and obsessive-compulsive disorder: evidence supporting a genetic relationship. Arch Gen Psychiatry 43:1180–1182, 1986

Pauls DL, Alsobrook JP 2nd, Goodman W, et al: A family study of obsessive-compulsive disorder. Am J Psychiatry 152:76–84, 1995

Perna G, Cocchi S, Bertani A, et al: Sensitivity to 35% $CO_2$ in healthy first-degree relatives of patients with panic disorder. Am J Psychiatry 152:623–625, 1995

Perna G, Bertani A, Caldirola D, et al: Family history of panic disorder and hypersensitivity to $CO_2$ in patients with panic disorder. Am J Psychiatry 153:1060–1064, 1996

Peyser CE, Folstein SE: Huntington's disease as a model for mood disorders: clues from neuropathology and neurochemistry. Mol Chem Neuropathol 12:99–119, 1990

Philibert RA, Nelson JJ, Sandhu HK, et al: Association of an exonic LDHA polymorphism with altered respiratory response in probands at high risk for panic disorder. Am J Med Genet B Neuropsychiatr Genet 117:11–17, 2003

Pine DS, Klein RG, Roberson-Nay R, et al: Response to 5% carbon dioxide in children and adolescents: relationship to panic disorder in parents and anxiety disorders in subjects. Arch Gen Psychiatry 62:73–80, 2005

Rasmussen SA, Eisen JL: The epidemiology and clinical features of obsessive compulsive disorder. Psychiatr Clin North Am 15:743–758, 1992

Rasmussen SA, Tsuang MT: The epidemiology of obsessive compulsive disorder. J Clin Psychiatry 45:450–457, 1984

Richard F, Amouyel P: Genetic susceptibility factors for Alzheimer's disease. Eur J Pharmacol 412:1–12, 2001

Robins LN, Helzer JE, Weissman MM, et al: Lifetime prevalence of specific psychiatric disorders in three sites. Arch Gen Psychiatry 41:949–958, 1984

Rosenthal D, Wender PH, Kety SS, et al: Schizophrenics' offspring reared in adoptive homes. J Psychiatr Res 6:377–391, 1968

Shumaker SA, Legault C, Rapp SR, et al: WHIMS Investigators: estrogen plus progestin and the incidence of dementia and mild cognitive impairment in postmenopausal women: the Women's Health Initiative Memory Study: a randomized controlled trial. JAMA 289:2651–2662, 2003

Skre I, Onstad S, Torgersen S, et al: A twin study of DSM-III-R anxiety disorders. Acta Psychiatr Scand 88:85–92, 1993

Sobin C, Blundell ML, Karayiorgou M: Phenotypic differences in early- and late-onset obsessive-compulsive disorder. Compr Psychiatry 41:373–379, 2000

Stern Y, Gurland B, Tatemichi TK, et al: Influence of education and occupation on the incidence of Alzheimer's disease [see comments]. JAMA 271:1004–1010, 1994

Swedo SE, Rapoport JL, Cheslow DL, et al: High prevalence of obsessive-compulsive symptoms in patients with Sydenham's chorea. Am J Psychiatry 146:246–249, 1989a

Swedo SE, Rapoport JL, Leonard H, et al: Obsessive-compulsive disorder in children and adolescents: clinical phenomenology of 70 consecutive cases. Arch Gen Psychiatry 46:335–341, 1989b

Swedo SE, Leonard HL, Mittleman BB, et al: Identification of children with pediatric autoimmune neuropsychiatric disorders associated with streptococcal infections by a marker associated with rheumatic fever. Am J Psychiatry 154:110–112, 1997

Swedo SE, Leonard HL, Garvey M, et al: Pediatric autoimmune neuropsychiatric disorders associated with streptococcal infections: clinical description of the first 50 cases [published erratum appears in Am J Psychiatry 155:578, 1998]. Am J Psychiatry 155:264–271, 1998

Tang MX, Maestre G, Tsai WY, et al: Effect of age, ethnicity, and head injury on the association between APOE genotypes and Alzheimer's disease. Ann N Y Acad Sci 802:6–15, 1996

Tienari P: Interaction between genetic vulnerability and family environment: the Finnish adoptive family study of schizophrenia. Acta Psychiatr Scand 84:460–465, 1991

Todd RD, Reich W, Reich T: Prevalence of affective disorder in the child and adolescent offspring of a single kindred: a pilot study. J Am Acad Child Adolesc Psychiatry 33:198–207, 1994

Todd RD, Reich W, Petti TA, et al: Psychiatric diagnoses in the child and adolescent members of extended families identified through adult bipolar affective disorder probands. J Am Acad Child Adolesc Psychiatry 35:664–671, 1996

Torgersen S: Genetic factors in anxiety disorders. Arch Gen Psychiatry 40:1085–1089, 1983

Tsuang MT, Faraone SV: The Genetics of Mood Disorders. Baltimore, MD, Johns Hopkins University Press, 1990

van Dyck CH, Seibyl JP, Malison RT, et al: Age-related decline in dopamine transporters: analysis of striatal subregions, nonlinear effects, and hemispheric asymmetries. Am J Geriatr Psychiatry 10:36–43, 2002

Wahlberg KE, Wynne LC, Oja H, et al: Gene-environment interaction in vulnerability to schizophrenia: findings from the Finnish Adoptive Family Study of Schizophrenia. Am J Psychiatry 154:355–362, 1997

Webber KM, Casadesus G, Marlatt MW, et al: Estrogen bows to a new master: the role of gonadotropins in Alzheimer pathogenesis. Ann N Y Acad Sci 1052:201–209, 2005

Weissman MM: Family genetic studies of panic disorder. J Psychiatr Res 27 (suppl 1):69–78, 1993

Weissman MM, Leckman JF, Merikangas KR, et al: Depression and anxiety disorders in parents and children: results from the Yale family study. Arch Gen Psychiatry 41:845–852, 1984

Weissman MM, Bland RC, Canino GJ, et al: The cross national epidemiology of obsessive compulsive disorder. The Cross National Collaborative Group. J Clin Psychiatry 55(suppl): 5–10, 1994

Weissman MM, Bland RC, Canino GJ, et al: Cross-national epidemiology of major depression and bipolar disorder. JAMA 276:293–299, 1996

Weissman MM, Bland RC, Canino GJ, et al: The cross-national epidemiology of panic disorder. Arch Gen Psychiatry 54:305–309, 1997

Wender PH, Kety SS, Rosenthal D, et al: Psychiatric disorders in the biological and adoptive families of adopted individuals with affective disorders. Arch Gen Psychiatry 43:923–929, 1986

Wexler NS, Lorimer J, Porter J, et al: Venezuelan kindreds reveal that genetic and environmental factors modulate Huntington's disease age of onset. Project US-VCR. Proc Natl Acad Sci USA 101:3498–3503, 2004

Zandi PP, Carlson MC, Plassman BL, et al; Cache County Memory Study Investigators: Hormone replacement therapy and incidence of Alzheimer disease in older women: the Cache County Study. JAMA 288:2123–2129, 2002

# 11

# The Psychiatric Interview and Mental Status Examination

LINDA B. ANDREWS, M.D.

FRED OVSIEW, M.D., F.A.N.P.A.

## Content of the Psychiatric Interview

The principal tasks for the therapist in conducting a psychiatric interview are summarized in Table 11–1.

TABLE 11–1. **Tasks for the therapist conducting a psychiatric interview**

1. Establish goals.
2. Establish rapport.
3. Develop a collaborative doctor–patient relationship.
4. Communicate empathically.
5. Maintain appropriate boundaries.
6. Communicate in a language that the patient understands, and avoid psychiatric jargon.
7. Monitor the emotional intensity of the interview and adjust as necessary.
8. Gather pertinent psychiatric history data.
9. Perform a mental status examination.
10. Assess patient reliability.
11. Assess patient safety.
12. Develop a plan for possible emergencies.
13. Review previous records and other available data.
14. Interview others as appropriate.
15. Document accurately.
16. Manage time.

The key points for the psychiatric interview are discussed below (see Table 11–2 for outline).

TABLE 11–2. **Outline of the psychiatric interview**

1. Chief complaint
2. History of present illness
3. Psychiatric history
4. Family psychiatric and medical history
5. Medical history
6. Social history
7. Developmental history
8. Review of systems

### Chief Complaint and History of Present Illness

It is usually best to begin the interview with a relatively open-ended, unstructured question to elicit the patient's chief complaint or primary concern. These types of questions allow the patient to direct the conversation initially and to decide what is discussed first between the patient and the doctor. If possible, the psychiatrist will allow the patient adequate time to present his or her chief complaint, or primary concern, in a relatively uninterrupted manner.

Using information learned initially from the patient, the psychiatric interviewer should slowly direct the questions to obtain more details about the chief complaint and allow the chief complaint to be expanded to include a more thorough discussion of the history of the present illness. The interviewer assumes, and this is usually the case, that the chief complaint and the history of the present illness will be linked in some important way. It is extremely important to spend adequate time and effort to flesh out considerable details about the history of the present illness. Otherwise, upon completing the interview, the psychiatrist will have an understanding of the patient that is simply based on a list of facts and data points without the important personal connecting thread to develop and create this patient's story at this point in time. Questions about the history of present illness should include a review of current psychiatric symptoms: their onset, frequency, intensity, duration, precipitating factors, relieving or aggravating factors, and associated symptoms.

## Psychiatric History

Expanding the history of the present illness to inquire whether such symptoms have ever occurred before will lead to questions about the patient's psychiatric history. This discussion should include past symptom frequency, intensity, and duration; precipitating, relieving, or aggravating factors; and associated symptoms. The review of the patient's psychiatric history should include questions about past treatment with medications, therapy, or electroconvulsive therapy; previous hospitalizations; previous treatment for alcohol or substance abuse or dependence; and previous suicidal or homicidal ideation or attempts. With respect to previous medications, the psychiatrist should ask the patient to list all previously taken medications, including their dosages, side effects, length of treatment, compliance with treatment, and, if relevant, reason(s) for stopping treatment. With respect to psychotherapy, the psychiatrist should ask the patient to describe all previous experiences in psychotherapy, including therapy type, format, frequency, duration, and adherence. With respect to treatment for substance abuse, the psychiatrist should ask the patient to describe his or her substance use history, including quantity; frequency; route of administration; pattern of use; functional, interpersonal, or legal consequences of use; tolerance or withdrawal phenomena; and experience in any previous addiction treatment programs, including type and duration of the program and the patient's compliance with or completion of any such addiction treatment program (Vergare et al. 2006). The psychiatric interviewer should try to understand the patient's opinion about the efficacy of all previous treatments. The psychiatrist should avoid recommending a treatment deemed by

the patient to have been previously unsuccessful. The psychiatrist should pay particular attention to treatments that have been successful in the past, because the patient is more likely to respond to such treatments again in the future. Family members' positive responses to a particular treatment also may predict a good response for the patient being evaluated.

## Family Psychiatric History

The interviewer should gather detailed information about the patient's family psychiatric history, including the presence or absence of psychiatric illnesses in parents, grandparents, siblings, aunts, uncles, cousins, and children. A patient should be made aware that his or her risk for developing certain psychiatric illnesses, including schizophrenia, bipolar disorder, major depressive disorder, obsessive-compulsive disorder, and panic disorder, increases if his or her family members have or have had these illnesses. The psychiatric interviewer may need to use less medical jargon when inquiring about the patient's family psychiatric history, because family stories and lore about family members' previous experiences with mental illness vary widely.

## Medical History

The interviewer must inquire about the patient's past and current medical problems. Specifically, the psychiatrist needs to know what medications the patient takes regularly and if the patient is allergic to any medications or other things. Inquiry about medications also should include over-the-counter medications, herbal or energy supplements, vitamins, and complementary or alternative medical treatments (Vergare et al. 2006). The patient should be asked about any history of side effects to medications taken. Even if the patient denies any medical problems, it is important for the psychiatrist to ask specific questions about several medical illnesses, such as diabetes mellitus, seizure disorder, hypo- or hyperthyroidism, and cardiac disease, because if a patient has any of these illnesses, the psychiatrist may alter his or her diagnostic impressions or treatment plans. The psychiatrist also should inquire about a family history of medical problems.

## Social History

The psychiatric interviewer should inquire about the patient's living situation:

- Does the patient have a stable place of residence that is safe and affordable?
- Has anything about the patient's living situation changed recently?
- Are any changes expected in the near future?
- Does the patient have a reliable source of income?
- Is the patient working?
- Does the patient rely on some sort of subsidy, such as Medicare, Medicaid, or Social Security disability, for financial resources?
- Does the patient have an adequate support system, including family, friends, neighbors, and so on?
- Is the patient's support system reliable and available in times of need?
- What is the patient's sexual orientation?
- Is the patient married, single, divorced, or separated?
- Does the patient have children?
- Does the patient have family nearby and available to help?
- What is the nature of the patient's relationship with his or her family—that is, is the family supportive and helpful or intrusive and difficult?

Understanding the family system and dynamics is particularly important. If prescribed treatment plans require the patient to change behaviors, the psychiatrist must understand how such behavior changes might affect other family members. Even if a patient wishes to change his or her problematic behaviors, the family's willingness to support such change will be critical. The family's resistance to such change may severely undermine the patient's efforts for change.

The psychiatrist should ask about the patient's level of education. It is wise to ask specific questions about the patient's level of education to ensure that the interviewer does not misinterpret a patient's answers as indicative of neuropsychiatric deficits when they really represent a lower level of education. Similarly, the interviewer should gather some information about the patient's ethnic and cultural beliefs because symptoms considered to be problematic and indicative of serious psychiatric illness in Western cultures are often believed to be normal behaviors in other cultures. The psychiatrist should ask the patient if he or she has strong connections to or receives support from a particular faith or spiritual group. Does the patient have any religious or other beliefs about psychiatry and psychiatric medications that might influence the efficacy of prescribed treatments?

The interviewer should ask the patient if he or she has any habits that could negatively affect the efficacy of any psychi-

atric treatments prescribed, such as tobacco use, alcohol use, or sexual promiscuity. When inquiring about these types of habits, the interviewer must ask specific questions to elicit meaningful answers. Patients do not generally easily or openly discuss behaviors about which they have some concern, embarrassment, or shame. The examiner should consider asking some of the following questions:

- Do you drink alcohol daily?
- How many drinks do you drink each night?
- Have you ever thought you should cut back on your drinking?
- Have you ever felt annoyed by people criticizing your drinking?
- Have you ever felt guilty about your drinking?
- Have you ever had to drink first thing in the morning to relieve a hangover?
- Have you ever blacked out from alcohol use?
- Have you ever had a legal problem, such as a DWI (driving while intoxicated), from drinking too much?

A similarly detailed series of questions should be asked if the examiner suspects other drug use or abuse. Tobacco use can alter the metabolism of several psychiatric medications, so the examiner should ask every patient about smoking. The interviewer also should ask the patient about any current or pending legal problems. The interviewer should ask whether the patient is now serving or has ever served in the military. If yes, the interviewer should ask the patient to describe his or her experiences in the military. Patients who serve or did serve in the military may be eligible for specialized medical and psychological services through the federal government. Questions about domestic violence should be covered at some time during the interview, and for many psychiatrists, doing so concurrently with discussions about the patient's social history seems most appropriate. As is the case with other sensitive topics, the psychiatric interviewer will likely need to ask very specific questions about domestic violence or other abusive relationships because many patients will be reticent to discuss this with the interviewer, especially during their first meeting. The psychiatric interviewer should consider asking some of the following questions:

- Is your home a safe place to live?
- Has anyone in your family ever hit you?
- Have you ever gone to an emergency department because you were injured during a fight with your spouse or partner?

- Has anyone in your family forced you to have sexual contact with him or her against your wishes?

## Developmental History

Gathering information about the patient's developmental history is another critical aspect of the psychiatric interview. Understanding a patient's development will greatly improve the likelihood that the psychiatrist will be able to contextualize the patient's current psychiatric symptoms accurately. A truly thorough developmental history will include questioning along a number of developmental continua, including motor, language, physical, sexual, emotional, and moral. The psychiatrist should ask about any unusual perinatal events and whether the patient achieved most developmental milestones, such as talking, walking, and reading, in a normal fashion. Sometimes a patient will not remember this information, but family members, especially parents or siblings, can be particularly helpful in obtaining a thorough and accurate developmental history. Psychiatrists often focus most on the patient's emotional development because problems in this arena most dramatically influence the patient's subsequent psychiatric symptomatology. In this regard, most psychiatric interviewers ask the patient some of the following questions:

- Who lived in the home with you in early childhood?
- Are both of your parents still living?
- Did your family unit seem safe and stable to you?

Also, the psychiatrist will try to ascertain the quality of the patient's attachments to parental figures, the patient's experiences of various separations in childhood, and the quality of the patient's peer relationships, considering issues of attachment, trust, and intimacy to be of critical importance. Many adult manifestations of personality health or disorder relate significantly to the presence or absence of and the quality of these early childhood relationships. The psychiatric interviewer should ask if the patient experienced any verbal, emotional, physical, or sexual abuse as a child or teenager.

Because development extends beyond the childhood years, the psychiatric interviewer should assess the patient's ongoing development through adolescence and early, middle, and late adulthood, as appropriate, including an assessment of patterns of response to normal life transitions and major life events as well as the quality of ongoing interpersonal relationships. Some important areas to consider include how the patient handled the fol-

lowing events: moving away from home for the first time, going to college, getting married, having children, losing a job, and losing a parent.

## Review of Systems

The psychiatric interviewer should complete this portion of the evaluation by reviewing any general medical systems or psychiatric illness categories that have not previously been discussed. The psychiatric interviewer should ask every patient about his or her sleep and appetite patterns, weight regulation, and sexual functioning (MacKinnon et al. 2006). The psychiatric interviewer also should ask every patient at least one or two questions about thought, mood, anxiety, substance use, and cognitive disorders, if these have not already been covered elsewhere.

# Mental Status Examination

## General Appearance

The psychiatric interviewer should observe the patient's general appearance throughout the interview. The interviewer's report should include some comment on the patient's posture, grooming, clothing, and body habitus. When reporting this portion of the mental status examination, the interviewer may simply state that the patient's general appearance is within normal limits or may include specific mention of any particular abnormality.

If the psychiatrist has been treating a patient over time, he or she should mention any changes in the patient's general appearance, particularly because these may correlate with changes in the patient's overall mental health.

## Orientation

When a psychiatrist interviews a patient for the first time, he or she should complete some formal assessment of orientation, asking the patient his or her full name, the full date (number, month, and year), and the place where the interview is occurring (city, state, building, floor, clinic name). In subsequent appointments with the same patient, the interviewer may decide to ask these very specific orientation questions again only if the patient's attention or focus seems to have changed from previous meetings.

# Speech

## Dysarthria

In pyramidal disorders, the speech output is slow, strained, and slurred. Often accompanying the speech disorder are other features of pseudobulbar palsy, including dysphagia, drooling, and disturbance of the expression of emotions. Usually, the causative lesions are bilateral. Bulbar, or flaccid, dysarthria is marked by breathiness and nasality, as well as impaired articulation. Signs of lower motor neuron involvement can be found in the bulbar musculature. The lesion is in the lower brain stem. Scanning speech is a characteristic sign of disease of the cerebellum and its connections; the rate of speech output is irregular, with equalized stress on the syllables. In parkinsonism and in depression, speech is hypophonic and monotonous, often tailing off with longer phrases.

Darley et al. (1975) described in detail a scheme for examining the motor aspects of speech. It begins with assessment of the elements of speech production (e.g., facial musculature, tongue, palate) at rest and during voluntary movement. The patient is asked to produce the vowel "ah" steadily for as long as possible; the performance is assessed for voice quality, duration, pitch, steadiness, and loudness. Production of strings of individual consonants (e.g., "puh-puh-puh-puh") and alternated consonants (e.g., "puh-tuh-kuh-puh-tuh-kuh") is assessed for rate and rhythm. Extended utterances also are examined to observe the effects of fatigue and context.

## Stuttering and Cluttering

The rhythm of speech is disturbed by the repetition, prolongation, or arrest of sounds. Acquired stuttering, subtly different from the developmental variety (Helm-Estabrooks 1999; Van Borsel and Taillieu 2001), is unusual but can be caused by stroke (Carluer et al. 2000; Ciabarra et al. 2000; Hamano et al. 2005; Kakishita et al. 2004), traumatic brain injury (Ardila et al. 1999), psychotropic drugs (Bär et al. 2004), and extrapyramidal disease (Benke et al. 2000; Leder 1996; Nicholas et al. 2005). Although ictal or postictal stuttering occurs rarely in epilepsy, the more common occurrence is in pseudoseizures (Chung et al. 2004; Michel et al. 2004; Vossler et al. 2004). In developmental but not acquired stuttering, involuntary movements of the face and head resembling those of cranial dystonia—such as excessive blinking, forced eye closure, clonic jaw movements, and head tilt—are characteristically seen (Kiziltan and Akalin 1996). Alternatively, such movements can be interpreted as being akin to tics; this view is supported by an increased prevalence of obsessive-compulsive behaviors in persons with developmental stuttering (Abwender et al. 1998). Rarely, developmental stuttering that has been overcome returns after a brain injury, or developmental stuttering disappears after a brain injury (Helm-Estabrooks 1999). Psychogenic stuttering—marked by dramatic response to psychological treatment, atypical or "bizarre" speech features, multiple concurrent pseudoneurological complaints, and variability or situation specificity in presentation—may occur with or without concomitant organic disease (Duffy and Baumgartner 1997).

Cluttering is a disorder of fluency in which discourse, rather than purely articulation, is disturbed by a range of deficits in speech pragmatics, motor control, and attention (Daly and Burnett 1999). Speech output is abnormal because of rapid rate, disturbed prosody, sound transpositions or slips of the tongue, poor narrative skills, and impaired management of the social interaction encompassing speech. Thoughts may be expressed in fragments; words or phrases may be repeated. In sharp contrast to developmental stuttering, patients with cluttering are characteristically unconcerned about their impairment.

## Aprosodia

Ross and Mesulam (1979), following the work of Heilman and his colleagues on "auditory affective agnosia" (Heilman et al. 1975; Tucker et al. 1977), reported cases in which right hemisphere lesions led to loss of the production or recognition of affective elements of speech. Analysis of the cases led to recognition of syndromes of loss of prosody in expression and of impaired decoding of prosodic information in speech. Ross (1981) later schematized these syndromes—the "aprosodias"—as mirror images of left hemisphere aphasic syndromes, although others failed to confirm this schema (Cancelliere and Kertesz 1990; Wertz et al. 1998).

Lesions of either the left or the right hemisphere may disturb prosody, the "melody of language," which conveys both propositional and affective information. Left hemisphere lesions may be marked by prosodic abnormality, along with aphasia and cortical dysarthria; right hemisphere lesions may produce alterations in the affective component of speech, sometimes with dysarthria as well (Wertz et al. 1998). Often, appropriate test materials also disclose disturbed recognition of the affective component of material presented visually to the right hemisphere patients. Unless the primary prosodic alteration is recognized, the abnormality may appear to lie in mood or social relatedness. The examiner should listen to spontaneous speech for prosodic elements; ask the patient to produce statements in various emotional tones, such as anger, sadness, surprise, and joy; produce such emotional phrasings himself or herself, using a neutral sentence (e.g., "I am going to the store") while turning his or her face away from the patient, and ask the patient to identify the emotion; and ask the patient to reproduce an emotional phrasing the examiner has generated (Ross 1993).

## Echolalia

In echolalia, the patient repeats the speech of another person automatically, without communicative intent or effect (Ford 1989). Often, the speech repeated is the examiner's and the phenomenon is immediately apparent without being specifically elicited. However, at times other verbalizations in the environment are repeated; for example, patients may repeat words overheard from the corridor or the television. Sometimes the patient repeats only the last portion of what he or she hears, beginning with a natural break in the utterance. Sometimes grammatical corrections are made when the examiner deliberately utters an ungrammatical sentence. The patient may reverse pronouns (e.g., "I" for "you") in the interlocutor's utterance, altering the sentence in a grammatically appropriate way. These corrections and alterations evince intactness of the patient's syntactic capabilities. The patient may automatically complete a well-known phrase uttered by the examiner (the completion phenomenon): "Roses are red," says the examiner. "Roses are red, violets are blue," responds the patient. Speaking to the patient in a foreign language may elicit obviously automatic echolalic speech.

Echolalia is a normal phenomenon in the learning of language in infancy (Lecours et al. 1983). Echolalia in transcortical aphasia marks the intactness of primary language areas in the frontal and temporal lobes, with syntax thus unimpaired but disconnected from control by other language functions (Hadano et al. 1998; Mendez 2002). Other underlying disorders include autism, Tourette's syndrome, dementia of the frontal type and other degenerative disorders, catatonia, and startle reaction disorders (McPherson et al. 1994). In all these situations, echolalia may represent an environmental-dependency reaction, in which verbal responding is tightly stimulus-bound, echolalia representing the converse of failure of normal initiation of speech much as perseveration represents the converse of impersistence.

## Palilalia

Palilalia is the patient's automatic repetition of his or her own word or phrase. Commonly, the volume of the pa-

tient's voice trails off and the rate of speech is festinant; less frequently, in *palilalie atonique*, repetitions of the utterance without acceleration alternate with silence (Benke and Butterworth 2001). Despite claims to the contrary, repetition need not be confined to elements at the end of the utterance (Van Borsel et al. 2001). Palilalia occurs with extrapyramidal diseases, including progressive supranuclear palsy (Kluin et al. 1993) and postencephalitic or idiopathic parkinsonism (Benke et al. 2000), but thalamic lesions (Dietl et al. 2003), general paresis (Geschwind 1964), Tourette's syndrome (Serra-Mestres et al. 1998; Van Borsel et al. 2004), traumatic brain injury (Ardila et al. 1999), and epilepsy (Linetsky et al. 2000; Yankovsky and Treves 2002) have been implicated as well.

## Mutism

The term *mutism* should be reserved for the situation "in which a person does not speak and does not make any attempt at spoken communication despite preservation of an adequate level of consciousness" (Departments of Psychiatry and Child Psychiatry, The Institute of Psychiatry, and The Maudsley Hospital London 1987, p. 33). The first order of business in assessing an alert patient who does not speak is to examine phonation, articulation, and nonspeech movements of the relevant musculature (e.g., swallowing and coughing) to determine whether the disorder is due to elementary sensorimotor abnormalities involving the apparatus of speech.

If an elementary disorder is not at fault, the examination proceeds to a search for specific disturbances of verbal communication. Does the patient make any spontaneous attempt at communication through means other than speech? Does the patient gesture? Can the patient write, or, if hemiplegic, can he or she write with the nondominant hand? Can he or she arrange cut-out paper letters or letters from a child's set of spelling toys? Or, if familiar with sign language, can he or she sign?

Some patients with acute vascular lesions restricted to the lower primary motor cortex and the adjacent frontal operculum have transient mutism and then recover through severe dysarthria without agrammatism, a disorder known as *aphemia* (Fox et al. 2001). The same syndrome can arise from right hemisphere disease, testifying to its nature as an articulatory rather than a language disorder (Mendez 2004; Vitali et al. 2004). Transcortical motor aphasia features a prominent disturbance of spontaneous speech, occasionally beginning as mutism (M.P. Alexander 1989). Damasio and Van Hoesen (1983) described such a patient with a lesion in the dominant supplementary motor area; after recovery, the patient reported that she lacked the urge to speak. Mutism commonly develops in patients with frontotemporal dementia or primary progressive aphasia (Snowden et al. 1992). A restricted disturbance of verbal communication must be distinguished from a more global disorder of the initiation of activity. At its extreme, the latter is the state of akinetic mutism. M.P. Alexander (1999) pointed out that mutism has its "lesser forms": long latencies, terseness, and simplification of utterances.

## Language and Praxis

### *Aphasia*

The term *aphasia* refers to acquired deficits in lexical and syntactic capacities. Goodglass and Kaplan (1983) presented a scheme for examination that has been widely adopted. Higher-level disorders of language, such as pragmatic deficits and thought disorder, are discussed elsewhere in this chapter.

**Spontaneous speech.** Although the clinician hears the patient's spontaneous speech during the interview, it is nonetheless essential to listen for a period of time with an ear to language abnormalities. One listens for fluency—melody, effortfulness, rate, and phrase length—and for errors, both of syntax and of word choice (lexicon).

**Repetition.** Language disorders with spared repetition (or even excessive echolalic repetition) and disproportionately impaired repetition both occur. Repetition is tested by offering the patient phrases of increasing length and grammatical complexity. For example, one may start with single words and continue with simple phrases, then invert the phrases into questions, and then use phrases made up of grammatical function words (e.g., "no ifs, ands, or buts").

**Naming.** Naming can be tested by using items at hand: a watch and its parts; parts of the body; shirt, sleeve, and cuff; and so on. Naming is dependent on the frequency of occurrence of the target word in the vocabulary, so testing must employ less frequently used items to detect mild but clinically meaningful deficits. Occasionally, alternative methods are required, as with a blind patient (or a patient with optic aphasia or visual agnosia), for whom tactile naming can be used. One also can ask the patient to name items based on a description (e.g., "What do you call the four-legged animal that barks?" "What is the vehicle that travels underwater?"). Some patients have extraordinary domain-specific dissociations in naming ability (category-

specific anomia); for example, the ability to name vegetables may be intact, but the ability to name animals is devastated (Gainotti 2000).

**Comprehension.** Preferably the output demands are minimized in testing comprehension, so motor responses should not be required. Asking yes-or-no questions of progressive difficulty (e.g., "Am I wearing a hat?" "Is there a tree in the room?" "Does lunch come before dinner?" "Is ice cream hotter than coffee?") is simple and is systematized in the Boston Diagnostic Aphasia Examination (Goodglass and Kaplan 1983). Patients with anterior aphasia often have mild disorders of comprehension of syntactically complex material. This can be observed by asking patients to interpret sentences in which the passive voice and similarly difficult constructions are used (e.g., "The lion was killed by the tiger. Which animal is dead?").

**Reading.** Reading comprehension can be tested conveniently by offering the same stimuli as were used orally. Before diagnosing alexia, one must establish the patient's premorbid literacy. Alexia can be present with no other abnormality of language (alexia without agraphia or pure alexia) (Coslett 2000).

**Writing.** Writing is most conveniently tested by asking the patient spontaneously to write a short paragraph about his or her illness or about being in the hospital. Agraphia is a constant accompaniment of aphasic syndromes, so the writing sample is a good screening test of language function (assuming premorbid literacy). It is a particularly sensitive test in identifying confusional states (Chédru and Geschwind 1972a, 1972b). One study found that delirious patients produce jagged, angular segments of letters that should be curved (Baranowski and Patten 2000). Similarly, agraphic errors can be seen in writing samples of patients with Alzheimer's disease earlier in the course than are aphasic errors in spontaneous speech (Faber-Langendoen et al. 1988; Horner et al. 1988). Isolated defects of writing ability (pure agraphia) also occur (Luzzi and Piccirilli 2003).

## Motor Activity

The mental status examination should include specific mention of the patient's motor behavior. This should include comment on the patient's gait and station, gestures, abnormal movements, tics, and overall general body movements as witnessed throughout the entire interview. Some psychiatric illnesses, such as bipolar disorder, manic phase, may produce a tendency toward exaggerated movements, whereas others, such as schizophrenia or major depressive disorder, may produce a tendency toward sluggish or diminished body movements. Monitoring changes in motor activity over time may help the clinician track the patient's illness progression over time, including compliance with and response to psychiatric medications.

The term *agitation* is often misused to refer to the behavior of aggression or the affect of anxiety. "The preferred definition of psychomotor agitation is of a disorder of motor activity associated with mental distress which is characterized by a restricted range of repetitive, nonprogressive ('to-and-fro'), non–goal directed activity" (Day 1999, p. 95). In distinction from akathisia, the excessive movement characteristically involves the upper extremities. Agitation in the verbal sphere is manifested in repetitive questioning or complaining, screaming, or attention seeking (Cohen-Mansfield and Libin 2005). In some patients with Alzheimer's disease, wandering is associated with depressive and anxiety symptoms and may represent agitation in this cognitively impaired population (Klein et al. 1999; Logsdon et al. 1998).

### Akathisia

Motor restlessness accompanied by an urge to move is referred to as *akathisia* (Sachdev 1995). Although akathisia is most familiar as a side effect of psychotropic drugs, the phenomenon occurs often in idiopathic Parkinson's disease (Comella and Goetz 1994) and occasionally with extensive destruction of the orbitofrontal cortex, as in traumatic brain injury (Stewart 1991) or herpes simplex encephalitis (Brazzelli et al. 1994). In a few cases, it has been associated with restricted basal ganglion lesions, even occurring unilaterally with a contralateral lesion (Carrazana et al. 1989; Hermesh and Munitz 1990; Stuppaeck et al. 1995). Akathisia also may occur after withdrawal from dopamine-blocking drugs or as a tardive movement disorder (Sachdev 1995).

Eliciting the account of subjective restlessness from a psychotic patient may be difficult. Complaints specifically referable to the legs are more characteristic of akathisia than of anxiety (Sachdev and Kruk 1994). Although by derivation the term refers to an inability to sit, its objective manifestations are most prominent when the patient attempts to stand still. The patient "marches in place," shifting weight from foot to foot. Seated, the patient may shuffle or tap his or her feet or repeatedly cross his or her legs. When the disorder is severe, the recumbent patient may show myoclonic jerks or a coarse tremor of the legs.

One patient with severe withdrawal akathisia caused an ulcer on the heel of her foot by constantly rubbing her heel against the bedsheets.

### Hypertonus

Three forms of increased muscle tone concern the neuropsychiatrist. In *spasticity*, tone is increased in flexors in the upper extremity and extensors in the lower but not in the antagonists. The hypertonus shows an increase in resistance followed by an immediate decrease (the clasp-knife phenomenon) and depends on the velocity of the passive movement. This is the typical hemiplegic pattern of hemisphere stroke, universally called pyramidal, which indicates a lesion actually not in the pyramidal tract but in the corticoreticulospinal tract (G.E. Alexander and DeLong 1992; Brodal 1981). In *rigidity*, tone is increased in both agonists and antagonists throughout the range of motion; the increase is not velocity dependent. This is the characteristic hypertonus of extrapyramidal disease.

In *paratonia*, or *gegenhalten*, increased tone is erratic and depends on the intensity of the imposed movement. This pattern of hypertonus is usually related to extensive brain dysfunction, typically with frontosubcortical involvement. The erratic quality is related to the presence of both oppositional and facilitatory aspects of the patient's motor performance. Beversdorf and Heilman (1998) described a test for "facilitory paratonia": the patient's arm is repeatedly flexed to 90° and extended to 180° at the elbow, then the examiner's hand is withdrawn at the point of arm extension. In the abnormal response, the patient lifts or even continues to flex and extend the arm. Sudo et al. (2002) described the same phenomenon under the designation "elbow flexion response." A cogwheel feel to increased muscle tone is not intrinsic to the hypertonus; the cogwheeling in parkinsonism is imparted by postural (not rest) tremor superimposed on rigidity (Findley et al. 1981). In delirium and dementia, the paratonia of diffuse brain dysfunction can be mistaken for extrapyramidal rigidity when the examiner feels cogwheeling, which actually indicates the additional presence of the common tremor of metabolic encephalopathy or postural tremor of some other etiology (Kurlan et al. 2000). Striking variability in muscle tone ("poikilotonia") can occur in the acute phase of parietal stroke (Ghika et al. 1998).

### Dystonia

*Dystonia* constitutes "sustained muscle contractions, frequently causing twisting and repetitive movements, or abnormal postures" (Fahn et al. 1987, p. 335). The contractions may be generalized or focal. Typically, the dystonic arm hyperpronates, with a flexed wrist and extended fingers; the dystonic lower extremity shows an inverted foot with plantar flexion. Several syndromes of focal dystonia are well recognized, such as torticollis, writer's cramp, and blepharospasm with jaw and mouth movements (Meige syndrome). A dystonic pattern of particular interest is oculogyric crisis, in which forced thinking or other psychological disturbance accompanies forced deviation of the eyes (Benjamin 1999; Leigh et al. 1987).

Dystonic movements characteristically worsen with voluntary action and may be evoked only by very specific action patterns. Dystonic movements, especially in an early stage or mild form of the illness, can produce apparently bizarre symptoms, such as a patient who cannot walk because of twisting feet and legs but who is able to run or a patient who can do everything with his or her hands except write. Adding to the oddness is the frequent capacity of the patient to reduce the involuntary movement by using "sensory tricks" (*le geste antagoniste*); in torticollis, for example, the neck contractions that are forceful enough to break restraining devices may yield to the patient's simply touching the chin with his or her own finger. Eliciting a history of such tricks or observing the patient's use of them is diagnostic.

## Tremor

Tremors are rhythmic, regular, oscillating movements. Three major forms of tremor are distinguished. In *rest tremor*, the movement is present distally when the limb is supported and relaxed; action reduces the intensity of the tremor. The frequency is usually low, about 4–8 cps. This is the well-known tremor of Parkinson's disease. Because the amplitude of the tremor diminishes with action, rest tremor is usually less disabling than it might appear. In *postural tremor*, the outstretched limb oscillates. At times, this can be better visualized by placing a piece of paper over the outstretched hand. Postural tremor is produced by anxiety, by certain drugs (e.g., caffeine, lithium, steroids, and adrenergic agonists), and by hereditary essential tremor. A coarse, irregular, postural tremor is frequently seen in metabolic encephalopathy (Young 2002). In *intention tremor* (also called *kinetic tremor*), the active limb oscillates more prominently as the limb approaches its target during goal-directed movements, but the tremor is present throughout the movement. *Rubral*, or *midbrain*, *tremor* is a low-frequency, large-amplitude, predominantly proximal, sometimes unilateral tremor with rest, postural, and intention components (Vidailhet et al. 1998). In a few reported cases, tardive tremor has had both rest and postural components (Tarsy and Indorf 2002).

Observing the patient with arms supported and fully at rest, then with arms outstretched, and then with arms abducted to 90° at the shoulders and bent at the elbows while the hands are held palms down with the fingers pointing at each other in front of the chest will identify most upper-extremity tremors (Jankovic and Lang 2004). A given patient's organic tremor may vary in amplitude, for example, with anxiety when the patient is aware of being observed. However, anxiety and other factors do not alter tremor frequency. Thus, if the patient's tremor slows or accelerates when the examiner asks him or her to tap slowly or quickly with the opposite limb, hysteria should be suspected (Koller et al. 1989).

## Stereotypy and Mannerisms

Stereotypies are purposeless and repetitive movements that may be performed in lieu of other motor activity for long periods (Lees 1988). Ridley (1994) distinguished stereotypy from perseveration, noting that in the former, the amount of one type of behavior is excessive, and in the latter, the range of behavior is reduced so that behavior is repetitive but not excessive. Stereotypies include movements such as crossing and uncrossing the legs, clasping and unclasping the hands, picking at clothes or at the nails or skin, head banging, and rocking. In schizophrenia, a delusional idea associated with stereotyped movements can sometimes, but not always, be elicited (Jones 1965).

Stereotyped movements are seen in schizophrenia, autism, mental retardation, Rett syndrome, Tourette syndrome, neuroacanthocytosis, congenital blindness (but not in those whose blindness is acquired late; Fazzi et al. 1999), and numerous other psychopathological states (Frith and Done 1990; Ridley and Baker 1982; Stein et al. 1998). They are particularly characteristic of frontotemporal dementia (Mendez et al. 2005; Nyatsanza et al. 2003). Nonautistic children may show repetitive complex movements. These are phenomenologically distinct from tics in that they are more rhythmic, patterned, and prolonged; lack premonitory urges or internal tension; are easily abolished by distraction but are not disturbing to the child and thus are not intentionally controlled; and start earlier, often before age 2 years (Mahone et al. 2004). They may persist into adulthood and may be associated with obsessive and compulsive symptoms (Niehaus et al. 2000). At times, especially in the mentally retarded, a distinction of stereotypies from epileptic events may be difficult (Paul 1997). Many of the abnormal movements of tardive dyskinesia (e.g., chewing movements and pelvic rocking) are patterned and repetitive, not random as is chorea, and are best described as stereotypies (Kaneko et al. 1993; Stacy et al. 1993).

Amphetamine intoxication is a well-recognized cause of stereotypy, known in this setting as *punding*, a Swedish word introduced during a Scandinavian epidemic of amphetamine abuse (Rylander 1972). Similarly, cocaine and levodopa can cause stereotyped movements (Evans et al. 2004). Stereotypies occur occasionally ipsilateral or contralateral to a motor deficit during the acute phase of stroke (Ghika et al. 1995; Ghika-Schmid et al. 1997) and rarely with other focal lesions (Edwards et al. 2004; Maraganore et al. 1991; McGrath et al. 2002). Manneristic movements are purposeful movements carried out in a bizarre way. They may result from the incorporation of stereotypies into goal-directed movements (Lees 1985, 1988).

## Affect

The interviewer should note if the patient's affect changes throughout the interview. If so, the interviewer should include comment about whether the changes are congruent to the interview content and appropriate for the interview setting. The interviewer also should note whether the affect changes occur gradually or abruptly. The lack of affective responsivity may occur in several psychiatric illnesses, such as depressive or thought disorders. Affective lability and instability may occur in other psychiatric illnesses, such as during a manic phase of bipolar disorder or alcohol intoxication. A patient's affect might also be inappropriate, such as when it does not match the expressed content of the current conversation—for example, when a patient laughs while recounting a friend's death. The psychiatric interviewer should note whether the patient's affect and affect changes are appropriate.

## Mood

Reporting the patient's mood is the only element of the mental status examination that actually is historical and not observed. The interviewer should ask the patient to report his or her mood for the past few days and weeks. The psychiatric interviewer can only know this by asking the patient. Information about mood cannot be obtained simply by observation during the psychiatric interview. Whenever possible, the psychiatric interviewer should use words directly reported by the patient, such as "The patient states that her mood has been gloomy over the past few weeks." It is helpful for the psychiatrist to compare the patient's reported mood with the psychiatrist's observation of the patient's affect during the psychiatric interview. Because a patient's affect is normally more fluid

and more likely to fluctuate in response to surrounding circumstances, the patient's reported mood and manifest affect may or may not be congruent at all times. However, if the patient's mood and affect never seem to be congruent, the psychiatrist might comment on this observation to gather the patient's perspective. Patients who use denial as the defense mechanism to avoid dealing with their problems or who have poor insight into their problems may not realize that their pleasant, even cheerful, outward affective expression does not match their reported depressed mood.

## Thought Production

*Thought process* or *thought production* describes how the patient's thoughts are expressed during the psychiatric interview. The psychiatric interviewer should comment on the patient's thought production rate and flow, including comments about whether the patient's thinking is logical, goal-directed, circumstantial, or tangential or shows loosening of associations or flight of ideas (i.e., ideas are not connected one to the next). A patient's flow of thought usually can be described somewhere on the continuum between goal-directed and disconnected. Disorganizing psychiatric illnesses, such as thought disorders and bipolar disorder, manic type, most commonly cause loosely connected or disorganized thought production. Stimulant intoxication or manic episodes also can cause excessively rapid thought production.

## Thought Content

A description of the patient's thought content should include mention of important themes and the presence or absence of delusional or obsessional thinking and suicidal or homicidal thoughts. *Delusional thinking* includes fixed false beliefs that are persecutory, erotomanic, grandiose, somatic, or jealous in content. Patients with delusions believe that their fixed false beliefs are reality. Thought disorders, such as schizophrenia or schizoaffective disorder, are the most likely causes of bizarre delusions over a long time. Alcohol or drug intoxication may cause acute changes in thought content, including paranoid ideation or even delusional thinking. *Obsessions* are defined as recurrent, persistent thoughts that intrude involuntarily into a person's thinking. Obsessions appear to be senseless and are not based in reality. They most commonly occur in obsessive-compulsive disorder but also may occur in eating disorders or other impulse-control disorders. Patients with obsessions recognize that their intrusive thoughts are not normal. A patient's awareness that these thoughts are senseless, as opposed to believing them to be reality, distinguishes obsessions from delusions.

## Perceptual Disturbances

The psychiatric interviewer must inquire about the patient's perceptual abilities. Asking questions about perceptual disturbances can be particularly challenging for the novice interviewer because the questions may seem strange and even intrusive to the psychiatric interviewer him- or herself. The interviewer must ask if the patient sees, hears, smells, or feels anything that is not based on an actual sensory stimulus. Of course, the interviewer probably should word the question more clearly to a patient, such as "Do you ever see things that other people don't see?" or "Do you ever hear voices talking to you and then realize that no one is actually in the room with you?" Perceptual disturbances such as hearing, seeing, smelling, or feeling things in the absence of an actual sensory stimulus are called *hallucinations*. Hallucinations most typically occur as part of a psychotic illness, such as schizophrenia, or during intoxication or withdrawal from alcohol or illicit drugs. During a psychiatric interview, the interviewer may be able to observe a patient who is responding to internal stimuli because the patient is answering a question even though a question has not been asked or is turning to talk to someone in a different part of the room when another person is not actually present. A patient may or may not acknowledge or admit to having such perceptual disturbances. Often the patient is so frightened by the auditory or visual hallucinations that he or she denies hearing voices or seeing things even when the psychiatric interviewer is convinced that the patient has such perceptual disturbances. Patients often will admit to these hallucinations only after establishing some sort of therapeutic relationship with the doctor, after several appointments together.

## Suicidal and Homicidal Ideation

A competently conducted psychiatric interview should always include an assessment of suicidality and homicidality. The suicide assessment is particularly critical for patients with a personal or family history of suicide attempts or a family history of completed suicide and should include exploring for the presence or absence of current suicidal ideation, intent, and plan. The homicide assessment is particularly critical for patients with a history of violence or trouble with the law. If, during a psychiatric interview, the psychiatrist learns that a patient is actively suicidal or homicidal, the psychiatrist must redirect his or her interviewing efforts to manage this acute situation. Such management might be to organize admission to a psychiatric hospital for an acutely suicidal patient or to call the police to get assistance with an acutely agitated or homicidal patient. The interviewer should be knowledgeable about state laws regarding the duty to warn, should a patient threaten to harm another person.

## Attention, Concentration, and Memory

As part of the mental status examination, the psychiatric interviewer should assess the patient's attention, concentration, and memory. Theoretically, this could be done without asking any specific questions but based solely on the patient's participation in the entire psychiatric interview. This is most possible for a patient whose memory is completely intact or for a more experienced clinician. However, most clinicians will ask at least a few testing questions before concluding that the patient's attention, concentration, and memory are within normal limits. Some tests include the following:

- "Please spell the word 'world' forward for me. Now spell the word 'world' backwards."
- "Start with the number 100, subtract 7, and continue to count backward by 7s until I tell you to stop."
- "Who is the current president of the United States? Who was president before him? Who were the previous four presidents of the United States before him?"

The psychiatric interviewer must carefully choose the questions to assess attention, concentration, and memory to ensure that the questions match the patient's educational level and cultural background. Patients with lower educational levels and with non-Western cultural backgrounds may be at particular risk to perform poorly on these questions. For patients who appear to have cognitive deficits, it is recommended that the psychiatric interview include a formal Mini-Mental State Examination (MMSE), which includes a specific set of questions whose answers are scored and compared with a 30-point maximum score. Patients with cognitive disorders as well as cognitive impairment secondary to other psychiatric disorders usually have lower MMSE scores (Folstein et al. 1975). Several psychiatric disorders, in addition to actual cognitive disorders, can cause attention, concentration, memory, and other cognitive changes. Such deficits caused by psychiatric disorders, such as attention-deficit disorder or major depressive disorder, may improve with appropriate treatment. Therefore, for patients who have lower MMSE scores, the psychiatrist should repeat the MMSE at each subsequent appointment and track the patient's performance over time to monitor for cognitive changes. Upon receiving appropriate consent, the psychiatric interviewer might choose to expand his or her understanding about the patient's apparent cognitive problems by speaking with family members who live with or near the patient.

## Abstract Thinking

Some psychiatric conditions, including serious thought disorders, traumatic brain injury, and chronic alcohol or substance abuse, can impair patients' ability to perform abstract thinking. Therefore, as part of the mental status examination, most psychiatrists perform some assessment of abstraction abilities. Most often, the psychiatric interviewer will ask the patient to interpret a proverb by saying something similar to the following: "Please tell me what this saying might mean, as if you were trying to explain its meaning to a small child: 'Don't cry over spilled milk' or 'People who live in glass houses shouldn't throw stones.'" Patients with less than an eighth-grade education or patients who have not yet fully acculturated into the Western culture may struggle with this type of question, regardless of any superimposed psychiatric illness. Therefore, a psychiatrist must be guarded in interpreting the meaning of a patient's concrete responses to this type of question. The psychiatrist should incorporate data from the entire interview when determining whether a patient's thinking is more concrete than would otherwise be expected for the patient's level of education or acculturation.

## Insight/Judgment

Toward the end of the psychiatric interview and mental status examination, the interviewer should consider the degree to which the patient understands and appreciates the effect of his or her psychiatric illness on the rest of the patient's life. Psychiatrists refer to this capacity to understand one's illness as *insight*. Patients with greater insight into their illnesses generally have greater compliance with treatment recommendations. Patients with poorer insight into their illnesses tend to comply less well with treatment recommendations. Compliance can also serve as a measure of judgment. Psychiatrists assume that patients with better judgment will be more compliant with treatment recommendations.

Some interviewers ask questions to assess judgment more formally. In the past, these questions would tend to be about hypothetical situations, such as "What would you do if you found a stamped, addressed envelope on the sidewalk?" or "What would you do if you were in a movie theater and smelled smoke?" However, asking questions that are pertinent and more probable in their likelihood of occurrence is probably a more helpful approach and will likely provide a better assessment of the patient's judgment. Suggested questions include "What would you do if you ran out of your medications 1 week before your next scheduled doctor's appointment?" or "What would you do if you developed severe diarrhea 2 days after starting a new medication for your depression?" These questions allow the physician to test the patient's judgment and also introduce an effective way to discuss important treatment issues such as compliance and medication side effects.

Throughout the interview, the psychiatrist must remain cognizant of time constraints. The psychiatric interviewer should have decided before beginning the interview whether he or she will make diagnostic and treatment recommendations during the first interview or whether these issues will be presented to and discussed with the patient at a subsequent visit. If the psychiatric interviewer plans to discuss diagnosis and treatment during the first appointment, then the interviewer should manage the interview to leave adequate time toward the end for patient questions and to discuss significant diagnostic and treatment issues. If the psychiatrist has decided to have this discussion at the next appointment, then he or she should leave a few minutes at the end of this appointment to allow the patient to ask questions and to schedule the next appointment together.

## Key Points: The Psychiatric Interview and Mental Status Examination

- Establish rapport and communicate respect. Introduce yourself, use patient's name, make eye contact, and limit interruptions.

- Use empathic connection to guide and adjust interview to match the particular patient and situation. Follow the patient's leads or cues whenever possible and use open-ended questions to increase depth of understanding and information gathered (fewer topics covered, greater depth). Use focused questions to increase breadth of understanding and information gathered (more topics covered, less depth). Increase focus of questions for patients with disturbances of thought content or production, perceptual disturbances, or cognitive deficits. Abbreviate the interview for acutely agitated, dangerous, or medically compromised patients. Use words that the patient can understand—avoid medical jargon; assess the patient's education, language, and cultural needs; and use a translator when necessary. Clarify and verify that the patient understands you and that you understand the patient.

- Assess the patient's safety, including assessment of suicide risk in every patient. Assess dangerousness early and often during an interview with a potentially dangerous patient.

- Take notes to record necessary data, but do not let note taking interfere with your ability to establish and maintain rapport with the patient. Review available medical records and test results before completing your assessment and developing your treatment plan. Interview other relevant persons in the patient's life.

- Cover all key elements of the psychiatric history and mental status examination. Psychiatric history includes chief complaint, history of present illness, past psychiatric history, past medical history, social history, developmental history, family psychiatric and medical history, and review of systems. For the mental status examination, observe or assess the following aspects of behavior and thought: general appearance; orientation; speech; motor activity; affect and mood; thought production; thought content; perceptual disturbances; suicidal or homicidal ideation; attention, concentration, and memory; abstract thinking; and insight/judgment.

- Formulate the data gathered during psychiatric interview and develop a biopsychosocial formulation and a thorough differential diagnosis, including information for all five DSM-IV-TR axes. Develop a treatment plan that includes appropriate biological, psychological, and social interventions and considers the patient's overall prognosis. Ensure that the patient understands the treatment goals and plan, and verify that the patient can afford the treatment recommendations. Document if the patient refuses treatment. Establish follow-up plans (e.g., next appointment, tests to complete).

## References

Abwender DA, Trinidad KS, Jones KR, et al: Features resembling Tourette syndrome in developmental stutterers. Brain Lang 62:455–464, 1998

Alexander GE, DeLong MR: Central mechanisms of initiation and control of movement, in Diseases of the Nervous System/Clinical Neurobiology, 2nd Edition, Vol 1. Edited by Asbury AK, McKhann GM, McDonald WI. Philadelphia, PA, WB Saunders, 1992, pp 285–308

Alexander MP: Frontal lobes and language. Brain Lang 37:656–691, 1989

Alexander MP: Disturbances in language initiation: mutism and its lesser forms, in Movement Disorders in Neurology and Psychiatry, 2nd Edition. Edited by Joseph AB, Young RR. Oxford, UK, Blackwell Science, 1999, pp 366–371

Ardila A, Rosselli M, Surloff C, et al: Transient paligraphia associated with severe palilalia and stuttering: a single case report. Neurocase 5:435–440, 1999

Bär KJ, Häger F, Sauer H: Olanzapine- and clozapine-induced stuttering: a case series. Pharmacopsychiatry 37:131–134, 2004

Baranowski SL, Patten SB: The predictive value of dysgraphia and constructional apraxia for delirium in psychiatric inpatients. Can J Psychiatry 45:75–78, 2000

Benjamin S: Oculogyric crisis, in Movement Disorders in Neurology and Neuropsychiatry, 2nd Edition. Edited by Joseph AB, Young RR. Boston, MA, Blackwell Scientific, 1999, pp 92–103

Benke T, Butterworth B: Palilalia and repetitive speech: two case studies. Brain Lang 78:62–81, 2001

Benke T, Hohenstein C, Poewe W, et al: Repetitive speech phenomena in Parkinson's disease. J Neurol Neurosurg Psychiatry 69:319–325, 2000

Beversdorf DQ, Heilman KM: Facilitory paratonia and frontal lobe functioning. Neurology 51:968–971, 1998

Brazzelli M, Colombo N, Della Sala S, et al: Spared and impaired cognitive abilities after bilateral frontal damage. Cortex 30:27–51, 1994

Brodal A: Neurological Anatomy in Relation to Clinical Medicine, 3rd Edition. New York, Oxford University Press, 1981

Cancelliere AEB, Kertesz A: Lesion localization in acquired deficits of emotional expression and comprehension. Brain Cogn 13:133–147, 1990

Carluer L, Marié R-M, Lambert J, et al: Acquired and persistent stuttering as the main symptom of striatal infarction. Mov Disord 15:343–346, 2000

Carrazana E, Rossitch E, Martinez J: Unilateral "akathisia" in a patient with AIDS and a toxoplasmosis subthalamic abscess. Neurology 39:449–450, 1989

Chédru F, Geschwind N: Disorders of higher cortical functions in acute confusional states. Cortex 8:395–411, 1972a

Chédru F, Geschwind N: Writing disturbances in acute confusional states. Neuropsychologia 10:343–353, 1972b

Chung SJ, Im JH, Lee JH, et al: Stuttering and gait disturbance after supplementary motor area seizure. Mov Disord 19:1106–1109, 2004

Ciabarra AM, Elkind MS, Roberts JK, et al: Subcortical infarction resulting in acquired stuttering. J Neurol Neurosurg Psychiatry 69:546–549, 2000

Cohen-Mansfield J, Libin A: Verbal and physical non-aggressive agitated behaviors in elderly persons with dementia: robustness of syndromes. J Psychiatr Res 39:325–332, 2005

Comella CL, Goetz CG: Akathisia in Parkinson's disease. Mov Disord 9:545–549, 1994

Coslett HB: Acquired dyslexia. Semin Neurol 20:419–426, 2000

Daly DA, Burnett ML: Cluttering: traditional views and new perspectives, in Stuttering and Related Disorders of Fluency, 2nd Edition. Edited by Curlee RF. New York, Thieme Medical Publishing, 1999, pp 222–254

Damasio AR, Van Hoesen GW: Emotional disturbances associated with focal lesions of the limbic frontal lobe, in Neuropsychology of Human Emotion. Edited by Heilman KM, Satz P. New York, Guilford, 1983, pp 85–110

Darley FL, Aronson AE, Brown JR: Motor Speech Disorders. Philadelphia, PA, WB Saunders, 1975

Day RK: Psychomotor agitation: poorly defined and badly measured. J Affect Disord 55:89–98, 1999

Departments of Psychiatry and Child Psychiatry, The Institute of Psychiatry, and The Maudsley Hospital London: Psychiatric Examination: Notes on Eliciting and Recording Clinical Information in Psychiatric Patients, 2nd Edition. Oxford, UK, Oxford University Press, 1987

Dietl T, Auer DP, Modell S, et al: Involuntary vocalisations and a complex hyperkinetic movement disorder following left side thalamic haemorrhage. Behav Neurol 14:99–102, 2003

Duffy JR, Baumgartner J: Psychogenic stuttering in adults with and without neurologic disease. J Med Speech Lang Pathol 5:75–96, 1997

Edwards MJ, Dale RC, Church AJ, et al: Adult-onset tic disorder, motor stereotypies, and behavioural disturbance associated with antibasal ganglia antibodies. Mov Disord 19:1190–1196, 2004

Evans AH, Katzenschlager R, Paviour D, et al: Punding in Parkinson's disease: its relation to the dopamine dysregulation syndrome. Mov Disord 19:397–405, 2004

Faber-Langendoen K, Morris JC, Knesevich JW, et al: Aphasia in senile dementia of the Alzheimer type. Neurology 23:365–370, 1988

Fahn S, Marsden CD, Calne DB: Classification and investigation of dystonia, in Movement Disorders 2. Edited by Marsden CD, Fahn S. London, Butterworths, 1987, pp 332–358

Fazzi E, Lanners J, Danova S, et al: Stereotyped behaviours in blind children. Brain Dev 21:522–528, 1999

Findley LJ, Gresty MA, Halmagyi GM: Tremor, the cogwheel phenomenon and clonus in Parkinson's disease. J Neurol Neurosurg Psychiatry 44:534–546, 1981

Folstein MF, Folstein SE, McHugh PR: "Mini-Mental State": a practical method for grading the cognitive state of patients for the clinician. J Psychiatr Res 12:189–198, 1975

Ford RA: The psychopathology of echophenomena. Psychol Med 19:627–635, 1989

Fox RJ, Kasner SE, Chatterjee A, et al: Aphemia: an isolated disorder of articulation. Clin Neurol Neurosurg 103:123–126, 2001

Frith CD, Done DJ: Stereotyped behaviour in madness and in health, in Neurobiology of Stereotyped Behaviour. Edited by Cooper SJ, Dourish CT. Oxford, UK, Clarendon Press, 1990, pp 232–259

Gainotti G: What the locus of brain lesion tells us about the nature of the cognitive defect underlying category-specific disorders: a review. Cortex 36:539–559, 2000

Geschwind N: Non-aphasic disorders of speech. Int J Neurol 4:207–214, 1964

Ghika J, Bogousslasvky J, van Melle G, et al: Hyperkinetic motor behaviors contralateral to hemiplegia in acute stroke. Eur Neurol 35:27–32, 1995

Ghika J, Ghika-Schmid F, Bogousslasvky J: Parietal motor syndrome: a clinical description in 32 patients in the acute phase of pure parietal strokes studied prospectively. Clin Neurol Neurosurg 100:271–282, 1998

Ghika-Schmid F, Ghika J, Regli F, et al: Hyperkinetic movement disorders during and after acute stroke: the Lausanne Stroke Registry. J Neurol Sci 146:109–116, 1997

Goodglass H, Kaplan E: The Assessment of Aphasia and Related Disorders, 2nd Edition. Philadelphia, PA, Lea & Febiger, 1983

Hadano K, Nakamura H, Hamanaka T: Effortful echolalia. Cortex 34:67–82, 1998

Hamano T, Hiraki S, Kawamura Y, et al: Acquired stuttering secondary to callosal infarction. Neurology 64:1092–1093, 2005

Heilman KM, Scholes R, Watson RT: Auditory affective agnosia: disturbed comprehension of affective speech. J Neurol Neurosurg Psychiatry 38:69–72, 1975

Helm-Estabrooks N: Stuttering associated with acquired neurological disorders, in Stuttering and Related Disorders of Fluency, 2nd Edition. Edited by Curlee RF. New York, Thieme Medical Publishers, 1999, pp 255–268

Hermesh H, Munitz H: Unilateral neuroleptic-induced akathisia. Clin Neuropharmacol 13:253–258, 1990

Horner J, Heyman A, Dawson D, et al: The relationship of agraphia to the severity of dementia in Alzheimer's disease. Arch Neurol 45:760–763, 1988

Jankovic J, Lang AE: Movement disorders: diagnosis and assessment, in Neurology in Clinical Practice, 4th Edition, Vol 1. Edited by Bradley WG, Daroff RB, Fenichel G, et al. Philadelphia, PA, Butterworth-Heinemann, 2004, pp 293–322

Jones IH: Observations on schizophrenic stereotypies. Compr Psychiatry 6:323–335, 1965

Kakishita K, Sekiguchi E, Maeshima S, et al: Stuttering without callosal apraxia resulting from infarction in the anterior corpus callosum. J Neurol 251:1140–1141, 2004

Kaneko K, Yuasa T, Miyatake T, et al: Stereotyped hand clasping: an unusual tardive movement disorder. Mov Disord 8:230–231, 1993

Kiziltan G, Akalin MA: Stuttering may be a type of action dystonia. Mov Disord 11:278–282, 1996

Klein DA, Steinberg M, Galik E, et al: Wandering behaviour in community-residing persons with dementia. Int J Geriatr Psychiatry 14:272–279, 1999

Kluin KJ, Foster NL, Berent S, et al: Perceptual analysis of speech disorders in progressive supranuclear palsy. Neurology 43:563–566, 1993

Koller W, Lang A, Vetere-Overfield B, et al: Psychogenic tremors. Neurology 39:1094–1099, 1989

Kurlan R, Richard IH, Papka M, et al: Movement disorders in Alzheimer's disease: more rigidity of definitions is needed. Mov Disord 15:24–29, 2000

Lecours AR, Lhermitte F, Bryans B: Aphasiology. London, Ballière Tindall, 1983

Leder SB: Adult onset of stuttering as a presenting sign in a parkinsonian-like syndrome: a case report. J Commun Disord 29:471–478, 1996

Lees AJ: Tics and Related Disorders. Edinburgh, Churchill Livingstone, 1985

Lees AJ: Facial mannerisms and tics. Adv Neurol 49:255–261, 1988

Leigh RJ, Foley JM, Remler BF, et al: Oculogyric crisis: a syndrome of thought disorder and ocular deviation. Ann Neurol 22:13–17, 1987

Linetsky E, Planer D, Ben-Hur T: Echolalia-palilalia as the sole manifestation of nonconvulsive status epilepticus. Neurology 55:733–734, 2000

Logsdon RG, Teri L, McCurry SM, et al: Wandering: a significant problem among community-residing individuals with Alzheimer's disease. J Gerontol B Psychol Sci Soc Sci 53:P294–P299, 1998

Luzzi S, Piccirilli M: Slowly progressive pure dysgraphia with late apraxia of speech: a further variant of the focal cerebral degeneration. Brain Lang 87:355–360, 2003

MacKinnon RA, Michels R, Buckley PJ: The Psychiatric Interview in Clinical Practice, 2nd Edition. Washington, DC, American Psychiatric Publishing, 2006

Mahone EM, Bridges D, Prahme C, et al: Repetitive arm and hand movements (complex motor stereotypies) in children. J Pediatr 145:391–395, 2004

Maraganore DM, Lees AJ, Marsden CD: Complex stereotypies after right putaminal infarction: a case report. Mov Disord 6:358–361, 1991

McGrath CM, Kennedy RE, Hoye W, et al: Stereotypic movement disorder after acquired brain injury. Brain Inj 16:447–451, 2002

McPherson SE, Kuratani JD, Cummings JL, et al: Creutzfeldt-Jakob disease with mixed transcortical aphasia: insights into echolalia. Behav Neurol 7:197–203, 1994

Mendez MF: Prominent echolalia from isolation of the speech area. J Neuropsychiatry Clin Neurosci 14:356–357, 2002

Mendez MF: Aphemia-like syndrome from a right supplementary motor area lesion. Clin Neurol Neurosurg 106:337–339, 2004

Mendez MF, Shapira JS, Miller BL: Stereotypical movements and frontotemporal dementia. Mov Disord 20:742–745, 2005

Michel V, Burbaud P, Taillard J, et al: Stuttering or reflex seizure? A case report. Epileptic Disord 6:181–185, 2004

Nicholas AP, Earnst KS, Marson DC: Atypical Hallervorden-Spatz disease with preserved cognition and obtrusive obsessions and compulsions. Mov Disord 20:880–886, 2005

Niehaus DJ, Emsley RA, Brink P, et al: Stereotypies: prevalence and association with compulsive and impulsive symptoms in college students. Psychopathology 33:31–35, 2000

Nyatsanza S, Shetty T, Gregory C, et al: A study of stereotypic behaviours in Alzheimer's disease and frontal and temporal variant frontotemporal dementia. J Neurol Neurosurg Psychiatry 74:1398–1402, 2003

Paul A: Epilepsy or stereotypy? Diagnostic issues in learning disabilities. Seizure 6:111–120, 1997

Ridley RM: The psychology of perseverative and stereotyped behaviour. Prog Neurobiol 44:221–231, 1994

Ridley RM, Baker HF: Stereotypy in monkeys and humans. Psychol Med 12:61–72, 1982

Ross ED: The aprosodias: functional-anatomic organization of the affective components of language in the right hemisphere. Arch Neurol 38:561–569, 1981

Ross ED: Nonverbal aspects of language. Neurol Clin 11:9–23, 1993

Ross ED, Mesulam M-M: Dominant language functions of the right hemisphere? Prosody and emotional gesturing. Arch Neurol 36:144–148, 1979

Rylander G: Psychoses and the punding and choreiform syndromes in addiction to central stimulant drugs. Psychiatr Neurol Neurochir 75:203–212, 1972

Sachdev P: Akathisia and Restless Legs. Cambridge, UK, Cambridge University Press, 1995

Sachdev P, Kruk J: Clinical characteristics and predisposing factors in acute drug-induced akathisia. Arch Gen Psychiatry 51:963–974, 1994

Serra-Mestres J, Robertson MM, Shetty T: Palicoprolalia: an unusual variant of palilalia in Gilles de la Tourette's syndrome. J Neuropsychiatry Clin Neurosci 10:117–118, 1998

Snowden JS, Neary D, Mann DM, et al: Progressive language disorder due to lobar atrophy. Ann Neurol 31:174–183, 1992

Stacy M, Cardoso F, Jankovic J: Tardive stereotypy and other movement disorders in tardive dyskinesias. Neurology 43:937–941, 1993

Stein DJ, Niehaus DJH, Seedat S, et al: Phenomenology of stereotypic movement disorder. Psychiatr Ann 28:397–412, 1998

Stewart JT: Akathisia following traumatic brain injury: treatment with bromocriptine. J Neurol Neurosurg Psychiatry 52:1200–1201, 1991

Stuppaeck CH, Miller CH, Ehrmann H, et al: Akathisia induced by necrosis of the basal ganglia after carbon monoxide intoxication. Mov Disord 10:229–231, 1995

Sudo K, Matsuyama T, Goto Y, et al: Elbow flexion response as another primitive reflex. Psychiatry Clin Neurosci 56:131–137, 2002

Tarsy D, Indorf G: Tardive tremor due to metoclopramide. Mov Disord 17:620–621, 2002

Tucker DM, Watson RT, Heilman KM: Discrimination and evocation of affectively intoned speech in patients with right parietal disease. Neurology 27:947–950, 1977

Van Borsel J, Taillieu C: Neurogenic stuttering versus developmental stuttering: an observer judgment study. J Commun Disord 34:385–395, 2001

Van Borsel J, Schelpe L, Santens P, et al: Linguistic features in palilalia: two case studies. Clin Linguist Phon 15:663–677, 2001

Van Borsel J, Goethals L, Vanryckeghem M: Disfluency in Tourette syndrome: observational study in three cases. Folia Phoniatr Logop 56:358–366, 2004

Vergare MJ, Binder RL, Cook IA, et al: Practice guideline for the psychiatric evaluation of adults, 2nd Edition. Am J Psychiatry 163:1–36, 2006

Vidailhet M, Jedynak CP, Pollak P, et al: Pathology of symptomatic tremors. Mov Disord 13 (suppl 3):49–54, 1998

Vitali P, Nobili F, Raiteri U, et al: Right hemispheric dysfunction in a case of pure progressive aphemia: fusion of multimodal neuroimaging. Psychiatry Res 130:97–107, 2004

Vossler DG, Haltiner AM, Schepp SK, et al: Ictal stuttering: a sign suggestive of psychogenic nonepileptic seizures. Neurology 63:516–519, 2004

Wertz RT, Henschel CR, Auther LL, et al: Affective prosodic disturbance subsequent to right hemisphere stroke: a clinical application. J Neurolinguistics 11:89–102, 1998

Yankovsky AE, Treves TA: Postictal mixed transcortical aphasia. Seizure 11:278–279, 2002

Young RR: What is a tremor? Neurology 58:165–166, 2002

# 12

# Laboratory Testing in Psychiatry

H. FLORENCE KIM, M.D.

PAUL E. SCHULZ, M.D.

ELISABETH A. WILDE, Ph.D.

STUART C. YUDOFSKY, M.D.

## Approach to Screening Laboratory and Diagnostic Testing of Psychiatric Patients

Table 12–1 lists some of the many medical and neurological illnesses that may present with prominent neuropsychiatric symptoms.

### Screening Laboratory Testing

Several studies have been conducted to investigate the utility of screening laboratory testing in the psychiatric patient, although most of these have been conducted in a retrospective manner, drawing from varied patient populations (Barnes et al. 1983; Catalano et al. 2001; Dolan and Mushlin 1985; Hall et al. 1980; Korn et al. 2000; Mookhoek and Sterrenburg-vdNieuwegiessen 1998; Sheline and Kehr 1990; White and Barraclough 1989; Willett and King 1977).

Based on these varied studies, it appears that patients with psychiatric complaints alone, without other medical problems or complaints, will benefit from a few screening tests such as serum glucose concentration, serum urea nitrogen concentration, creatinine clearance, and urinalysis (Anfinson and Kathol 1992). Screening of female psychiatric patients older than 50 years, especially those with mood symptoms, may be justified because of a high prevalence of hypothyroidism in the patients.

### Screening Electroencephalograms

The electroencephalogram (EEG) can be very useful when a patient has altered mental status, such as delirium or encephalopathy. It can be useful for distinguishing between possible diagnoses. For example, it can diagnose complex partial status epilepticus. It can also be useful for diagnosing metabolic encephalopathy, which is generally due to a systemic illness that is having an effect on the nervous system. The EEG is also useful for distinguishing some specific etiologies of encephalopathy. For example, it might show the di- and triphasic waves characteristic of renal failure, hepatic failure, or anoxia. In the patient who is frankly comatose, the EEG can be very valuable for identifying the level of nervous system impairment. For example, it can show an alpha coma pattern or a theta coma pattern characteristic of brain stem lesions producing coma or may show a delta coma pattern characteristic of bihemispheric disease. In the patient who appears to be obtunded, the EEG can be useful for determining whether a patient is catatonic, and hence has a normal, awake-looking EEG, versus encephalopathic, where there might be diffuse slowing or triphasic waves (metabolic encephalopathy).

**TABLE 12–1.  Selected medical conditions with psychiatric manifestations**

Neurological

Cerebrovascular disease

Multiple sclerosis

Multiple systems atrophy

Parkinson's disease

Progressive supranuclear palsy

Alzheimer's disease

Frontotemporal dementias

Dementia associated with Lewy bodies

Seizure disorder

Huntington's disease

Traumatic brain injury

Anoxic brain injury

Migraine headache

Sleep disorders (narcolepsy, sleep apnea)

Normal-pressure hydrocephalus

Neoplastic

Central nervous system tumors, primary and metastatic

Pancreatic carcinoma

Paraneoplastic syndromes

Endocrine tumors

Pheochromocytoma

Infectious

HIV

Neurosyphilis

Creutzfeldt-Jakob disease

Systemic viral and bacterial infections

Viral and bacterial meningitis and encephalitis

Tuberculosis

Infectious mononucleosis

Pediatric autoimmune neuropsychiatric disorder associated with streptococcal infections (PANDAS)

Nutritional

Vitamin deficiencies

$B_{12}$: pernicious anemia

Folate: megaloblastic anemia

Nicotinic acid deficiency: pellagra

Thiamine deficiency: Wernicke-Korsakoff syndrome

Trace mineral deficiency (zinc, magnesium)

**TABLE 12–1.  Selected medical conditions with psychiatric manifestations (continued)**

Autoimmune

Systemic lupus erythematosus

Sarcoidosis

Sjögren's syndrome

Behçet's syndrome

Endocrine/metabolic

Wilson's disease

Fluid and electrolyte disturbances (syndrome of inappropriate antidiuretic hormone [SIADH], central pontine myelinolysis)

Porphyrias

Uremias

Hypercapnia

Hepatic encephalopathy

Hyper-/hypocalcemia

Hyper-/hypoglycemia

Thyroid and parathyroid disease

Diabetes mellitus

Pheochromocytoma

Pregnancy

Gonadotropic hormonal disturbances

Panhypopituitarism

Drugs and toxins

Environmental toxins: organophosphates, heavy metals, carbon monoxide

Drug or alcohol intoxication/withdrawal

Adverse effects of prescription and over-the-counter medications

*Source.*  Adapted from Ringholz 2001; Sadock and Sadock 2007; Wallach 2000.

# Laboratory Approach to Specific Clinical Situations in Psychiatry

Table 12–2 presents a list of screening laboratory tests that clinicians often use during the initial evaluation of the patient with psychiatric complaints.

## New-Onset Psychosis

Routine screening tests often include serum chemistries, such as sodium, potassium, chloride, carbon dioxide, serum urea nitrogen, and creatinine; liver function tests;

**TABLE 12–2. Useful screening laboratory tests in the workup of the neuropsychiatric patient**

| Test | Reference range | Indication | Comments |
|---|---|---|---|
| **Hematological studies** | | | |
| Coombs test, direct and indirect | Positive/negative | Hemolytic anemias secondary to psychiatric medications | Evaluation of drug-induced hemolytic anemias, such as those secondary to chlorpromazine, phenytoin, levodopa, and methyldopa |
| Ferritin (serum) | 20–323 ng/mL 16–283 ng/mL | Cognitive/neuropsychiatric workup | Decreased: iron-deficiency anemia; most-sensitive test Elevated: anemias other than iron-deficiency |
| Folate Plasma Red cell | 3.1–12.4 ng/mL 186–645 ng/mL | Alcohol abuse | Used in vitamin $B_{12}$ deficiencies associated with psychosis, paranoia, fatigue, agitation, dementia, delirium |
| Hemoglobin | Male: 13.8–17.2 g/dL Female: 12.1–15.1 g/dL | Cognitive/neuropsychiatric workup | Decreased: alcohol abuse, cirrhosis, liver disease |
| Hematocrit | Male: 40.7%–50.3% Female: 44.3%–63.1% | Cognitive/neuropsychiatric workup | |
| Iron (serum) | 45–160 µg/dL 30–160 µg/dL | Cognitive/neuropsychiatric workup | Decreased: iron-deficiency anemia, other normochromic anemias |
| Iron-binding capacity | 220–420 µg/dL | Cognitive/neuropsychiatric workup | Decreased: hemochromatosis, liver cirrhosis, thalassemia Elevated: iron-deficiency anemia, acute and chronic blood loss, acute liver damage |
| Mean corpuscular volume | $87 \pm 5$ µm$^3$ | Alcohol abuse | Elevated: alcoholism and vitamin $B_{12}$ and folate deficiency |
| Partial thromboplastin time | 21–32 secs | Treatment with antipsychotics, heparin | Monitor anticoagulant therapy; elevated: in presence of lupus anticoagulant and anticardiolipin antibodies |
| Platelets | $1.8$–$6.6 \times 10^3$/µL $140$–$144 \times 10^3$/µL | Use of psychotropic medications | Decreased by certain psychotropic medications (carbamazepine, clozapine, phenothiazines) |
| Porphobilinogen deaminase (erythrocyte uroporphyrinogen I synthase) | 2.1–4.3 mU/g Hgb | Porphyrias | Decreased: porphyria synthesizing enzyme in red blood cells (RBCs) in patients with acute intermittent porphyria |
| Prothrombin time | 8.2–10.3 sec | Cognitive/medical workup | Elevated: significant liver damage (cirrhosis) |

**TABLE 12–2.    Useful screening laboratory tests in the workup of the neuropsychiatric patient (continued)**

| Test | Reference range | Indication | Comments |
| --- | --- | --- | --- |
| **Hematological studies (continued)** | | | |
| Reticulocyte count | 0.5%–1.5% | Cognitive/medical workup | Decreased: megaloblastic or iron-deficiency anemia and anemia of chronic disease, alcoholism. Indicator of effective RBC production |
| White blood cell (WBC) count | $3.8–9.8 \times 10^3/\mu L$ | Use of psychiatric medications | Leukopenia and agranulocytosis associated with certain psychotropic medications, such as phenothiazines, carbamazepine, clozapine. Leukocytosis associated with lithium and neuroleptic syndrome |
| **Serum chemistries/vitamins** | | | |
| Acid phosphatase | 0–0.7 IU/L | Cognitive/medical workup | Elevated: prostate cancer, benign prostatic hypertrophy, excessive platelet destruction, bone disease |
| Alanine transaminase (ALT)/serum glutamate pyruvate transaminase (SGPT) | 7–53 IU/L | Neuropsychiatric workup | Elevated: hepatitis, cirrhosis, liver metastasis. Decreased: $B_6$/pyridoxine deficiency |
| Albumin | 3.6–5.0 g/dL | Cognitive/medical workup | Elevated: dehydration |
| Alkaline phosphatase | 38–126 IU/L | Cognitive/neuropsychiatric workup; Use of psychiatric medications | Elevated: Paget's disease, hyperparathyroidism, hepatic disease, liver metastases, heart failure, phenothiazine use. Decreased: pernicious anemia (vitamin $B_{12}$ deficiency) |
| Ammonia | 11–35 μmol/L | Cognitive/neuropsychiatric workup | Elevated: hepatic encephalopathy, liver failure, Reye's syndrome; increases with gastrointestinal hemorrhage and severe congestive heart failure |
| Amylase | 25–115 IU/L | Eating disorders | May be elevated in bulimia nervosa |
| Aspartate aminotransferase (AST)/serum glutamic oxaloacetic transaminase (SGOT) | 11–47 IU/L | Cognitive/neuropsychiatric workup | Elevated: heart failure, hepatic disease, pancreatitis, eclampsia, cerebral damage, alcoholism. Decreased: pyridoxine (vitamin $B_6$) deficiency, terminal stages of liver disease |
| Bicarbonate | 21–29 mEq/L | Panic disorder; Eating disorder | Decreased: hyperventilation syndrome, panic disorder, anabolic steroid abuse. May be elevated in patients with bulimia nervosa, in laxative abuse, psychogenic vomiting |

**TABLE 12–2.  Useful screening laboratory tests in the workup of the neuropsychiatric patient** (*continued*)

| Test | Reference range | Indication | Comments |
|---|---|---|---|
| *Serum chemistries/vitamins (continued)* | | | |
| Bilirubin | 0.3–1.1 mg/dL | Cognitive/neuropsychiatric workup | Elevated: hepatic disease |
| Blood urea nitrogen | 7–35 mg/dL | Delirium | Elevated: renal disease, dehydration |
| Calcium | 8.6–10.3 mg/dL | Cognitive/neuropsychiatric workup<br>Mood disorders<br>Psychosis<br>Eating disorders | Elevated: hyperparathyroidism, bone metastases<br>Elevation associated with delirium, depression, psychosis<br>Decreased: hypoparathyroidism, renal failure<br>Decrease associated with depression, irritability, delirium, chronic laxative abuse |
| Chloride | 97–110 mmol/L | Eating disorder<br>Panic disorder | Decreased: patients with bulimia, psychogenic vomiting<br>Mild elevation in hyperventilation syndrome, panic disorder |
| $CO_2$ content (plasma) | 22–32 mmol/L | Cognitive/neuropsychiatric workup<br>Delirium | |
| Creatine phosphokinase (CPK) | ≤150 U/L | Delirium | Elevated: neuroleptic malignant syndrome, intramuscular injection rhabdomyolysis (secondary to substance abuse), patients in restraint, patients experiencing dystonic reactions; asymptomatic elevations with use of antipsychotic drugs |
| Creatinine | 0.8–1.8 g/day | Cognitive/neuropsychiatric workup | Elevated: renal disease (see blood urea nitrogen) |
| Gamma-glutamyl transpeptidase (serum) | 11–50 IU/L<br>7–32 IU/L | Alcohol abuse | Elevated: alcohol abuse, cirrhosis, liver disease |
| Glucose | 65–109 mg/dL | Panic attacks<br>Anxiety<br>Delirium<br>Depression | Very high fasting blood sugar associated with delirium<br>Very low fasting blood sugar associated with delirium, agitation, panic attacks, anxiety, depression |
| Lactate dehydrogenase | 100–250 IU/L | Cognitive/neuropsychiatric workup | Elevated: myocardial infarction, pulmonary infarction, hepatic disease, renal infarction, seizures, cerebral damage, megaloblastic (pernicious) anemia<br>Factitious elevations secondary to rough handling of blood specimen tube |

**TABLE 12–2.** Useful screening laboratory tests in the workup of the neuropsychiatric patient (*continued*)

| Test | Reference range | Indication | Comments |
|---|---|---|---|
| **Serum chemistries/vitamins (*continued*)** | | | |
| Magnesium (serum) | 65–109 mg/dL | Alcohol abuse | Decreased: alcoholism; low levels associated with agitation, delirium, seizures |
| Phosphorus (serum) | 2.5–4.5 mg/dL | Cognitive/neuropsychiatric workup | Increased: acute porphyria |
| Potassium | 3.3–4.9 mmol/L | Cognitive/neuropsychiatric workup Eating disorders | Increased: hyperkalemic acidosis |
| | | | Increase associated with anxiety in cardiac arrhythmia |
| | | | Decreased: cirrhosis, metabolic alkalosis, laxative abuse, diuretic abuse |
| | | | Decrease common in bulimic patients and in psychogenic vomiting, anabolic steroid abuse |
| Protein (total) | 6.5–8.5 g/dL | Cognitive/neuropsychiatric workup | Increased: multiple myeloma, myxedema, lupus |
| Sodium | 135–145 mmol/L | Cognitive/neuropsychiatric workup | Decreased: water intoxication; SIADH; use of carbamazepine; myxedema, congestive heart failure, diarrhea, polydipsia, renal failure |
| | | | Increased: diabetes insipidus; anabolic steroids |
| Vitamin A (serum) | 360–1,200 mg/L | Depression Delirium | Hypervitaminosis A is associated with a variety of mental status changes, headache |
| Vitamin B$_{12}$ (serum) | 200–1,100 pg/mL | Cognitive/neuropsychiatric workup Dementia Mood disorder | Part of workup of megaloblastic anemia and dementia B$_{12}$ deficiency associated with psychosis, paranoia, fatigue, agitation, dementia, delirium Often associated with chronic alcohol abuse |
| Zinc (serum) | 75–120 µg/dL | Cognitive/neuropsychiatric workup | |
| **Endocrine studies** | | | |
| Beta-human chorionic gonadotropin | Negative | Pregnancy test | Prior to initiation of teratogenic psychotropic medications |
| Catecholamines, urinary and plasma Homovanillic acid, vanillylmandelic acid | <540 µg/day | Panic attacks Anxiety | Elevated: pheochromocytoma |
| Corticotropin | <60 pg/mL | Cognitive/neuropsychiatric workup | Changes with steroid abuse; may be elevated in seizures, psychosis, Cushing's disease, and in response to stress |
| Cortisol | 6–30 mg/dL | Cognitive/neuropsychiatric workup Mood disorders | Excess levels may indicate Cushing's disease; associated with anxiety, depression, and variety of other conditions |

**TABLE 12–2.** Useful screening laboratory tests in the workup of the neuropsychiatric patient (*continued*)

| Test | Reference range | Indication | Comments |
|---|---|---|---|
| **Endocrine studies** (*continued*) | | | |
| Estrogens (total) | Male: 29–127 pg/mL<br>Female: 35–650 pg/mL (varies over menstrual cycle) | Mood disorder | Decreased: menopausal depression and premenstrual syndrome; variable changes in anxiety |
| Follicle-stimulating hormone | Male: 1.1–13.5 mIU/mL<br>Female: 0.4–22.6 mIU/mL (varies over menstrual cycle) | Depression | High normal in anorexia nervosa, higher values in postmenopausal women; low levels in patients with panhypopituitarism |
| Growth hormone | Male: <1 ng/mL<br>Female: <10 ng/mL | Depression<br>Anxiety<br>Schizophrenia | Blunted response to insulin-induced hypoglycemia in depressed patients; increased response to dopamine agonist challenge in schizophrenic patients; elevated in some anorexic patients |
| Luteinizing hormone | Male: 1.4–7.7 mIU/mL<br>Female: 1.6–62.0 mIU/mL (varies over menstrual cycle) | Depression | Decreased: patients with panhypopituitarism<br>Decrease associated with depression |
| Parathyroid hormone | 12–72 pg/mL | Anxiety<br>Cognitive/neuropsychiatric workup | Low level causes hypocalcemia and anxiety<br>Dysregulation associated with wide variety of organic mental disorders |
| Prolactin | Male: 1.6–18.8 ng/mL<br>Female: 1.4–24.2 ng/mL | Use of antipsychotic medications<br>Cocaine use<br>Pseudoseizures | Antipsychotics, by decreasing dopamine, increase prolactin synthesis and release, especially in women<br>Elevated: cocaine withdrawal<br>Lack of prolactin elevation after seizure suggestive of pseudoseizure |
| Testosterone (serum) | Male: 270–1,070 ng/dL<br>Female: 6–86 ng/dL | Impotence<br>Inhibited sexual desire | Elevated: anabolic steroid abuse<br>May be decreased in impotence and inhibited sexual desire<br>Used in follow-up of sex offenders treated with medroxyprogesterone<br>Decreased: medroxyprogesterone treatment |
| **Thyroid function tests** | | | |
| Thyrotropin | 2–11 μU/mL | Cognitive/neuropsychiatric workup<br>Depression | Detection of hypo- or hyperthyroidism<br>Abnormalities can be associated with depression, anxiety, psychosis, dementia, delirium, lithium treatment |
| Thyroxine (T$_4$) | 4–11 μg/dL | | |

**TABLE 12–2. Useful screening laboratory tests in the workup of the neuropsychiatric patient (continued)**

| Test | Reference range | Indication | Comments |
|---|---|---|---|
| **Endocrine studies (continued)** | | | |
| Thyroid function tests (continued) | | | |
| Triiodothyronine ($T_3$) | 75–220 ng/dL | | |
| Thyroxine-binding globulin capacity | 12–28 µg/dL | | |
| $T_3$ resin uptake | 25%–35% | | |
| **Autoimmune studies** | | | |
| Antinuclear antibody | Negative at 1:10 dilution | Cognitive/neuropsychiatric workup | Most sensitive test for systemic lupus erythematosus (SLE; detects up to 95% of cases); specificity is low in rheumatic diseases in general (50%) — Elevated: SLE and drug-induced lupus (e.g., secondary to phenothiazines, anticonvulsants); SLE can be associated with delirium, psychosis, mood disorders |
| Anti-DNA antibody | None detected | Cognitive/neuropsychiatric workup | Positive in 40%–80% of SLE patients — High titers characteristic of SLE; low titers in other rheumatic diseases |
| Erythrocyte sedimentation rate | <20 mm/hour | Cognitive/neuropsychiatric workup | Elevated: nonspecific indicator of infectious, inflammatory, autoimmune, or malignant disease; sometimes recommended in the evaluation of anorexia nervosa |
| Lupus anticoagulant | Negative | Use of phenothiazines | An antiphospholipid antibody that has been described in some patients using phenothiazines, especially chlorpromazine; often associated with elevated partial thromboplastin time; associated with anticardiolipin antibodies |
| Rheumatoid factor | 0.0–20.0 IU/mL | Neuropsychiatric workup | Use in evaluation of stroke in young person or in cases of vasculitis |
| **Cerebrospinal fluid (CSF) studies** | | | |
| Acid-fast bacilli stain | None detected | Neuropsychiatric workup | Useful for diagnosis of tuberculous meningitis |
| Cell count (CSF) | 0–2 WBCs / 0–5 RBCs | Neuropsychiatric workup | Lymphocytes present in tuberculous meningitis — Polymorphonuclear leukocytes present in bacterial meningitis |
| Culture and sensitivities | | Neuropsychiatric workup | For evaluation of bacterial meningitis/encephalitis |

**TABLE 12–2.** Useful screening laboratory tests in the workup of the neuropsychiatric patient (*continued*)

| Test | Reference range | Indication | Comments |
|---|---|---|---|
| **Cerebrospinal fluid (CSF) studies** (*continued*) | | | |
| Glucose (CSF) | 65–109 mg/dL | Neuropsychiatric workup | Decreased: bacterial, tuberculous and fungal meningitis |
| Immunoglobulin (Ig) G | <4 mg/dL | Neuropsychiatric workup | Elevated in 70% of multiple sclerosis (MS) patients |
| Myelin basic protein | 0.07–4.10 ng/mL | Neuropsychiatric workup | Elevated in 70%–90% of MS patients during an acute exacerbation; also elevated in other demyelinating diseases |
| Protein electrophoresis (CSF and serum) | | Neuropsychiatric workup | Oligoclonal bands positive in 85%–95% of patients with definite MS; most sensitive marker of MS |
| Prealbumin | 2%–7% | | Use in evaluation of inflammatory and hypercoagulable states |
| Albumin | 56%–76% | | |
| Alpha-1 globulin | | | |
| Alpha-2 globulin | | | |
| Beta globulin | | | |
| Gamma globulin | | | |
| Opening pressure | <7 mm Hg (100 mm water) | Neuropsychiatric workup | Elevated: in pseudotumor cerebri, meningitis, subarachnoid hemorrhage or other head trauma |
| Protein (CSF) | 6.5–8.5 g/dL | Neuropsychiatric workup | Elevated: bacterial, tuberculous, and fungal meningitis Must obtain serum protein levels as reference |
| **Serological studies** | | | |
| Cytomegalovirus (CMV) (serum and CSF) | Positive/negative | Altered mental status/neuropsychiatric workup | CMV can produce anxiety, confusion, mood disorders CMV IgG and IgM |
| Epstein-Barr virus (EBV) (serum and CSF) | Positive/negative | Cognitive/neuropsychiatric workup Anxiety Mood disorders | Part of herpes virus group EBV is causative agent for infectious mononucleosis, which can present with depression, fatigue, and personality change EBV may be associated with chronic mononucleosis-like syndrome associated with chronic depression and fatigue |

**TABLE 12–2.   Useful screening laboratory tests in the workup of the neuropsychiatric patient (continued)**

| Test | Reference range | Indication | Comments |
|---|---|---|---|
| **Serological studies (continued)** | | | |
| Hepatitis A viral antigen (serum) | Positive/negative | Mood disorders<br>Cognitive/neuropsychiatric workup | Less severe, better prognosis than hepatitis B; may present with anorexia, depression |
| Hepatitis B surface antigen<br>Hepatitis B core antigen | Positive/negative | Mood disorders<br>Cognitive/neuropsychiatric workup | Active hepatitis B infection indicates greater degree of infectivity and of progression to chronic liver disease |
| Hepatitis C core antibody | Positive/negative | Mood disorders<br>Cognitive/neuropsychiatric workup | High rates of depression related to interferon treatment |
| HIV-1 p24 antigen (serum) | Positive/negative | Altered mental status/neuropsychiatric workup | Positive ELISA confirmed via Western blot or immunofluorescence assay |
| Lyme titer (serum) | | Altered mental status | Evaluation of meningitis due to Lyme disease (*Borrelia burgdorferi*)<br>Elevated: IgM and IgG antibodies<br>Suspected cause of meningitis with elevated lymphocytes, elevated protein and IgG oligoclonal bands in CSF |
| Syphilis test (rapid plasma reagin test, Venereal Disease Research Laboratory slide test) (serum and CSF) | Nonreactive | Neuropsychiatric workup | Positive in syphilis |
| **Urine tests** | | | |
| Myoglobin | 0–1 mg/L | Phenothiazine use<br>Substance abuse<br>Use of restraints | Elevated: neuroleptic malignant syndrome; phencyclidine (PCP), cocaine, or lysergic acid diethylamide (LSD) intoxication; and in patients in restraints |
| Urinalysis<br>  Specific gravity<br>  pH<br>  Protein<br>  Glucose<br>  Occult blood<br>  Ketones<br>  Bilirubin<br>  Nitrite | 1.005–1.030<br>5.0–8.5<br>Negative<br>Negative<br>Negative<br>Negative<br>Negative<br>Negative | Cognitive/neuropsychiatric workup<br>Pretreatment workup of lithium<br>Drug screening | Provides clues to cause of various cognitive disorders (assessing general appearance, pH, specific gravity, bilirubin, glucose, blood, ketones, protein, etc.); specific gravity may be affected by lithium |

**TABLE 12–2.** Useful screening laboratory tests in the workup of the neuropsychiatric patient *(continued)*

| Test | Reference range | Indication | Comments |
|---|---|---|---|
| **Urine tests** *(continued)* | | | |
| *Urinalysis (continued)* | | | |
| Urobilinogen | 0.1–1.0 | | |
| Microscopic | ≤2 WBC/high-power field (hpf), ≤2 RBC/hpf | | |
| Urine porphyrins | | Altered mental status | Elevated: acute intermittent porphyria, especially during acute attack |
| Uroporphyrin | 0–4 μmol/mol Cr | | |
| Coproporphyrin | 0–22 μmol/mol Cr | | |
| Porphobilinogen | 0–8.8 μmol/L | | |
| Urine catecholamines, metanephrines, vanillylmandelic acid | 0.0–7.0 | Altered mental status, anxiety | Elevated: pheochromocytoma; metanephrines most reliable screening test for pheochromocytoma |
| **Toxicology** | | | |
| Alcohol | | Altered mental status | Elevated blood alcohol level varies by state law (>0.08%–0.15%) |
| | | Anxiety | Tolerance likely if blood alcohol level >0.10% but intoxication symptoms absent |
| | | | Elevated gamma-glutamyltransferase and liver function test results |
| | | | Detectable for up to 12 hours in urine |
| Amphetamines | Positive/negative | Altered mental status | Detectable for up to 48 hours in urine |
| Barbiturates | Positive/negative | Altered mental status | |
| Benzodiazepines | Positive/negative | Altered mental status Suicide attempts | Detectable for up to 3 days in urine |
| Caffeine | Positive/negative | Anxiety/panic disorder | Evaluation of patients with suspected caffeinism |
| Cannabis | Positive/negative | Altered mental status | Detectable for up to 4 weeks in chronic users |
| Cocaine | Positive/negative | Altered mental status | Elevated levels of benzoylecgonine (metabolite) present |
| | | | Detectable for up to 48 hours in urine |
| Inhalants | | Altered mental status | |
| Nicotine | Positive/negative | Anxiety Nicotine addiction | Evaluation of anxiety in smokers Elevated levels of cotinine (metabolite) can be detected in blood, saliva, or urine |

**TABLE 12–2.** Useful screening laboratory tests in the workup of the neuropsychiatric patient *(continued)*

| Test | Reference range | Indication | Comments |
|---|---|---|---|
| **Toxicology** *(continued)* | | | |
| Opiates/narcotics | Positive/negative | Altered mental status | |
| Phencyclidine (PCP) | Positive/negative | Altered mental status | Elevated AST and CPK<br>Detectable for up to 8 days in urine |
| Salicylates | | Organic hallucinosis<br>Suicide attempts | Toxic levels may be seen in suicide attempts; high levels may cause organic hallucinosis |
| **Other diagnostic tests/procedures** | | | |
| $CO_2$ inhalation, sodium bicarbonate infusion | | Anxiety/panic disorder | Provocative test<br>Panic attacks induced in subgroup of patients |
| Doppler ultrasound | | Impotence<br>Cognitive/neuropsychiatric workup | Carotid occlusion, transient ischemic attack, reduced penile blood flow in impotence |
| Echocardiogram | | Panic disorder | 10%–40% of patients with panic disorder have mitral valve prolapse |
| Electroencephalogram | | Cognitive/neuropsychiatric workup | Evaluation of seizures, brain death, lesions<br>Shortened REM latency in depression<br>High-voltage activity in excitement; functional nonorganic cases (e.g., dissociative states); alpha activity present in the background, which responds to auditory and visual stimuli<br>Biphasic or triphasic slow bursts seen in dementia of Creutzfeldt-Jakob disease |
| Holter monitor | | Panic disorder | Evaluation of panic disorder patients with palpitations and other cardiac symptoms |
| Nocturnal penile tumescence | | Impotence | Quantification of penile circumference changes, penile rigidity, frequency of penile tumescence<br>Evaluation of erectile function during sleep<br>Erections associated with REM sleep<br>Helpful in differentiation between organic and functional causes of impotence |

*Note.* Reference values given in conventional units; may vary between laboratories; Cr=creatinine; ELISA=enzyme-linked immunosorbent assay; REM=rapid eye movement; SIADH=syndrome of inappropriate antidiuretic hormone.

*Source.* Adapted from Alpay and Park 2000; Anfinson and Stoudemire 2000; Fadem and Simring 1998; Methodist Health Care System 2001; Sadock and Sadock 2007; Wallach 2000.

**TABLE 12–3. Recommended diagnostic workup for a patient with new-onset psychosis**

**Routine screening**

Complete blood count with differential and platelets

Serum chemistries, including liver and renal function tests

Thyrotropin

Rapid plasma reagin

HIV serology

Erythrocyte sedimentation rate

Serum alcohol level

Urine toxicology screen

Head computed tomography or brain magnetic resonance imaging scan

Electroencephalogram

Urine pregnancy test

Baseline electrocardiogram

Therapeutic drug levels

**Consider per clinical suspicion**

Antinuclear antibody

Rheumatoid factor

Blood cultures

Serum B$_{12}$ and folate levels

Metal assays: serum and urine copper, serum ceruloplasmin; lead; mercury; manganese

Cerebrospinal fluid analysis: red blood cell count; white blood cell count; protein; glucose; opening pressure; bacterial cultures; cryptococcal antigen; viral serologies

Urine porphyrins

complete blood count (CBC) with platelets and differential; thyrotropin; a rapid plasma reagin for syphilis; HIV serology; serum alcohol level; urinalysis; and a urine toxicology screen for drugs of abuse. Other tests to consider during the initial workup include structural neuroimaging (head computed tomography [CT] or brain magnetic resonance imaging [MRI]) and electroencephalography. If appropriate, the clinician also should consider ordering a urine pregnancy test and baseline electrocardiogram, especially if he or she is planning to initiate or change antipsychotic medication. If these initial tests do not immediately yield an etiology, the clinician also may consider a lumbar puncture to analyze cerebrospinal fluid (CSF) for the presence of red and white blood cells, protein, and glucose; opening pressure; and bacterial culture, cryptococcal antigen, and viral serologies. Antinuclear antibodies,

rheumatoid factor, erythrocyte sedimentation rate, urine porphyrins, blood cultures, and assays for heavy metals (manganese and mercury) and bromides are other tests to consider. Table 12–3 summarizes some of the recommended tests in the diagnostic approach to a patient with new-onset psychosis.

## Mood Disturbance: Depressive or Manic Symptoms

A thorough laboratory screening is also recommended for the evaluation of adult patients with new-onset mood symptoms such as depression or mania. Tests might include thyrotropin, serum chemistries, CBC, urinalysis, and a urine toxicology screen for drugs of abuse. If appropriate, the clinician also should consider ordering a urine pregnancy test and electrocardiogram, especially if he or she is considering starting a mood-stabilizing medication (Wallach 1992). Serum trough levels of mood stabilizers such as lithium, valproate, or carbamazepine and tricyclic antidepressants (TCAs) can be obtained to monitor therapeutic response in accordance with therapeutic levels.

Neuroimaging and electroencephalography are often helpful as well in understanding the etiology of a patient's mood symptoms. The diagnostic approach to a patient with new-onset depressive or manic symptoms is summarized in Table 12–4.

**TABLE 12–4. Recommended diagnostic workup for patient with new-onset depressive or manic symptoms**

**Routine screening**

Complete blood count with differential and platelets

Serum chemistries, including liver and renal function tests

Thyrotropin

Rapid plasma reagin

HIV serology

Urinalysis

Urine toxicology screen

Serum alcohol level (if suspected)

Urine pregnancy test

Electrocardiogram

Therapeutic drug levels (if patient is already taking psychiatric medications)

**Consider per clinical suspicion**

Structural neuroimaging (brain magnetic resonance imaging)

Electroencephalogram

**TABLE 12–5.  Recommended diagnostic workup for a patient with new-onset anxiety symptoms**

**Routine screening**

Serum chemistries, including liver and renal function tests

Serum glucose

Thyrotropin

Referral for cardiac evaluation: electrocardiogram, Holter monitoring, stress test, and/or echocardiogram

**Consider per clinical suspicion**

Referral for respiratory evaluation: chest radiograph, pulmonary function tests

Electroencephalogram

Urine porphyrins and vanillylmandelic acid levels

Urine metanephrines

Blood gas

## Anxiety

The initial workup for anxiety symptoms should include serum chemistries, serum glucose, thyrotropin, and other endocrine measures (Table 12–5). Cardiac workup is important because cardiac symptoms may masquerade as panic attacks and are often misdiagnosed as such, especially in female patients. Therefore, electrocardiography, Holter monitoring, a stress test, and/or echocardiography may be necessary. Respiratory function also should be evaluated with a chest radiograph or pulmonary function tests to rule out chronic obstructive pulmonary disease as a contributory factor. Other tests to consider if one has clinical suspicion include electroencephalography, urine porphyrins, and urine vanillylmandelic acid.

## Altered Mental Status

Patients with a fluctuating mental status of acute onset most likely will have one or more underlying medical or neurological causes for their impaired consciousness. Many medical and neurological disorders can cause impairment in mental status, including seizures, central nervous system and systemic infection, kidney or liver failure, cardiac arrhythmias, stroke, myocardial infarction, and substance intoxication and withdrawal. This often constitutes a medical emergency, and comprehensive laboratory and diagnostic testing is indicated on an emergency basis, as summarized in Table 12–6. In addition to a complete physical examination and as much history as can be

**TABLE 12–6.  Recommended diagnostic workup for a patient with altered mental status**

**Routine screening**

Serum chemistries, including liver and renal function tests

Complete blood count

Erythrocyte sedimentation rate

HIV serology

Antinuclear antibody

Rheumatoid factor

$B_{12}$

Folate

Rapid plasma reagin

Urinalysis

Urine toxicology

Serum alcohol level

Therapeutic drug levels

Electrocardiogram

Chest radiograph

Head computed tomography scan

Electroencephalogram

**Consider per clinical suspicion**

Cerebrospinal fluid analysis: red blood cell count; white blood cell count; protein; glucose; opening pressure; bacterial cultures; cryptococcal antigen; viral serologies

Urine porphyrins

Serum ammonia level

Brain magnetic resonance imaging

Arterial blood gases

Blood cultures

obtained from the patient and ancillary sources, the clinician should order serum chemistries, CBC, erythrocyte sedimentation rate, HIV serology, urinalysis and urine toxicology, electrocardiogram, and chest radiograph. A CT scan, blood cultures, lumbar puncture with CSF analysis, and an EEG can be helpful as well, if clinically indicated.

## Cognitive Decline: Dementias

The current American Academy of Neurology (2007) practice recommendations for evaluation of reversible causes of dementia include testing for vitamin $B_{12}$ deficiency and hypothyroidism. These laboratory tests are recommended in addition to structural imaging (noncontrast head CT or MRI studies) and evaluation of depression to rule out so-called pseudodementia, or dementia-like symptoms that stem from depression. Syphilis serology screening is necessary only in patients with dementia who are at risk for neurosyphilis. Table 12–7 lists the laboratory and diagnostic tests that would be included in the workup of a patient with cognitive impairment.

## Substance Abuse

Laboratory testing for substance abuse can be conducted with blood and urine specimens or with saliva and hair samples. Urine specimens are typically preferred because the detectable length of time that a particular drug of abuse and its metabolites are present is longer in urine than in blood. However, some substances, such as alcohol or barbiturates, are best detected in blood specimens. Table 12–8 reviews common substances of abuse, toxic levels, and length of detection time.

The length of time that a drug of abuse is detectable in the urine varies based on the amount and duration of substance consumed, kidney and liver function, and the specific drug itself. Laboratory methodologies vary. If the screening tests yield a positive result, follow-up with more specific tests, including quantitative analyses, can be ordered for confirmation.

# Medication Monitoring and Maintenance

## Mood Stabilizers

Most experts recommend screening during the use of mood stabilizers every 3–6 months; however, some experts recommend that clinical monitoring of signs of toxicity may be more effective than periodic screening. A potential set of guidelines, which most authors appear to support, is listed in Table 12–9.

## Tricyclic Antidepressants

Four TCAs—imipramine, nortriptyline, desipramine, and amitriptyline—have been well studied, and generalizations can be made about the relation of drug levels to therapeutic response. For imipramine, optimal response rates occur as blood levels reach 200–250 ng/mL, and levels greater than 250 ng/mL often produce more side effects but no change in antidepressant response (American

**TABLE 12–7. Recommended diagnostic workup for a patient with cognitive decline**

**Routine screening**

Complete blood count with differential and platelets

Serum chemistries, including liver and renal function tests

Erythrocyte sedimentation rate

Antinuclear antibody

Rheumatoid factor

$B_{12}$ and folate levels

Thyrotropin

Structural neuroimaging studies (head computed tomography or brain magnetic resonance imaging scan)

**Consider per clinical suspicion**

Rapid plasma reagin

HIV serology

C-reactive protein

Cerebrospinal fluid (CSF) analysis: red blood cell count; white blood cell count; protein; glucose; opening pressure; bacterial cultures; cryptococcal antigen; viral serologies; CSF 14–3–3 protein immunoassay (if Creutzfeldt-Jakob disease is suspected); CSF tau and Aβ amyloid 42 levels for frontotemporal dementia vs. Alzheimer's disease

Urine porphyrins

Functional neuroimaging studies (single photon emission computed tomography or positron emission tomography)

Electroencephalogram

Apolipoprotein E genotyping

Neuropsychological testing

Fasting lipids, triglycerides, and blood sugar when a vascular etiology is suspected

Psychiatric Association Task Force on the Use of Laboratory Tests in Psychiatry 1985). Nortriptyline, in contrast, appears to have a specific therapeutic window between 50 and 150 ng/mL, and poor clinical response occurs both above and below that window. Desipramine also appears to have a linear relation between drug concentration and clinical outcome, with plasma concentrations greater than 125 ng/mL being significantly more effective. Amitriptyline has been fairly well studied; however, some studies have found a linear relation similar to that of imipramine, others have found a curvilinear relation, and oth-

TABLE 12–8.    Substances of abuse

| Agent | Toxic level | Urine detection time |
|---|---|---|
| Alcohol | 300 mg/dL at any time or >100 g ingested | 7–12 hours |
| Amphetamines | | 48 hours |
| Barbiturates | >6 μg/mL | 24 hours (short-acting) |
| | | 3 weeks (long-acting) |
| Benzodiazepines | Varies with medication | 3 days |
| | Lorazepam: >25–100 mg | |
| | Diazepam: >250 mg | |
| Cannabis | 50–200 μg/kg | 4–6 weeks |
| Cocaine | >1.2 g | 6–8 hours |
| | | 2–4 days (metabolites) |
| Opiates | Varies with medication | 2–3 days |
| | Heroin: >100–250 mg | |
| | Codeine: >500–1,000 mg | |
| | Morphine: >50–100 μg/kg | |
| Phencyclidine (PCP) | >10–20 mg | 1–2 weeks |

*Source.*    Adapted from Wallach 2000.

ers have found no relation between blood levels and clinical outcomes (American Psychiatric Association Task Force on the Use of Laboratory Tests in Psychiatry 1985) (see Table 12–9).

## Antipsychotics

Blood level monitoring may be useful to confirm the presence of the antipsychotic when adherence is a concern. It may be used to ascertain the presence of drug interactions in a patient who has relapsed or experienced an exacerbation of symptoms after a period of stabilization and who has been taking drugs that may interact with antipsychotics, such as carbamazepine or fluoxetine. It also may be helpful to obtain drug levels in patients who develop excessive side effects to moderate dosages of antipsychotics (Bernardo et al. 1993).

In patients who are older than 50, or who have preexisting cardiac disease, a screening electrocardiogram should be ordered before institution of antipsychotic medications, such as thioridazine, quetiapine, risperidone, or ziprasidone, that may cause prolongation of the QTc interval (a marker for potentially life-threatening cardiac arrhythmias such as torsades de pointes). Follow-up electrocardiograms should be ordered for any patient receiving treatment with antipsychotic medications in whom symptoms indicative of cardiac compromise appear. It is also recommended that

screening laboratory studies be performed at regular intervals (every 6 months) to test for glucose and metabolic dysregulation (hyperlipidemias, diabetes, hypothyroidism), which are often associated with atypical antipsychotic medications (see Table 12–9).

## Pharmacogenetics and Pharmacogenomics

Most psychiatric drugs are metabolized by microsomal enzymes called the cytochrome P450 (CYP) enzyme system. The CYP enzymes are a superfamily of more than 20 related enzymes, although only 6 metabolize more than 90% of all medications (Streetman 2000). These six enzymes that are important to human drug metabolism are CYP1A2, CYP2C9, CYP2C19, CYP2D6, CYP2E1, and CYP3A. Enzymes are identified by numbers and letters that identify the family and subfamily grouping. For example, CYP2D6 is in family 2 and subfamily 2D and is structurally related to CYP2C19 in the same family, but it is not similar to CYP3A, which is in a different family (Streetman 2000).

The majority of CYP enzyme metabolism occurs in the liver, although metabolism can occur elsewhere in the body, such as the small intestine (CYP3A4), the brain (CYP2D6), and the lung (CYP1A1). The CYP enzyme

TABLE 12–9.  Medication monitoring

| Medication type | Medication | Therapeutic range | Toxic level | Recommended screening |
|---|---|---|---|---|
| Mood stabilizers | Lithium | 0.8–1.2 mEq/L | >1.5 mEq/L | Initiation: sodium, potassium, calcium, phosphate, blood urea nitrogen, creatinine, thyrotropin, $T_4$, CBC, urinalysis, beta-HCG if appropriate; ECG for patients older than 50 or with preexisting cardiac disease |
| | | | | Maintenance: thyrotropin, blood urea nitrogen/creatinine recommended every 6 months; ECGs as needed in patients older than 40 or with preexisting cardiac disease |
| | Valproate | 50–150 µg/mL | >150 µg/mL | Initiation: CBC with platelets, LFTs; beta-HCG if appropriate |
| | | | | Maintenance: LFTs, CBC recommended every 6 months |
| | Carbamazepine | 8–12 µg/mL | >12 µg/mL | Initiation: CBC with platelets, LFTs, blood urea nitrogen/creatinine |
| | | | | Maintenance: CBC with platelets, LFTs, blood urea nitrogen/creatinine |
| TCAs | Imipramine + desipramine[a] | 125–250 ng/mL | >500 ng/mL or >1 g ingested | Initiation: ECG in patients older than 40 years or with preexisting cardiac disease for all TCAs |
| | Doxepin + metabolite desmethyl-doxepin | 100–275 ng/mL | >500 ng/mL | Initiation: ECG in patients older than 40 years or with preexisting cardiac disease for all TCAs |
| | Amitriptyline + nortriptyline | 75–225 ng/mL | >500 ng/mL | Initiation: ECG in patients older than 40 years or with preexisting cardiac disease for all TCAs |
| | Nortriptyline only | 50–150 ng/mL | >50 ng/mL | Initiation: ECG in patients older than 40 years or with preexisting cardiac disease for all TCAs |
| Antipsychotics | Olanzapine, quetiapine, risperidone, ziprasidone | | | Fasting serum glucose Triglycerides |

*Note.*  CBC=complete blood count; ECG=electrocardiogram; HCG=human chorionic gonadotropin; LFT=liver function test; $T_4$=thyroxine; TCA=tricyclic antidepressant.
[a]Desipramine is metabolite of imipramine.
*Source.*  Adapted from Hyman et al. 1991; Wallach 2000.

system, in addition to metabolizing drugs, metabolizes exogenous substances, such as environmental toxins and dietary nutrients, and endogenous substances, such as steroids and prostaglandins. Through drug metabolism, a medication is made more hydrophilic or water soluble in order to be excreted by the kidneys. Table 12–10 lists many of the psychiatric drugs that are metabolized by selected CYP enzymes (substrates) as well as those that may decrease enzyme activity (inhibitors). CYP drug metabolism is highly variable as a result of several factors, including genetic polymorphisms, effects of concomitant medications (inhibition or induction of enzymes), physiological or disease status, and environmental or exogenous factors such as toxins and diet (Ingelman-Sundberg et al. 1999).

*Pharmacogenetics* is the study of genetic variation as it relates to drug response and metabolism. Research in pharmacogenetics to date has focused largely on genes that encode receptors targeted by drugs such as the serotonin and dopamine receptor subtypes or those that encode CYP enzymes. Research on the latter has been significantly more helpful to our understanding of the genetic basis of variability in medication response than the former.

The pharmacokinetic effects of the CYP enzyme system, specifically CYP2D6 and CYP2C19 polymorphisms, on psychiatric medications have been studied extensively. The allele sequence that produces a normally functioning enzyme is coded by the wild-type gene (given the suffix "*1"). Thereafter, differing genetic sequence polymorphisms are numbered sequentially (i.e.,*2, *3). Thus, multiple copies of a functional CYP enzyme gene can occur, resulting in enzyme overactivity. Conversely, polymorphisms may be inactivating, resulting in decreased CYP enzyme activity or even a complete loss of activity.

Four general phenotypes have been used to describe the outcomes of these CYP genetic polymorphisms (see Table 12–11): ultrarapid metabolizers, extensive metabolizers, intermediate metabolizers, and poor metabolizers. Extensive metabolizers have the normal two copies of fully active CYP enzyme alleles for a particular microsomal enzyme. Poor metabolizers do not have the active enzyme gene allele, resulting in increased concentrations of medications because of reduced metabolism, and may have more adverse effects at usual, recommended dosages. In contrast, ultrarapid metabolizers will have multiple copies of the functional enzyme allele, resulting in increased rate of drug metabolism, and medications may not reach therapeutic concentrations at the recommended dosage.

**TABLE 12–10.    Psychiatric drug metabolism by specific P450 enzymes**

| Enzyme | CYP2D6 | CYP2C19 |
|---|---|---|
| Substrates (drugs metabolized by specific enzyme) | Antidepressants<br>  Amitriptyline<br>  Desipramine<br>  Duloxetine<br>  Imipramine<br>  Fluoxetine<br>  Fluvoxamine<br>  Nortriptyline<br>  Paroxetine<br>  Sertraline<br>  Trazodone<br>  Venlafaxine<br>Antipsychotics<br>  Aripiprazole<br>  Clozapine<br>  Haloperidol<br>  Fluphenazine<br>  Perphenazine<br>  Olanzapine<br>  Risperidone<br>  Thioridazine<br>Other drugs<br>  Donepezil<br>  Methadone | Antidepressants<br>  Citalopram<br>  Escitalopram<br>  Amitriptyline<br>  Clomipramine<br>  Imipramine<br>Other drugs<br>  Diazepam |
| Inhibitors | Antidepressants<br>  Amitriptyline<br>  Bupropion<br>  Desipramine<br>  Fluoxetine<br>  Paroxetine<br>  Sertraline<br>Antipsychotics<br>  Thioridazine<br>  Clomipramine<br>  Clozapine | Amitriptyline<br>Citalopram<br>Clomipramine<br>Fluvoxamine<br>Fluoxetine |

*Source.*    Data adapted from Kirchheiner et al. 2001; Streetman 2000.

In general, dosages of TCAs are reduced by 50% for poor metabolizers of CYP2D6 or CYP2C19 substrates, with less dramatic dosage reductions for selective serotonin reuptake inhibitors (de Leon 2006; Kirchheiner et al. 2001). A very small proportion of poor metabolizers are lacking both CYP2D6 and CYP2C19 functional alleles.

TABLE 12–11. Drug metabolizer phenotype classification

| Type | Number of active enzyme gene alleles | Expected response to substrate drug |
|---|---|---|
| Poor metabolizer | None | Reduced metabolism of drug may result in increased concentrations and more adverse effects |
| Intermediate metabolizer | 1 active and 1 inactive allele, or 2 gene alleles with reduced activity | Lesser degree of adverse effects related to reduced metabolism |
| Extensive metabolizer (normal) | 2 | Expected response to standard medication dosage |
| Ultrarapid metabolizer | >2 | Rapid clearance of medications, so may not reach therapeutic concentrations at recommended dosages |

*Source.* Adapted from Ingelman-Sundberg et al. 1999; Mrazek 2006.

These patients are likely to have adverse reactions to most available antidepressant medications. Thus, the use of antidepressant medications such as bupropion and mirtazapine, which are not dependent on these metabolic pathways, would be prudent in these patients (de Leon et al. 2006).

## Cerebrospinal Fluid Studies

CSF studies are often used in the secondary evaluation of a psychiatric patient when a neurological and possibly reversible cause is suspected, including infections, such as encephalitis or meningitis, which may be caused by bacteria; acid-fast bacilli (e.g., tuberculosis); spirochetes (e.g., syphilis, Lyme disease); viruses (e.g., herpes simplex, cytomegalovirus, Epstein-Barr virus, West Nile virus); prions (e.g., Creutzfeldt-Jakob disease); or fungi (e.g., *Cryptococcus*). CSF analysis also can identify subarachnoid hemorrhage, which can present with altered mental status, headache, coma, and/or focal findings.

Spinal fluid analysis also can be useful for investigating inflammatory etiologies for neuropsychiatric complaints. These include autoimmune demyelinating disorders (e.g., multiple sclerosis or acute demyelinating encephalomyelitis) and autoimmune neuronal disorders (systemic lupus erythematosus). CSF analysis also can detect disorders of CSF production that produce elevated (e.g., pseudotumor cerebri) or low pressure. Finally, CSF analysis can be very useful for identifying neoplastic processes

within the nervous system, including direct tumor invasion (e.g., lymphoma), carcinomatous meningitis (e.g., prostate cancer), and a paraneoplastic syndrome.

## Electrophysiological Testing

### Standard Electroencephalogram

An EEG would be prudent to obtain in a patient with new-onset psychosis, episodic behavioral disturbance, or altered mental status. In a patient with altered mental status, the EEG can be diagnostically useful because it can differentiate between a diffuse encephalopathy, nonmotoric status epilepticus, and focal lesion (Boutros and Struve 2004). A normal electroencephalographic result does not exclude seizure disorder from the differential diagnosis because 20% of patients with epilepsy will have normal electroencephalographic findings, and 2% of patients without epilepsy will have spike and wave formations (Engel 1992). The diagnosis of epilepsy is a clinical one, based on observation of the patient or the report of someone who has observed the patient having a seizure. Although the EEG can support the diagnosis, it cannot exclude it.

Several techniques can be implemented to increase the diagnostic yield of the EEG, including sleep deprivation, serial EEGs, 24-hour electroencephalographic monitoring, or adjustments in electrode placement, including nasopharyngeal, sphenoidal, and anterior temporal electrodes.

## Key Points: Laboratory Testing in Psychiatry

- Laboratory testing of the psychiatric patient in the past has been used mainly to uncover medical or neurological causes of psychiatric symptoms.

- The consensus of studies evaluating the role and value of laboratory testing is that patients who have psychiatric signs and symptoms but who do not have other physical complaints or symptoms will benefit from a small screening battery that includes serum glucose concentration, blood urea nitrogen concentration, creatinine clearance, and urinalysis. Female patients older than 50 years will also benefit from a screening thyrotropin test regardless of the presence or absence of mood symptoms.

- More extensive laboratory screening may be necessary for psychiatric patients who do have concomitant physical complaints or findings on physical examination or for patients who are of higher risk, such as elderly or institutionalized patients or those with low socioeconomic status, self-neglect, alcohol or drug dependence, or cognitive impairment.

- Newer laboratory testing methods such as pharmacogenetic testing and testing for investigational genetic and biological markers have the potential to transform and dramatically increase the importance of laboratory testing in the workup of the psychiatric patient.

## References

Alpay M, Park L: Laboratory tests and diagnostic procedures, in Psychiatry: Update and Board Preparation. Edited by Stern TA, Herman JB. New York, McGraw-Hill, 2000, pp 251–266

American Academy of Neurology: American Academy of Neurology practice guidelines for dementia. Continuum 13(2):Appendix A, 2007

American Psychiatric Association Task Force on the Use of Laboratory Tests in Psychiatry: Tricyclic antidepressants: blood level measurements and clinical outcome. An APA Task Force report. Am J Psychiatry 142:155–162, 1985

Anfinson TJ, Kathol RG: Screening laboratory evaluation in psychiatric patients: a review. Gen Hosp Psychiatry 14:248–257, 1992

Anfinson TJ, Stoudemire A: Laboratory and neuroendocrine assessment in medical-psychiatric patients, in Psychiatric Care of the Medical Patient, 2nd Edition. Edited by Stoudemire S, Fogel BS, Greenberg D. New York, Oxford University Press, 2000, pp 119–145

Barnes RF, Mason JC, Greer C, et al: Medical illness in chronic psychiatric outpatients. Gen Hosp Psychiatry 5:191–195, 1983

Bernardo M, Palao DJ, Araúxo A, et al: Monitoring plasma level of haloperidol in schizophrenia. Hosp Community Psychiatry 44:115, 118, 1993

Boutros N, Struve F: Electrophysiological testing, in Neuropsychiatric Assessment. Edited by Yudofsky SC, Kim HF (Review of Psychiatry Series; Oldham JM and Riba MB, series eds). Washington, DC, American Psychiatric Publishing, 2004, pp 69–104

Catalano G, Catalano MC, O'Dell KJ, et al: The utility of laboratory screening in medically ill patients with psychiatric symptoms. Ann Clin Psychiatry 13:135–140, 2001

de Leon J: Psychopharmacological treatment based on individual drug metabolism: CYP2D6 poor metabolizers. CNS Spectr 11:8–12, 2006

de Leon J, Armstrong S, Cozza KL: Clinical guidelines for psychiatrists for the use of pharmacogenetic testing for CYP450 2D6 and CYP450 2C19. Psychosomatics 47:75–85, 2006

Dolan JG, Mushlin AI: Routine laboratory testing for medical disorders in psychiatric inpatients. Arch Intern Med 145:2085–2088, 1985

Engel J Jr: The epilepsies, in Cecil Textbook of Medicine, 19th Edition, Vol 2. Edited by Wyngaarden JB, Smith LH Jr, Bennett JC. Philadelphia, PA, WB Saunders, 1992, pp 2202–2213

Fadem B, Simring S: High Yield Psychiatry. Baltimore, MD, Williams & Wilkins, 1998

Hall RC, Gardner ER, Stickney SK, et al: Physical illness manifesting as psychiatric disease, II: analysis of a state hospital inpatient population. Arch Gen Psychiatry 37:989–995, 1980

Ingelman-Sundberg M, Oscarson M, McLellan RA: Polymorphic human cytochrome P450 enzymes: an opportunity for individualized drug treatment. Trends Pharmacol Sci 20:342–349, 1999

Kirchheiner J, Brosen K, Dahl ML, et al: CYP2D6 and CYP2C19 genotype–based dose recommendations for antidepressants: a first step towards subpopulation-specific dosages. Acta Psychiatr Scand 104:173–192, 2001

Korn CS, Currier GW, Henderson SO: "Medical clearance" of psychiatric patients without medical complaints in the emergency department. J Emerg Med 18:173–176, 2000

Methodist Health Care System: Laboratory Medicine Handbook, 4th Edition. Hudson, OH, Lexi-Comp, 2001

Mookhoek EJ, Sterrenburg-vdNieuwegiessen IM: Screening for somatic disease in elderly psychiatric patients. Gen Hosp Psychiatry 20:102–107, 1998

Mrazek DA: The context of genetic testing in clinical psychiatric practice. CNS Spectr 11:3–4, 2006

Ringholz GR: Differential Diagnosis. Lecture presented at Current Neurology conference, Houston, TX, November 2001

Sadock BJ, Sadock VA: Laboratory tests in psychiatry, in Kaplan and Sadock's Synopsis of Psychiatry, 10th Edition. Baltimore, MD, Lippincott Williams & Wilkins, 2007, pp 255–267

Sheline Y, Kehr C: Cost and utility of routine admission laboratory testing for psychiatric inpatients. Gen Hosp Psychiatry 12:329–334, 1990

Streetman DS: Metabolic basis of drug interactions in the intensive care unit. Crit Care Nurs Q 22:1–13, 2000

Wallach J: Interpretation of Diagnostic Tests. Boston, MA, Little, Brown, 1992

Wallach J: Interpretation of Diagnostic Tests, 7th Edition. Philadelphia, PA, Lippincott Williams & Wilkins, 2000

White AJ, Barraclough B: Benefits and problems of routine laboratory investigations in adult psychiatric admissions. Br J Psychiatry 155:65–72, 1989

Willett AB, King T: Implementation of laboratory screening procedures on a short-term psychiatric inpatient unit. Dis Nerv Syst 38:867–870, 1977

# 13

# Clinical and Functional Neuroimaging

ROBIN A. HURLEY, M.D., F.A.N.P.A.

RONALD E. FISHER, M.D., Ph.D.

KATHERINE H. TABER, Ph.D., F.A.N.P.A.

Currently, brain imaging is divided into two categories: structural and functional (Table 13–1).

## General Principles of Structural Imaging

Indications for imaging are shown in Table 13–2.

## Magnetic Resonance Imaging

### Safety and Contraindications

There are important contraindications to the use of magnetic resonance imaging (MRI) (see Table 13–3 for summary). The magnetic field can damage electrical, mechanical, or magnetic devices implanted in or attached to the patient. Pacemakers can be damaged by programming changes, possibly inducing arrhythmias. Currents can develop within the wires, leading to burns, fibrillation, or movement of the wires or the pacemaker unit itself. Cochlear implants, dental implants, magnetic stoma plugs, bone-growth stimulators, and implanted medication-infusion pumps can all be demagnetized or injure the patient by movement during exposure to the scanner's magnetic field. In addition, metallic implants, shrapnel, bullets, or metal shavings within the eye (e.g., from welding) can conduct a current and/or move, injuring the eye. All of these devices distort the magnetic resonance image locally and may decrease diagnostic accuracy. Metallic objects near the magnet can be drawn into the magnet at high speed, injuring the patient or staff (Price 1999; Shellock 1991, 2002; Shellock and Crues 2004).

### Magnetic Resonance Imaging Versus Computed Tomography

The choice of imaging modality should be based on the anatomy and/or pathology that one desires to view (see Table 13–3).

Computed tomography (CT) is used as an inexpensive screening examination. Also, a few conditions are best viewed with CT, including calcification, acute hemorrhage, and any bone injury, because these pathologies are not yet reliably imaged with MRI (Figure 13–1). However, in the vast majority of cases, MRI is the preferred modality (Figure 13–2). The anatomical detail is much better, more types of pathology are visible, and the brain can be imaged in any plane of section.

For example, subcortical lesions are consistently better visualized with MRI because of the greater gray-white contrast and the ability to image in planes other than axial. Thus, most temporal lobe structures, especially the

TABLE 13–1.    Brain imaging modalities

| Type of imaging | Parameter measured |
| --- | --- |
| **Anatomical and pathological** | |
| Computed tomography (CT) | Tissue density |
| Magnetic resonance imaging (MRI) | Many properties of tissue (T1 and T2 relaxation times, spin density, magnetic susceptibility, water diffusion, blood flow) |
| **Functional (resting brain activity, brain activation, neurotransmitter receptors)** | |
| Positron emission tomography (PET) | Radioactive tracers in blood or tissue |
| Single-photon emission computed tomography (SPECT) | Radioactive tracers in tissue |
| Xenon-enhanced computed tomography (Xe/CT) | Xenon concentration in blood |
| Functional magnetic resonance imaging (fMRI) | Deoxyhemoglobin levels in blood |
| Magnetoencephalography (MEG) | Magnetic fields induced by neuronal discharges |
| Magnetic resonance spectroscopy (MRS) | Metabolite concentrations in tissue |

TABLE 13–2.    Indications for imaging

**Diagnosis or medical condition**

Traumatic brain injury

Significant alcohol abuse

Seizure disorders with psychiatric symptoms

Movement disorders

Autoimmune disorders

Eating disorders

Poison or toxin exposure

Delirium

**Clinical signs and symptoms**

Dementia or cognitive decline

New-onset mental illness after age 50

Initial psychotic break

Presentation at an atypical age for diagnosis

Focal neurological signs

Catatonia

Sudden personality changes

hippocampal formation and amygdala, are most easily evaluated with the coronal and sagittal planes of section rather than axial. Demyelination resulting from poison exposure or from autoimmune disease (such as multiple sclerosis) is also better visualized on MRI, especially when many small lesions are present (see Figure 13–3). MRI does not produce the artifacts from bone that are seen in

CT, so all lesions near bone (e.g., brain stem, posterior fossa, pituitary, hypothalamus) are better visualized on MRI.

# Nuclear Brain Imaging: Single-Photon Emission Computed Tomography and Positron Emission Tomography

Both single-photon emission computed tomography (SPECT) and positron emission tomography (PET) involve intravenous injection of a radioactive compound that distributes in the brain and emits (indirectly, in the case of PET) photons that are detected and used to form an image. The tracer is a molecule whose chemical properties determine its distribution in the body (e.g., fluorodeoxyglucose distributes in cells in proportion to their glucose metabolic rate) and which contains one radioactive atom, called a *radionuclide*. Depending on what compound is injected, the distribution of radioactivity indicates regional blood flow, metabolism, number of available neurotransmitter receptors, and so forth. Regional cerebral metabolism and cerebral perfusion are tightly linked under most physiological and pathophysiological conditions (Raichle 2003).

Both types of imaging studies provide very similar functional information. Tracers are most useful in research, but clinical applications for some are under development.

**TABLE 13–3.** Factors considered when choosing computed tomography (CT) or magnetic resonance imaging (MRI) examination

| Clinical considerations | CT | MRI |
|---|---|---|
| Availability | Universal | Limited |
| Sensitivity | Good | Superior |
| Resolution | 1.0 mm | 1.0 mm |
| Average examination time | 4–5 minutes | 30–35 minutes |
| Plane of section | Axial only | Any plane of section |
| Conditions for which it is the preferred procedure | Screening examination | All subcortical lesions |
| | Acute hemorrhage | Poison or toxin exposure |
| | Calcified lesions | Demyelinating disorders |
| | Bone injury | Eating disorders |
| | | Examination requiring anatomical detail, especially temporal lobe or cerebellum |
| | | Any condition best viewed in nonaxial plane |
| Contraindications | History of anaphylaxis or severe allergic reaction (contrast-enhanced CT) | Any magnetic metal in the body, including surgical clips and sutures |
| | Creatinine≥1.5 mg/dL (contrast-enhanced CT) | Implanted electrical, mechanical, or magnetic devices |
| | Metformin administration on day of scan (contrast-enhanced CT) | Claustrophobia |
| | | History of welding (requires skull films before MRI) |
| | | Pregnancy (legal contraindication) |
| Medicare reimbursement per scan without contrast medium | ~$240 | ~$540 |
| Medicare reimbursement with and without contrast medium[a] | ~$380 | ~$1,150 |

[a]A scan without contrast media is always acquired before the contrast-enhanced scan.

## Safety and Contraindications

The only contraindication to a nuclear medicine scan (SPECT) is pregnancy, and even this is only a relative indication. If the brain scan can be postponed until after delivery, a small radiation dose to the fetus can be avoided.

The safety considerations and contraindications to PET are the same as for SPECT above.

## SPECT Versus PET

PET has the advantages of higher spatial resolution and true attenuation correction (nearly eliminating attenuation artifacts). SPECT has the advantages of being more widely available, less expensive, and reimbursable for most conditions. Reimbursement for brain PET in the United States is currently limited to distinguishing frontotemporal dementia from Alzheimer's disease, doing presurgical evaluation of intractable epilepsy (seizure focus localization), and distinguishing radiation necrosis from recurrent brain tumors. SPECT imaging is considered a standard clinical investigative tool for neuropsychiatric evaluation. However, PET scanners are rapidly becoming more commonplace, and reimbursement for other indications is likely to occur in the near future. The old requirement for an on-site cyclotron has been obviated by the establishment of numerous commercial cyclotrons throughout the United States, from many of which a fluorine 18 ([18]F) tracer (110-minute half-life) can be delivered great distances by airplane. Virtually any hospital in the United States with a PET scanner can have [[18]F]fluorode-

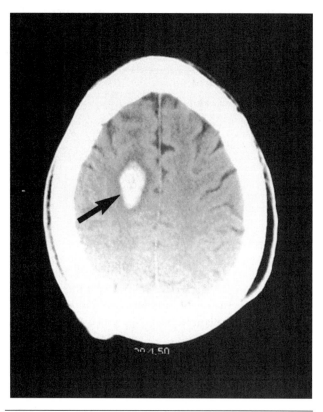

FIGURE 13–1.    **Computed tomography is the preferred imaging method for acute head injury.** This axial image is from a 56-year-old man taking warfarin who presented with left-sided weakness a few hours after being involved in a motorcycle accident. He experienced a brief loss of consciousness following the accident. Note the well-visualized area of hyperdense hemorrhage (*arrow*).

oxyglucose delivered relatively inexpensively. Tracers that use carbon 11 (20-minute half-life), oxygen 15 (2-minute half-life), or nitrogen 13 (10-minute half-life) require an on-site cyclotron facility.

## Clinical Applications

Common nuclear medicine findings in selected clinical conditions are discussed in the following subsections.

### Primary Dementias

Dementia is the most common clinical reason for nuclear brain imaging. Scanning is particularly helpful in the evaluation of patients with atypical clinical presentations. It is expected to play a more significant role as better treatment options become available for different etiolo-

gies. For Alzheimer's disease, bilateral, symmetrical posterior temporoparietal decreased perfusion or metabolism is the classic pattern. However, this is seen in about one-third of the patients with Alzheimer's disease. Frequently, the abnormalities are asymmetrical and may initially involve only temporal or parietal cortex. As the disease progresses, the frontal (and occasionally occipital) lobes become involved, with decreased perfusion. Uptake in the subcortical structures, primary visual cortex, and primary sensorimotor cortex is usually preserved even in late-stage disease. The defects are always diffuse, over a large area of cortex, and easily recognizable as neurodegenerative in origin, although not necessarily specific to Alzheimer's disease.

Clinical SPECT and PET findings in dementia with Lewy bodies (DLB) overlap those of Alzheimer's disease, although the abnormalities are more likely to be asymmetrical and to involve the occipital cortex. Dopamine transporter imaging has shown more promise in distinguishing the two entities. The loss of dopamine neurons is significant in DLB, resulting in striking abnormalities in the striatum in these patients compared with those who have Alzheimer's disease (Walker et al. 2002).

SPECT or PET scanning shows reduced perfusion of the frontal and/or anterior temporal cortex (usually bilaterally) in frontotemporal dementia (e.g., Pick's disease), which is usually readily distinguished from Alzheimer's disease and DLB. Parkinson's patients often develop dementia that may be etiologically distinct from DLB, but the SPECT and PET appearance has not been well characterized and likely overlaps significantly with both Alzheimer's disease and DLB. Clinical SPECT and PET imaging in Creutzfeldt-Jakob disease identifies large areas of severely reduced perfusion. These are usually symmetrical. This appearance overlaps with Alzheimer's disease and DLB, so clinical correlation is needed. Sequential SPECT and PET scans (performed about 2 months apart) often show dramatic progression (Taber et al. 2002). In Huntington's disease, SPECT and PET imaging show characteristic reduced perfusion to the basal ganglia, especially the head of the caudate, often early in the course of the illness. Nuclear imaging is quite sensitive and reasonably specific but is rarely used for diagnosis (diagnosis is made very accurately by sequence analysis of the Huntington's disease gene). It may be useful in predicting progression of disease (Hurley et al. 1999). As dementia progresses, many patients develop large regions of reduced cortical perfusion or metabolism on SPECT and PET in a pattern similar to that for other neurodegenerative diseases.

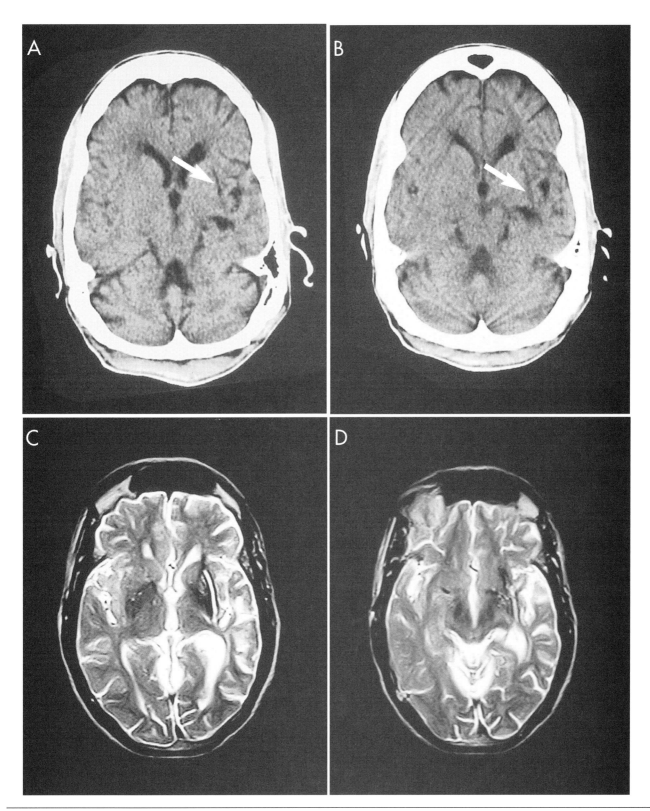

**FIGURE 13–2.** **Many types of pathology are more easily seen on magnetic resonance imaging (MRI) than on computed tomographic (CT) imaging.**

These axial images are from a 69-year-old man who presented status post a generalized tonic-clonic seizure. Abnormal areas indicative of subcortical ischemia are evident on (*A, B*) the conventional CT images (*arrows*). Areas of ischemic injury and old hemorrhage as well as normal anatomy are much better visualized on (*C, D*) T2-weighted MRI.

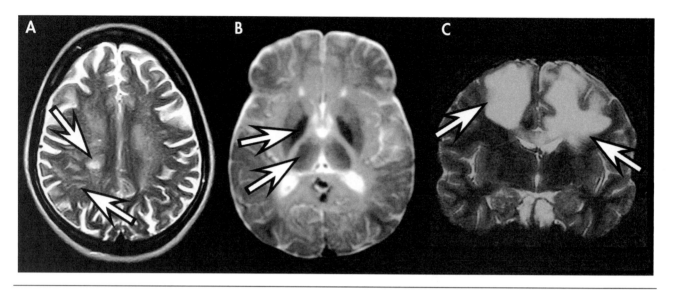

**FIGURE 13–3.    Magnetic resonance imaging (MRI) has many clinical applications.**
(*A*) Multiple sclerosis is characterized by ovoid hyperintense demyelinating lesions parallel to the subependymal veins (*arrows*) on T2-weighted MRI. (*B*) Chronic toluene abuse causes hypointensity in the basal ganglia and thalamus on both T1- and T2-weighted (*arrows*) images. (*C*) Acute disseminated encephalomyelitis causes extensive white matter damage, resulting in areas of hyperintensity (*arrows*) on T2-weighted images.

## Vascular Disease

Although multi-infarct dementia is commonly diagnosed by structural imaging, the pattern of SPECT and PET abnormalities is often quite distinctive, with multiple moderate-sized perfusion defects that have well-defined boundaries. Small vessel disease (e.g., Binswanger's disease) is not associated with a specific SPECT or PET pattern, although basal ganglia and frontal cortex lesions often have been reported (Hurley et al. 2000). Areas of cerebral infarction are easily identified on clinical SPECT, but it is rarely clinically useful in this regard. In acute stroke, the essential information that is needed from neuroimaging is whether the stroke is hemorrhagic prior to initiating thrombolytic therapy. CT scanning is much quicker to obtain and is quite accurate in this regard. SPECT is superior to CT and MRI in predicting outcome of acute stroke and defining the size of viable but at-risk tissue but not sufficiently as to warrant routine clinical use (Barthel et al. 2001; Guadagno et al. 2003). Areas of compromised vascular reserve (partially occluded vessels), which often appear normal on a resting SPECT scan, can be visualized on a SPECT scan performed following intravenous injection of acetazolamide. Acetazolamide raises blood carbon dioxide levels, causing normal arterioles to dilate. Arterioles distal to an arterial stenosis or obstruction are already fully dilated as a

physiological compensatory mechanism and cannot dilate further in response to acetazolamide. Brain regions supplied by such arterioles thus appear relatively hypoperfused, compared with normal tissue, on a postacetazolamide SPECT perfusion scan indicating decreased vascular reserve. Such findings are thought to predict impending ischemic events that may warrant therapeutic intervention (e.g., carotid endarterectomy), although well-controlled studies with long-term clinical follow-up are not available (Martí-Fàbregas et al. 2001).

## Traumatic Brain Injury

Many studies have reported that SPECT is more sensitive than CT or MRI for traumatic brain injury. SPECT often shows abnormal findings (areas of reduced perfusion) in symptomatic patients even when structural imaging shows negative results (Anderson et al. 2005). It must always be borne in mind, however, that many nonimpaired subjects have some limited areas of mildly reduced perfusion. Patient motion during imaging also can produce abnormalities. False-positive studies are an important concern because almost any abnormality, even relatively small or mild ones, would have to be called positive in the scenario of traumatic brain injury. Perhaps the most useful result at this time is that a few studies have indicated that a negative (normal) brain SPECT result after mild traumatic brain injury predicts an excellent long-term neurological outcome (Anderson et al. 2005; Bonne et al. 2003).

# Functional Magnetic Resonance Imaging

Functional MRI (fMRI) is based on modulation of image intensity by the oxygenation state of blood. Deoxygenated hemoglobin (deoxyhemoglobin) is highly paramagnetic. It distorts the local magnetic field in its immediate vicinity. This causes a loss of magnetic resonance signal, particularly on gradient-echo and other susceptibility-weighted pulse sequences. Thus, it is a natural magnetic resonance contrast agent. Image intensity is dependent on the local balance between oxygenated and deoxygenated hemoglobin. This is the origin of the acronym BOLD (blood oxygen level dependent) for the fMRI technique (Taber et al. 2003; Turner and Jones 2003).

An area of brain suddenly becomes more active when it is participating in a cognitive task. The increase in local blood flow is larger than is required to meet the activity-related increase in oxygen consumption. As a result, the venous blood becomes slightly *more* oxygenated. This decrease in local deoxyhemoglobin concentration causes a slight (1%–5%) increase in signal intensity in the activated area of brain on the magnetic resonance image. The change is too small to see by eye. It is measured by comparing the signal intensity under a baseline (resting or control) condition with the signal intensity under an activated condition. Unlike PET, SPECT, or xenon-enhanced CT, all of the fMRI measures depend on comparison of two conditions (e.g., baseline and activated).

Activations will be seen in many areas when a subject performs a task in a scanner. Defining and creating a baseline state for comparison can be a considerable challenge. Ideally, the subject is scanned under two conditions that differ only in the cognitive function under study. For example, to identify the brain regions involved in verbal short-term memory, the subject might be scanned while viewing words projected onto a screen and then clicking with a mouse on those recently seen (test scan). For comparison, the same subject might be scanned while viewing words and clicking on all words beginning with a particular letter (control scan). When the areas of activity on the control scan are subtracted from the areas of activity on the test scan, the remaining areas of activation should primarily reflect verbal short-term memory. However, if a brain area of interest is abnormally active under the baseline (control) condition, further activation may not be measurable, resulting in an apparent absence of activation when the image sets are analyzed.

fMRI has several advantages over other methods of imaging brain activity. Most important, it is totally noninvasive and requires no ionizing radiation or radiopharmaceuticals. Minimal risk makes it appropriate for use in both children and adults and for use in longitudinal studies requiring multiple scanning sessions for each subject. High-resolution structural images are acquired in the same session, providing much better localization of areas of interest than is possible with PET or SPECT. In addition, most clinical MRI scanners can be modified without great expense to enable fMRI. However, fMRI is neither simple nor easy to implement and analyze, which may limit its clinical usefulness. At present, it should be considered a research technique.

# Key Points: Clinical and Functional Neuroimaging

| Testing modality | Indications | Caveats |
|---|---|---|
| **Structural neuroimaging** | | |
| Computed tomography (CT) | Screening examination | *Contraindications for use of contrast enhancement:* |
| | Acute hemorrhage | History of anaphylaxis or severe allergic reaction |
| | Calcified lesions | Creatinine level ≥ 15 mg/dL |
| | Bone injury | Metformin administration on day of scan |
| Magnetic resonance imaging (MRI) | Sustained confusion/delirium | *Contraindications for use of MRI:* |
| | Subtle cognitive deficits | Any magnetic metal in the body, including surgical clips and sutures |
| | Unusual age at symptom onset or evolution | Implanted electrical, mechanical, or magnetic devices |
| | Atypical clinical findings | Claustrophobia |
| | Abrupt personality changes with accompanying neurological signs or symptoms | History of welding (requires skull films before MRI) |
| | Following poison or toxin exposures (including significant alcohol abuse) | Pregnancy (legal contraindication) |
| | Following brain injuries of any kind (traumatic or "organic") | |
| **Functional neuroimaging** | | |
| Positron emission tomography (PET) | Particularly useful for identification of "hidden" lesions (areas that are dysfunctional but do not look abnormal on structural imaging) | Reimbursement limited to dementia, presurgical evaluation of epilepsy, and distinguishing radiation necrosis from recurrent brain tumors |
| | Particularly useful also for patients whose clinical symptoms do not fit the classic historical picture for the working diagnosis | |
| | Evaluation of resting state has shown potential for prediction of treatment response in some conditions | |
| | PET has the advantages of higher spatial resolution than SPECT and true attenuation correction (nearly eliminating attenuation artifacts) | |
| Single-photon emission computed tomography (SPECT) | Same indications as for PET | Lower spatial resolution, more artifacts |
| | SPECT has the advantages of being more widely available than PET, less expensive, and reimbursable for most conditions | |

# References

Anderson KE, Taber KH, Hurley RA: Functional imaging, in Textbook of Traumatic Brain Injury. Edited by Silver JM, McAllister TW, Yudofsky SC. Washington, DC, American Psychiatric Publishing, 2005, pp 107–133

Barthel H, Hesse S, Dannenberg C, et al: Prospective value of perfusion and X-ray attenuation imaging with single-photon emission and transmission computed tomography in acute cerebral ischemia. Stroke 32:1588–1597, 2001

Bonne O, Gilboa A, Louzoun Y, et al: Cerebral blood flow in chronic symptomatic mild traumatic brain injury. Psychiatry Res 124:141–152, 2003

Guadagno JV, Calautti C, Baron JC: Progress in imaging stroke: emerging clinical applications. Br Med Bull 65:145–157, 2003

Hurley RA, Jackson EF, Fisher RE, et al: New techniques for understanding Huntington's disease. J Neuropsychiatry Clin Neurosci 11:173–175, 1999

Hurley RA, Tomimoto H, Akiguchi I, et al: Binswanger's disease: an ongoing controversy. J Neuropsychiatry Clin Neurosci 12:301–304, 2000

Martí-Fàbregas JA, Catafau AM, Marí C, et al: Cerebral perfusion and haemodynamics measured by SPET in symptom-free patients with transient ischaemic attack: clinical implications. Eur J Nucl Med 28:1828–1835, 2001

Price RR: The AAPM/RSNA physics tutorial for residents: MR imaging safety considerations. Radiological Society of North America. Radiographics 19:1641–1651, 1999

Raichle ME: Functional brain imaging and human brain function. J Neurosci 23:3959–3962, 2003

Shellock FG: Bioeffects and safety considerations, in Magnetic Resonance Imaging of the Brain and Spine. Edited by Atlas SW. New York, Raven, 1991, pp 87–107

Shellock FG: Magnetic resonance safety update 2002: implants and devices. J Magn Reson Imaging 16:485–496, 2002

Shellock FG, Crues JV: MR procedures: biologic effects, safety, and patient care. Radiology 232:635–652, 2004

Taber KH, Cortelli P, Staffen W, et al: Expanding the role of imaging in prion disease. J Neuropsychiatry Clin Neurosci 14:371–376, 2002

Taber KH, Rauch SL, Lanius RA, et al: Functional magnetic resonance imaging: application to posttraumatic stress disorder. J Neuropsychiatry Clin Neurosci 15:125–129, 2003

Turner R, Jones T: Techniques for imaging neuroscience. Br Med Bull 65:3–20, 2003

Walker Z, Costa DC, Walker RW, et al: Differentiation of dementia with Lewy bodies from Alzheimer's disease using a dopaminergic presynaptic ligand. J Neurol Neurosurg Psychiatry 73:134–140, 2002

# Section II

# Psychiatric Disorders

Biederman J, Newcorn J, Sprich S: Comorbidity of attention deficit hyperactivity disorder with conduct, depressive, anxiety, and other disorders. Am J Psychiatry 148:564–577, 1991

Biederman J, Milberger S, Faraone SV, et al: Associations between childhood asthma and ADHD: issues of psychiatric comorbidity and familiality. J Am Acad Child Adolesc Psychiatry 33:842–848, 1994

Biederman J, Swanson JM, Wigal SB, et al: A comparison of once-daily and divided doses of modafinil in children with attention-deficit/hyperactivity disorder: a randomized, double blind, and placebo-controlled study. J Clin Psychiatry 67:727–735, 2006

Bruun RD, Budman CL: Natural history of Gilles de la Tourette's syndrome, in Handbook of Tourette's Syndrome and Related Tic Behavioral Disorders. Edited by Kurlan R. New York, Marcel Dekker, 1994, pp 27–43

Castellanos FX, Sharp WS, Gottesman RF, et al: Anatomic brain abnormalities in monozygotic twins discordant for attention deficit hyperactivity disorder. Am J Psychiatry 160:1693–1696, 2003

Chandola CA, Robling MR, Peters TJ, et al: Pre and perinatal factors and the risk of subsequent referral for hyperactivity. J Child Psychol Psychiatry 33:1077–1090, 1992

Chappell PB, Riddle MA, Scahill L, et al: Guanfacine treatment of comorbid attention-deficit hyperactivity disorder and Tourette's syndrome: preliminary clinical experience. J Am Acad Child Adolesc Psychiatry 34:1140–1146, 1995

Charach A, Figueroa M, Chen S, et al: Stimulant treatment over 5 years: effects on growth. J Am Acad Child Adolesc Psychiatry 45:415–421, 2006

Cobham VE, Dadds MR, Spence SH: The role of parental anxiety in the treatment of childhood anxiety. J Consult Clin Psychol 66:893–905, 1998

Coccaro EF, Siever LJ: Pathophysiology and treatment of aggression, in Neuropsychopharmacology: The Fifth Generation of Progress. Edited by Davis KL, Charney D, Coyle JT, et al. Baltimore, MD, Lippincott Williams & Wilkins, 2002, pp 1709–1724

Costello EJ, Mustillo S, Erkanli A, et al: Prevalence and development of psychiatric disorders in childhood and adolescence. Arch Gen Psychiatry 60:837–844, 2003

de Groot CM, Bornstein RA: Obsessive characteristics in subjects with Tourette's syndrome are related to characteristics in their parents. Compr Psychiatry 35:248–251, 1994

Eapen V, Yakeley JW, Robertson MM: Gilles de la Tourette's syndrome and obsessive-compulsive disorder, in Neuropsychiatry, 2nd Edition. Edited by Schiffer RB, Rao SM, Fogel BS. Baltimore, MD, Lippincott Williams & Wilkins, 2003, pp 947–990

Elia J, Gulotta C, Rose SR, et al: Thyroid function and attention deficit hyperactivity disorder. J Am Acad Child Adolesc Psychiatry 33:169–172, 1994

Fergusson DM, Lynskey MT, Horwood LJ: The effect of maternal depression on maternal ratings of child behavior. J Abnorm Child Psychol 21:245–269, 1993

Filipek PA, Semrud-Clikeman M, Steingard RJ, et al: Volumetric MRI analysis comparing subjects having attention deficit hyperactivity disorder with normal controls. Neurology 48:589–601, 1997

Fombonne E, Zakarian R, Bennett A, et al: Pervasive developmental disorders in Montreal, Quebec, Canada: prevalence and links with immunizations. Pediatrics 118:e139–e150, 2006

Gershorn J: A meta-analytic review of gender differences in ADHD. J Atten Disord 5:143–154, 2002

Gillberg C, Wing L: Autism: not an extremely rare disorder. Acta Psychiatr Scand 99:399–406, 1999

Goldstein S, Reynolds CR: Handbook of Neurodevelopmental and Genetic Disorders in Children. New York, Guilford, 1999

Griffiths DM, Gardner WI, Nugent JA: Behavioral Supports and Community Living. Kingston, NY, NADD Press, 1998

Guthrie E, Mast J, Engel M: Diagnosing genetic anomalies by inspection. Child Adolesc Psychiatr Clin N Am 8:777–790, 1999

Harris JC: Behavioral phenotypes of neurodevelopmental disorders: portals into the developing brain, in Neuropsychopharmacology: The Fifth Generation of Progress. Edited by Davis KL, Charney D, Coyle JT, et al. Baltimore, MD, Lippincott Williams & Wilkins, 2002, pp 625–638

Harris JC: Intellectual Disability: Understanding Its Development, Causes, Classification, Evaluation and Treatment. New York, Oxford University Press, 2006

Hechtman L: Genetic and neurobiological aspects of attention deficit hyperactivity disorder: a review. J Psychiatry Neurosci 19:193–201, 1994

Hendren RL, Mullen DJ: Conduct disorder and oppositional defiant disorder, in Essentials of Child and Adolescent Psychiatry. Edited by Dulcan MK, Wiener JM. Washington, DC, American Psychiatric Publishing, 2006, pp 357–387

Hynd GW, Semrud-Clikeman M, Lorys AR, et al: Corpus callosum morphology in attention deficit-hyperactivity disorder: morphometric analysis of MRI. J Learn Disabil 24:141–146, 1991

Iida J, Sakiyama S, Iwasaka H, et al: The clinical features of Tourette's disorder with obsessive-compulsive symptoms. Psychiatry Clin Neurosci 50:185–189, 1996

Jankovic J, DeLeon ML: Basal ganglia and behavioral disorders, in Neuropsychiatry, 2nd Edition. Edited by Schiffer RB, Rao SM, Fogel BS. Baltimore, MD, Lippincott Williams & Wilkins, 2002, pp 934–945

Jensen PS, Shervette RE, Xenakis SN, et al: Anxiety and depressive disorders in attention deficit disorder with hyperactivity: new findings. Am J Psychiatry 150:1203–1209, 1993

Joy SP, Lord JS, Green L, et al: Mental retardation and developmental disabilities, in Neuropsychiatry, 2nd Edition. Edited by Schiffer RB, Rao SM, Fogel BS. Baltimore, MD, Lippincott Williams & Wilkins, 2003, pp 552–604

Kanner L: Autistic disturbances of affective contact. Nerv Child 2:217–250, 1943

Kelly DP, Kelly BJ, Jones MI, et al: Attention deficits in children and adolescents with hearing loss: a survey. Am J Dis Child 147:737–741, 1993

King RA, Scahill L, Lombroso P, et al: Tourette's syndrome and other tic disorders, in Pediatric Psychopharmacology. Edited by Martin A, Scahill L, Charney DS, et al. New York, Oxford University Press, 2003, pp 526–542

Labellarte M, Ginsburg G: Anxiety disorders, in Pediatric Psychopharmacology. Edited by Martin A, Scahill L, Charney DS, et al. New York, Oxford University Press, 2003, pp 497–510

Leckman JF, Yeh C-B, Lombroso PJ: Neurobiology of tic disorders, in Pediatric Psychopharmacology. Edited by Martin A, Scahill L, Charney DS, et al. New York, Oxford University Press, 2003, pp 164–174

Loeber R, Green SM, Keenan K, et al: Which boys will fare worse? Early predictors for the onset of conduct disorder in a six-year longitudinal study. J Am Acad Child Adolesc Psychiatry 34:499–509, 1995

McCracken JT, McGough J, Shah B, et al: Risperidone in children with autism and serious behavioral problems. N Engl J Med 347:314–321, 2002

McDougle CJ, Scahill L, Aman MG, et al: Risperidone for the core symptom domains of autism: results from the study by the autism network of the research units on pediatric psychopharmacology. Am J Psychiatry 162:1142–1148, 2005

McGee R, Stanton WR, Sears MR: Allergic disorders and attention deficit disorder in children. J Abnorm Child Psychol 21:79–88, 1993

Mendlowitz SL, Manassis K, Bradley S, et al: Cognitive-behavioral group treatments in childhood anxiety disorders: the role of parental involvement. J Am Acad Child Adolesc Psychiatry 38:1223–1229, 1999

Motofsky SH, Reiss AL, Lockhart P, et al: Evaluation of cerebellar size in attention-deficit hyperactivity disorder. J Child Neurol 13:434–439, 1998

Multimodal Treatment of ADHD Cooperative Group: A 14-month randomized clinical trial of treatment strategies for attention-deficit/hyperactivity disorder. Multimodal Treatment Study of Children with ADHD. Arch Gen Psychiatry 56:1073–1086, 1999

Newcorn JH, Halperin JM: Comorbidity among disruptive behavior disorders: impact on severity, impairment, and response to treatment. Child Adolesc Psychiatr Clin N Am 3:227–252, 1994

Ornoy A, Uriel L, Tennenbaum A: Inattention, hyperactivity and speech delay at 2–4 years of age as a predictor for ADD-ADHD syndrome. Isr J Psychiatry Relat Sci 30:155–163, 1993

Pelham WE Jr, Gnagy EM, Greenslade KE, et al: Teacher ratings of DSM-III-R symptoms for the disruptive behavior disorders. J Am Acad Child Adolesc Psychiatry 31:210–218, 1992

Piven J, Palmer P, Landa R, et al: Personality and language characteristics in parents from multiple-incidence autism families. Am J Med Genet 74:398–411, 1997

Popper CW, Elliott GR: Sudden death and tricyclic antidepressants: clinical considerations for children. J Child Adolesc Psychopharmacol 1:125–132, 1990

Posey DJ, Erickson CA, Stigler KA, et al: The use of selective serotonin reuptake inhibitors in autism and related disorders. J Child Adolesc Psychopharmacol 16:181–186, 2006

Potenza MN, Hollander E: Pathological gambling and impulse control disorders, in Neuropsychopharmacology: The Fifth Generation of Progress. Edited by Davis KL, Charney DS, Coyle JT, et al. Baltimore, MD, Lippincott Williams & Wilkins, 2002, pp 1725–1742

Riddle MA, Nelson JC, Kleinman CS, et al: Sudden death in children receiving Norpramin: a review of three reported cases and commentary. J Am Acad Child Adolesc Psychiatry 30:104–108, 1991

Rizwan S, Manning JT, Brabin BJ: Maternal smoking during pregnancy and possible effects of in utero testosterone: evidence from the 2D:4D finger length ratio. Early Hum Dev 83:87–90, 2007

Robertson MM: Tourette's syndrome, associated conditions, and the complexities of treatment. Brain 23:425–463, 2000

Robins LN, Ratcliff KS: Risk factors in the continuation of childhood antisocial behavior into adulthood. Int J Ment Health 7:96–111, 1979

Rutter M: Concepts of autism: a review of research. J Child Psychol Psychiatry 9:1–25, 1968

Saint-Cyr JA, Taylor AE, Nicholson K: Behavior and the basal ganglia. Adv Neurol 28:273–281, 1995

Santangelo SI, Pauls DL, Goldstein JM, et al: Tourette's syndrome: what are the influences of gender and comorbid obsessive-compulsive disorders? J Am Acad Child Adolesc Psychiatry 33:785–804, 1994

Saxena S, Bota RG, Brody AI: Brain behavior relationships in obsessive-compulsive disorders. Semin Clin Neuropsychiatry 6:82–101, 2001

Scahill L, Schwab-Stone M: Epidemiology of ADHD in school-age children. Child Adolesc Psychiatr Clin N Am 9:541–555, 2000

Scahill L, Chappell PB, Kim YS, et al: A placebo-controlled study of guanfacine in the treatment of children with tic disorders and attention deficit hyperactivity disorder. Am J Psychiatry 158:1067–1074, 2001

Sechzer JA, Faro MD, Windle WF: Studies of monkeys asphyxiated at birth: implications for minimal cerebral dysfunction. Semin Psychiatry 5:19–34, 1973

Smyke AT, Dumitrescu A, Zeanah CH: Attachment disturbances in young children, I: the continuum of caretaking casualty. J Am Acad Child Adolesc Psychiatry 41:972–982, 2002

Speiser Z, Korczyn AD, Teplitzky I, et al: Hyperactivity in rats following postnatal anoxia. Behav Brain Res 7:379–382, 1983

Spencer TJ, Biederman J, Steingard R, et al: Bupropion exacerbates tics in children with attention-deficit hyperactivity disorder and Tourette's syndrome. J Am Acad Child Adolesc Psychiatry 32:211–214, 1993

Spencer TJ, Biederman J, Wilens TE: Attention-deficit/hyperactivity disorder and comorbidity. Pediatr Clin North Am 46:915–927, 1999

Spencer TJ, Faraone SV, Biederman J, et al: Does prolonged therapy with a long-acting stimulant suppress growth in children with ADHD? J Am Acad Child Adolesc Psychiatry 45:527–537, 2006

Stein DJ, Zohar J, Simeon D: Compulsive and impulsive aspects of self-injurious behavior, in Neuropsychopharmacology: The Fifth Generation of Progress. Edited by Davis KL, Charney D, Coyle JT, et al. Baltimore, MD, Lippincott Williams & Wilkins, 2002, pp 1743–1758

Swanson JM, McBurnett K, Wigal T, et al: Effect of stimulant medication on children with attention deficit disorder: "a review of reviews." Except Child 60:154–162, 1993

Swedo SE, Pine DS: Anxiety. Child Adolesc Psychiatr Clin N Am 14:xv–xviii, 2005

Tcheremissine OV, Lieving LM: Pharmacological aspects of the treatment of conduct disorder in children and adolescents. CNS Drugs 20:549–565, 2006

Tsai LY: Autistic disorder, in The American Psychiatric Publishing Textbook of Child and Adolescent Psychiatry, 3rd Edition. Edited by Weiner JM, Dulcan MK. Washington, DC, American Psychiatric Publishing, 2004, pp 261–315

Vaccarino FM, Leckman JF: Overview of brain development, in Pediatric Psychopharmacology. Edited by Martin A, Scahill L, Charney DS, et al. New York, Oxford University Press, 2003, pp 3–19

Vitiello B, Stoff D, Atkins M, et al: Soft neurological signs and impulsivity in children. J Dev Behav Pediatr 11:112–115, 1990

Volkmar FR, Klin A, Siegel B, et al: Field trial for autistic disorder in DSM-IV. Am J Psychiatry 151:1361–1367, 1994

Walkup JT, Mink JW, Hollenbeck PJ: Advances in Neurology, Vol 99. Baltimore, MD, Lippincott Williams & Wilkins, 2006

Whitaker AH, Van Rossen R, Feldman JF, et al: Psychiatric outcomes in low-birth-weight children at age 6 years: relation to neonatal cranial ultrasound abnormalities. Arch Gen Psychiatry 54:847–856, 1997

Wigal S, Swanson JM, Feifel D, et al: A double-blind, placebo-controlled trial of dexmethylphenidate hydrochloride and d,l-threo-methylphenidate hydrochloride in children with attention-deficit/hyperactivity disorder. J Am Acad Child Adolesc Psychiatry 43:1406–1414, 2004

Wilens TE, Dodson W: A clinical perspective of attention-deficit/hyperactivity disorder into adulthood. J Clin Psychiatry 65:1301–1313, 2004

Wolraich M, Hannah J, Pinnock T, et al: Comparison of diagnostic criteria for attention-deficit/hyperactivity disorder in a country-wide sample. J Am Acad Child Adolesc Psychiatry 35:319–324, 1996

Zachor DA, Roberts AW, Hodgens JB, et al: Effects of long-term psychostimulant medication on growth of children with ADHD. Res Dev Disabil 27:162–174, 2006

Zeanah CH: Disturbances of attachment in young children adopted from institutions. J Dev Behav Pediatr 21:230–236, 2000

Zeanah CH, Smyke AT, Dumitrescu A: Attachment disturbances in young children, II: indiscriminant behavior and institutional care. J Am Acad Child Adolesc Psychiatry 41:983–989, 2002

Zeanah CH, Smyke AT, Koga SF, et al: Attachment in institutionalized and community children in Romania. Child Dev 76:1015–1028, 2005

CHAPTER

# 15

# Delirium, Dementia, and Amnestic and Other Cognitive Disorders

JAMES A. BOURGEOIS, O.D., M.D., F.A.P.M.

JEFFREY S. SEAMAN, M.S., M.D.

MARK E. SERVIS, M.D.

## Delirium

### DSM-IV-TR Diagnosis of Delirium

The DSM-IV-TR (American Psychiatric Association 2000) diagnostic criteria for delirium (Table 15–1) require a disturbance in *consciousness/attention* and a change in *cognition* that develop *acutely* and *tend* to fluctuate. Lipowski (1983, 1987) characterized delirium as a disorder of attention, wakefulness, cognition, and motor behavior. The disruption of attention is often considered the core symptom. Sleep and wake cycles are disrupted as well, with patients frequently having grossly fragmented sleep and loss of normal circadian rhythm. The impairment in cognition can be across a wide spectrum—from subtle to overt and from focal to global. Deficits can occur in perception, memory, language, processing speed, and executive functioning.

The ranges of reported frequencies for clinical features are poor attention/vigilance (100%), memory impairment (64%–100%), clouding of consciousness (45%–100%), disorientation (43%–100%), acute onset (93%), disorganized thinking/thought disorder (59%–95%), diffuse cognitive impairment (77%), language disorder (41%–93%), sleep disturbance (25%–96%), delusions (18%–68%),

mood lability (43%–63%), psychomotor changes (38%–55%), and perceptual changes/hallucinations (17%–55%) (Meagher and Trzepacz 1998; Voyer et al. 2006).

### Delirium Subtypes

Consistent with the ancient descriptions of phrenitis and lethargus, hyperactive and hypoactive subtypes of delirium have been reported. Liptzin and Levkoff (1992) first characterized delirious patients with restlessness, hypervigilance, rapid speech, irritability, and combativeness as *hyperactive*, whereas those showing slowed speech and kinetics, apathy, and reduced alertness were designated *hypoactive*. The mixed type vacillated or included elements of the two other subtypes. Hypoactive patients tend to be older (McCusker et al. 2001; Peterson et al. 2006), to have more severe cognitive disturbances (Koponen et al. 1989c), to be less likely to be diagnosed (Inouye et al. 2001), and to have a poorer prognosis (Andrew et al. 2005; Liptzin and Levkoff 1992).

### Etiopathogenesis

One key to sustained progress in understanding delirium is a *refutation* of the misleading model wherein delirium is

221

**TABLE 15–1.   DSM-IV-TR diagnostic criteria for delirium due to...*[indicate the general medical condition]***

A.  Disturbance of consciousness (i.e., reduced clarity of awareness of the environment) with reduced ability to focus, sustain, or shift attention.

B.  A change in cognition (such as memory deficit, disorientation, language disturbance) or the development of a perceptual disturbance that is not better accounted for by a preexisting, established, or evolving dementia.

C.  The disturbance develops over a short period of time (usually hours to days) and tends to fluctuate during the course of the day.

D.  There is evidence from the history, physical examination, or laboratory findings that the disturbance is caused by the direct physiological consequences of a general medical condition.

**Coding note:**   If delirium is superimposed on a preexisting vascular dementia, indicate the delirium by coding 290.41 vascular dementia, with delirium.

**Coding note:**   Include the name of the general medical condition on Axis I, e.g., 293.0 delirium due to hepatic encephalopathy; also code the general medical condition on Axis III (see DSM-IV-TR Appendix G for codes).

believed to be *caused* by the comorbid systemic disease. We suggest instead that comorbid disease states, environmental stressors, and certain medications may *precipitate* delirium in vulnerable patients. The vast number and disparate nature of the identified precipitants (Elie et al. 1998) innately argue against most of them having *direct* causality for delirium.

### Neuronal Integrity

Engel and Romano's (1959) recommendation to examine the functional integrity of the neuron and brain energy metabolism during delirium is still valid. Nonetheless, several hypotheses seeking to elucidate the causative cascade for delirium have been advanced in recent years and are presented in brief.

### Role of Oxygen

The clinical importance of oxygen in the pathogenesis of delirium has been reported in several studies. Among *healthy young* adults, concentration and short-term learning are degraded when the partial pressure of oxygen ($PaO_2$) drops to 45–60 mm Hg, and frank delirium reliably occurs at a $PaO_2$ of 35–45 mm Hg (Gibson et al. 1981).

In one retrospective analysis of intensive care unit (ICU) patients, three measures of oxygenation (hemoglobin, hematocrit, pulse oximetry) and two of metabolic stress (sepsis, pneumonia) were worse in patients prior to developing delirium, despite no difference in illness severity between groups (Seaman et al. 2006).

### *Cardiovascular and Respiratory Reserves*

A broad decline in cardiovascular and respiratory reserves occurs with age. By age 85 years, vital capacity is reduced by 30%–40% and the arterial–alveolar gradient widens; by age 90 years, basal $PaO_2$ drops to 70 mm Hg, the ventilatory response to acute hypoxia is blunted, and maximum heart rate and cardiac output are decreased (Pack and Millman 1988).

### *Oxygen Demand and Anemia*

Brown (2000) noted the hospitalized patient's homeostasis is threatened by the increased $O_2$ demand from acute illness and fever (Fink 1997). Anemia is also commonly encountered among hospitalized patients, which can further limit $O_2$ delivery to the brain. Although the "baseline minimum" hematocrit may be enough to keep the brain alive and to avoid watershed strokes, it may *not be enough* to support normal function, particularly for the patient with limited cerebral reserve.

### *Anoxia*

A proposed causal link between metabolic derangements and the development of delirium has been presented by Brown (2000) and Bourgeois et al. (2003) and is summarized in Figure 15–1.

### *Additional Selective Mechanisms*

In one hypoxic encephalopathy model, dopamine release was shown to increase 500-fold, whereas γ-aminobutyric acid (GABA) release was increased only 5-fold (Globus et al. 1988). This massive increase in dopamine results from a breakdown in adenosine triphosphate–dependent transporters (decreased reuptake) during anoxic depolarization (Pulsinelli and Duffy 1983) as well as decreases in metabolism through the reduced activity of the $O_2$-dependent catechol-*O*-methyltransferase (Gibson et al. 1981).

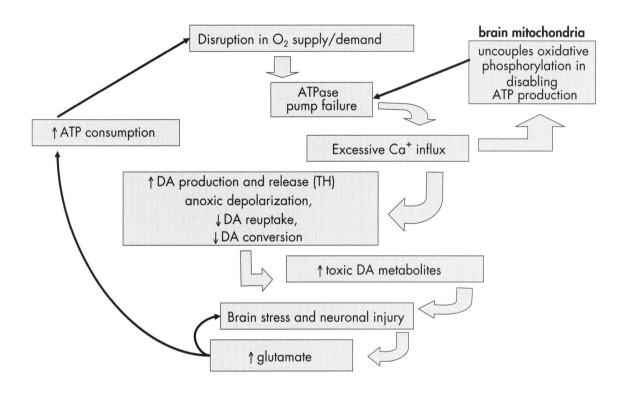

**FIGURE 15–1.** **Hypothesized delirium cascade: dopamine–oxygen link.**
ATP=adenosine triphosphate; Ca⁺=calcium; DA=dopamine; $O_2$=oxygen; TH=tyrosine hydroxylase.

### Neurotransmitter Roles

Regarding specific changes in neurotransmitters in delirium, the two most accepted are a reduction in acetylcholine activity and an excess of dopamine activity (Trzepacz 2000). Acetylcholine has long been known to be decreased in delirium (Itil and Fink 1966) as well as in hypoxia (Gibson and Blass 1976). Arousal, the sleep–wake cycle, attention, learning, and memory are heavily dependent on acetylcholine via its nicotinic and muscarinic receptors (Picciotto and Zoli 2002; Trzepacz 2000). It is important to note GABAergic interactions with acetylcholine appear critical in serving cognitive and attentional processes (Picciotto and Zoli 2002).

Dopamine is considered to have important roles in attention, mood, motor activity, perception, and executive functioning. Dopamine may be particularly valuable in facilitating cortical circuit activity during times of change, stress, or disequilibrium (Grace 2002). Excess dopamine activity can lead to delirium, as seen with drugs such as L-dopa or cocaine. Moreover, interplay between dopamine and acetylcholine exists, as evidenced experimentally by the finding that $D_2$ antagonists enhance acetylcholine release

(Ikarashi et al. 1997) and clinically by the utility of antipsychotics in reversing anticholinergic-precipitated delirium (Itil and Fink 1966).

## Epidemiology: Inpatient Studies

Inpatient studies have reported a delirium prevalence of 12%–40% among geriatric patients (Francis and Kapoor 1992; Inouye and Charpentier 1996; Inouye et al. 1998; O'Keeffe and Lavan 1997), 10%–15% across patients of all ages (Cameron et al. 1987), and 37% among postoperative patients (Dyer et al. 1995).

## Clinical Evaluation

### History

A thorough history provides the majority of the diagnostic information (Table 15–2). The referral problem is frequently characterized as psychosis, depression, noncompliance, or unruly behavior.

Central to the history gathering is establishing what the patient's premorbid baseline was, whether a recent change

| TABLE 15–2. | Evaluation of delirium |
| --- | --- |

**Standard**

Vital signs

Complete history

Medication review: recent past and current

Neurological examination

Bedside testing: months of the year backward (5), verbal Trails B (10), clock drawing, A test for vigilance

**As clinically warranted**

Laboratory work: complete blood count, electrolytes, blood urea nitrogen, creatinine, glucose, calcium, pulse oximetry or arterial blood gas, urinalysis, drug screen, liver function test with serum albumin, cultures, HIV screening, cerebrospinal fluid examination

Tests: chest X ray, electrocardiogram, brain imaging, electroencephalogram

occurred, and when. Not only is this information key in distinguishing delirium from dementia, but it may also serve to identify precipitants.

## Medication Review

Every delirium evaluation warrants a medication review inclusive of current and recently discontinued drugs, whether prescription, over-the-counter, herbal, or illicit. Medications with anticholinergic properties should be avoided as possible. The potential for drug–drug interactions should be reviewed. Adverse interactions include both pharmacodynamic (e.g., toxic synergies) and pharmacokinetic (e.g., cytochrome P450 system induction/inhibition, competition for serum protein binding, decreased clearance in renal or hepatic disease) effects.

## Interview and Observation

The interview itself should focus on establishing a global image of the patient's cognitive functioning. It is helpful to observe the patient for decreased attention capacity, psychosis, short-term memory deficits, disorientation, executive dysfunction, and changes in mood or kinetics. Bedside examinations (e.g., the A test for vigilance) and tests sensitive to frontal lobe dysfunction (Royall et al. 1998) are quick and easy to administer.

In regard to the Mini-Mental State Exam (MMSE), one study (C. A. Ross et al. 1991) reported that the mean MMSE score was 14.3 for delirious patients, versus 29.6

for control subjects. The first elements of the MMSE in their relatively young cohort to show deficits were the reverse calculation, orientation, and recall items. A single MMSE is not sensitive (33%) for identifying delirium, however, and is incapable of discriminating delirium from dementia (Trzepacz et al. 1986). Serial MMSEs, on the other hand, can help identify improvement or worsening of delirium (O'Keeffe et al. 2005; Tune and Folstein 1986) and assist in delirium screening when baseline MMSE scores are clearly known (Fayers et al. 2005).

## Rating Scales

Diagnostic and rating tools are critical for objectifying and unifying diagnostic and research efforts in delirium. The most cited and most validated instruments are the Delirium Rating Scale and the Delirium Rating Scale—Revised–98 (Trzepacz et al. 1988, 2001), the Confusion Assessment Method (Inouye et al. 1990), and the Memorial Delirium Assessment Scale (Breitbart et al. 1997).

## Neurological Examination

Unexplained or new focal neurological signs beyond cognitive disturbances are atypical in delirium and warrant discussion with a neurologist. Neuroimaging should be considered for patients with head injuries, focal findings, cancer, stroke risk, AIDS, or atypical presentations (e.g., young, healthy, lack of identifiable precipitants). Nonspecific abnormalities visible on neuroimaging such as periventricular white matter disease, varying degrees of generalized atrophy, and ventricular enlargement are common among the delirious elderly (Koponen et al. 1989a). In line with this, the degree of generalized cortical atrophy has been more closely linked to delirium risk than has the presence of focal cortical lesions alone (Tsai and Tsuang 1979).

## Laboratory Tests

Evaluations may include a complete blood count, electrolytes, blood urea nitrogen, creatinine, glucose, calcium, pulse oximetry or arterial blood gas, and urinalysis (see Table 15–2). Other tests commonly obtained are urine drug screens, liver function tests with serum albumin, cultures, chest X ray, and electrocardiogram. Cerebrospinal fluid examination also should be considered for cases in which meningitis or encephalitis is suspected as well as for atypical cases of delirium.

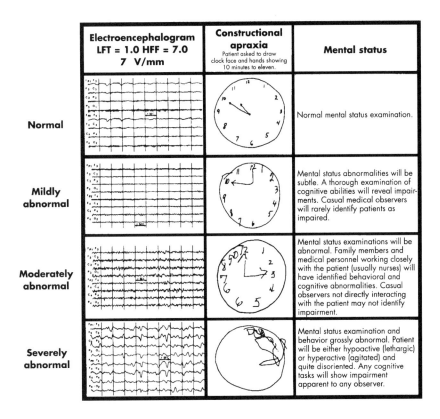

**FIGURE 15–2.** Comparison of electroencephalogram, constructional apraxia, and mental status in delirium.

## Electroencephalography

Romano and Engel (1944) were the first investigators to use electroencephalography to show that delirious patients had progressive disorganization of rhythms and generalized slowing (Figure 15–2). Delirious patients specifically have slowing of the peak and average frequencies in addition to increased theta and delta but decreased alpha rhythms (Koponen et al. 1989b).

## Differential Diagnosis

Delirium needs to be distinguished most frequently from dementia (Table 15–3). Dementia has an insidious rather than an acute onset, features chronic memory and executive disturbances, and—unless it is Lewy body dementia (LBD) or there is a superimposed delirium—tends not to fluctuate. A nondelirious dementia patient typically has intact attention and alertness. Other possibilities to consider in the differential diagnosis include conditions listed in Table 15–4.

**TABLE 15–3.** Delirium versus dementia

| Feature | Delirium | Dementia |
|---|---|---|
| Onset | Acute | Insidious |
| Cognitive dysfunction | Acute/acutely worse | Chronic |
| Attention | Disrupted | Intact (except Lewy body dementia and end-stage disease) |
| Fluctuation | Common | No (except Lewy body dementia) |
| Speech | Disorganized/confused | Impoverished |

TABLE 15–4. Delirium differential beyond dementia

| Diagnosis | Similarities | Differences |
|---|---|---|
| Depression | Withdrawn, hypoactive | Intact attention, insidious, EEG |
| Catatonia | Hypo- or hyperactive, odd behavior, limited or no speech | Motor findings, resolves with lorazepam/ECT, EEG |
| Bell's mania | Hyperactive, confused | Responsive to ECT, other manic symptoms and history, EEG |
| First-break schizophrenia | Disorganized, poor attention, diffuse cognitive dysfunction | Young age, no precipitants, persistent psychotic symptoms after confusion clears, EEG |
| Drug/alcohol intoxication or withdrawal | Hypo- or hyperactive, hallucinations, poor attention | Positive drug screen or history, EEG |

*Note.* ECT=electroconvulsive therapy; EEG=electroencephalogram.

### Risk Factors: Precipitants and Baseline Vulnerability

The term *precipitant* can be justifiably used to subsume risk factors that are generally transient or acute (e.g., a urinary tract infection). Similarly, *baseline vulnerability* is a term coined by Inouye to describe the risk factors that are, by definition, chronic and innate to the patient (e.g., cerebral atrophy).

Inouye and Charpentier (1996) eloquently supported this concept in their landmark 1996 study. They separated out baseline risks present at admission (e.g., prior cognitive impairment) from precipitants affecting the patient after admission (e.g., new-onset respiratory insufficiency). Robust patients with less baseline vulnerability ("more cerebral reserve") were more resilient to new precipitants after admission. The reverse was true as well.

Numerous medications across many classes have been noted to precipitate delirium (Brown and Stoudemire 1998). The commonly used benzodiazepine lorazepam has been shown to independently increase delirium development in ICU patients (Pandharipande et al. 2006). Importantly, the capacity of a medication to exert anticholinergic activity has been shown to correlate with its propensity to trigger delirium (L. Han et al. 2001).

Prospective studies have identified many other precipitants and baseline risks for delirium (Table 15–5). Two of the most frequently reported are preexisting cognitive decline and advanced age. On the basis of these risk factors, standardized intervention protocols often are effective treatments (e.g., Inouye et al. 1999).

## Prognosis

### Mortality

Seven studies have been published that used multivariate and logistic regression analyses to establish that delirium *independently* increased mortality risk in their groups. A group from Taiwan (Lin et al. 2004) found a hazard ratio of 2.6 and an odds ratio of 13 for delirium's effect on ICU patient mortality. Ely et al. (2004; Figure 15–3) uncovered a 6-month mortality hazard ratio of 3.2 for ICU patients who had been delirious while on the ventilator. Leslie et al. (2005) strengthened this claim further by reporting that death rates increased in step with delirium severity during the index hospitalization 1 year after hospitalization. A large study from Finland tracked a combined elderly sample (most subjects older than 85 years) from nursing homes and geriatric hospital wards for 2 years. In this group, delirium was an independent predictor of death at 1 and 2 years (Pitkala et al. 2005).

### Morbidity

Delirium also often portends poor clinical outcomes. The length of hospital stay is longer (Ely et al. 2004; Thomason et al. 2005), the readmission rate higher (Marcantonio et al. 2005), and the loss of independent living more common (Adamis et al. 2006; Bourdel-Marchasson et al. 2004; Francis and Kapoor 1992; Pitkala et al. 2005) among patients who have been delirious. Overall, a meta-analysis (Cole and Primeau 1993) found that patients with delirium had a mean length of hospital stay of 20.7 days (vs. 8.9 days for control subjects) and a reduced rate of independent living 6 months after admission of 56.8% (vs. 91.7% in control subjects).

TABLE 15–5.  Risk factors for delirium

| Baseline type (less modifiable) | Precipitant type (more modifiable) |
|---|---|
| Dementia | Blood urea nitrogen/creatinine >18 |
| Preexisting cognitive impairment | Abnormal Na$^+$, K$^+$, or blood glucose levels |
| Age | Anticholinergics |
| Cerebral atrophy | Hypoxia |
| Illness severity | Windowless intensive care unit |
| Vision or hearing impairment | Malnutrition |
| Impaired functional status | Hyper- or hypothermia |
| Orthopedic, thoracic, or aortic aneurysm surgery | Infection |
| Fracture | Uremia |
| Lower education level | Preoperative depression |
| Smoking history | Perioperative and intraoperative hypotension |
| Previous delirium | Anemia |
| Previous stroke | Disseminated intravascular coagulation |
| Diabetes mellitus | More than three new medications begun |
| Vascular depression? | Benzodiazepines >2 mg lorazepam equivalents |
| | Corticosteroids >15 mg dexamethasone equivalents |
| | Opioids >90 mg morphine equivalents |
| | Many chemotherapy and immunosuppressive agents |
| | Many medications with strong anticholinergic activity |
| | Several Parkinson's disease medications |
| | Numerous isolated reports of varying medications |

*Source.*   Benoit et al. 2005; Brown and Stoudemire 1998; Centeno et al. 2004; Culp et al. 2004; Edlund et al. 2001; Foy et al. 1995; Francis et al. 1990; Gaudreau et al. 2005; Gustafson et al. 1988; Henon et al. 1999; Inouye and Charpentier 1996; Inouye et al. 1993; Leung et al. 2005; Lundström et al. 2003; Marcantonio et al. 1994; Minden et al. 2005; Pompei et al. 1994; Rockwood 1989; Rogers et al. 1989; Schor et al. 1992; Williams-Russo et al. 1992; Wilson 1972.

### Permanent Cognitive Dysfunction: Clinical Studies

Several groups have reported MMSE score decreases or increased dementia rates for older patients who were tracked for 1 year (Katz et al. 2001; Koponen et al. 1989b), 2 years (Dolan et al. 2000; Francis and Kapoor 1992; Rahkonen et al. 2000; Wacker et al. 2006), 3 years (Rahkonen et al. 2001), and 5 years (Lundström et al. 2003) after an index hospitalization with delirium versus comparison groups.

### Duration

Average delirium episodes of 3–13 days are typically reported, although 20 days was the mean in a sample of patients with "beclouded" dementia (Koponen et al. 1989c). Persistence beyond 30 days has been described to occur in as many as 13%–50% of delirious elderly (Marcantonio et al. 2000). Patients with hypoactive delirium have been shown to have longer episodes than do those with the mixed or hyperactive subtypes (Kelly et al. 2001).

## Treatment and Prevention

Modifiable precipitants may be an undetected urinary tract infection, pneumonia, organ failure, sepsis, select medications, or a host of other variables (see Table 15–5). Anticholinergics, benzodiazepines, corticosteroids, powerful dopamine agonists, and some opioids are best limited when feasible (Morita et al. 2005), although uncertainty remains in this arena (Gaudreau et al. 2005). The fundamental goal of treating delirium is not to control agitation or hallucinations alone; *it is to prevent and reverse the delirium and thus mitigate associated morbidity and mortality risks.*

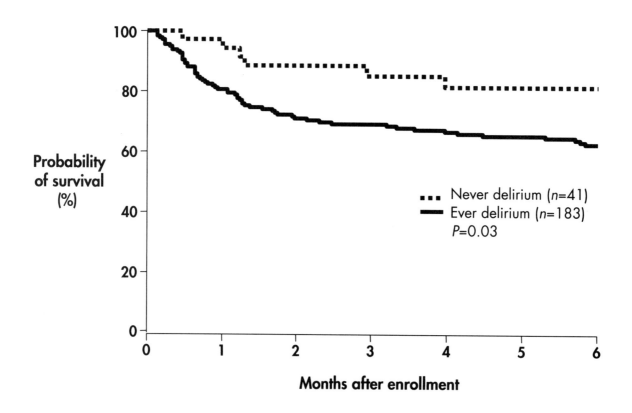

FIGURE 15–3.   **Delirium and mortality in intensive care unit patients.**
*Source.* Ely et al. 2004.

## Pharmacotherapy

The American Psychiatric Association (1999) practice guideline supported haloperidol as a first-line agent for delirium because of its minimal anticholinergic effects, minimal orthostasis, limited sedation, and flexibility in dosing and administration with oral, intramuscular, and intravenous routes. Both oral and intravenous forms have been used for more than 40 years and have an extensive track record of safety and efficacy in even the most ill medical and surgical patients (Cassem and Sos 1978). Haloperidol also has been proven clearly superior to benzodiazepines given alone in delirium (Breitbart et al. 1996).

The recommended dosage of haloperidol (American Psychiatric Association 1999) is 1–2 mg every 2–4 hours as needed, with further titration until desired effects are seen. Once stabilized, patients are often transitioned to a twice-daily or a daily bedtime oral dose, which is then continued or slowly tapered until the delirium has resolved.

In severe delirium refractory to boluses, continuous haloperidol infusions of 3–25 mg/hour have been used safely (Riker et al. 1994), although the practice guideline suggested a ceiling of 5–10 mg/hour. Electrocardiographic monitoring is recommended with continuous infusion because of concerns about torsades de pointes, although no specific dosage threshold has been designated (American Psychiatric Association 1999; Sharma et al. 1998). Awareness and management of risk factors for QTc prolongation are advised (Gury et al. 2000). Prolonged QTc intervals beyond 450 msec or 25% above baseline should prompt a cardiology consultation, a dosage reduction, or discontinuation of the antipsychotic agent (American Psychiatric Association 1999).

At least 19 English-language reports are available regarding atypical antipsychotics for delirium. The advantages are the lowered risk of extrapyramidal symptoms or electrocardiographic abnormalities (Titier et al. 2004), the mood-modulating effects, and possibly the enhanced efficacy in select patients. These agents also may exert their effectiveness via blockade at serotonin type 2A (5-HT$_{2A}$), D$_4$, and $\alpha_1$ receptors and agonism at 5-HT$_{1A}$ (Meltzer 2002).

### Cholinergic Modulation

Tune et al. (1992) have shown that numerous commonly used medications have anticholinergic effects. Furthermore, there appears to be a substantial interplay between acetylcholine systems in the brain and anesthetic agents (Pratico et al. 2005).

With this knowledge to go on, there has been a resurgent interest in using procholinergic agents in delirium, specifically acetylcholinesterase/butyrylcholinesterase inhibitors. Recently, there have been several case reports and small case series noting improvements in beclouded dementia (Wengel et al. 1998), opioid-precipitated delirium (Slatkin and Rhiner 2004; Slatkin et al. 2001), postsurgical delirium (Gleason 2003; Liptzin et al. 2005), and antipsychotic-resistant delirium (Dautzenberg et al. 2004; Wengel et al. 1999).

### Prevention

Several studies have identified and tracked risk factors with which to develop predictive instruments, also called risk-stratification models (Freter et al. 2005; Inouye and Charpentier 1996; Marcantonio et al. 1994). Four risk factors—vision impairment, severe illness, preexisting cognitive impairment, and dehydration—were used in one predictive model (Inouye et al. 1993). Nine percent of the low-risk patients (i.e., those with none of the four factors) later developed delirium compared with 23% of those with one or two factors and 83% of those with three or four factors.

# Dementia

## Clinical Features

### DSM-IV-TR Classification of Dementias

According to DSM-IV-TR, core features of the dementias include multiple cognitive deficits (anterograde and/or retrograde memory impairment and aphasia, apraxia, agnosia, or disturbance in executive functioning) that cause impairment in role functioning and represent a significant decline (American Psychiatric Association 2000). Dementia subtypes specified in DSM-IV-TR are shown in Table 15–6.

**TABLE 15–6. Diagnostic features of the dementias**

**Features common to all dementias**

Multiple cognitive deficits that do not occur exclusively during the course of delirium, including memory impairment and aphasia, apraxia, agnosia, or disturbed executive functioning, and that represent a decline from previous level of functioning and impair role functioning

**Dementia of the Alzheimer's type, additional features**

Gradual onset and continuing cognitive decline; deficits are not due to other central nervous system, systemic, or substance-induced conditions and are not better attributed to another Axis I disorder

**Vascular dementia, additional features**

Focal neurological signs and symptoms or laboratory/radiological evidence indicative of cerebrovascular disease etiologically related to deficits

**Dementia due to other general medical conditions, additional features**

Clinical evidence that cognitive disturbance is direct physiological consequence of one of the following: HIV, head trauma, Parkinson's disease, Huntington's disease, Pick's disease, Creutzfeldt-Jakob disease, or another general medical condition (includes Lewy body dementia)

**Substance-induced persisting dementia, additional features**

Deficits persist beyond usual duration of substance intoxication or withdrawal, with clinical evidence that deficits are etiologically related to the persisting effects of substance use

**Dementia due to multiple etiologies, additional feature**

Clinical evidence that the disturbance has more than one etiology

**Dementia not otherwise specified, additional feature**

Dementia that does not meet criteria for one of the specified types above

*Source.* Adapted from American Psychiatric Association 2000.

### Cortical Versus Subcortical Dementias

A distinction is made between dementias with primarily cortical and those with primarily subcortical pathology (Table 15–7). Whereas all dementias have the same core clinical features, cortical and subcortical dementias often

**TABLE 15–7.    Cortical and subcortical dementia types**

**Cortical dementias**

Dementia of the Alzheimer's type (DAT)

Frontotemporal dementia, including dementia due to Pick's disease

Dementia due to Creutzfeldt-Jakob disease

Dementia due to chronic subdural hematoma

**Subcortical dementias**

Dementia due to HIV

Dementia due to Parkinson's disease

Dementia due to Huntington's disease

Dementia due to multiple sclerosis

**Dementias with cortical and subcortical features**

Vascular dementia (formerly multi-infarct dementia)[a]

Vascular dementia (poststroke dementia)[a]

Mixed dementia (DAT + vascular dementia)

Lewy body variant of Alzheimer's disease[a]

Lewy body dementia[a]

Dementia due to fragile X–associated tremor/ataxia syndrome

Dementia due to normal-pressure hydrocephalus

[a]Relative amount of cortical and subcortical features is dependent on location of neuropathology.

**TABLE 15–8.    Established and proposed risk factors for dementia of the Alzheimer's type**

Increased age

Female gender

Head trauma

Small head size

Family history

Low childhood intelligence

Limited education

Childhood rural residence

Large sibships

Smoking

Never having married

Depression

Diabetes mellitus

Increased total cholesterol

Vascular disease

Hypertension

Increased platelet membrane fluidity

Apolipoprotein E (APOE) ε4 allele on chromosome 19

Abnormalities on chromosomes 1, 6, 12, 14, and 21

Trisomy 21

differ in their specific clinical presentation. Cortical dementia is characterized by prominent memory impairment (recall *and* recognition), language deficits, apraxia, agnosia, and visuospatial deficits (Doddy et al. 1998; Paulsen et al. 1995). Subcortical dementia features greater impairment in recall memory, decreased verbal fluency without anomia, bradyphrenia (slowed thinking), depressed mood, affective lability, apathy, and decreased attention/concentration (Doddy et al. 1998; Paulsen et al. 1995). Cortical dementias generally lack prominent motor signs, whereas subcortical dementias typically feature such signs (Geldmacher and Whitehouse 1997).

### Cortical Dementias

Dementia of the Alzheimer's type (DAT), the most common dementia, is estimated to affect nearly 2 million white Americans (Hy and Keller 2000). There is an important conceptual and semantic distinction between the DSM-IV-TR diagnoses of DAT and Alzheimer's disease (AD) (Rabins et al. 1997). DAT is a clinical diagnosis, based on the findings of insidious onset and gradual, steady progression of cognitive deficits. Because symptoms and signs consistent with DAT may be present with other types of neuropathology, a clinical diagnosis of AD should be made only after medical evaluation fails to identify other causes for the dementia symptoms (Rabins et al. 1997). Established and proposed risk factors for DAT are shown in Table 15–8 (Blennow et al. 2006; Moceri et al. 2000).

The noncognitive symptoms in dementia are also referred to as the behavioral and psychological symptoms of dementia (Lawlor 2004). These include psychiatric symptoms and behavioral manifestations that cross the boundaries of DSM-IV-TR categories of psychiatric disorders. Over the course of a case of dementia, the symptoms tend to fluctuate as the patient's cognitive status changes. Mood symptoms that occur before cognitive deficits may represent a prodromal state (Berger et al. 1999). Depressive disorders have been reported in up to 86% of patients with DAT, with a median estimate of 19% (Aalten et al. 2003; Zubenko et al. 2003). Apathy is common and may occur in the absence of full-syndrome depression; apathy, agitation, dysphoria, and aberrant motor behavior all increase with illness progression and increasing cognitive impairment (Aalten et al. 2003; Lyketsos et al. 2002). Disinhibited social and sexual behavior, assaultiveness, and inappropriate laughter or tearfulness are common. Evening agitation ("sundowning") may be a notably disruptive symptom and has been linked to disturbed circadian rhythms and a phase delay of body temperature in DAT (Volicer et al. 2001). Psychosis is common in DAT; the early appearance of psychosis correlates with more rapid cognitive decline (Ropacki and Jeste 2005; Wilkosz et al. 2006). Visual hallucinations are the most common perceptual disturbance (Class et al. 1997). The prevalence of delusions in DAT is as high as 73%; delusions of persecution, theft, reference, and jealousy are common (Rao and Lyketsos 1998; Ropacki and Jeste 2005).

The neuropathology of AD includes β-amyloid deposits, neuritic plaques, and neurofibrillary tangles (Felician and Sandson 1999; Jellinger 1996). Amyloid precursor protein (APP, coded on chromosome 21) is cleaved by proteases (β and γ secretases), producing insoluble β-amyloid (Haass and De Strooper 1999; Jellinger 1996). APP processing may be partially controlled by cholinergic mechanisms (Small 1998b). Inhibition of β and γ secretases and presenilin proteins 1 and 2 (proteins coded for on chromosomes 1 and 14, respectively, which appear to modulate secretase activity) may decrease cleavage of APP, thereby decreasing production of insoluble β-amyloid (Haass and De Strooper 1999).

The apolipoprotein E (APOE) ε4 allele on chromosome 19 affects the rate of β-amyloid production and the clinical manifestations of AD in a dose-dependent fashion; homozygotes have a higher risk, earlier onset, and faster rate of decline than do heterozygotes and noncarriers (Blennow et al. 2006; Caselli et al. 1999; Craft et al. 1998). Adults without dementia who carried the APOE ε4 allele were found to have decreased verbal memory performance and minor hippocampal damage (Bottino and Almeida 1997; Small et al. 1999). The APOE ε2 allele may confer protection against AD, whereas the APOE ε3 allele appears to not change AD risk (Rebeck and Hyman 1999).

Frontotemporal dementia (FTD), including dementia due to Pick's disease, features an earlier age at onset than DAT, executive dysfunction, attentional deficits, loss of insight, aphasia, and personality changes (typically increased extroversion), with relatively spared memory and visuospatial functions (Boeve 2006; Kertesz and Munoz 2002; Mendez et al. 2006). Patients may show "childlike" exuberance, "catastrophic" reactions to trivial events, decreased social awareness, disinhibition, distractibility,

aphasia, perseveration, carbohydrate cravings, and frontal lobe release signs and may have a poorer response to cholinesterase inhibitors than do patients with AD (Duara et al. 1999; Kertesz and Munoz 2002). Neuropathological findings in FTD are restricted to the frontal and anterior temporal lobes and include characteristic Pick inclusion bodies, neurofibrillary tangles, and ballooned cells, all containing tau protein (Jellinger 1996; Kertesz and Munoz 2002).

Dementia due to chronic subdural hematoma may present with focal neurological signs, personality changes, various cognitive impairments (including decreased memory, language disturbances, difficulty with abstraction, problems with calculation, and poor social judgment), lethargy, and/or agitation (G.W. Ross and Bowen 2002). The syndrome may have a relatively sudden onset and may show fluctuation in clinical status; a history of trauma may be absent in one-third of affected patients (G.W. Ross and Bowen 2002).

### Subcortical Dementias

Dementia due to HIV initially manifests as decreases in psychomotor and information processing speed, verbal memory, learning efficiency, and fine motor function, with later cortical symptoms of decreased executive function, aphasia, apraxia, and agnosia (Maldonado et al. 2000). In advanced stages, ataxia, spasticity, increased muscle tone, and incontinence may develop (Maldonado et al. 2000). Dementia has been reported in up to 30% of HIV-positive patients, may present early in the course of illness, increases suicide risk, and may compromise compliance with antiviral regimens (Cohen and Jacobson 2000; Maldonado et al. 2000). More recent estimates of the incidence of dementia due to HIV are somewhat lower, possibly because of the neuroprotective effects of early, aggressive antiviral treatment (d'Arminio Monforte et al. 2000; Goodkin et al. 2001).

Dementia due to Parkinson's disease (PD) is seen in as many as 60% of patients with PD and features bradyphrenia, apathy, poor retrieval memory, decreased verbal fluency, and attention deficits (Levy and Cummings 2000; Marsh 2000). Increased age, greater severity of neurological symptoms, and the APOE ε2 allele have been associated with an increased risk of dementia in patients with PD (Harhangi et al. 2000; Hughes et al. 2000). Cognition may improve with treatment for the common comorbid mood disorders (Levy and Cummings 2000). Psychosis can be induced by antiparkinsonian treatment of the motor symptoms of PD. Dementia due to PD features deposition of α-synuclein or tau protein in the substantia nigra and commonly involves Lewy bodies in the substantia nigra, cortex, and subcortex, with resulting deficits in dopaminergic, noradrenergic, cholinergic, and serotonergic neurotransmission (Levy and Cummings 2000; Marsh 2000).

Dementia due to Huntington's disease features abulia and impairments in retrieval memory, cognitive speed, concentration, verbal learning, and cognitive flexibility (Boeve 2006; Ranen 2000). With progression, more global impairment in memory, visuospatial function, and executive function may follow (Ranen 2000). Comorbid mood disturbance, anxiety (including obsessive-compulsive symptoms), and psychotic symptoms are common (Boeve 2006; Tost et al. 2004). These patients have a high risk for personality change, irritability, aggressive behavior, and suicide (Ranen 2000; Rosenblatt and Leroi 2000). The dementia results from cell loss in primary sensory and association areas, entorhinal cortex, caudate nucleus, and putamen (Jellinger 1996; Ranen 2000).

Dementia due to multiple sclerosis is seen in as many as 65% of multiple sclerosis patients (Schwid et al. 2000). Clinical features include deficits in memory, attention, information processing speed, learning, and executive functions; language and verbal intelligence are relatively spared (Schwid et al. 2000). Cognitive impairment may present early in the course of multiple sclerosis, and progression is roughly proportional to the number of central nervous system (CNS) demyelinating lesions (Schwid et al. 2000).

### Dementias With Cortical and Subcortical Features

Vascular dementia (VaD) broadly includes dementias resulting from vascular pathology that have as a final common pathway the loss of functional cortex. Because VaD exists on a continuum extending from the essentially subcortical pathology formerly described as "multi-infarct dementia" to the primarily cortical pathology in "poststroke dementia" (i.e., dementia following a single stroke), it is problematic to attempt to fit all VaDs (thus inclusively defined) into the "cortical versus subcortical" dichotomy.

Multi-infarct VaD is characterized by abrupt onset, decreased executive functioning, gait disturbance, affective lability, and parkinsonian symptoms (Choi et al. 2000; Patterson et al. 1999). Risk factors include increased age, hypertension, diabetes mellitus, atherosclerotic heart disease, hypertriglyceridemia, and hyperlipidemia (Curb et al. 1999; G.W. Ross et al. 1999). Because the cognitive deficits follow a series of discrete lesions, progression is "stepwise," with relative stability of cognitive status between vascular insults as opposed to the gradual progression of deficits seen in AD. The progression of multi-infarct VaD may be affected by risk factor modification and antiplatelet therapy (Rabins et al. 1997). Lesions are generally located in the subcortical nuclei, frontal lobe white matter, thalamus, and internal capsule and are associated with a characteristic appearance on magnetic resonance imaging (MRI) of periventricular hyperintensities on the T2 images (Choi et al. 2000).

Poststroke VaD—dementia occurring as the acute or subacute consequence of a single stroke—may be difficult to clearly distinguish from multi-infarct VaD that follows a series of vascular events. Poststroke dementia is associated with apraxia, neglect, hemianopsia, facial paralysis, and extremity weakness (de Koning et al. 1998). Major dominant-hemisphere stroke, left hemisphere location, internal carotid artery distribution, diabetes mellitus, prior cerebrovascular accident (CVA), older age, less education, and nonwhite race were found to be risk factors for poststroke dementia (Desmond et al. 2000). Major depression is common with poststroke dementia, with anterior left hemisphere stroke posing the highest risk (Robinson 1998). Deficits in orientation, language, visuoconstruction, and executive functions are common but may improve with treatment of the poststroke depression (Robinson 1998).

Lewy body variant (LBV) of AD and LBD have a significant degree of phenomenological overlap and may be difficult to differentiate clinically (Leverenz and McKeith 2002). Clinically, LBV and LBD share the common features of fluctuation of mental status, well-formed visual hallucinations, delusions, depression, apathy, anxiety, and extrapyramidal symptoms (Heyman et al. 1999; Lopez et al. 2000). Visual hallucinations occur early in the course of illness, even with mild levels of cognitive impairment (Ballard et al. 2001; Leverenz and McKeith 2002). In comparison with AD, LBV is associated with greater deficits in attention, verbal fluency, and visuospatial functioning and increased parkinsonian symptoms (Lopez et al. 2000; McKeith et al. 2000). LBV has also been associated with more rapid cognitive decline, earlier institutionalization, and shorter survival time (Lopez et al. 2000; Serby et al. 2003). LBD also features impaired executive functioning, disinhibited social behavior, syncope, and increased sensitivity to antipsychotic agents (manifested by drowsiness, further cognitive decline, and neuroleptic malignant syndrome) (Aarsland et al. 2005; McKeith et al. 2000). Progression is usually more rapid in LBD than in AD, although psychotic symptoms in

LBV and LBD may be improved by treatment with cholinesterase inhibitors, whereas psychotic symptoms may paradoxically worsen with antipsychotic agents (Ballard et al. 2001; Leverenz and McKeith 2002; Levy and Cummings 2000). LBV and LBD are also associated with neuroleptic sensitivity, characterized by sedation, immobility, rigidity, postural instability, falls, and decreased cognitive status (Baskys 2004).

## Epidemiology

The risk of dementia increases exponentially with age, from 1% for those younger than 65 years to 25%–50% for those older than 85 years (Jorm and Jolley 1998). Reported estimates of the relative frequency of the different dementia types in study populations of dementia patients are 50%–90% for DAT, 8%–20% for VaD, and 7%–26% for LBD, with other subtypes less common (Lyketsos et al. 2000; Roman 2002). Reversible dementias are estimated to account for 1%–10% of dementias; examples of potentially reversible dementias are shown in Table 15–9 (Gliatto and Caroff 2001; Tager and Fallon 2001).

## Comorbidity and Differential Diagnosis

The patient with cognitive impairment may have psychiatric illnesses other than or in addition to dementia. Clinical history and examination need to be focused to consider these other diagnostic possibilities. The psychiatric differential diagnosis of dementia is shown in Table 15–10.

**TABLE 15–10. Psychiatric differential diagnosis of dementia**

Mild cognitive impairment

Delirium

Mood disorders

Amnestic disorders

Substance use disorders

Psychotic disorders

Mental retardation

## Clinical Evaluation

### *History*

A clinical history should first be obtained from the patient directly, initially without the presence of other family members. History taking should address recent cognitive

**TABLE 15–9. Potentially reversible etiologies of dementia**

**Structural central nervous system factors**

Vascular dementia

Head trauma

Subdural hematoma

Normal-pressure hydrocephalus

Multiple sclerosis

**Psychiatric illnesses**

Major depression

Substance dependence

**Systemic/metabolic factors**

Hypothyroidism

Hypercalcemia

Hypoglycemia

Thiamine, niacin, $B_{12}$ deficiency

Renal failure

Hepatic failure

Medications

**Infectious diseases**

HIV

Central nervous system infection

function; examples include function at work, at home, while driving, and while performing other high-risk activities (Patterson et al. 1999). A complaint of memory loss may be predictive of a later diagnosis of DAT, even without demonstrable memory deficits on initial clinical examination (Geerlings et al. 1999). A personal and family history of psychiatric illness should be obtained, specifically to include dementia and neurological illness with high risk for dementia. Because the patient is most reliable in the early stages of illness, the physician should then separately interview family members and synthesize the separate histories obtained to derive the most balanced view of the patient's functioning.

The medical history should address all chronic systemic illnesses, with particular attention to conditions that increase risk for DAT, VaD, and other dementia types. Specific examples of such systemic illnesses include hypertension, diabetes mellitus, hyperlipidemia, PD, multiple sclerosis, and prior CVA (Geldmacher and Whitehouse 1997). The medication history should address both psychotropic and nonpsychotropic medications taken before the onset of the cognitive and behavioral symptoms (Doraiswamy et al. 1998). The use of nonprescription medications (especially antihistamines and sedatives) and herbal preparations also needs to be explored.

The social history should address the patient's living circumstances, presence of supportive family members and/or of other significant persons living nearby, financial and insurance resources, participation in social activities, and personal relationships. Collateral history obtained from family members should focus on concerns about the patient's cognitive function and overt behavior. Problematic symptoms such as paranoia, agitation, physical violence, and inattentive and dangerous operation of dangerous machinery need to be addressed, as well as access to weapons and any threats made to self or others. Any complaint of neglect or abuse, or any physical examination findings suggestive of inappropriate care, should be reported promptly to the agency responsible for performing on-site evaluation of neglect or abuse of adults. Aggressive and/or delusional patients may be at greatest risk for such maltreatment (Cummings and Masterman 1998).

### Mental Status Examination

Formal assessment of cognitive function must be added to routine evaluation of mood and affect, level of consciousness, psychomotor activity, speech production, thought content, and thought processes. It is recommended that the clinician use a cognitive assessment instrument such as the MMSE. A score of 24 or less on the MMSE, when correlated with clinical findings, is highly suggestive of dementia (Patterson et al. 1999). A cutoff score of 22 is advised in the elderly nursing home population; the MMSE may overestimate dementia in patients with less education, age older than 85, or a history of depression (Dufouil et al. 2000). Serial administrations of the MMSE can quantify the progress or stability of dementia; a typical decline in MMSE scores in DAT is 2–4 points per year in untreated patients (Folstein et al. 1975; Rabins et al. 1997). Adjunctive tests of cognitive function include clock drawing, category generation (e.g., having the patient name as many animals as possible in 1 minute; 16 is a cutoff score), and the "go, no-go" test (the patient is instructed to tap once if the examiner taps once, and to not tap if the examiner taps twice). The Neuropsychiatric Inventory is a 12-item behavioral rating scale used to assess noncognitive symptoms of dementia (Aalten et al. 2003). A series of structured questions administered to the patient's caregiver are used to assess the following behavioral domains: delusions, hallucinations, agitation/aggression, dysphoria/depression, anxiety, apathy, irritability, euphoria, dis-

inhibition, aberrant motor behavior, nighttime behavioral disturbance, and appetite/eating abnormalities (Aalten et al. 2003). Depression rating scales are recommended to assist in distinguishing dementia from depression and in monitoring response to antidepressants (Katz 1998). Suicide risk increases in the elderly population, and clinical assessment of other suicide risk factors (e.g., substance abuse, isolation, past suicidal behavior, access to weapons) needs to be integrated into the physician's clinical examination.

### Physical Examination

Relative sensory deprivation due to uncorrected vision and/or hearing deficits can cause spuriously poor performance on formal cognitive testing. Loss of visual acuity and severe cognitive impairment in patients with DAT can increase visual hallucinations (Chapman et al. 1999). Neurological examination should include assessment of gait, frontal lobe release signs, movement disorders, sensory function, and focal neurological deficits (Doraiswamy et al. 1998). Physical examination should address blood pressure, orthostatic hypotension, cardiovascular disease, cerebrovascular disease, signs of metabolic illnesses, marginal hygiene, poor nutritional status, weight loss, and dehydration. Treatment of vascular risk factors has been shown to decrease the risk of dementia, including DAT and VaD (Alagiakrishnan et al. 2006; Peila et al. 2006).

### Laboratory Tests

The usual laboratory tests that should be obtained to evaluate dementia are shown in Table 15–11.

### Neuroimaging

Neuroimaging is increasingly routine in the evaluation of dementia. In cases of suspected DAT, hippocampal atrophy may serve as a sensitive early marker for cognitive decline (Jack et al. 2000; Petersen et al. 2000).

Cortical atrophy and ventriculomegaly do not by themselves confirm dementia and, in isolation, are not specific findings (Doraiswamy et al. 1998; Small 1998a). If initial neuroimaging shows hippocampal and/or cortical atrophy that correlates with the clinical presentation and gradual course of DAT, then serial neuroimaging to follow progress is not routinely necessary. Periventricular hyperintensities on MRI may be seen in DAT as well as in VaD; their significance in DAT is unclear because they may not correlate independently with cognitive changes (Doddy et al. 1998; Smith et al. 2000). Decreased white

**TABLE 15–11.** Laboratory tests for dementia workup

Electrolytes, blood urea nitrogen, creatinine, calcium

Liver-associated enzymes

Glucose

Complete blood count

Thyroid profile with thyrotropin assay

Erythrocyte sedimentation rate, antinuclear antibody panel

Prothrombin time/partial thromboblastin time

$B_{12}$ and folate

Syphilis serology

Urinalysis and urine toxicology

Pulse oximetry

Medication levels (e.g., tricyclic antidepressants, anticonvulsants, digitalis, antiarrhythmics)

HIV

---

matter volume has been associated with DAT (Smith et al. 2000). If initial imaging shows white matter lesions typical of VaD that correlate with clinical findings, a follow-up computed tomography (CT) or MRI scan could be considered if the patient later presents with an abrupt decrease in mental status suggestive of delirium and/or a new CVA. Diffusion-weighted MRI, which has been shown to be more sensitive than CT in imaging the ischemic small-vessel disease in VaD, may be used to monitor progression of these patients (Choi et al. 2000). Functional neuroimaging (e.g., single photon emission computed tomography, positron emission tomography (PET) scanning, and in vivo proton magnetic resonance spectroscopy), although not currently widely available, holds promise in the evaluation of the cortical pathology of dementia, particularly when combined with genetic assessment of patients at risk for clinical dementia (Weiss et al. 2003). Functional neuroimaging techniques may detect a specific pattern of parietal and temporal deficits in DAT that could lead the physician to consider earlier treatment with antidementia pharmacotherapy (Small and Leiter 1998).

## Management

### Clinical Management

Early frank discussion of diagnosis, prognosis, and management, with clinical follow-ups scheduled at least every 3 months, is advised. Every visit should include an evalu-

ation of whether the patient can still safely live at home. More frequent visits should be scheduled to monitor response and side effects when psychotropic medications are prescribed. Supportive psychotherapy may assist the patient in dealing with grief and loss. Admission to a psychiatry inpatient unit skilled in dealing with dementia patients may be needed for severely regressed, suicidal, violent, or psychotic patients, especially if complex psychopharmacological regimens or electroconvulsive therapy (ECT) is considered (Rabins et al. 1997).

Psychoeducation can be very valuable, especially for family caregivers (Grossberg and Lake 1998). *The 36-Hour Day: A Family Guide to Caring for Persons With Alzheimer's Disease, Related Dementing Illnesses, and Memory Loss in Later Life* (Mace and Rabins 1981) is often helpful to both patients and families. Support and advocacy groups are available through the Alzheimer's Association (1-800-621-0379; www.alz.org) (Rabins et al. 1997). The Alzheimer's Association can facilitate patient enrollment in the Safe Return Program, a nationwide program that assists in the identification and return of dementia patients who wander. The patient should always carry and/or wear identification (e.g., a MedicAlert bracelet) and can be registered with the local police department. Physicians should inform caregivers of the increased risk of depression in primary caregivers of dementia patients and facilitate respite opportunities for caregivers (Grossberg and Lake 1998).

A recent major review of the psychological approaches to the neuropsychiatric disturbances in dementia found that behavior management strategies, caregiver and residential staff education, and (possibly) cognitive stimulation techniques had an adequate evidence base supporting their prolonged effectiveness (Livingston et al. 2005). Environmental and behavioral management may include provision of adequate lighting, music, access to pets, and appropriate levels of psychological stimulation. Because of the decreased psychological flexibility of the dementia patient, the home should be organized to allow for simplicity of routines, with prominent display of calendars, schedules, and the photographs and names of people close to the patient. Events that trigger problematic behaviors should be identified and minimized (Parnetti 2000). For safety, childproofing devices may be considered. Vehicle keys, power tools, and sharp household objects should be secured. Weapons should be removed from the home or at least be secured in a locked cabinet.

Legal issues should be addressed early in the course of the illness, while the patient can still direct his or her wishes. These matters include the completion of medicolegal documents such as living wills, durable powers of attorney, and advance directives (Grossberg and Lake 1998). The physician may be asked to comment on the patient's capacity to make legally binding decisions. Neuropsychological testing may be of help. The capacity for medical decision making needs to be considered as well. The physician is advised to evaluate the patient's clinical status thoroughly at the time a medical decision is needed, to ensure that the patient understands the implications of his or her medical choices. The capacity to vote is generally preserved in mild DAT, whereas patients with moderate disease may require specific assessment of this capacity (Applebaum et al. 2005).

Driving or the operation of other dangerous machinery is often a point of great contention. Many patients will maintain the motor skills for driving despite showing substantial cognitive deficits on the clinical interview and on formal mental status testing (Rabins 1998). Even in mild dementia, the statistical risk of motor vehicle accidents is increased (Dubinsky et al. 2000). Physicians are advised to acquaint themselves with the disclosure laws regarding notification of dementia diagnoses to state motor vehicle departments. A road competency test may be advisable. A useful clinical guideline to consider is that driving is not advised whenever a dementia diagnosis leads the clinician to institute pharmacotherapy for dementia and/or when the MMSE score is less than 24. Other contraindications could be the presence of paranoia, agitation, or assaultive behavior.

Institutional placement is often a painful decision. To many patients, the loss of the home environment, even when clearly necessary to preserve safety, is a devastating experience that usually leads to further confusion, behavioral regression, and increased risk of depression. The lack of or loss of a primary caregiver may predict earlier institutionalization (Patterson et al. 1999). The physician should make every reasonable effort to maintain the patient in his or her home environment. An important intervention is respite care for caregivers. Various respite models to consider include in-home caregivers (e.g., the visiting nurse model) and adult day care centers/senior centers (in which the patient attends a supervised therapeutic environment for the business day and returns home at night).

However, the patient may ultimately regress to a point at which life without 24-hour supervision is not safe. Specific examples of behaviors that cannot safely be managed at home include exhibiting assaultive or threatening behavior; leaving dangerous appliances on inappropriately; continuing to drive despite prohibitions; and being un-

able to maintain feeding, drinking, dressing, and toileting functions. When placement is necessary, an institution that specializes in the care of dementia patients is advised. A secured unit may be required to prevent wandering. Treatment models emphasizing behavioral modification can decrease agitated behavior and minimize the need for pharmacological therapy and physical restraint (Teri et al. 2000). Physicians and family members should clarify with nursing home facilities what degree of medical morbidity can be managed in these institutions, because medical illnesses may lead to more frequent changes in care setting, promoting further behavioral regression with each change of venue.

### Pharmacotherapy

Anticholinesterase agents act through inhibition of acetylcholinesterase, increasing the net amount of synaptic acetylcholine available for neurotransmission (Table 15–12). Anticholinesterase agents are advised early in the course of DAT and may reduce the rate of cognitive decline (Blennow et al. 2006). Once initiated and well tolerated at the highest recommended dosages, anticholinesterase agents should be continued indefinitely, with regular monitoring of cognitive, emotional, and functional behavioral status.

Anticholinesterase agents also should be considered (along with antipsychotics) in managing dementia-related psychotic symptoms (Rao and Lyketsos 1998). These agents also can be safely combined with antidepressants, which may lead to greater symptomatic improvement, given that catecholamine abnormalities may be related to some of the symptoms of dementia (Tune and Sunderland 1998). Cholinergic side effects seen with anticholinesterase agents include nausea, abdominal discomfort, vomiting, loose stools, muscle cramps, muscle weakness, increased sweating, and bradycardia. Acetylcholinesterase inhibitors should be discontinued before surgery in which succinylcholine may be used, because of the risk of prolonged paralysis.

Memantine is an $N$-methyl-D-aspartate (NMDA) antagonist that blocks glutamate-mediated excitotoxicity (Winblad and Poritis 1999). Physiological receptor activation is not affected, but pathological excitotoxicity is inhibited (Reisberg et al. 2003). Dosages start at 5 mg/day and are increased to 10 mg twice a day for moderate to severe DAT to reduce clinical behavioral disturbances and to reduce caregiver distress, and this may delay institutionalization (Reisberg et al. 2003; Wimo et al. 2003). Side effects reported include dizziness, headache, constipation, falls, and confusion (Hartman and Mobius 2003;

| TABLE 15–12.  Dementia pharmacotherapy | | | |
|---|---|---|---|
| **Medication class** | **Target symptom(s)** | **Starting dosage** | **High dosage** |
| **Cholinesterase inhibitors** | Decreased cognition, delusions, hallucinations | | |
| Tacrine | | 10 mg/day | 40 mg/day |
| Donepezil | | 5 mg/day | 10 mg/day |
| Rivastigmine | | 1.5 mg bid | 6 mg bid |
| Galantamine | | 4 mg bid | 12 mg bid |
| **NMDA antagonist** | Decreased cognition | | |
| Memantine | | 5 mg/day | 10 mg bid |
| **Antioxidants** | | | |
| α-Tocopherol | | 1,000 IU bid | |
| Selegiline | | 5 mg/day | 10 mg/day |
| **Antidepressants** | Depression, irritability, anxiety | | |
| Fluoxetine | | 10 mg/day | 40 mg/day |
| Paroxetine | | 10 mg/day | 40 mg/day |
| Sertraline | | 25 mg/day | 200 mg/day |
| Citalopram | | 10 mg/day | 40 mg/day |
| Escitalopram | | 5 mg/day | 20 mg/day |
| Venlafaxine (extended release) | | 37.5 mg/day | 350 mg/day |
| Mirtazapine | | 7.5 mg/day hs | 45 mg/day hs |
| Duloxetine | | 20 mg bid | 30 mg bid |
| Trazodone | | 25 mg/day hs | 400 mg/day hs |
| Bupropion | | 37.5 mg bid | 200 mg bid |
| **Anxiolytic** | Anxiety, irritability | | |
| Buspirone | | 5 mg tid | 20 mg tid |
| **Anticonvulsants** | Irritability, agitation | | |
| Carbamazepine | | 100 mg/day | —[a] |
| Valproate | | 125 mg/day | —[b] |
| Oxcarbazepine | | 150 mg bid | 600 mg bid |
| **Antipsychotics** | Delusions, hallucinations, disorganized thoughts, agitation | | |
| Risperidone | | 0.25 mg/day hs | 3 mg/day hs |
| Olanzapine | | 2.5 mg/day hs | 10 mg/day hs |
| Quetiapine | | 25 mg/day hs | 150 mg bid |
| Ziprasidone | | 20 mg/day hs | 40 mg bid |
| Aripiprazole | | 5 mg/day | 15 mg/day |
| Clozapine | | 25 mg bid | 100 mg bid |

**Additional medications** (consider as adjunctive therapy on case-by-case basis)

| | | | |
|---|---|---|---|
| Beta-blockers | Antiplatelet agents | Statins | Hormones |
| Psychostimulants | Antihypertensives | Warfarin | HAART |
| NSAIDs | Calcium channel blockers | Neuroprotective agents | |

*Note.*  bid=twice a day; HAART=highly active antiretroviral therapy; hs=at bedtime; NMDA=*N*-methyl-D-aspartate; NSAID= nonsteroidal anti-inflammatory drug; tid=three times a day.
[a]Upper limit of dosage to give serum drug level of 8–12 ng/mL.
[b]Upper limit of dosage to give serum drug level of 50–60 ng/mL.

Tariot et al. 2004). Memantine is usually used in concert with a cholinesterase inhibitor; this combination is generally well tolerated (Hartman and Mobius 2003). Memantine also has been shown to benefit cognitive function in VaD (Mobius and Stoffler 2003).

Antidepressants should be used for comorbid depressive disorders, depressive and anxiety symptoms that do not qualify for a full depressive or anxiety disorder diagnosis, sleep disturbances, and agitation. Because of their generally benign side-effect profile and their effectiveness, selective serotonin reuptake inhibitors are the preferred class of antidepressants in dementia patients and should be started at lower dosages than in healthy adults. Other antidepressants to consider include bupropion, trazodone, mirtazapine, duloxetine, and venlafaxine extended release. Blood pressure must be monitored in patients taking venlafaxine, because of the risk of hypertension. Tricyclics should be used with caution in dementia because of the cognitive toxicity that may result from anticholinergic side effects. "Pseudodementia" due to depression should be managed with antidepressants and follow-up cognitive assessment.

Psychostimulants as adjunctive therapy with antidepressants may be considered for refractory mood symptoms and/or apathy; methylphenidate 2.5–5 mg/day is a recommended starting dosage (Rabins et al. 1997). An alternative agent is modafinil, with dosages starting at 100 mg to a maximum of 400 mg in the morning. ECT should be considered for cases of treatment-refractory depression; however, because of the risk for post-ECT delirium and amnesia, ECT treatments should be given no more frequently than twice per week, with unilateral electrode placement (Rabins et al. 1997).

Anxiolytics may be used for anxiety or agitation. Because of the high risk of further memory impairment, sedation, and falls, physicians should avoid the use of benzodiazepines in dementia patients (Rabins et al. 1997). The clinician might consider buspirone, 5 mg three times a day, and increase dosage gradually to an upper limit of 20 mg three times a day (Alexopoulos et al. 1998).

Anticonvulsants may be indicated for agitated and aggressive behavior or for emotional lability (Class et al. 1997). A recommended starting dosage of carbamazepine for the elderly patient with dementia is 100 mg/day, which can be titrated to achieve a serum drug level of 8–12 ng/mL (Rabins et al. 1997). Side effects include ataxia, sedation, confusion, and (rarely) bone marrow suppression (Rabins et al. 1997).

Divalproex sodium can be started at 125 mg/day and titrated upward to yield a serum drug level of 50–60 ng/mL

(Rabins et al. 1997). Divalproex sodium is associated with gastrointestinal distress, ataxia, and (less frequently) hyperammonemia, hepatotoxicity, or bone marrow suppression (Rabins et al. 1997). Monitoring of complete blood count and of liver-associated enzymes is recommended with the use of carbamazepine and valproate (Rabins et al. 1997). Oxcarbazepine may be a safer alternative to carbamazepine; initial dosages of 150 mg twice a day may be gradually increased to a maximum of 600 mg as needed.

Antipsychotics are indicated for paranoid thinking, hallucinations, delirium, and agitation. Initial dosages in elderly patients with dementia should be less than those used in younger patients because of the risks of sedation and further cognitive decline. Although conventional antipsychotic agents are often used as first-line treatment for agitation, they are associated with frequent adverse side effects in patients with dementia (Alexopoulos et al. 1998; Daniel 2000).

The atypical antipsychotics have been associated with weight gain, increased serum glucose, emergence of diabetes mellitus, and hyperlipidemia. This risk is particular high for olanzapine and clozapine (Keys and DeWald 2005b). Use of these medications for dementia should be accompanied by monitoring for these conditions (Keys and DeWald 2005a).

Recent concern has been raised over the increased risk of both CVA and death in dementia patients taking atypical antipsychotics; there does not seem to be a differential risk among the agents of this class (Schneider et al. 2005; Sink et al. 2005). This increased risk of adverse cerebrovascular events with atypical antipsychotics has not been seen in all studies (Herrmann et al. 2004; Liperoti et al. 2005). Risk for these complications may be greater in the immediate post-CVA period (Keys and De Wald 2005b). Speculation of causality of this finding has included the atypical antipsychotics' effect on arrhythmia potential (Titier et al. 2004), serotonin blood vessels, thrombus formation, and orthostasis (Keys and DeWald 2005a). This concern has led to a 2005 health advisory warning from the U.S. Food and Drug Administration (Sink et al. 2005). As a result, physicians should consider avoiding indefinite treatment with atypical antipsychotics for dementia-related psychosis and agitation and discontinue these medications promptly if clinical improvement is not seen (Sink et al. 2005). The risk of death from haloperidol was similar to that from the atypical antipsychotics; thus, renewed use of the typical antipsychotics may not be a viable alternative to mitigate this risk (Sink et al. 2005).

Follow-up monitoring should include examination for medication-induced movement disorders with the Abnormal Involuntary Movement Scale. If problems with compliance lead the physician to consider depot antipsychotics, reduced dosages (e.g., fluphenazine decanoate, 1.25–3.75 mg intramuscularly monthly) can be considered. In the United States, the use of antipsychotic medication in nursing home patients with dementia is regulated by the Omnibus Budget Reconciliation Act of 1987, which requires clear documentation of clinical indications and consideration of alternative interventions (Rabins et al. 1997). Dosage decreases or trial discontinuations of antipsychotics should be considered as the illness progresses. Highly active antiretroviral therapy for underlying HIV infection is an essential part of the management of HIV dementia and can reverse cognitive losses (Cohen and Jacobson 2000; McDaniel et al. 2000). The cognitive effects of this therapy may be further enhanced in combination with ibuprofen (Gendelman et al. 1998). Psychostimulants may be helpful in HIV-associated fatigue and decreased concentration and memory (Maldonado et al. 2000; McDaniel et al. 2000).

# Amnestic and Other Cognitive Disorders

## Amnestic Disorders

Amnestic disorders are characterized by a loss of memory due to the direct physiological effects of a general medical condition or due to the persisting effects of a substance. The amnestic disorders share a common symptom presentation of memory impairment but are differentiated by etiology. Amnestic disorders are secondary syndromes caused by systemic medical illness, primary cerebral disease or trauma, substance use disorders, or adverse medication effects. The impairment must be sufficient to compromise social and occupational functioning, and it should represent a significant decline from the previous level of functioning.

### *Epidemiology*

Limited data are available on the prevalence and incidence of amnestic disorders (Harper et al. 1995). Memory impairment due to head trauma is probably the most common etiology, with more than 500,000 patients hospitalized annually in the United States for head injury. Alcohol abuse and associated thiamine deficiency are historically common etiologies, but some studies suggest that the incidence of alcohol-induced amnestic disorders is decreasing, whereas that of amnestic disorders due to head trauma is increasing (Kopelman 1995).

### *Etiology*

The DSM-IV-TR diagnostic classification for amnestic disorders is based on etiology. Amnestic disorders can be diagnosed as resulting from a general medical condition (Table 15–13), as due to the effects of a substance (Table 15–14), or as "not otherwise specified." The most common etiologies are listed in Table 15–15 and usually involve bilateral damage to areas of the brain involved in memory. These areas include the dorsomedial and midline thalamic nuclei, the hippocampus, the amygdala, the fornix, and the mammillary bodies. Unilateral damage may sometimes be sufficient to produce memory impairment, particularly in the case of left-sided temporal lobe and thalamic structures (Benson 1978). Several iatrogenic causes, such as medication effects, ECT, and the ICU setting, lack clearly identified neuroanatomical damage (Jones et al. 2000).

### *Clinical Features*

Patients with amnestic disorders either are impaired in their ability to learn and recall new information (anterograde amnesia) or are unable to recall previously learned material (retrograde amnesia). The deficits in short-term or recent memory seen in anterograde amnesia can be assessed by asking the patient to recall three objects after a 5-minute distraction. Whereas anterograde amnesia is nearly always present, retrograde amnesia is more variable and depends on the location and severity of brain damage. Both immediate recall (as tested by digit span) and remote memory for distant past events are usually preserved. Memory for the physical traumatic event that caused the deficit is often lost. Orientation may be impaired because it is dependent on the ability to store information regarding time, date, location, and circumstance. The patient may therefore present as confused and disoriented but without the fluctuation in level of consciousness associated with delirium. Orientation to self is nearly always preserved in amnestic disorders.

Most patients with amnestic disorders lack insight into their deficits and may vehemently deny the presence of memory impairment despite clear evidence to the contrary. This lack of insight may lead to anger, accusations, and occasionally agitation. More commonly, patients present with apathy, lack of initiative, and diminished affective expression suggestive of altered personality function.

**TABLE 15–13.   DSM-IV-TR diagnostic criteria for amnestic disorder due to…_[indicate the general medical condition]_**

A.  The development of memory impairment as manifested by impairment in the ability to learn new information or the inability to recall previously learned information.

B.  The memory disturbance causes significant impairment in social or occupational functioning and represents a significant decline from a previous level of functioning.

C.  The memory disturbance does not occur exclusively during the course of a delirium or a dementia.

D.  There is evidence from the history, physical examination, or laboratory findings that the disturbance is the direct physiological consequence of a general medical condition (including physical trauma).

   _Specify_ if:

   **Transient:**   if memory impairment lasts for 1 month or less

   **Chronic:**   if memory impairment lasts for more than 1 month

**Coding note:**   Include the name of the general medical condition on Axis I, e.g., 294.0 amnestic disorder due to head trauma; also code the general medical condition on Axis III (see DSM-IV-TR Appendix G for codes).

Confabulation is often associated with amnestic disorders. Confabulation is characterized by responses to questions that not only are inaccurate but also are often so bizarre and unrealistic as to appear psychotic. Historically, confabulation was considered to represent an attempt by these patients to "cover up" their deficits in memory, but this explanation is probably overly simplistic. The presence and degree of confabulation are usually correlated not with the severity of memory deficits but rather with the loss of self-corrective and monitoring functions, as seen in bifrontal lobe disease (Mercer et al. 1977).

Confabulation in amnestic disorders is usually seen during the early stages of the illness and tends to disappear over time.

**TABLE 15–14.   DSM-IV-TR diagnostic criteria for substance-induced persisting amnestic disorder**

A.  The development of memory impairment as manifested by impairment in the ability to learn new information or the inability to recall previously learned information.

B.  The memory disturbance causes significant impairment in social or occupational functioning and represents a significant decline from a previous level of functioning.

C.  The memory disturbance does not occur exclusively during the course of a delirium or a dementia and persists beyond the usual duration of substance intoxication or withdrawal.

D.  There is evidence from the history, physical examination, or laboratory findings that the memory disturbance is etiologically related to the persisting effects of substance use (e.g., a drug of abuse, a medication).

_Code_ [specific substance]–induced persisting amnestic disorder: (291.1 alcohol; 292.83 sedative, hypnotic, or anxiolytic; 292.83 other [or unknown] substance)

**TABLE 15–15.   Causes of amnestic disorders**

Head trauma
Wernicke-Korsakoff syndrome
Alcohol-induced blackouts
Benzodiazepines
Barbiturates
Intrathecal methotrexate
Methylenedioxymethamphetamine (MDMA; "Ecstasy")
Seizures
Herpes simplex encephalopathy
Klüver-Bucy syndrome
Electroconvulsive therapy
Carbon monoxide poisoning
Heavy metal poisoning
Hypoxia
Hypoglycemia
Cerebrovascular disorders
Cerebral neoplasms

## Selected Amnestic Disorders

**Head injury.**   Severe neurological and psychiatric symptoms can result from head injury, even in the absence of radiological evidence of structural damage. Amnesia after head injury typically includes both anterograde (or ongoing) amnesia and retrograde amnesia for a period ranging from a few minutes to several years before the injury. As anterograde amnesia fades and the patient regains the ability to learn and recall new information, retrograde amnesia "shrinks," usually remaining only for the very short period (seconds to minutes) before the injury. A prolonged retrograde amnesia is an indication of ongoing anterograde amnesia, whereas a short period of retrograde amnesia is associated with recovery (Benson and McDaniel 1991). Severe injuries may result in permanent deficits, although some recovery of memory function can be seen up to 24 months after head trauma.

**Korsakoff's syndrome.**   Korsakoff's syndrome is an amnestic disorder caused by thiamine deficiency, usually associated with excessive, prolonged ingestion of alcohol. It can occur in other malnourished conditions, such as marasmus, gastric carcinoma, and HIV (Kopelman 1995). Korsakoff's syndrome is associated with an acute phase of illness—known as Wernicke's encephalopathy—that presents with ophthalmoplegia, peripheral neuropathy, ataxia, nystagmus, and delirium. Although these acute neurological symptoms respond to aggressive thiamine repletion, a residual, persistent amnestic syndrome usually remains. The associated neuroanatomical abnormalities in Korsakoff's syndrome include bilateral sclerosis of the mammillary bodies (Benson 1978) and punctate lesions of the gray nuclei in the periventricular regions of the third and fourth ventricles and the sylvian aqueduct (Victor et al. 1989).

Some investigators have questioned whether there are distinctive pathophysiological differences between Wernicke-Korsakoff syndrome and the cognitive impairment and dementia due to chronic alcohol neurotoxicity (Blansjaar and Van Dijk 1992). Given the high prevalence of missed diagnoses of Wernicke-Korsakoff syndrome and the insidious, progressive course of the illness, in which each episode gives rise to cumulative damage, all alcohol-dependent patients should be treated with thiamine.

**Transient global amnesia.**   Transient global amnesia (TGA) is a form of amnestic disorder characterized by an abrupt episode of profound anterograde amnesia and a variable inability to recall events that occur during the episode. These episodes typically last for only a few minutes or hours, ending with a rapid, spontaneous restoration of intact cognitive function. Mean duration of the amnestic period is 4.2 hours; periods greater than 12 hours are exceptional. The patient's level of consciousness and orientation to self are unaffected during the episode (Shuping et al. 1980). Patients are often bewildered and confused during the episodes and may ask repeated questions about their circumstances. No data are available to suggest that TGA is associated with focal neurological features or with any comorbid psychiatric illness. TGA is more common in men and usually occurs after age 50. In women, episodes are often associated with anxiety and an emotional precipitating event. In younger patients, a history of headaches may constitute an important risk factor (Quinette et al. 2006). The etiology is unclear, but most experts believe that it is associated with cerebrovascular disease and episodic vascular insufficiency of the mesial temporal lobe. Other etiologies of TGA, including brain tumors, cardiac arrhythmias, migraine, thyroid disorders, general anesthesia, sexual intercourse, polycythemia vera, epilepsy, and myxomatous mitral valve disease, also have been reported (Hodges and Warlow 1990a; Pai and Yang 1999). The most common angiographic findings are in the vertebrobasilar system, specifically occlusion or stenosis of the posterior cerebral artery. TGA generally has a good prognosis, with only 8% of patients experiencing a second episode (Hodges and Warlow 1990b).

## Differential Diagnosis

Memory deficits seen in amnestic syndromes are frequently a feature of delirium and dementia. In delirium, the memory disturbance is accompanied by a disturbed level of consciousness and usually fluctuates with time. More pervasive signs of cerebral dysfunction, such as difficulty focusing or sustaining attention, are present. In dementia, memory impairment is accompanied by additional cognitive impairments such as aphasia, apraxia, agnosia, and disturbances in executive functioning.

In dissociative or psychogenic forms of amnesia, the memory loss usually does not involve deficits in learning and recalling new information. Patients typically present with a circumscribed inability to recall previously learned and personal information, often regarding the patients' own identity or a traumatic or stressful event. These deficits persist even as the patient continues to function normally in the present. Interestingly, changes in limbic function are observed on PET in patients with psychogenic amnesia (Yasuno et al. 2000). Patients with malingering or factitious disorders can present with amnestic symptoms that also fit the profile for dissociative amnesia.

Systematic memory testing of these patients will often yield inconsistent results.

### *Treatment*

As in delirium and dementia, the primary goal of treatment in amnestic disorders is to identify and treat the underlying cause or pathological process. There are no definitively effective treatments for amnestic disorder that are specifically aimed at reversing apparent memory deficits. Fortunately, these deficits are often temporary—as in transient amnestic syndromes—or are partially or completely reversible—as in head trauma, thiamine deficiency, or anoxia.

Acute management should include continuous reorientation of the patient by means of verbal redirection, clocks, calendars, and familiar stimuli. Individual supportive psychotherapy for the patient, and family counseling to assist and educate caregivers, is also helpful. Chronic reversible amnestic syndromes may be managed with cognitive rehabilitation and therapeutic milieus intended to promote recovery from brain injury. More severe and permanent deficits may require supervised living environments to ensure appropriate care.

## Mild Cognitive Impairment

Mild cognitive impairment (MCI) is a clinical syndrome defined as cognitive decline that is greater than expected for a patient's age and education level but that does not interfere with normal functioning. A classification has been proposed that differentiates between amnestic or single memory MCI, multiple-domain MCI, and single nonmemory MCI (Petersen 2004). Prevalence in population-based epidemiological studies ranges from 3% to 19% in adults older than 65 years (Gauthier et al. 2006; G.W. Ross and Bowen 2002). Some patients with MCI remain stable or return to normal over time, but more than half progress to dementia within 5 years. The amnestic subtype in particular has a high probability of progressing to DAT (Ganguli et al. 2004) and could constitute a prodro-mal stage of this disorder, although the multiple-domain subtype has higher sensitivity for both DAT and VaD (Rasquin et al. 2005). The rate of progression to DAT may be predicted by the severity of memory impairment at baseline, the severity of hippocampal atrophy, and the presence of an ε4 allele of the *APOE* gene (Geda et al. 2006). Comorbid depression with MCI more than doubles the risk of developing DAT, and patients with a poor response to antidepressants appear to be at an even greater risk (Modrego and Ferrández 2004).

## Postconcussion Syndrome

Postconcussion syndrome is defined as a condition arising from traumatic brain injury that produces deficits in three areas of CNS function: somatic, psychological, and cognitive. The most common somatic symptom is headache, but fatigue, dizziness, blurred vision, and photophobia can also occur. Psychological symptoms include anxiety, depression, apathy, and emotional lability. Cognitive symptoms include decreased concentration, decreased verbal fluency, and impairments in working memory. The American Psychiatric Association's current criteria for postconcussional disorder, a similar diagnosis in Appendix B of DSM-IV-TR, require that there be an "acquired impairment in cognitive functioning, accompanied by specific neurobehavioral symptoms, that occurs as a consequence of closed head injury of sufficient severity to produce a significant cerebral concussion" (American Psychiatric Association 2000, p. 760).

The most important differential diagnosis is usually malingering, and several psychiatric and neurological tests are available to assist the clinician. The Halstead-Reitan battery is reported to be 93.8% reliable in detecting patients who are intentionally trying to fake cognitive symptoms of head trauma (Mittenberg et al. 1996). Additional psychological testing that can be helpful includes the Minnesota Multiphasic Personality Inventory–2, the Dissimulation Scale, the Ego Strength Scale, and the Fake Bad Scale (Hall et al. 2005).

# Key Points: Delirium, Dementia, and Amnestic and Other Cognitive Disorders

## Delirium

- Delirium is an acute brain disorder manifested by a syndromal array of neuropsychiatric symptoms.

- Delirium is epidemic among hospitalized patients, especially in the elderly.

- Numerous and widely varying precipitants can activate delirium in vulnerable patients.

- Delirium likely exerts an independent mortality risk for select populations and serves as a "medical alarm" for many others.

- Delirium can resolve completely, resolve gradually, or lead to a permanent cognitive disorder.

- The fundamental goal of treating delirium is to prevent and reverse delirium and thus mitigate associated morbidity and mortality risks.

## Dementia

- Dementia is characterized by amnesia and one or more other impairment in cognition.

- Cortical dementias feature notable aphasia, apraxia, agnosia, and visuospatial deficits plus amnesia that is not helped by cueing, whereas subcortical dementias feature apathy, affective lability, depressed mood, bradyphrenia, and decreased attention/concentration plus amnesia that is helped by cueing.

- Compared with dementia of the Alzheimer's type (DAT), frontotemporal dementia is characterized by executive dysfunction, disinhibition, attentional deficits, and personality changes, with relatively preserved memory and visuospatial function.

- Lewy body dementia and Lewy body variant are characterized by fluctuations in mental status, well-formed visual hallucinations, delusions, depression, apathy, anxiety, extrapyramidal symptoms, and neuroleptic sensitivity.

- Patients with mild cognitive impairment (MCI) have memory symptoms validated by clinical examination and/or testing that are significantly less impairing than full-spectrum dementia; whether this condition warrants medication treatment for cognitive symptoms is controversial.

- Neuroimaging is a routine expectation in the workup of dementia.

- A common clinical combination of medications for DAT is an anticholinesterase agent with memantine.

## Amnestic and Other Cognitive Disorders

- Amnestic disorders are characterized by an inability to learn and recall new information (anterograde amnesia) or an inability to recall previously learned information (retrograde amnesia).

- Common causes of amnestic disorder include head injury, transient global amnesia, and benzodiazepines.

- MCI is defined as cognitive decline greater than expected for a patient's age and education level but without the deficits in normal functioning associated with dementia.

- MCI is a risk state for dementia, with more than half of patients with the amnestic subtype of MCI progressing to dementia within 5 years.

- Postconcussion syndrome is a constellation of somatic, psychological, and cognitive symptoms resulting from head trauma that usually resolve within 1 month, although persistent symptoms may continue for 1 year in 7%–15% of patients.

# References

Aalten P, de Vugt ME, Lousberg R, et al: Behavioral problems in dementia: a factor analysis of the Neuropsychiatric Inventory. Dement Geriatr Cogn Disord 15:99–105, 2003

Aarsland D, Perry R, Larsen JP, et al: Neuroleptic sensitivity in Parkinson's disease and parkinsonian dementias. J Clin Psychiatry 66:633–637, 2005

Adamis D, Treloar A, Martin FC, et al: Recovery and outcome of delirium in elderly medical inpatients. Arch Gerontol Geriatr 43:289–298, 2006

Alagiakrishnan K, McCracken P, Feldman H: Treating vascular risk factors and maintaining vascular health: is this the way towards successful cognitive ageing and preventing cognitive decline? Postgrad Med J 82:101–105, 2006

Alexopoulos GS, Silver JM, Kahn DA, et al: Treatment of Agitation in Older Patients With Dementia: Postgraduate Medicine Special Report. Minneapolis, MN, McGraw-Hill, 1998, pp 1–88

American Psychiatric Association: Practice guideline for the treatment of patients with delirium. Am J Psychiatry 156(suppl): 1–20, 1999

American Psychiatric Association: Diagnostic and Statistical Manual of Mental Disorders, 4th Edition, Text Revision. Washington, DC, American Psychiatric Association, 2000

Andrew MK, Freter SH, Rockwood K: Incomplete functional recovery after delirium in elderly people: a prospective cohort study. BMC Geriatr 5:5, 2005

Applebaum PS, Bonnie RJ, Karlawish JH: The capacity to vote of persons with Alzheimer's disease. Am J Psychiatry 162:2094–2100, 2005

Ballard CG, O'Brien JT, Swann AG, et al: The natural history of psychosis and depression in dementia with Lewy bodies and Alzheimer's disease: persistence and new cases over 1 year of follow-up. J Clin Psychiatry 62:46–49, 2001

Baskys A: Lewy body dementia: the litmus test for neuroleptic sensitivity and extrapyramidal symptoms. J Clin Psychiatry 65 (suppl 11):16–22, 2004

Benoit AG, Campbell BI, Tanner JR, et al: Risk factors and prevalence of perioperative cognitive dysfunction in abdominal aneurysm patients. J Vasc Surg 42:884–890, 2005

Benson DF: Amnesia. South Med J 71:1221–1227, 1231, 1978

Benson DF, McDaniel KD: Memory disorders, in Neurology in Clinical Practice, Vol 2. Edited by Bradley WG, Daroff RB, Fenichel GM, et al. Boston, MA, Butterworth-Heinemann, 1991, pp 1389–1406

Berger A-K, Fratiglioni L, Frosell Y, et al: The occurrence of depressive symptoms in the preclinical phase of AD: a population-based study. Neurology 53:1998–2002, 1999

Blansjaar BA, Van Dijk JG: Korsakoff minus Wernicke syndrome. Alcohol Alcohol 27:435–437, 1992

Blennow K, de Leon MJ, Zetterberg H: Alzheimer's disease. Lancet 368:387–403, 2006

Boeve BF: A review of the non-Alzheimer dementias. J Clin Psychiatry 67:1983–2001, 2006

Bottino CM, Almeida OP: Can neuroimaging techniques identify individuals at risk of developing Alzheimer's disease? Int Psychogeriatr 9:389–403, 1997

Bourdel-Marchasson I, Vincent S, Germain C, et al: Delirium symptoms and low dietary intake in older patients are independent predictors of institutionalization: a 1-year prospective population-based study. J Gerontol A Biol Sci Med Sci 59A:350–354, 2004

Bourgeois JA, Seaman JS, Servis ME: Delirium, dementia, and amnestic disorders, in The American Psychiatric Publishing Textbook of Clinical Psychiatry, 4th Edition. Edited by Hales RE, Yudofsky SC. Washington, DC, American Psychiatric Publishing, 2003, pp 259–308

Breitbart W, Marotta R, Platt MM, et al: A double-blind trial of haloperidol, chlorpromazine, and lorazepam in the treatment of delirium in hospitalized AIDS patients. Am J Psychiatry 153:231–237, 1996

Breitbart W, Rosenfeld B, Roth A, et al: The Memorial Delirium Assessment Scale. J Pain Symptom Manage 13:128–137, 1997

Breitbart W, Tremblay A, Gibson C: An open trial of olanzapine for the treatment of delirium in hospitalized cancer patients. Psychosomatics 43:175–182, 2002

Brown TM: Basic mechanisms in the pathogenesis of delirium, in Psychiatric Care of the Medical Patient, 2nd Edition. Edited by Stoudemire A, Fogel BS, Greenberg DB. New York, Oxford University Press, 2000, pp 571–580

Brown TM, Stoudemire A: Psychiatric Side Effects of Prescription and Over-the-Counter Medications. Washington, DC, American Psychiatric Press, 1998

Cameron DJ, Thomas RI, Mulvihill M, et al: Delirium: a test of the Diagnostic and Statistical Manual III criteria on medical inpatients. J Am Geriatr Soc 35:1007–1010, 1987

Caselli RJ, Graff-Radford NR, Reiman EM, et al: Preclinical memory decline in cognitively normal apolipoprotein E epsilon4 homozygotes. Neurology 53:201–207, 1999

Cassem NH, Sos J: Intravenous use of haloperidol for acute delirium in intensive care settings. Paper presented at the 131st annual meeting of the American Psychiatric Association, Washington, DC, May 1978

Centeno C, Sanz A, Bruera E: Delirium in advanced cancer patients. Palliat Med 18:184–194, 2004

Chapman FM, Dickinson J, McKeith I, et al: Association among visual hallucinations, visual acuity, and specific eye pathologies in Alzheimer's disease: treatment implications. Am J Psychiatry 156:1983–1985, 1999

Choi SH, Na DL, Chung CS, et al: Diffusion-weighted MRI in vascular dementia. Neurology 54:83–89, 2000

Class CA, Schneider L, Farlow MR: Optimal management of behavioural disorders associated with dementia. Drugs Aging 10:95–106, 1997

Cohen MAA, Jacobson JM: Maximizing life's potential in AIDS: a psychopharmacological update. Gen Hosp Psychiatry 22:375–388, 2000

Cole MG, Primeau FJ: Prognosis of delirium in elderly hospital patients. CMAJ 149:41–46, 1993

Craft S, Teri L, Edland SD, et al: Accelerated decline in apolipoprotein E-epsilon4 homozygotes with Alzheimer's disease. Neurology 51:149–153, 1998

Culp KR, Wakefield B, Dyck MJ, et al: Bioelectric impedance analysis and other hydration parameters as risk factors for delirium in rural nursing home residents. J Gerontol A Biol Sci Med Sci 59:813–817, 2004

Cummings JL, Masterman DL: Assessment of treatment-associated changes in behavior and cholinergic therapy of neuropsychiatric symptoms in Alzheimer's disease. J Clin Psychiatry 59 (suppl 13):23–30, 1998

Curb JD, Rodriguez BL, Abbott RD, et al: Longitudinal association of vascular and Alzheimer's dementias, diabetes, and glucose tolerance. Neurology 52:971–975, 1999

Daniel DG: Antipsychotic treatment of psychosis and agitation in the elderly. J Clin Psychiatry 61 (suppl 14):49–52, 2000

d'Arminio Monforte A, Duca PG, Vago L, et al: Decreasing incidence of CNS AIDS-defining events associated with antiretroviral therapy. Neurology 54:1856–1859, 2000

Dautzenberg PLJ, Mulder LJ, Olde Rikkert MGM, et al: Adding rivastigmine to antipsychotics in the treatment of a chronic delirium. Age Ageing 33:516–517, 2004

de Koning I, van Kooten F, Dippel DW, et al: The CAMCOG: a useful screening instrument for dementia in stroke patients. Stroke 29:2080–2086, 1998

Desmond DW, Moroney JT, Paik MC, et al: Frequency and clinical determinants of dementia after ischemic stroke. Neurology 54:1124–1131, 2000

Doddy RS, Massman PJ, Mawad M, et al: Cognitive consequences of subcortical magnetic resonance imaging changes in Alzheimer's disease: comparison to small vessel ischemic vascular dementia. Neuropsychiatry Neuropsychol Behav Neurol 11:191–199, 1998

Dolan MM, Hawkes WG, Zimmerman SI, et al: Delirium on hospital admission in aged hip fracture patients: prediction of mortality and 2-year functional outcomes. J Gerontol A Biol Sci Med Sci 55:M527–M534, 2000

Doraiswamy PM, Steffens DC, Pitchumoni S, et al: Early recognition of Alzheimer's disease: What is consensual? What is controversial? What is practical? J Clin Psychiatry 59(suppl):6–18, 1998

Duara R, Barker W, Luis CA: Frontotemporal dementia and Alzheimer's disease: differential diagnosis. Dement Geriatr Cogn Disord 10(suppl):37–42, 1999

Dubinsky RM, Stein AC, Lyons K: Practice parameter: risk of driving and Alzheimer's disease (an evidence-based review). Neurology 54:2205–2211, 2000

Dufouil C, Clayton D, Brayne C, et al: Population norms for the MMSE in the very old: estimates based on longitudinal data. Mini-Mental State Examination. Neurology 55:1609–1613, 2000

Dyer CB, Ashton CM, Teasdale TA: Postoperative delirium: a review of 80 primary data-collection studies. Arch Intern Med 155:461–465, 1995

Edlund A, Lundström M, Brännström B, et al: Delirium before and after operation for femoral neck fracture. J Am Geriatr Soc 49:1335–1340, 2001

Elie M, Cole MG, Primeau FJ, et al: Delirium risk factors in elderly hospitalized patients. J Gen Intern Med 13:204–212, 1998

Ely EW, Shintani A, Truman B, et al: Delirium as a predictor of mortality in mechanically ventilated patients in the intensive care unit. JAMA 291:1753–1762, 2004

Engel GL, Romano J: Delirium: a syndrome of cerebral insufficiency. J Chronic Dis 9:260–277, 1959

Fayers PM, Hjermstad MJ, Ranhoff AH, et al: Which Mini-Mental State Exam items can be used to screen for delirium and cognitive impairment? J Pain Symptom Manage 30:41–50, 2005

Felician O, Sandson TA: The neurobiology and pharmacotherapy of Alzheimer's disease. J Neuropsychiatry Clin Neurosci 11:19–31, 1999

Fink M: Cytopathic hypoxia in sepsis. Acta Anaesthesiol Scand 110(suppl):87–95, 1997

Folstein MF, Folstein SE, McHugh PR: "Mini-Mental State": a practical method for grading the cognitive state of patients for the clinician. J Psychiatr Res 12:189–198, 1975

Foy A, O'Connell D, Henry D, et al: Benzodiazepine use as a cause of cognitive impairment in elderly hospital inpatients. J Gerontol A Biol Sci Med Sci 50A:M99–M106, 1995

Francis J, Kapoor WN: Prognosis after hospital discharge of older medical patients with delirium. J Am Geriatr Soc 40:601–606, 1992

Francis J, Martin D, Kapoor WN: A prospective study of delirium in hospitalized elderly. JAMA 263:1097–1101, 1990

Freter SH, Dunbar MJ, MacLeod H, et al: Predicting postoperative delirium in elective orthopaedic patients: Delirium Elderly At-Risk (DEAR) instrument. Age Ageing 34:169–171, 2005

Ganguli M, Dodge HH, Shen C, et al: Mild cognitive impairment, amnestic type: an epidemiologic study. Neurology 63:115–121, 2004

Gaudreau JD, Gagnon P, Harel F, et al: Fast, systematic, and continuous delirium assessment in hospitalized patients: the Nursing Delirium Screening Scale. J Pain Symptom Manage 29:368–375, 2005

Gauthier S, Reisberg B, Zaudig M, et al: Mild cognitive impairment. Lancet 367:1262–1270, 2006

Geda YE, Knopman DS, Mrazek DA, et al: Depression, apolipoprotein E genotype, and the incidence of mild cognitive impairment: a prospective cohort study. Arch Neurol 63:435–440, 2006

Geerlings MI, Jonker C, Bouter LM, et al: Association between memory complaints and incident Alzheimer's disease in elderly people with normal baseline cognition. Am J Psychiatry 156:531–537, 1999

Geldmacher DS, Whitehouse PJ Jr: Differential diagnosis of Alzheimer's disease. Neurology 48 (5 suppl):S2–S9, 1997

Gendelman HE, Zheng J, Coulter CL, et al: Suppression of inflammatory neurotoxins by highly active antiretroviral therapy in human immunodeficiency virus–associated dementia. J Infect Dis 178:1000–1007, 1998

Gibson GE, Blass JP: Impaired synthesis of acetylcholine in brain accompanying mild hypoxia and hypoglycemia. J Neurochem 27:37–42, 1976

Gibson GE, Pulsinelli W, Blass JP, et al: Brain dysfunction in mild to moderate hypoxia. Am J Med 70:1247–1254, 1981

Gleason OC: Donepezil for postoperative delirium. Psychosomatics 44:437–438, 2003

Gliatto MF, Caroff SN: Neurosyphilis: a history and clinical review. Psychiatr Ann 31:153–161, 2001

Globus MY, Busto R, Dietrich WD, et al: Effect of ischemia on the in vivo release of striatal dopamine, glutamate, and gamma-aminobutyric acid studied by intracerebral microdialysis. J Neurochem 51:1455–1464, 1988

Goodkin K, Baldewicz TT, Wilkie FL, et al: Cognitive-motor impairment and disorder in HIV-1 infection. Psychiatr Ann 31:37–44, 2001

Grace AA: Dopamine, in Neuropsychopharmacology: The Fifth Generation of Progress. Edited by Davis KL, Charney D, Coyle JT, et al. Philadelphia, PA, Lippincott Williams & Wilkins, 2002, pp 119–132

Grossberg GT, Lake JT: The role of the psychiatrist in Alzheimer's disease. J Clin Psychiatry 59 (suppl 9):3–6, 1998

Gupta N, Sharma P, Prabhakar S: Olanzapine for delirium in parkinsonism: therapeutic benefits in lieu of adverse consequences. Neurol India 52:274–275, 2004

Gury C, Canceil O, Iaria P: Antipsychotic drugs and cardiovascular safety: current studies of prolonged QT interval and risk of ventricular arrhythmia [in French]. Encephale 26:62–72, 2000

Gustafson K, Berggren D, Brännström B, et al: Acute confusional states in elderly patients treated for femoral neck fracture. J Am Geriatr Soc 36:525–530, 1988

Haass C, De Strooper B: The presenilins in Alzheimer's disease: proteolysis holds the key. Science 286:916–919, 1999

Hall R, Hall R, Chapman M: Definition, diagnosis, and forensic implications of postconcussional syndrome. Psychosomatics 46:195–202, 2005

Han CS, Kim YK: A double-blind trial of risperidone and haloperidol for the treatment of delirium. Psychosomatics 45:297–301, 2004

Han L, McCusker J, Cole M, et al: Use of medications with anticholinergic effect predicts clinical severity of delirium symptoms in older medical inpatients. Arch Intern Med 161:1099–1105, 2001

Harhangi BS, de Rijk MC, van Duijn CM, et al: APOE and the risk of PD with or without dementia in a population-based study. Neurology 54:1272–1276, 2000

Harper C, Fornes P, Duyckaerts C, et al: An international perspective on the prevalence of the Wernicke-Korsakoff syndrome. Metab Brain Dis 10:17–24, 1995

Hartman S, Mobius HJ: Tolerability of memantine in combination with cholinesterase inhibitors in dementia therapy. Int Clin Psychopharmacol 18:81–85, 2003

Henon H, Lebert F, Durieu I, et al: Confusional state in stroke: relation to preexisting dementia, patient characteristics, and outcome. Stroke 30:773–779, 1999

Herrmann N, Mamdani M, Lanctôt KL: Atypical antipsychotics and risk of cerebrovascular accidents. Am J Psychiatry 161:1113–1115, 2004

Heyman A, Fillenbaum GG, Gearing M, et al: Comparison of Lewy body variant of Alzheimer's disease with pure Alzheimer's disease. Neurology 52:1839–1844, 1999

Hodges JR, Warlow CP: Syndromes of transient global amnesia: towards a classification: a study of 153 cases. J Neurol Neurosurg Psychiatry 53:834–843, 1990a

Hodges JR, Warlow CP: The aetiology of transient global amnesia: a case-control study of 114 cases with prospective follow-up. Brain 113 (pt 3):639–657, 1990b

Horikawa N, Yamazaki T, Miyamoto K, et al: Treatment for delirium with risperidone: results of a prospective open trial with 10 patients. Gen Hosp Psychiatry 25:289–292, 2003

Hughes TA, Ross HF, Musa S, et al: A 10-year study of the incidence of and factors predicting dementia in Parkinson's disease. Neurology 54:1596–1602, 2000

Hy LX, Keller DM: Prevalence of AD among whites: a summary by levels of severity. Neurology 55:198–204, 2000

Ikarashi Y, Takahashi A, Ishimura H, et al: Regulation of dopamine D1 and D2 receptors on striatal acetylcholine release in rats. Brain Res Bull 43:107–115, 1997

Inouye SK, Charpentier PA: Precipitating factors for delirium in hospitalized elderly persons: predictive model and interrelationship with baseline vulnerability. JAMA 275:852–857, 1996

Inouye SK, van Dyck CH, Alessi CA, et al: Clarifying confusion: the confusion assessment method: a new method for detection of delirium. Ann Intern Med 113:941–948, 1990

Inouye SK, Viscoli CM, Horwitz RI, et al: A predictive model for delirium in hospitalized elderly medical patients based on admission characteristics. Ann Intern Med 119:474–481, 1993

Inouye SK, Rushing JT, Foreman MD, et al: Does delirium contribute to poor hospital outcomes? A three-site epidemiologic study. J Gen Intern Med 13:234–242, 1998

Inouye SK, Bogardus ST Jr, Charpentier PA, et al: A multicomponent intervention to prevent delirium in hospitalized older patients. N Engl J Med 340:669–676, 1999

Inouye SK, Foreman MD, Mikon LC, et al: Nurses' recognition of delirium and its symptoms: comparison of nurse and researcher ratings. Arch Intern Med 161:2467–2473, 2001

Itil T, Fink M: Anticholinergic drug–induced delirium: experimental modification, quantitative EEG and behavioral correlations. J Nerv Ment Dis 6:492–507, 1966

Jack CR, Petersen RC, Xu YC, et al: Prediction of AD with MRI-based hippocampal volume in mild cognitive impairment. Neurology 54:1397–1403, 2000

Jellinger KA: Structural basis of dementia in neurodegenerative disorders. J Neural Transm 47(suppl):1–29, 1996

Jones C, Griffiths R, Humphris G: Disturbed memory and amnesia related to intensive care. Memory 8:79–94, 2000

Jorm AF, Jolley D: The incidence of dementia: a meta-analysis. Neurology 51:728–733, 1998

Katz IR: Diagnosis and treatment of depression in patients with Alzheimer's disease and other dementias. J Clin Psychiatry 59 (suppl 9):38–44, 1998

Katz IR, Curyto KJ, TenHave T, et al: Validating the diagnosis of delirium and evaluating its association with deterioration over a one-year period. Am J Geriatr Psychiatry 9:148–159, 2001

Kelly KG, Zisselman M, Cutillo-Schmitter T, et al: Severity and course of delirium in medically hospitalized nursing facility residents. Am J Geriatr Psychiatry 9:72–77, 2001

Kertesz A, Munoz DG: Frontotemporal dementia. Med Clin North Am 86:501–518, 2002

Keys MA, DeWald C: Clinical perspective on choice of atypical antipsychotics in elderly patients with dementia, part I. Annals of Long-Term Care: Clinical Care and Aging 13(2):26–32, 2005a

Keys MA, DeWald C: Clinical perspective on choice of atypical antipsychotics in elderly patients with dementia, part II. Annals of Long-Term Care: Clinical Care and Aging 13(3):30–38, 2005b

Kim JY, Jung IK, Han C, et al: Antipsychotics and dopamine transporter gene polymorphisms in delirium patients. Psychiatry Clin Neurosci 59:183–188, 2005

Kim KS, Pae CU, Chae JH, et al: An open pilot trial of olanzapine for delirium in the Korean population. Psychiatry Clin Neurosci 55:515–519, 2001

Kim KY, Bader GM, Kotlyar V, et al: Treatment of delirium in older adults with quetiapine. J Geriatr Psychiatry Neurol 16:29–31, 2003

Kopelman MD: The Korsakoff syndrome. Br J Psychiatry 166:154–173, 1995

Koponen H, Hurri L, Stenback U, et al: Computed tomography findings in delirium. J Nerv Ment Dis 177:226–231, 1989a

Koponen H, Partanen J, Paakkonen A, et al: EEG spectral analysis in delirium. J Neurol Neurosurg Psychiatry 52:980–985, 1989b

Koponen H, Stenback U, Mattila E, et al: Delirium among elderly persons admitted to a psychiatric hospital: clinical course during the acute stage and one-year follow-up. Acta Psychiatr Scand 79:579–585, 1989c

Lawlor BA: Behavioral and psychological symptoms in dementia: the role of atypical antipsychotics. J Clin Psychiatry 65(suppl):5–10, 2004

Lee KU, Won WY, Lee HK, et al: Amisulpride versus quetiapine for the treatment of delirium: a randomized, open prospective study. Int Clin Psychopharmacol 20:311–314, 2005

Leslie DL, Zhang Y, Holford TR, et al: Premature death associated with delirium at 1-year follow-up. Arch Intern Med 165:1657–1662, 2005

Leung JM, Sands LP, Mullen EA, et al: Are preoperative depressive symptoms associated with postoperative delirium in geriatric surgical patients? J Gerontol A Biol Sci Med Sci 60:1563–1568, 2005

Leverenz JB, McKeith IG: Dementia with Lewy bodies. Med Clin North Am 86:519–535, 2002

Levy ML, Cummings JL: Parkinson's disease, in Psychiatric Management in Neurological Disease. Edited by Lauterbach EC. Washington, DC, American Psychiatric Press, 2000, pp 41–70

Lin SM, Liu CY, Wang CH, et al: The impact of delirium on the survival of mechanically ventilated patients. Crit Care Med 32:2254–2259, 2004

Liperoti R, Gambassi G, Lapane KL, et al: Cerebrovascular events among elderly nursing home patients treated with conventional or atypical antipsychotics. J Clin Psychiatry 66:1090–1096, 2005

Lipowski ZJ: Transient cognitive disorders (delirium, acute confusional states) in the elderly. Am J Psychiatry 140:1426–1436, 1983

Lipowski ZJ: Delirium (acute confusional states). JAMA 258:1789–1792, 1987

Liptzin B, Levkoff SE: An empirical study of delirium subtypes. Br J Psychiatry 161:843–845, 1992

Liptzin B, Laki A, Garb JL, et al: Donepezil in the prevention and treatment of postsurgical delirium. Am J Geriatr Psychiatry 13:1100–1106, 2005

Liu CY, Juang YY, Liang HY, et al: Efficacy of risperidone in treating the hyperactive symptoms of delirium. Int Clin Psychopharmacol 19:165–168, 2004

Livingston G, Johnston K, Katona C, et al: Systematic review of psychological approaches to the management of neuropsychiatric symptoms of dementia. Am J Psychiatry 162:1996–2021, 2005

Lopez OL, Wisniewski S, Hamilton RL, et al: Predictors of progression in patients with AD and Lewy bodies. Neurology 54:1774–1779, 2000

Lundström M, Edlund A, Bucht G, et al: Dementia after delirium in patients with femoral neck fractures. J Am Geriatr Soc 51:1002–1006, 2003

Lyketsos CG, Steinberg M, Tschanz JT, et al: Mental and behavioral disturbances in dementia: findings from the Cache County Study on Memory in Aging. Am J Psychiatry 157:708–714, 2000

Lyketsos CG, Lopez O, Jones B, et al: Prevalence of neuropsychiatric symptoms in dementia and mild cognitive impairment: results from the Cardiovascular Health Study. JAMA 288:1475–1483, 2002

Mace NL, Rabins PV: The 36-Hour Day: A Family Guide to Caring for Persons With Alzheimer's Disease, Related Dementing Illnesses, and Memory Loss in Later Life. Baltimore, MD, Johns Hopkins University Press, 1981

Maldonado JL, Fernandez F, Levy JK: Acquired immunodeficiency syndrome, in Psychiatric Management in Neurological Disease. Edited by Lauterbach EC. Washington, DC, American Psychiatric Press, 2000, pp 271–295

Marcantonio ER, Goldman L, Mangione CM, et al: A clinical predictive rule for delirium after elective noncardiac surgery. JAMA 271:134–139, 1994

Marcantonio ER, Flacker JM, Michaels M, et al: Delirium is independently associated with poor functional recovery after hip fracture. J Am Geriatr Soc 48:618–624, 2000

Marcantonio ER, Kiely DK, Simon SE, et al: Outcomes of older people admitted to postacute facilities with delirium. J Am Geriatr Soc 53:963–969, 2005

Marsh L: Neuropsychiatric aspects of Parkinson's disease. Psychosomatics 41:15–23, 2000

McCusker J, Cole M, Dendukuri N, et al: Delirium in older medical inpatients and subsequent cognitive and functional status: a prospective study. CMAJ 165:575–583, 2001

McDaniel JS, Chung JY, Brown L, et al: Practice guideline for the treatment of patients with HIV/AIDS. Work Group on HIV/AIDS. American Psychiatric Association. Am J Psychiatry 157(suppl):1–62, 2000

McKeith IG, Ballard CG, Perry RH, et al: Prospective validation of consensus criteria for the diagnosis of dementia with Lewy bodies. Neurology 54:1050–1058, 2000

Meagher DJ, Trzepacz PT: Delirium phenomenology illuminates pathophysiology, management, and course. J Geriatr Psychiatry Neurol 11:150–156, 1998

Meltzer HY: Mechanism of action of atypical antipsychotic drugs, in Neuropsychopharmacology: Fifth Generation of Progress. Edited by Davis KL, Charney D, Coyle JT, et al. Philadelphia, PA, Lippincott Williams & Wilkins, 2002, pp 819–831

Mendez MF, Chen AK, Shapiro JS, et al: Acquired extroversion with bitemporal variant of frontotemporal dementia. J Neuropsychiatry Clin Neurosci 18:100–107, 2006

Mercer B, Wepner W, Gardner H, et al: A study of confabulation. Arch Neurol 34:429–433, 1977

Minden SL, Carbone LA, Barsky A, et al: Predictors and outcomes of delirium. Gen Hosp Psychiatry 27:209–214, 2005

Mittal D, Jimerson NA, Neely EP, et al: Risperidone in the treatment of delirium: results from a prospective open-label trial. J Clin Psychiatry 65:662–667, 2004

Mittenberg W, Rotholc A, Russell E, et al: Identification of malingered head injury on the Halstead-Reitan battery. Arch Clin Neuropsychol 11:271–281, 1996

Mobius HJ, Stoffler A: Memantine in vascular dementia. Int Psychogeriatr 15(suppl):207–213, 2003

Moceri VM, Kukull WA, Emanuel I, et al: Early life risk factors and the development of Alzheimer's disease. Neurology 54:415–420, 2000

Modrego PJ, Ferrández J: Depression in patients with mild cognitive impairment increases the risk of developing dementia of Alzheimer type: a prospective cohort study. Arch Neurol 61:1290–1293, 2004

Morita T, Takigawa C, Onishi H, et al: Opioid rotation from morphine to fentanyl in delirious cancer patients: an open-label trial. J Pain Symptom Manage 30:96–103, 2005

O'Keeffe ST, Lavan J: The prognostic significance of delirium in older hospital patients. J Am Geriatr Soc 45:174–178, 1997

O'Keeffe ST, Mulkerrin EC, Nayeem K, et al: Use of serial Mini-Mental Status Examinations to diagnose and monitor delirium in elderly hospital patients. J Am Geriatr Soc 53:867–870, 2005

Pack AI, Millman RP: The lungs in later life, in Pulmonary Diseases and Disorders, 2nd Edition. Edited by Fishman AP. New York, McGraw-Hill, 1988, pp 80–90

Pae CU, Lee SJ, Lee CU, et al: A pilot trial of quetiapine for the treatment of patients with delirium. Hum Psychopharmacol 19:125–127, 2004

Pai M, Yang S: Transient global amnesia: a retrospective study of 25 patients. Chin Med J (Engl) 62:140–144, 1999

Pandharipande P, Shintani A, Peterson J, et al: Lorazepam is an independent risk factor for transitioning to delirium in intensive care unit patients. Anesthesiology 104:21–26, 2006

Parellada E, Baeza I, de Pablo J, et al: Risperidone in the treatment of patients with delirium. J Clin Psychiatry 65:348–353, 2004

Parnetti L: Therapeutic options in dementia. J Neurol 247:163–168, 2000

Patterson CJS, Gauthier S, Bergman H, et al: The recognition, assessment, and management of dementing disorders: conclusions from the Canadian Consensus Conference on Dementia. CMAJ 160:S1–S14, 1999

Paulsen JS, Butters N, Sadek JR, et al: Distinct cognitive profiles of cortical and subcortical dementia in advanced illness. Neurology 45:951–956, 1995

Peila R, White LR, Masaki K, et al: Reducing the risk of dementia: efficacy of long-term treatment of hypertension. Stroke 37:1165–1170, 2006

Petersen RC: Mild cognitive impairment as a diagnostic entity. J Intern Med 256:183–194, 2004

Petersen RC, Jack CR, Xu Y-C, et al: Memory and MRI-based hippocampal volumes in aging and AD. Neurology 54:581–587, 2000

Peterson JF, Pun BT, Dittus RS, et al: Delirium and its motoric subtypes: a study of 624 critically ill patients. J Am Geriatr Soc 54:479–484, 2006

Picciotto MR, Zoli M: Nicotinic receptors in aging and dementia. J Neurobiol 53:641–655, 2002

Pitkala KH, Laurila JV, Strandberg TE, et al: Prognostic significance of delirium in frail elderly people. Dement Geriatr Cogn Disord 19:158–163, 2005

Pompei P, Foreman M, Rudberg MA, et al: Delirium in hospitalized older persons: outcomes and predictors. J Am Geriatr Soc 42:809–815, 1994

Pratico C, Quattrone D, Lucanto T, et al: Drugs of anesthesia acting on central cholinergic system may cause postoperative cognitive dysfunction and delirium. Med Hypotheses 65:972–982, 2005

Pulsinelli WA, Duffy TE: Regional energy balance in rat brain after transient forebrain ischemia. J Neurochem 40:1500–1503, 1983

Quinette P, Guillery-Girard B, Dayan J, et al: What does transient global amnesia really mean? Review of the literature and thorough study of 142 cases. Brain 129:1640–1658, 2006

Rabins PV: Alzheimer's disease management. J Clin Psychiatry 59 (suppl 13):36–38, 1998

Rabins PV, Blacker D, Bland A, et al: Practice guideline for the treatment of patients with Alzheimer's disease and other dementias of late life. American Psychiatric Association. Am J Psychiatry 154(suppl):1–39, 1997

Rahkonen T, Luukkainen-Markkula R, Paanila S, et al: Delirium episode as a sign of undetected dementia among community dwelling elderly subjects: a 2 year follow up study. J Neurol Neurosurg Psychiatry 69:519–521, 2000

Rahkonen T, Eloniemi-Sulkava U, Halonen P, et al: Delirium in the nondemented oldest old in the general population: risk factors and prognosis. Int J Geriatr Psychiatry 16:415–421, 2001

Ranen NG: Huntington's disease, in Psychiatric Management in Neurological Disease. Edited by Lauterbach EC. Washington, DC, American Psychiatric Press, 2000, pp 71–92

Rao V, Lyketsos CG: Delusions in Alzheimer's disease: a review. J Neuropsychiatry Clin Neurosci 10:373–382, 1998

Rasquin SM, Lodder J, Visser PJ, et al: Predictive accuracy of MCI subtypes for Alzheimer's disease and vascular dementia in subjects with mild cognitive impairment: a 2-year follow-up study. Dement Geriatr Cogn Disord 19:113–119, 2005

Rebeck GW, Hyman BT: Apolipoprotein and Alzheimer's disease, in Alzheimer's Disease, 2nd Edition. Edited by Terry RD, Katzman R, Bick KL, et al. Philadelphia, PA, Lippincott Williams & Wilkins, 1999, pp 339–346

Reisberg B, Doody R, Stoffler A, et al: Memantine in moderate-to-severe Alzheimer's disease. N Engl J Med 348:1333–1341, 2003

Riker RR, Fraser GL, Cox PM: Continuous infusion of haloperidol controls agitation in critically ill patients. Crit Care Med 22:433–440, 1994

Robinson RG: The Clinical Neuropsychiatry of Stroke: Cognitive, Behavioral, and Emotional Disorders Following Vascular Brain Injury. New York, Cambridge University Press, 1998

Rockwood K: Acute confusion in elderly medical patients. J Am Geriatr Soc 37:150–154, 1989

Rogers MP, Liang MH, Daltroy LH, et al: Delirium after elective orthopedic surgery: risk factors and natural history. Int J Psychiatry Med 19:109–121, 1989

Roman GC: Vascular dementia revisited: diagnosis, pathogenesis, treatment, and prevention. Med Clin North Am 86:3477–3499, 2002

Romano J, Engel GL: Delirium, part 1: electroencephalographic data. Arch Neurol Psychiatry 51:356–377, 1944

Ropacki SA, Jeste DV: Epidemiology of and risk factors for psychosis of Alzheimer's disease: a review of 55 studies published from 1990 to 2003. Am J Psychiatry 162:2022–2030, 2005

Rosenblatt A, Leroi I: Neuropsychiatry of Huntington's disease and other basal ganglia disorders. Psychosomatics 41:24–30, 2000

Ross CA, Peyser CE, Shapiro I, et al: Delirium: phenomenological and etiologic subtypes. Int Psychogeriatr 3:135–147, 1991

Ross GW, Bowen JD: The diagnosis and differential diagnosis of dementia. Med Clin North Am 86:455–476, 2002

Ross GW, Petrovitch H, White LR, et al: Characterization of risk factors for vascular dementia: the Honolulu–Asia Aging Study. Neurology 53:337–343, 1999

Royall DR, Cordes JA, Polk M: CLOX: an executive clock drawing task. J Neurol Neurosurg Psychiatry 64:588–594, 1998

Sasaki Y, Matsuyama T, Inoue S, et al: A prospective, open-label, flexible-dose study of quetiapine in the treatment of delirium. J Clin Psychiatry 64:1316–1321, 2003

Schneider LS, Dagerman KS, Insel P: Risk of death with atypical antipsychotic drug treatment for dementia: meta-analysis of randomized placebo-controlled trials. JAMA 294:1934–1943, 2005

Schor JD, Levkoff SE, Lipsitz LA, et al: Risk factors for delirium in hospitalized elderly. JAMA 267:827–831, 1992

Schwartz TL, Masand PS: Treatment of delirium with quetiapine. Prim Care Companion J Clin Psychiatry 2:10–12, 2000

Schwid SR, Weinstein A, Wishart HA, et al: Multiple sclerosis, in Psychiatric Management in Neurological Disease. Edited by Lauterbach EC. Washington, DC, American Psychiatric Press, 2000, pp 249–270

Seaman J, Schillerstrom J, Carroll D, et al: Impaired oxidative metabolism precipitates delirium: a study of 101 ICU patients. Psychosomatics 47:56–61, 2006

Serby M, Brickman AM, Haroutunian V: Cognitive burden and excess Lewy-body pathology in the Lewy-body variant of Alzheimer's disease. Am J Geriatr Psychiatry 11:371–374, 2003

Sharma ND, Rosman HS, Padhi D, et al: Torsades de pointes associated with intravenous haloperidol in critically ill patients. Am J Cardiol 81:238–240, 1998

Shuping JR, Rollinson RD, Toole JF: Transient global amnesia. Ann Neurol 7:281–285, 1980

Sink KM, Holden KF, Yaffe K: Pharmacological treatment of neuropsychiatric symptoms of dementia: a review of the evidence. JAMA 293:596–608, 2005

Sipahimalani A, Masand PS: Use of risperidone in delirium: case reports. Ann Clin Psychiatry 9:105–107, 1997

Skrobik YK, Bergeron N, Dumont M, et al: Olanzapine vs haloperidol: treating delirium in a critical care setting. Intensive Care Med 30:444–449, 2004

Slatkin N, Rhiner M: Treatment of opioid-induced delirium with acetylcholinesterase inhibitors: a case report. J Pain Symptom Manage 27:268–273, 2004

Slatkin N, Rhiner M, Bolton TM: Donepezil in the treatment of opioid-induced sedation: report of six cases. J Pain Symptom Manage 21:425–438, 2001

Small GW: Differential diagnosis and early detection of dementia. Am J Geriatr Psychiatry 6 (2 suppl 1):S26–S33, 1998a

Small GW: The pathogenesis of Alzheimer's disease. J Clin Psychiatry 59 (suppl 9):7–14, 1998b

Small GW, Leiter F: Neuroimaging for diagnosis of dementia. J Clin Psychiatry 59 (suppl 11):4–7, 1998

Small GW, Chen ST, Komo S, et al: Memory self-appraisal in middle-aged and older adults with the apolipoprotein E-4 allele. Am J Psychiatry 156:1035–1038, 1999

Smith CD, Snowdon DA, Wang H, et al: White matter volumes and periventricular white matter hyperintensities in aging and dementia. Neurology 54:838–842, 2000

Straker D: Aripiprazole for the treatment of delirium. Webb Fellow Presentation at the 52nd annual meeting of the Academy of Psychosomatic Medicine, Santa Ana Pueblo, NM, November 2005

Tager FA, Fallon BA: Psychiatric and cognitive features of Lyme disease. Psychiatr Ann 31:173–181, 2001

Tariot PN, Farlow MR, Grossberg GT: Memantine treatment in patients with moderate to severe Alzheimer's disease already receiving donepezil. JAMA 291:317–324, 2004

Teri L, Logsdon RG, Peskind E, et al: Treatment of agitation in AD: a randomized, placebo-controlled clinical trial [published erratum appears in Neurology 56:426, 2001]. Neurology 55:1271–1278, 2000

Thomason JW, Shintani A, Peterson JF, et al: Intensive care unit delirium is an independent predictor of longer hospital stay: a prospective analysis of 261 non-ventilated patients. Crit Care 9:R375–R381, 2005

Titier K, Canal M, Deridet E, et al: Determination of myocardium to plasma concentration ratios of five antipsychotic drugs: comparison with their ability to induce arrhythmia and sudden death in clinical practice. Toxicol Appl Pharmacol 199:52–60, 2004

Toda H, Kusumi I, Sasaki Y, et al: Relationship between plasma concentration levels of risperidone and clinical effects in the treatment of delirium. Int Clin Psychopharmacol 20:331–333, 2005

Torres R, Mittal D, Kennedy R: Use of quetiapine in delirium: case reports. Psychosomatics 42:347–349, 2001

Tost H, Wendt CS, Schmitt A, et al: Huntington's disease: phenomenological diversity of a neuropsychiatric condition that challenges traditional concepts in neurology and psychiatry. Am J Psychiatry 161:28–34, 2004

Trzepacz PT: Is there a final common neural pathway in delirium? Focus on acetylcholine and dopamine. Semin Clin Neuropsychiatry 5:132–148, 2000

Trzepacz PT, Maue FR, Coffman G, et al: Neuropsychiatric assessment of liver transplantation candidates: delirium and other psychiatric disorders. Int J Psychiatry Med 7:101–111, 1986

Trzepacz PT, Baker RW, Greenhouse J: A symptom rating scale for delirium. Psychiatry Res 23:89–97, 1988

Trzepacz PT, Mittal D, Torres R, et al: Validation of the Delirium Rating Scale—Revised–98: comparison with the delirium rating scale and cognitive test for delirium. J Neuropsychiatry Clin Neurosci 13:229–242, 2001

Tsai L, Tsuang MT: The Mini-Mental State test and computerized tomography. Am J Psychiatry 136:436–439, 1979

Tune LE, Folstein MF: Postoperative delirium. Adv Psychosom Med 15:51–68, 1986

Tune LE, Sunderland T: New cholinergic therapies: treatment tools for the psychiatrist. J Clin Psychiatry 59 (suppl 13):31–35, 1998

Tune LE, Carr S, Hoag E, et al: Anticholinergic effects of drugs commonly prescribed for the elderly: potential means for assessing risk of delirium. Am J Psychiatry 149:1393–1394, 1992

Victor M, Adams RD, Collins GH: The Wernicke-Korsakoff Syndrome and Related Neurologic Disorders Due to Alcoholism and Malnutrition, 2nd Edition. Philadelphia, PA, FA Davis, 1989

Volicer L, Harper DG, Manning BC, et al: Sundowning and circadian rhythms in Alzheimer's disease. Am J Psychiatry 158:704–711, 2001

Voyer P, Cole MG, McCusker J, et al: Prevalence and symptoms of delirium superimposed on dementia. Clin Nurs Res 15:46–66, 2006

Wacker P, Nunes PV, Cabrita H, et al: Postoperative delirium is associated with poor cognitive outcome and dementia. Dement Geriatr Cogn Disord 21:221–227, 2006

Weiss U, Bacher R, Vonbank H, et al: Cognitive impairment: assessment with brain magnetic resonance imaging and proton mass spectroscopy. J Clin Psychiatry 64:235–242, 2003

Wengel SP, Roccaforte WH, Burke WJ: Donepezil improves symptoms of delirium in dementia: implications for future research. J Geriatr Psychiatry Neurol 11:159–161, 1998

Wengel SP, Burke WJ, Roccaforte WH: Donepezil for postoperative delirium associated with Alzheimer's disease. J Am Geriatr Soc 47:379–380, 1999

Wilkosz PA, Miyahara S, Lopez OL, et al: Prediction of psychosis onset in Alzheimer disease: the role of cognitive impairment, depressive symptoms, and further evidence of psychosis subtypes. Am J Geriatr Psychiatry 14:352–360, 2006

Williams-Russo P, Urquhart BL, Sharrock NE, et al: Postoperative delirium: predictors and prognosis in elderly orthopedic patients. J Am Geriatr Soc 40:759–767, 1992

Wilson LM: Intensive care delirium: the effect of outside deprivation in a windowless unit. Arch Intern Med 130:225–226, 1972

Wimo A, Winblad B, Stoffler A, et al: Resource utilization and cost analysis of memantine in patients with moderate to severe Alzheimer's disease. Pharmacoeconomics 21:327–340, 2003

Winblad B, Poritis N: Memantine in severe dementia: results of the 9M-Best Study (Benefit and efficacy in severely demented patients during treatment with memantine). Int J Geriatr Psychiatry 14:135–146, 1999

Yasuno F, Nishikawa T, Nakagawa Y, et al: Functional anatomical study of psychogenic amnesia. Psychiatry Res 99:43–57, 2000

Zubenko GS, Zubenko WN, McPherson S: A collaborative study of the emergence and clinical features of the major depressive syndrome of Alzheimer's disease. Am J Psychiatry 160:857–866, 2003

# 16

# Substance-Related Disorders

MARTIN H. LEAMON, M.D.

TARA M. WRIGHT, M.D.

HUGH MYRICK, M.D.

## Classification Systems

DSM-IV-TR defines *substance* as "a drug of abuse, a medication, or a toxin" (American Psychiatric Association 2000, p. 191) and classifies disorders attributable to substance use according to the schema in Table 16–1. Eleven classes of substances that include the commonly recognized abusable drugs are described, and then other medications or toxins that could cause disorders are grouped into the class of "other or unknown." The specific substance-related disorders are the substance-induced disorders of *intoxication* and *withdrawal* and the substance use disorders of *abuse* and *dependence* (Tables 16–2, 16–3, 16–4, and 16–5).

Other substance-induced disorders are classified with their phenomenologically similar disorders; for example, substance-induced mood disorder is included in the DSM-IV-TR mood disorders section. Not all types of disorders are recognized for all classes of substances (Table 16–6). The ICD-10 (World Health Organization 2006) classification is shown in Table 16–7.

A word on terminology is in order. The words *dependence*, *abuse*, *addiction*, and others are often used with different meanings when discussing psychoactive substance use, potentially leading to confusion and misunderstanding (O'Brien et al. 2006). For the purposes of this chapter, the uncapitalized terms *dependence* and *addiction* are used interchangeably, and the uncapitalized term *abuse* is used

**TABLE 16–1.** **DSM-IV-TR classification of substance-related disorders**

Substance-related disorders
Substance use disorders
    Dependence
    Abuse
Substance-induced disorders
    Intoxication
    Withdrawal
    Others (see Table 16–6)

to refer to substance use that leads to problems at any level. In DSM-IV-TR, the diagnoses are capitalized, thus leading to the commonly encountered but somewhat paradoxical situation in which Substance Dependence and Substance Abuse are both forms of substance abuse. It is also important to keep in mind the potential differences between lay, pharmacological, and psychiatric meanings of the term *intoxication*—the psychiatric disorder requires the effect of the substance to be "clinically significant" and "maladaptive." Last, many clinicians and patients consider treatment for substance dependence to be a process that involves a reorientation of all areas of a patient's life—a process termed *recovery*. At times, this chapter uses the terms *recovery* and *treatment* synonymously. Shown in

---

**TABLE 16–2.  DSM-IV-TR diagnostic criteria for substance intoxication**

A.  The development of a reversible substance-specific syndrome due to recent ingestion of (or exposure to) a substance.  **Note:** Different substances may produce similar or identical syndromes.

B.  Clinically significant maladaptive behavioral or psychological changes that are due to the effect of the substance on the central nervous system (e.g., belligerence, mood lability, cognitive impairment, impaired judgment, impaired social or occupational functioning) and develop during or shortly after use of the substance.

C.  The symptoms are not due to a general medical condition and are not better accounted for by another mental disorder.

---

Table 16–8 are recommended maximum alcohol consumption goals for low-risk drinking. Table 16–9 shows the percentage of past-year substance users with abuse or dependence by substance.

# Neurobiology

A number of different neuronal circuits and neurotransmitters have been implicated in the process of addiction. Recent theories suggest that the process of becoming addicted to a substance includes a usurpation of the brain circuits involved in the pursuit and acquisition of normal "survival-relevant natural goals…[or] 'rewards,'" such as food or mating opportunities (Hyman 2005). The firing of dopamine-releasing neurons, with cell bodies in the ventral tegmental area and axon terminals in the nucleus accumbens, serves to mark the importance or salience of a reward as well as signaling that a rewarding event is about to occur. Many, if not all, addictive substances produce a measure of firing that is much greater than that produced by more mundane survival-relevant ones.

Further processing of the stimulus by prefrontal cortical areas leads to associative learning that attributes an unduly high level of significance to the substance effect and substance use–related cues (Kalivas and Volkow 2005).

In addition to dopamine, the neurotransmitters glutamate, γ-aminobutyric acid (GABA), and opioid neuropeptides are important in this circuitry.

---

**TABLE 16–3.  DSM-IV-TR diagnostic criteria for substance withdrawal**

A.  The development of a substance-specific syndrome due to the cessation of (or reduction in) substance use that has been heavy and prolonged.

B.  The substance-specific syndrome causes clinically significant distress or impairment in social, occupational, or other important areas of functioning.

C.  The symptoms are not due to a general medical condition and are not better accounted for by another mental disorder.

---

**TABLE 16–4.  DSM-IV-TR diagnostic criteria for substance abuse**

A.  A maladaptive pattern of substance use leading to clinically significant impairment or distress, as manifested by one (or more) of the following, occurring within a 12-month period:

(1)  recurrent substance use resulting in a failure to fulfill major role obligations at work, school, or home (e.g., repeated absences or poor work performance related to substance use; substance-related absences, suspensions, or expulsions from school; neglect of children or household)

(2)  recurrent substance use in situations in which it is physically hazardous (e.g., driving an automobile or operating a machine when impaired by substance use)

(3)  recurrent substance-related legal problems (e.g., arrests for substance-related disorderly conduct)

(4)  continued substance use despite having persistent or recurrent social or interpersonal problems caused or exacerbated by the effects of the substance (e.g., arguments with spouse about consequences of intoxication, physical fights)

B.  The symptoms have never met the criteria for substance dependence for this class of substance.

---

# Approach to the Patient

A patient with a substance use disorder may present in several different ways, and in a general psychiatric practice he or she may present with complaints of mood problems, anxiety, sleep difficulties, or symptoms of another Axis I or Axis II psychiatric disorder. For this reason, all patients

**TABLE 16–5.   DSM-IV-TR diagnostic criteria for substance dependence**

A maladaptive pattern of substance use, leading to clinically significant impairment or distress, as manifested by three (or more) of the following, occurring at any time in the same 12-month period:

(1) tolerance, as defined by either of the following:

   (a) a need for markedly increased amounts of the substance to achieve intoxication or desired effect

   (b) markedly diminished effect with continued use of the same amount of the substance

(2) withdrawal, as manifested by either of the following:

   (a) the characteristic withdrawal syndrome for the substance (refer to Criteria A and B of the criteria sets for withdrawal from the specific substances)

   (b) the same (or a closely related) substance is taken to relieve or avoid withdrawal symptoms

(3) the substance is often taken in larger amounts or over a longer period than was intended

(4) there is a persistent desire or unsuccessful efforts to cut down or control substance use

(5) a great deal of time is spent in activities necessary to obtain the substance (e.g., visiting multiple doctors or driving long distances), use the substance (e.g., chain-smoking), or recover from its effects

(6) important social, occupational, or recreational activities are given up or reduced because of substance use

(7) the substance use is continued despite knowledge of having a persistent or recurrent physical or psychological problem that is likely to have been caused or exacerbated by the substance (e.g., current cocaine use despite recognition of cocaine-induced depression, or continued drinking despite recognition that an ulcer was made worse by alcohol consumption)

should be routinely and consistently screened for substance use disorders. A number of instruments exist, and different ones may be used depending on the specific clinical setting (Dyson et al. 1998; McPherson and Hersch 2000; Workgroup on Substance Use Disorders 2006). One such instrument is the CAGE-D; the patient's answers to the questions (about need to Cut down drinking or drug use, Annoyance about criticism of use, Guilt over drinking or drug use, and use of drink or drugs as Eye-opener in morning) can serve as a springboard into further discussion of substance use (Dyson et al. 1998). One should inquire about all classes of substances (e.g., alcohol, opioids, sedative-hypnotics, stimulants, cannabis, nicotine), including prescription medications as well as legal and illegal substances, because a patient may not regard abuse of some substances to be as significant as that of others.

There is a large societal stigma against people with substance use disorders, and patients may be quite averse to acknowledging substance-related problems. Additionally, patients may be hesitant to disclose illegal activities. Questions must be asked with nonjudgmental empathy and caring professional interest. Confrontational challenging is not always useful and may disrupt therapeutic rapport (Miller et al. 1993). The basic areas of inquiry are listed in Table 16–10. Obtaining information from collateral sources with the patient's consent and repeated assessments and history taking over time may be necessary to gain a sufficiently detailed picture of the patient's use to make accurate treatment recommendations.

# Treatment: General Principles

## Intoxication and Withdrawal

Severe intoxications can be life threatening and may require emergent general medical care. Detailed discussion of such care is beyond the scope of this chapter, and the interested reader is referred to specialized emergency medicine texts. When necessary, treatment of withdrawal is generally accomplished by one or a combination of two general methods (Center for Substance Abuse Treatment 2006). In the first, a cross-tolerant, less harmful, and usually longer-acting medication is substituted for the drug of abuse (e.g., methadone for heroin, nicotine for tobacco smoke, diazepam for alcohol). The dosage is adjusted until withdrawal symptoms are minimized, and then the medication is gradually tapered off. In the second method, non-cross-tolerant medications are used to reduce withdrawal-associated symptoms (e.g., clonidine for opioid withdrawal, bupropion for nicotine withdrawal). Treatment of substance withdrawal alone does little to improve outcomes for patients with substance use disorders. The time during the treatment of withdrawal also should be used to enhance motivation and initiate treatment for abuse or dependence.

**TABLE 16–6. DSM-IV-TR diagnoses associated with class of substances**

| | Dependence | Abuse | Intoxication | Withdrawal | Intoxication delirium | Withdrawal delirium | Dementia | Amnestic disorder | Psychotic disorders | Mood disorders | Anxiety disorders | Sexual dysfunctions | Sleep disorders |
|---|---|---|---|---|---|---|---|---|---|---|---|---|---|
| Alcohol | X | X | X | X | X | X | X | X | X | X | X | X | X |
| Amphetamines | X | X | X | X | X | | | | X | X | X | X | X |
| Caffeine | | | X | | | | | | | | X | | X |
| Cannabis | X | X | X | | X | | | | X | | X | | |
| Cocaine | X | X | X | X | X | | | | X | X | X | X | X |
| Hallucinogens | X | X | X | | X | | | | X[a] | X | X | | |
| Inhalants | X | X | X | | X | | X | | X | X | X | | |
| Nicotine | X | | | X | | | | | | | | | |
| Opioids | X | X | X | X | X | | | | X | X | | X | X |
| Phencyclidine | X | X | X | | X | | | | X | X | X | | |
| Sedatives, hypnotics, or anxiolytics | X | X | X | X | X | X | X | X | X | X | X | X | X |
| Polysubstance | X | | | | | | | | | | | | |
| Other | X | X | X | X | X | X | X | X | X | X | X | X | X |

*Note.* X indicates that the disorder is recognized in DSM-IV-TR.
[a]Includes hallucinogen persisting perception disorder (flashbacks).
*Source.* Adapted from American Psychiatric Association 2000, p. 193.

**TABLE 16–7.** **ICD-10 classification of substance use disorders**

Mental and behavioral disorders due to psychoactive substance use (F10–F19)

**Acute intoxication**

**Harmful use**

"A pattern of psychoactive substance use that is causing damage to health. The damage may be physical (e.g., hepatitis from self-administration of injected psychoactive substances) or mental (e.g., episodes of depressive disorder secondary to heavy consumption of alcohol)" (World Health Organization 2006).

**Dependence syndrome**

**Withdrawal state**

**Others** (e.g., withdrawal state with delirium, psychotic disorder, amnesic syndrome)

## Substance Use Disorders

The Stages of Change model is useful for conceptualizing a patient's motivation to address substance use problems. The model, derived from research on tobacco cessation, divides the recovery process into sequential stages, with stage-specific goals to achieve before progression (Table 16–11) (Prochaska and DiClemente 1992). The practitioner matches interventions to the patient's stage to enhance commitment to change and to increase the probability of successful change in substance use. Accordingly, a patient with severe addiction who is in the Contemplation stage is less likely to respond to strong recommendations to enter intensive treatment (which may provoke refusal and rejection of further attempts to help) and is more likely to develop motivation for treatment if initially engaged in specific discussion about the advantages and disadvantages of recovery as contrasted with continued substance use and an addicted lifestyle.

A patient sufficiently motivated is ideally enrolled in a treatment program of an intensity commensurate with his or her level of problems. The Patient Placement Criteria algorithm developed by the American Society of Addiction Medicine assigns a patient within five levels of care (with sublevels) based on six dimensions (Table 16–12) (Mee-Lee et al. 2001). Patients matched to treatment placements based on this algorithm have been shown to have better outcomes than mismatched patients, and although further research continues, it already has been widely implemented (Magura et al. 2003). A number of professional psychosocial interventions and psychotherapies have been shown

**TABLE 16–8.** **Maximum alcohol consumption for low-risk drinking**

For healthy men up to age 65 years

No more than 4 drinks in a day *and*

No more than 14 drinks in a week

For healthy women up to age 65 years

No more than 3 drinks in a day *and*

No more than 7 drinks in a week

For healthy adults older than 65 years

No more than 1 drink in a day *and*

No more than 7 drinks in a week

Recommend lower limits or abstinence as medically indicated; for example, for patients who

Take medications that interact with alcohol

Have a health condition exacerbated by alcohol

Are pregnant (advise abstinence)

*Source.* Adapted from National Institute on Alcohol Abuse and Alcoholism 2005. Public domain.

in large studies to be effective for substance use disorder treatment (see Table 16–17 later in this chapter).

### *Psychotherapies*

The most prevalent and widely used psychosocial interventions are the mutual self-help groups based on the 12 Steps of Alcoholics Anonymous (AA) (Table 16–13) (Peter D. Hart Research Associates 2001; Substance Abuse and Mental Health Services Administration 2005).

### *Outcomes*

In general, the optimal goal for the individual patient with substance dependence is abstinence from all non–medically supervised substance use. Treatment, however, may need to focus sequentially on intermediate objectives, such as moving into the Preparation stage (see Table 16–11), decreased psychiatric hospitalizations, and more drug-free urine tests.

# Alcohol

## Epidemiology

Based on combined data from the 2002–2004 National Surveys on Drug Use and Health, it is estimated that 7.6%

**TABLE 16–9.    Percentage of past-year substance users with abuse or dependence, by substance: 2004**

| Substance | Percentage of users with abuse or dependence |
|---|---|
| Heroin | 67.8 |
| Cocaine | 27.8 |
| Marijuana | 17.6 |
| Alcohol | 11.9 |
| Hallucinogens | 11.6 |
| Inhalants | 10.3 |

*Source.*   Substance Abuse and Mental Health Services Administration 2005.

**TABLE 16–10.    Basic components of substance use disorder evaluation**

1. Chronology of substance use: onset, fluctuations over time, development of tolerance, episodes of withdrawal, periods of abstinence, resumption of use, most recent use

2. History of formal substance abuse treatment, attendance at self-help meetings or groups

3. Perceptions of substance-related difficulties, problems, or complications

4. Full psychiatric and general medical histories, including medication history

5. Legal history, including substance-related legal problems

6. Family and social histories, including psychiatric or substance-related disorders in family members, diagnosed/treated or not

7. General psychiatric examination, including screening for other psychiatric disorders, and a mental status examination

8. General physical examination

9. Laboratory studies, as indicated by substances used

*Source.*   Adapted from Workgroup on Substance Use Disorders: *Practice Guideline for the Treatment of Patients With Substance Use Disorders*, 2nd Edition. Washington, DC, American Psychiatric Publishing, 2006. Used with permission.

(18.2 million) of persons age 12 years or older met the criteria for alcohol dependence or abuse in the past year. Data from the national Epidemiologic Catchment Area (ECA) study of the late 1980s indicate that lifetime prevalence of alcohol dependence is as high as 14.7% (Regier et al. 1990).

## Intoxication

Table 16–14 lists blood alcohol levels and typical corresponding clinical features of intoxication in an individual who has not developed any tolerance. A blood alcohol level of 0.4 g/dL is associated with a 50% mortality risk in nonalcoholic persons. In determining how quickly a person's blood alcohol level will decrease, a rule of thumb is that the body metabolizes approximately one drink (approximately 0.015 g/dL) per hour.

## Withdrawal

Alcohol withdrawal typically begins 6–8 hours after the last drink, peaks 24–28 hours after the last drink, and generally resolves within 7 days (Myrick and Anton 2004). The spectrum of alcohol withdrawal symptoms is wide, and the more common presentations are outlined in Table 16–15. Only about 5% of individuals with alcohol dependence will develop more than mild to moderate withdrawal symptoms.

Alcohol hallucinosis occurs in 3%–10% of patients with severe alcohol withdrawal. It can present as auditory, visual, or tactile hallucinations in the presence of a clear sensorium. Delirium tremens (DT), or alcohol withdrawal delirium, is characterized by agitation and tremulousness, autonomic instability, fevers, auditory and visual hallucinations, and disorientation. DT usually develops 2–4 days from the person's last drink, and the average duration is less than 1 week. DT has been estimated to occur in 5% of patients admitted for alcohol withdrawal (Mayo-Smith et al. 2004). It must be considered a medical emergency because the mortality rate can be as high at 20% without prompt and adequate treatment of the severe withdrawal.

Seizures, another complication of alcohol withdrawal, are estimated to occur in 5%–15% of patients. They usually occur in the first 24 hours from last drink, but they can occur any time in the first 5 days. Alcohol withdrawal seizures are usually grand mal in type. Persons with a history of alcohol withdrawal seizures are at increased risk for seizures in subsequent episodes of alcohol withdrawal.

## Diagnosis

Several questionnaires are available for the detection of drinking-related problems. A positive response to any of the questions on the CAGE should lead the clinician to investigate problem drinking with the patient further. The Alcohol Use Disorders Identification Test is another

**TABLE 16–11.** Stages of change

| Stage | Patient presentation | Stage task | Change strategy |
|---|---|---|---|
| Precontemplation | No intention of changing In "denial" or resistant | Increase doubt and awareness of problem | Nonjudgmental, respectful assessments<br>Consciousness-raising, provide information<br>Low intensity of interaction |
| Contemplation | Aware of problem Ambivalent about change | Tip the decisional balance | Acknowledge the ambivalence<br>Weigh pros and cons of change vs. risks and benefits of problem<br>Reinforce advantages of change<br>Responsibility for change lies with the patient |
| Preparation | Intends to change Confusion about best way to do so | Determine best course of action | Offer menu of choices, co-create plan<br>Demystify change process<br>Inspire realistic hope |
| Action | Actual behavior change "Treatment" | Implement collaborative, realistic plan | Monitor progress<br>Reinforce incremental success<br>Problem-solve |
| Maintenance | Behavior changed | Develop new lifestyle<br>Avoid relapse | Watch for overblown expectations<br>Be alert for "seemingly irrelevant decisions"<br>Support realistic hopes |

*Source.* Prochaska and DiClemente 1992.

10-item questionnaire used for the screening of alcohol use disorders.

Laboratory data and biological markers can be clues to an alcohol use disorder in a patient. Table 16–16 illustrates possible laboratory abnormalities in the setting of alcohol abuse or dependence.

## Treatment

### Acute Withdrawal

The general management strategies in alcohol detoxification include adjunctive treatment of comorbid medical problems, rehydration, and correction of electrolyte abnormalities (including hypomagnesemia, hypophosphatemia, and hypokalemia). Because nutritional deficiencies are common in individuals with chronic alcoholism, oral multivitamin preparations containing folic acid are routinely administered to early abstinent individuals.

The replacement of thiamine, particularly before giving glucose, is especially important to prevent Wernicke's encephalopathy, precipitated by depletion of thiamine reserves.

Benzodiazepines have historically been considered the gold standard for the treatment of alcohol withdrawal. They can be administered either via fixed dosage and taper or on an as-needed basis. The Clinical Institute Withdrawal Assessment Scale for Alcohol—Revised is a short test rating the severity of alcohol withdrawal as observed by a health care professional.

### Relapse Prevention

Once an individual has been successfully detoxified from alcohol, maintenance of the abstinence is the next goal. The maintenance of abstinence can be a very difficult goal to achieve; it has been estimated that approximately 50% of alcoholic individuals relapse within 3 months of com-

**TABLE 16–12.    American Society of Addiction Medicine Patient Placement Criteria levels and dimensions**

**Patient assessment dimensions**

1. Intoxication/withdrawal potential
2. Biomedical conditions and complications
3. Emotional, behavioral, or cognitive conditions and complications
4. Readiness to change
5. Relapse, continued use, or continued problem potential
6. Recovery environment

**Levels of care[a]**

Level 0.5    Early intervention

Level I    Outpatient treatment

Level II    Intensive outpatient treatment/ partial hospitalization

Level III    Residential/inpatient treatment

Level IV    Medically managed intensive inpatient treatment

[a]Within each general level of care are a number of more refined sublevels.
*Source.*    Mee-Lee et al. 2001.

**TABLE 16–13.    Twelve-Step group Web sites**

| | |
|---|---|
| Alcoholics Anonymous | www.aa.org |
| Narcotics Anonymous | www.na.org |
| Cocaine Anonymous | www.ca.org |
| Marijuana Anonymous | www.marijuana-anonymous.org |
| Crystal Meth Anonymous (methamphetamine) | www.crystalmeth.org |
| Dual Recovery Anonymous (co-occurring substance abuse and other psychiatric disorders) | www.draonline.org |

*Note.*    Sites were accessed July 9, 2006.

**TABLE 16–14.    Blood alcohol level and corresponding symptoms of intoxication in the nontolerant patient**

| Blood alcohol level (mg/dL) | Clinical presentation |
|---|---|
| 30 | Attention difficulties (mild), euphoria |
| 50 | Coordination problems, driving is legally impaired |
| 100 | Ataxia, drunk driving |
| 200 | Confusion, decreased consciousness |
| >400 | Anesthesia, possible coma, possible death |

*Source.*    Adapted from Mack et al. 2003.

pletion of treatment. Psychosocial support remains the cornerstone in achieving this goal, and recent advances in pharmacotherapy have been a valuable addition. Research has shown that three forms of individual behavioral treatment (cognitive-behavioral therapy [CBT], motivational enhancement, and 12-Step facilitation [see Table 16–17]) contribute to sustained abstinence and reduced drinking.

As of July 2007, there were only four medications with U.S. Food and Drug Administration (FDA) approval for the maintenance treatment of alcohol dependence: disulfiram, naltrexone, a long-acting intramuscular formulation of naltrexone, and acamprosate. Table 16–18 offers a comparison of these medications.

## Medical Complications

Heavy alcohol consumption results in serious health sequelae over time, with many cases ultimately resulting in death. It is known to elevate blood pressure and increase the risk of myocardial infarction. There is an increased risk of cancer, particularly esophageal, head, neck, liver, stomach, colon, and lung. Long-term alcoholism results in damage to the liver, with the end point being cirrhosis and

death. Esophageal varices resulting from the long-term abuse of alcohol can also be life threatening because they can rupture, leading to rapid, profuse bleeding.

Wernicke-Korsakoff syndrome is a result of thiamine deficiency in alcoholism. The syndrome can be precipitated by the administration of glucose to asymptomatic individuals with thiamine deficiency. It is therefore of utmost importance to be sure that alcohol-dependent individuals receive supplemental thiamine before administration of glucose in an acute setting. Early symptoms include decreased concentration, apathy, mild agitation, and depressed mood. Confusion, amnesia, and confabulation are late signs of severe and prolonged thiamine deficit.

Fetal alcohol syndrome results from a mother consuming alcohol during her pregnancy; no amount of alcohol can be considered safe during pregnancy. In this syndrome, mental retardation is common (44% of children with fetal alcohol syndrome have an IQ of 79 or below). Other congenital defects include wide-set eyes, short

**TABLE 16–15. DSM-IV-TR diagnostic criteria for alcohol withdrawal**

A. Cessation of (or reduction in) alcohol use that has been heavy and prolonged.

B. Two (or more) of the following, developing within several hours to a few days after Criterion A:
 (1) autonomic hyperactivity (e.g., sweating or pulse rate greater than 100)
 (2) increased hand tremor
 (3) insomnia
 (4) nausea or vomiting
 (5) transient visual, tactile, or auditory hallucinations or illusions
 (6) psychomotor agitation
 (7) anxiety
 (8) grand mal seizures

C. The symptoms in Criterion B cause clinically significant distress or impairment in social, occupational, or other important areas of functioning.

D. The symptoms are not due to a general medical condition and are not better accounted for by another mental disorder.

*Specify* if: **With perceptual disturbances**

**TABLE 16–16. Laboratory abnormalities associated with harmful levels of drinking**

Measurable blood alcohol level
 Legal limit for driving is <0.08 mg/mL
 Levels >0.3 mg/mL with minimal intoxication may indicate tolerance
Elevated mean corpuscular volume >94 fL
Elevated liver transaminases
 Gamma-glutamyltransferase >65 IU/L
 Less specific
  Aspartate aminotransferase >38 IU/L
  Alanine aminotransferase >45 IU/L
Elevated relative percent in serum of carbohydrate-deficient transferrin >2.5%
Decreased platelets <140 K/mm$^3$

palpebral fissure, short and broad-bridged nose, hypoplastic philtrum, thinned upper lip, and flattened midface. Maternal alcohol use with breast-feeding has been shown to impair a child's motor, but not mental, development.

# Cannabis

## Epidemiology

Cannabis, whether as leaves/flowers (marijuana) or resin (hashish), is the most commonly used illicit drug worldwide (United Nations Office on Drugs and Crime 2005). In 2004, 6.1% of subjects in the National Household Survey on Drug Use and Health reported past-month use of marijuana, with about 35% of those using other illicit drugs as well (Substance Abuse and Mental Health Services Administration 2005).

## Intoxication and Withdrawal

Intoxication (Table 16–19) has been associated with increased risk of automobile accidents. No specific treatment is generally indicated. A cannabis withdrawal syndrome has recently been described (Table 16–20). It begins 2–3 days after cessation of use and is generally mild, but the duration has been variable in studies, from 12 to 115 days.

## Diagnosis and Treatment

Patients often use cannabis in addition to other substances, and careful history taking may be required to determine a diagnosis of abuse or dependence. The comparatively milder symptoms of cannabis intoxication and withdrawal can lead patients to thinking its use is not "serious" or that abstinence is not necessary.

## Medical Complications

Chronic marijuana use has long been associated with increased risk of paranoia, but there is growing evidence (and debate) about associations between early onset of marijuana use and psychosis or schizophrenia (Moore et al. 2007). Additionally, as would be expected in a product that is burned and smoked, there is an increased risk of certain cancers and pulmonary complications.

Women considering becoming pregnant or who are already so should be strongly advised not to use cannabis. Fetal growth decreases, and subsequent cognitive and behavioral impairments and psychiatric symptoms in the child appear to be epidemiologically related to cannabis abuse during pregnancy (Workgroup on Substance Use Disorders 2006).

**TABLE 16–17. Empirically based psychosocial interventions**

| Type | Summary | Example |
|---|---|---|
| Motivational enhancement therapy | Directive client-centered approach that focuses on uncovering and resolving ambivalence about changing substance use in a manner that increases the patient's internal motivation for and commitment to change; avoids confronting resistance. | Miller WR, Zweben A, DiClemente CC, et al.: *Motivational Enhancement Therapy Manual.* Rockville, MD, U.S. Department of Health and Human Services, 1994 |
| Cognitive-behavioral therapy | Focuses on relapse prevention and the reversing of maladaptive thoughts and beliefs that support substance use. | Kadden R, Carroll KM, Donovan D, et al.: *Cognitive-Behavioral Coping Skills Therapy Manual.* Rockville, MD, U.S. Department of Health and Human Services, 1994<br>Carroll KM: *A Cognitive-Behavioral Approach: Treating Cocaine Addiction.* Rockville, MD, U.S. Department of Health and Human Services, 1998 |
| 12-Step facilitation therapy | Reinforces the Alcoholics/Narcotics Anonymous approach to abstinence. Outside participation in 12-Step groups essential. May include couples sessions. | Nowinski J, Baker S, Carroll KM: *Twelve Step Facilitation Therapy Manual.* Rockville, MD, U.S. Department of Health and Human Services, 1995 |
| Network therapy | Cognitive-behavioral approach combined with sessions with support network (e.g., family, friends). May be combined with disulfiram. | Galanter M: *Network Therapy for Alcohol and Drug Abuse.* New York, Guilford, 1999 |
| Matrix model | A combination of cognitive-behavioral therapy groups, family education groups, social support groups, individual counseling, regular drug testing, and optional 12-Step attendance. | Rawson RA, Marinelli-Casey P, Anglin MD, et al.: "A Multi-Site Comparison of Psychosocial Approaches for the Treatment of Methamphetamine Dependence." *Addiction* 99:708–717, 2004 |
| Contingency management | Reinforces the achievement of interim goals (e.g., drug-free urine tests) with intermittent tangible rewards of increasing value. | Budney AJ, Higgins ST: *A Community Reinforcement Plus Vouchers Approach: Treating Cocaine Addiction.* Rockville, MD, U.S. Department of Health and Human Services, 1998<br>Petry NM, Peirce JM, Stitzer ML, et al.: "Effect of Prize-Based Incentives on Outcomes in Stimulant Abusers in Outpatient Psychosocial Treatment Programs: A National Drug Abuse Treatment Clinical Trials Network Study." *Archives of General Psychiatry* 62:1148–1156, 2005 |

**TABLE 16–17.**   **Empirically based psychosocial interventions** *(continued)*

| Type | Summary | Example |
|---|---|---|
| Brief advice or intervention | 5- to 15-minute motivational/educational office-based intervention; may include one or more in-person or telephone follow-up contacts. | National Institute on Alcohol Abuse and Alcoholism: *Helping Patients Who Drink Too Much: A Clinician's Guide.* Rockville, MD, U.S. Department of Health and Human Services, 2005<br><br>Fiore MC, Bailey WC, Cohen SJ, et al.: *Treating Tobacco Use and Dependence: Quick Reference Guide for Clinicians.* Rockville, MD, U.S. Department of Health and Human Services, 2000 |
| Group and individual drug counseling | Strong emphasis on abstinence, preventing relapses, problem-solving, and involvement in 12-Step groups. | Boren JJ, Onken LS, Carroll KM (eds.): *Approaches to Drug Abuse Counseling.* Rockville, MD, U.S. Department of Health and Human Services, 2000 |
| Integrated treatment | A service delivery model for patients with chronic mental illness and substance abuse in which the same provider team delivers both mental health and substance abuse treatment. | Bellack AS, Bennett ME, Gearon JS, et al.: "A Randomized Clinical Trial of a New Behavioral Treatment for Drug Abuse in People With Severe and Persistent Mental Illness." *Archives of General Psychiatry* 63:426–432, 2006<br><br>Mueser KT, Noorksy DL, Drake RE, et al.: *Integrated Treatment for Dual Disorders: A Guide to Effective Practice.* New York, Guilford, 2003 |
| Couples and family therapies | A number of different models. | Reviewed in Carroll KM, Onken LS: "Behavioral Therapies for Drug Abuse." *American Journal of Psychiatry* 162:1452–1460, 2005 |

*Note.*   This listing is intended to be more representative than comprehensive. For general reviews, see Carroll and Onken 2005 or Woody 2003.

TABLE 16–18.    Comparison of U.S. Food and Drug Administration–approved medications for the treatment of alcohol dependence

| | Disulfiram | Acamprosate | Naltrexone | Extended-release naltrexone injection |
|---|---|---|---|---|
| Mechanism of action | Alcohol deterrent | Reduces craving | Reduces craving | Reduces craving |
| | Inhibits alcohol dehydrogenase | Restores balance between excitatory glutamate and inhibitory γ-amino-butyric acid neuro-transmitter systems | Opioid receptor antagonist | Opioid receptor antagonist |
| Interactions with alcohol | Causes adverse reaction, including flushing, nausea, and vomiting | None | None | None |
| Major advantages | Physical reaction is a strong disincentive to drinking while taking medication | Generally well tolerated, few drug interactions, is not processed through liver | Generally well toler-ated, recent large multisite study supports efficacy | Once-a-month injection can greatly enhance compliance |
| Major disadvantages | Cannot use in the setting of liver failure | Dosing is two tablets three times daily | Cannot use in the setting of liver failure | Cannot use in the setting of liver failure |
| | Patient must avoid *all* products containing alcohol | | Cannot use concurrently with opioid analgesics | Cannot use concurrently with opioid analgesics |

TABLE 16–19.    Symptoms of cannabis intoxication

Lower doses

Relaxation

Euphoria

Altered time and sensory perception

Increased appetite

Higher doses

Hypervigilance or paranoia

Anxiety or panic

Derealization or depersonalization

Hallucinations (auditory or visual)

TABLE 16–20.    Cannabis withdrawal symptoms

Most frequently seen

Cannabis craving

Anxiety, restlessness, and/or irritability

Insomnia

Changes in appetite

Boredom

Improved memory

Less frequently seen

Tremor

Diaphoresis (sweating)

Tachycardia

Gastrointestinal disturbances, including nausea, vomiting, and diarrhea

Change in libido

Depression

*Source.*   Center for Substance Abuse Treatment 2006; Coper-sino et al. 2006.

# Stimulants

## Epidemiology

The category of stimulants includes cocaine, amphetamine, and amphetamine-like substances. According to the National Survey on Drug Use and Health, there were an estimated 1 million new cocaine users in 2004, and about 1% of the U.S. population age 12 years or older had used cocaine within the past 30 days (Substance Abuse and Mental Health Services Administration 2005). Amphetamine-type substances come in several different forms. Powdered methamphetamine hydrochloride ("speed," "meth," or "crank") can be snorted, injected, or dissolved in beverages. Pills can be prescription medications such as dexamphetamine or clandestinely manufactured tablets of powdered methamphetamine. Freebase methamphetamine (sometimes called "ice") can be vaporized in a pipe or on aluminum foil and insufflated (smoked), producing as rapid a high as with injection but without having to use needles (Maxwell 2005).

Alarmingly, although the total number of past-year and past-month methamphetamine users did not change significantly between 2002 and 2004, the number of past-month methamphetamine users *who met criteria for abuse or dependence* increased from 27.5% in 2002 to 59.3% in 2004 (Substance Abuse and Mental Health Services Administration 2005).

## Intoxication

Cocaine and amphetamine intoxication have similar symptoms (Table 16–21). The differences in clinical presentation are due to the respective half-lives of the drugs, which are approximately 40–60 minutes for cocaine and 6–12 hours for methamphetamine. Chronic administration of either drug can induce a paranoid psychotic state. There is some evidence that methamphetamine-induced psychosis can be long lasting and may recur in the absence of further drug use. Individuals may be at risk of acting violently in response to frightening delusions common in induced paranoia.

## Withdrawal

As with intoxication, the symptoms of cocaine and amphetamine withdrawal are similar, distinguished primarily by time course (Table 16–22). Methamphetamine withdrawal may be more protracted and less abrupt than cocaine withdrawal. Not uncommonly, clinically significant

---

**TABLE 16–21. DSM-IV-TR diagnostic criteria for cocaine or amphetamine intoxication**

A. Recent use of cocaine, amphetamine, or a related substance (e.g., methylphenidate).

B. Clinically significant maladaptive behavioral or psychological changes (e.g., euphoria or affective blunting; changes in sociability; hypervigilance; interpersonal sensitivity; anxiety, tension, or anger; stereotyped behaviors; impaired judgment; or impaired social or occupational functioning) that developed during, or shortly after, use of cocaine, amphetamine, or a related substance.

C. Two (or more) of the following, developing during, or shortly after, cocaine, amphetamine, or a related substance use:

(1) tachycardia or bradycardia
(2) pupillary dilation
(3) elevated or lowered blood pressure
(4) perspiration or chills
(5) nausea or vomiting
(6) evidence of weight loss
(7) psychomotor agitation or retardation
(8) muscular weakness, respiratory depression, chest pain, or cardiac arrhythmias
(9) confusion, seizures, dyskinesias, dystonias, or coma

D. The symptoms are not due to a general medical condition and are not better accounted for by another mental disorder.

*Specify* if: **With perceptual disturbances**

---

depressive symptoms can accompany the withdrawal. During the late withdrawal phase, a person may experience brief periods of intense, cue-induced drug craving.

## Treatment

Psychosocial and behavioral approaches are the mainstays of treatment in stimulant-dependent individuals. There are currently no medications with FDA approval for the treatment of cocaine- or amphetamine-dependent individuals. Several lines of pharmacotherapy have been investigated, including antidepressant agents (e.g., selective serotonin reuptake inhibitors [SSRIs], tricyclics), dopaminergic agents (e.g., pergolide [withdrawn from U.S. market], antipsychotics), and anticonvulsant agents (e.g., carbamazepine).

---

**TABLE 16–22.    DSM-IV-TR diagnostic criteria for cocaine or amphetamine withdrawal**

A.  Cessation of (or reduction in) cocaine or amphetamine (or a related substance) use that has been heavy and prolonged.

B.  Dysphoric mood and two (or more) of the following physiological changes, developing within a few hours to several days after Criterion A:

    (1)  fatigue

    (2)  vivid, unpleasant dreams

    (3)  insomnia or hypersomnia

    (4)  increased appetite

    (5)  psychomotor agitation or retardation

C.  The symptoms in Criterion B cause clinically significant distress or impairment in social, occupational, or other important areas of functioning.

D.  The symptoms are not due to a general medical condition and are not better accounted for by another mental disorder.

---

Behavior therapies, including CBT and supportive-expressive psychotherapy, have been shown to help retain people in treatment and can lead to abstinence. Positive contingency management procedures also have been shown to help an individual achieve initial abstinence. More recently, the Matrix model has received attention as an effective treatment for stimulant disorders. The Matrix model is a 16-week manualized outpatient treatment that combines CBT materials and techniques, educational materials for patient and family on the effects of stimulants, 12-Step program participation, and positive reinforcement for behavior change and treatment compliance.

## Medical Complications

Cocaine-related myocardial ischemia and infarction are the most serious complications of cocaine abuse. Cocaine produces a powerful sympathetic effect via inhibition of presynaptic uptake of norepinephrine and dopamine. Chest pain is the most common symptom in cocaine users presenting to the emergency department, and therefore, individuals presenting with chest pain should be asked about cocaine use. Seven percent to 25% of patients presenting to emergency departments with nontraumatic chest pain will screen positive for cocaine in their urine, and approximately 6% of these individuals will have en-

zymatic evidence of myocardial infarction. It has been estimated that cocaine use acutely increases the risk of acute myocardial infarction by a factor of 24 in otherwise healthy individuals (Mittleman et al. 1999).

Acute coronary syndrome and cardiac arrhythmias are common in individuals presenting to emergency departments after the use of methamphetamine (Turnipseed et al. 2003). Methamphetamine use is also a risk factor for stroke, likely because use of this drug can lead to elevations in blood pressure, vasculitis, and vasoconstriction.

Of particular concern has been increased methamphetamine use among men of all sexual orientations with an accompanying increased risk of HIV infection. Methamphetamine, and "ice" in particular, is associated with increases in sex drive, decreases in sexual inhibition, and increases in risky behaviors.

# Opioids

## Epidemiology

The 2004 National Survey on Drug Use and Health estimated that 118,000 persons had used heroin for the first time within the past 12 months (Substance Abuse and Mental Health Services Administration 2005).

## Intoxication

The pleasurable sensation derived from the ingestion of an opioid drug is referred to as a "rush." The onset, duration, and intensity of the rush are dependent on the particular drug that is used, how much is used, and the route of administration (oral ingestion, inhalation, intravenous injection). The characteristic symptoms of intoxication are listed in Table 16–23. Nausea, vomiting, and severe itching also can occur. After the initial rush, sedation can last for the next several hours.

Overdose involving opioid drugs is a life-threatening situation. Fatal respiratory depression can occur as a result of direct suppression of respiratory centers in the midbrain and medulla. Obtaining a urine drug screen can be crucial to identify not only the presence of an opioid but also that of other unsuspected drugs. Treatment of an opioid overdose includes general supportive management in addition to the use of naloxone, a pure opioid antagonist that can reverse the central nervous system effects of opioid intoxication and overdose. Table 16–24 reviews the steps necessary in the management of an opioid overdose (Zimmerman 2003).

**TABLE 16–23. DSM-IV-TR diagnostic criteria for opioid intoxication**

A. Recent use of an opioid.

B. Clinically significant maladaptive behavioral or psychological changes (e.g., initial euphoria followed by apathy, dysphoria, psychomotor agitation or retardation, impaired judgment, or impaired social or occupational functioning) that developed during, or shortly after, opioid use.

C. Pupillary constriction (or pupillary dilation due to anoxia from severe overdose) and one (or more) of the following signs, developing during, or shortly after, opioid use:

(1) drowsiness or coma

(2) slurred speech

(3) impairment in attention or memory

D. The symptoms are not due to a general medical condition and are not better accounted for by another mental disorder.

*Specify* if: **With perceptual disturbances**

## Withdrawal

Table 16–25 outlines the most common signs and symptoms of opioid withdrawal. The timing of the withdrawal is dependent on the type of opioid used. With cessation of chronic heroin use, withdrawal symptoms begin about 8–12 hours after the last dose, peak between 36 and 72 hours, and subside over about 5 days. With methadone, which has a much longer half-life than heroin, the peak of the withdrawal syndrome is usually between days 4 and 6, with acute symptoms persisting for 14–21 days. With any opioid, after acute withdrawal symptoms have subsided, a protracted abstinence syndrome, including disturbances of mood and sleep, can persist for 6–8 months.

## Treatment

Management of acute opioid withdrawal involves a combination of general supportive measures in conjunction with pharmacotherapy. There are several options (see also Table 16–26).

Methadone has long been considered the gold standard for maintenance treatment. In late 2002, the FDA also approved buprenorphine for both detoxification and maintenance treatment of opioid dependence. Potential advantages of buprenorphine over methadone include a longer half-life, which decreases the frequency of clinic

**TABLE 16–24. Management of acute opioid overdose**

1. Establish and maintain airway. Intubation and mechanical ventilation may be necessary.

2. Naloxone 0.4–0.8 mg may be administered intravenously, intramuscularly, by sublingual injection, or via endotracheal tube to reverse toxic effects.

(a) Onset of action with intravenous administration is approximately 2 minutes.

(b) If initial doses of naloxone restore adequate respiration and further therapy is needed, repeat boluses, or a continuous infusion of naloxone can be used.

(c) The infusion dose is typically one-half to two-thirds of the initial amount of naloxone that reversed the respiratory depression, administered on an hourly basis.

(d) If the patient has been intubated, a naloxone infusion is not necessary.

3. Monitor for development of pulmonary edema

**TABLE 16–25. Signs and symptoms of opioid withdrawal**

| Early to moderate | Moderate to advanced |
| --- | --- |
| Anorexia | Abdominal cramps |
| Anxiety | Broken sleep |
| Craving | Hot or cold flashes |
| Dysphoria | Increased blood pressure |
| Fatigue | Increased pulse |
| Headache | Low-grade fever |
| Irritability | Muscle and bone pain |
| Lacrimation | Muscle spasm ("kicking |
| Mydriasis (mild) | the habit") |
| Perspiration | Mydriasis (with fixed, |
| Piloerection (gooseflesh; | dilated pupils at the |
| "cold turkey") | peak) |
| Restlessness | Nausea and vomiting |
| Rhinorrhea | |
| Yawning | |

*Source.* Adapted from Collins and Kleber 2004.

---

**TABLE 16–26.    Opioid detoxification medication protocols**

**Methadone substitution and taper**

*Day 1:* Start with a dose of 10–20 mg. If withdrawal symptoms persist 1 hour after dosing, an additional 5–10 mg of methadone can be given. The initial dose should not exceed 30 mg, and the total 24-hour dose should not exceed 40 mg in the first few days unless there is clear documentation of the patient using opioids in excess of 40-mg methadone equivalents per day.

*Days 2–4:* Maintain a stable dose for 2–3 days.

*Day 5–Completion:* Slowly taper dose by 10%–15% per day.

**Buprenorphine substitution and taper**

*Day 1:* Administer buprenorphine 4 mg sublingually after the emergence of mild to moderate withdrawal symptoms. If withdrawal symptoms persist after 1 hour, another 4-mg dose may be given.

*Days 2–4:* On subsequent days, 8–12 mg may be sufficient to relieve withdrawal symptoms, although higher dosages may be required.

*Day 5–Completion:* A slow taper has been shown to be superior to rapid tapers in some studies, although the rate of taper is not clearly defined.

**Clonidine taper**

*Day 1:* 0.1–0.2 mg orally every 4–6 hours up to 1 mg.

*Days 2–4:* 0.2–0.4 mg orally every 4–6 hours up to 1.2 mg.

*Day 5–Completion:* Reduce total daily dose by 0.2 mg daily, given in two to three divided doses (the nighttime dose should be reduced last).

Adjunctive therapy, including nonsteroidal anti-inflammatory drugs for myalgias, benzodiazepines for insomnia, antiemetics, antimotility drugs for intestinal cramping, and muscle relaxants, may be necessary.

*Note.* For clonidine–naltrexone protocols, consult one of the "Suggested Readings" texts listed at the end of the chapter.

---

visits, and a high safety profile with less risk of respiratory depression in overdose. Training programs are available for physicians to become certified to prescribe buprenorphine in office-based settings, not just in the traditional methadone maintenance treatment program.

## Medical Complications

One cohort study in South London estimated a standardized morality ratio of 17 for both male and female heroin users (Hickman et al. 2003). The risk of transmission of HIV, particularly in intravenous opioid users, is a major concern, and an estimated 85% of patients receiving methadone maintenance for opioid dependence in the United States are infected with the hepatitis C virus. Opioid users also can experience decreased immune function, hyperalgesia, and bacterial infections (particularly with intravenous drug use), including abscesses and cellulitis of the skin. Endocarditis with intravenous drug use is another serious concern: more than 50% of these cases will be right-sided, most often involving the tricuspid valve. Sequelae of right-sided endocarditis will often involve the lungs as well.

# Nicotine

## Epidemiology

Approximately 42.4% of U.S. adults have ever smoked cigarettes, with half of those (20.9%) being current smokers (Centers for Disease Control and Prevention 2005). The prevalence is higher among men and the poor and decreases with increasing educational levels.

## Intoxication and Abuse

Although one can certainly feel ill from too much acute tobacco use (e.g., nausea, dizziness, tachycardia), because there are rarely prolonged maladaptive or clinically significant social sequelae, nicotine intoxication is not a recognized substance-induced disorder.

## Diagnosis

Although the diagnosis of nicotine dependence is made according to DSM-IV-TR criteria, other rating scales may be useful in treating the disorder. The number of cigarettes smoked per day correlates negatively with ease in quitting and, in many studies, with response to formal treatment.

## Treatment and Withdrawal

Given that tobacco use is legal, and its acute use causes minimal behavioral disruption, treatment of nicotine dependence focuses on managing withdrawal and cravings (Table 16–27) and developing other behaviors that promote abstinence and prevent relapse.

**TABLE 16–27.  DSM-IV-TR diagnostic criteria for nicotine withdrawal**

A.  Daily use of nicotine for at least several weeks.

B.  Abrupt cessation of nicotine use, or reduction in the amount of nicotine used, followed within 24 hours by four (or more) of the following signs:

   (1)  dysphoric or depressed mood

   (2)  insomnia

   (3)  irritability, frustration, or anger

   (4)  anxiety

   (5)  difficulty concentrating

   (6)  restlessness

   (7)  decreased heart rate

   (8)  increased appetite or weight gain

C.  The symptoms in Criterion B cause clinically significant distress or impairment in social, occupational, or other important areas of functioning.

D.  The symptoms are not due to a general medical condition and are not better accounted for by another mental disorder.

---

Although the long-term (e.g., 12-month) quit rates for a single attempt are less than 10%, the lifetime long-term quit rate is approximately 50%. Accordingly, one of the tasks for the treatment provider is to help the patient deal with relapse and maintain a sense of hope and self-efficacy.

Evidence-based clinical practice guidelines for nicotine dependence are readily available (e.g., Fiore et al. 2000), as are self-help Web sites and telephone lines (Table 16–28). Nicotine treatment includes 1) offering treatment to all patients who use tobacco and, for patients attempting cessation, 2) providing practical counseling and social support as part of treatment, and helping patients secure support outside of treatment; and 3) providing adjunctive pharmacotherapy unless contraindicated (U.S. Department of Health and Human Services 2000). Pharmacotherapeutic treatment principles are listed in Table 16–29.

## Medical Complications

One pharmacological complication especially relevant to psychiatric practice is the induction of hepatic enzymes and drug metabolism by the nonnicotine components (probably polycyclic aromatic hydrocarbons) of tobacco smoke. Nicotine-dependent patients hospitalized on non-smoking units who are stabilized on medications such as haloperidol, valproate, clozapine, oxazepam, and others will experience decreased blood levels of the medications once discharged if they resume smoking.

**TABLE 16–28.  Smoking cessation information Web sites**

- Smokefree.gov (http://www.smokefree.gov): Tobacco Control Research Branch of the National Cancer Institute, National Institutes of Health. A handheld computer intervention tool software program is available through this site.

- ACS Guide to Quitting Smoking (http://www.cancer.org/docroot/PED/content/PED_10_13X_Guide_for_Quitting_Smoking.asp): American Cancer Society

- Smoking & Tobacco Use (http://www.cdc.gov/tobacco): Office on Smoking and Health of National Center for Chronic Disease Prevention and Health Promotion, Centers for Disease Control and Prevention

- Treatobacco.net (http://www.treatobacco.net): Society for Research on Nicotine and Tobacco, World Bank, Cochrane Group, and others

- "Clinical Practice Guideline: Treating Tobacco Use and Dependence" (http://www.ncbi.nlm.nih.gov/books/bv.fcgi?rid=hstat2.chapter.28163): Agency for Healthcare Research and Quality, U.S. Department of Health and Human Services

*Note.*  Sites accessed March 4, 2009.

# Sedative-Hypnotics

## Epidemiology

Just over 12% of individuals older than 12 years report lifetime abuse of sedative-hypnotic medications (Substance Abuse and Mental Health Services Administration 2005).

## Intoxication

Signs and symptoms of intoxication are similar to those of alcohol intoxication and can include slurred speech, ataxia, and incoordination. At more severe levels of intoxication, stupor and coma may develop. With the older nonbenzodiazepine agents, tolerance may develop to a drug's therapeutic effects but not to its toxicity, and a barbiturate overdose can be fatal. An overdose on benzodiazepines alone virtually never leads to death. When they are ingested along with alcohol, major tranquilizers, or opioids, however, the polysubstance overdose can be fatal.

TABLE 16–29.  First-line pharmacotherapies approved for use for smoking cessation by the U.S. Food and Drug Administration[a]

| Agent | Precautions/ contraindications | Side effects | Dosage | Duration | Availability |
|---|---|---|---|---|---|
| Bupropion SR | History of seizure History of eating disorders | Insomnia Dry mouth | 150 mg every morning for 3 days, then 150 mg twice daily. (Begin treatment 1–2 weeks before quitting.) | 7–12 weeks, maintenance up to 6 months | Zyban (prescription only) |
| Nicotine gum | | Mouth soreness Dyspepsia | 1–24 cigarettes/day: 2-mg gum (up to 24 pieces/day) 25+ cigarettes/day: 4-mg gum (up to 24 pieces/day) | Up to 12 weeks | Nicorette, different flavors (OTC only) |
| Nicotine inhaler | | Local irritation of mouth and throat | 6–16 cartridges/day | Up to 6 months | Nicotrol Inhaler (prescription only) |
| Nicotine nasal spray | | Nasal irritation | 8–40 doses/day | 3–6 months | Nicotrol NS (prescription only) |
| Nicotine patch | | Local skin reaction Insomnia | 21 mg/24 hours 14 mg/24 hours 7 mg/24 hours 15 mg/16 hours | 4 weeks then 2 weeks then 2 weeks 8 weeks | Nicoderm CQ, (OTC only) Generic patches (prescription and OTC) Nicotrol (OTC only) |
| Varenicline | | Nausea Sleep disturbance Constipation | Taper up to 1 mg twice a day by day 8. (Begin treatment 1 week prequitting.) | 12–24 weeks | Chantix (prescription only) |

*Note.* The information contained within this table is not comprehensive. Please see package inserts for the individual medications for additional information. OTC=over the counter; SR=sustained release.
[a]Other agents such as rimonabant (cannabinoid-1 receptor antagonist) and selegiline (irreversible monoamine oxidase B inhibitor) are under investigation.
*Source.*  Adapted from Agency for Healthcare Research and Quality 2001.

## Withdrawal

The withdrawal symptoms that occur with benzodiazepines, barbiturates, and nonbarbiturate/nonbenzodiazepine agents are similar to one another as well as to the withdrawal symptoms of alcohol. Table 16–30 identifies the most common signs and symptoms seen in sedative-hypnotic withdrawal. The time course and intensity of withdrawal symptoms depend on the particular drug on which the individual is dependent. With short-acting sedative-

hypnotics and benzodiazepines, symptoms can begin between 12 and 24 hours after the last dose and reach peak intensity between 24 and 72 hours. With long-acting drugs, withdrawal symptoms may not peak until the fifth to eighth day.

For patients who were initially prescribed benzodiazepines for the treatment of psychiatric symptoms, those target symptoms may reemerge during withdrawal. Symptom rebound is a brief, intensified return of the target symptoms and is the most common consequence of pro-

**TABLE 16–30. DSM-IV-TR diagnostic criteria for sedative-hypnotic withdrawal**

A. Cessation of (or reduction in) sedative, hypnotic, or anxiolytic use that has been heavy and prolonged.

B. Two (or more) of the following, developing within several hours to a few days after Criterion A:

   (1) autonomic hyperactivity (e.g., sweating or pulse rate greater than 100)

   (2) increased hand tremor

   (3) insomnia

   (4) nausea or vomiting

   (5) transient visual, tactile, or auditory hallucinations or illusions

   (6) psychomotor agitation

   (7) anxiety

   (8) grand mal seizures

C. The symptoms in Criterion B cause clinically significant distress or impairment in social, occupational, or other important areas of functioning.

D. The symptoms are not due to a general medical condition and are not better accounted for by another mental disorder.

*Specify* if: **With perceptual disturbances**

longed benzodiazepine use. Rebound symptoms usually resolve within a few weeks after discontinuation of the benzodiazepine. Signs and symptoms of withdrawal can occur for weeks to months and consist of slowly abating symptoms of withdrawal as noted in Table 16–30.

## Treatment

Management of severe benzodiazepine overdose includes careful monitoring of the patient's airway and ventilatory support when necessary. Repeated doses of activated charcoal may be particularly helpful in barbiturate or other nonbenzodiazepine ingestions. Flumazenil, a competitive antagonist at the benzodiazepine receptor, may be useful, but if it is not used carefully, the abruptly induced severe withdrawal can induce seizures in patients dependent on benzodiazepines.

Four general strategies can be used for the management of sedative-hypnotic withdrawal, including benzodiazepines. The first option gradually reduces the dosage of the sedative-hypnotic on which the patient is dependent. The second option substitutes a long-acting benzo-

diazepine (such as chlordiazepoxide) for the agent to which the person is dependent and then tapers the substituted agent. The third option substitutes a long-acting barbiturate (usually phenobarbital) and then tapers that. A fourth option is to use valproate or carbamazepine.

The phenobarbital substitution option has the broadest use for sedative-hypnotic withdrawal and can be used for barbiturate, benzodiazepine, or combined alcohol/sedative-hypnotic withdrawals. Phenobarbital is long-acting, has little variation in blood levels between doses, and has both a low abuse potential and a high therapeutic index. The signs of toxicity (e.g., sustained nystagmus, slurred speech, or ataxia) are reliable and easily observable. The patient's average daily sedative-hypnotic dosage is calculated (Table 16–31) and then divided into three doses spread out over the day. Before each dose of phenobarbital, the patient is checked for signs of toxicity, and if any are present, the dose is withheld. If minimal or no signs or symptoms of withdrawal occur, the phenobarbital dosage is decreased by 30 mg each day. If objective signs of withdrawal develop, the daily dosage of phenobarbital is increased by 50%, and the patient is restabilized before continuing the withdrawal.

# Hallucinogens

## Epidemiology

The family of hallucinogens includes drugs that induce a distortion of reality in the user, including alterations of sensory perceptions of sight and sounds as well as changes in emotions. Lysergic acid diethylamide (LSD) is the prototypical hallucinogen. It is an odorless and tasteless synthetic chemical, usually ingested as a solution or dissolved on paper or sugar cubes. Typical hallucinogenic doses are 25–75 µg.

Analogous lysergic acid derivatives can be extracted from morning glory seeds and ergot, a rye fungus. In 2005, the annual use among twelfth graders was 1.8%. Among tenth graders, annual use was 1.5% (National Institute on Drug Abuse 2005).

## Intoxication

LSD interferes with serotonin neurotransporters. The drug typically induces euphoria in addition to delusions and visual hallucinations; however, the psychological effects it induces can be unpredictable.

The experience of LSD can be significantly influenced by the user's preintoxication mind set and also by the set-

**TABLE 16–31.    Sedative-hypnotics and their phenobarbital withdrawal equivalents**

| Generic name | Trade name | Common therapeutic uses | Therapeutic dosage range (mg/day) | Dose equal to 30 mg phenobarbital for withdrawal, mg[a] |
|---|---|---|---|---|
| **Benzodiazepines** | | | | |
| Alprazolam | Xanax | Sedative, antipanic | 0.75–6 | 1 |
| Chlordiazepoxide | Librium | Sedative | 15–100 | 25 |
| Clonazepam | Klonopin | Anticonvulsant | 0.5–4 | 2 |
| Clorazepate | Tranxene | Sedative | 15–60 | 7.5 |
| Diazepam | Valium | Sedative | 4–40 | 10 |
| Estazolam | ProSom | Hypnotic | 1–2 | 1 |
| Flunitrazepam[b] | Rohypnol[b] | Hypnotic | 0.5–1 | 0.5 |
| Flurazepam | Dalmane | Hypnotic | 15–30 | 15 |
| Halazepam | Paxipam | Sedative | 60–160 | 40 |
| Lorazepam | Ativan | Sedative | 1–6 | 2 |
| Midazolam | Versed | Intravenous sedation | 2.5–7 | 2.5 |
| Nitrazepam[b] | Mogadon[b] | Hypnotic | 5–10 | 5 |
| Oxazepam | Serax | Sedative | 10–120 | 10 |
| Temazepam | Restoril | Hypnotic | 15–30 | 15 |
| Triazolam | Halcion | Hypnotic | 0.125–0.50 | 0.25 |
| **Barbiturates** | | | | |
| Butabarbital | Butisol | Sedative | 45–120 | 100 |
| Butalbital | Fiorinal, Sedapap | Sedative/analgesic[c] | 100–300 | 100 |
| Pentobarbital | Nembutal | Hypnotic | 50–100 | 100 |
| Secobarbital | Seconal | Hypnotic | 50–100 | 100 |
| **Other sedative-hypnotics** | | | | |
| Zaleplon | Sonata | Hypnotic | 5–20 | 5 |
| Zolpidem | Ambien | Hypnotic | 5–10 | 5 |

[a]Phenobarbital withdrawal conversion equivalence is not the same as therapeutic dose equivalency. Withdrawal equivalence is the amount of the drug that 30 mg of phenobarbital will substitute for and that will prevent serious high-dose withdrawal signs and symptoms.
[b]Although not marketed in the United States, these benzodiazepines are commonly used in many countries.
[c]Butalbital is usually available in combination with opioid and nonopioid analgesics.
*Source.*    Adapted from Smith and Wesson 2004.

ting in which the drug is used. "Bad trips" can be marked by feelings of intense fear with avoidant responses. Physical effects include increased body temperature, heart rate, and blood pressure; sleeplessness; and a loss of appetite.

## Withdrawal

Although hallucinogen withdrawal is not a recognized disorder, withdrawal symptoms of minimal clinical signifi-

cance (including fatigue, irritability, and anhedonia) are reported by approximately 10% of hallucinogen users.

## Treatment

The treatment of acute intoxication with hallucinogens is largely supportive. Providing reassurance, support, and a calm, quiet environment is the mainstay of treatment. For patients with extreme feelings of panic or fear, the use of a benzodiazepine may be warranted.

## Medical Complications

A potential complication of hallucinogen use is hallucinogen persisting perception disorder, or "flashbacks." The etiological mechanism underlying flashbacks is not clearly understood, but they have reportedly been precipitated by SSRIs. Flashbacks are spontaneous experiences of the same effects that occurred while a person was intoxicated with a hallucinogen in the past. LSD users may also manifest relatively long-lasting psychoses, such as schizophrenia or severe depression, although such severe reactions are not common.

## Phencyclidine and Ketamine

### Epidemiology

Phencyclidine (PCP), commonly referred to as "angel dust," inhibits catecholamine reuptake in neurons, leading to adrenergic potentiation (Greydanus and Patel 2003). It can be used as a liquid, tablet, or powder and can also be sprinkled on a cigarette. Results from the Monitoring the Future survey found that in 2005, 2.4% of high school seniors reported a lifetime use of PCP (National Institute on Drug Abuse 2005).

Ketamine is a derivative of PCP. It is less potent, shorter-acting, and used as a dissociative anesthetic in humans as well as animals. Ketamine is commonly referred to on the street as "Special K," "Vitamin K," "Kit Kat," and "cat Valium."

### Intoxication

Both PCP and ketamine cause anesthesia and behavioral effects, at least in part by selectively reducing the excitatory actions of glutamate on central nervous system neurons mediated by the *N*-methyl-D-aspartate (NMDA) receptor complex. Acute PCP intoxication can manifest as behavior changes, including impulsiveness, unpredictability, psychomotor agitation, impaired judgment, and assaultiveness. Physical findings include hypertension, tachycardia, diminished pain sensation, ataxia, dysarthria, muscle rigidity, and seizures. PCP is the only drug that causes a vertical nystagmus, although it can also cause horizontal or rotatory nystagmus.

The spectrum of behavioral effects of ketamine intoxication appears to be similar to that of PCP, although less has been published on the treatment of ketamine intoxication.

### Withdrawal

Although there is not a specifically defined PCP withdrawal syndrome, about 25% of heavy PCP users report withdrawal symptoms, including depression, anxiety, irritability, hypersomnolence, diaphoresis, and tremor.

### Treatment

The management of acute intoxication with PCP includes providing a calm environment with minimal stimuli. Objects that can be used to harm oneself or others should be removed from the patient's access. Diazepam or haloperidol may be useful for the management of PCP-induced agitation. Physical restraints should be avoided because of the risk of increasing the likelihood of rhabdomyolysis, which may occur on its own during PCP intoxication.

### Medical Complications

With PCP intoxication, death can occur secondary to severe hypertension or hypotension, hypothermia, seizures, or psychotic delirium.

## Polysubstance Use

Polysubstance use is common; 56% of patients admitted to publicly funded treatment programs in 2002 reported abuse of more than one substance, and more than 70% smoked cigarettes (Office of Applied Studies 2005). If undetected, polysubstance use can complicate the treatment of intoxication and withdrawal (see Table 16–32 for DSM-IV-TR diagnostic criteria).

---

**TABLE 16–32.** **DSM-IV-TR diagnostic criteria for polysubstance dependence**

---

Over the same 12-month period, three or more substances (other than nicotine or caffeine) are repeatedly used.

The diagnostic criteria for substance dependence are not met for any single substance but are met when the substances are considered together.

**Note.** When multiple substances are used and the criteria for substance dependence are met by each of the substances individually, then each substance dependence diagnosis is listed separately.

---

# Co-occurring Substance Use Disorders and Other Psychiatric Disorders

Substance use disorders and other psychiatric disorders commonly co-occur, and the relation is complex and bidirectional. The National Institute of Mental Health's ECA study and the National Comorbidity Survey (NCS) are two large epidemiological surveys that have evaluated the prevalence of comorbid psychiatric and substance use disorders in community samples. In the ECA study, 45% of the individuals with alcohol use disorders and 72% of the individuals with a drug use disorder had at least one co-occurring psychiatric disorder (Regier et al. 1990). Likewise, in the NCS, 78% of the alcohol-dependent men and 86% of the alcohol-dependent women met lifetime criteria for another psychiatric disorder, including drug dependence (Kessler et al. 1994).

## Diagnostic Considerations

Accurate diagnosis and differentiation between substance-induced states and primary psychiatric diagnoses is one of the more difficult tasks in assessing patients with co-occurring psychiatric symptoms and substance use disorders. The complex relations between psychiatric and substance-induced symptoms can often lead to diagnostic uncertainty for several reasons. Some individuals with psychiatric disorders may abuse substances in an attempt to ameliorate psychiatric symptoms. Chronic and excessive use of some substances may precipitate, trigger, or unmask other latent psychiatric illness. Symptoms of intoxication, withdrawal, or other substance-induced disorders can mimic other psychiatric disorders. Some substances, such as methamphetamine, PCP, and LSD, can cause psychiatric symptoms that persist long after the substance has been measurably eliminated from the body. Individuals in acute distress may present with combined symptoms, some attributable to substance abuse and some attributable to another psychiatric disorder.

Screening patients presenting at either substance abuse or psychiatric treatment settings for both substance use disorders and other psychiatric disorders is essential. Prompt diagnosis and treatment can reduce morbidity, increase treatment efficiency, and improve treatment outcomes. Brief screening tools for substance use disorders that have been found useful in psychiatric settings include the Alcohol Use Disorders Identification Test, the Michigan Alcoholism Screening Test (Selzer 1971), and the Drug Abuse Screening Test (Skinner 1982). The Symptom Checklist has been found to have moderate specificity and high sensitivity in screening for anxiety and mood disorders in substance use patients (Kennedy et al. 2001). The Psychiatric Research Interview for Substance and Mental Disorders (Hasin et al. 1996) also can be used to facilitate determination of the chronological relations between psychiatric symptoms and substance abuse.

## Treatment Considerations

### Psychosocial Treatments

Although the treatments for psychiatric and substance abuse disorders have historically largely consisted of separate clinical services, the integration of services results in better treatment for individuals with co-occurring disorders (see Table 16–17). Programs often include a mix of group and individual therapies. CBTs are among the most efficacious treatments for anxiety and depressive disorders as well as for the treatment of substance use disorders. Behavioral therapies such as relaxation and breathing techniques, biofeedback, and meditation are often used in substance abuse treatment facilities and can also be effective in decreasing psychiatric symptoms. Individuals with co-occurring substance abuse and other psychiatric disorders can also benefit from participation in 12-Step groups such as Dual Recovery Anonymous (see Table 16–13).

### Pharmacological Treatments

The ideal approach to the pharmacological treatment of these co-occurring conditions would be to use an agent that has no abuse potential, is safe and well tolerated, and is efficacious in both disorders. The benzodiazepines, SSRIs, tricyclic antidepressants, monoamine oxidase inhibitors, antipsychotics, and anticonvulsant agents have all been found to be efficacious in treatment studies of specific psychiatric disorders. Unfortunately, there are sparse data in the co-occurring population. Data support the use of SSRI agents in the treatment of co-occurring alcohol dependence and major depression. Higher dosages of SSRIs and tricyclic antidepressants may be required if alcohol use has induced hepatic microsomal enzyme activity. The use of SSRIs in the treatment of particular subtypes of patients with alcohol dependence shows promise, but much work remains to be done. Mirtazapine may be of interest in a population with comorbid alcoholism and depression because of its antagonism of serotonin type 3 receptors, a property that it shares with ondansetron. Although lithium is accepted as the gold standard agent in the treatment of bipolar disorder, anticonvulsant agents have shown some promise in the treatment of co-occurring bipolar and substance use disorders (Myrick et al. 2004). Research investi-

gating the use of psychiatric medications in combination with alcoholism treatment medications such as naltrexone and acamprosate would be of interest.

## Key Points: Substance-Related Disorders

- Worldwide drug and alcohol use disorders, excluding tobacco, are the sixth leading cause of disease burden in adults, whereas tobacco use and exposure to tobacco smoke are the leading preventable causes of death.

- Physicians should inquire about all classes of substances (e.g., alcohol, opioids, sedative-hypnotics, stimulants, cannabis, nicotine), including prescription medications, as well as legal and illegal substances, because a patient may not regard abuse of some substances to be as significant as that of others.

- Although psychosocial and behavioral approaches are the cornerstones of treatment for substance dependence, medications are increasingly used to augment the treatment of alcohol, opioid, and nicotine dependence. Developing medications for the treatment of stimulant dependence is a federal research priority.

- There are currently four medications with FDA approval for the maintenance treatment of alcohol dependence: disulfiram, naltrexone, a long-acting intramuscular formulation of naltrexone, and acamprosate.

- The use of buprenorphine for detoxification or maintenance treatment in opioid dependence is increasingly common, in part because buprenorphine can be prescribed in a physician's office with up to 1 month's prescription at a time.

- Although it may take several tries, the overall success rate in helping patients quit smoking is relatively good. The long-term (e.g., 12 months) quit rates for a single attempt are less than 10%, whereas the lifetime long-term quit rate is approximately 50%.

- Polysubstance abuse is common; 56% of patients admitted to publicly funded treatment programs in 2002 reported abuse of more than one substance, and more than 70% smoked cigarettes. If undetected, polysubstance abuse can complicate the treatment of substance intoxication, withdrawal, abuse, or dependence.

- Substance use disorders and other psychiatric disorders commonly co-occur, and the relationship is complex and bidirectional.

- The recent increase in the rates of nonmedical use of prescription pain killers (specifically opioids) in adolescents is notable and concerning.

## Suggested Readings

American Journal of Psychiatry, Vol 162, Issue 8, 2005, contains 8 review articles on different aspects of substance use disorders.

Galanter M, Kleber HD (eds): The American Psychiatric Publishing Textbook of Substance Abuse Treatment, 3rd Edition. Washington, DC, American Psychiatric Publishing, 2004

Graham AW, Schultz TK, Mayo-Smith MF, et al (eds): Principles of Addiction Medicine, 3rd Edition. Chevy Chase, MD, American Society of Addiction Medicine, 2003

Kleber HD, Weiss RD, Anton RF Jr, et al: Practice Guidelines for the Treatment of Patients With Substance Use Disorders, 2nd Edition. Washington, DC, American Psychiatric Publishing, 2006

Lowinson JH, Ruiz P, Millman RB, et al (eds): Substance Abuse: A Comprehensive Textbook, 4th Edition. Philadelphia, PA, Lippincott Williams & Wilkins, 2005

Nature Neuroscience, Vol 8, Issue 11, 2005, contains 10 review articles and commentaries. The issue is available online at: http://www.nature.com/neuro/focus/addiction/index.html. Accessed July 2006.

# References

Agency for Healthcare Research and Quality: Suggestions for the Clinical Use of Pharmacotherapies for Smoking Cessation. Rockville, MD, U.S. Public Health Service, 2001. Available at: http://www.ahrq.gov/clinic/tobacco/clinicaluse.htm. Accessed July 7, 2006.

American Psychiatric Association: Diagnostic and Statistical Manual of Mental Disorders, 4th Edition, Text Revision. Washington, DC, American Psychiatric Association, 2000

Carroll KM, Onken LS: Behavioral therapies for drug abuse. Am J Psychiatry 162:1452–1460, 2005

Center for Substance Abuse Treatment: Detoxification and Substance Abuse Treatment: Treatment Improvement Protocol (TIP) Series 45. DHHS Publ No (SMA) 06-4131. Rockville, MD, Substance Abuse and Mental Health Services Administration, 2006

Centers for Disease Control and Prevention: Cigarette Smoking Among Adults—United States, 2004. MMWR Morb Mortal Wkly Rep 54:1121–1124, 2005

Collins ED, Kleber HD: Opioids: detoxification, in The American Psychiatric Publishing Textbook of Substance Abuse Treatment, 3rd Edition. Edited by Galanter M, Kleber HD. Washington, DC, American Psychiatric Publishing, 2004, pp 265–289

Copersino M, Boyd SJ, Tashkin D, et al: Cannabis withdrawal among non-treatment-seeking adult cannabis users. Am J Addict 15:8–14, 2006

Dyson V, Appleby L, Altman E, et al: Efficiency and validity of commonly used substance abuse screening instruments in public psychiatric patients. J Addict Dis 17:57–76, 1998

Fiore MC, Bailey WC, Cohen SJ, et al: Treating Tobacco Use and Dependence. Quick Reference Guide for Clinicians. Rockville, MD, Department of Health and Human Services, U.S. Public Health Service, 2000

Greydanus DE, Patel DR: Substance abuse in adolescents: a complex conundrum for the clinician. Pediatr Clin North Am 50:1179–1223, 2003

Hasin DS, Trautman KD, Miele GM, et al: Psychiatric Research Interview for Substance and Mental Disorders (PRISM): reliability for substance abusers. Am J Psychiatry 153:1195–1201, 1996

Hickman M, Carnwath Z, Madden P, et al: Drug-related mortality and fatal overdose risk: pilot cohort study of heroin users recruited from specialist drug treatment sites in London. J Urban Health 80:274–287, 2003

Hyman SE: Addiction: a disease of learning and memory. Am J Psychiatry 162:1414–1422, 2005

Kalivas PW, Volkow ND: The neural basis of addiction: a pathology of motivation and choice. Am J Psychiatry 162:1403–1413, 2005

Kennedy BL, Morris RL, Pedley LL, et al: The ability of the Symptom Checklist SCL-90 to differentiate various anxiety and depressive disorders. Psychiatr Q 72:277–288, 2001

Kessler RC, McGonagle KA, Zhao S, et al: Lifetime and 12-month prevalence of DSM-III-R psychiatric disorders in the United States: results from the National Comorbidity Survey. Arch Gen Psychiatry 51:8–19, 1994

Mack A, Franklin JE Jr, Frances RJL: Substance use disorders, in The American Psychiatric Publishing Textbook of Clinical Psychiatry, 4th Edition. Edited by Hales RE, Yudofsky SC. Washington, DC, American Psychiatric Publishing, 2003, pp 309–378

Magura S, Staines G, Kosanke N, et al: Predictive validity of the ASAM Patient Placement Criteria for naturalistically matched vs. mismatched alcoholism patients. Am J Addict 12:386–397, 2003

Maxwell JC: Emerging research on methamphetamine. Curr Opin Psychiatry 18:235–242, 2005

Mayo-Smith MF, Beecher LH, Fischer TL, et al: Management of alcohol withdrawal delirium: an evidence-based practice guideline. Arch Intern Med 164:1405–1412, 2004

McPherson TL, Hersch RK: Brief substance use screening instruments for primary care settings: a review. J Subst Abuse Treat 18:193–202, 2000

Mee-Lee D, Shulman G, Fishman M, et al (eds): ASAM Patient Placement Criteria for the Treatment of Substance-Related Disorders, 2nd Edition, Revised. Chevy Chase, MD, American Society of Addiction Medicine, 2001

Miller WR, Benefield RG, Tonigan JS: Enhancing motivation for change in problem drinking: a controlled comparison of two therapist styles. J Consult Clin Psychol 61:455–461, 1993

Mittleman MA, Mintzer D, Maclure M, et al: Triggering of myocardial infarction by cocaine. Circulation 99:2737–2741, 1999

Moore THM, Zammit S, Lingford-Hughes A, et al: Cannabis use and risk of psychotic or affective mental health outcomes: a systematic review. Lancet 370:319–328, 2007

Myrick H, Anton R: Recent advances in the pharmacotherapy of alcoholism. Curr Psychiatry Rep 6:332–338, 2004

Myrick H, Cluver J, Swavely S, et al: Diagnosis and treatment of co-occurring affective disorders and substance use disorders. Psychiatr Clin North Am 27:649–659, 2004

National Institute on Alcohol Abuse and Alcoholism: Helping Patients Who Drink Too Much: A Clinician's Guide. Rockville, MD, U.S. Dept of Health and Human Services, 2005

National Institute on Drug Abuse: NIDA InfoFacts: High School and Youth Trends. Bethesda, MD, National Institute on Drug Abuse, 2005. Available at: http://www.drugabuse.gov/infofacts/HSYouthtrends.html. Accessed May 26, 2006.

O'Brien CP, Volkow N, Li TK: What's in a word? Addiction versus dependence in DSM-V. Am J Psychiatry 163:764–765, 2006

Office of Applied Studies: The DASIS Report: Polydrug Admissions: 2002. Rockville, MD, Office of Applied Studies, Substance Abuse and Mental Health Services Administration, 2005. Available at: http://www.drugabusestatistics.samhsa.gov/2k5/polydrugTX/polydrugTX.pdf. Accessed June 15, 2006.

Peter D. Hart Research Associates: The Face of Recovery. Washington, DC, Peter D. Hart Research Associates, 2001. Available at: http://www.facesandvoicesofrecovery.org/pdf/hart_research.pdf. Accessed May 22, 2006

Prochaska JO, DiClemente CC: Stages of change in the modification of problem behaviors. Prog Behav Modif 28:183–218, 1992

Regier DA, Farmer ME, Rae DS, et al: Comorbidity of mental disorders with alcohol and other drug abuse: results from the Epidemiologic Catchment Area (ECA) Study. JAMA 264:2511–2518, 1990

Selzer ML: The Michigan Alcoholism Screening Test (MAST): the quest for a new diagnostic instrument. Am J Psychiatry 127:1653–1658, 1971

Skinner HA: The Drug Abuse Screening Test. Addict Behav 7:363–371, 1982

Smith DE, Wesson DR: Benzodiazepines and other sedative-hypnotics, in The American Psychiatric Publishing Textbook of Substance Abuse Treatment, 3rd Edition. Edited by Galanter M, Kleber HK. Washington, DC, American Psychiatric Publishing, 2004, pp 243–244

Substance Abuse and Mental Health Services Administration: Results From the 2004 National Survey on Drug Use and Health: National Findings. Rockville, MD, Substance Abuse and Mental Health Services Administration, 2005. Available at: http://www.drugabusestatistics.samhsa.gov/nsduh/2k4nsduh/2k4Results/2k4Results.htm#toc. Accessed July 7, 2006.

Turnipseed SD, Richards JR, Kirk JD, et al: Frequency of acute coronary syndrome in patients presenting to the emergency department with chest pain after methamphetamine use. J Emerg Med 24:369–373, 2003

United Nations Office on Drugs and Crime: World Drug Report 2005. Vienna, Austria, United Nations, 2005

U.S. Department of Health and Human Services: Agency for Health Care Policy and Research Supported Clinical Practice Guidelines: Treating Tobacco Use and Dependence (Revised 2000). Rockville, MD, U.S. Department of Health and Human Services, Public Health Service, 2000. Available at: http://www.ncbi.nlm.nih.gov/books/bv.fcgi?rid=hstat2.chapter.7644. Accessed July 1, 2006.

Woody GE: Research findings on psychotherapy of addictive disorders. Am J Addict 12(suppl):S19–S26, 2003

Workgroup on Substance Use Disorders: Practice Guideline for the Treatment of Patients With Substance Use Disorders, 2nd Edition. Washington, DC, American Psychiatric Publishing, 2006

World Health Organization: International Statistical Classification of Diseases and Related Health Problems, 10th Revision, Version for 2006. Geneva, Switzerland, World Health Organization, 2006. Available at: http://www.who.int/classifications/apps/icd/icd10online. Accessed May 18, 2006.

Zimmerman JL: Poisonings and overdoses in the intensive care unit: general and specific management issues. Crit Care Med 31:2794–2801, 2003

# 17

# Schizophrenia

MICHAEL J. MINZENBERG, M.D.

JONG H. YOON, M.D.

CAMERON S. CARTER, M.D.

## Clinical Features

Schizophrenia is operationally defined by a large set of signs and symptoms cutting across diverse domains of behavior and mental processes. The variability of clinical features over time for any particular patient with schizophrenia further adds to this complexity. Although active debate continues on the relative merits and validity of the various symptom classification systems that have been proposed, in this chapter we mostly rely on a scheme that segregates clinical findings into positive, negative, and disorganized symptoms (Table 17–1). This system is simple and has received empirical validation in factor analytic studies (Bilder et al. 1985; Liddle 1987). The term *positive symptom* refers to the *presence* of abnormal mental processes, whereas *negative symptom* refers to the *absence* of normal mental function. The *disorganized* category refers to the linguistic and behavioral abnormalities. In addition to the three symptom clusters, we have included two additional groups of symptoms—the cognitive deficits and soft neurological signs—in recognition of the importance of these clinical features of the illness.

## Positive Symptoms

Three positive symptoms of schizophrenia are generally recognized: hallucinations, delusions, and disorganized speech or behavior (often referred to as *thought disorder*).

The fact that the presence of certain types of hallucinations and delusions satisfies Criterion A of the DSM-IV-TR (American Psychiatric Association 2000) criteria for schizophrenia (Table 17–2) reflects the relative importance placed on these two symptoms.

### Hallucinations

Although hallucinations are encountered in a diverse range of conditions, they have traditionally been viewed as one of the core clinical features of schizophrenia. *Hallucinations* are defined as the perception of a real sensory process in the absence of an external source (e.g., hearing a voice when no one is talking). The perceptual qualities of hallucinations are variable. In some cases, hallucinations are perceived to be indistinguishable from real sensory experiences, whereas in other cases, they are described as only approximating real sensory experiences. It is important to keep in mind that this discussion about the perceptual aspects of hallucinations is distinct from the question of insight. With sufficient insight, a patient may realize that a hallucinatory experience is in fact not real, even if the hallucination fully replicates the sensory qualities of a true sensory experience.

Hallucinations are most frequently reported in the auditory domain. Auditory hallucinations are manifest as voices or other common sounds in the environment such as dogs barking or objects clanging. The presence of a hallucination in other sensory domains is generally more characteristic of other conditions, such as delirium in the

**TABLE 17–1.  Major symptoms in schizophrenia**

| | | |
|---|---|---|
| **Positive** | Hallucinations | Perception of a real sensory experience in the absence of an external source |
| | | Most commonly auditory but can occur in all sensory modalities<br>Common attributes of auditory hallucinations:<br>External source<br>Commentary on patient's actions or thoughts<br>Running dialogue between two or more voices |
| | Delusions | Fixed false beliefs<br>Common types:<br>Paranoid<br>Grandiose<br>Somatic<br>Ideas of reference |
| **Negative** | Affect | Diminished expression of emotions (e.g., blunted affect)<br>Apathy or amotivation |
| | Social | Withdrawal<br>Lack of interest in social contacts |
| | Cognitive | Alogia/poverty of speech |
| **Disorganized** | Speech | Formal thought disorder (e.g., tangentiality) |
| | Behavior | Purposeless movements or sequence of actions |

case of visual hallucinations and seizures in the case of olfactory hallucinations. However, note that hallucinations can occur in all sensory modalities in schizophrenia, including visual, olfactory, gustatory, and tactile (Goodwin et al. 1971).

## Delusions

The second core positive symptom is *delusions*, which are defined as fixed false beliefs. A belief is fixed when the individual cannot be dissuaded from believing in its veracity with contradictory evidence or arguments pointing out its implausibility. Another important feature of delusional thinking is the illogical manner in which a conviction is inferred. Delusions also may be vague or poorly formed, such as having a foreboding sense that others have ill intentions or are plotting, or may be highly crystallized, such as the specific examples given later in this subsection. The content of delusions also can be quite variable and may involve almost any subject. However, in general, delusions can be grouped into the following common types on the basis of their content: paranoid or persecutory, grandiose, religious, and somatic.

Paranoid or persecutory delusions are perhaps the single most common variety. They involve the conviction that individuals, institutions, or forces are intending the patient harm. The degree of harm can be quite variable—from simply being monitored to being ostracized or singled out for poor treatment to believing that death or torture is imminent.

*Grandiose delusions* refers to self-aggrandizing beliefs (e.g., that the patient has special powers or abilities), often but not necessarily of a bizarre or an unrealistic nature. Religious delusions involve religious themes or concepts such as being the son of God.

*Somatic delusions* refers to false beliefs about the patient's own body parts or internal organs. Somatic delusions also can include idiosyncratic beliefs about a body part's function. These false beliefs usually involve more than just subjective perceptions (e.g., certainty that one's nose is unattractive), such as specific convictions about the body part that is part of a more elaborate delusional system. Somatic delusions sometimes can tragically lead patients to commit grotesque self-injurious acts on the involved body part.

A special class of delusions, ideas of reference, deserves special attention because of its high prevalence and historical importance. Patients with ideas of reference misperceive communications from other persons or entities to be referring to them.

TABLE 17–2.    **DSM-IV-TR diagnostic criteria for schizophrenia**

A.  *Characteristic symptoms:* Two (or more) of the following, each present for a significant portion of time during a 1-month period (or less if successfully treated):

(1)  delusions

(2)  hallucinations

(3)  disorganized speech (e.g., frequent derailment or incoherence)

(4)  grossly disorganized or catatonic behavior

(5)  negative symptoms, i.e., affective flattening, alogia, or avolition

**Note:**   Only one Criterion A symptom is required if delusions are bizarre or hallucinations consist of a voice keeping up a running commentary on the person's behavior or thoughts, or two or more voices conversing with each other.

B.  *Social/occupational dysfunction:* For a significant portion of the time since the onset of the disturbance, one or more major areas of functioning such as work, interpersonal relations, or self-care are markedly below the level achieved prior to the onset (or when the onset is in childhood or adolescence, failure to achieve expected level of interpersonal, academic, or occupational achievement).

C.  *Duration:* Continuous signs of the disturbance persist for at least 6 months. This 6-month period must include at least 1 month of symptoms (or less if successfully treated) that meet Criterion A (i.e., active-phase symptoms) and may include periods of prodromal or residual symptoms. During these prodromal or residual periods, the signs of the disturbance may be manifested by only negative symptoms or two or more symptoms listed in Criterion A present in an attenuated form (e.g., odd beliefs, unusual perceptual experiences).

D.  *Schizoaffective and mood disorder exclusion:* Schizoaffective disorder and mood disorder with psychotic features have been ruled out because either (1) no major depressive, manic, or mixed episodes have occurred concurrently with the active-phase symptoms; or (2) if mood episodes have occurred during active-phase symptoms, their total duration has been brief relative to the duration of the active and residual periods.

E.  *Substance/general medical condition exclusion:* The disturbance is not due to the direct physiological effects of a substance (e.g., a drug of abuse, a medication) or a general medical condition.

F.  *Relationship to a pervasive developmental disorder:* If there is a history of autistic disorder or another pervasive developmental disorder, the additional diagnosis of schizophrenia is made only if prominent delusions or hallucinations are also present for at least 1 month (or less if successfully treated).

*Classification of longitudinal course* (can be applied only after at least 1 year has elapsed since the initial onset of active-phase symptoms):

**Episodic with interepisode residual symptoms** (episodes are defined by the reemergence of prominent psychotic symptoms); *also specify if:*   **With prominent negative symptoms**

**Episodic with no interepisode residual symptoms**

**Continuous** (prominent psychotic symptoms are present throughout the period of observation); *also specify if:*
**With prominent negative symptoms**

**Single episode in partial remission;** *also specify if:*   **With prominent negative symptoms**

**Single episode in full remission**

**Other or unspecified pattern**

# Negative Symptoms

The negative symptoms of schizophrenia refer to clinical features putatively resulting from the absence of normal mental functions. These include deficits in affective, so-cial, and cognitive realms. Although the positive symptoms have traditionally garnered more attention in the clinical assessment and treatment of schizophrenia, negative symptoms have been long recognized as a core feature of this disorder.

## Affective Deficits

One of the most apparent clinical manifestations of negative symptoms in patients with schizophrenia is the disturbance of normal affective processes. *Blunting of affect* is a term describing the decrease in the amount and range of affective expressivity. This term usually refers to facial expressions in which the normal expressions associated with emotional states are diminished or absent. Other related descriptors are *flat* and *constricted affect*, which are defined, respectively, as a total absence of, and a moderate decrease in, affective expressivity.

Another common affective deficit is apathy, or apparent indifference of the patient to the consequences of his or her own or others' actions and decisions. This can manifest as lack of motivation to initiate or maintain activity. For example, patients with apathy spend an inordinate amount of time at home alone, unable to initiate and engage in a planned activity. Another common manifestation of this deficit may be evident in the patient's lack of interest in events around him or her, such as the clinical interview.

## Social Deficits

Deficits in the domain of social functioning are increasingly recognized as important aspects of schizophrenia. *Social withdrawal* describes the common situation in which the patient has little interest in participating in social events and interacting with people. Patients often describe not needing to spend much time with other people and preferring to be by themselves. They appear to have decreased social drive in that they do not derive pleasure from social interactions that most people experience.

## Cognitive Deficits

*Alogia* or *poverty of speech* describes the significant decrease in the amount of unprompted speech given by a patient. Patients with poverty of speech give very short and unelaborated responses to questions. The interviewer often finds himself or herself having to guide the patient with numerous explicit questions to obtain responses with sufficient detail.

# Disorganization

The third symptom cluster is disorganization in language or other behavior. The phrase *formal thought disorder* has been defined in a variety of ways, but here we use a more restricted definition of this term, as in the disorganization of the form or flow of thoughts as evident in language output. Various terms can be used in the psychiatric mental status examination to describe formal thought disorder, including (in the order of increasing severity) *circumstantiality, derailment, tangentiality*, and *word salad*.

These terms attempt to capture the disruption of the normal processes that govern the logical, syntactic, or semantic ordering or association of words and ideas. *Circumstantiality* refers to the preservation of a logical link between each consecutive sentence concomitant with a progressive drifting of ideas away from the original topic. *Derailment* describes a process in which a patient's response is initially topical and logical but then becomes not obviously related. *Tangentiality* refers to the immediate loss of connection between the patient's response and the initial question. Finally, *word salad* describes the highly remarkable phenomenon characterized by a complete absence of a logical link between adjacent words in an utterance. Other common manifestations of formal thought disorder are distractibility, echolalia, clang associations, perseverations, blocking, and neologisms.

# Cognitive Impairment

As a group, patients with schizophrenia show a range of impaired higher cognitive functions, including problems with attention, long-term memory, working memory, abstraction and planning, and language comprehension and production. These cognitive deficits present significant barriers to maintaining occupational and everyday function. Research has shown that cognitive deficits may be the best predictor of functionality, over and above other symptom clusters (Green 1996).

One of the most clinically apparent cognitive deficits is in the domain of attention. In addition to the internal preoccupation and preoccupation associated with hallucinatory and delusional experiences, an individual with schizophrenia experiences difficulty maintaining focused attention on relevant tasks or events. Attentional problems also may manifest in patients as an inability to shift their focus of attention in an appropriate manner, expressed clinically as *perseveration*.

Working memory, the ability to store and manage information temporarily to rapidly guide thoughts and behavior, has been proposed as a fundamental cognitive deficit in schizophrenia. These theories suggest that many of the clinical features of schizophrenia are manifestations of working memory deficits. For example, thought disorder can be conceived of as the inability to maintain a linguistic goal in mind. Problems with multitasking, distractibility, and planning also may involve working memory problems.

Long-term declarative memory deficits have been noted to be an important source of disability in schizophrenia. Although memory problems may not be progressive or as profound as in Alzheimer's dementia, they are nonetheless readily apparent. Common and clinically relevant manifestations of this impairment include forgotten appointments or medication directions, which may directly affect the treatment and stability of the patient.

# Soft Neurological Signs

Interestingly, before the age of pharmacological treatments, early schizophrenia researchers noted a heightened prevalence of neurological abnormalities, particularly movement disturbances, in individuals who later developed schizophrenia. In modern research, substantial and growing evidence now indicates a higher prevalence of subtle neurological deficits—most notably, the so-called soft neurological signs (e.g., motor dyscoordination)—in patients with schizophrenia (Bombin et al. 2005).

# Subtypes of Schizophrenia

Table 17–3 lists the various subtypes of schizophrenia.

## Paranoid Schizophrenia

The hallmark of paranoid schizophrenia is the relative prominence of paranoid delusions and auditory hallucinations compared with the other symptoms of schizophrenia. Most important is that the presence of disorganized behavior or speech, catatonia, or flat or inappropriate affect precludes this diagnosis. This subtype has received perhaps the most validation in research, which has suggested that these patients have better premorbid functioning, an older age at onset, higher social and occupational functioning after illness onset, and fewer cognitive and affective deficits.

## Disorganized Schizophrenia

According to DSM-IV-TR, all of the following must be prominent to diagnose this subtype: disorganized speech,

| TABLE 17–3. | DSM-IV-TR subtypes of schizophrenia |
| --- | --- |
| **Paranoid** | Prominent hallucinations and delusions |
| | Absence of prominent disorganization, flat or inappropriate affect, or catatonia |
| **Disorganized** | All of the following: |
| | disorganized speech |
| | disorganized behavior |
| | flat or inappropriate affect |
| | Diagnostic criteria for catatonic schizophrenia should not be met |
| **Catatonic** | Catatonia is the most prominent clinical feature |
| | At least two of the following: |
| | immobility (cataplexy or stupor) |
| | motor hyperactivity without purpose or external influence |
| | extreme negativism or mutism |
| | peculiar voluntary movement or postures |
| | stereotyped movements or prominent mannerisms or grimacing |
| | echophenomena (echolalia or echopraxia) |
| **Undifferentiated** | Criterion A for schizophrenia |
| | Diagnostic criteria for the paranoid, disorganized, or catatonic subtypes are not met |
| **Residual** | Persistence of negative symptoms or two or more Criterion A symptoms in attenuated form |
| | Absence of prominent delusions, hallucinations, disorganized speech, and grossly disorganized or catatonic behavior |

disorganized behavior, and flat or inappropriate affect. Additionally, diagnostic criteria for catatonic schizophrenia should not be met. This subtype is thought to represent a more severe form of schizophrenia, with earlier onset, low levels of social and occupational functioning, and poor long-term prognosis. The presence of delusions or hallucinations does not exclude the diagnosis of this subtype, but these symptoms play a less prominent role in psychopathology. The older term *hebephrenic schizophrenia* is synonymous with the disorganized subtype.

## Catatonic Schizophrenia

The term *catatonia* refers to extreme motor states of either stupor or overexcitement that can occur independently of schizophrenia. In catatonic stupor, the patient maintains one body position for a very long time without talking or reacting to others. In this state, some patients may have waxy flexibility, in which a limb or body part is maintained in a posture that is passively positioned by another individual. In catatonic excitement, the patient engages in a series of apparently aimless and exaggerated rapid movements, which also may include acts of minimally directed violent behavior. Note that many clinicians have recognized a significant decrease in the prevalence of catatonic states in recent years such that it is now relatively rare to find classic cases of catatonia. The diagnosis of catatonic schizophrenia is made when catatonia is the most prominent clinical feature, and requires the presence of at least two of the following: immobility (cataplexy or stupor); motor hyperactivity without purpose or external influence; extreme negativism or mutism; peculiar voluntary movement or postures, stereotyped movements, or prominent mannerisms or grimacing; and echophenomena (echolalia or echopraxia).

## Undifferentiated Schizophrenia

Undifferentiated schizophrenia encompasses cases in which no one cluster of symptoms constituting the paranoid, disorganized, or catatonic subtypes predominates the clinical picture.

## Residual Schizophrenia

The residual subtype is thought to represent a relatively attenuated state of schizophrenia in which the positive symptoms are relatively quiescent or less symptomatic. Like undifferentiated schizophrenia, this is a subtype diagnosis made by exclusion. The diagnosis is made when negative symptoms persist or two or more symptoms listed in DSM-IV-TR Criterion A for schizophrenia (see Table 17-2) are present in an attenuated form, and prominent delusions, hallucinations, disorganized speech, and grossly disorganized or catatonic behavior are absent. Many patients achieve this relatively remitted clinical subtype after sustained effective treatment.

## Diagnosis

In DSM-IV-TR, the diagnostic manual currently in use in the United States, the emphasis on both cross-sectional and longitudinal criteria continues (see Table 17-2), with a 6-month minimum duration. However, clinical courses that are episodic in manner, including single-episode cases that are followed by full remission, are now recognized. The positive symptom criteria reflect the influence of Schneider's first-rank symptoms as exemplars. The negative and disorganized symptom criteria reflect a renewed prominence given to features originally emphasized by Bleuler. The DSM-IV-TR criteria identify an individual as having schizophrenia if he or she experiences characteristic positive, negative, and/or disorganized symptoms for a significant portion of time during at least 1 month, unless the symptoms are successfully treated; these Criterion A symptoms are referred to as *active-phase symptoms*. The patient must have impairment in psychosocial function (work, interpersonal relationships, or self-care). Continuous signs of disturbance must be evident for at least 6 months; this must include at least 1 month of active-phase symptoms but may include periods of prodromal or residual symptoms, which appear as attenuated Criterion A symptoms. The longitudinal course is classified as episodic, continuous, or single episode, with remission, residual symptoms, and prominent negative symptoms further specified. In addition, subtypes are specified as outlined in the "Subtypes of Schizophrenia" section earlier in this chapter.

## Differential Diagnosis

The diagnosis of schizophrenia continues to rest solely on the history of illness and a thorough mental status examination (Table 17-4). Along with the history taking and mental status examination, a full physical examination usually should be performed, particularly for new-onset cases, because medical causes of psychotic illness are varied. This list includes intracranial processes such as infections and neoplastic, epileptic, and hypoxic or ischemic disorders; metabolic disorders; and endocrine disorders. The dementias, such as Alzheimer's disease, frontotemporal dementia, Parkinson's disease, Pick's disease, and Huntington's disease, are often associated with psychotic features. Illicit substance use is also quite common in the community and can frequently lead to psychotic symptoms, not only with acute intoxication but also in an intermittent or even a persistent manner with chronic use,

**TABLE 17–4.** Differential diagnosis of schizophrenia

| Other disorders | Common clinical features | Distinctions from schizophrenia |
|---|---|---|
| **Axis I diagnoses** | | |
| Schizoaffective disorder | Criterion A for schizophrenia, plus at least one lifetime major mood episode (unipolar and bipolar types) | On average, higher function but higher suicide risk; history of major mood episode not found in schizophrenia |
| Mood disorders with psychosis | Multiple symptoms of mood changes, vegetative symptoms, mood-congruent ideation, and other cognitive changes, with acute or subacute onset and often in response to psychosocial stressors | Mood symptoms are more enduring; more complete interepisodic recovery; psychosis only with severe mood episodes; fuller response to psychotherapy |
| Delusional disorder | Prominent delusions, with other cognitions and behavior organized around delusion but no other significant psychosis | Psychosis confined to one or more delusions, usually nonbizarre; function largely intact; minimal decline in function or change in symptoms over time; more refractory to treatment |
| Schizophreniform disorder | Duration of Criterion A met for more than 1 month but less than 6 months | Shorter duration than schizophrenia; many ultimately receive schizophrenia diagnosis |
| Brief psychotic disorder | Psychosis with abrupt onset and duration less than 1 month; often in response to acute stressor | No prodrome; cognition generally intact; better prognosis |
| Drug-related psychosis | Significant history of drug use, with abuse and often dependence criteria met; associated cyclic impulsivity and interpersonal, occupational, and legal history | Psychosis typically during active periods of drug use, particularly psychostimulants; more complete recovery with sustained abstinence; characteristic medical comorbidity with chronic abuse |
| **Axis II (personality) disorders** | | |
| Cluster A: schizotypal, paranoid, schizoid personality disorders | Subpsychotic (positive and/or negative) symptoms with mild to moderate cognitive and social impairment | Less functional decline than schizophrenia; cognition more intact, and rare impulsivity or need for hospitalization |
| Cluster B: borderline personality disorder | Instability in mood, impulse control, and interpersonal relationships | Less functional decline than schizophrenia; symptoms more sensitive to interpersonal factors; more unstable over time; psychosis only with significant stress |
| **Axis III (medical) disorders** | | |
| Dementias (cortical and subcortical) | Slow onset in middle to late adulthood, with progressive cognitive decline; some with prominent motor symptoms | Later onset; cognitive deficits more prominent compared with other symptoms; psychosis primarily in late stages |

**TABLE 17–4.    Differential diagnosis of schizophrenia _(continued)_**

| Other disorders | Common clinical features | Distinctions from schizophrenia |
|---|---|---|
| **Axis III (medical) disorders _(continued)_** | | |
| Acute confusional states (delirium; varied etiologies) | Abrupt onset with risk factors for neurological illness; clouded sensorium; transient psychosis can be in various sensory modes | Premorbid function intact; acute onset; psychotic symptoms less formed; full recovery possible with medical treatment |
| Iatrogenic psychosis (e.g., steroids, antibiotics, anticholinergics, antiparkinsonian medications) | Acute onset; transient psychosis can be in various sensory modes | Stable premorbid function; acute onset; psychotic symptoms less formed; associated somatic effects of medications; full recovery possible with medical treatment |

particularly with stimulant drugs. Many commonly prescribed medications can also cause psychosis, particularly those with direct effects on the brain, such as steroids, anticholinergics, and medications prescribed for Parkinson's disease. Those cases that present with atypical clinical features, such as late age at onset, clouding of the sensorium (i.e., confusional states), or findings on history or physical examination suggestive of concurrent medical problems, should prompt the clinician to pursue alternative causes of illness. Routine laboratory tests that may aid the clinician in ruling out these etiologies include a complete blood count, renal and metabolic panels, liver enzymes, thyroid function, urinalysis, and serological tests for syphilis and HIV. Brain imaging such as magnetic resonance imaging (MRI) or computed tomography (CT) and electroencephalography may be indicated in atypical cases or when the history suggests the need to rule out intracranial pathology unrelated to psychiatric illness.

Although care should be taken to rule out medical causes of psychosis confidently, the major task in differential diagnosis is distinguishing schizophrenia from a range of other psychiatric disorders that also may involve psychotic symptoms. These conditions include schizoaffective disorder; major mood disorders that can present with psychotic features, such as major depression and acute mania among bipolar affective disorder type I patients; delusional disorder; and personality disorders, particularly those in the A or B clusters. To rule out the major mood disorders or schizoaffective disorder, the active phase of psychosis should occur in the absence of an acute mood disorder episode, or alternatively, the mood episodes should be relatively brief in relation to the total duration of the psychotic episode. Most mood disorder patients also maintain or recover significant levels of psychosocial

function in between episodes of illness because they do not experience continuous psychotic symptoms or persistently severe mood disturbance. Delusional disorder is distinguished by the lack of other psychotic symptoms, and the content of delusions tends not to be the bizarre thoughts or beliefs often observed in schizophrenia, such as beliefs that monitoring devices are implanted in the patient's body or that the patient is communicating with other species. Individuals with this disorder also tend to maintain a higher level of function because they largely experience only the circumscribed delusions that meet the criteria for the disorder. Schizophreniform disorder and brief psychotic disorder are also characterized by overt psychotic symptoms. In some cases, a clinician may encounter the patient relatively early in the active psychotic phase of illness, and as a result, one of these diagnoses (both with a briefer duration criterion than that for schizophrenia) is most appropriate to assign initially. However, if psychotic symptoms persist beyond 6 months, then the diagnosis of schizophrenia is most appropriate. It remains to be determined what percentage of individuals with schizophreniform disorder represent patients early in the course of schizophrenia (see section "Related Psychotic Disorders" later in this chapter for discussion of schizoaffective disorder, delusional disorder, schizophreniform disorder, and brief psychotic disorder).

Cluster A ("odd") personality disorders (i.e., schizoid, schizotypal, and paranoid) are often referred to as _schizophrenia spectrum disorders_ and may be characterized by subthreshold or attenuated psychotic symptoms related to those of schizophrenia. Patients with these personality disorders may show symptoms of social withdrawal, anhedonia, and flat affect quite similar to, but more mild than, the negative symptoms of schizophrenia. However, overt psychotic symptoms are rare (and transient) in these individuals, and their level of function is typically higher, with gainful employment and independent living being the norm. Borderline personality disorder may present with acute, overt psychotic symptoms; however, in this personality disorder, in contrast to schizophrenia, interpersonal stressors are common precipitants of acute psychosis, emotional dysregulation (with lability, multiple negative mood states, and overt antagonism) is nearly ubiquitous, and behavioral impulsivity is present, often including dangerous or hazardous acts such as self-injury and aggressive behavior. Other disorders such as depersonalization disorder, panic disorder, and obsessive-compulsive disorder may present with feelings of unreality or bizarre behavior; however, in each of these disorders, reality testing and social function are preserved, and overt delusions or hallucinations are rare. Finally, factitious disorder and malingering can be found in many clinical settings; the degree to which the clinical picture diverges from well-established profiles found in schizophrenia, along with the identification of secondary gains (e.g., material reward or avoidance of incarceration) attainable as a result of a psychiatric diagnosis or treatment, may call attention to the possibility of these last diagnoses.

# Clinical Course

## Premorbid Functioning

Any description of the clinical course of schizophrenia should address periods of development occurring well before the onset of overt psychotic symptoms, especially given the neurodevelopmental perspective on this illness.

## Prodrome to Schizophrenia

During adolescence, however, those who later develop schizophrenia often begin to undergo changes that are discernible to others, with the onset of significant behavioral and other overt psychiatric symptoms. These include symptoms of depression, social withdrawal, irritability, and antagonistic thoughts and behavior. In this period, these adolescents often come to the attention of school and community clinicians for conduct problems and academic decline. These symptoms may be retrospectively identified as heralding the onset of the so-called prodrome of schizophrenia, a period of variable duration (usually lasting from several months to a few years) that precedes the onset of schizophrenia in most

cases (Phillips et al. 2005). Several clinical signs that can be observed during this period have a high positive predictive value for the later onset of schizophrenia. These symptoms may include suspiciousness or perceptual distortions that do not qualify as overtly psychotic. Reality testing is often intact at this stage because many individuals will doubt the veracity of these experiences. Many of these individuals, in adolescence or early adulthood, will at this clinical stage qualify for the diagnosis of schizotypal personality disorder.

## Early Period of Psychotic Illness in Schizophrenia

The onset of psychosis can be insidious or abrupt, and those who experience a rapid onset tend to have a more favorable prognosis. This active phase of initial psychotic symptoms is often referred to informally as the *first break*. Patients during this phase will experience florid symptoms of hallucinations, delusions, and occasionally disorganized thought and behavior and agitation. At this point, the distress experienced by the patient, family, or both often increases dramatically, prompting entry into treatment. Less often, the patient comes to the attention of the mental health system for involuntary evaluation, as the result of public disturbances or behaviors that are dangerous to the self or others. As treatment for first-episode psychosis proceeds, overt psychotic symptoms commonly abate in the days to few months thereafter. Ample evidence indicates that those patients who experience significant treatment delays have a worse prognosis, even when illness severity at presentation is taken into account.

Longitudinal studies of first-episode psychosis leading to a schizophrenia diagnosis find considerable heterogeneity at follow-up. One review found that approximately one-third of these patients (across 13 prospective studies) experienced a benign course, in contrast to the two-thirds who relapsed, failed to recover, or were rehospitalized, in the first 2 years after a first hospitalization for psychosis (Ram et al. 1992). More recent, longer-term prospective follow-up studies have found considerable heterogeneity in clinical (Bromet and Fennig 1999) and functional status among these patients; significant numbers achieve adequate social and occupational function and quality of life in the several years after onset of psychosis, whereas others experience a decline in these measures (Malla and Payne 2005). For patients who do receive adequate treatment, a *residual phase* follows, during which the range and severity of symptoms can be quite similar to those seen in the prodrome. Psychotic symptoms may persist during this period, although with less intensity and less attendant distress. Over time, most patients will experience a series of acute exacerbations of symptoms occurring episodically as they go into and out of active-phase psychosis. These episodes are often precipitated by environmental stressors, substance abuse, or treatment discontinuation. The degree of remission between these episodes may vary, and there is a tendency in the early phase (the first 5–10 years after onset) of the overt illness for patients to progressively fail to attain the level of function observed prior to each episode (Lieberman et al. 2001). The chronology, number of acute episodes, and rate of decline during this period do vary considerably among patients. Following this period, however, patients appear to attain a measure of stability in the severity of symptoms, rate of relapse, treatment responsivity, and general level of function.

## Long-Term Outcome

Several studies have now been reported in which patients with schizophrenia were identified with contemporary diagnostic criteria and follow-up was obtained over at least 10 years (Jobe and Harrow 2005). The Iowa 500 study followed up 500 psychiatric patients admitted to the Iowa State Psychiatric Hospital between 1934 and 1944 and used the Feighner criteria to identify schizophrenia patients, of whom 200 were followed up an average of 35 years from the index hospitalization (Tsuang and Winokur 1975). In this study, the patients with schizophrenia were observed to have poorer outcome on all measures, relative to other psychiatric patients and nonpsychiatric surgical patients: 54% had incapacitating symptoms, 67% had never married, 18% were living in institutions, and more than 10% had committed suicide (Tsuang and Winokur 1975). The Chestnut Lodge study followed up 532 patients discharged from this private hospital between 1950 and 1975, for an average of 15 years. Patients were diagnosed by less restrictive DSM-III (American Psychiatric Association 1980) criteria, yet the findings were broadly similar to those of the Iowa 500. The 163 schizophrenia patients as a group had the following outcomes: 6% recovered, 8% good, 22% moderate, 23% marginal, and 41% continuously incapacitated (McGlashan 1984). A study conducted at the New York State Psychiatric Institute included 552 patients who underwent treatment with psychoanalytically oriented psychotherapy, of whom 99 met DSM-III criteria for schizophrenia. With follow-up between 10 and 23 years, the patients with schizophrenia showed poorer outcome compared with other psychiatric patients, had an average DSM Global Assessment of Functioning score of 39, and had a completed suicide rate of 10% (Stone 1986).

Although these studies largely emphasized the relatively poor prognosis of most patients with schizophrenia, other follow-up studies identified subgroups with better outcomes. These studies include Vaillant's study in Boston, Massachusetts, in which the patients identified as completely remitted from an earlier study were then followed up prospectively for 4–16 years. He found that 61% of these patients remained in remission. A study in Edmonton, Alberta, Canada, found that 58% of 92 patients with DSM-II (American Psychiatric Association 1968) schizophrenia experienced full recovery, despite 45% of the full sample having discontinued their psychiatric medication in the 10 months after the index hospitalization. When this same sample was narrowed by using stricter Feighner diagnostic criteria, the percentage of those considered fully recovered was halved (Bland et al. 1978).

Only two long-term follow-up studies were fully prospective in design. The Chicago Follow-Up Study included 73 schizophrenia patients followed up to 20 years. This study found that patients with schizophrenia generally fluctuated between moderate and severe disability, but more than 40% showed periods of recovery that often lasted for several years (Harrow and Jobe 2005). Some of these patients were able to function without the benefit of continuous antipsychotic treatment and had tended to have better premorbid function. In addition, a large percentage of the full sample of schizophrenia patients (65%) also had experienced at least one depressive syndrome at 20-year follow-up; the completed suicide rate was 10% at 10 years and higher than 12% at 20 years. The other long-term prospective study of schizophrenia patients, conducted by Carpenter and Strauss (1991), followed up 55 DSM-III-identified schizophrenia patients for 11 years and found no change in their relatively poorer outcome status at 5 and 10 years.

## Etiology and Pathophysiology

Modern psychiatric research has produced an abundance of evidence supporting the notion that schizophrenia is a disorder primarily related to brain dysfunction. Consequently, the term *functional brain disorder*, which was once commonly used to distinguish schizophrenia and other psychiatric conditions from structurally evident brain disorders found in neurological conditions, has become antiquated.

## Genetics

That schizophrenia has a strong genetic component is a readily accepted notion (see Chapter 4 in this volume, "Genetics," by Choudary and Knowles). The degree of risk is proportional to the degree of shared genes (Gottesman 1991). A review of twin studies showed concordance rates between 25% and 50% (Gottesman 1991). Adoption studies showed an elevated risk for schizophrenia among the offspring of mothers with schizophrenia (Kety et al. 1971).

The exact manner in which schizophrenia is heritable and the identity of the specific genes that may give rise to schizophrenia, however, remain topics of significant debate and uncertainty. It is very evident that schizophrenia does not follow simple Mendelian principles of inheritance (McGue and Gottesman 1989). Complex diseases involve several genes, each with a modest effect on heritability, acting in concert, in either a linear or a synergistic manner, to confer an overall disease risk (Risch 1990). Additional complexity may arise from partial penetrance of these genes, interactions between genes, and epigenetic neurodevelopmental or environmental factors.

The potential complexity of genetic and nongenetic factors in schizophrenia is illustrated by twin adoption studies. Several have been published, and on the whole, they have been remarkably consistent in reporting approximately 50% concordance rate for monozygotic twins. This result accentuates the importance of both the genetic and the nongenetic factors in conferring disease risk.

In the past 10 years, with the development of novel study designs and high throughput methods, we have witnessed a tremendous proliferation in the number of putative schizophrenia risk genes. An interesting aspect of this list is that many of these genes are related to neurodevelopmental processes involved in the establishment of neural networks (e.g., neuronal migration and synapse formation or the regulation of synaptic transmission).

## Environmental Factors

The idea that fetal neural development represents an especially vulnerable period for the genesis of schizophrenia is supported by observations of higher incidence of obstetric and perinatal complications in patients with schizophrenia in several studies. A recent meta-analytic review categorized these events as 1) complications of pregnancy, 2) abnormal fetal growth and development, and 3) complications of delivery (Cannon et al. 2002).

The Dutch Famine study examined the prevalence of schizophrenia among a cohort of births that occurred during the winter of 1944–1945, a period of severe malnutrition for most citizens in a region of the Netherlands (Susser et al. 1996). The study showed a twofold increased risk for schizophrenia associated with extreme prenatal malnutrition.

Seasonal variation in the prevalence of births leading to schizophrenia has been identified, with an excess of births in winter and spring months (Davies et al. 2003).

## Neurochemical Factors

### Dopamine

The serendipitous discovery of the usefulness of chlorpromazine in schizophrenia led ultimately to the development of the dopamine hypothesis, one of the most influential theories on the etiology of schizophrenia. It posits that the symptoms of this illness are the by-products of dysfunction of dopamine neurotransmission. Carlsson and Lindqvist (1963) determined that the administration of phenothiazines in animals blocks the behavioral effects of dopamine agonists (such as amphetamine) and results in increased turnover of dopamine. Conversely, the administration of amphetamine, which was known to increase synaptic levels of dopamine, resulted in behavioral abnormalities and symptoms reminiscent of schizophrenia. Later work further specified that the most important dopamine receptor may be the $D_2$ subtype in that clinical potency is best correlated with binding to this receptor subtype (Creese et al. 1976).

The challenge to the dopamine hypothesis comes from primarily two lines of evidence. First, the dopamine hypothesis does not account for negative symptoms, which are now acknowledged to be essential components of this illness. Dopamine-blocking agents have not been shown to be effective in treating negative symptoms, nor have dopaminergic agents been shown to induce negative symptoms. The second challenge to the dopamine hypothesis comes from the efficacy of the so-called atypical antipsychotics, medications that are thought to act through multiple neurotransmitter systems, with dopamine being only one of the monoamines involved).

### Other Monoamines

The observations that the prototypical atypical neuroleptic—clozapine—is often effective in patients who have symptoms refractory to the traditional $D_2$ receptor-blocking agents and has high affinity for diverse monoaminergic receptors, including serotonergic, histaminergic, muscarinic, and $\alpha$-adrenergic receptors, in addition to the $D_2$ receptor, have led to the hypothesis that other neurotransmitter systems may be involved in the pathophysiology of schizophrenia. One of the most important of these other neurotransmitters is serotonin. Serotonin has been implicated by the clinical efficacy of the many atypical agents with high affinity for its receptors. There are 14 known serotonin receptor subtypes, but some of the most important for schizophrenia include the $5\text{-HT}_{2C}$, $5\text{-HT}_{2A}$, and $5\text{-HT}_{1A}$ subtypes.

The acetylcholine system was implicated in the pathophysiology of schizophrenia initially on the basis of the observation that patients with schizophrenia have high rates of use of tobacco products. This led to the hypothesis that the nicotine in tobacco provides some amelioration of symptoms through its action on the acetylcholine system. This hypothesis has received some support by work examining the effects of nicotine on early sensory deficits that were well documented in schizophrenia; nicotine normalized measures of deficient auditory gating in schizophrenia (Adler et al. 1992).

### *Glutamate and* N-*Methyl-*D-*Aspartate*

Glutamate is the most prevalent excitatory neurotransmitter in the brain. The involvement of the glutamate system in the pathophysiology of schizophrenia is inferred primarily from the observation that people intoxicated with agents acting on the glutamate receptor, such as phencyclidine (PCP) and ketamine, often have a behavioral syndrome mimicking schizophrenia. Interestingly, this syndrome can include both positive and negative symptoms of schizophrenia (Javitt and Zukin 1991). PCP and ketamine bind to the N-methyl-D-aspartate (NMDA) class of glutamate receptors, and consequently the main focus of glutamate research has been on this receptor. NMDA receptor regulation is highly complex, with numerous sites of allosteric modulation. One of the most important in terms of psychopathology appears to be the glycine site. Several clinical trials have examined partial (D-cycloserine) and full (glycine, D-serine, and D-alanine) agonists of this site. The pharmacodynamics of cycloserine with the NMDA receptor are complex, with cycloserine acting as an agonist at low and an antagonist at high concentrations.

### *Gamma-Aminobutyric Acid*

The potential role for $\gamma$-aminobutyric acid (GABA) in the pathophysiology of schizophrenia follows two separate but related lines of research involving inhibitory interneurons. In the first line of research, the psychotomimetic effects of NMDA antagonists, such as PCP, are thought to be mediated through their action on GABA release. NMDA receptors are found on GABAergic inhibitory interneurons. Activation of these NMDA receptors results in increased GABA release, which then causes suppression of glutamate release from glutamatergic cells. The binding of an antagonist on the NMDA receptor on the inhibitory neurons ultimately results in a hyperglutamatergic state, which is presumed to cause symptoms of psychosis.

In the second line of research, alterations in the neural circuitry of the prefrontal cortex, involving GABA, are thought to give rise to the higher-order cognitive deficits in schizophrenia. Theories on GABA dysfunction in schizophrenia center on the parvalbumin-containing group of inhibitory interneurons. Studies showing a reduction in the number of parvalbumin cells and underexpression of glutamic acid decarboxylase, a key enzyme in GABA synthesis (Akbarian et al. 1995; Volk et al. 2000), point to a functional deficit in GABA in the prefrontal cortex.

## Anatomical and Histological Studies

The study of structural abnormalities in the brains of individuals with schizophrenia was once considered a "graveyard" for neuropathologists. The emergence of modern neuroimaging and molecular techniques has led to a renewed interest in this field. Neuroimaging studies have shown consistent evidence of whole-brain volume deficits, and modern neuropathology studies have uncovered provocative clues pointing to alterations in the microscopic neuroanatomy in schizophrenia.

CT studies documenting significant enlargement of cerebral ventricles and decreases in overall brain volume in subjects with schizophrenia (relative to healthy control subjects) have provided the first compelling neuroimaging results indicating that schizophrenia is a brain-based disorder (Johnstone et al. 1976). These results remain the most reliable and consistent volumetric findings in schizophrenia, with a median reduction in ventricular volume estimated to be 40% (Lawrie and Abukmeil 1998). More recent MRI volumetric studies have confirmed the results of these earlier CT studies. They also have identified several specific regions of decreased volume, including the prefrontal and medial temporal structures and lateral temporal cortex and thalamus (Harrison 1999). A recent meta-analysis of MRI studies involving first-episode subjects showed highly significant reductions in total brain volume and increased ventricular volume (Steen et al. 2006), suggesting that these findings are not just the result of disease chronicity or medication exposure.

## Cognitive and Information Processing Deficits

Emil Kraepelin referred to schizophrenia as *dementia praecox*, or premature dementia, to describe the prominent cognitive deficits that he thought formed the core of this condition. The interest in cognition waned in the intervening years as other aspects of the illness became the focal point of research interest. However, in the last 20 years, there has been renewed interest in studying cognitive dysfunction in schizophrenia as a way to understand its pathophysiology.

Dysfunction in higher-order cognitive processes has now been firmly established; however, another line of research is investigating the hypothesis that deficits in early sensory processing are a fundamental aspect of schizophrenia. Some have proposed that these early sensory deficits may contribute to higher-order cognitive deficits and have significant effects on the functional status of the affected individuals (Brenner et al. 2002; Javitt et al. 1997; Saccuzzo and Braff 1981).

## Affect Processing

With the recognition of the importance of negative symptoms in schizophrenia, increasing attention is being paid to the study of affect and related processes in schizophrenia. In the last 10 years, we have witnessed an exponential increase in the number of studies focusing on this aspect of the illness. These affect studies can be further categorized as those focusing on emotional expression, recognition of emotional signals, and the subjective experiencing of emotions.

## Social Cognition

A strong argument can be made that the social deficits of schizophrenia constitute a core feature of this illness because abnormalities in social functions often occur during the prodromal phase (Davidson et al. 1999), at the time of initial diagnosis, and throughout the course of illness (Addington and Addington 2000).

Studies on social cognition have identified two general areas of abnormality in schizophrenia: theory of mind and social perceptions (Pinkham et al. 2003). *Theory of mind* refers to the capacity to 1) understand that the mental state (beliefs, intentions, and perspectives) of others is separate and distinct from one's own and 2) make inferences about another's intentions.

Studies have shown that patients with schizophrenia lack theory of mind skills (Corcoran et al. 1995; Frith and Corcoran 1996). *Social perception*, the ability to recognize information governing appropriate social behavior, also consistently has been shown to be abnormal in schizophrenia. It is thought that deficits in affect recognition are the cause of patients' inability to decode the emotional state of others.

# Intervention and Management

## Antipsychotic Medications

### Mechanism of Action

First-generation antipsychotics (typified by haloperidol) all have in common a high affinity for $D_2$ receptors, and the clinical efficacy of these medications is strongly related to binding affinity for these receptors (Seeman et al. 1976). Studies in which positron emission tomography was used found that clinical antipsychotic effects occurred at doses at which striatal $D_2$ receptor occupancy was 65%–70%, whereas $D_2$ receptor occupancy greater than 80% was associated with a significantly increased incidence of extrapyramidal side effects (EPS) (Remington and Kapur 1999). These studies also have found that at therapeutic doses, first-generation antipsychotics block $D_2$-like receptors to an equal degree in limbic cortical areas and the striatum, which is also consistent with the relatively narrow range of antipsychotic efficacy in the absence of EPS (Xiberas et al. 2001).

In contrast, the six second-generation antipsychotics that are currently available in the United States are more heterogeneous in their profile of dopamine receptor antagonism. Risperidone, for example, has $D_2$ antagonism that is within the range of that for first-generation antipsychotics and, consequently, at therapeutic doses is associated with rates of EPS intermediate between first-generation antipsychotics and other second-generation antipsychotics. Other second-generation antipsychotics, such as clozapine and quetiapine, show minimal $D_2$ receptor binding at therapeutic doses (Miyamoto et al. 2005). These medications (including the other available second-generation antipsychotics olanzapine, ziprasidone, and aripiprazole) show very heterogeneous profiles of binding at other dopamine receptors.

**TABLE 17–5.    Relative neurotransmitter receptor affinities for antipsychotics at therapeutic doses**

| Receptor | Clozapine | Risperidone | Olanzapine | Quetiapine | Ziprasidone | Sertindole | Sulpiride | Amisulpride | Zotepine | Aripiprazole | Haloperidol |
|---|---|---|---|---|---|---|---|---|---|---|---|
| $D_1$ | + | + | ++ | − | + | ++ | − | − | + | − | + |
| $D_2$ | + | +++ | ++ | + | +++ | +++ | ++++ | ++++ | ++ | ++++ | ++++ |
| $D_3$ | + | ++ | + | − | ++ | ++ | ++ | ++ | ++ | ++ | +++ |
| $D_4$ | ++ | − | ++ | − | ++ | + | − | − | + | + | +++ |
| $5\text{-}HT_{1A}$ | − | − | − | − | +++ | | | | ++ | ++ | − |
| $5\text{-}HT_{1D}$ | − | + | − | − | +++ | | | | | + | − |
| $5\text{-}HT_{2A}$ | +++ | ++++ | +++ | ++ | ++++ | ++++ | − | − | +++ | +++ | + |
| $5\text{-}HT_{2C}$ | ++ | ++ | ++ | − | ++++ | ++ | − | − | ++ | + | |
| $5\text{-}HT_6$ | ++ | − | ++ | − | + | | | | ++ | + | − |
| $5\text{-}HT_7$ | ++ | +++ | − | − | ++ | | | | ++ | ++ | − |
| $\alpha_1$ | +++ | +++ | ++ | +++ | ++ | ++ | − | − | ++ | + | +++ |
| $\alpha_2$ | + | ++ | + | − | − | + | − | − | ++ | + | |
| $H_1$ | +++ | − | +++ | ++ | − | + | − | − | ++ | + | − |
| $M_1$ | ++++ | − | +++ | ++ | − | − | − | − | + | − | − |
| DA transporter | ++ | | ++ | | | | | | | − | |
| NA transporter | + | | ++ | | ++ | | | | ++ | − | |
| 5-HT transporter | | | | | ++ | | | | | − | |

*Note.*    −=weak; +=moderate; ++=good; +++=strong; ++++=shown by meta-analysis. DA=dopamine; NA=noradrenaline.
*Source.*    Adapted from Miyamoto et al. 2005.

A leading current hypothesis (the "fast-off" hypothesis) suggests that the relative lack of EPS stemming from the use of these medications may be a result of the relatively faster rate of dissociation of these agents from $D_2$ receptors. In contrast, a competing hypothesis of what constitutes "atypicality" emphasizes the serotonergic receptor activity ($5\text{-}HT_{2A}$ and $5\text{-}HT_{2C}$ antagonism and $5\text{-}HT_{1A}$ agonism) that is found among second-generation antipsychotics. These actions are associated with enhanced dopamine and glutamate in prefrontal relative to subcortical areas, and in particular, the ratio of $5\text{-}HT_{2A}$ to $D_2$ blockade may prevent EPS and remediate negative symptoms of schizophrenia in a manner superior to the first-generation antipsychotics (Meltzer et al. 2003). In addition, aripiprazole is unique as a $D_2$ partial agonist, which may stabilize elevated rates of dopamine transmission while avoiding a degree of dopamine blockade necessary for EPS.

It also should be emphasized here that all antipsychotics (first- and second-generation antipsychotics) have high-affinity binding at a range of other monoamine receptors in the brain, which may be partly responsible for their efficacy but is well established as the basis for many of their side effects. This includes antagonism at muscarinic, histaminergic, and α-adrenergic receptors, with predictable autonomic effects. In addition, the monoaminergic transporter–blocking effects and $5\text{-}HT_{1A}$ receptor partial agonism or antagonism shown by some second-generation antipsychotics suggest that these medications may exert antidepressant and anxiolytic effects as well (Table 17–5).

## Clinical Comparison of Second-Generation Antipsychotics With First-Generation Antipsychotics

Second-generation antipsychotics appear to have efficacy in treatment of positive symptoms that is comparable to that of first-generation antipsychotics (Miyamoto et al.

2005). However, they are consistently superior to first-generation antipsychotics (and placebo) in the treatment of negative symptoms. In addition, results from the recent Clinical Antipsychotic Trials of Intervention Effectiveness (CATIE) suggested that olanzapine in particular may be more effective than perphenazine (an intermediate-potency first-generation antipsychotic), as well as the other second-generation antipsychotics risperidone, quetiapine, and ziprasidone, in the maintenance of successful treatment of chronic schizophrenia, including the reduction of symptoms and rates of hospital readmission (Lieberman et al. 2005). Some evidence indicates that second-generation antipsychotics (clozapine in particular) show greater efficacy in patients with treatment-refractory schizophrenia (McEvoy et al. 2006; Miyamoto et al. 2005).

At present, the empirical literature strongly indicates that second-generation antipsychotics are superior to first-generation antipsychotics in the lower incidence of EPS resulting from their use. It appears likely that the incidence of tardive dyskinesia will be lower with second-generation antipsychotics. Other side effects of first-generation antipsychotic treatment that are lessened or nonexistent with second-generation antipsychotics include hyperprolactinemia and ocular effects in the lens and retina. In contrast, the second-generation antipsychotics as a group have been increasingly associated with significant weight gain, hyperlipidemia, insulin resistance and diabetes mellitus onset, prolonged QTc interval, and other cardiovascular complications (Newcomer 2004).

## Treatment of Acute Psychosis

The mainstay of treatment involves the use of first-generation antipsychotics, often at higher doses than those needed for maintenance treatment of schizophrenia. Repeated doses of first-generation antipsychotics are often necessary in the short term in inpatient settings; however, the literature indicates that either rapid loading or sustained high-dose antipsychotic treatment regimens do not confer added benefit and increase the risk of adverse side effects. Adjunctive medications such as benzodiazepines are frequently used both for their sedating effects and to permit the use of relatively lower doses of antipsychotics. Prophylaxis of EPS with the use of anticholinergic medications is also often indicated, particularly because the incidence of EPS is higher in younger patients and EPS are a common cause of early nonadherence to antipsychotics.

An increasingly used alternative to the first-generation antipsychotics in acute psychosis is the second-generation antipsychotics, particularly those for which therapeutic blood levels can be quickly attained (e.g., olanzapine, risperidone) or those for which parenteral formulations are available (olanzapine, ziprasidone). Current evidence indicates that these medications are probably as effective in acute psychosis as the first-generation antipsychotics and are much better tolerated, suggesting that the second-generation antipsychotics may replace the first-generation antipsychotics for this indication in the future.

## Treatment of First-Episode Psychosis

An individual with a first-episode psychosis presenting as an agitated acute psychosis frequently settles into lower doses of either first-generation antipsychotics or second-generation antipsychotics as the inpatient hospital course proceeds (often by increasing the time interval between doses throughout the day), often with adjunct benzodiazepines discontinued prior to discharge. In this setting, or in a first presentation to an outpatient clinic, the relative merits of first-generation antipsychotics versus second-generation antipsychotics must be considered. An increasingly common approach in the outpatient setting is to initiate low to moderate doses of second-generation antipsychotics, primarily in light of the improved patient satisfaction and compliance that may be largely a function of reduced rates of EPS. It should be recalled that this approach largely trades the higher long-term risk of tardive dyskinesia for lower but significant metabolic and cardiovascular risks.

The clinical response rates to both first- and second-generation antipsychotics are high in a first psychotic episode, up to 75% (Robinson et al. 2005). A large percentage of first-episode patients respond within the first week of treatment, with response rates reaching a plateau in the subsequent 3 months.

## Maintenance Treatment in Schizophrenia

Once the diagnosis of schizophrenia is certain, antipsychotic medication should be continued indefinitely, in a manner analogous to the lifelong pharmacological treatment indicated for disorders such as diabetes mellitus and hypertension. In addition to minimizing relapse, sustained treatment with antipsychotics may modify the long-term course of this illness.

## Treatment-Refractory Schizophrenia

The overall rates of clinical response of schizophrenia patients to antipsychotic medications are within the range observed for outpatients with mood disorders undergoing antidepressant medication treatment. Nonetheless, a significant percentage of patients with schizophrenia (up to 40%) can be considered to be poorly responsive to standard antipsychotic medications (Kane et al. 1988). Treatment-refractory states indicate poor response of positive symptoms to antipsychotic medications, with these symptoms may increase over time in these patients. In contrast, refractory negative symptoms and cognitive impairment are usually present at the first episode (Meltzer and Pringuey 1998).

The available evidence favors clozapine as the most effective antipsychotic for treatment-refractory schizophrenia, although treatment-resistant schizophrenia may respond to other second-generation antipsychotics as well (possibly at lower response rates relative to clozapine) (Conley and Kelly 2001). In addition, most clinicians and experts in this area would agree that previous treatment trials should have included at least one second-generation antipsychotic before clozapine is considered, primarily because of the added burden of frequent clinical monitoring necessary for the early detection of agranulocytosis, which occurs in approximately 1% of those taking clozapine. Unfortunately, as many as 40%–70% of patients with treatment-refractory schizophrenia also experience an inadequate response to clozapine. These patients, who have been referred to as "ultra-refractory," have been increasingly studied in clinical trials of antipsychotic augmentation strategies. At present, among U.S. Food and Drug Administration–approved medications that are widely available in the United States, promising initial results have been obtained for the clinical response of these patients to the addition of lamotrigine and lithium (for schizoaffective patients) (Kontaxakis et al. 2005).

## Other Adjunctive Biological Treatments for Schizophrenia

Anticholinergic medications are a mainstay of treatment, serving as effective prophylaxis for EPS found in response to not only first-generation antipsychotics but occasionally second-generation antipsychotics (especially risperidone). Some second-generation antipsychotics, such as clozapine and olanzapine, have significant intrinsic anticholinergic activity, which may be partly responsible for their lower rates of EPS and obviates the need for a second, anticholinergic agent. Benzodiazepines are also well used in the treatment of acute psychosis and effective in treating akathisia associated with antipsychotics. They are often used in maintenance treatment of psychotic symptoms

and in the treatment of anxiety and insomnia commonly found in these patients. Other adjunctive treatments that target co-occurring symptoms in patients with schizophrenia include anticonvulsants (Hosak and Libiger 2002), beta-blockers and lithium for aggressive and impulsive behaviors, and antidepressants for both depressive and anxiety disorders that are commonly found in schizophrenia (Escamilla 2001).

Electroconvulsive therapy (ECT) is another treatment modality that may continue to have a role in the rapid treatment of acute and subacute states that are refractory to pharmacological intervention, particularly catatonia (Tharyan and Adams 2005). Nevertheless, access to ECT is limited in many treatment settings, and ECT has no apparent advantage over pharmacological treatment in the maintenance phase of schizophrenia.

## Psychosocial Treatments for Schizophrenia

### Case Management and Assertive Community Treatment

Case management is fundamentally a method of coordinating services for the patient in the community. In this model, an individual case manager (typically, a licensed social worker) serves a role somewhat analogous to that of a primary care physician, assessing and prioritizing the needs of the patient, developing an integrated care plan, arranging for provision of this care, and serving as the patient's primary point of contact in the mental health system. Case managers interact with both social service agencies and clinicians to achieve and maintain access to entitlements, social services, and clinical care.

One particularly successful form of case management is referred to in the United States as Assertive Community Treatment (ACT). Candidates for this care are typically identified in community mental health settings as those with the highest service needs (e.g., the most frequent users of emergency or inpatient services) and referred to a multidisciplinary team, often composed of the case manager (licensed social worker or psychologist), psychiatric nurse, psychiatrist, and other psychiatric support staff. These teams have a fixed caseload and a high staff-to-patient ratio, delivering care when and where the patient requires it, including at the patient's residence, clinics and hospitals, and social service agencies, 24 hours a day.

### Cognitive-Behavioral Therapy

Cognitive-behavioral therapy (CBT) was used to treat schizophrenia in the United Kingdom during a period

(1970s–1980s) when clinicians in the United States used it primarily for treatment of depression, and CBT remains more popular in the United Kingdom for the treatment of schizophrenia (Turkington et al. 2006). Several features of CBT techniques are highly modified for use with schizophrenia patients. For instance, a relatively greater emphasis is placed on development of the therapeutic alliance as it arises from the patient's perspective. The clinician also works to identify and develop alternative explanations of symptoms that are acceptable to both patient and therapist. Another technique involves the use of "peripheral questioning," in which the therapist facilitates the patient to elaborate on the belief system, and a related approach of "inference chaining," in which the personalized meaning and string of logic underlying a delusional structure are identified. Cognitive-behavioral therapists attempt to normalize the patient's experience when it is appropriate and in general reduce the effect of positive symptoms. CBT is probably not advisable when the patient is too paranoid, withdrawn, or cognitively impaired to engage in treatment.

## Cognitive Remediation and Rehabilitation

Cognitive remediation and rehabilitation emphasize the cognitive deficits that are readily evident in schizophrenia and are associated with functional impairment. Techniques include training exercises that have been successfully used in diverse clinical populations such as focal brain-injured and learning-disabled individuals. Computer-based or "pencil-and-paper" tasks guide patients through successive levels of skill in performing cognitive tasks of attention, memory, cognitive flexibility, problem solving, and other functions that are impaired in these patients. Treatment courses typically extend from 1 to 6 months with multiple sessions each week. The evidence to date suggests that certain cognitive functions (such as problem solving) may improve with this type of treatment, and modest effects on social function have been observed in some studies (Bellack et al. 1999).

## Social Skills–Based Therapies

Social skills have been defined by Bellack and Mueser (1993) as "specific response capabilities necessary for effective social performance." Social skills training aims to improve social function in patients by training the behavioral repertoire called on in social settings. One form of training, the basic model, decomposes complex social sequences into simpler components, with subsequent corrective training in which role-playing is used, and the settings should be as naturalistic as possible. In contrast, the social problem-solving model emphasizes improvements in cognitive functions that are thought to underlie social dysfunction. Deficits in receptive and expressive communicatory functions are addressed in the context of treatment adherence, basic social interactions, recreation, and general self-care.

## Vocational Rehabilitation

The rate of continuous employment in a competitive setting (outside of a rehabilitation or "sheltered" work setting) among patients with schizophrenia is probably much lower than 20% in most communities (Lehman 1995). Sheltered work settings provide an environment for patients in which the work and social demands are manageable and the interpersonal environment is accepting of limitations caused by the patient's illness. The long-term goal for many patients will be attaining employment in competitive settings in the community.

## Family Therapy

Interventions that involve working with the families of those with schizophrenia emphasize that the the family is the primary environment in which the disease is expressed and modified in a reciprocal manner and, for most patients, the first line of support. Intact, adequately functioning family environments offer an important buffer for the symptoms of schizophrenia and are associated with a relatively better prognosis for the patient. Reducing family distress and fostering a collaborative approach to treatment involving the patient, family, and treatment team are important goals for patients at all stages of illness. Earlier studies and models of interaction in families of patients with schizophrenia were focused on the construct of expressed emotion, in which high rates of expressions critical of the patient were associated with elevated relapse rates. Approaches to these families often include psychoeducation and psychological support, which aid family members in anticipation of the patient's illness expression, and response strategies that help both patient and relatives optimally cope with the patient's illness.

## Individual Psychotherapy

At present, individual psychotherapy is generally considered to elevate the risk for psychotic decompensation, probably because of the unstructured and anxiety-provoking nature of this treatment. In contrast, supportive therapy approaches appear to be superior to treatment as usual in studies in which the primary focus is on relative efficacy of CBT. Supportive therapy is a diverse set of approaches to the patient, yet all have in common the goal of providing reassurance, guidance, and an interpersonal environment that is stable, predictable, and tolerant of the patient's expression, symptoms, and problems in living. It is generally less systematic and less symptom-focused than CBT. One particular approach has been termed *personal therapy*, which was developed by Hogarty et al. (1995). It uses techniques that are individualized for the patient, with progressive focus on stress reduction first, followed by cognitive reframing, and later vocational rehabilitation, as the emphasis follows the patient's stage of recovery.

# Related Psychotic Disorders

## Schizoaffective Disorder

The construct of schizoaffective disorder addresses individuals who have prominent features of both schizophrenia and major mood disorders. The current DSM-IV-TR diagnostic criteria for schizoaffective disorder require an uninterrupted period of illness during which Criterion A for schizophrenia is met, along with criteria for depressive, manic, or mixed mood episode. During this same period, either delusions or hallucinations must be present for at least 2 weeks in the absence of prominent mood symptoms. This criterion is the major distinction from psychotic mood episodes. The base prevalence may be less than 1% in the community, although the disorder is found at much higher rates in clinical settings. The relatives of patients with schizoaffective disorder have an elevated risk for both schizophrenia and mood disorders. Conversely, children with family histories of either schizophrenia or bipolar disorders develop schizoaffective disorder at an elevated rate (Berrettini 2000; Gershon et al. 1988). Individuals with schizoaffective disorder have an elevated rate of winter and spring births compared with the community, like those with schizophrenia or bipolar disorder (Torrey et al. 1997). A significant percentage of these patients show a deteriorating clinical course with persistent psychosis, although many others show a clinical course more similar to that of bipolar disorder patients (Benabarre et al. 2001).

Overall, the prognosis for schizoaffective patients is intermediate between that for patients with schizophrenia and that for patients with mood disorders. Predictors of poor prognosis in schizoaffective disorder include many of those also established for schizophrenia, including a family history of schizophrenia, poor premorbid function, insidious onset, early age at onset, lack of a clear precipitating factor, predominance of psychotic symptoms, and poor recovery between episodes.

## Delusional Disorder

Delusional disorder is characterized by the presence of one or more nonbizarre delusions in the relative absence of other symptoms of psychosis (it is also required that Criterion A for schizophrenia has not been met). This is the central DSM-IV-TR diagnostic criterion and the only one that requires the presence of a particular symptom or sign. The delusions tend to be systematized, with associated affect that is consistent with the delusional belief. However, cognitive function and personality features tend to remain intact (although the delusional belief itself may have circumscribed effects on interpersonal function). This diagnosis requires adequate exclusion of other, more common psychotic disorders, such as schizophrenia, mood disorders, and dementia, and other medical etiologies. Thus, the DSM-IV-TR criteria require that any associated auditory hallucinations, or affective symptoms, not be prominent, and behavior not be odd or bizarre.

The predominant theme of the delusional ideation is used to identify subtypes, such as persecutory, jealous, erotomanic, somatic, grandiose, mixed, and unspecified. The lifetime risk is approximately 0.05%–0.10%, as defined by DSM-IV-TR, with onset in middle to late adulthood. The diagnostic stability of delusional disorder may be relatively low because many patients will develop other psychotic symptoms, leading to the diagnosis of schizophrenia. However, the pattern of clinical features and familial aggregation suggest that delusional disorder should not be classified as a subtype of schizophrenia or other psychotic disorders (Cardno and McGuffin 2006).

The pathophysiology of delusional disorder remains obscure, although some preliminary evidence indicates that polymorphisms in genes coding for dopamine receptors (*DRD3* and *DRD4*) are associated with the disorder (Cardno and McGuffin 2006). Most delusional disorder patients experience the delusional belief as *ego-syntonic*, which means that the delusional thought is experienced as consistent with the patients' expectations, sense of self, and sense of reality in general. This sharply limits the capacity for insight into the nature of the belief, and as a result, patients generally do not have any incentive to enter mental health treatment because the subjective distress they feel is attributed to a rigid sense of the "state of affairs" in their environment rather than a psychological state in need of remediation. In addition, patients generally do not come to the attention of the mental health system because aggressive behavior or decline in self-care (which would prompt intervention from law enforcement, emergency medical, or social services) is not typical. However, a small percentage of these patients may be at significant risk for aggressive behavior, particularly those with persecutory delusions, which may prompt them to "defend" or retaliate against the perceived source of malevolence. Violent behavior also may result from the relentless pursuit observed in some jealous or erotomanic subtypes of delusional patients. The empirical evidence for antipsychotic use in delusional disorder remains scant, and treatment of delusions in this disorder largely proceeds on the basis of established efficacy against delusions in schizophrenia (Smith and Buckley 2006).

## Schizophreniform Disorder and Brief Psychotic Disorder

In DSM-IV-TR, the criteria for schizophreniform disorder are largely coincident with those for schizophrenia, except that the duration of symptoms in Criterion A is shorter—in this case, longer than 1 month but less than 6 months. It appears likely that at the time of diagnosis with this disorder, patients in general are early in the course of

overt illness, experiencing psychotic symptoms but without the duration criterion met for schizophrenia. The relatively better prognosis for these patients as a group, compared with patients identified as having schizophrenia at first encounter, may reflect the percentage who go on to identified mood disorders and also that, as a group, these patients have not endured repeated or sustained psychotic episodes and steady functional decline, as would a percentage of any group with a clearly established diagnosis of schizophrenia.

Brief psychotic disorder, on the other hand, is distinguished from schizophrenia as a DSM-IV-TR diagnostic category by the abrupt onset of overt psychotic symptoms (the same set of positive psychotic symptoms as in Criterion A for schizophrenia), but the symptoms last for less than 1 month. Individuals whose symptoms meet the criteria for this disorder do not have a history of functional decline or signs that may be retrospectively attributed to a prodrome. In addition, the psychotic symptoms associated with the diagnosis tend to be precipitated more commonly by acute stressors, be associated with acute mood changes, and generally respond well to treatment. These patients as a group also have minimal negative symptoms and a significantly better long-term prognosis than do patients with schizophrenia (on average).

# Key Points: Schizophrenia

- Among medical illnesses, schizophrenia is one of the most serious for the afflicted individual, the family of the patient, and society at large.

- Schizophrenia, like psychiatric illness in general, occurs as a function of both a genetic predisposition and environmental factors.

- Schizophrenia is characterized by cognitive, perceptual, behavioral, and social disturbances and has profound consequences for the individual's capacity for autonomy and function in the community.

- Schizophrenia is currently conceived of as a neurodevelopmental disorder, with disturbances in development across a range of epochs, from early gestation through late adolescence.

- The pathophysiology of schizophrenia involves several anatomical regions and neurotransmitters and other functional systems in the brain.

- The various symptoms and problems in living that patients with schizophrenia experience can be treated with the full range of treatment modalities currently available in psychiatry, including pharmacological and psychosocial approaches.

- Although many patients with schizophrenia endure relapsing and remitting periods of illness, with a significant decline in function over the early period of illness, many can retain a measure of well-being, symptom control, and autonomy in the community.

- Research into the causes, clinical course, and treatment of schizophrenia has shown considerable progress in recent times and shows promise for significant advances in the future treatment of this disorder.

## Suggested Readings

Andreasen NC: Schizophrenia: the fundamental questions. Brain Res Brain Res Rev 31:106–112, 2000

Compton WM, Guze SB: The neo-Kraepelinian revolution in psychiatric diagnosis. Eur Arch Psychiatry Clin Neurosci 245:196–201, 1995

Lewis DA, Levitt P: Schizophrenia as a disorder of neurodevelopment. Annu Rev Neurosci 25:409–432, 2002

Miyamoto S, Duncan GE, Marx CE, et al: Treatments for schizophrenia: a critical review of pharmacology and mechanisms of action of antipsychotic drugs. Mol Psychiatry 10:79–104, 2005

Mueser KT, McGurk SR: Schizophrenia. Lancet 363:2063–2072, 2004

## Online Resources

Schizophrenia.com (http://www.schizophrenia.com; general site, appropriate for families and lay public)

Schizophrenia Research Forum (http://www.schizophreniaforum.org; research-oriented site)

## References

Addington J, Addington D: Neurocognitive and social functioning in schizophrenia: a 2.5 year follow-up study. Schizophr Res 44:47–56, 2000

Adler LE, Hoffer LJ, Griffith J, et al: Normalization by nicotine of deficient auditory sensory gating in the relatives of schizophrenics. Biol Psychiatry 32:607–616, 1992

Akbarian S, Kim JJ, Potkin SG, et al: Gene expression for glutamic acid decarboxylase is reduced without loss of neurons in prefrontal cortex of schizophrenics. Arch Gen Psychiatry 52:258–266, 1995

American Psychiatric Association: Diagnostic and Statistical Manual of Mental Disorders, 2nd Edition. Washington, DC, American Psychiatric Association, 1968

American Psychiatric Association: Diagnostic and Statistical Manual of Mental Disorders, 3rd Edition. Washington, DC, American Psychiatric Association, 1980

American Psychiatric Association: Diagnostic and Statistical Manual of Mental Disorders, 4th Edition, Text Revision. Washington, DC, American Psychiatric Association, 2000

Bellack AS, Mueser KT: Psychosocial treatment for schizophrenia. Schizophr Bull 19:317–336, 1993

Bellack AS, Gold JM, Buchanan RW: Cognitive rehabilitation for schizophrenia: problems, prospects, and strategies. Schizophr Bull 25:257–274, 1999

Benabarre A, Vieta E, Colom F, et al: Bipolar disorder, schizoaffective disorder and schizophrenia: epidemiologic, clinical and prognostic differences. Eur Psychiatry 16:167–172, 2001

Berrettini WH: Are schizophrenic and bipolar disorders related? A review of family and molecular studies. Biol Psychiatry 48:531–538, 2000

Bilder RM, Mukherjee S, Rieder RO, et al: Symptomatic and neuropsychological components of defect states. Schizophr Bull 11:409–419, 1985

Bland RC, Parker JH, Orn H: Prognosis in schizophrenia: prognostic predictors and outcome. Arch Gen Psychiatry 35:72–77, 1978

Bombin I, Arango C, Buchanan RW: Significance and meaning of neurological signs in schizophrenia: two decades later. Schizophr Bull 31:962–977, 2005

Brenner CA, Lysaker PH, Wilt MA, et al: Visual processing and neuropsychological function in schizophrenia and schizoaffective disorder. Psychiatry Res 111:125–136, 2002

Bromet EJ, Fennig S: Epidemiology and natural history of schizophrenia. Biol Psychiatry 46:871–881, 1999

Cannon M, Jones PB, Murray RM: Obstetric complications and schizophrenia: historical and meta-analytic review. Am J Psychiatry 159:1080–1092, 2002

Cardno AG, McGuffin P: Genetics and delusional disorder. Behav Sci Law 24:257–276, 2006

Carlsson A, Lindqvist M: Effect of chlorpromazine or haloperidol on formation of 3methoxytyramine and normetanephrine in mouse brain. Acta Pharmacol Toxicol (Copenh) 20:140–144, 1963

Carpenter WT Jr, Strauss JS: The prediction of outcome in schizophrenia, IV: eleven-year follow-up of the Washington IPSS cohort. J Nerv Ment Dis 179:517–525, 1991

Conley RR, Kelly DL: Management of treatment resistance in schizophrenia. Biol Psychiatry 50:898–911, 2001

Corcoran R, Mercer G, Frith CD: Schizophrenia, symptomatology and social inference: investigating "theory of mind" in people with schizophrenia. Schizophr Res 17:5–13, 1995

Creese I, Burt DR, Snyder SH: Dopamine receptor binding predicts clinical and pharmacological potencies of antischizophrenic drugs. Science 192:481–483, 1976

Davidson M, Reichenberg A, Rabinowitz J, et al: Behavioral and intellectual markers for schizophrenia in apparently healthy male adolescents. Am J Psychiatry 156:1328–1335, 1999

Davies G, Welham J, Chant D, et al: A systematic review and meta-analysis of Northern Hemisphere season of birth studies in schizophrenia. Schizophr Bull 29:587–593, 2003

Escamilla MA: Diagnosis and treatment of mood disorders that co-occur with schizophrenia. Psychiatr Serv 52:911–919, 2001

Frith CD, Corcoran R: Exploring "theory of mind" in people with schizophrenia. Psychol Med 26:521–530, 1996

Gershon ES, DeLisi LE, Hamovit J, et al: A controlled family study of chronic psychoses: schizophrenia and schizoaffective disorder. Arch Gen Psychiatry 45:328–336, 1988

Goodwin DW, Alderson P, Rosenthal R: Clinical significance of hallucinations in psychiatric disorders: a study of 116 hallucinatory patients. Arch Gen Psychiatry 24:76–80, 1971

Gottesman II: Schizophrenia Genesis: The Origins of Madness. New York, WH Freeman, 1991

Green MF: What are the functional consequences of neurocognitive deficits in schizophrenia? Am J Psychiatry 153:321–330, 1996

Harrison PJ: The neuropathology of schizophrenia: a critical review of the data and their interpretation. Brain 122 (pt 4): 593–624, 1999

Harrow M, Jobe TH: Longitudinal studies of outcome and recovery in schizophrenia and early intervention: can they make a difference? Can J Psychiatry 50:879–880, 2005

Hogarty GE, Kornblith SJ, Greenwald D, et al: Personal therapy: a disorder-relevant psychotherapy for schizophrenia. Schizophr Bull 21:379–393, 1995

Hosak L, Libiger J: Antiepileptic drugs in schizophrenia: a review. Eur Psychiatry 17:371–378, 2002

Javitt DC, Zukin SR: Recent advances in the phencyclidine model of schizophrenia. Am J Psychiatry 148:1301–1308, 1991

Javitt DC, Strous RD, Grochowski S, et al: Impaired precision, but normal retention, of auditory sensory ("echoic") memory information in schizophrenia. J Abnorm Psychol 106:315–324, 1997

Jobe TH, Harrow M: Long-term outcome of patients with schizophrenia: a review. Can J Psychiatry 50:892–900, 2005

Johnstone EC, Crow TJ, Frith CD, et al: Cerebral ventricular size and cognitive impairment in chronic schizophrenia. Lancet 2:924–926, 1976

Kane JM, Honigfeld G, Singer J, et al: Clozapine in treatment-resistant schizophrenics. Psychopharmacol Bull 24:62–67, 1988

Kety SS, Rosenthal D, Wender PH, et al: Mental illness in the biological and adoptive families of adopted schizophrenics. Am J Psychiatry 128:302–306, 1971

Kontaxakis VP, Ferentinos PP, Havaki-Kontaxakis BJ, et al: Randomized controlled augmentation trials in clozapine-resistant schizophrenic patients: a critical review. Eur Psychiatry 20:409–415, 2005

Lawrie SM, Abukmeil SS: Brain abnormality in schizophrenia: a systematic and quantitative review of volumetric magnetic resonance imaging studies. Br J Psychiatry 172:110–120, 1998

Lehman AF: Vocational rehabilitation in schizophrenia. Schizophr Bull 21:645–656, 1995

Liddle PF: The symptoms of chronic schizophrenia: a re-examination of the positive-negative dichotomy. Br J Psychiatry 151:145–151, 1987

Lieberman JA, Perkins D, Belger A, et al: The early stages of schizophrenia: speculations on pathogenesis, pathophysiology, and therapeutic approaches. Biol Psychiatry 50:884–897, 2001

Lieberman JA, Stroup TS, McEvoy JP, et al: Effectiveness of antipsychotic drugs in patients with chronic schizophrenia. N Engl J Med 353:1209–1223, 2005

Malla A, Payne J: First-episode psychosis: psychopathology, quality of life, and functional outcome. Schizophr Bull 31:650–671, 2005

McEvoy JP, Lieberman JA, Stroup TS, et al: Effectiveness of clozapine versus olanzapine, quetiapine, and risperidone in patients with chronic schizophrenia who did not respond to prior atypical antipsychotic treatment. Am J Psychiatry 163:600–610, 2006

McGlashan TH: The Chestnut Lodge follow-up study, II: long-term outcome of schizophrenia and the affective disorders. Arch Gen Psychiatry 41:586–601, 1984

McGue M, Gottesman II: A single dominant gene still cannot account for the transmission of schizophrenia. Arch Gen Psychiatry 46:478–480, 1989

Meltzer HY, Pringuey D: Treatment-resistant schizophrenia: the importance of early detection and treatment. Introduction. J Clin Psychopharmacol 18 (2 suppl 1):1S, 1998

Meltzer HY, Li Z, Kaneda Y, et al: Serotonin receptors: their key role in drugs to treat schizophrenia. Prog Neuropsychopharmacol Biol Psychiatry 27:1159–1172, 2003

Miyamoto S, Duncan GE, Marx CE, et al: Treatments for schizophrenia: a critical review of pharmacology and mechanisms of action of antipsychotic drugs. Mol Psychiatry 10:79–104, 2005

Newcomer JW: Metabolic risk during antipsychotic treatment. Clin Ther 26:1936–1946, 2004

Phillips LJ, McGorry PD, Yung AR, et al: Prepsychotic phase of schizophrenia and related disorders: recent progress and future opportunities. Br J Psychiatry Suppl 48:S33–S44, 2005

Pinkham AE, Penn DL, Perkins DO, et al: Implications for the neural basis of social cognition for the study of schizophrenia. Am J Psychiatry 160:815–824, 2003

Ram R, Bromet EJ, Eaton WW, et al: The natural course of schizophrenia: a review of first-admission studies. Schizophr Bull 18:185–207, 1992

Remington G, Kapur S: D2 and 5-HT2 receptor effects of antipsychotics: bridging basic and clinical findings using PET. J Clin Psychiatry 60 (suppl 10):15–19, 1999

Risch N: Genetic linkage and complex diseases, with special reference to psychiatric disorders. Genet Epidemiol 7:3–16; discussion 17–45, 1990

Robinson DG, Woerner MG, Delman HM, et al: Pharmacological treatments for first-episode schizophrenia. Schizophr Bull 31:705–722, 2005

Saccuzzo DP, Braff DL: Early information processing deficit in schizophrenia: new findings using schizophrenic subgroups and manic control subjects. Arch Gen Psychiatry 38:175–179, 1981

Seeman P, Lee T, Chau-Wong M, et al: Antipsychotic drug doses and neuroleptic/dopamine receptors. Nature 261:717–719, 1976

Smith DA, Buckley PF: Pharmacotherapy of delusional disorders in the context of offending and the potential for compulsory treatment. Behav Sci Law 24:351–367, 2006

Steen RG, Mull C, McClure R, et al: Brain volume in first-episode schizophrenia: systematic review and meta-analysis of magnetic resonance imaging studies. Br J Psychiatry 188:510–518, 2006

Stone MH: Exploratory psychotherapy in schizophrenia-spectrum patients: a reevaluation in the light of long-term follow-up of schizophrenic and borderline patients. Bull Menninger Clin 50:287–306, 1986

Susser E, Neugebauer R, Hoek HW, et al: Schizophrenia after prenatal famine: further evidence. Arch Gen Psychiatry 53:25–31, 1996

Tharyan P, Adams CE: Electroconvulsive therapy for schizophrenia. Cochrane Database Syst Rev (2):CD000076, 2005

Torrey EF, Miller J, Rawlings R, et al: Seasonality of births in schizophrenia and bipolar disorder: a review of the literature. Schizophr Res 28:1–38, 1997

Tsuang MT, Winokur G: The Iowa 500: field work in a 35-year follow-up of depression, mania, and schizophrenia. Can Psychiatr Assoc J 20:359–365, 1975

Turkington D, Kingdon D, Weiden PJ: Cognitive behavior therapy for schizophrenia. Am J Psychiatry 163:365–373, 2006

Volk DW, Austin MC, Pierri JN, et al: Decreased glutamic acid decarboxylase67 messenger RNA expression in a subset of prefrontal cortical gamma-aminobutyric acid neurons in subjects with schizophrenia. Arch Gen Psychiatry 57:237–245, 2000

Xiberas X, Martinot JL, Mallet L, et al: Extrastriatal and striatal D(2) dopamine receptor blockade with haloperidol or new antipsychotic drugs in patients with schizophrenia. Br J Psychiatry 179:503–508, 2001

# 18

# Mood Disorders

JOHN A. JOSKA, M.D., M.MED.(PSYCH.), F.C.PSYCH.(S.A.)

DAN J. STEIN, M.D., Ph.D.

## Phenomenology of Mood Disorders

### Subtypes and Forms of Mood Disorders

Assessment of mood disorders requires both a cross-sectional and a longitudinal review. Figure 18–1 summarizes mood disorders according to episode features and specifiers.

### Clinical Features of Depression

#### Mental State Examination

Certain features of depression may be present on the mental state examination. These include a downcast appearance, poor eye contact, and diminished or increased psychomotor activity. Speech may be slow and monotonous, with delays in the production of speech (so-called speech latency or speech pause time). The patient with depression may describe a low mood or may represent it by using particular cultural idioms. Affective expression in depression varies from bland and restricted to anxious, dysphoric, and agitated. Thought may be altered in depression—ranging from slowed flow to poverty of ideation. In psychotic depression, the patient may have loosening of associations, delusions of nihilism ("I am worthless"; "I will be dying shortly"), perceptual disturbances (defamatory and command-type auditory hallucinations are commonest), and visual hallucinations. Cognitive impairment can occur, with disturbed memory, attention, and executive functions.

#### Depressed Mood and Anhedonia

Together with low mood, a loss of pleasure—anhedonia—is the other essential feature of a DSM-IV-TR (American Psychiatric Association 2000a) diagnosis of depression. Factor analytic studies have established that low mood and anhedonia are consistently present in individuals with depression and, as such, are critical to its diagnosis (Nelson and Charney 1981). Qualitative differences in mood are seen in depressive disorders: an inability to experience a lifting of mood in the presence of typically rewarding events is a key feature of melancholia (lack of "mood reactivity"). This subtype of depression includes the problems of early-morning awakening and diurnal variation in mood (see Figure 18–1).

#### Cognitive, Neurovegetative, and Behavioral Symptoms

Cognitive impairment in depression includes the errors in information processing and distortions described by a cognitive-behavioral model. These errors and distortions include negative thoughts about the self, the world, and the future. These negative thoughts may begin with vague negative thoughts about the self and the future but ultimately lead to the emergence and expression of suicidal thoughts. Neuropsychological disturbances in depression include poor performance on tests of memory, concentration, and executive functions. In the elderly, this may lead to inappropriate diagnosis of cognitive disorders such as dementia (a condition known as "pseudodementia").

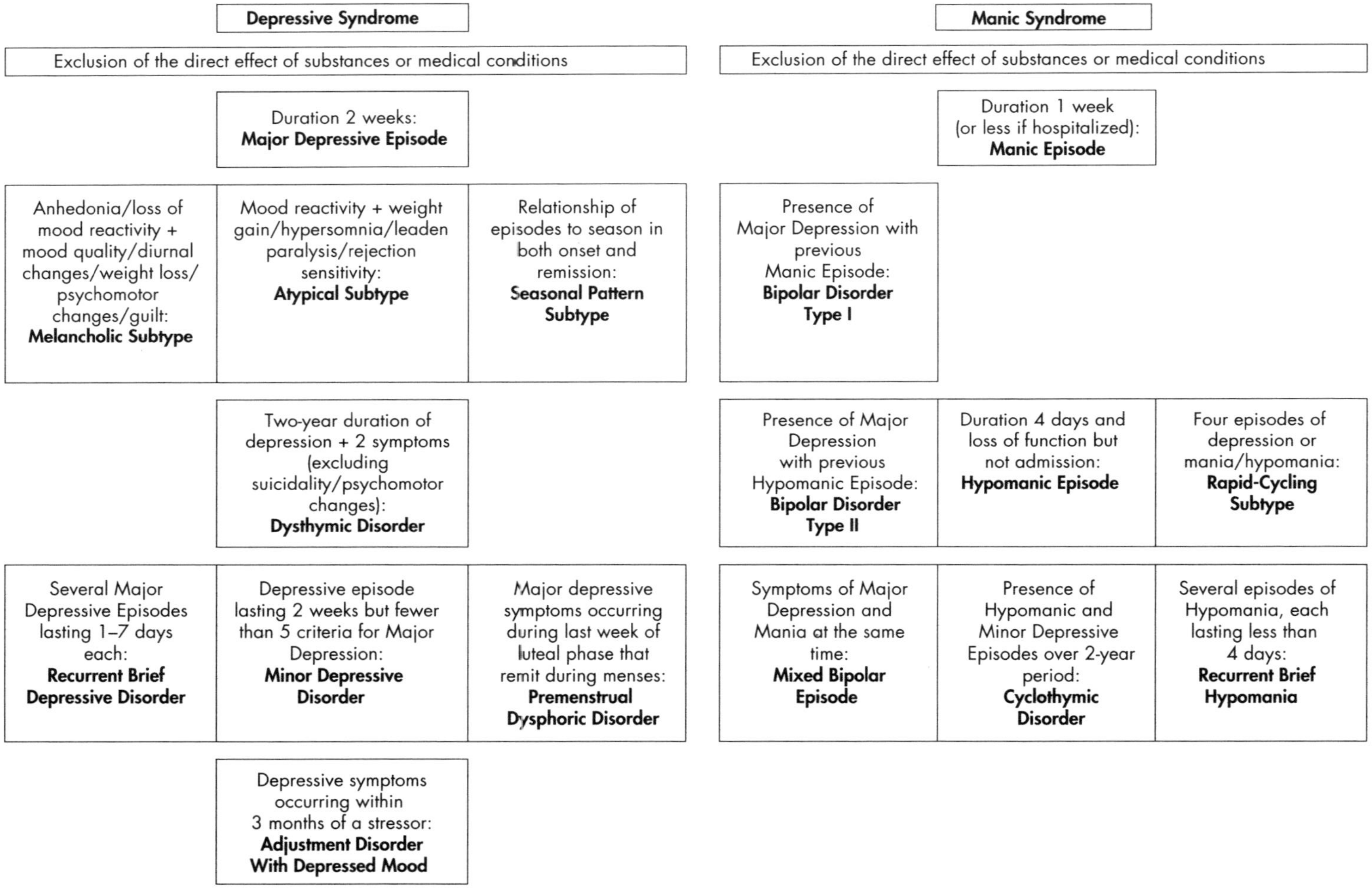

**Manic Syndrome**

Exclusion of the direct effect of substances or medical conditions

- Duration 1 week (or less if hospitalized): **Manic Episode**
- Presence of Major Depression with previous Manic Episode: **Bipolar Disorder Type I**
- Duration 4 days and loss of function but not admission: **Hypomanic Episode**
- Presence of Major Depression with previous Hypomanic Episode: **Bipolar Disorder Type II**
- Four episodes of depression or mania/hypomania: **Rapid-Cycling Subtype**
- Symptoms of Major Depression and Mania at the same time: **Mixed Bipolar Episode**
- Presence of Hypomanic and Minor Depressive Episodes over 2-year period: **Cyclothymic Disorder**
- Several episodes of Hypomania, each lasting less than 4 days: **Recurrent Brief Hypomania**

**Depressive Syndrome**

Exclusion of the direct effect of substances or medical conditions

- Duration 2 weeks: **Major Depressive Episode**
- Anhedonia/loss of mood reactivity + mood quality/diurnal changes/weight loss/psychomotor changes/guilt: **Melancholic Subtype**
- Mood reactivity + weight gain/hypersomnia/leaden paralysis/rejection sensitivity: **Atypical Subtype**
- Relationship of episodes to season in both onset and remission: **Seasonal Pattern Subtype**
- Two-year duration of depression + 2 symptoms (excluding suicidality/psychomotor changes): **Dysthymic Disorder**
- Several Major Depressive Episodes lasting 1–7 days each: **Recurrent Brief Depressive Disorder**
- Depressive episode lasting 2 weeks but fewer than 5 criteria for Major Depression: **Minor Depressive Disorder**
- Major depressive symptoms occurring during last week of luteal phase that remit during menses: **Premenstrual Dysphoric Disorder**
- Depressive symptoms occurring within 3 months of a stressor: **Adjustment Disorder With Depressed Mood**

FIGURE 18–1.   **Summary of mood disorders, specifiers, and relationships.**

Disturbances of sleep, appetite, and sexual behavior are sometimes referred to as "neurovegetative." Patients describe different sleep patterns in depression, but the presence of terminal insomnia, or early-morning awakening, may be a particularly severe symptom. Appetite is often diminished and, if persistent, will be followed by a significant loss of weight. Sexual interest and activity are also reduced. A small proportion of individuals sleep and eat excessively (hypersomnia and hyperphagia); these symptoms are part of the syndrome of atypical depression (see Figure 18–1).

### *Duration, Intensity, and Specifiers*

Assessment of the depressive episode includes evaluation of the duration of the current episode, the intensity of the episode, and any episode specifiers. The diagnosis of major depression requires depressive symptoms to be present for most days over a 2-week period. When symptoms have been present for a shorter period, a diagnosis of depressive disorder not otherwise specified or recurrent brief depression may be considered. When depression lasts 2 years or more, the diagnosis of dysthymic disorder is possible.

Although the characterization of an episode as mild, moderate, or severe may seem overly broad, it potentially helps inform management by suggesting which episode may require intensive, combined, or inpatient treatments. In addition, more severe depressive episodes have a tendency to recur more frequently and may require a longer duration of treatment (Kessler et al. 1994).

DSM-IV-TR includes several episode specifiers. Some, which have been mentioned earlier, include subtype specifiers, such as depression with melancholia, atypical features, or catatonic features. Other specifiers indicate when depression occurs: postpartum onset (occurring within 4 weeks of childbirth) or seasonal onset (occurring during a particular season, usually winter). The presence of psychotic symptoms also should be specified.

## Major Depressive Disorder

### *Diagnostic Criteria*

The DSM-IV-TR diagnostic criteria for major depressive episode are listed in Table 18–1.

### *Single-Episode Versus Recurrent Major Depression*

Recurrence only follows a previously remitted episode and should not be diagnosed in the presence of residual symptoms of an inadequately treated episode. The use of rating scales such as the Hamilton Rating Scale for Depression may be useful (Hamilton 1960). Symptom scores of less than 75% of baseline, for example, are considered to indicate remission.

## Other Depressive Disorders

### *Dysthymic Disorder*

Dysthymic disorder is a common depressive condition, with a lifetime prevalence of up to 6% of the population (Moore and Bona 2001). It is characterized by milder depressive symptoms than in major depression that persist for at least 2 years, with a symptom-free period of only 2 months in each year (Table 18–2).

### *Psychotic Depression*

The presence of psychotic symptoms in depression is an indication of severity and a tendency to recurrence (Coryell 1996). Inpatient treatment is usually required because of associated risk. Nihilistic or somatic delusions, together with auditory hallucinations, constitute the commonest psychotic symptoms in major depression. Significant impairment, distress, and sometimes suicide accompany this syndrome. The differential diagnosis includes schizophrenia and schizoaffective disorder.

### *Seasonal Affective Disorder*

Seasonal affective disorder (SAD) is classified as a mood disorder specifier—with seasonal pattern. In major depressive disorder, a seasonal pattern may occur in up to one-third of cases (Table 18–3). Research into the pathophysiology of SAD has focused on the effect of light. Possible derangements include melatonin dysregulation, disrupted circadian rhythm, neurotransmitter dysfunction, and visual sensitivity (Lewy et al. 1988). In addition to the usual treatments for depression, light therapy has been shown to be effective.

### *Premenstrual Dysphoric Disorder*

Premenstrual mood symptoms are common, and about 3%–9% of women meet criteria for premenstrual dysphoric disorder (PMDD) (Halbreich et al. 2003). PMDD is characterized by the onset of severe symptoms, with at least one mood symptom, in the late luteal phase of the menstrual cycle, with remission during the early follicular phase (Table 18–4). The association between depression and derangements of the hypothalamic-pituitary-gonadal

**TABLE 18–1.    DSM-IV-TR diagnostic criteria for major depressive episode**

A.  Five (or more) of the following symptoms have been present during the same 2-week period and represent a change from previous functioning; at least one of the symptoms is either (1) depressed mood or (2) loss of interest or pleasure.

   **Note:**   Do not include symptoms that are clearly due to a general medical condition, or mood-incongruent delusions or hallucinations.

   (1)  depressed mood most of the day, nearly every day, as indicated by either subjective report (e.g., feels sad or empty) or observation made by others (e.g., appears tearful).   **Note:** In children and adolescents, can be irritable mood.

   (2)  markedly diminished interest or pleasure in all, or almost all, activities most of the day, nearly every day (as indicated by either subjective account or observation made by others)

   (3)  significant weight loss when not dieting or weight gain (e.g., a change of more than 5% of body weight in a month), or decrease or increase in appetite nearly every day.   **Note:** In children, consider failure to make expected weight gains.

   (4)  insomnia or hypersomnia nearly every day

   (5)  psychomotor agitation or retardation nearly every day (observable by others, not merely subjective feelings of restlessness or being slowed down)

   (6)  fatigue or loss of energy nearly every day

   (7)  feelings of worthlessness or excessive or inappropriate guilt (which may be delusional) nearly every day (not merely self-reproach or guilt about being sick)

   (8)  diminished ability to think or concentrate, or indecisiveness, nearly every day (either by subjective account or as observed by others)

   (9)  recurrent thoughts of death (not just fear of dying), recurrent suicidal ideation without a specific plan, or a suicide attempt or a specific plan for committing suicide

B.  The symptoms do not meet criteria for a mixed episode.

C.  The symptoms cause clinically significant distress or impairment in social, occupational, or other important areas of functioning.

D.  The symptoms are not due to the direct physiological effects of a substance (e.g., a drug of abuse, a medication) or a general medical condition (e.g., hypothyroidism).

E.  The symptoms are not better accounted for by bereavement, i.e., after the loss of a loved one, the symptoms persist for longer than 2 months or are characterized by marked functional impairment, morbid preoccupation with worthlessness, suicidal ideation, psychotic symptoms, or psychomotor retardation.

---

(HPG) axis has been established, but the precise nature of the link is unclear. Treatment of PMDD with gonadal hormones has limited effectiveness, whereas intermittent treatment with selective serotonin reuptake inhibitors (SSRIs) is the current pharmacotherapy of choice (Dimmock et al. 2000).

## Differential Diagnosis of Depressive Disorders

### Medical Disorders

Many medical conditions may be associated with depression (Peveler et al. 2002). Some of these conditions are listed in Table 18–5.

### Depression Secondary to Substance Use

The most widespread substance of abuse, alcohol, is a common and independent cause of depressive illness. Other causes of depression secondary to substance and medication use are listed in Table 18–6.

## Clinical Features of Mania

### Mental State Examination

Central to mania, hypomania, or mixed episodes is the presence of either elevated, irritable, or expansive mood. Mania may manifest in obvious ways (e.g., catatonic stupor; violent and aggressive behavior) or in more subtle ways (e.g., dressing in brighter clothing; agitated psycho-

**TABLE 18–2.   DSM-IV-TR diagnostic criteria for dysthymic disorder**

A.  Depressed mood for most of the day, for more days than not, as indicated by either subjective account or observation by others, for at least 2 years.   **Note:** In children and adolescents, mood can be irritable and duration must be at least 1 year.

B.  Presence, while depressed, of two (or more) of the following:

   (1)  poor appetite or overeating

   (2)  insomnia or hypersomnia

   (3)  low energy or fatigue

   (4)  low self-esteem

   (5)  poor concentration or difficulty making decisions

   (6)  feelings of hopelessness

C.  During the 2-year period (1 year for children or adolescents) of the disturbance, the person has never been without the symptoms in Criteria A and B for more than 2 months at a time.

D.  No major depressive episode has been present during the first 2 years of the disturbance (1 year for children and adolescents); i.e., the disturbance is not better accounted for by chronic major depressive disorder, or major depressive disorder, in partial remission.   **Note:** There may have been a previous major depressive episode provided there was a full remission (no significant signs or symptoms for 2 months) before development of the dysthymic disorder. In addition, after the initial 2 years (1 year in children or adolescents) of dysthymic disorder, there may be superimposed episodes of major depressive disorder, in which case both diagnoses may be given when the criteria are met for a major depressive episode.

E.  There has never been a manic episode, a mixed episode, or a hypomanic episode, and criteria have never been met for cyclothymic disorder.

F.  The disturbance does not occur exclusively during the course of a chronic psychotic disorder, such as schizophrenia or delusional disorder.

G.  The symptoms are not due to the direct physiological effects of a substance (e.g., a drug of abuse, a medication) or a general medical condition (e.g., hypothyroidism).

H.  The symptoms cause clinically significant distress or impairment in social, occupational, or other important areas of functioning.

   *Specify* if:

   **Early onset:**   if onset is before age 21 years

   **Late onset:**   if onset is age 21 years or older

   *Specify* (for most recent 2 years of dysthymic disorder):

   **With atypical features**

motor function). Speech may be pressured. Expansive mood may be elicited when the person describes his or her social interactions; a sense of being connected to the world is often expressed. Affect is often euphoric but may be labile or hostile. Problems with thought include excessive flow of ideas ("flight of ideas"); grandiose, religious, or persecutory delusions; and sometimes bizarre delusions. Perceptual disturbances range from auditory hallucinations (such as hearing the voice of God) to visions of religious and grandiose significance. These mood-congruent symptoms are most common, but incongruent psychosis has been described. Cognitive disturbances include distractibility, poor attention, and executive dysfunction (Table 18–7).

### Mood Disturbance in Mania

Establishing the presence of a disturbed mood in mania is critical to distinguishing mania from other psychiatric conditions. Dysphoria is distinct from depression in that it describes a subjective sense of negative, labile, or irritable mood in the absence of persistently low mood and anhedonia. Questions around the nature of social relationships, work productivity, and plans for the future may be useful to establish changes in goal-directed behavior.

**TABLE 18–3.  DSM-IV-TR criteria for seasonal pattern specifier**

*Specify* if:

**With seasonal pattern** (can be applied to the pattern of major depressive episodes in bipolar I disorder, bipolar II disorder, or major depressive disorder, recurrent)

A. There has been a regular temporal relationship between the onset of major depressive episodes in bipolar I or bipolar II disorder or major depressive disorder, recurrent, and a particular time of the year (e.g., regular appearance of the major depressive episode in the fall or winter).   **Note:** Do not include cases in which there is an obvious effect of seasonal-related psychosocial stressors (e.g., regularly being unemployed every winter).

B. Full remissions (or a change from depression to mania or hypomania) also occur at a characteristic time of the year (e.g., depression disappears in the spring).

C. In the last 2 years, two major depressive episodes have occurred that demonstrate the temporal seasonal relationships defined in Criteria A and B, and no nonseasonal major depressive episodes have occurred during that same period.

D. Seasonal major depressive episodes (as described above) substantially outnumber the nonseasonal major depressive episodes that may have occurred over the individual's lifetime.

Collateral informants may offer insight into whether mood has been irritable, with interactions characterized by friction and disagreement out of keeping with usual relating. DSM-IV-TR specifies that mood disturbance may be present for only a short time—1 week, or a shorter duration if the person requires hospitalization.

### Cognitive, Neurovegetative, and Behavioral Symptoms

Cognitive disturbance in mania includes the nature and content of thinking. The problem of distractibility is listed as a diagnostic criterion in DSM-IV-TR. This phenomenon may be the result of excessive thought flow or a primary disturbance of information processing and attention. Impairments in memory, executive function, judgment, and visuospatial integration are also frequently encountered (Osuji and Cullum 2005).

Neurovegetative symptoms are usual in mania. Sleep disturbance is characterized by a decreased need for sleep.

Libido and appetite are both often increased. Two types of behavior problems in mania may occur: increase in goal-directed behavior and behavior with potential for harm. In some cases, goal-directed behavior leads to increased productivity, increased self-esteem, and even an increase in earnings. This can hinder the patient's insight into the behavior as being abnormal. Harmful behaviors may include excessive spending, gambling, sexual promiscuity, traveling, drug use, or other risk-taking behavior.

### Duration, Intensity, and Specifiers

Determining the duration of elevated mood episodes is key to establishing diagnosis. Short-lived episodes may reflect cyclothymic disturbance or rapid cycling, whereas longer episodes may result from treatment resistance or ongoing substance abuse. A life chart may be useful in depicting the nature and extent of mood episodes. Other specifiers include whether the episode was single or recurrent, whether it was postpartum in onset, and whether it was associated with psychosis.

## Bipolar I Disorder

### Diagnostic Criteria

The diagnostic criteria for bipolar I disorder are listed in Table 18–8. The presence of any past or present manic episode is sufficient to meet criteria. The diagnosis of bipolar disorder should be considered in any patient who presents with depressive symptoms. Certain features may suggest bipolarity: earlier age at onset of symptoms, family history of bipolarity, and presence of atypical depressive symptoms (Perlis et al. 2006).

### Single Versus Recurrent Manic Episodes

The recurrence of mania requires a careful reevaluation of contributory factors, such as substance use, poor medication adherence, psychosocial stressors, and medical problems. In addition, a diagnosis of rapid-cycling bipolar disorder should be considered; this diagnosis requires the presence of at least four discrete mood episodes in a 12-month period.

## Other Bipolar Disorders

### Bipolar II Disorder

A diagnosis of bipolar II disorder requires the presence of hypomanic and major depressive episodes (Table 18–9). It is most usual for patients to present with severe depression.

---

**TABLE 18-4.** **DSM-IV-TR research criteria for premenstrual dysphoric disorder**

A. In most menstrual cycles during the past year, five (or more) of the following symptoms were present for most of the time during the last week of the luteal phase, began to remit within a few days after the onset of the follicular phase, and were absent in the week postmenses, with at least one of the symptoms being either (1), (2), (3), or (4):

   (1) markedly depressed mood, feelings of hopelessness, or self-deprecating thoughts

   (2) marked anxiety, tension, feelings of being "keyed up" or "on edge"

   (3) marked affective lability (e.g., feeling suddenly sad or tearful or increased sensitivity to rejection)

   (4) persistent and marked anger or irritability or increased interpersonal conflicts

   (5) decreased interest in usual activities (e.g., work, school, friends, hobbies)

   (6) subjective sense of difficulty in concentrating

   (7) lethargy, easy fatigability, or marked lack of energy

   (8) marked change in appetite, overeating, or specific food cravings

   (9) hypersomnia or insomnia

  (10) a subjective sense of being overwhelmed or out of control

  (11) other physical symptoms, such as breast tenderness or swelling, headaches, joint or muscle pain, a sensation of "bloating," weight gain

**Note:** In menstruating females, the luteal phase corresponds to the period between ovulation and the onset of menses, and the follicular phase begins with menses. In nonmenstruating females (e.g., those who have had a hysterectomy), the timing of luteal and follicular phases may require measurement of circulating reproductive hormones.

B. The disturbance markedly interferes with work or school or with usual social activities and relationships with others (e.g., avoidance of social activities, decreased productivity and efficiency at work or school).

C. The disturbance is not merely an exacerbation of the symptoms of another disorder, such as major depressive disorder, panic disorder, dysthymic disorder, or a personality disorder (although it may be superimposed on any of these disorders).

D. Criteria A, B, and C must be confirmed by prospective daily ratings during at least two consecutive symptomatic cycles. (The diagnosis may be made provisionally prior to this confirmation.)

---

### *Cyclothymia*

Cyclothymia is characterized by a 2-year history of changing mood, with both depressive and hypomanic symptoms (Table 18–10). It occurs in about 0.5% of the general population (Weissman and Myers 1978). Some will later develop manic episodes (6%), and a quarter will go on to develop major depression (Akiskal et al. 1979).

## Differential Diagnosis of Bipolar Disorders

### *Medical Disorders*

The emergence of mania or hypomania in the presence of a medical disorder may result from the disorder itself or the associated treatment (Table 18–11). The emergence of a manic episode in an individual older than 35 years should raise the level of suspicion for an underlying medical cause (Larson and Richelson 1988).

### *Mania Secondary to Substance Use*

The use of substances early in the course of bipolar disorder is common (Table 18–12).

## Comorbidity of Mood Disorders

### *Anxiety Disorders*

Nearly 50% of individuals with depression will develop a lifetime anxiety disorder (de Graaf et al. 2003), and anxiety disorders are also commonly comorbid with bipolar disorders (M.P. Freeman et al. 2002).

The association between mania and anxiety also may be heterogeneous in nature. When an anxious individual has used substances as self-medication for the condition, a manic state may be induced.

**TABLE 18–5.   Some medical conditions that may cause depression**

**Neurological disorders**

Epilepsies

Parkinson's disease

Multiple sclerosis

Alzheimer's disease

Cerebrovascular disease

**Infectious disorders**

Neurosyphilis

HIV/AIDS

**Cardiac disorders**

Ischemic heart disease

Cardiac failure

Cardiomyopathies

**Endocrine and metabolic disorders**

Hypothyroidism

Diabetes mellitus

Vitamin deficiencies

Parathyroid disorders

**Inflammatory disorders**

Collagen-vascular diseases

Irritable bowel syndrome

Chronic liver disorders

**Neoplastic disorders**

Central nervous system tumors

Paraneoplastic syndromes

**TABLE 18–6.   Some substances and medications that may cause depression**

**Central nervous system depressants**

Alcohol

Barbiturates

Benzodiazepines

Clonidine

**Central nervous system medications**

Amantadine

Bromocriptine

Levodopa

Phenothiazines

Phenytoin

**Psychostimulants**

Amphetamines

**Systemic medications**

Corticosteroids

Digoxin

Diltiazem

Enalapril

Ethionamide

Isotretinoin

Mefloquine

Methyldopa

Metoclopramide

Quinolones

Reserpine

Statins

Thiazides

Vincristine

## Schizophrenia

The presence of mood disorders in the context of schizophrenia is important. The coexistence of depression significantly increases the risk of suicide, with rates of up to 10%. When a major mood disturbance has been present throughout the psychosis, then a mood disorder with psychotic features must be diagnosed. If the patient has had a short (2-week) period of psychosis in the absence of mood symptoms within this disturbance, then DSM-IV-TR schizoaffective disorder should be diagnosed. Other clinical symptoms that may assist in differentiating mood disorders with psychotic features from schizophrenia include bizarreness of delusions and severe thought disorder in schizophrenia and mood congruency of delusions and hallucinations in mood disorders.

## Personality Disorders

Personality disorders are commonly associated with mood disorders. Indeed, Cluster B personality disorders, particularly borderline personality disorder, may be characterized by a core disturbance in affect, with both decreased and elevated mood at times. In Cluster A and C personalities, depression may be more common than mania.

| | |
|---|---|

**TABLE 18–7.  DSM-IV-TR diagnostic criteria for manic episode**

A.  A distinct period of abnormally and persistently elevated, expansive, or irritable mood, lasting at least 1 week (or any duration if hospitalization is necessary).

B.  During the period of mood disturbance, three (or more) of the following symptoms have persisted (four if the mood is only irritable) and have been present to a significant degree:

(1)  inflated self-esteem or grandiosity

(2)  decreased need for sleep (e.g., feels rested after only 3 hours of sleep)

(3)  more talkative than usual or pressure to keep talking

(4)  flight of ideas or subjective experience that thoughts are racing

(5)  distractibility (i.e., attention too easily drawn to unimportant or irrelevant external stimuli)

(6)  increase in goal-directed activity (either socially, at work or school, or sexually) or psychomotor agitation

(7)  excessive involvement in pleasurable activities that have a high potential for painful consequences (e.g., engaging in unrestrained buying sprees, sexual indiscretions, or foolish business investments)

C.  The symptoms do not meet criteria for a mixed episode.

D.  The mood disturbance is sufficiently severe to cause marked impairment in occupational functioning or in usual social activities or relationships with others, or to necessitate hospitalization to prevent harm to self or others, or there are psychotic features.

E.  The symptoms are not due to the direct physiological effects of a substance (e.g., a drug of abuse, a medication, or other treatment) or a general medical condition (e.g., hyperthyroidism).

**Note:**  Manic-like episodes that are clearly caused by somatic antidepressant treatment (e.g., medication, electroconvulsive therapy, light therapy) should not count toward a diagnosis of bipolar I disorder.

# Epidemiology

## Epidemiology of Mood Disorders

### Current and Lifetime Prevalence Rates

Selected studies assessing the current and lifetime prevalence of depression and bipolar disorder in the general population are tabulated (Table 18–13). The 1-year prevalence rates of major depression in these studies range from 2.7% in the Epidemiologic Catchment Area (ECA) study to 10.3% in the National Comorbidity Survey (NCS). The lifetime prevalence rates for the same disorder range from 7.8% to 17.1%.

Fewer data are available for bipolar disorder. The ECA study found a prevalence of bipolar disorder type I of 0.7%. Bijl et al. (1998) reported a 1-year prevalence of 1.1% and a lifetime prevalence of 1.8%. When validation studies used the Structured Clinical Interview for DSM-IV, adjusted rates of 0.9% were found (R.D. Goodwin et al. 2006).

### Sociodemographic Correlates

The mean age at onset of major depression has been found to be in the late 20s: 27.4 years in the ECA study and 29.9 years reported by de Graaf et al. (2003) in the Netherlands Mental Health Survey and Incidence Study (NEMESIS). In the replication of the National Comorbidity Survey (NCS-R), the median age at onset for mood disorders was 30 years (Kessler et al. 2003). People with bipolar disorder tend to develop symptoms in a bimodal distribution from ages 18 to 44 years (Kessler and Walters 1998).

Depression is twice as common in women (Kessler and Walters 1998). This finding emerges only after adolescence; before this period, rates are similar. In contrast, the rates of bipolar disorder among men and women appear to be similar (Kessler et al. 1994).

Kessler et al. (2003) reported that never having been married was associated with a lower rate of depression than having been divorced or widowed. These findings are similar for bipolar disorder. Higher rates of depression in ethnic minorities have been reported, but this effect has been attributed to higher rates of other factors (such as poverty and lack of resources) in these groups. Low socioeconomic status consistently has been shown to be associated with an increased rate of depression (Kessler et al. 1994).

---

**TABLE 18-8.** **DSM-IV-TR diagnostic criteria for bipolar I disorder, single manic episode**

A. Presence of only one manic episode and no past major depressive episodes.

    **Note:** Recurrence is defined as either a change in polarity from depression or an interval of at least 2 months without manic symptoms.

B. The manic episode is not better accounted for by schizoaffective disorder and is not superimposed on schizophrenia, schizophreniform disorder, delusional disorder, or psychotic disorder not otherwise specified.

    *Specify* if:

    **Mixed:** if symptoms meet criteria for a mixed episode

    If the full criteria are currently met for a manic, mixed, or major depressive episode, *specify* its current clinical status and/or features:

    **Mild, moderate, severe without psychotic features/severe with psychotic features**

    **With catatonic features**

    **With postpartum onset**

    If the full criteria are not currently met for a manic, mixed, or major depressive episode, *specify* the current clinical status of the bipolar I disorder or features of the most recent episode:

    **In partial remission, in full remission**

    **With catatonic features**

    **With postpartum onset**

---

## Risk Factors for Mood Disorders

Early childhood trauma and adverse life events are associated with an increased risk for developing depression, particularly severe types. Other types of trauma, such as loss of a parent, also have been associated with the development of depression. Some evidence indicates that other types of trauma, such as neglect, predispose to anxiety and other disorders rather than depression (Brown and Eales 1993). In adulthood, the presence of a negative life event has been shown consistently to be a risk factor for major depression. The categories of loss and humiliation appear to predict the onset of depression (Kendler et al. 2003), whereas entrapment and danger may precede anxiety problems.

The risk of developing major depression is significantly higher in relatives of patients with depression. Fur-

thermore, a family history of major depression appears to confer a risk of developing severe, recurrent, and possibly early-onset major depression. Rates of depression among people in the community who have experienced a negative life event are significantly higher in those with a family history (Kendler 1998). Independent of family history, the most consistent sociodemographic risk factor for the development of depression is female gender (R.D. Goodwin et al. 2006).

## Course of Mood Disorders

### *Course of Major Depression*

Current evidence has shown that depression usually begins by age 30 (Oldehinkel et al. 1999). The presence of other conditions, such as anxiety and other depressive disorders, may result in an earlier age at onset (Bittner et al. 2004). Major depression tends to recur—figures range from 72.3% in the NCS (Kessler et al. 1994) to 40%–50% in the NEMESIS (Spijker et al. 2002). Factors that may affect the course of depression include family history, presence of comorbid anxiety, and the age at onset.

### *Course of Bipolar Disorder*

Data have consistently shown that bipolar disorder usually manifests in the early 20s. In retrospective studies, both manic and depressive episodes have been reported to occur between ages 14 and 15 years, suggesting an earlier age at onset than originally thought. Following the development of a first hypomanic or manic episode, bipolar disorder tends to be recurrent (Coryell and Winokur 1992).

# Pathogenesis of Mood Disorders

## Genetics and Inherited Factors

### *Family Studies*

Studies have shown that first-degree relatives of patients who have recurrent unipolar depression have a two- to four-times higher risk of depression compared with control subjects (Gershon et al. 1982; Sullivan and Kendler 2001). Factors that confer a greater degree of heritability (i.e., that yield an increased risk of depression in relatives) are age at onset before 30 years, recurrence, presence of psychotic symptoms, and presence of certain comorbidities (such as panic disorder).

---

**TABLE 18–9.  DSM-IV-TR diagnostic criteria for bipolar II disorder**

A. Presence (or history) of one or more major depressive episodes.

B. Presence (or history) of at least one hypomanic episode.

C. There has never been a manic episode or a mixed episode.

D. The mood symptoms in criteria A and B are not better accounted for by schizoaffective disorder and are not superimposed on schizophrenia, schizophreniform disorder, delusional disorder, or psychotic disorder not otherwise specified.

E. The symptoms cause clinically significant distress or impairment in social, occupational, or other important areas of functioning.

*Specify* current or most recent episode:

**Hypomanic:**  if currently (or most recently) in a hypomanic episode

**Depressed:**  if currently (or most recently) in a major depressive episode

If the full criteria are currently met for a major depressive episode, *specify* its current clinical status and/or features:

**Mild, moderate, severe without psychotic features/severe with psychotic features  Note:** Fifth-digit codes specified on DSM-IV-TR p. 413 cannot be used here because the code for bipolar II disorder already uses the fifth digit.

**Chronic**

**With catatonic features**

**With melancholic features**

**With atypical features**

**With postpartum onset**

If the full criteria are not currently met for a hypomanic or major depressive episode, specify the clinical status of the bipolar II disorder and/or features of the most recent major depressive episode (only if it is the most recent type of mood episode):

**In partial remission, in full remission  Note:**  Fifth-digit codes cannot be used here because the code for bipolar II disorder already uses the fifth digit.

**Chronic**

**With catatonic features**

**With melancholic features**

**With atypical features**

**With postpartum onset**

*Specify:*

**Longitudinal course specifiers (with and without interepisode recovery)**

**With seasonal pattern** (applies only to the pattern of major depressive episodes)

**With rapid cycling**

---

In families of bipolar patients, a spectrum of bipolar and unipolar disorders is found (Baron et al. 1983). These include bipolar I and II disorder, schizoaffective disorder, and recurrent major depression. There does not appear to be a risk of schizophrenia in relatives of bipolar probands. However, first-degree relatives of schizophrenic patients are at increased risk for schizoaffective disorder and recurrent major depression (Gershon 1988).

### Twin Studies

Twin studies of recurrent major depression indicate that heritability is approximately 37%. The effect of the individual environment and the interaction between genes and the said environment probably account for a large portion of the remaining risk. In bipolar disorder, concordances range from 65.1% in monozygotic twins to 14.0% in dizy-

## TABLE 18–10.  DSM-IV-TR diagnostic criteria for cyclothymic disorder

A.  For at least 2 years, the presence of numerous periods with hypomanic symptoms and numerous periods with depressive symptoms that do not meet criteria for a major depressive episode.  **Note:** In children and adolescents, the duration must be at least 1 year.

B.  During the above 2-year period (1 year in children and adolescents), the person has not been without the symptoms in Criterion A for more than 2 months at a time.

C.  No major depressive episode, manic episode, or mixed episode has been present during the first 2 years of the disturbance.

   **Note:**  After the initial 2 years (1 year in children and adolescents) of cyclothymic disorder, there may be superimposed manic or mixed episodes (in which case both bipolar I disorder and cyclothymic disorder may be diagnosed) or major depressive episodes (in which case both bipolar II disorder and cyclothymic disorder may be diagnosed).

D.  The symptoms in Criterion A are not better accounted for by schizoaffective disorder and are not superimposed on schizophrenia, schizophreniform disorder, delusional disorder, or psychotic disorder not otherwise specified.

E.  The symptoms are not due to the direct physiological effects of a substance (e.g., a drug of abuse, a medication) or a general medical condition (e.g., hyperthyroidism).

F.  The symptoms cause clinically significant distress or impairment in social, occupational, or other important areas of functioning.

## TABLE 18–11.  Some conditions that may cause mania

**Neurological disorders**
Epilepsies
Traumatic brain injury
Multiple sclerosis
Cerebrovascular disease

**Infectious disorders**
Neurosyphilis
HIV/AIDS

**Neoplastic disorders**
Central nervous system tumors
Paraneoplastic syndromes
Traumatic brain injury

**Endocrine disorders**
Hypo- and hyperthyroidism
Diabetes mellitus
Hypercortisolemia
Vitamin deficiencies

**Inflammatory disorders**
Collagen-vascular diseases

gotic twins. Estimates of heritability of bipolar disorder in monozygotic twins are about 80% (McGuffin et al. 2003).

### Adoption Studies

The risk of developing bipolar or unipolar disorder was found to be about 31% in adopted relatives of bipolar patients (Mendlewicz and Rainer 1977). This is similar to the risk of 26% seen in first-degree relatives of affected individuals who have not been adopted.

### Molecular Linkage Studies

Molecular linkage genetic studies examine the tendency of two genes to be inherited together in families more fre-

quently than by chance. No major loci have been found, but about 10 minor or susceptibility loci have been identified. In meta-analyses, three areas appear to contribute to the development of bipolar disorder: 13q32, 22q11–13, and the pericentromeric region of 18 (Badner and Gershon 2002; Segurado et al. 2003). Linkage studies of recurrent major depression are less consistent.

### Linkage Disequilibrium Studies

Although not all data are consistent, evidence indicates that people with one or more copies of the short allele of the serotonin transporter (5-HTT) promoter polymorphism are more likely to develop depression or suicidality if they experience stressful life events.

## Neurochemistry

### Serotonin System

Serotonin (5-hydroxytryptamine [5-HT]) is synthesized from the essential amino acid tryptophan. Serotonin is metabolized by monoamine oxidase (MAO) to 5-hydroxyindoleacetic acid (5-HIAA). Synaptic serotonin is trans-

**TABLE 18–12.  Some substances and medications that may cause mania**

Central nervous system depressants

Alcohol

Psychostimulants

Amphetamines

Cocaine

Methylphenidate

Pseudoephedrine

Central nervous system medications

Amantadine

Antidepressants

Baclofen

Bromocriptine

Systemic medications

Anabolic steroids

Chloroquine

Corticosteroids

Dapsone

Isoniazid

Metoclopramide

Theophylline

ported back into the neuron by a reuptake pump. Descending serotonergic projections innervate the spinal cord to modulate pain, whereas ascending fibers project to the limbic system and thalamus. The 5-HT$_2$, 5-HT$_4$, 5-HT$_6$, and 5-HT$_{2C}$ receptors appear to be particularly significant in mood disorders. Most of these are found presynaptically, but some are located postsynaptically. Serotonin has an important modulatory effect on dopamine (DA), mainly in the mesolimbic region (Di Matteo et al. 2001). Functions of the serotonin system in the brain include regulating neurovegetative functions, such as sleep, pain sensitivity, sexual function, and appetite (Maes and Meltzer 1995).

**Genetics.**  Functional variants in the 5-HTT promoter region have been isolated. The so-called short allele of one of the key variants may predispose to depression when environmental stressors are experienced (Caspi et al. 2003).

**Biochemistry.**  Decreased 5-HIAA in the cerebrospinal fluid (CSF) is associated with aggression, impulsivity, and violent suicide (Asberg et al. 1976).

**Challenge tests.**  The release of serotonin facilitates the release of prolactin and corticotrophin. A blunted release of prolactin in response to intravenous tryptophan or clomipramine has been shown to occur in depression (Delgado et al. 1992). Compounds that deplete serotonin or tryptophan are likely to produce depression.

**Postmortem findings.**  5-HTT density has been found to be low in frontal cortex, hippocampus, and occipital cortex. Other postmortem findings include reductions in the 5-HT$_{1A}$ receptors in the dorsal and median raphe (Arango et al. 2001).

### Norepinephrine System

Norepinephrine (NE) or noradrenaline is synthesized from tyrosine via phenylalanine and DA in neuronal vesicles. NE is released into the synapse in a calcium-dependent process. Removal of released NE is by reuptake pumps for either NE or DA (into dopaminergic neurons) (Torres et al. 2003). NE then may be either reused in vesicles or metabolized by MAO into 3-methoxy-4-hydroxymandelic acid. NE neurons originate from several brain-stem nuclei, including the locus coeruleus (Grant and Redmond 1981), and project to fore- and midbrain, cerebellum, and lumbar spinal cord. The effects of NE are modulated in the postsynaptic neuron by metabotropic G protein–linked receptors. These include β$_1$- and β$_2$-adrenergic receptors (stimulatory) and α$_1$-, α$_{2A}$-, α$_{2B}$-, and α$_{2C}$-adrenergic types (Bylund 1988). The NE system is responsible for modulating behavior and attention, together with the prefrontal cortex. Firing of the locus coeruleus is stimulated by certain stressful situations. Together with the amygdala, NE neurons impart an emotional component to memory (Cahill et al. 2001). This may improve recall of emotionally charged material, but it also may provoke inappropriate memory cueing.

**Biochemistry.**  Investigation of CSF, plasma, and urine for NE and its metabolites in depression has not identified specific correlates of depression.

**Challenge tests.**  The daily use of α-methyl-*p*-tyrosine (AMPT) in depressed patients who are taking an adrenergic antidepressant is likely to produce a return of depressive symptoms (Delgado et al. 1993).

### Dopamine System

DA is synthesized in DA neurons from tyrosine, via two enzymatic steps. Synaptic DA is taken up by both NE and DA reuptake pumps (Torres et al. 2003). DA neurons

**TABLE 18–13. Studies of current and lifetime prevalence of mood disorders**

| Study | Authors | Time frame | Site | N | Instrument | Age (years) | Total | Major depression | Bipolar disorder |
|---|---|---|---|---|---|---|---|---|---|
| ECA | Weissman et al. 1991 | 1 year | United States | 18,572 | DIS | >18 | 3.7 | 2.7 | 0.7 (bipolar I) |
| | | Lifetime | | | | | 7.8 | | |
| NCS | Kessler et al. 1994 | 1 year | United States | 8,098 | CIDI | 15–54 | 11.3 | 10.3 | |
| | | Lifetime | | | | | 19.3 | 17.1 | |
| NEMESIS | Bijl et al. 1998 | 1 year | Netherlands | 7,076 | CIDI | 18–64 | 7.6 | 5.8 | 1.1 |
| | | Lifetime | | | | | 19 | 15.4 | 1.8 |
| ODIN | Ayuso-Mateos et al. 2001 | Point | Europe | 8,764 | SCAN | 18–64 | | 6.6 | |
| ANMHS | Andrews et al. 2001 | 1 year | Australia | 10,641 | CIDI | >18 | | 6.3 | |
| NCS-R | Kessler et al. 2003 | 1 year | United States | 9,090 | CIDI | >18 | | 6.6 | |
| | | Lifetime | | | | | | 16.2 | |
| WHO WMHSC | Demyttenaere et al. 2004 | 1 year | Nigeria | 4,985 | WMH-CIDI | >18 | 0.8 | | |
| | | | Japan | 1,663 | WMH-CIDI | >18 | 3.1 | | |

*Note.* ANMHS=Australian National Mental Health Survey; CIDI=Composite International Diagnostic Interview; DIS=Diagnostic Interview Schedule; ECA=Epidemiologic Catchment Area study; NCS=National Comorbidity Survey; NCS-R=National Comorbidity Survey Replication; NEMESIS=Netherlands Mental Health Survey and Incidence Study; ODIN study=European Outcome of Depression International Network study; SCAN=Schedule for Clinical Assessment in Neuropsychiatry; WHO WMHSC=World Health Organization World Mental Health Survey Consortium; WMH-CIDI=World Mental Health CIDI.

project mainly from the ventral mesencephalon or from the pituitary gland. Important tracts include the nigrostriatal, mesolimbic, and mesocortical pathways. DA receptors are grouped into the stimulatory $D_1$-like (including $D_1$ and $D_5$) and the inhibitory $D_2$-like ($D_2$, $D_3$, and $D_4$). The $D_2$-like receptors are found mainly in limbic brain, whereas $D_1$-like receptors are widespread and especially rich in the striatum. The DA projections are involved in modulating higher centers: nigrostriatal fibers affect motor function, mesolimbic fibers (together with the nucleus accumbens) affect reward and motivation, and mesocortical fibers affect memory and attention (Chen and Zhuang 2003).

**Biochemistry.** DA plays a role in reward processing and may be dysregulated in depression (Hasler et al. 2004) and mania. The role of DA in mania has been suggested by the manic illness following DA agonist use (e.g., amphetamine compounds). Similarly, DA releasers may be useful in depression, and DA antagonists are effective in treating mania.

### Neuropeptides in Mood Disorders

Many neuropeptides are cotransmitters; they are located and released together with a neurotransmitter. Neuropeptide release from large vesicles is usually slower than neurotransmitter release (Baraban and Tallent 2004). Reduced levels of somatostatin and neuropeptide Y have been found in the CSF of depressed patients (Heilig and Widerlov 1995).

### Neuroplasticity and Neurotrophic Factors

Reduction in hippocampal volumes and other structures in depression suggests that maladaptive neuroplastic changes occur during depressive episodes (Campbell et al. 2004).

## Psychoneuroendocrinology

### Hypothalamic-Pituitary-Adrenal Axis

Hypothalamic-pituitary-adrenal (HPA) axis stimulation modulates metabolism, reproduction, inflammation, immunity, and hippocampal neurogenesis (Plotsky et al. 1998). A state of reversible depression is induced in more than half of the people with hypercortisolemic conditions, with nearly 10% developing suicidality or psychosis. Conversely, patients with major depression have elevated plasma, CSF, and urine cortisol levels, as well as elevated corticotropin-releasing hormone (CRH). In addition, the

dexamethasone suppression test (DST) (failure to suppress cortisol release) is blunted in depression. The test is 90% sensitive to detecting depression but only 30%–50% specific (Copolov et al. 1989).

### Thyroid Physiology in Depression

Hyperthyroid states are documented to produce emotional lability, irritability, insomnia, anxiety, weight loss, and agitation (Demet et al. 2002). Hypothyroidism typically induces fatigue, memory impairment, irritability, and loss of libido (Chueire et al. 2003). In established depression, approximately a quarter of individuals have thyroid dysfunction—most commonly, an increase in free thyroxine ($T_4$) (Rubin 1989). Hypofunction of the hypothalamic-pituitary-thyroid (HPT) axis has been linked to poor antidepressant response and earlier recurrence (Joffe and Marriott 2000). HPT axis abnormalities also have been reported in rapid-cycling bipolar disorder, although most first-line mood stabilizers decrease thyroid hormone levels (Baumgartner et al. 1995). The addition of thyroid hormone to tricyclic antidepressants (TCAs) may induce remission in some individuals with depression (Joffe 1997) and stabilize some patients with refractory bipolar disorder (Whybrow et al. 1992).

### Hypothalamic-Pituitary-Gonadal Axis

The use of testosterone is controversial—in hypogonadal men, use appears to be associated with improvement in mood (Wang et al. 2004), whereas the effects of replacement in older men seem to be associated with only improvement in sexual function (Gray et al. 2005). Exogenous testosterone does not appear to have direct antidepressant properties (Seidman 2006).

In menopausal women, population-based studies have not shown an increase in major depression (Avis et al. 1997). In menopausal women who have established depression, the HPG axis appears to be abnormal—in the early phases, axis activity is increased (high luteinizing hormone and follicle-stimulating hormone), and in the subsequent phases, activity is decreased (O'Toole and Rubin 1995).

Two neuroendocrine theories have been proposed to explain the higher prevalence of depression in women: 1) estrogen release sensitizes neurotransmitter systems (Steiner et al. 2003), and 2) the cyclical release causes ongoing changes in neurotransmitter systems that make women more vulnerable to depression (Rubinow et al. 2002). In premenopausal women with major depression, the HPG axis appears to be normal (Amsterdam et al.

1995). PMDD occurs during the luteal phase and remits during menses. However, no clear luteal-phase-specific physiological changes have been confirmed (Rubinow et al. 2002). Postpartum depression affects 10% of women and is more likely in those with a prior episode (Rubinow et al. 2002). HPG axis function appears to be normal in this state, whereas the HPA axis may be abnormal. Menopausal women often report irritability, crying, mood lability, fatigue, loss of libido, loss of motivation, and anxiety (Steiner et al. 2003). These symptoms may be a result of changes in and withdrawal from estrogens.

## Cognitive Processing Models of Depression

### *Cognitive Deficits in Depression*

A range of cognitive changes have been described in studies of depression. These include the speed of cognitive processing, impaired attention, and the bias toward negative stimuli (Williams 1997). Memory problems are also seen in depressed individuals. Delayed recall is impaired more than recognition. Immediate recall seems to be relatively spared. Mood-congruent memory—the phenomenon whereby depressed individuals more readily recall memories when they are matched to negative emotional valence—is also affected. People with depression recall more negative memories (Matt et al. 1992).

Kindling and sensitization are important depressive phenomena. In kindling, people with prior depressive episodes are thought to be more likely to carry depressive thoughts and therefore activate subsequent episodes more readily (Post 1992). This theory is supported by evidence that people with recurrent depression develop subsequent episodes despite the absence of a stressor (Kendler et al. 2000).

### *Cognitive Features of Depression*

A common feature of studies of cognition in depression is the bias toward negative information, emotions, and memories. Negative thoughts and beliefs that prevail during depressive episodes are reinforced by underlying structures that have already been defined by previous negative experiences. More specifically, the person will ruminate on negative thoughts and the potential personal negative consequences: a depressed and self-referent bias. This mode of thinking usually is not disrupted by positive or other external stimuli and leads to a closed loop (Teasdale and Barnard 1993). The ability to shift focus from this negative loop may be a key strategy in treatment. The

process whereby the depressed patient accesses negative information from the environment and the inner world could be seen as a selective filter. One strategy in cognitive therapy is to highlight this problem and challenge its use. The individual is then taught to focus on neutral or even positive information.

# Somatic Interventions for Mood Disorders

## Antidepressants

Antidepressants are classified according to their activity at monoamine receptors (Table 18–14).

### *Tricyclics, Tetracyclics, and Monoamine Oxidase Inhibitors*

The TCAs act by reuptake inhibition at both NE and serotonin transporters. This combined effect is probably mediated by active metabolites of the TCAs as much as by primary drug. However, other receptors are also antagonized by the TCAs: adrenergic, histaminergic, muscarinic, and dopaminergic receptors. These produce many of the undesirable side effects. The anticholinergic side effects (dry mouth and constipation), together with hypotension, somnolence, and cardiac arrhythmias, make these medications less widely used. Other side effects include confusion, urinary retention, and blurred vision in the elderly; and increased appetite and weight gain.

Some drug interactions of the TCAs need to be taken into account. Generally, these result from induced or impaired metabolism by the liver microsomal cytochrome P450 system. Care should be taken when any other drug with potential anticholinergic, antiadrenergic, or monoamine inhibition is given. The TCAs generally should be administered in a slow, upward dose titration. The measurement of plasma levels may be indicated in suspected overdose or poor adherence and to establish a minimum effective dose.

The monoamine oxidase inhibitors (MAOIs) act by the inhibition of the presynaptic enzyme MAO. This produces an increase in synaptic concentrations of all monoamines. The two isoforms are MAO-A and MAO-B. The MAOIs are classified according to the degree of reversibility of binding to MAO and by their binding to the respective isoforms. Tranylcypromine and phenelzine are irreversible inhibitors of both isoforms; selegiline is more selective for MAO-B; moclobemide is a reversible inhib-

**TABLE 18–14.  Currently available antidepressants: activity, indications, adverse effects, and dosing**

| Antidepressant | Examples | Primary activity | Indications | Adverse effects | Dosing |
|---|---|---|---|---|---|
| Tricyclic antidepressants (TCAs) | Amitriptyline, desipramine, imipramine | SRI, NRI, Ach-M, Hist, $\alpha_1$ | Major depression, enuresis | Dry mouth, constipation, urinary retention, blurred vision, hypotension, cardiac toxicity, sedation | Commence at 25 mg; increase to 100–200 mg/day |
| Selective serotonin reuptake inhibitors (SSRIs) | Fluoxetine, paroxetine, sertraline | SRI | Major depression, anxiety disorders, impulse-control disorders, bulimia nervosa | Agitation, insomnia, headache, nausea and vomiting, sexual dysfunction, hyponatremia | Usually 20 mg/day (fluoxetine); may increase to 60 mg/day |
| Monoamine oxidase inhibitors (MAOIs) | Tranylcypromine, moclobemide | MAOI | Major depression, social phobia | Hypertensive crises for older agents, insomnia, nausea, agitation, confusion | Moclobemide: 150–600 mg twice daily after food |
| Serotonin-norepinephrine reuptake inhibitors (SNRIs) | Venlafaxine, duloxetine | NRI, SRI | Major depression, generalized anxiety disorder | Hypertension (venlafaxine), nausea, insomnia, dry mouth, sedation, sweating, agitation, headache, sexual dysfunction | Venlafaxine: commence at 75 mg/day; increase to 225 mg/day as needed |
| Norepinephrine-dopamine reuptake inhibitors (NDRIs) | Bupropion | NRI, DRI | Major depression, smoking cessation | Agitation, insomnia, headache, nausea and vomiting, seizures (0.4%) | 150 mg twice daily |
| Serotonin antagonist and reuptake inhibitor (SARI) | Nefazodone | SRI, 5-HT$_2$, $\alpha_1$, NRI | Major depression | Sedation, hepatotoxicity, dizziness, hypotension, paresthesias; priapism (trazodone) | 100–300 mg twice daily |
| Norepinephrine and serotonin specific antidepressant (NASSA) | Mirtazapine | $\alpha_2$, 5-HT$_3$, 5-HT$_{2A}$, 5-HT$_{2C}$, Hist | Major depression | Weight gain, sedation, dizziness, headache; sexual dysfunction is rare | 15–45 mg/day at night |
| Norepinephrine reuptake inhibitor (NRI) | Reboxetine, atomoxetine | NRI | ?Major depression, attention-deficit/hyperactivity disorder | Insomnia, sweating, dizziness, dry mouth, constipation, urinary hesitancy, tachycardia | Reboxetine: 4–6 mg twice daily |

*Note.*  Ach-M=muscarinic anticholinergic; $\alpha_1$=alpha-1 adrenergic blockade; $\alpha_2$=alpha-2 adrenergic blockade; DRI=dopamine reuptake inhibition; Hist=histamine blockade; 5-HT$_2$=serotonin type 2 receptor antagonism; 5-HT$_3$=serotonin type 3 receptor antagonism; 5-HT$_{2A}$=serotonin type 2A receptor antagonism; 5-HT$_{2C}$=serotonin type 2C receptor antagonism; NRI=norepinephrine reuptake inhibition; SRI=serotonin reuptake inhibition.

itor of MAO-A (not available in the United States). The inhibition of MAO-A leads to an increase in NE, which may precipitate a hypertensive crisis. For this reason, a diet free of the precursor tyramine is mandatory in patients taking these drugs. Problems in the use of MAOIs have curtailed their use, but a transdermal preparation of selegiline may offer a novel approach to depression, particularly depression with atypical features. Transdermal selegiline has the advantage over older MAOIs in that it does not irreversibly inhibit gut or liver MAO-A, while binding to both forms of MAO in the brain. This preparation may therefore be better tolerated and provide the therapeutic effects of the MAOIs sought by clinicians (Thase 2006). Other adverse effects of the MAOIs include anticholinergic effects, dizziness, nausea, forgetfulness, and myoclonic jerks. Weight gain, muscle cramps,

sexual dysfunction, and hypoglycemia are late effects. The MAOIs may interact with a range of medications. Prescribers should be particularly aware of any other medications that may increase adrenergic tone or increase serotonin or DA concentrations to dangerous levels. The MAOIs are useful in bipolar depression or atypical depression, but they are not commonly used in view of dietary restrictions and adverse events.

### Selective Serotonin Reuptake Inhibitors

The SSRIs are a group of drugs with similar but not identical effects. They are safer in overdose than are TCAs. Activities and dosing are shown in Table 18–15. In general, antidepressant response rates across studies vary from 60% to 75%.

**TABLE 18–15.** Selective serotonin reuptake inhibitors (SSRIs): activity, prescribing notes, and dosing

| SSRI | Activity | Indications | Notes | Dosing |
|---|---|---|---|---|
| Fluoxetine | SRI, weak NRI and 5-HT$_{2C}$ | Major depression, anxiety disorders, impulse-control disorders, bulimia nervosa | Long half-life (2 weeks), requires long washout before switching; highly protein bound | Usual dose 20 mg/day; increase gradually to 80 mg/day. Start 10 mg in young and old. |
| Paroxetine | SRI, weak ACh, Hist, and NRI | Major depression, panic disorder, generalized anxiety disorder, OCD | Produces sedation and anticholinergic effects; short half-life; discontinuation a problem | Start 20 mg/day; may increase to 60 mg/day |
| Sertraline | SRI, weak NRI and DRI | Major depression, PTSD | | Start 50 mg/day; may increase to 200 mg/day |
| Fluvoxamine | NRI, SRI | OCD, depression | | Start 50 mg/day; may increase to 200 mg/day |
| Citalopram | SRI, NRI (weak) | Major depression, panic disorder, agoraphobia | Low inhibition of cytochrome P450 system; useful when drug interactions may be a problem | Start 20 mg/day; may increase to 60 mg/day |
| Escitalopram | SRI, NRI (weak) | Major depression, panic disorder, agoraphobia | Low inhibition of cytochrome P450 system; useful when drug interactions may be a problem | Start 10 mg/day; may increase to 30 mg/day |

*Note.* ACh=anticholinergic; DRI=dopamine reuptake inhibition; 5-HT$_{2C}$=serotonin type 2C receptor antagonism; Hist=histamine blockade; NRI=norepinephrine reuptake inhibition; OCD=obsessive-compulsive disorder; PTSD=posttraumatic stress disorder; SRI=serotonin reuptake inhibition.

### Serotonin-Norepinephrine Reuptake Inhibitors

Venlafaxine is an inhibitor of serotonin and NE transporters. It is prescribed in the dosage range of 75–225 mg/day. The extended-release preparation may be administered once daily (Gutierrez et al. 2003). Some elevation of blood pressure may be seen at higher doses, and this should be monitored in patients with a history of hypertension. Duloxetine is a more newly introduced serotonin-norepinephrine reuptake inhibitor that is given in dosages ranging from 20 to 80 mg/day.

### Other Antidepressants

Bupropion is an inhibitor of both NE and DA reuptake. It also may facilitate presynaptic release of these monoamines. It may spare depressed individuals from the sexual side effects commonly seen with serotonergic agents. It is regarded as having a lower tendency to induce rapid cycling or to induce mania compared with other antidepressants (Stoll et al. 1994). Bupropion is also approved for the treatment of smoking cessation. Adverse effects include anxiety, agitation, dizziness, and nausea. The risk of seizures may be significantly increased, and bupropion should be used with caution in individuals with any predisposing factors for seizures. Dosages should not exceed 400 mg/day.

Mirtazapine is a novel tetracyclic that antagonizes the NE $\alpha_2$ receptor, as well as the 5-$HT_{2A}$ receptor (norepinephrine and serotonin specific antidepressant) (de Boer et al. 1996). In addition, it blocks 5-$HT_2$ and 5-$HT_3$ receptors, which contribute to anxiolysis. Antihistaminic effects include weight gain and sedation. Patients are given dosages between 15 and 45 mg/day.

## Mood Stabilizers

### Lithium

In acute mania, lithium remains effective across a range of domains of the illness (Hirschfeld et al. 2002). Treatment response usually can be seen within 5–14 days. Some evidence suggests that lithium is most effective when used in classic or euphoric mania or when the patient has had few lifetime episodes (Bowden 1995). In addition, efficacy appears to be accelerated when dose titration is rapid (Keck et al. 2001). Plasma monitoring is essential in lithium treatment. A range of 0.6–1.2 mEq/L is regarded as therapeutic. Levels greater than that may raise the risk of toxicity, with nausea, vomiting, confusion, myoclonus, seizures, hyperreflexia, and coma. Lower levels may increase the risk of relapse. Other adverse effects of lithium treat-ment include tremor, cognitive dulling, nausea, weight gain, and sedation.

In the maintenance phase of bipolar illness, lithium has been shown to reduce the risk of relapse (Burgess et al. 2001). More recent studies have confirmed lithium's effectiveness in this regard but also have shown that most patients require more than one drug to achieve stability (Grof 2003). In one study, the combination of lithium and valproate resulted in a significantly lower rate of relapse, compared with monotherapy (Solomon et al. 1997).

Lithium also has been shown to reduce the risk of suicide independently of its mood-stabilizing properties (Baldessarini et al. 2003). In acute bipolar depression, lithium is superior to placebo, although response is usually partial (Zornberg and Pope 1993). This finding often provokes the concomitant use of antidepressants. As for acute mania, plasma levels of lithium need to be greater than 0.8 mEq/L. In unipolar depression, lithium has proven useful in treatment-refractory cases. Rates of improvement of 56%–96% have been reported (M.P. Freeman et al. 2004).

### Valproate and Carbamazepine

In the late 1980s, valproate (sodium valproate or divalproex) was found to be superior to placebo in the treatment of acute mania (Bowden et al. 1994). Although studies have failed to show differences in efficacy among agents, the presence of depressive symptoms, impulsivity, hyperactivity, and multiple prior episodes may be associated with a better treatment response for valproate than for lithium (T.W. Freeman et al. 1992; Swann et al. 2002). The usual dose of valproate is 20 mg/kg but can be increased to 30 mg/kg. Adverse effects include sedation, tremor, nausea and vomiting, hair loss, and weight gain. Rare problems include hepatotoxicity and pancreatitis.

Carbamazepine has been shown in recent studies to be effective in acute mania (Weisler et al. 2004). Adverse effects of carbamazepine include diplopia, blurred vision, ataxia, sedation, and nausea. Rarer problems such as blood dyscrasias, hepatic failure, pancreatitis, and exfoliative dermatitis have been reported. Small studies have shown some effects of carbamazepine in acute bipolar and unipolar depression, but these were in treatment-refractory cases (Kramlinger and Post 1989). Oxcarbazepine is a similar agent with a lower incidence of side effects, but data on its efficacy are limited.

### Other Anticonvulsants

Several newer anticonvulsants have been studied in bipolar illness, including gabapentin, lamotrigine, and topiramate.

To date, no trials have conclusively shown that any of these agents is effective in acute mania (Keck and McElroy 2006). In maintenance treatment, lamotrigine has been shown to reduce the incidence of depressive episodes but not manic ones (Bowden et al. 2003). Lamotrigine also has proven effective in acute bipolar depression (Calabrese et al. 1999). Adverse effects of lamotrigine include headache, nausea, and xerostomia. The risk of serious (but rare) rash is reduced with careful dose titration.

## Antipsychotic Medications

In the United States, several antipsychotic agents are registered for use in acute mania: olanzapine, risperidone, quetiapine, ziprasidone, aripiprazole, and chlorpromazine. In addition, olanzapine and aripiprazole are approved for the maintenance treatment of bipolar disorder, and olanzapine is approved for acute bipolar depression. Almost all the antipsychotics are useful in acute mania. Likewise, the second-generation agents have been subjected to several controlled trials, and all were found to be effective in acute mania (Strakowski 2003). In addition to being effective primary agents, the second-generation agents seem to increase the rate and degree of antimanic effect when used in combination with a mood stabilizer (Strakowski 2003).

In the maintenance phase, only the medications listed in the previous paragraph are approved in the United States. The first-generation antipsychotics, although widely used in this setting, have not proven effective (Keck et al. 2000). The problem of depression in the long-term course of bipolar disorder has prompted the use of second-generation agents in this phase. To date, olanzapine, aripiprazole, and quetiapine have been studied and have been found to be effective in preventing relapse in bipolar disorder (Marcus et al. 2003; Tohen et al. 2003). In unipolar depression, the first-generation agents have been used chiefly when psychotic symptoms are present. However, effective augmentation of antidepressants in nonpsychotic depression recently has been shown with some of the second-generation agents.

An emerging role for second-generation agents has been found in treatment-resistant depression (Shelton et al. 2001). Risperidone is effective in combination with SSRIs in treatment-resistant unipolar depression. Olanzapine in combination with fluoxetine is safe and effective in patients with bipolar depression and those with fluoxetine-resistant depression. Ziprasidone and aripiprazole augmentation of SSRIs have been reported to be effective in treatment-resistant depression in open-label studies.

# Psychotherapy for Mood Disorders

## Cognitive-Behavioral Therapy: Strategies and Techniques

Cognitive-behavioral therapy (CBT) is essentially a brief, structured, and collaborative therapeutic intervention. A therapy may last from 12 to 20 sessions. Each session is structured to include a period of symptom review, intervention performance, and homework setting. Collaboration requires that the patient appreciate the need to give and receive feedback and that the patient–therapist team tackle assignments in a scientific and interactive manner. As the therapy develops, the patient takes on a greater role and ultimately will manage assignments independently. Psychoeducation is a crucial early component and usually makes use of a personally informed explanation of the condition and the therapy. Compliance with homework is associated with a greater treatment response (Burnes and Spangler 2000). Assignments should be described and performed during sessions and then recorded into a book, which is used as a manual. During assessment and early therapy, a record is made of negative automatic thoughts. The therapist may use some during initial feedback but must soon begin to help the patient recognize them. The goal is to identify these thoughts and then begin to challenge their assumed truth in order to modify them. In a patient's workbook, stressors or situations should be recorded. These should include the patient's associated feelings and negative thoughts. As the patient learns to challenge the thoughts, recorded entries may include weighting of the degree to which he or she believed the thought before and after modification. The Socratic technique offers an approach to challenge negative thoughts by means of reasoned inquiry (Beck et al. 1979). The therapist may go on to assist the patient in constructing a case for and a case against these thoughts. An opportunity to provide a reasonable alternative to the negative thought may then follow. For some, the use of imagery or role-playing may better elicit negative automatic thoughts and allow the therapist to analyze and challenge them.

As the therapy progresses, a pattern of thinking may emerge that belies a series of underlying themes. In the same way, these formative beliefs can be challenged. In some instances, they may be related to early experiences. The linking of a current belief system to a past experience may allow a patient to understand the source of negative feelings and thoughts. The introduction of behavioral techniques is particularly important when behavioral inactivation is present (Rehm 1977). Strategies aimed at improving a sense of competence through mastery by offering a series of graded exercises may be included. Similarly, depressed patients have reduced hedonic capacity, and the guided introduction of pleasurable activities may break a negative behavioral cycle. These behavioral tasks should be included in the patient's workbook and feedback about tasks sought at each session.

## Interpersonal Psychotherapy

### Theory

Interpersonal therapy (IPT) has its roots in the attachment theory of Bowlby. Building on this approach, the interpersonal theorists noted that social events may be protective and also destructive, if negative in nature. Klerman et al. (1984) described interpersonal events in the social world as complicated bereavement, role disputes (relationship difficulties), role transitions (a loss of any kind), and interpersonal deficits (when social isolation is encountered). These events, when identified by the therapist, form the content of IPT. They need not be causative, merely proximal to the condition. IPT differs from CBT in that it does not make use of homework assignments and differs from psychodynamic therapy in that the therapeutic relationship is not a focus of therapy. IPT has a wide range of indications within mood disorders, all of which have a strong evidence base. IPT has been shown to reduce depressive symptoms in several different settings of major depression, including acute and recurrent major depression (Frank et al. 1990), depression in adolescents and elderly persons (Mufson et al. 1999), depression associated with HIV (Markowitz et al. 1998), depression in primary care (Schulberg et al. 1996), and dysthymia (Markowitz 2003).

### Technique

IPT is a brief, structured, and collaborative therapy that usually lasts between 12 and 20 sessions. It is conventionally separated into early, middle, and termination phases. Central to the early phase are psychiatric assessment and formulation, which take changes in the interpersonal world into account. A clear diagnosis is made, followed by feedback and psychoeducation. The focus is always on depression being a medical condition that is not the patient's fault. The analysis of the patient's interpersonal world is discussed, taking into account recent changes, patient expectations, and relationships that are proximal to the current depressive episode. In the middle phase, the therapist uses the selected interpersonal focus area (see "Interper-

sonal Therapy Theory" earlier in this section) and applies strategies to address it. These may include examining the patient's expectations of the relationship, exploring options in relationships, and role-playing to practice tactics. Each session brings current relationship experiences to the fore. During termination, the patient's competencies are reinforced, and an approach to identifying future depressive triggers is explored. IPT continues to be explored as an effective therapy for various psychiatric conditions.

## Psychodynamic Psychotherapy: Psychodynamic and Psychoanalytic Approach to Depression

In psychodynamic therapy for the treatment of depression, the therapist must listen carefully to experiences and themes that may have developed into depression. These may include ideas that the patient has internalized anger, has an overdeveloped superego or sense of responsibility, or feels helpless and dependent. Out of these thoughts and feelings, a range of defense mechanisms may have evolved. These include repression, denial, projection, and reaction formation. During the patient's account, patterns of relating may emerge. A core relationship theme may become prominent (Luborsky 1984). This conflict usually will repeat itself within the therapeutic relationship. This affords the therapist the opportunity to understand the patient's contribution to the conflict and a means by which to point out maladaptive defenses. The transference must be understood and brought into the therapy. The termination of psychodynamic therapy inevitably evokes earlier feelings of loss, and the therapist must deal with the unconscious sense of responsibility and anger.

## Psychotherapy for Bipolar Disorder

Psychotherapy for bipolar disorder has lagged behind pharmacotherapy, partly because of the pronounced effects that medication alone has on many aspects of the condition. In the past, psychotherapies focused mainly on the depressive episodes and psychological consequences of bipolar disorder. The manic patient's absence of insight and lack of motivation to understand precluded benefit from psychodynamic therapy.

### Psychoeducation

A brief, focused psychoeducational therapy aimed at remitted patients with bipolar disorder is effective in reducing relapse rates (Perry et al. 1999). A psychoeducational program should include education about the illness and medication, training in recognition of the signs of early relapse, information about the value of seeking help, and promotion of regular sleep–wake cycles.

### Cognitive-Behavioral Therapy

CBT for bipolar disorder has made use of mood diaries, examination of negative thoughts about the illness, and addressing of barriers to treatment adherence. When this type of CBT was added to routine care, the CBT group had fewer bipolar episodes, reduced episode duration, and reduced hospitalizations (Lam et al. 2003). CBT appears to have a greater advantage for depressive episodes than for manic episodes (Scott et al. 2001).

### Family Therapy

Family therapy for bipolar disorder has been developed as a family-focused therapy. This therapy, offered as 21 sessions over 9 months, makes use of psychoeducation, communication skills, and problem-solving skills (Miklowitz and Hooley 1998).

### Interpersonal and Social Rhythm Therapy

The utility of IPT has been studied in bipolar disorder, and some data support its efficacy. In particular, IPT and social rhythm therapy have been integrated. The combined therapy makes use of the following principles: identifying and managing affective symptoms, linking mood and life events, maintaining regular daily rhythms, linking interpersonal factors to rhythm dysregulation, and mourning the lost healthy self (Frank et al. 2000).

## Integrative Management of Mood Disorders

### Major Depressive Disorder

#### Treatment Guidelines in Major Depression

Practice guidelines for the treatment of major depression include those published by the American Psychiatric Association (2000b). The Texas Medication Algorithm Project (Crismon et al. 1999), the Sequenced Treatment Alternatives to Relieve Depression (STAR*D) study (Fava et al. 2003), and the National Institute of Clinical Excellence (www.nice.org.uk/page.aspx?o=mental) have all provided algorithms for the treatment of depression. The Texas Medication Algorithm Project strategies for the treatment of nonpsychotic major depression are shown in Figure 18–2 (Trivedi et al. 2004).

Because no consistent evidence distinguishes between initial monotherapies at this time, a selection strategy might rather use other guides, such as a previously effective agent for that person or a first-degree relative or an agent with effectiveness for a comorbid condition. The goal of treatment is to achieve remission (absence of symptoms) rather than merely response (reduction of at least 50% of symptoms).

The duration of a first treatment trial is often debated. A response should be seen by 10 weeks. When response is partial, an augmentation or a combination strategy may be used. Fair evidence for lithium, thyroid hormone, and buspirone exists in this regard, and some of the atypical antipsychotics are showing promise as augmenting agents in major depression (Ostroff and Nelson 1999; Shelton et al. 2001). Augmentation should result in response from 4 weeks. If response is adequate, then the strategy should be continued for 4–9 months.

### Combined Medication and Psychotherapeutic Approaches

There is empirical evidence for the effectiveness of CBT, IPT, and a cognitive-behavioral analysis system of psychotherapy in the treatment of depression. The combination of medication and psychotherapy is indicated in chronic depressive conditions (Keller et al. 2000). Psychotherapy, particularly a cognitive-behavioral analysis system of psychotherapy, may be considered at stage 1 of the treatment algorithm shown in Figure 18–2 if an individual with chronic depression presents for treatment (Schatzberg et al. 2005). Evidence indicates that individuals with chronic depression and a history of parental loss or abuse in childhood may respond well to psychotherapy (Nemeroff 2003).

### Medication Combination and Augmentation

To date, the most evidence on medication combination exists for a combination of TCA and SSRI, but other combinations are used. The evidence is good for the addition of lithium and thyroid hormone and fair for the use of tryptophan (Fava et al. 1994; Joffe and Singer 1990; S. Smith 1998). Other strategies include using ECT (see stage 6 of the depression treatment algorithm in Figure 18–2) and high-dose venlafaxine (D. Smith et al. 2002).

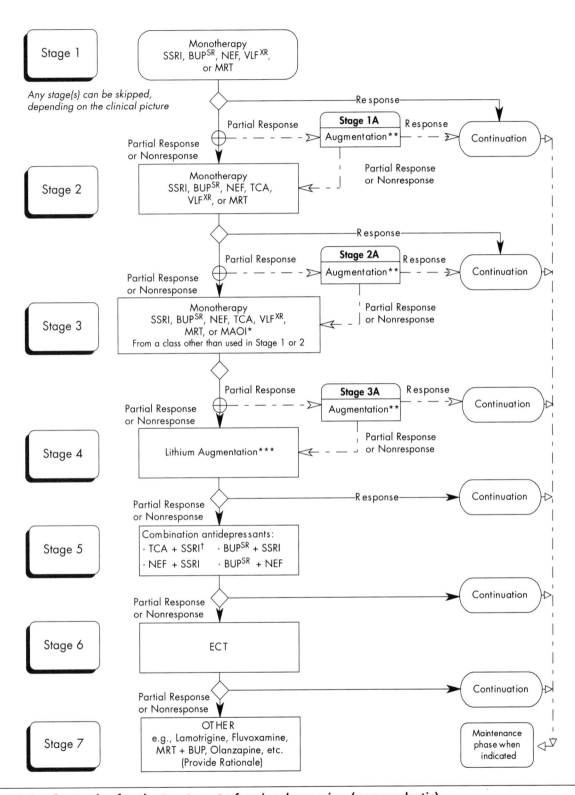

**FIGURE 18–2.** **Strategies for the treatment of major depression (nonpsychotic).**

*Note.* BUP^SR = bupropion sustained release; ECT = electroconvulsive therapy; MAOI = monoamine oxidase inhibitor; MRT = mirtazapine; NEF = nefazodone; SSRI = selective serotonin reuptake inhibitor (fluoxetine, sertraline, paroxetine, citalopram); TCA = tricyclic antidepressant; VLF^XR = venlafaxine extended release.

*Consider TCA/VLF if not tried. **Lithium, thyroid, buspirone. ***Skip if lithium augmentation has already failed. †Most studied combination.

*Source.* Trivedi et al. 2004. Algorithms are revised as new data become available; consult the Texas Implementation of Medication Algorithms (TIMA) Web site (http://www.dshs.state.tx.us/mhprograms/TIMA.shtm) for the most recent versions.

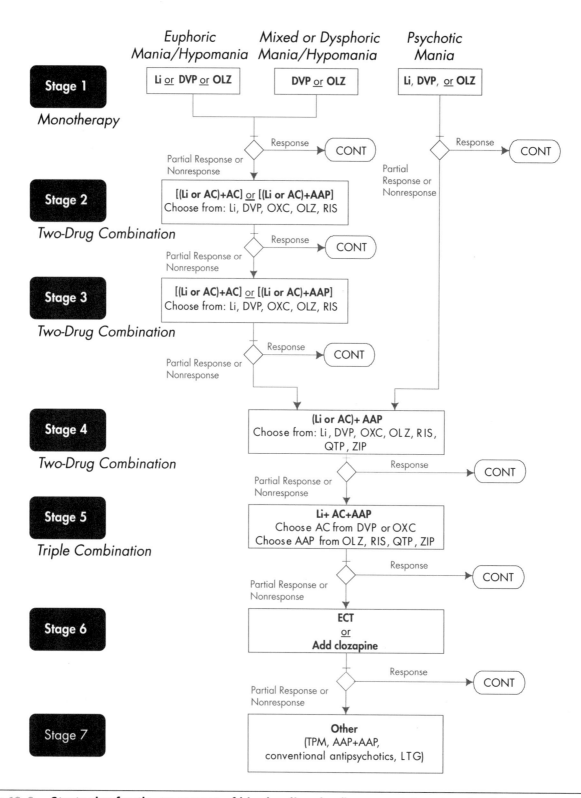

**FIGURE 18–3.    Strategies for the treatment of bipolar disorder (hypomanic/manic episode).**

*Note.*    AAP=atypical antipsychotic; AC=anticonvulsant; CONT=continuation treatment; DVP=divalproex; ECT = electroconvulsive therapy; Li=lithium; LTG=lamotrigine; OLZ=olanzapine; OXC=oxcarbazepine; QTP=quetiapine; RIS=risperidone; TPM=topiramate; VPA=valproate; ZIP=ziprasidone.

*Source.*    Suppes et al. 2001. Algorithms are revised as new data become available; consult the Texas Implementation of Medication Algorithms (TIMA) Web site (http://www.dshs.state.tx.us/mhprograms/TIMA.shtm) for the most recent versions.

## Bipolar Disorder

An integrative approach demands that the clinician appreciate the longitudinal course of the illness, the tendency of the illness to recur, and the prominence of depressive episodes. It is useful to understand the management of bipolar disorder from acute-episode and maintenance-phase perspectives.

### Treatment Guidelines in Bipolar Disorder

Currently available guidelines include the practice guideline for the treatment of patients with bipolar disorder published by the American Psychiatric Association (2002), the guidelines published by the British Association for Psychopharmacology (G.M. Goodwin et al. 2003), and the Texas Medication Algorithm Project treatment algorithm for patients with bipolar disorder (Suppes et al. 2001). The Texas Medication Algorithm Project treatment strategies for hypomania/mania in bipolar disorder are presented in Figure 18–3. In addition, the prescriber must take into account whether the patient's symptoms have previously responded to an agent, whether rapid cycling is present (use an anticonvulsant), and whether psychotic symptoms are present. The recommended duration of a trial of monotherapy is unclear. A response should be noted by 7–14 days, but remission may take considerably longer. Guidelines for the maintenance phase of the illness are less clear. Common practice and consensus suggest that most clinicians will continue the mood stabilizer that the patient's symptoms responded to in the acute phase and will discontinue any antipsychotics that were used (Bowden et al. 2000).

In acute bipolar depression, the use of antidepressants alone generally should be avoided because of the risk of inducing rapid cycling. Fair evidence indicates that the prescriber should select one of three treatment strategies: lithium, lamotrigine, or a fluoxetine–olanzapine combination. If the episode is severe, combinations of mood stabilizers, ECT, or an antidepressant–mood stabilizer combination may be used. In all cases, thyroid abnormalities and comorbid substance abuse should be ruled out. In the maintenance phase of bipolar depression, there is good evidence for the effectiveness of lamotrigine when depressive episodes are recurrent (Bowden et al. 2003) and for lithium when both manic and depressive episodes recur (Prien et al. 1984). Long-term antidepressant use is associated with a higher risk of recurrence of mania.

### Treatment of Bipolar Disorder in Women of Childbearing Age

The clinician must pay special attention to a broad range of needs in women of childbearing age. It is best for women to plan pregnancies to allow for the possible withdrawal of mood stabilizers. In all instances, the clinician must make treatment decisions on the basis of benefits and risks to the fetus. All mood stabilizers are potentially teratogenic, and some may be harmful during lactation (American Psychiatric Association 2002). If drug therapy is considered essential, several strategies may be used to reduce risk to the fetus: using monotherapy at the lowest effective dose, using concomitant folate therapy, and avoiding medication during the first trimester of pregnancy (Iqbal et al. 2001).

## Key Points: Mood Disorders

- The causes of depression are multifactorial and usually include genetic and environmental contributions.
- Bipolar disorders can be difficult to diagnose because of the inability to detect past and future episodes.
- The clinical features of depression across cultures may vary, including expressions such as loneliness and somatic complaints.
- Major depression is common, with a lifetime prevalence of about 10%. It also causes about twice as much disability as any other medical condition.
- Major depression is a chronic and recurring illness, with relapses occurring in at least half of patients.
- Treatment of major depression consists of selecting an appropriate antidepressant and giving consideration to an effective psychotherapy.
- Bipolar disorders should be treated with mood stabilizers first, with the addition of other agents if response is unsatisfactory.

## Suggested Readings

Butler A, Chapman J, Forman E, et al: The empirical status of cognitive-behavioral therapy: a review of meta-analyses. Clin Psychol Rev 26:17–31, 2006

Caspi A, Sugden K, Moffitt T, et al: Influence of life stress on depression: moderation by a polymorphism in the 5HTT gene. Science 301:386–389, 2003

Fava M, Rush AJ, Trivedi M, et al; for the STAR*D Investigators Group: Background and rationale for the Sequenced Treatment Alternatives to Relieve Depression (STAR*D) study. Psychiatr Clin North Am 26:457–494, 2003

Kessler RC, Berglund P, Demler O, et al: The epidemiology of major depressive disorder: results from the National Comorbidity Survey Replication (NCS-R). JAMA 289:3095–3105, 2003

Manji H, Drevets W, Charney D: The cellular neurobiology of depression. Nat Med 5:541–547, 2001

Stein DJ, Kupfer DJ, Schatzberg AF (eds): The American Psychiatric Publishing Textbook of Mood Disorders. Washington, DC, American Psychiatric Publishing, 2006

## Online Resources

American Psychiatric Association Practice Guidelines (http://www.psych.org/psych_pract/treatg/pg/prac_guide.cfm)

National Comorbidity Survey (http://www.hcp.med.harvard.edu/ncs/ncs_data.php)

National Institute of Clinical Excellence, UK (http://www.nice.org.uk/guidance/index.jsp?action=byTopic&o=7281&set=true)

Texas Medication Algorithm Project (http://www.dshs.state.tx.us/mhprograms/TMAPover.shtm)

## References

Akiskal HS, Rosenthal RH, Rosenthal TL, et al: Differentiation of primary affective illness from situational, symptomatic, and secondary depressions. Arch Gen Psychiatry 36:635–643, 1979

American Psychiatric Association: Diagnostic and Statistical Manual of Mental Disorders, 4th Edition, Text Revision. Washington, DC, American Psychiatric Association, 2000a

American Psychiatric Association: Practice Guideline for the Treatment of Patients With Major Depressive Disorder, 2nd Edition. Washington, DC, American Psychiatric Association, 2000b

American Psychiatric Association: Practice guideline for the treatment of patients with bipolar disorder (revision). Am J Psychiatry 159 (4 suppl):1–50, 2002

Amsterdam JD, Maislin G, Rosenzweig M, et al: Gonadotropin (LH and FSH) response after submaximal GnRH stimulation in depressed premenopausal women and healthy controls. Psychoneuroendocrinology 20:311–321, 1995

Andrews G, Henderson S, Hall W: Prevalence, comorbidity, disability and service utilisation: overview of the Australian National Mental Health Survey. Br J Psychiatry 178:145–153, 2001

Arango V, Underwood MD, Boldrini M, et al: Serotonin 1A receptors, serotonin transporter binding and serotonin transporter mRNA expression in the brainstem of depressed suicide victims. Neuropsychopharmacology 25:892–903, 2001

Asberg M, Traskman L, Thoren P: 5-HIAA in the cerebrospinal fluid: a biochemical suicide predictor? Arch Gen Psychiatry 33:1193–1197, 1976

Avis NE, Crawford SL, McKinlay SM: Psychosocial, behavioral, and health factors related to menopause symptomatology. Womens Health 3:103–120, 1997

Ayuso-Mateos JL, Vasques-Barquero JL, Dowrick C, et al: Depressive disorders in Europe: prevalence figures from the ODIN study. Br J Psychiatry 179:308–316, 2001

Badner JA, Gershon ES: Meta-analysis of whole-genome linkage scans of bipolar disorder and schizophrenia. Mol Psychiatry 7:405–411, 2002

Baldessarini RJ, Tondo L, Hennen J: Lithium treatment and suicide risk in major affective disorders: update and new findings. J Clin Psychiatry 64 (suppl 5):44–52, 2003

Baraban SC, Tallent MK: Interneuron Diversity series: Interneuronal neuropeptides—endogenous regulators of neuronal excitability. Trends Neurosci 27:135–142, 2004

Baron M, Gruen R, Anis L, et al: Schizoaffective illness, schizophrenia and affective disorders: morbidity risk and genetic transmission. Acta Psychiatr Scand 65:253–262, 1983

Baumgartner A, von Stuckrad M, Müller-Oerlinghausen B, et al: The hypothalamic-pituitary-thyroid axis in patients maintained on lithium prophylaxis for years: high triiodothyronine serum concentrations are correlated to the prophylactic efficacy. J Affect Disord 34:211–218, 1995

Beck AT, Rush AJ, Shaw BF, et al: Cognitive Therapy of Depression. New York, Guilford, 1979

Bijl RV, Ravelli A, van Zessen G: Prevalence of psychiatric disorder in the general population: results of the Netherlands Mental Health Survey and Incidence Study (NEMESIS). Soc Psychiatry Psychiatr Epidemiol 33:587–595, 1998

Bittner A, Goodwin RD, Wittchen HU, et al: What characteristics of primary anxiety disorders predict subsequent major depressive disorder? J Clin Psychiatry 65:618–626, 2004

Bowden CL: Predictors of response to divalproex and lithium. J Clin Psychiatry 56 (suppl 2):25–30, 1995

Bowden CL, Brugger AM, Swann AC, et al: Efficacy of divalproex vs lithium and placebo in the treatment of mania. The Depakote Mania Study Group. JAMA 271:918–924, 1994

Bowden CL, Calabrese JR, McElroy SL, et al: Efficacy of divalproex versus lithium and placebo in maintenance treatment of bipolar disorder. Arch Gen Psychiatry 57:481–489, 2000

Bowden CL, Calabrese JR, Sachs GS, et al: A placebo-controlled 18-month trial of lamotrigine and lithium maintenance treatment in recently manic or hypomanic patients with bipolar I disorder. Arch Gen Psychiatry 60:392–400, 2003

Brown G, Eales M: Etiology of anxiety and depressive disorders in an inner-city population. Psychol Med 23:155–165, 1993

Burgess S, Geddes J, Hawton K, et al: Lithium for maintenance treatment of mood disorders. Cochrane Database Syst Rev (3):CD003013, 2001

Burnes DD, Spangler DL: Does psychotherapy homework lead to improvements in depression in cognitive-behavioral therapy or does improvement lead to increased homework compliance? J Consult Clin Psychol 68:46–56, 2000

Bylund DB: Subtypes of alpha 2-adrenoceptors: pharmacological and molecular biological evidence converge. Trends Pharmacol Sci 9:356–361, 1988

Cahill L, McGaugh JL, Weinberger NM: The neurobiology of learning and memory: some reminders to remember. Trends Neurosci 24:578–581, 2001

Calabrese JR, Bowden CL, Sachs GS, et al: A double-blind placebo-controlled study of lamotrigine monotherapy in outpatients with bipolar I depression. Lamictal 602 Study Group. J Clin Psychiatry 60:79–88, 1999

Campbell S, Marriott M, Nahmias C, et al: Lower hippocampal volume in patients suffering from depression: a meta-analysis. Am J Psychiatry 161:598–607, 2004

Caspi A, Sugden K, Moffitt TE, et al: Influence of life stress on depression: moderation by a polymorphism in the 5-HTT gene. Science 301:386–389, 2003

Chen L, Zhuang X: Transgenic mouse models of dopamine deficiency. Ann Neurol 54 (suppl 6):S91–S102, 2003

Chueire VB, Silva ET, Perotta E, et al: High serum TSH levels are associated with depression in the elderly. Arch Gerontol Geriatr 36:281–288, 2003

Copolov DL, Rubin RT, Stuart GW, et al: Specificity of the salivary cortisol dexamethasone suppression test across psychiatric diagnoses. Biol Psychiatry 25:879–893, 1989

Coryell W: Psychotic depression. J Clin Psychiatry 57 (suppl 3): 27–31; discussion 49, 1996

Coryell W, Winokur G: Course and outcome, in Handbook of Affective Disorders, 2nd Edition. Edited by Paykel ES. New York, Guilford, 1992, pp 89–108

Crismon ML, Trivedi M, Pigott TA, et al: The Texas Medication Algorithm Project: report of the Texas Consensus Conference Panel on Medication Treatment of Major Depressive Disorder. J Clin Psychiatry 60:142–156, 1999

de Boer TH, Nefkens F, van Helvoirt A, et al: Differences in modulation of noradrenergic and serotonergic transmission by the alpha-2 adrenoceptor antagonists, mirtazapine, mianserin and idazoxan. J Pharmacol Exp Ther 277:852–860, 1996

de Graaf R, Bijl RV, Spijker J, et al: Temporal sequencing of lifetime mood disorders in relation to comorbid anxiety and substance use disorders—findings from the Netherlands Mental Health Survey and Incidence Study. Soc Psychiatry Psychiatr Epidemiol 38:1–11, 2003

Delgado PL, Price LH, Heninger GR, et al: Neurochemistry of affective disorders, in Handbook of Affective Disorders, 2nd Edition. Edited by Paykel ES. Edinburgh, UK, Churchill Livingstone, 1992, pp 219–253

Delgado PL, Miller HL, Salomon RM, et al: Monoamines and the mechanism of antidepressant action: effects of catecholamine depletion on mood of patients treated with antidepressants. Psychopharmacol Bull 29:389–396, 1993

Demet MM, Ozmen B, Deveci A, et al: Depression and anxiety in hyperthyroidism. Arch Med Res 33:552–556, 2002

Demyttenaere K, Bruffaerts R, Rosada-Villa J, et al; WHO World Mental Health Survey Consortium: Prevalence, severity, and unmet need for treatment of mental disorders in the World Health Organization World Mental Health Surveys. JAMA 291:2581–2590, 2004

Di Matteo V, De Blasi A, Di Giulio C, et al: Role of 5-HT(2C) receptors in the control of central dopamine function. Trends Pharmacol Sci 22:229–232, 2001

Dimmock PW, Wyatt KM, Jones PW, et al: Efficacy of selective serotonin reuptake inhibitors in premenstrual syndrome: a systematic review. Lancet 356:1131–1136, 2000

Fava M, Rosenbaum JF, McGrath PJ, et al: Lithium and tricyclic augmentation of fluoxetine treatment for resistant major depression: a double-blind, controlled study. Am J Psychiatry 151:1372–1374, 1994

Fava M, Rush AJ, Trivedi M, et al; for the STAR*D Investigators Group: Background and rationale for the Sequenced Treatment Alternatives to Relieve Depression (STAR*D) study. Psychiatr Clin North Am 26:457–494, 2003

Frank E, Kupfer DJ, Perel JM, et al: Three-year outcomes for maintenance therapies in recurrent depression. Arch Gen Psychiatry 47:1093–1099, 1990

Frank E, Swartz HA, Kupfer DJ: Interpersonal and social rhythm therapy: managing the chaos of bipolar disorder. Biol Psychiatry 48:593–604, 2000

Freeman MP, Freeman SA, McElroy SL: The comorbidity of bipolar and anxiety disorders: prevalence, psychobiology, and treatment issues. J Affect Disord 68:1–23, 2002

Freeman MP, Wiegand C, Gelenberg AJ: Lithium, in The American Psychiatric Publishing Textbook of Psychopharmacology, 3rd Edition. Edited by Schatzberg AF, Nemeroff CB. Washington, DC, American Psychiatric Publishing, 2004, pp 547–565

Freeman TW, Clothier JL, Pazzaglia P, et al: A double-blind comparison of valproate and lithium in the treatment of acute mania. Am J Psychiatry 149:108–111, 1992

Gershon ES: Genetics, in Manic-Depressive Illness. Edited by Goodwin FK, Jamison KR. London, Oxford University Press, 1988, pp 373–401

Gershon ES, Hamovit J, Guroff JJ, et al: A family study of schizoaffective, bipolar I, bipolar II, unipolar, and normal control probands. Arch Gen Psychiatry 39:1157–1167, 1982

Goodwin GM; for the Consensus Group of the British Association for Psychopharmacology: Evidence-based guidelines for treating bipolar disorder: recommendations from the British Association for Psychopharmacology. J Psychopharmacol 17:149–173, 2003

Goodwin RD, Jacobi F, Bittner A, et al: Epidemiology of mood disorders, in The American Psychiatric Publishing Textbook of Mood Disorders. Edited by Stein DJ, Kupfer DJ, Schatzberg AF. Washington, DC, American Psychiatric Publishing, 2006, pp 33–54

Grant SJ, Redmond DE Jr: The neuroanatomy and pharmacology of the nucleus locus coeruleus. Prog Clin Biol Res 71:5–27, 1981

Gray PB, Singh AB, Woodhouse LJ, et al: Dose-dependent effects of testosterone on sexual function, mood, and visuospatial cognition in older men. J Clin Endocrinol Metab 90:3838–3846, 2005

Grof P: Selecting effective long-term treatment for bipolar patients: monotherapy and combinations. J Clin Psychiatry 64 (suppl 5):53–61, 2003

Gutierrez MA, Stimmel GL, Aiso JY: Venlafaxine: a 2003 update. Clin Ther 25:2138–2154, 2003

Halbreich U, Borenstein J, Pearlstein T, et al: The prevalence, impact, and burden of premenstrual dysphoric disorder. Psychoneuroendocrinology 28 (suppl 3):1–23, 2003

Hamilton M: A rating scale for depression. J Neurol Neurosurg Psychiatry 23:56–62, 1960

Hasler G, Drevets W, Manji H, et al: Discovering endophenotypes for major depression. Neuropsychopharmacology 29:1765–1781, 2004

Heilig M, Widerlov E: Neurobiology and clinical aspects of neuropeptide Y. Crit Rev Neurobiol 9:115–136, 1995

Hirschfeld RM, Bowden CL, Gitlin MJ, et al: Practice guideline for the treatment of patients with bipolar disorder (revision). Am J Psychiatry 159:1–50, 2002

Iqbal MM, Gunlapalli SP, Ryan WG, et al: Effects of antimanic mood-stabilizing drugs on fetuses, neonates, and nursing infants. South Med J 94:304–322, 2001

Joffe RT: Refractory depression: treatment strategies, with particular reference to the thyroid axis. J Psychiatry Neurosci 22:327–331, 1997

Joffe RT, Marriott M: Thyroid hormone levels and recurrence of major depression. Am J Psychiatry 157:1689–1691, 2000

Joffe RT, Singer W: A comparison of triiodothyronine and thyroxine in the potentiation of tricyclic antidepressants. Psychiatry Res 32:241–251, 1990

Keck PE Jr, McElroy SL: Lithium and mood stabilizers, in The American Psychiatric Publishing Textbook of Mood Disorders. Edited by Stein DJ, Kupfer DJ, Schatzberg AF. Washington, DC, American Psychiatric Publishing, 2006, pp 281–290

Keck PE Jr, Strakowski SM, McElroy SL: The efficacy of atypical antipsychotics in the treatment of depressive symptoms, hostility, and suicidality in patients with schizophrenia. J Clin Psychiatry 61 (suppl 3):4–9, 2000

Keck PE Jr, Strakowski SM, Hawkins JM, et al: Rapid lithium administration in the treatment of acute mania. Bipolar Disord 3:68–72, 2001

Keller MB, McCullough JP, Klein DN, et al: A comparison of nefazodone, the cognitive behavioral-analysis system of psychotherapy, and their combination for the treatment of chronic depression. N Engl J Med 342:1462–1470, 2000

Kendler KS: Major depression and the environment: a psychiatric genetic perspective. Pharmacopsychiatry 31:5–9, 1998

Kendler KS, Thornton LM, Gardner CO: Stressful life events and previous episodes in the etiology of major depression in women: an evaluation of the "kindling" hypothesis. Am J Psychiatry 157:1243–1251, 2000

Kendler KS, Prescott CA, Myers JK, et al: The structure of genetic and environmental risk factors for common psychiatric and substance use disorders in men and women. Arch Gen Psychiatry 60:929–937, 2003

Kessler RC, Walters EE: Epidemiology of DSM-III-R major depression and minor depression among adolescents and young adults in the National Comorbidity Survey. Depress Anxiety 7:3–14, 1998

Kessler RC, McGonagle KA, Zhao S, et al: Lifetime and 12-month prevalence of DSM-III-R psychiatric disorders in the United States: results from the National Comorbidity Survey. Arch Gen Psychiatry 51:8–19, 1994

Kessler RC, Berglund P, Demler O, et al: The epidemiology of major depressive disorder: results from the National Comorbidity Survey Replication (NCS-R). JAMA 289:3095–3105, 2003

Klerman GL, Weissman MM, Rounsaville BJ, et al: Interpersonal Psychotherapy of Depression. New York, Basic Books, 1984

Kramlinger KG, Post RM: The addition of lithium to carbamazepine. Arch Gen Psychiatry 46:794–800, 1989

Lam DH, Watkins ER, Hayward P, et al: A randomized controlled study of cognitive therapy for relapse prevention for bipolar affective disorder: outcome of the first year. Arch Gen Psychiatry 60:145–152, 2003

Larson EW, Richelson E: Organic causes of mania. Mayo Clin Proc 63:906–912, 1988

Lewy AJ, Sack RL, Singer CM, et al: Winter depression and the phase-shift hypothesis for bright light's therapeutic effects: history, theory, and experimental evidence. J Biol Rhythms 3:121–134, 1988

Luborsky L: Principles of Psychoanalytic Psychotherapy: A Manual for Supportive Expressive Treatment. New York, Basic Books, 1984

Maes M, Meltzer HY: The serotonin hypothesis of major depression, in Psychopharmacology: The Fourth Generation of Progress. Edited by Bloom FE, Kupfer DJ, Bunney BS, et al. New York, Raven, 1995, pp 933–944

Marcus R, Carson W, McQuada R, et al: Long-term efficacy of aripiprazole in the maintenance treatment of bipolar disorder. Paper presented at the 42nd annual meeting of the American College of Neuropsychopharmacology, San Juan, PR, December 7–11, 2003

Markowitz JC: Interpersonal psychotherapy for chronic depression. J Clin Psychol 59:847–858, 2003

Markowitz JC, Kocsis JH, Fishman B, et al: Treatment of HIV-positive patients with depressive symptoms. Arch Gen Psychiatry 55:452–457, 1998

Matt GE, Vazquez C, Campbell WK: Mood-congruent recall of affectively toned stimuli: a meta-analytic review. Clin Psychol Rev 12:227–255, 1992

McGuffin P, Rijsdijk S, Andrew M, et al: The heritability of bipolar affective disorder and the genetic relationship to unipolar depression. Arch Gen Psychiatry 60:497–502, 2003

Mendlewicz J, Rainer JD: Adoption study supporting genetic transmission in manic-depressive illness. Nature 368:327–329, 1977

Miklowitz DJ, Hooley JM: Developing family psychoeducational treatments for patients with bipolar and other severe psychiatric disorders: a pathway from basic research to clinical trials. J Marital Fam Ther 24:419–435, 1998

Moore JD, Bona JR: Depression and dysthymia. Med Clin North Am 85:631–644, 2001

Mufson L, Weissman MM, Moreau D, et al: Efficacy of interpersonal psychotherapy for depressed adolescents. Arch Gen Psychiatry 56:573–579, 1999

Nelson JC, Charney DS: The symptoms of major depressive illness. Am J Psychiatry 138:1–13, 1981

Nemeroff C: The neurobiological consequences of child abuse. Paper presented at the 156th annual meeting of the American Psychiatric Association, San Francisco, CA, May 19, 2003

Oldehinkel AJ, Wittchen HU, Schuster P: Prevalence, 20-month incidence and outcome of unipolar depressive disorders in a community sample of adolescents. Psychol Med 29:655–668, 1999

Ostroff RB, Nelson JC: Risperidone augmentation of selective serotonin reuptake inhibitors in major depression. J Clin Psychiatry 60:256–259, 1999

Osuji IJ, Cullum CM: Cognition in bipolar disorder. Psychiatr Clin North Am 28:427–441, 2005

O'Toole SM, Rubin RT: Neuroendocrine aspects of primary endogenous depression, XIV: gonadotropin secretion in female patients and their matched controls. Psychoneuroendocrinology 20:603–612, 1995

Perlis RH, Brown E, Baker RW, et al: Clinical features of bipolar depression versus major depressive disorder in large multicenter trials. Am J Psychiatry 163:225–231, 2006

Perry A, Tarrier N, Morriss R, et al: Randomised controlled trial of efficacy of teaching patients with bipolar disorder to identify early symptoms of relapse and obtain treatment. BMJ 318:149–153, 1999

Peveler R, Carson A, Rodin G: Depression in medical patients. BMJ 325:149–152, 2002

Plotsky PM, Owens MJ, Nemeroff CB: Psychoneuroendocrinology of depression: hypothalamic-pituitary-adrenal axis. Psychiatr Clin North Am 21:293–307, 1998

Post RM: Transduction of psychosocial stress into the neurobiology of recurrent affective disorder. Am J Psychiatry 149:999–1010, 1992

Prien RF, Kupfer DJ, Mansky PA, et al: Drug therapy in the prevention of recurrences in unipolar and bipolar affective disorders: report of the NIMH Collaborative Study Group comparing lithium carbonate, imipramine, and a lithium carbonate-imipramine combination. Arch Gen Psychiatry 41:1096–1104, 1984

Rehm LP: A self-control model of depression. Behav Ther 8:787–804, 1977

Rubin RT: Pharmacoendocrinology of major depression. Eur Arch Psychiatry Neurol Sci 238:259–267, 1989

Rubinow DR, Schmidt PJ, Roca CA, et al: Gonadal hormones and behavior in women: concentrations versus context, in Hormones, Brain and Behavior. Edited by Pfaff D, Arnold AP, Etgen AM, et al. New York, Academic Press, 2002, pp 37–73

Schatzberg AF, Rush AJ, Arnow BA, et al: Chronic depression: medication (nefazodone) or psychotherapy (CBASP) is effective when the other is not. Arch Gen Psychiatry 62:513–520, 2005

Schulberg HC, Block MR, Madonia MJ, et al: Treating major depression in primary care practice: eight-month clinical outcomes. Arch Gen Psychiatry 53:913–919, 1996

Scott J, Garland A, Moorhead S: A pilot study of cognitive therapy in bipolar disorders. Psychol Med 31:459–467, 2001

Segurado R, Detera-Wadleigh SD, Levinson DF, et al: Genome scan meta-analysis of schizophrenia and bipolar disorder, part III: bipolar disorder. Am J Hum Genet 73:49–62, 2003

Seidman SN: Psychoneuroendocrinology of mood disorders, in The American Psychiatric Publishing Textbook of Mood Disorders. Edited by Stein DJ, Kupfer DJ, Schatzberg AF. Washington, DC, American Psychiatric Publishing, 2006, pp 117–130

Shelton RC, Tollefson GD, Tohen M, et al: A novel augmentation strategy for treating resistant major depression. Am J Psychiatry 158:131–134, 2001

Smith D, Dempster C, Glanville J, et al: Efficacy and tolerability of venlafaxine compared with selective serotonin reuptake inhibitors and other antidepressants: a meta-analysis. Br J Psychiatry 180:396–404, 2002

Smith S: Tryptophan in the treatment of resistant depression: a review. Pharm J 261:819–821, 1998

Solomon DA, Ryan CE, Keitner GI: A pilot study of lithium carbonate plus divalproex sodium for the continuation and maintenance treatment of patients with bipolar I disorder. J Clin Psychiatry 58:95–99, 1997

Spijker J, de Graaf R, Bijl RV, et al: Duration of major depressive episodes in the general population: results from the Netherlands Mental Health Survey and Incidence Study. Br J Psychiatry 181:208–213, 2002

Steiner M, Dunn E, Born L: Hormones and mood: from menarche to menopause and beyond. J Affect Disord 74:67–83, 2003

Stoll AL, Mayer PV, Kolbrener M, et al: Antidepressant-associated mania: a controlled comparison with spontaneous mania. Am J Psychiatry 151:1642–1645, 1994

Strakowski SM: Clinical update in bipolar disorders: second-generation antipsychotics in the maintenance therapy of bipolar disorder. Available at: http://www.medscape.com/viewprogram/2496. Release date June 26, 2003.

Sullivan P, Kendler K: Genetic case-control studies in neuropsychiatry. Arch Gen Psychiatry 58:1015–1024, 2001

Suppes T, Swann AC, Dennehy EB, et al: Texas Medication Algorithm Project: development and feasibility testing of a treatment algorithm for patients with bipolar disorder. J Clin Psychiatry 62:439–447, 2001

Swann AC, Bowden CL, Calabrese JR, et al: Pattern of response to divalproex, lithium, or placebo in four naturalistic subtypes of mania. Neuropsychopharmacology 26:530–536, 2002

Teasdale JD, Barnard PJ: Affect, Cognition and Change: Remodeling Depressive Thought. Hove, East Sussex, UK, Lawrence Erlbaum, 1993

Thase ME: Novel transdermal delivery formulation of the monoamine oxidase inhibitor selegiline nearing release for treatment of depression. J Clin Psychiatry 67:671–672, 2006

Tohen M, Bowden CL, Calabrese JR, et al: Olanzapine versus placebo for relapse prevention in bipolar disorder. Paper presented at the 156th annual meeting of the American Psychiatric Association, San Francisco, CA, May 17–22, 2003

Torres GE, Gainetdinov RR, Caron MG: Plasma membrane monoamine transporters: structure, regulation and function. Nat Rev Neurosci 4:13–25, 2003

Trivedi MH, Rush AJ, Crismon ML, et al: Clinical results for patients with major depressive disorder in the Texas Medication Algorithm Project. Arch Gen Psychiatry 61:669–680, 2004

Wang C, Cunningham G, Dobs A, et al: Long-term testosterone gel (AndroGel) treatment maintains beneficial effects on sexual function and mood, lean and fat mass, and bone mineral density in hypogonadal men. J Clin Endocrinol Metab 89:2085–2098, 2004

Weisler RH, Kalali AH, Ketter TA; the SPD417 Study Group: A multicenter, randomized, double-blind, placebo-controlled trial of beaded carbamazepine extended-release capsules (beaded-ERC-CBZ; SPD417) as monotherapy for bipolar patients with manic or mixed episodes. J Clin Psychiatry 65:478–484, 2004

Weissman MM, Myers J: Affective disorders in a US urban community: the use of research diagnostic criteria in an epidemiological survey. Arch Gen Psychiatry 35:1304–1311, 1978

Weissman MM, Bruce LM, Leaf PJ, et al: Affective disorders, in Psychiatric Disorders in America: The Epidemiologic Catchment Area Study. Edited by Robins LN, Regier DA. New York, Free Press, 1991, pp 53–80

Whybrow PC, Bauer MS, Gyulai L: Thyroid axis considerations in patients with rapid cycling affective disorder. Clin Neuropharmacol 15 (suppl 1, pt A):391A–392A, 1992

Williams JMG: Depression, in Science and Practice of Cognitive Behavior Therapy. Edited by Clark DM, Fairburn CG. Oxford, England, Oxford University Press, 1997, pp 259–283

Zornberg GL, Pope HG Jr: Treatment of depression in bipolar disorder: new directions for research. J Clin Psychopharmacol 13:397–408, 1993

CHAPTER

# 19

# Anxiety Disorders

ERIC HOLLANDER, M.D.

DAPHNE SIMEON, M.D.

Anxiety disorders are the most common of all psychiatric illnesses and result in considerable functional impairment and distress.

Table 19–1 presents a summary overview of the prevalence, gender ratio, and comorbidities of the major anxiety disorders. Figure 19–1 shows a diagnostic decision tree for the anxiety disorders.

TABLE 19–1.  **Approximate lifetime prevalence, gender ratio, and common comorbidities for the major anxiety disorders**

| Disorder | Prevalence (%) | Females: Males | Comorbidity |
|---|---|---|---|
| Panic disorder | 2–4 | 2+:1 | Depression, other anxiety disorders |
| Generalized anxiety disorder | 5–7 | 2:1 | Overall, 90%; 50%–60% for major depression or other anxiety disorder |
| Social phobia | 13–16 | 1+:1 | Twofold risk for alcohol dependence, three- to sixfold risk of mood disorders |
| Specific phobias | 10 | 2:1 | Depression and somatoform disorders |
| Agoraphobia | 6 | 2:1 | |
| Obsessive-compulsive disorder | 2–3 | 1:1 | Anxiety, depression, tics, hypochondriasis, eating disorder, body dysmorphic disorder (childhood-onset more common in males) |
| Posttraumatic stress disorder | 7–9 | 2:1 | Depression, obsessive-compulsive disorder, panic, phobias |

## Panic Disorder

### Definition

The DSM-IV-TR (American Psychiatric Association 2000)

definition of a *panic attack* is presented in Table 19–2. Panic disorder is subdivided into panic disorder with and without agoraphobia, as in DSM-III-R (American Psychiatric Association 1987), depending on whether there is any secondary phobic avoidance (see Table 19–3).

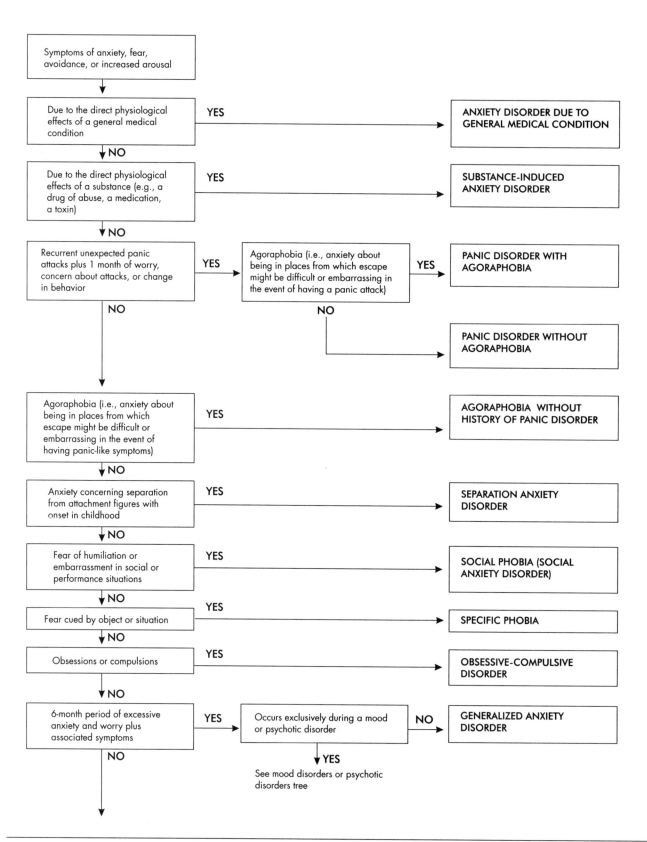

**FIGURE 19–1.   Diagnostic decision tree for anxiety disorders.**

Patients may have more than one disorder and thus must be evaluated for each disorder.

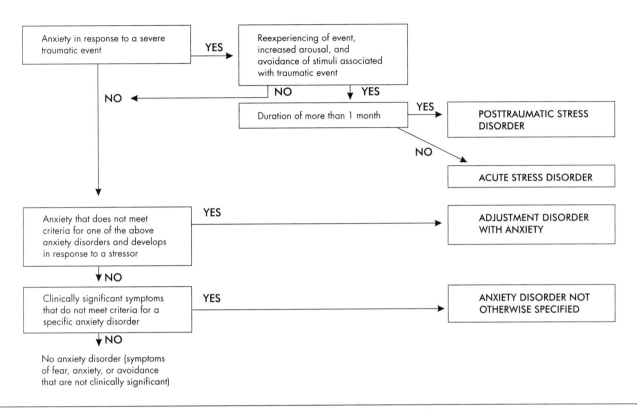

**FIGURE 19–1.** Diagnostic decision tree for anxiety disorders *(continued)*.

Patients may have more than one disorder and thus must be evaluated for each disorder.

---

**TABLE 19–2. DSM-IV-TR criteria for panic attack**

**Note:** A panic attack is not a codable disorder. Code the specific diagnosis in which the panic attack occurs (e.g., 300.21 panic disorder with agoraphobia).

A discrete period of intense fear or discomfort, in which four (or more) of the following symptoms developed abruptly and reached a peak within 10 minutes:

(1) palpitations, pounding heart, or accelerated heart rate

(2) sweating

(3) trembling or shaking

(4) sensations of shortness of breath or smothering

(5) feeling of choking

(6) chest pain or discomfort

(7) nausea or abdominal distress

(8) feeling dizzy, unsteady, lightheaded, or faint

(9) derealization (feelings of unreality) or depersonalization (being detached from oneself)

(10) fear of losing control or going crazy

(11) fear of dying

(12) paresthesias (numbness or tingling sensations)

(13) chills or hot flushes

**TABLE 19–3.  DSM-IV-TR diagnostic criteria for panic disorder with or without agoraphobia**

**Diagnostic criteria for panic disorder without agoraphobia**

A.  Both (1) and (2):

  (1)  recurrent unexpected panic attacks

  (2)  at least one of the attacks has been followed by 1 month (or more) of one (or more)
    of the following:

    (a)  persistent concern about having additional attacks

    (b)  worry about the implications of the attack or its consequences (e.g., losing control, having a heart attack,
      "going crazy")

    (c)  a significant change in behavior related to the attacks

B.  Absence of agoraphobia.

C.  The panic attacks are not due to the direct physiological effects of a substance (e.g., a drug of abuse, a medication)
  or a general medical condition (e.g., hyperthyroidism).

D.  The panic attacks are not better accounted for by another mental disorder, such as social phobia
  (e.g., occurring on exposure to feared social situations), specific phobia (e.g., on exposure to a
  specific phobic situation), obsessive-compulsive disorder (e.g., on exposure to dirt in someone with
  an obsession about contamination), posttraumatic stress disorder (e.g., in response to stimuli associated
  with a severe stressor), or separation anxiety disorder (e.g., in response to being away from home or
  close relatives).

**Diagnostic criteria for panic disorder with agoraphobia**

A.  Both (1) and (2):

  (1)  recurrent unexpected panic attacks

  (2)  at least one of the attacks has been followed by 1 month (or more) of one (or more) of the following:

    (a)  persistent concern about having additional attacks

    (b)  worry about the implications of the attack or its consequences (e.g., losing control, having a heart attack,
      "going crazy")

    (c)  a significant change in behavior related to the attacks

B.  The presence of agoraphobia.

C.  The panic attacks are not due to the direct physiological effects of a substance (e.g., a drug of abuse, a medication)
  or a general medical condition (e.g., hyperthyroidism).

D.  The panic attacks are not better accounted for by another mental disorder, such as social phobia (e.g., occurring
  on exposure to feared social situations), specific phobia (e.g., on exposure to a specific phobic situation), obsessive-
  compulsive disorder (e.g., on exposure to dirt in someone with an obsession about contamination), posttraumatic
  stress disorder (e.g., in response to stimuli associated with a severe stressor), or separation anxiety disorder (e.g.,
  in response to being away from home or close relatives).

## Clinical Description

### Onset

Patients experiencing their first panic attack generally fear they are having a heart attack or losing their mind. Such patients often rush to the nearest emergency department, where routine laboratory tests, electrocardiography, and physical examination are performed. All that is found is an occasional case of sinus tachycardia, and the patients are reassured and sent home. These patients may indeed feel reassured, and at this point the diagnosis of panic disorder would be premature. However, perhaps a few days or even weeks later they will again have the sudden onset of severe anxiety with all of the associated physical symptoms. Again they seek emergency medical treatment. At this point, they may be told the problem is psychological, be given a prescription for a benzodiazepine tranquilizer, or be referred for extensive medical workup.

## Symptoms

Typically, during a panic attack, a patient will be engaged in a routine activity when he or she will experience the sudden onset of overwhelming fear, terror, apprehension, and a sense of impending doom. Several of a group of associated symptoms, mostly physical, are also experienced: dyspnea, palpitations, chest pain or discomfort, choking or smothering sensations, dizziness or unsteady feelings, feelings of unreality (derealization and/or depersonalization), paresthesias, hot and cold flashes, sweating, faintness, trembling and shaking, and a fear of dying, going crazy, or losing control of oneself. It is clear that most of the physical sensations of a panic attack represent massive overstimulation of the autonomic nervous system.

Attacks usually last from 5 to 20 minutes and rarely as long as an hour. Patients who claim they have attacks that last a whole day may fall into one of four categories. Some patients continue to feel agitated and fatigued for several hours after the main portion of the attack has subsided. At times, attacks occur, subside, and occur again in a wave-like manner. Alternatively, the patient with so-called long panic attacks often has some other form of pathological anxiety, such as severe generalized anxiety, agitated depression, or obsessional tension states. Finally, in some cases, such severe anticipatory anxiety may develop with time in expectation of future panic attacks that the two may blend together in the patient's description and be difficult to distinguish.

Agoraphobia frequently develops in response to panic attacks, leading to the DSM-IV-TR diagnosis of panic disorder with agoraphobia. The clinical picture in agoraphobia consists of multiple and varied fears and avoidance behaviors that center around three main themes: 1) fear of leaving home, 2) fear of being alone, and 3) fear of being away from home in situations where one can feel trapped, embarrassed, or helpless. According to DSM-IV-TR, the fear is one of developing distressing symptoms in such situations where escape is difficult or help is unavailable.

Typical agoraphobic fears are of using public transportation (e.g., buses, trains, subways, airplanes); being in crowds, theaters, elevators, restaurants, supermarkets, or department stores; waiting in line; or traveling a distance from home. In severe cases, patients may be completely housebound, fearful of leaving home without a companion or even of staying home alone.

Most cases of agoraphobia begin with a series of spontaneous panic attacks. If the attacks continue, the patient usually develops a constant anticipatory anxiety characterized by continued apprehension about the possible occasion and consequences of the next attack. Agoraphobic symptoms represent a tertiary phase in the illness. Many patients will causally relate their panic attacks to the particular situation in which the attacks have occurred. They then avoid these situations in an attempt to prevent further panic attacks (Figure 19–2).

## Epidemiology

The National Institute of Mental Health Epidemiologic Catchment Area (ECA) study examined the population prevalence of DSM-III-diagnosed (American Psychiatric Association 1980) panic disorder using the Diagnostic Interview Schedule (Regier et al. 1988). The 1-month, 6-month, and lifetime prevalence rates for panic disorder at all five study sites combined were 0.5%, 0.8%, and 1.6%, respectively. Women had a 1-month prevalence rate of 0.7%, which was significantly higher than the 0.3% rate found among men; women also tended to have a greater rise in panic disorder in the age range of 25–44 years, and their attacks tended to continue longer into older age (Regier et al. 1988).

More recently, the 2001–2002 National Epidemiologic Survey on Alcohol and Related Conditions (or NESARC), which included about 43,000 participants, revealed 1-year and lifetime prevalence of panic disorder of 2.1% and 5.1%, respectively (Grant et al. 2006); rates for panic disorder without agoraphobia were 1.6% and 4.0%, respectively, exceeding those of panic disorder with agoraphobia (0.6% and 1.1%, respectively). Being female, Native American, middle-aged, widowed/separated/divorced, and of low income increased risk for panic disorder, whereas being Asian, African American, or Hispanic decreased risk. Subjects with agoraphobia had an earlier age at onset, more severe symptoms, greater disability, and greater Axis I and II comorbidity compared with subjects without agoraphobia and were more likely to seek treatment early on.

## Etiology

### Biological Theories

Biological models for panic disorder are summarized in Table 19–4.

**The sympathetic system.** The locus coeruleus also has been implicated in the pathogenesis of panic attacks. This nucleus is located in the pons and contains more than 50% of all noradrenergic neurons in the entire central

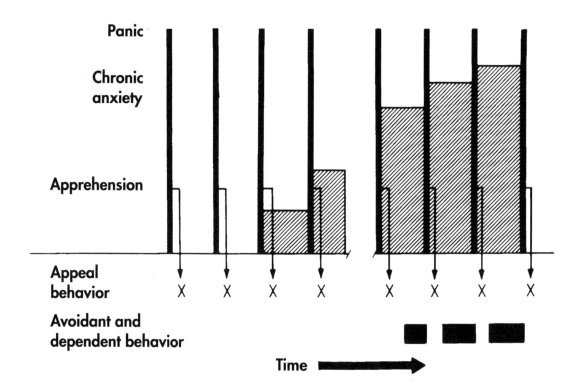

FIGURE 19–2.  **Development of agoraphobia.**

After onset of unexpected panic attacks (*solid bars*), patient develops acute help-seeking behavior (**X**), then apprehension culminating in chronic anxiety (*shaded areas*), and finally agoraphobic behavior (*black blocks*).

TABLE 19–4.  **Biological models of panic disorder**

Hyperreactivity of the locus coeruleus

Dysregulated serotonergic modulation

Decreased γ-aminobutyric acid (GABA)–
benzodiazepine receptor complex binding

Hypersensitive brain stem carbon dioxide
chemoreceptors

Hypersensitive conditioned fear network centered
in the amygdala

Moderate genetic component

nervous system. It sends afferent projections to a wide area of the brain, including the hippocampus, amygdala, limbic lobe, and cerebral cortex. In humans, drugs known to be capable of increasing locus coeruleus discharge in animals are anxiogenic, whereas many drugs that curtail locus coeruleus firing and decrease central noradrenergic turnover are antianxiety agents.

Yohimbine challenge was reported to induce greater anxiety and a greater increase in plasma 3-methoxy-4-hydroxyphenylglycol (MHPG), a major noradrenergic metabolite, in patients who had frequent panic attacks compared with patients who had panic attacks less frequently or healthy control subjects. Such a finding is suggestive of heightened central noradrenergic activity in panic (Charney et al. 1984).

**The panicogen sodium lactate.**  Having been replicated on numerous occasions under proper experimental conditions, the finding that 10 mL/kg of 0.5 molar sodium lactate infused over 20 minutes will provoke a panic attack in most patients with panic disorder but not in control subjects without panic disorder is now a well-accepted fact.

**The GABA–benzodiazepine system.**  Another area of inquiry that may relate to the biology of panic is the γ-aminobutyric acid (GABA)–benzodiazepine receptor complex; the benzodiazepine receptor is linked to a receptor for the inhibitory neurotransmitter GABA. Binding of a benzodiazepine to the benzodiazepine receptor facilitates the action of GABA, effectively slowing neural transmission. One series of compounds, the β-carbolines, which are inverse agonists of this receptor complex, produces an acute anxiety syndrome when administered to laboratory animals or to normal human volunteers. On the other hand, benzodiazepines have long been known to be a highly efficacious treatment for panic.

**The serotonergic system.** Although the serotonergic system has not been as extensively investigated in panic as other neurochemical systems, it is widely thought that it may be one of the systems that at least indirectly modulate dysregulated responses in the disorder. It has recently been proposed that serotonergic medications may act by desensitizing the brain's fear network via projections from the raphe nuclei to the locus coeruleus, inhibiting noradrenergic activation; to the periaqueductal gray region, inhibiting freeze/flight responses; and to the hypothalamus, inhibiting corticotropin-releasing factor (CRF) release; and possibly directly at the level of the amygdala, inhibiting excitatory pathways from the cortex and the thalamus (Gorman et al. 2000).

**Hypothalamic-pituitary-adrenal axis.** The hypothalamic-pituitary-adrenal (HPA) system, which is central to an organism's response to stress, would clearly be of interest in panic disorder, in which increased early-life stressful events such as separations, losses, and abuse have been described (M.B. Stein et al. 1996). However, HPA findings in panic have been very contradictory and have not consistently supported HPA axis dysregulation in the disorder.

**Carbon dioxide hypersensitivity theory.** Controlled hyperventilation and respiratory alkalosis do not routinely provoke panic attacks in most patients with panic disorder. Surprisingly, however, giving these patients a mixture of 5% $CO_2$ in room air to breathe causes panic almost as often as does a sodium lactate infusion (Gorman et al. 1984).

**Neurocircuitry of fear.** The neurocircuitry of fear model integrates neurochemical, imaging, and treatment findings in the disorder coupled with human and animal studies in the neurobiology of conditioned fear responses (Gorman et al. 2000). The model proposes that panic at-

tacks are analogous to animal fear and avoidance responses and may be manifestations of dysregulation in the brain circuits underlying conditioned fear responses. Panic is speculated to originate in an abnormally sensitive fear network, centered in the amygdala. Input into the amygdala is modulated by both thalamic input and prefrontal cortical projections, and there are amygdalar projections to several areas involved in various aspects of the fear response, such as the locus coeruleus and arousal, the brain stem and respiratory activation, the hypothalamus and activation of the HPA stress axis, and the cortex and cognitive interpretations.

**Genetics.** Crowe et al. (1983) found a morbidity risk for panic disorder of 24.7% among relatives of patients with panic disorder compared with only 2.3% among normal control subjects. Torgersen (1983) completed a study of 32 monozygotic and 53 dizygotic twins and found panic attacks to be five times more frequent in the former. However, the absolute concordance rate in monozygotic twins was 31%, suggesting that nongenetic factors also play an important role in the development of the illness.

### Psychodynamic Theories

**Freud's first theory of anxiety neurosis (id or impulse anxiety).** In his earliest concept of anxiety formation, Freud (1895[1894]/1962) postulated that anxiety stems from the direct physiological transformation of libidinal energy into the somatic symptoms of anxiety, without the mediation of psychic mechanisms. He found evidence for this process in the sexual practices and experiences of patients with anxiety, which were characterized by disturbed sexual arousal and continence and coitus interruptus. He termed such anxiety an "actual neurosis" as opposed to a psychoneurosis because of the postulated absence of psychic processes. Such anxiety, originating from overwhelming instinctual urges, would today be referred to as *id* or *impulse anxiety.*

**Structural theory and intrapsychic conflict.** By 1926, with the advent of the structural theory of the mind, Freud's theory of anxiety had undergone a major transformation (Freud 1926/1959).

According to Freud, anxiety is an affect belonging to the ego and acts as a signal alerting the ego to internal danger. The danger stems from intrapsychic conflict between instinctual drives from the id, superego prohibitions, and external reality demands. Anxiety acts as a signal to the ego for the mobilization of repression and other defenses to counteract the threat to intrapsychic equilibrium. Inhibitions and neurotic symptoms develop as measures designed to avoid the dangerous situation and to allow only partial gratification of instinctual wishes, thus warding off signal anxiety. In the revised theory, then, anxiety leads to repression, instead of the reverse.

### Learning Theories

Behavior or learning theorists hold that anxiety is conditioned by the fear of certain environmental stimuli. If every time a laboratory animal presses a bar it receives a noxious electric shock, the pressing of the lever becomes a conditioned stimulus that precedes the unconditioned stimulus (i.e., the shock). The conditioned stimulus releases a conditioned response in the animal, anxiety, that leads the animal to avoid contact with the lever, thereby avoiding the shock. Successful avoidance of the unconditioned stimulus, the shock, reinforces the avoidant behavior. This leads to a decrease in anxiety level.

### Traumatic Antecedents

Childhood interpersonal trauma also appears to make a contribution to the likelihood that individuals will manifest panic disorder. In a clinical cross-sectional study comparing panic disorder and psychiatrically healthy subjects, severe traumatic events during childhood and unfavorable parental attitudes were associated with panic disorder (Bandelow et al. 2002). Similarly, examination of trauma rates in the National Comorbidity Survey community sample, after disaggregating the effect of comorbid posttraumatic stress disorder (PTSD), found that 24% of females and 5% of males with panic disorder reported histories of sexual molestation, suggesting the latter could be one risk factor for developing panic disorder (Leskin and Sheikh 2002). In a large prospective birth cohort studied to the age of 21 years, exposure to childhood physical and sexual abuse was associated with increased risk of later panic attacks and disorder, even after adjusting for prospectively assessed confounding factors. Exposure to interparental violence was not a factor (Goodwin et al. 2005).

**TABLE 19–5. Course and prognosis of panic disorder**

**Course**

Variable, typically with periods of exacerbations and remissions

**Outcome**

About 33% recover, 50% have limited impairment, 20% or less have major impairment

**Predictors of worse prognosis**

More severe initial panic attacks

More severe initial agoraphobia

Longer duration of illness

Comorbid depression

History of separation from parent (e.g., death, divorce)

High interpersonal sensitivity

Single marital status

## Course, Prognosis, Morbidity, and Mortality

The course of illness without treatment is highly variable and is summarized in Table 19–5.

A possible association between panic disorder and increased suicide risk has received extensive attention and does not appear to hold up based on extensive epidemiological analyses. Epidemiological data further supported this finding in the ECA study, in which the lifetime rate of suicide attempts in persons with uncomplicated panic disorder was 7%, about the same as the 7.9% rate for uncomplicated major depression (Johnson et al. 1990). However, in a reanalysis of the ECA data, controlling for all comorbidity rather than one disorder at a time, an association between panic and suicide attempts could no longer be shown (Hornig and McNally 1995).

Similarly, a 5-year prospective study concluded that there was no association between panic and suicide risk in the absence of other risk factors (Warshaw et al. 2000). Finally, reanalysis of the National Comorbidity Survey data found that in the absence of comorbidity, panic disorder responders were not at heightened risk for self-reported suicide attempts (Vickers and McNally 2004).

# Diagnosis

## Physical Signs and Behavior

The diagnosis of panic disorder is made when a patient experiences recurrent panic attacks that are discrete and unexpected and followed by a month of persistent anticipatory anxiety or behavior change. These panic attacks are characterized by a sudden crescendo of anxiety and fearfulness, in addition to the presence of at least four physical symptoms. Finally, these attacks are not secondary to a known organic factor or due to another mental disorder. However, these diagnoses are not always obvious, and several other psychiatric and medical disorders may mimic these conditions (Table 19–6).

# Differential Diagnosis

## Other Psychiatric Illnesses

Patients with depression often manifest signs of anxiety and may even have frank panic attacks. On the other hand, patients with panic disorder, if untreated for significant amounts of time, routinely become demoralized as the effect of the illness progressively restricts their ability to enjoy a normal life.

The order of developing symptoms also differentiates depression from anxiety. In cases of panic disorder. anxiety symptoms usually precede any seriously altered mood. Patients can generally recall having anxiety attacks first, then becoming gradually more disgusted with life, and then feeling depressed. In depression, patients usually experience dysphoria first, with anxiety symptoms coming later.

Patients with somatization disorder complain of a variety of physical ailments and discomforts, none of which are substantiated by physical or laboratory findings. Unlike panic disorder patients, somatizing patients present with physical problems that do not usually occur in episodic attacks but are virtually constant.

Undoubtedly some patients with anxiety disorders abuse alcohol and drugs, such as sedatives, in attempts at self-medication. In one study, after successful detoxification, a group of alcoholic patients with a history of panic disorder were treated with medication to block spontaneous panic attacks (Quitkin and Babkin 1982). These patients did not resume alcohol consumption once their panic attacks were eliminated.

**TABLE 19–6. Differential diagnosis of panic disorder**

Anxious depression

Somatization with panic-like physical complaints

Social phobia with socially cued panic attacks

Generalized anxiety with severe symptoms or during peak periods

Posttraumatic stress disorder with intense physiological response to reminders of the trauma

Agoraphobia secondary to conditions other than panic (depression, posttraumatic stress, paranoia, psychosis)

Obsessional anxiety of near-panic severity

Depersonalization disorder

Personality disorder with anxiety symptoms

Hyperthyroidism

Hypothyroidism

Mitral valve prolapse

Pheochromocytoma

## Hyperthyroidism and Hypothyroidism

Both hyper- and hypothyroidism can present with anxiety unaccompanied by other signs or symptoms. For this reason, it is imperative that all patients complaining of anxiety undergo routine thyroid function tests.

## Cardiac Disease

Although patients with mitral valve prolapse occasionally complain of palpitations, chest pain, light-headedness, and fatigue, symptoms of a full-blown panic attack are rare. A comparison of symptoms in mitral valve prolapse and panic disorder is provided in Table 19–7. Panic patients with and without mitral valve prolapse are similar in several important ways. Treatment for panic attacks works regardless of the presence of the prolapsed valve, and patients with both mitral valve prolapse and panic disorder are just as sensitive to sodium lactate as are those with panic disorder alone.

# Treatment

## Pharmacotherapy

**Antidepressants.** The central feature in the treatment of panic disorder is the pharmacological blockade of the spontaneous panic attacks. Several classes of medications have been shown to be effective in accomplishing this goal, and a summary of the pharmacological treatment of panic disorder is presented in Table 19–8.

TABLE 19–7.  Comparison of symptoms of mitral valve prolapse and panic disorder

| Symptoms | Mitral valve prolapse | Panic disorder |
|---|---|---|
| Fatigue | + | – |
| Dyspnea | + | ++ |
| Palpitations | ++ | ++ |
| Chest pain | ++ | + |
| Syncope | + | – |
| Choking | – | ++ |
| Dizziness | – | ++ |
| Derealization | – | ++ |
| Hot/cold flashes | – | ++ |
| Sweating | – | ++ |
| Fainting | – | ++ |
| Trembling | – | ++ |
| Fear of dying, going crazy, losing control | – | ++ |

*Note.*  +=occasionally; ++=often present; –=rarely present.

A standard tricyclic antidepressant (TCA) regimen is to start the patient at a dosage of 10 mg of imipramine at bedtime and increase the dosage by 10 mg every other night until 50 mg is reached. Because 50 mg is usually inadequate for full panic blockade, the dosage can then be raised by 25-mg increments every 3 days or by 50-mg increments weekly to as high as 300 mg. Most patients need at least 150 mg daily of TCAs, and unfortunately, underdosage commonly occurs. On "high" imipramine dosing of around 200 mg/day, more than 80% of patients show a marked response in panic attacks (Mavissakalian and Perel 1989).

Some controlled treatment trials have now shown that the potent serotonin reuptake blockers are highly effective in the treatment of panic. Given their higher safety, tolerability, and ease of administration compared with TCAs, they constitute the first line in the treatment of panic disorder, either alone or in combination with a benzodiazepine when needed. As a first-line treatment, they also offer the advantage that they are effective for several of the commonly comorbid disorders, such as depression, social phobia, generalized anxiety disorder (GAD), and obsessive-compulsive disorder (OCD). Although paroxetine and sertraline are the only U.S. Food and Drug Administration (FDA)–approved selective serotonin reuptake inhibitors (SSRIs) for this indication, all SSRIs

have comparable efficacy in treating panic. A head-on comparison of paroxetine (40–60 mg/day) with sertraline (50–150 mg/day) reported similar efficacy for the two medications (Bandelow et al. 2004).

A meta-analysis of 43 treatment studies compared the short-term efficacy of SSRIs and TCAs and reported no differences in effect sizes in reducing panic symptoms, agoraphobic avoidance, anxiety, depressive symptoms, or the proportion of patients free of panic attacks at end point; however, the dropout rate was significantly lower in those treated with SSRIs (18%) versus TCAs (31%) (Bakker et al. 2002). Like the TCAs, SSRIs can cause uncomfortable overstimulation in panic patients if started at the usual dosages. It is therefore suggested that treatment be started gingerly at 5–10 mg/day for fluoxetine, paroxetine, and citalopram and 25 mg/day for sertraline and fluvoxamine. The dosage can then be gradually increased to an average dosage through weekly adjustments. A moderate or lower daily dosage is usually adequate for most patients, as in the trials just described, and high dosages are generally not needed and less tolerated.

Venlafaxine is also effective in treating panic disorder. A large multisite, placebo-controlled trial of venlafaxine extended-release in 361 adult patients, using a flexible dosage range of 75–225 mg/day for 10 weeks, reported better response and remission rates than with placebo, with a greater improvement in number of panic attacks, anticipatory anxiety, fear, and avoidance (Bradwejn et al. 2005). An open trial of mirtazapine administered at 30 mg/day for 3 months to 45 panic disorder patients also showed a pronounced decline in panic attacks and anticipatory anxiety, coupled with a very low 6% discontinuation rate (Sarchiapone et al. 2003). Although one small open trial reported significant improvement in panic with bupropion (Simon et al. 2003), controlled data and clinical lore do not support its use.

Monoamine oxidase inhibitors (MAOIs) are equally as effective as the TCAs and the SSRIs in treating panic. Both phenelzine and tranylcypromine successfully treat panic. Phenelzine can be started at 15 mg daily in the morning. The dosage is then increased by 15 mg every 4–7 days as tolerated, up to a maximum of 60–90 mg daily. If sedation or weight gain is of concern, tranylcypromine may be tried, starting at 10 mg in the morning and increasing by 10 mg every 4 days to a maximum of 80 mg daily. TCAs and serotonin reuptake inhibitors are typically preferred over MAOIs because they are better tolerated and obviate the need for dietary restrictions and the risk of hypertensive crises. Furthermore, patients who do not respond to a TCA or a serotonin reuptake inhibitor

---

**TABLE 19-8.** **Pharmacological treatment of panic disorder**

---

**Selective serotonin reuptake inhibitors and serotonin-norepinephrine reuptake inhibitors**

*General indications:* First-line, alone or in combination with benzodiazepines if needed. Also first choice with comorbid obsessive-compulsive disorder, generalized anxiety disorder, depression, and social phobia. Start with very low dosages and increase; response seen with low to moderate dosages.

*Sertraline, paroxetine:* FDA approved

*Fluvoxamine, fluoxetine, citalopram, escitalopram:* similarly efficacious

*Venlafaxine extended-release:* FDA approved

**Tricyclic antidepressants**

*General indications:* Established efficacy, second-line if SSRIs fail or are not tolerated.

*Imipramine:* well studied

*Clomipramine:* high efficacy but not easily tolerated

*Desipramine:* if low tolerance to anticholinergic side effects

*Nortriptyline:* if prone to orthostatic hypotension, elderly

**Monoamine oxidase inhibitors**

*General indications:* Poor response or tolerance to other antidepressants; comorbid atypical depression or social phobia.

*Phenelzine:* most studied

*Tranylcypromine:* less sedation

**High-potency benzodiazepines**

*General indications:* Poor response or tolerance to antidepressants; prominent anticipatory anxiety or phobic avoidance; initial treatment phase until antidepressant begins to work.

*Clonazepam:* longer-acting, less frequent dosing, less withdrawal, first choice

*Alprazolam:* well studied but short-acting

*Alprazolam extended-release:* once-daily dosing

**Other medications**

*General indications:* Particularly as augmentation in patients whose illness is refractory or who are intolerant of the above medications, not well tested to date.

*Pindolol:* effective augmentation in one controlled trial

*Valproic acid:* open trials only

*Inositol:* open trials only

*Clonidine:* initial response tends to fade in open trials

*Atypical antipsychotics:* open trials

---

*Note.* FDA=U.S. Food and Drug Administration; SSRI=selective serotonin reuptake inhibitor.

---

alone may respond to a combination of the two. However, MAOIs are an option to consider for patients who fail to tolerate or to respond well to other antidepressants.

Full remission of panic attacks with antidepressants usually requires 4–12 weeks of treatment. The disorder can probably best be characterized as chronic, with an exacerbating and remitting course. Therefore, complete agreement has not been reached regarding the recommended course of treatment. In a controlled prospective study, a very high relapse rate for panic was found when imipramine was discontinued after 6 months of acute treatment (Mavissakalian and Perel 1992). Thus, a reasonable

recommendation in treating panic disorder is to continue full-dosage medication for at least 6 months to prevent early relapse. Afterward, patients can be tapered to half-dosage medication and be followed up to ensure that clinical improvement is maintained.

**Benzodiazepines.** Although clinicians prefer to use antidepressants for the first-line treatment of panic, high-potency benzodiazepines are also highly effective in treating the condition. In one study (Pecknold et al. 1988), 82% of patients treated acutely with alprazolam showed at least moderate improvement in panic, compared with

43% given placebo. Onset of response was rapid, with significant improvement occurring in the first couple weeks of treatment, and the mean final dosage was 5.7 mg/day. After 8 weeks of acute treatment, patients were tapered off medication over 4 weeks; 27% experienced rebound panic attacks, and 35% had withdrawal symptoms. Clonazepam appears equally promising in the acute treatment of panic, according to a large multicenter trial (Rosenbaum et al. 1997). In the acute treatment of panic attacks, the lowest dosage of 0.5 mg/day was least efficacious, but dosages of 1.0 mg/day or higher (2, 3, and 4 mg/day) were equally efficacious, and the lower dosages of 1–2 mg/day were better tolerated. Long-term efficacy, possible tolerance and dependency, and difficulties in discontinuing the medication are the main areas of concern when choosing benzodiazepine treatment. Naturalistic follow-up studies of long-term benzodiazepine treatment appear generally optimistic because most patients maintain their therapeutic gains without increasing their benzodiazepine dosage over time.

Clonazepam should generally be preferred as a first choice because it is longer-acting and thus has the advantage of less frequent twice-daily or even once-daily dosing and less risk of withdrawal symptoms than alprazolam. It should generally be started at 0.5 mg twice a day and increased only if needed, usually to a maximum dosage of 4 mg/day. Alprazolam is usually started at 0.5 mg four times a day and is gradually increased to an average dosage of 4 mg/day and a range of 2–10 mg/day according to the individual patient. Treatment of at least 6 months is recommended, as with the antidepressants. In a controlled study, one-third of patients were unable to tolerate a 4-week taper off alprazolam after 8 months of maintenance treatment; the strongest predictor of taper failure was initial severity of panic attacks rather than alprazolam dosage (Rickels et al. 1993).

**Other medications.** Buspirone is a serotonin type 1A (5-HT$_{1A}$) receptor agonist, nonbenzodiazepine antianxiety agent and has not been found effective in treating panic. Similarly, there is no evidence that β-adrenergic-blocking drugs, such as propranolol, are effective in blocking spontaneous panic attacks. If panic attacks occur in a specific social context, such as public speaking, a trial of β-blockers would be indicated.

Clonidine, which inhibits locus coeruleus discharge, would seem for theoretical reasons to be a good antipanic drug. Although some patients may initially respond to clonidine, the therapeutic effect tends to be lost in a matter of weeks because of receptor habituation. This loss of response, plus a number of bothersome side effects, makes clonidine a poor initial choice for treatment of panic disorder. However, one controlled study found clonidine to be efficacious for both panic disorder and GAD (Hoehn-Saric et al. 1993).

Valproic acid also may have some beneficial effects in the treatment of panic attacks (Keck et al. 1993). In one open trial, all 12 patients were moderately to markedly improved after 6 weeks of treatment, and 11 continued the medication and maintained their gains after 6 months (Woodman and Noyes 1994). Controlled trials, however, have not been reported. A fairly large controlled trial of another mood stabilizer, gabapentin, at flexible dosages of 600–3,600 mg daily, showed it to be no better than placebo in treating panic disorder (Pande et al. 2000), although a post hoc analysis showed it to have some efficacy in the more severely symptomatic patients, suggesting that an augmentation study in refractory panic might be worthwhile.

Atypical antipsychotics also have received attention in recent years. In one study, patients who previously had not responded to SSRI monotherapy were treated openly for 12 weeks with 5 mg/day of olanzapine added to an SSRI, resulting in 82% of patients rated as responders by the end of the trial (Sepede et al. 2006). Similarly, another open trial of 10 patients with refractory panic disorder treated for 8 weeks with flexible-dose olanzapine at an average dosage of 12 mg/day resulted in an approximately 75% decrease in panic attacks and anticipatory anxiety (Hollifield et al. 2005).

### Psychotherapy

**Psychodynamic psychotherapy.** Systematic studies examining the efficacy of psychodynamically oriented psychotherapy in panic disorder are few but promising. Psychodynamically oriented clinicians tend to agree that psychological factors do not appear to be significant in a proportion of patients with panic, and emphasize the importance of conducting a psychodynamic assessment to determine whether a particular patient will benefit from a psychodynamic treatment component (Gabbard 1990). Cooper (1985) emphasized that in patients with a predominant biological component to their illness, insistence on dynamic understanding and on responsibility for one's symptoms may, in the long run, be not only useless but also potentially harmful, leading to further damage in self-esteem and strengthened masochistic defenses. However, it is also clear that there are case reports of patients who were successfully treated for panic with psychodynamic therapy or psychoanalysis.

**Supportive psychotherapy.** Despite adequate treatment of panic attacks with medication, phobic avoidance may remain. Supportive psychotherapy and education about the illness are necessary to urge the patient to confront the phobic situation. Patients who fail to respond may then need additional psychotherapy, either dynamic or behavioral. Encouragement from other patients with similar conditions is often quite helpful. Yet supportive psychotherapy alone is not an effective enough treatment for panic disorder.

**Cognitive-behavioral therapy.** In recent years, interest in cognitive-behavioral therapy (CBT) for panic has surged, and it has become firmly established as a first-line treatment for this disorder and found to be comparable in effectiveness to first-line medication treatments (Table 19–9).

The major behavioral techniques for the treatment of panic attacks are breathing retraining, to control both acute and chronic hyperventilation; exposure to somatic cues, usually involving a hierarchy of exposure to feared sensations through imaginal and behavioral exercises; and relaxation training. Cognitive treatment of panic involves cognitive restructuring, so as to give the uncomfortable affects and physical sensations associated with panic a more benign interpretation. These techniques can be administered in various combinations. The pure cognitive view is that panic attacks consist of normal physical sensations (e.g., palpitations, slight dizziness) to which panic disorder patients grossly overreact with catastrophic cognitions. A more middle-of-the-road view is that panic patients do have extreme physical sensations, such as bursts of tachycardia, but can still significantly help themselves by changing their interpretation of the event from "I am going to die of a heart attack" to "There go my heart symptoms again."

### *Treatment of the Agoraphobic Component of Panic Disorder*

There continues to be some disagreement in the literature regarding the best method of treatment for agoraphobia with panic attacks. Antipanic medication is given to block the occurrence of panic attacks, and its efficacy in this regard is well documented. However, medication alone is often not adequate treatment in patients with significant agoraphobic avoidance; it is generally accepted that some means of exposing agoraphobic patients to the feared situations is necessary for overall improvement. This may be achieved through various nonspecific methods, such as psychoeducation, reassurance, and supportive therapy.

**TABLE 19–9.** Cognitive and behavioral approaches to treating panic disorder

Interoceptive exposure (to the somatic cues of panic attacks)

Situational exposure (to the settings that are phobically avoided)

Cognitive restructuring

Breathing retraining

Applied relaxation training

However, focused CBT is, on the whole, more successful than nonspecific techniques in reducing agoraphobic avoidance.

### *Treatment With Combined Medication and Psychotherapy*

A recent meta-analytic study, based on 23 randomized comparisons involving about 1,700 participants, found that combined treatment was superior to antidepressant pharmacotherapy and to psychotherapy alone. However, after termination of acute-phase treatment, combination therapy was more effective than pharmacotherapy alone but as effective as psychotherapy, suggesting a more lasting effect of psychotherapy (Furukawa et al. 2006).

## Generalized Anxiety Disorder

### Definition and Clinical Description

DSM-IV-TR sharpened the distinction of GAD from "normal" anxiety by specifying that in GAD the worry must be clearly excessive, pervasive, difficult to control, and associated with marked distress or impairment (Table 19–10).

GAD is the main diagnostic category for prominent and chronic anxiety in the absence of panic disorder. The essential feature of this syndrome, according to DSM-IV-TR, is persistent anxiety lasting at least 6 months. The symptoms of this type of anxiety fall within two broad categories: apprehensive expectation and worry, and physical symptoms. Patients with GAD are constantly worried over minor matters, fearful, and anticipating the worst. Muscle tension, restlessness, a "keyed up" feeling, difficulty concentrating, insomnia, irritability, and fatigue are typical signs of GAD and became the symptom criteria for the disorder in DSM-IV (American Psychiatric Association 1994) after a number of studies attempted to

**TABLE 19–10.  DSM-IV-TR diagnostic criteria for generalized anxiety disorder**

A. Excessive anxiety and worry (apprehensive expectation), occurring more days than not for at least 6 months, about a number of events or activities (such as work or school performance).

B. The person finds it difficult to control the worry.

C. The anxiety and worry are associated with three (or more) of the following six symptoms (with at least some symptoms present for more days than not for the past 6 months).  **Note:** Only one item is required in children.

   (1) restlessness or feeling keyed up or on edge
   (2) being easily fatigued
   (3) difficulty concentrating or mind going blank
   (4) irritability
   (5) muscle tension
   (6) sleep disturbance (difficulty falling or staying asleep, or restless unsatisfying sleep)

D. The focus of the anxiety and worry is not confined to features of an Axis I disorder, e.g., the anxiety or worry is not about having a panic attack (as in panic disorder), being embarrassed in public (as in social phobia), being contaminated (as in obsessive-compulsive disorder), being away from home or close relatives (as in separation anxiety disorder), gaining weight (as in anorexia nervosa), having multiple physical complaints (as in somatization disorder), or having a serious illness (as in hypochondriasis), and the anxiety and worry do not occur exclusively during posttraumatic stress disorder.

E. The anxiety, worry, or physical symptoms cause clinically significant distress or impairment in social, occupational, or other important areas of functioning.

F. The disturbance is not due to the direct physiological effects of a substance (e.g., a drug of abuse, a medication) or a general medical condition (e.g., hyperthyroidism) and does not occur exclusively during a mood disorder, a psychotic disorder, or a pervasive developmental disorder.

single out the physical symptoms that are the most distinctive and characteristic of GAD. Motor tension and hypervigilance better differentiate GAD from other anxiety states than does autonomic hyperactivity. The diagnosis of GAD is made when a patient experiences at least 6 months of chronic anxiety and excessive worry. At least three of six physical symptoms must also be present.

## Epidemiology and Comorbidity

One epidemiological study using DSM-IV (American Psychiatric Association 1994) criteria (Carter et al. 2001) found a 1.5% 1-year prevalence for threshold GAD and a 3.6% 1-year prevalence for subthreshold GAD. Higher rates of the disorder were found in women (2.7%) and the elderly (2.2%). A high degree of comorbidity was again confirmed: 59% for major depression and 56% for other anxiety disorders. The NESARC reported 1-year and lifetime DSM-IV GAD prevalences of 2.1% and 4.1%, respectively, with rates higher in female, middle-aged, widowed/separated/divorced, and low-income individuals (Grant et al. 2005b).

## Etiology

### Biological Theories

Although the neurobiology of GAD is among the least investigated in the anxiety disorders, advances are now being made (a summary is presented in Table 19–11).

**TABLE 19–11.  Biological models of generalized anxiety disorder**

Abnormalities of the γ-aminobutyric acid (GABA)–benzodiazepine receptor

Hypersensitive conditioned fear network centered in the amygdala

Noradrenergic activation

Serotonergic dysregulation

Modest genetic component

Recent work has focused on brain circuits underlying the neurobiology of fear in animal models and in humans and on how inherited and acquired vulnerabilities in these circuits might underlie a variety of anxiety disorders. It is speculated that alterations in the structure and function of the amygdala, which are central to fear-related behaviors, may be associated with GAD.

Abnormalities of the GABA–benzodiazepine receptor complex also have been implicated in GAD. One series of compounds, the β-carbolines, which are inverse agonists of this receptor complex, produce an acute anxiety syndrome when administered to laboratory animals or to nonanxious human volunteers. Accordingly, benzodiazepines are well established as an efficacious treatment of GAD. GAD subjects have been found to have decreased benzodiazepine receptor density in peripheral blood cells as well as decreased transcriptional mRNA encoding for the receptor, both of which return to normal values with treatment and reduction in anxiety levels (Ferrarese et al. 1990; Rocca et al. 1998).

The evidence for noradrenergic dysregulation in GAD has been mixed. Abelson et al. (1991) reported a blunted growth hormone response to clonidine in GAD compared with responses in control subjects without GAD. Plasma norepinephrine and its metabolite were found to be elevated, and $\alpha_2$ adrenoreceptors decreased, in GAD patients compared with healthy control subjects (Sevy et al. 1989). Other studies of the noradrenergic system have had negative results (Mathew et al. 1981). There is also some evidence of serotonergic dysregulation in GAD, such as heightened anxiety responses to the partial serotonin agonist *meta*-chlorophenylpiperazine (*m*-CPP) compared with control subjects (Germine et al. 1992).

There appears to be a genetic component to GAD, albeit relatively modest. Kendler et al. (1992) studied GAD in female twins and determined that the familial component of the disorder was almost entirely genetic, with a modest heritability of about 30%. Twin studies have reported about 20%–33% overlap in genetic influences between GAD and neuroticism, whereas environmental influences on GAD and neuroticism were largely unshared (Hettema et al. 2004).

## Psychological Theories

With regard to the origins of GAD, it has been proposed that insecure attachment relationships and ambivalence toward caregivers, as well as parental overprotection and lack of emotional warmth, may all contribute to later development of anxiety. Regarding mechanisms that may perpetuate GAD, three are summarized. First, worry is used as a strategy for avoiding intense negative affects. Second, worry about unlikely and future threat removes the need to deal with more proximal and realistic threats and limits the capacity to find solutions to more immedi-

ate conflicts. Finally, individuals with GAD engage in a certain degree of magical thinking and believe that their worry helped prevent a feared outcome, thus leading to a negative reinforcement of the process of worrying. In terms of the etiology of GAD, cognitive theory speculates a relation to early cognitive schemas born from negative experiences of the world as a dangerous place (Barlow 1988) or insecure, anxious early attachments to important caregivers (Cassidy 1995).

## Course and Prognosis

In contrast with panic disorder, no overwhelming single event prompts the patient with GAD to seek help. Such patients seem only over time to develop the recognition that their experience of chronic tension, hyperactivity, worry, and anxiety is excessive. Often they will state that there has never been a time in their lives, as long as they can remember, that they were not anxious. Patients with GAD experience substantial interference with their lives and have a high degree of professional help seeking and a high use of medications (Wittchen et al. 1994).

In clinical samples, GAD is commonly comorbid with major depression and other anxiety disorders but still emerges as a clearly distinct entity (Wittchen et al. 2000). Abuse of alcohol, barbiturates, and antianxiety medications is also common. Comorbid avoidant and dependent personality disorders appear to lessen the likelihood of remission from GAD (Massion et al. 2002). Contrary to panic disorder, which declines with old age, GAD appears to account for a lot of the anxiety states in late life, often occurring comorbidly with medical illnesses (Flint 1994).

## Differential Diagnosis

The differential diagnosis of GAD is summarized in Table 19–12.

## Treatment

### *Pharmacotherapy*

The pharmacological treatment of GAD is summarized in Table 19–13.

**Benzodiazepines.** In past years, benzodiazepines were the first-line treatment of GAD. Currently, however, newer medication choices such as buspirone, SSRIs, and serotonin and norepinephrine reuptake inhibitors (SNRIs)

## TABLE 19–12. Differential diagnosis of generalized anxiety disorder

Anxious depression

Panic attacks or anticipatory anxiety

Social anxiety

Posttraumatic stress disorder–related hyperarousal symptoms

Obsessional fearfulness

Hypochondriasis

Paranoid anxiety associated with psychosis or personality disorder

---

have replaced the benzodiazepines as first-line treatments. There is some evidence that benzodiazepines may be more effective in treating the physical symptoms of anxiety, whereas antidepressants, whether TCAs or SSRIs, may be more effective in treating the psychic symptoms (Rocca et al. 1998).

Although benzodiazepines are generally safe, with side effects limited mainly to sedation and slowed mentation, there is a concern that some patients may become tolerant or even addicted to these medications. However, available data indicate that the concern over benzodiazepine abuse in chronically anxious populations is overestimated, and in reality most patients continue to derive clinical benefits without developing abuse or dependence (Romach et al. 1995).

**Buspirone.** Buspirone is a 5-HT$_{1A}$ agonist, nonbenzodiazepine antianxiety agent that may have similar efficacy to the benzodiazepines in treating GAD. Its advantages are a different side-effect profile without sedation and the absence of tolerance and withdrawal. Its disadvantage is a slower rate of onset (Rickels et al. 1988), which can lead to early patient noncompliance.

Treatment with buspirone is usually started at 5 mg three times a day, and the dosage can be increased until a maximum dosage of 60 mg/day is reached. A twice-daily regimen is probably as efficacious as a thrice-daily regimen and easier to comply with. There is recent evidence, via a controlled trial (Rickels et al. 2000), that in long-term benzodiazepine users, a successful strategy may be to start buspirone or an antidepressant for 1 month prior to undertaking a gradual 4- to 6-week taper of the benzodiazepine. Other independent predictors of successful benzodiazepine taper were lower initial dosages and less severe and chronic anxiety symptoms.

## TABLE 19–13. Pharmacological treatment of generalized anxiety disorder

**Venlafaxine extended-release**

*General indications:* First-line treatment; approved by FDA, with proven efficacy in large controlled trials; generally well tolerated; once-daily dosing; recommended starting dosage is 75 mg/day, which may be adequate for a number of patients.

**Selective serotonin reuptake inhibitors (SSRIs)**

*General indications:* First-line treatment; paroxetine is FDA approved; generally well tolerated; once-daily dosing; recommended starting dosage is 20 mg/day, which may be adequate for many patients; other SSRIs also efficacious.

**Benzodiazepines**

*General indications:* Well-known efficacy and widely used; all appear similarly efficacious; issues with dependence and withdrawal in certain patients; may be more effective for the physical rather than cognitive symptoms of generalized anxiety disorder.

**Buspirone**

*General indications:* Proven efficacy; well tolerated; a trial is generally indicated in all patients; compared with benzodiazepines, takes longer to take action and is not associated with a "high"; may have less efficacy and compliance with very recent benzodiazepine use.

**Tricyclic antidepressants (TCAs)**

*General indications:* Demonstrated efficacy in few trials; more side effects than benzodiazepines, buspirone, and newer antidepressants; delayed action compared with benzodiazepines; may be more effective for cognitive rather than physical symptoms of anxiety.

*Imipramine:* demonstrated efficacy

*Trazodone:* demonstrated efficacy

**Other medications**

*Clonidine:* tends to lose initial response

*Propranolol:* may be useful adjuvant in patients with pronounced palpitations and tremor

*Atypical antipsychotics*

*Riluzole:* open trials

*Tiagabine:* randomized controlled trial, mixed results

*Pregabalin:* not marketed in United States

*Note.* FDA=U.S. Food and Drug Administration.

**Antidepressants.** Several large controlled trials to date have established the efficacy of extended-release venlafaxine, an SNRI, in treating GAD (Davidson et al. 1999; Gelenberg et al. 2000; Rickels et al. 2000). Venlafaxine has been found effective in dosages ranging from 75 to 225 mg/day. Response rate is approximately 70%, with benefits appearing as early as the first 2 weeks of treatment. Venlafaxine is generally well tolerated, with nausea, somnolence, and dry mouth being the most common side effects. Studies have not found consistent differences in efficacy as a function of dosing, suggesting that it can be started at 75 mg/day for GAD and subsequently be increased if clinical improvement is not adequate and side effects permit.

The SSRI paroxetine has been studied in several controlled trials. One trial showed paroxetine at fixed dosages of both 20 mg and 40 mg daily to be superior to placebo over an 8-week treatment period, with approximately two-thirds of patients considered responders (Bellew et al. 2000). Another large flexible-dosing trial showed that paroxetine at dosages ranging from 20 to 50 mg daily was superior to placebo in treating GAD over an 8-week period (Pollack et al. 2001). In a paroxetine trial using dosages of 20–40 mg/day, an approximately 65% response rate and 33% remission rate were reported (Rickels et al. 2003). Sertraline also has been found to be superior to placebo in decreasing both the psychic and the somatic symptoms of GAD during a 12-week treatment (Dahl et al. 2005) at flexible dosages of 50–150 mg/day (Allgulander et al. 2004), and one study showed comparable efficacy and tolerability for paroxetine and sertraline (Ball et al. 2005). Three pooled similar placebo-controlled trials of the SSRI escitalopram, administered for 8 weeks at a dosage of 10–20 mg/day, reported significant improvement in GAD with good tolerability in more than 800 patients (Goodman et al. 2005).

In one controlled study comparing imipramine and alprazolam in treating GAD, similar efficacy was found for the two medications, with imipramine acting more on negative affects and cognitions and alprazolam acting more on somatic symptoms (Hoehn-Saric et al. 1988).

### Psychotherapy

Research into the psychotherapy of GAD has not been as extensive as for other anxiety disorders. Still, a number of studies exist that clearly show that a variety of psychotherapies are helpful in treating GAD (Table 19–14).

CBT is superior to general nondirective or supportive therapy in treating GAD (Chambless and Gillis 1993) and possibly superior to behavior therapy alone (Bork-

**TABLE 19–14. Cognitive and behavioral approaches to treating generalized anxiety disorder**

Exposure
Cognitive restructuring
Breathing retraining
Applied relaxation training

ovec and Costello 1993). Cognitive therapy alone may have an edge over behavior therapy alone, according to some studies (Butler et al. 1991) but not others (Ost and Breitholtz 2000). In a study that compared four conditions—behavior therapy alone, cognitive therapy alone, combined CBT, and a wait-list control group—all three active treatments were similarly efficacious and superior to the control condition during an up to 2-year follow-up period; however, the combined CBT group had a much lower dropout rate than the other groups (Barlow et al. 1992). Cognitive therapy and applied relaxation were found to have similar effectiveness during a 12-week treatment and at a 6-month follow-up (Arntz 2003). Another randomized study compared cognitive, analytic, and behavioral management in treating GAD (Durham et al. 1994). Cognitive therapy emerged as superior, with some edge over behavioral management alone and a significantly better result than analytic treatment. A "well-being" component aimed at restoring overall function may be a useful addition to usual CBT (Fava et al. 2005).

### Combined Pharmacotherapy and Psychotherapy

In a meta-analysis of 65 CBT and pharmacological treatment studies of GAD, overall similar efficacy was reported for the two treatment approaches, with lower attrition rates for psychotherapy (Mitte 2005). There are minimal data on the use of combined psychotherapy and medication in the treatment of GAD.

## Social Phobia (Social Anxiety Disorder)

### Definition and Clinical Description

DSM-IV-TR criteria for social phobia are presented in Table 19–15.

---

**TABLE 19–15.    DSM-IV-TR diagnostic criteria for social phobia**

A.  A marked and persistent fear of one or more social or performance situations in which the person is exposed to unfamiliar people or to possible scrutiny by others. The individual fears that he or she will act in a way (or show anxiety symptoms) that will be humiliating or embarrassing.   **Note:** In children, there must be evidence of the capacity for age-appropriate social relationships with familiar people and the anxiety must occur in peer settings, not just in interactions with adults.

B.  Exposure to the feared social situation almost invariably provokes anxiety, which may take the form of a situationally bound or situationally predisposed panic attack.   **Note:** In children, the anxiety may be expressed by crying, tantrums, freezing, or shrinking from social situations with unfamiliar people.

C.  The person recognizes that the fear is excessive or unreasonable.   **Note:** In children, this feature may be absent.

D.  The feared social or performance situations are avoided or else are endured with intense anxiety or distress.

E.  The avoidance, anxious anticipation, or distress in the feared social or performance situation(s) interferes significantly with the person's normal routine, occupational (academic) functioning, or social activities or relationships, or there is marked distress about having the phobia.

F.  In individuals under age 18 years, the duration is at least 6 months.

G.  The fear or avoidance is not due to the direct physiological effects of a substance (e.g., a drug of abuse, a medication) or a general medical condition and is not better accounted for by another mental disorder (e.g., panic disorder with or without agoraphobia, separation anxiety disorder, body dysmorphic disorder, a pervasive developmental disorder, or schizoid personality disorder).

H.  If a general medical condition or another mental disorder is present, the fear in Criterion A is unrelated to it, e.g., the fear is not of stuttering, trembling in Parkinson's disease, or exhibiting abnormal eating behavior in anorexia nervosa or bulimia nervosa.

*Specify* if:

**Generalized:**   if the fears include most social situations (also consider the additional diagnosis of avoidant personality disorder)

---

Socially phobic individuals fear and/or avoid a variety of situations in which they would be required to interact with others or to perform a task in front of other people. Typical social phobias are of speaking, eating, or writing in public; using public lavatories; and attending parties or interviews. In addition, a common fear of socially phobic individuals is that other people will detect and ridicule their anxiety in social situations. An individual may have one, limited, or numerous social fears. Social phobia is described as generalized if the social fear encompasses most social situations as opposed to being present in circumscribed ones. Generalized social phobia is overall a more serious and impairing condition. Generalized social phobia can be reliably diagnosed as a subtype; it has an earlier onset, and affected individuals are more often single and have more interactional fears and greater comorbidity with atypical depression and alcoholism (Mannuzza et al. 1995).

## Epidemiology and Comorbidity

In the National Comorbidity Survey (Kessler et al. 1994; Magee et al. 1996), which used DSM-III-R criteria, social phobia had a lifetime occurrence of 13.3%, 1-year incidence of 7.9%, and 1-month incidence of 4.5% and was somewhat more common in women than in men (lifetime, 15.5% vs. 11.1%). Of those affected, about one-third reported exclusively public speaking fears. About one-third had multiple fears qualifying for the generalized type of social phobia, which was found to be more persistent, impairing, and comorbid than the specific public speaking type. The NESARC found a 1-year and lifetime prevalence of DSM-IV social anxiety disorder of 2.8% and 5.0%, respectively (Grant et al. 2005a). Mean age at onset was 15 years. The disorder was chronic; mean age at first treatment was about 12 years later, and 80% had never received treatment. There was significant comorbidity with other psychiatric disorders, especially GAD, bipolar I, and avoidant and dependent personality disorders.

Epidemiological studies have consistently found significant comorbidity between lifetime social phobia and various mood disorders, with an approximately three- to sixfold higher risk for dysthymia, depression, and bipolar disorder (Kessler et al. 1999).

Social phobia can be associated with a variety of personality disorders, particularly avoidant personality disorder. Indeed, a review of the literature comparing generalized social phobia, avoidant personality disorder, and shyness concluded that all three may exist on a continuum (Rettew 2000) or may even be alternative conceptualizations of the same underlying condition (Ralevski et al. 2005).

## Etiology

### *Psychosocial Theories*

A number of mechanisms are proposed in learning theories as contributors to the pathogenesis of social phobia (Stemberger et al. 1995), and risk factors for social anxiety are summarized in Table 19–16.

Risk factors include direct exposure to socially related traumatic events, vicarious learning through observing others engaged in such traumatic situations, and information transfer (i.e., things that one hears in various contexts regarding social interactions).

There is a significant familial component to social phobia, part of which is thought to be heritable and part acquired. Parents, whether socially anxious themselves or not, might rear socially anxious children through various mechanisms, such as lack of adequate exposure to social situations and development of social skills, overprotectiveness, controlling and critical behavior, modeling of socially anxious behaviors, and fearful information conveyed about social situations (Hudson and Rapee 2000).

**TABLE 19–16.  Risk factors for social anxiety**

Parental psychiatric history (especially social phobia, other anxiety disorders, depression)

Parental marital conflict

Parental overprotection or rejection

Childhood abuse

Childhood lack of close relationship with an adult

Not being firstborn for males

Frequent moves in childhood

Poor school performance

Running away from home

**TABLE 19–17.  Biological models of social anxiety disorder**

Hypersensitive conditioned fear network centered in the amygdala

Abnormalities of the γ-aminobutyric acid (GABA)–benzodiazepine receptor

Noradrenergic activation

Decreased dopaminergic tone

Altered serotonin availability

Modest to moderate genetic component

## Biological Theories

Biological theories of social phobia are summarized in Table 19–17.

**Neurochemistry.**  Patients with social phobia show a blunted growth hormone response to clonidine challenge, suggesting underlying noradrenergic dysfunction (Tancer et al. 1993), but this was not replicated in a subsequent study (Tancer et al. 1994). GABA–benzodiazepine receptor involvement is unclear.

**Genetics.**  First-degree relatives of probands with generalized social phobia have an approximately 10-fold higher risk for generalized social phobia or avoidant personality disorder.

## Course and Prognosis

Social phobia has its onset mainly in adolescence and early adulthood, earlier than with agoraphobia, and the course of illness is very chronic. Onset of symptoms is sometimes acute after a humiliating social experience but is usually insidious over months or years and without a clear-cut precipitant. Interestingly, in clinical studies, men are equally as affected as (or even more commonly affected than) women, in distinction to other anxiety disorders.

Social phobia is clearly a chronic and potentially highly impairing condition; course and prognosis are summarized in Table 19–18.

## Diagnosis and Differential Diagnosis

Differential diagnosis of social anxiety disorder is summarized in Table 19–19.

### TABLE 19–18.    Course and prognosis of social anxiety disorder

**Course**

Typically early onset at or before adolescence and very chronic course

**Outcome**

About one-half found to be recovered after 25 years of illness

**Predictors of poorer prognosis**

Onset before age 8–11 years

Psychiatric comorbidity

Lower educational status

More symptoms at baseline

Comorbid health problems

---

### TABLE 19–19.    Differential diagnosis of social anxiety disorder

Personality disorder, such as avoidant, schizoid, paranoid

Axis I paranoid disorder such as paranoid schizophrenia or paranoid delusional disorder

Depression-related social withdrawal secondary to anhedonia or feelings of defectiveness

Obsessive-compulsive disorder–related fears exacerbated in social settings (e.g., contamination)

Panic disorder with phobic avoidance not limited to social situations

Deficits/impaired social skills associated with schizophrenia and related disorders

## Treatment

### *Pharmacotherapy*

The pharmacological treatment of social anxiety disorder is summarized in Table 19–20.

**Beta-blockers.**  In performance-type social phobia, several analogue studies have shown beta-blocker efficacy, particularly when these agents are used acutely prior to a performance. Although a variety of beta-blockers have been used in studies and are probably efficacious for performance anxiety, the most common ones used are propranolol, 20 mg, or atenolol, 50 mg, taken about 45 minutes before a performance. It also seems that they are more

### TABLE 19–20.    Pharmacological treatment of social anxiety disorder

**Selective serotonin reuptake inhibitors (SSRIs)**

*General indications:* First-line treatment; shown efficacy; well tolerated; once-daily dosing; effective for comorbid depression, panic, generalized anxiety disorder, or obsessive-compulsive disorder.

*Paroxetine:* best studied in large controlled trials; FDA approved; average dosage 40 mg/day

*Other SSRIs:* also efficacious

*Venlafaxine:* also efficacious

*Mirtazapine:* also efficacious, fewer data

**Benzodiazepines**

*General indications:* Clinically widely used and reportedly efficacious in open trials; generally well tolerated; concerns about dependence and withdrawal in certain patients.

*Clonazepam:* long-acting; efficacy demonstrated in controlled trial

**Beta-blockers**

*General indications:* Highly effective for performance anxiety, taken on an as-needed basis about 1 hour before event. For the most part not helpful in patients with generalized social phobia.

*Propranolol, atenolol*

**Monoamine oxidase inhibitors (MAOIs)**

*General indications:* Demonstrated high effectiveness; may be difficult to tolerate and require dietary restrictions; effective for several comorbid conditions, including atypical depression, social phobia, and panic; well worth trying in patients with otherwise refractory illness.

*Phenelzine:* most studied

*Tranylcypromine:* also effective

**Other medications**

*Gabapentin:* effective in one controlled trial

*Buspirone:* well tolerated; effective in open but not in controlled trial

*Bupropion:* effective in open trial

*Topiramate:* open trial

*Pregabalin:* controlled trial

*Atypical neuroleptics:* open trials

D-*Cycloserine:* used in conjunction with exposure therapy

*Note.*  FDA=U.S. Food and Drug Administration.

effective in controlling stage fright than are benzodiazepines, which may decrease subjective anxiety but not optimize performance and may have an adverse effect on "sharpness."

**Newer antidepressants.** In the past decade, newer antidepressants have been tested and have shown efficacy in treating social phobia, resulting in the SSRIs becoming the first-line treatment for the disorder. They are generally well tolerated, easy to dispense and monitor, and used in standard dosages comparable with those used in depression. Paroxetine is FDA approved for treating social phobia, with efficacy shown in several controlled trials (Baldwin et al. 1999; M.B. Stein et al. 1998).

Fluvoxamine, given at 150 mg/day for 12 weeks, resulted in substantial improvement in 46% of patients compared with a 7% improvement among subjects given placebo in one controlled trial (van Vliet et al. 1994), replicated in a subsequent larger study with a comparable mean dosage of 200 mg/day and a response rate of 43% (M.B. Stein et al. 1999). Efficacy for sertraline at dosages of 50–200 mg/day was shown in one placebo-controlled study (Katzelnick et al. 1995). Similar responses were found in an open trial of fluoxetine (Van Ameringen et al. 1993) and an open trial of citalopram (Bouwer and Stein 1998). A 12-week placebo-controlled trial of escitalopram, 10–20 mg/day, reported efficacy with a 54% responder rate, good tolerability, and significant improvement in work and social impairment (Kasper et al. 2005).

A 12-week extended-release venlafaxine study, using dosages of 75–225 mg/day, showed significant benefit over placebo in social anxiety symptoms and social impairment, with good tolerability (Rickels et al. 2004). A placebo-controlled trial of mirtazapine in 66 women with social phobia also reported efficacy (Muehlbacher et al. 2005). Bupropion is the least studied antidepressant to date, but it may have some efficacy in social phobia (Emmanuel et al. 1991).

**Benzodiazepines.** Benzodiazepines can also be helpful in treating generalized social phobia, despite the usual concerns about their chronic use. Several open trials have reported positive results, and in one controlled study clonazepam at dosages of 0.5–3.0 mg/day (mean dosage = 2.4 mg/day) was found to be superior to placebo, with a response rate of 78% and improvement in social anxiety, avoidance, performance, and negative self-evaluation (Davidson et al. 1993). Alprazolam also has been found to be superior to placebo, with results comparable with those for phenelzine and CBT. The benzodiazepines

would not be considered a first-line treatment for social phobia.

**Monoamine oxidase inhibitors.** Liebowitz et al. (1992) conducted a controlled study comparing phenelzine, atenolol, and placebo in the treatment of DSM-III social phobia. About two-thirds of the patients had a marked response to phenelzine, at dosages of 45–90 mg/day, whereas atenolol was not superior to placebo. Tranylcypromine in dosages of 40–60 mg/day was also associated with significant improvement in about 80% of patients with DSM-III social phobia treated openly for 1 year (Versiani et al. 1988).

### Cognitive and Behavioral Therapies

Three major cognitive-behavioral techniques are used in the treatment of social phobia: exposure, cognitive restructuring, and social skills training (Table 19–21).

---

**TABLE 19–21. Cognitive and behavioral approaches to treating social anxiety disorder**

Exposure (imaginal and/or in vivo)

Cognitive restructuring

Social skills training (modeling, rehearsal, role-playing, practice)

Virtual reality exposure

Exposure preceded by D-cycloserine administration

---

Exposure, cognitive restructuring, and social skills training may all be of significant benefit to patients with social phobia. In addition, these techniques appear superior to nonspecific supportive therapy, as shown in a randomized controlled study comparing supportive therapy with initial individual cognitive therapy followed by group social skills training (Cottraux et al. 2000). The success of CBTs appears to be mediated, at least in part, by a decrease in self-focused attention (Woody et al. 1997). Decreases in negative self-focused thoughts and social anxiety symptoms were significantly intercorrelated in patients treated with CBT but not with exposure, despite the comparable improvement of the two groups (Hofmann et al. 2004). Attempts to correlate patient type (social skills deficits vs. phobic anxiety/avoidance) with preferred treatment modality (social skills training vs. exposure) have not always been fruitful (Wlazlo et al. 1990). Heimberg et al. (1990) compared cognitive-behavioral group treatment with a credible psychoeducational-supportive control intervention in patients with DSM-III social phobia; both groups got better, but the cognitive-behavioral group showed more improvement, especially in patients' self-appraisal.

### Other Types of Psychotherapy

The successful use of medication and/or behavioral treatments has resulted in psychodynamic therapy for phobias falling out of favor (Gabbard 1990). However, in those patients in whom underlying conflicts associated with phobic anxiety and avoidance can be identified by the clinician and are amenable to insightful exploration, psychodynamic therapy can be of benefit.

### Combination Treatment

It appears that medication alone compared with CBT alone has comparable results in the acute treatment of social phobia (Heimberg et al. 1998; Otto et al. 2000). In a recent study, treatment outcome was compared for medication alone (fluoxetine 10–60 mg/day), CBT alone, combined medication and CBT, CBT and placebo, and placebo (Davidson et al. 2004). The response rate was about 50% for both monotherapies and for combined treatment, significantly better than the 32% response rate for placebo alone, leading to the conclusion that combined treatment did not offer any advantage during the acute phase of treatment.

## Specific Phobias

### Definition and Clinical Description

Specific phobias are circumscribed fears of specific objects, situations, or activities. In DSM-IV, for the first time, types of specific phobias were adopted: natural environment (e.g., storms); animal (e.g., insects); blood-injection-injury; situational (e.g., cars, elevators, bridges); and other (e.g., choking, vomiting). The diagnostic criteria for specific phobia are presented in Table 19–22.

### Epidemiology

In the National Comorbidity Survey (Magee et al. 1996), which used DSM-III-R criteria, specific phobias had a lifetime prevalence of 11.3%, with a median age at illness onset of 15, and women were affected more than twice as often as men.

---

**TABLE 19–22.   DSM-IV-TR diagnostic criteria for specific phobia**

A.  Marked and persistent fear that is excessive or unreasonable, cued by the presence or anticipation of a specific object or situation (e.g., flying, heights, animals, receiving an injection, seeing blood).

B.  Exposure to the phobic stimulus almost invariably provokes an immediate anxiety response, which may take the form of a situationally bound or situationally predisposed panic attack.   **Note:** In children, the anxiety may be expressed by crying, tantrums, freezing, or clinging.

C.  The person recognizes that the fear is excessive or unreasonable.   **Note:** In children, this feature may be absent.

D.  The phobic situation(s) is avoided or else is endured with intense anxiety or distress.

E.  The avoidance, anxious anticipation, or distress in the feared situation(s) interferes significantly with the person's normal routine, occupational (or academic) functioning, or social activities or relationships, or there is marked distress about having the phobia.

F.  In individuals under age 18 years, the duration is at least 6 months.

G.  The anxiety, panic attacks, or phobic avoidance associated with the specific object or situation are not better accounted for by another mental disorder, such as obsessive-compulsive disorder (e.g., fear of dirt in someone with an obsession about contamination), posttraumatic stress disorder (e.g., avoidance of stimuli associated with a severe stressor), separation anxiety disorder (e.g., avoidance of school), social phobia (e.g., avoidance of social situations because of fear of embarrassment), panic disorder with agoraphobia, or agoraphobia without history of panic disorder.

*Specify* type:

**Animal type**

**Natural environment type** (e.g., heights, storms, water)

**Blood-injection-injury type**

**Situational type** (e.g., airplanes, elevators, enclosed places)

**Other type** (e.g., fear of choking, vomiting, or contracting an illness; in children, fear of loud sounds or costumed characters)

## Etiology

### *Psychodynamic Theory*

With the 1909 publication of the case of "Little Hans," Freud started to develop a psychological theory of phobic symptom formation (Freud 1909/1955). Little Hans was a 5-year-old boy who developed a phobia of horses. Through an analysis of the boy's conversations with his parents over a period of months, Freud hypothesized that Little Hans's unconscious and forbidden sexual feelings for his mother and aggressive, rivalrous feelings for his father, blocked from discharge because of repression, became physiologically transformed into anxiety, which was then displaced onto a symbolic object, in this case horses, the avoidance of which partly relieved Little Hans's anxiety. Freud later reconceptualized the case of Little Hans in the context of his evolving structural theory. Freud hypothesized that phobic symptoms occur as part of the resolution of intrapsychic conflict between instinctual impulses, superego prohibitions, and external reality constraints. Signal anxiety is experienced by the ego when such unconscious impulses threaten to break through. Such anxiety serves to mobilize not only further repression but also, in the case of phobia formation, projection and displacement of the conflict onto a symbolic object, which can then be avoided as a neurotic solution to the original conflict. In the case of Little Hans, sexual feelings for his mother, aggressive feelings toward his father, and the guilty fear of retribution and castration by his father generated anxiety as a signal of oedipal conflict. The conflict became displaced and projected onto an avoidable object, horses, which Little Hans consequently feared would bite him. According to Freud, such a phobic symptom had two advantages. It avoided the ambivalence inherent in Little Hans's original conflict because he not only hated but also loved his father. It also allowed his ego to cease generating anxiety as long as he could avoid the sight of horses. The cost of this compromise was that Little Hans had become housebound. Psychodynamic work with phobias, then, focuses on the symbolic meanings that the phobic object carries for any individual and the conflicts that it serves to avoid.

### *Behavioral Theories*

In learning theory, phobic anxiety is thought to be a conditioned response acquired through association of the phobic object (i.e., the conditioned stimulus) with a noxious experience (i.e., the unconditioned stimulus). Initially, the noxious experience (e.g., an electric shock) pro-duces an unconditioned response of pain, discomfort, and fear. If the individual frequently receives an electric shock when in contact with the phobic object, then by contiguous conditioning the appearance of the phobic object alone may come to elicit an anxiety response (i.e., conditioned response). Avoidance of the phobic object prevents or reduces this conditioned anxiety and is therefore perpetuated through drive reduction. This classical learning theory model of phobias has received much reinforcement from the relative success of behavioral (i.e., deconditioning) techniques in the treatment of many patients with specific phobias. However, it has also been criticized on the grounds that it is not consistent with a number of empirically observed aspects of phobic behavior in humans.

### *Biological Theories*

The brain circuits mediating conditioned fear responses have emerged as central to the pathogenesis of a number of anxiety disorders, and there is increasing evidence that the model also applies to specific phobias. Studies exposing specific phobia subjects to masked stimuli—that is, very brief stimuli that can only be perceived implicitly—have lent partial support to the notion that phobic stimuli, even when not consciously registered, can elicit a subjective or objectively measured fearful response (Van Den Hout et al. 1997).

## Course and Prognosis

Animal phobias usually begin in early childhood, whereas situational phobias tend to start later, in adolescence or early adulthood. A recent study followed up specific phobia patients 10–16 years after an initial treatment and found that even among responders with complete initial recovery, about half were clinically symptomatic at follow-up, and none of the patients who had not improved with the initial treatment were any better at follow-up (Lipsitz et al. 1999).

## Treatment

The treatment of choice for specific phobias is exposure, aimed at fear extinction. The method of exposure in both the in vivo and the imaginal techniques can be graded or ungraded. Graded exposure uses a hierarchy of anxiety-provoking events varying from least to most stressful. The patient begins at the least stressful level and then gradually progresses up the hierarchy. Ungraded exposure begins with the patients confronting the most stressful items in the hierarchy. Exposure can be accompanied by varying degrees and types of cognitive interventions that decatastrophize the phobic stimulus and encourage risk taking.

TCAs, benzodiazepines, and β-blockers generally do not appear useful for specific phobias, based on the limited number of studies available to date. One recent small controlled trial, in which 11 patients were randomly assigned to take either placebo or paroxetine up to 20 mg/day for 4 weeks, reported that 1 of 6 patients responded to placebo and 3 of 5 to paroxetine (Benjamin et al. 2000). Similarly, dramatic success with SSRIs was reported in three cases of childhood refractory choking phobia that had not responded to other interventions (Banerjee et al. 2005).

There has been a recent surge in interest in the combination of medication and exposure therapy, traditional or virtual reality, in treating anxiety and fear, including specific phobias. In this treatment paradigm, a 50-mg dose of D-cycloserine, a glutamatergic agent that at low dosages has N-methyl-D-aspartate receptor agonist effects and facilitates new learning, is combined with exposure to further promote extinction. In a treatment study of 28 patients with acrophobia (fear of heights), all subjects received two virtual reality exposure sessions and were premedicated with either D-cycloserine or placebo. The combination treatment group manifested significantly greater improvement, which persisted at 3-month follow-up (Ressler et al. 2004).

# Obsessive-Compulsive Disorder

## Definition

The essential features of OCD are obsessions or compulsions. DSM-IV-TR criteria for OCD are presented in Table 19–23.

There are several presentations of OCD based on symptom clusters. One group includes patients with obsessions about dirt and contamination, whose rituals center around compulsive washing and avoidance of contaminated objects. A second group includes patients with pathological counting and compulsive checking. A third group includes purely obsessional patients with no compulsions. Primary obsessional slowness is evident in another group, in whom slowness is the predominant symptom. Patients may spend many hours every day washing, getting dressed, and eating breakfast, and life

goes on at an extremely slow speed. Some OCD patients, called "hoarders," are unable to throw anything out for fear they might someday need something they discarded.

## Clinical Description

### Onset

OCD usually begins in adolescence or early adulthood but can begin prior to that time; 31% of first episodes occur between ages 10 and 15 years, with 75% developing OCD by age 30. In most cases, no particular stress or event precipitates the onset of OCD symptoms, and after an insidious onset there is a chronic and often progressive course. However, some patients describe a sudden onset of symptoms. This is particularly true of patients with a neurological basis for their illness. There is evidence of OCD associated with the 1920s encephalitis epidemic, abnormal birth events, and onset following head injury or seizures. Of interest are reports of new onset of OCD during pregnancy (Neziroglu et al. 1992).

### Symptoms

**Obsessions.** An *obsession* is an intrusive, unwanted mental event usually evoking anxiety or discomfort. Obsessions may be thoughts, ideas, images, ruminations, convictions, fears, or impulses and are often of an aggressive, sexual, religious, disgusting, or nonsensical content. Obsessional ideas are repetitive thoughts that interrupt the normal train of thinking, whereas obsessional images are often vivid visual experiences. Much obsessive thinking involves horrific ideas. The person may think of doing the worst possible thing (e.g., blasphemy, rape, murder, child molestation). Obsessional convictions are often characterized by an element of magical thinking, such as "step on the crack, break your mother's back." Obsessional ruminations may involve prolonged, excessive, and inconclusive thinking about metaphysical questions. Obsessional fears often involve dirt or contamination and differ from phobias because they are present in the absence of the phobic stimulus. Other common obsessional fears involve harm coming to oneself or to others as a consequence of the patient's misdoings, such as one's home catching on fire because the stove was not checked or running over a pedestrian because of careless driving. Obsessional impulses may be aggressive or sexual, such as intrusive impulses of stabbing one's spouse or raping one's child.

**TABLE 19–23.  DSM-IV-TR diagnostic criteria for obsessive-compulsive disorder**

A.  Either obsessions or compulsions:

*Obsessions as defined by (1), (2), (3), and (4):*

(1)  recurrent and persistent thoughts, impulses, or images that are experienced, at some time during the disturbance, as intrusive and inappropriate and that cause marked anxiety or distress

(2)  the thoughts, impulses, or images are not simply excessive worries about real-life problems

(3)  the person attempts to ignore or suppress such thoughts, impulses, or images, or to neutralize them with some other thought or action

(4)  the person recognizes that the obsessional thoughts, impulses, or images are a product of his or her own mind (not imposed from without as in thought insertion)

*Compulsions as defined by (1) and (2):*

(1)  repetitive behaviors (e.g., hand washing, ordering, checking) or mental acts (e.g., praying, counting, repeating words silently) that the person feels driven to perform in response to an obsession, or according to rules that must be applied rigidly

(2)  the behaviors or mental acts are aimed at preventing or reducing distress or preventing some dreaded event or situation; however, these behaviors or mental acts either are not connected in a realistic way with what they are designed to neutralize or prevent or are clearly excessive

B.  At some point during the course of the disorder, the person has recognized that the obsessions or compulsions are excessive or unreasonable.   **Note:** This does not apply to children.

C.  The obsessions or compulsions cause marked distress, are time consuming (take more than 1 hour a day), or significantly interfere with the person's normal routine, occupational (or academic) functioning, or usual social activities or relationships.

D.  If another Axis I disorder is present, the content of the obsessions or compulsions is not restricted to it (e.g., preoccupation with food in the presence of an eating disorder; hair pulling in the presence of trichotillomania; concern with appearance in the presence of body dysmorphic disorder; preoccupation with drugs in the presence of a substance use disorder; preoccupation with having a serious illness in the presence of hypochondriasis; preoccupation with sexual urges or fantasies in the presence of a paraphilia; or guilty ruminations in the presence of major depressive disorder).

E.  The disturbance is not due to the direct physiological effects of a substance (e.g., a drug of abuse, a medication) or a general medical condition.

*Specify* if:

**With poor insight:**   if, for most of the time during the current episode, the person does not recognize that the obsessions and compulsions are excessive or unreasonable

Attributing these obsessions to an internal source, the patient resists or controls them to a variable degree, and significant impairment in functioning can result. *Resistance* is the struggle against an impulse or intrusive thought, and *control* is the patient's actual success in diverting his or her thinking. Obsessions are usually accompanied by compulsions but may also occur as the main or only symptom. Approximately 10%–25% of OCD patients are purely obsessional or predominantly experience obsessions (Akhtar et al. 1975; Rachman and Hodgson 1980).

**Compulsions.**  A *compulsive ritual* is a behavior that usually reduces discomfort but is carried out in a pressured or rigid fashion. Such behavior may include rituals involving washing, checking, repeating, avoiding, striving for completeness, and being meticulous. "Washers" represent about 25%–50% of most OCD samples (Akhtar et al. 1975; Rachman and Hodgson 1980). These individuals are concerned with dirt, contaminants, or germs and may spend many hours a day washing their hands or showering. They may also attempt to avoid contaminating themselves with feces, urine, or vaginal secretions.

"Checkers" have pathological doubt and thus compulsively check to see if they have, for example, run over someone with their car or left the door unlocked. Checking often fails to resolve the doubt and, in some cases, may actually exacerbate it. In the DSM-IV field trial, washing and checking were the two most common groups of compulsions.

Mental compulsions are also quite common and should be inquired about directly because they could go undetected if the clinician only asks about behavioral rituals. Such patients, for example, may replay over and over in their minds past conversations with others to make sure they did not somehow incriminate themselves. In the DSM-IV OCD field trial, 80% of patients had both behavioral and mental compulsions, and mental compulsions were the third most common type after checking and washing.

### *Character Traits*

Psychoanalytic theorists have suggested that there is a continuum between compulsive personality and OCD. Janet (1908) stated that all obsessional patients have a premorbid personality that is causally related to the disorder. Freud (1913/1958) noted an association between obsessional neurosis (i.e., OCD) symptoms and personality traits such as obstinacy, parsimony, punctuality, and orderliness.

However, phenomenological and epidemiological evidence suggests that OCD is frequently distinct from obsessive-compulsive personality disorder. OCD symptoms are ego-dystonic, whereas obsessive-compulsive personality traits are ego-syntonic and do not involve a sense of compulsion that must be resisted against. Epidemiological studies show that obsessive-compulsive character pathology is neither necessary nor sufficient for the development of OCD symptoms.

## Epidemiology

The ECA study (described earlier in this chapter) suggested that OCD is quite common, with a 1-month prevalence of 1.3%, a 6-month prevalence of 1.5%, and a lifetime rate of 2.5% (Regier et al. 1988). In clinical samples of adult OCD, there is a roughly equal ratio of men to women (A. Black 1974). However, in childhood-onset OCD, about 70% of the patients are male (Swedo et al. 1989b).

Twin and family studies have found a greater degree of concordance for OCD (defined broadly to include obsessional features) among monozygotic twins compared with dizygotic twins (Carey and Gottesman 1981), suggesting that some predisposition to obsessional behavior is inherited. Studies of first-degree relatives of OCD patients show a higher-than-expected incidence of a variety of psychiatric disorders, including obsessive-compulsive symptoms, anxiety disorders, and depression (D.W. Black et al. 1992; Carey and Gottesman 1981). Family studies suggest a genetic link between OCD and Tourette's syndrome (Nee et al. 1982).

## Etiology

### *Psychodynamic Theory*

Psychodynamic theory views OCD as residing on a continuum with obsessive-compulsive character pathology and suggests that OCD develops when defense mechanisms fail to contain the obsessional character's anxiety.

**Isolation.**    Isolation is an attempt to separate the feelings or affects from the thoughts, fantasies, or impulses associated with them.

**Undoing.**    Undoing is an attempt to magically reverse a psychological event, such as a word, thought, or gesture. A real or imagined act can be undone by evoking its opposite, such as turning on and then turning off a light switch.

**Reaction formation.**    The defense of reaction formation substitutes an unacceptable unconscious impulse with its opposite. Thus, a patient who has sadistic impulses to hurt people might behave in a passive or masochistic manner or excessively pronounce his love at moments of heightened anger.

**Regression.**    In OCD, regression is theorized to take place from the genital oedipal phase to the earlier pregenital anal-sadistic phase, which has not been fully relinquished. This regression helps the patient avoid genital conflicts and the anxiety associated with them.

**Ambivalence.**    In OCD, strong aggressive impulses are thought to reemerge toward love objects, resulting in displaced ambivalence and paralyzing doubts. In addition, the characteristic thought omnipotence results in magical ideation and lack of certainty, such that thoughts of harming someone become confused with action and may lead to a sense of uncertainty over actually having harmed someone.

### *Cognitive and Behavioral Theories*

A prominent behavioral model of the acquisition and maintenance of obsessive-compulsive symptoms derives from the two-stage learning theory of Mowrer (1939). In Stage 1, anxiety is classically conditioned to a specific environmental event (i.e., classical conditioning). The person then engages in compulsive rituals (escape/avoidance responses) in order to decrease anxiety. If the individual is successful in reducing anxiety, the compulsive behavior is more likely to occur in the future (Stage 2: operant conditioning). Higher-order conditioning occurs when other neutral stimuli such as words, images, or thoughts are associated with the initial stimulus and the associated anxiety is diffused. Ritualized behavior preserves the fear response because the person avoids the eliciting stimulus and thus avoids extinction. Likewise, anxiety reduction after the ritual preserves the compulsive behavior.

### Biological Theories

Although OCD used to be viewed as having a psychological etiology, a wealth of biological findings that have emerged over the past few decades have rendered OCD one of the most elegantly elaborated psychiatric disorders from a biological standpoint (Table 19–24).

---

**TABLE 19–24.  Biological models of obsessive-compulsive disorder**

---

Serotonergic dysregulation

Additional dopaminergic dysregulation, at least in subgroup of patients

Neuropeptide abnormalities (oxytocin, vasopressin, somatostatin)

Hyperactive orbitofrontal–limbic–basal ganglia circuitry

Autoimmune streptococcal-related component in some individuals

Genetic component, ? polymorphisms of the catechol-*O*-methyltransferase and serotonin transporter genes

---

The association of OCD with a variety of neurological conditions or more subtle neurological findings has been known for some time. Such findings include the onset of OCD following head trauma or von Economo's disease; a high incidence of neurological premorbid illnesses in OCD; an association of OCD with birth trauma; abnormalities on the electroencephalogram, in auditory evoked potentials, and in ventricular brain ratio on computed tomography scan; an association with diabetes insipidus; and the presence of significantly more neurological soft signs in OCD patients compared with healthy control subjects. Basal ganglia abnormalities were partic-

ularly suspected in the pathogenesis of OCD, given that OCD is closely associated with Tourette's syndrome (Pauls et al. 1986), in which basal ganglia dysfunction results in abnormal involuntary movements, as well as with Sydenham's chorea, another disorder of the basal ganglia (Swedo et al. 1989a).

A certain form of OCD with childhood onset is believed to be related to an autoimmune process secondary to streptococcal infection. In such children, enlarged basal ganglia have been found on magnetic resonance imaging scans, which is consistent with an autoimmune hypothesis (Giedd et al. 2000). A particular B lymphocyte antigen, which can be identified by the monoclonal antibody D8/17, is expressed in nearly all patients with rheumatic fever and is thought to be a trait marker for susceptibility to group A streptococcal infection complications. Children with OCD and without a history of rheumatic fever or Sydenham's chorea have now been found to have significantly greater B cell D8/17 expression than do control children, suggesting that D8/17 may serve as a marker for susceptibility to childhood-onset OCD (Murphy et al. 1997). More recently, such children also have been found to have elevated anti–basal ganglia antibodies compared with pediatric autoimmune, neurological, or streptococcal control subjects (Dale et al. 2005).

## Course and Prognosis

Studies of the natural course of the illness suggest that 24%–33% of patients have a fluctuating course, 11%–14% have a phasic course with periods of complete remission, and 54%–61% have a constant or progressive course (A. Black 1974; Table 19–25). Although prognosis of OCD has traditionally been considered to be poor, with new developments in behavioral and pharmacological treatments, this prognosis is now considerably improved. The disorder usually has a major effect on daily functioning, with some patients spending many waking hours consumed with their obsessions and rituals.

## Diagnosis

DSM-IV-TR defines OCD as the presence of either obsessions or compulsions that cause marked distress, are time-consuming, or interfere with social or occupational functioning. Although all other Axis I disorders are allowed to be comorbidly present, the OCD symptoms must not be just secondary to another disorder (e.g., thoughts about food in the presence of an eating disorder or guilty thoughts in the presence of major depression).

---

**TABLE 19–25.　Course and prognosis of obsessive-compulsive disorder**

**Course**

Less than 15% phasic with periods of complete remission

One-fourth to one-third have fluctuating course

Half (50%) have constant or progressive illness

**Outcome**

80% improve over 40 years

**Predictors of worse prognosis**

Early age at onset

Longer duration of illness

Presence of both obsessions and compulsions

Poorer baseline social functioning

Magical thinking

---

The diagnosis is usually clear-cut, but occasionally it can be more difficult to distinguish OCD from depression, psychosis, phobias, or severe obsessive-compulsive personality disorder.

## Differential Diagnosis

The differential diagnosis of OCD is summarized in Table 19–26.

---

**TABLE 19–26.　Differential diagnosis of obsessive-compulsive disorder**

Eating disorder with obsessions surrounding food and weight

Body dysmorphic disorder with obsessions about body appearance other than weight

Hypochondriasis with obsessions related to feared illnesses

Panic disorder or generalized anxiety (if obsessional anxiety is severe)

Obsessive ruminations of depressions (typically mood congruent)

Severe obsessive-compulsive personality disorder

Paranoid psychosis (e.g., delusions of poisoning rather than contamination fears)

Social phobia (if avoiding social situations because they exacerbate illness)

---

### Schizophrenia

In some cases, the course of OCD may more closely resemble that of schizophrenia, with chronic debilitation, decline, and profound impairment in social and occupational functioning.

### Depression

Patients with psychotic depression, agitated depression, or premorbid obsessional features prior to depression are particularly likely to develop obsessions. These "secondary" obsessions often involve aggressive themes, but the distinction between primary and secondary obsessions rests on the order of occurrence.

### Phobic Disorders

OCD patients who are compulsive cleaners appear very similar to phobic individuals and are often mislabeled "germ phobics." Both have avoidant behavior, both show intense subjective and autonomic responses to focal stimuli, and both are said to respond to similar behavioral interventions.

## Treatment

### Pharmacotherapy

The pharmacological approach to treatment of OCD is summarized in Table 19–27.

**Serotonin reuptake inhibitors.** The most extensively studied medication for the treatment of OCD is clomipramine, a potent serotonin reuptake inhibitor with weak norepinephrine reuptake blockade. A series of well-controlled, double-blind studies have indisputably documented the efficacy of clomipramine in reducing OCD symptoms. The largest of these was a multicenter trial comparing clomipramine with placebo in more than 500 patients with OCD. On an average dosage of 200–250 mg/day of clomipramine, the average reduction in OCD symptoms was about 40%, and about 60% of all patients were clinically much or very much improved (Clomipramine Collaborative Study Group 1991). Patients should typically be started on 25 mg of clomipramine at nighttime, and the dosage then should be gradually increased by 25 mg every 4 days or 50 mg every week until a maximum dosage of 250 mg is reached. Improvement with clomipramine is relatively slow, with maximal response occurring after 5–12 weeks of treatment. Some of the more common side effects reported by

---

**TABLE 19-27. Pharmacological treatment of obsessive-compulsive disorder**

**Serotonin reuptake inhibitors**

*General indications:* First-line treatments; moderate to high dosages.

*Fluoxetine, fluvoxamine, sertraline:* efficacy shown in large controlled trials

*Paroxetine, citalopram:* less studied, similar efficacy

*Clomipramine:* efficacy shown in multiple controlled trials; may have small superiority over SSRIs; however, typically not used until at least two SSRIs have failed secondary to side-effect profile; can be used in low dosages in combination with SSRIs in patients with more refractory illness; clomipramine plus desmethylclomipramine levels must be closely followed for toxicity

*Venlafaxine, mirtazapine:* less studied

**Augmentation strategies**

*General indications:* Partial response to serotonin reuptake inhibitors; presence of other target symptoms.

*Atypical antipsychotics:* several studies show additional benefit

*Pindolol:* effective in controlled trial

*Clonazepam:* effective in controlled trial; comorbid very high anxiety

*Buspirone:* one positive trial, three negative

*Lithium:* ineffective in controlled trial

*Trazodone:* ineffective in controlled trial

*Monoamine oxidase inhibitors:* hardly any evidence; possibly phenelzine in symmetry obsessions

*Topiramate*

*Riluzole*

**Other medications**

*Intravenous clomipramine:* efficacy in controlled trial in oral clomipramine–refractory patients

*Plasma exchange and intravenous immunoglobulin:* effective in children with streptococcus-related obsessive-compulsive disorder

*Note.* SSRI=selective serotonin reuptake inhibitor.

---

patients are dry mouth, tremor, sedation, nausea, and ejaculatory failure in men. The seizure risk is comparable with that of TCAs and is acceptable for dosages up to 250 mg/day in the absence of prior neurological history. Controlled studies have also reported that clomipramine is effective in treating OCD when other antidepressants, such as amitriptyline, nortriptyline, desipramine, and the

MAOI clorgyline, have no therapeutic effect. This finding strongly suggests that improvement in OCD symptoms is mediated through the blockade of serotonin reuptake.

Numerous controlled trials since the early 1990s have documented the efficacy of all SSRIs for OCD. Fluoxetine has been shown to be superior to placebo in treating OCD at dosages of 20–60 mg/day, with greater efficacy at higher dosages (Montgomery et al. 1993; Tollefson et al. 1994).

Fluvoxamine also has been found to have a significant antiobsessional effect in several controlled studies (Hollander et al. 2003b; Jenike et al. 1990). The required daily dosage is titrated up to a maximum of 300 mg.

Sertraline is another serotonin reuptake blocker whose efficacy for OCD has been established at daily dosages ranging from 50 to 200 mg (Greist et al. 1995a; Kronig et al. 1999). Response began to appear as early as the third week of treatment and was firmly apparent by the eighth week (Kronig et al. 1999).

Paroxetine and citalopram are also efficacious in treating OCD, generally at dosages of 20–60 mg/day.

One issue with SSRI treatment is how high to push the dosage, beyond the standard recommended OCD treatment dosage, in an attempt to get a response. One study examined this question in subjects who did not respond to 16 weeks of treatment with sertraline 200 mg/day and found that increasing to a mean dosage of 350 mg/day did result in some symptom improvement but no change in responder status (Ninan et al. 2006).

The SNRI venlafaxine also appears effective in treating OCD. An open trial of venlafaxine in 39 patients, about two-thirds of whom had not responded to SSRIs, reported that about two-thirds responded to venlafaxine at a mean dosage of about 225 mg/day (Hollander et al. 2003a). Open-trial monotherapy followed by double-blind discontinuation of mirtazapine, in dosages of 30–60 mg/day, showed preliminary evidence of efficacy that awaits larger replication (Koran et al. 2005).

**Medication combination and augmentation.** It is important to keep in mind that the medication response in OCD is not as dramatic as in, for example, major depression: a considerable number of patients show a negligible or partial response to the first-line medications. As a helpful rule of thumb, it is useful to remember that approximately 40%–60% of OCD patients improve by about 30%–60% with a first-line drug. The most commonly used augmenting agents in OCD are buspirone, clonazepam, atypical antipsychotics, inositol, and glutamatergic agents.

Although an initial small study reported similar efficacy for clomipramine alone versus buspirone alone in treating OCD (Pato et al. 1991), three other studies failed to show a significant benefit to buspirone augmentation in clomipramine-treated (Pigott et al. 1992), fluoxetine-treated (Grady et al. 1993), or fluvoxamine-treated (McDougle et al. 1993b) patients. If buspirone is tried, higher dosages of 30–60 mg/day should be targeted. A controlled crossover study showed clonazepam to be effective in 40% of OCD subjects who failed to respond to clomipramine trials (Hewlett et al. 1992), and clonazepam also may be helpful with the very high anxiety levels frequently associated with OCD.

Antipsychotics are the main medication class used to augment partial response to serotonin reuptake blockers in OCD. McDougle et al. (1990) first reported that about 50% of OCD patients improved noticeably when pimozide was added to fluvoxamine; comorbid tic disorders or schizotypal personality predicted a good response. OCD patients with comorbid tic disorders may actually be less responsive to SSRI monotherapy (McDougle et al. 1993a) and appear to respond well to haloperidol augmentation (McDougle et al. 1994). In more recent years, atypical antipsychotics have received increasing attention as a major augmentation strategy for OCD, regardless of comorbid tics or schizotypy, and such a strategy is now supported by controlled trials.

The combination of clomipramine with an SSRI is also a commonly used strategy for treating refractory symptoms and is generally well tolerated, although lower dosages of clomipramine should be used, and blood levels should be monitored, to avoid toxicity, because clomipramine levels can become markedly elevated.

**Other somatic treatment options.**  In extreme cases of severely impaired patients with refractory OCD, neurosurgery can be considered. Guidelines for the use of neurosurgical techniques in the treatment of severe refractory OCD, including selection, documented failed treatments, indications, contraindications, benefits, risks, and workup, have been thoroughly reviewed elsewhere (Mindus and Jenike 1992).

**Maintenance treatment.**  Long-term continuation of medication treatment generally maintains a good treatment response; this is widely supported in clinical treatment and has been validated by a 1-year double-blind sertraline maintenance study at dosages of 50–200 mg/day (Greist et al. 1995b).

## Cognitive-Behavioral Therapy

Behavioral treatments of OCD (Table 19–28) can be highly effective and involve two main components: 1) exposure procedures that aim to decrease the anxiety associated with obsessions and 2) response prevention techniques that aim to decrease the frequency of rituals or obsessive thoughts. Exposure techniques range from systematic desensitization with brief imaginal exposure to flooding, in which prolonged exposure to the real-life ritual-evoking stimuli causes profound discomfort. Exposure techniques aim to ultimately decrease the discomfort associated with the eliciting stimuli through habituation. In exposure therapy, the patient is assigned homework exercises that must be adhered to, and he or she may require assistance from the therapist (in a home visit) or from family members to achieve exposure at home. Response prevention involves having patients face feared stimuli (e.g., dirt, chemicals) without excessive hand washing or tolerate doubt (e.g., "Is the door really locked?") without excessive checking. Initial work may involve delaying performance of the ritual, but ultimately the patient works to fully resist the compulsions. The psychoeducation and support of family members can be pivotal to the success of the behavior therapy because family dysfunction is very prevalent, and most parents or spouses accommodate to or are involved in the patients' rituals, possibly as a way to reduce the anxiety or anger that patients may direct at their family members.

---

**TABLE 19–28.  Cognitive and behavioral approaches to treating obsessive-compulsive disorder**

Graded exposure (imaginal and/or in vivo)

Flooding

Response prevention

Cognitive restructuring

---

Cognitive therapy also has been more recently advocated and is efficacious in the treatment of OCD, centering on cognitive reformulation of themes related to the perception of danger, estimation of catastrophe, expectations about anxiety and its consequences, excessive responsibility, thought–action fusion, and illogical inferences. Several studies have directly compared cognitive with behavior therapy for OCD in randomized trials and have reported similar efficacy (Cottraux et al. 2001; van Oppen et al. 1995; Whittal et al. 2005).

*Combination Pharmacotherapy and Psychotherapy*

A common approach used in clinical practice, especially by psychiatrists, is to start out with medication, attain a degree of clinical improvement that will allow better use of CBT, and then possibly attempt some degree of medication taper once CBT has been mastered and been effective. In a study testing this commonly used paradigm, it appeared quite effective. Patients who remained symptomatic with a 12-week course of an SSRI were entered into a course of exposure and ritual prevention and subsequently showed a 50% decrease in their OCD symptoms (Simpson et al. 1999). Similarly, in a wait-list controlled trial of CBT in OCD patients who had failed to adequately respond to multiple serotonin reuptake inhibitor medications, about 50% showed clinically significant improvement, and most maintained it at 6-month follow-up; poor insight and low CBT effort predicted lesser gains (Tolin et al. 2004).

# Posttraumatic Stress Disorder

## Definition

PTSD was first introduced in DSM-III, spurred in part by the increasing recognition of posttraumatic conditions in veterans of the Vietnam War. The current DSM-IV-TR diagnostic criteria for PTSD are presented in Table 19–29.

## Clinical Description

The characteristic features that may develop after traumatic events include psychic numbing, reexperiencing of the trauma, and increased autonomic arousal. The trauma is reexperienced in recurrent painful and intrusive recollections, daydreams, or nightmares. Dissociative states may occur, lasting from minutes to days, in which there is a dreamlike, unreal state with hazy memory and a distorted sense of time. Psychic numbing or emotional anesthesia is manifest by diminished responsiveness to the external world, with feelings of being detached from other people, loss of interest in usual activities, and inability to feel emotions such as intimacy, tenderness, or sexual interest. Symptoms of excessive autonomic arousal may include hyperactivity and irritability, an exaggerated startle response, difficulty concentrating, and sleep abnormalities. Rape or mugging victims sometimes become afraid to venture forth alone for variable periods of time. Situations reminiscent of the original trauma may be systematically avoided.

Other symptoms may include guilt about having survived, guilt about not having prevented the traumatic experience, depression, anxiety, panic attacks, shame, and rage. There may be prolonged episodes of intense affect; increased irritability; explosive, hostile behavior; and impulsive behavior. Other accompanying or complicating symptoms associated with PTSD may include substance abuse, self-injurious behavior and suicide attempts, occupational impairment, and interference with interpersonal relationships.

## Epidemiology

Although there are marked individual differences in how people react to stress, when stressors become extreme, such as in concentration camp situations or in extended combat, the rate of morbidity rapidly increases. In a large randomized community survey of young adults, the lifetime prevalence of PTSD was found to be 9.2% (Breslau et al. 1991). The prevalence was higher in women (11.3%) than in men (6%). In the National Comorbidity Survey, the lifetime prevalence of PTSD was similarly found to be 7.8%, and the prevalence was again higher in women. The most common stressors were combat exposure in men and sexual assault in women (Kessler et al. 1995).

The gender difference in PTSD prevalence, higher in women, has been consistent across several studies. It appears that women are more likely to develop PTSD than are men with comparable exposure to traumatic events, especially if exposure is before age 15 (Breslau et al. 1997).

In the Breslau et al. (1991) survey, a high comorbidity risk was found for OCD, agoraphobia, panic, and depression, whereas the association with drug or alcohol abuse was weaker. The comorbidity of PTSD with depression is a very consistent one, and the nature of the relation between the two conditions is controversial. Epidemiological analyses suggest that in trauma victims the vulnerabilities for PTSD and depression are not separate, but rather the risk for depression is highly elevated in just those trauma victims who manifest PTSD (Breslau et al. 2000).

## Etiology

The severity of the stressor in PTSD differs in magnitude from that found in adjustment disorder, in which the stressor is usually less severe and within the range of common life experience. However, this relation between the severity of the stressor and the type of subsequent symp-

**TABLE 19–29.    DSM-IV-TR diagnostic criteria for posttraumatic stress disorder**

A.  The person has been exposed to a traumatic event in which both of the following were present:

    (1)  the person experienced, witnessed, or was confronted with an event or events that involved actual or threatened death or serious injury, or a threat to the physical integrity of self or others

    (2)  the person's response involved intense fear, helplessness, or horror.    **Note:** In children, this may be expressed instead by disorganized or agitated behavior.

B.  The traumatic event is persistently reexperienced in one (or more) of the following ways:

    (1)  recurrent and intrusive distressing recollections of the event, including images, thoughts, or perceptions.    **Note:** In young children, repetitive play may occur in which themes or aspects of the trauma are expressed.

    (2)  recurrent distressing dreams of the event.    **Note:** In children, there may be frightening dreams without recognizable content.

    (3)  acting or feeling as if the traumatic event were recurring (includes a sense of reliving the experience, illusions, hallucinations, and dissociative flashback episodes, including those that occur on awakening or when intoxicated).    **Note:** In young children, trauma-specific reenactment may occur.

    (4)  intense psychological distress at exposure to internal or external cues that symbolize or resemble an aspect of the traumatic event

    (5)  physiological reactivity on exposure to internal or external cues that symbolize or resemble an aspect of the traumatic event

C.  Persistent avoidance of stimuli associated with the trauma and numbing of general responsiveness (not present before the trauma), as indicated by three (or more) of the following:

    (1)  efforts to avoid thoughts, feelings, or conversations associated with the trauma

    (2)  efforts to avoid activities, places, or people that arouse recollections of the trauma

    (3)  inability to recall an important aspect of the trauma

    (4)  markedly diminished interest or participation in significant activities

    (5)  feeling of detachment or estrangement from others

    (6)  restricted range of affect (e.g., unable to have loving feelings)

    (7)  sense of a foreshortened future (e.g., does not expect to have a career, marriage, children, or a normal life span)

D.  Persistent symptoms of increased arousal (not present before the trauma), as indicated by two (or more) of the following:

    (1)  difficulty falling or staying asleep

    (2)  irritability or outbursts of anger

    (3)  difficulty concentrating

    (4)  hypervigilance

    (5)  exaggerated startle response

E.  Duration of the disturbance (symptoms in Criteria B, C, and D) is more than 1 month.

F.  The disturbance causes clinically significant distress or impairment in social, occupational, or other important areas of functioning.

*Specify* if:

    **Acute:**    if duration of symptoms is less than 3 months
    **Chronic:**    if duration of symptoms is 3 months or more

*Specify* if:

    **With delayed onset:**    if onset of symptoms is at least 6 months after the stressor tomatology is not always predictable. In effect, it has generally been underestimated that in the average community setting, common events such as sudden loss of a spouse are a much more frequent cause for PTSD than are assault and violence (Breslau et al. 1998).

Nevertheless, events such as sexual assault or armed robbery, which are interpersonal insults to integrity, self-esteem, and security, are particularly likely to lead to PTSD. When stressors become extreme (e.g., rape, extended combat, torture, or concentration camp experiences), the rate of morbidity significantly increases. As an average, it is estimated that approximately one-fourth of all individuals who experience major trauma develop PTSD (Breslau et al. 1991).

## Risk Factors and Predictors

There is agreement that a variety of premorbid risk factors predispose to the development of PTSD (Table 19–30).

---

**TABLE 19–30.  Risk factors for posttraumatic stress disorder (PTSD)**

History of trauma prior to the index trauma

History of PTSD

History of depression

History of anxiety disorders

Comorbid Axis II disorders (predictive of greater chronicity)

Family history of anxiety (including parental PTSD)

Disrupted parental attachments

Severity of exposure to trauma (more predictive of acute symptoms)

High premorbid intelligence may be protective

---

The greater the amount of previous trauma experienced by an individual, the more likely he or she is to develop symptoms after a stressful life event (Horowitz et al. 1980). In addition, individuals with prior traumatic experiences are more likely to become exposed to future traumas because they can be prone to behaviorally reenact the original trauma (van der Kolk 1989).

Early predictors of PTSD after a traumatic event also have received great attention because of their obvious potential significance for early intervention and prevention. The occurrence of acute stress disorder in the first month after trauma is a very strong predictor of later PTSD.

## Cognitive and Behavioral Theories

A cognitive model has been proposed for the persistence of PTSD symptoms, suggesting that PTSD becomes persistent when individuals process the trauma in a way that leads to a sense of serious and current threat. This occurs through excessively negative appraisals of the trauma or its consequences and a disturbance of autobiographical memory so that there is poor contextualization and strong associative memory (Ehlers and Clark 2000).

Behavioral theory suggests that there is a disturbance of conditioned responses in PTSD. Autonomic responses to both innocuous and aversive stimuli are elevated, with larger responses to unpaired cues and reduced extinction of conditioned responses (Peri et al. 2000). It has been proposed that PTSD individuals have higher sympathetic system arousal at the time of conditioning and therefore are more conditionable than trauma-exposed individuals without PTSD (Orr et al. 2000).

## Biological Theories

Biological models for PTSD are summarized in Table 19–31.

---

**TABLE 19–31.  Biological models of posttraumatic stress disorder**

Limbic hyperactivity (amygdala, cingulate) and cortical hyporesponsivity (prefrontal, Broca's area) to traumatic stimuli

Hypothalamic-pituitary-adrenal axis dysregulation

Noradrenergic activation

Heightened physiological responses

Endogenous opioid dysregulation

Dysregulated serotonergic modulation

Hippocampal toxicity, decreased volumes

---

### *Sympathetic System*

The neurobiological response to acute stress and trauma involves the release of various stress hormones that allow the organism to respond adaptively to stress. These releases include heightened secretion of catecholamines and cortisol. When PTSD develops under severe or repeated trauma, the stress response becomes dysregulated, and chronic autonomic hyperactivity sets in. This manifests itself in the "positive" symptoms of PTSD—that is, the hyperarousal and intrusive recollections. The noradrenergic system, originating in the locus coeruleus, regulates arousal. Long-standing increases in the urinary catecholamines norepinephrine and epinephrine have been found in PTSD patients, as well as elevated plasma norepinephrine (Spivak et al. 1999). Elevated cerebrospinal fluid (CSF) norepinephrine also has been identified in men with chronic PTSD compared with control subjects (Geracioti et al. 2001). A decrease in the number and sensitivity of $\alpha_2$-adrenergic receptors, possibly as a consequence of chronic noradrenergic hyperactivity, has been reported (Perry et al. 1987).

In patients with PTSD, heightened physiological responses to stressful stimuli, such as in blood pressure, heart rate, respiration, galvanic skin responses, and electromyographic activity, have long been documented (Kolb 1987; Pitman et al. 1987). Studies of the startle response in PTSD have reported heightened amplitude of startle in some samples but not in others (Lipschitz et al. 2005).

### Serotonergic System

The serotonergic system also has been implicated in the symptomatology of PTSD (van der Kolk and Saporta 1991), although such work is still in its infancy. The septohippocampal brain system contains serotonergic pathways and mediates behavioral inhibition and constraint. Thus, the irritability and outbursts seen in patients with PTSD may be related to serotonergic deficit. The partial serotonin agonist *m*-CPP induces an increase in PTSD symptoms suggestive of a sensitized serotonergic system, and interestingly, this appears to be a separate subgroup of PTSD subjects from the ones with noradrenergic sensitization (Southwick et al. 1997). The efficacy of SSRIs in PTSD is also indirectly supportive of dysregulated serotonergic modulation in PTSD.

### Hypothalamic-Pituitary-Adrenal Axis

Several findings in PTSD have implicated a chronic dysregulation of HPA axis functioning that is highly characteristic of this disorder and distinct from that seen in other psychiatric disorders such as depression. The findings include elevated CSF corticotropin-releasing hormone (Bremner et al. 1997), low urinary cortisol (Mason et al. 1986) and an elevated urinary norepinephrine-to-cortisol ratio (Mason et al. 1988), a blunted corticotropin response to CRF (Smith et al. 1989), enhanced suppression of cortisol after dexamethasone administration, and a decrease in lymphocyte glucocorticoid receptor number.

### Genetics

A large study of Vietnam veteran twins found that genetic factors accounted for 13%–34% of the variance in liability to the various PTSD symptom clusters, whereas no etiological role was found for shared environment (True et al. 1993). Molecular genetic studies of PTSD are very few.

## Course and Prognosis

The course and prognosis of PTSD are summarized in Table 19–32.

---

**TABLE 19–32.  Course and prognosis of posttraumatic stress disorder (PTSD)**

**Course**

80% longer than 3 months

75% longer than 6 months

50% 2 years' duration

**Outcome**

Minority can remain symptomatic for years or decades

**Predictors of worse outcome**

Greater number of PTSD symptoms

Psychiatric history of other anxiety and mood disorders

Higher numbing or hyperarousal to stressors

Comorbid medical illnesses

Female sex

Childhood trauma

Alcohol abuse

---

Scrignar (1984) divided the clinical course of PTSD into three stages. Stage I involves the response to trauma. Nonsusceptible persons may experience an adrenergic surge of symptoms immediately after the trauma but do not dwell on the incident. Predisposed persons have higher levels of anxiety and dissociation at baseline, an exaggerated response to the trauma, and an obsessive preoccupation with it following the trauma. If symptoms persist beyond 4–6 weeks, the patient enters Stage II, or acute PTSD. Feelings of helplessness and loss of control, symptoms of increased autonomic arousal, reliving of the trauma, and somatic symptoms may occur. The patient's life becomes centered around the trauma, with subsequent changes in lifestyle, personality, and social functioning. Phobic avoidance, startle responses, and angry outbursts may occur. In Stage III, chronic PTSD develops, with disability, demoralization, and despondency. The patient's emphasis changes from preoccupation with the actual trauma to preoccupation with the physical disability resulting from the trauma. Somatic symptoms, chronic anxiety, and depression are common complications at this time, as are substance abuse, disturbed family relationships, and unemployment. Some patients may focus on compensation and lawsuits.

## Diagnosis

The diagnosis of PTSD is usually not difficult if there is a clear history of exposure to a traumatic event, followed by symptoms of intense anxiety lasting at least 1 month, with arousal and stimulation of the autonomic nervous system, numbing of responsiveness, and avoidance or reexperiencing of the traumatic event.

## Differential Diagnosis

The differential diagnosis of PTSD is described in Table 19–33.

---

**TABLE 19–33.  Differential diagnosis of posttraumatic stress disorder (PTSD)**

Depression after trauma (numbing and avoidance may be present, but not hyperarousal and intrusive symptoms)

Panic disorder if the panic attacks are not limited to reminders/triggers of the trauma

Generalized anxiety (may have similar symptoms to PTSD hyperarousal)

Agoraphobia (if avoidance not directly trauma related)

Specific phobia (if avoidance not directly trauma related)

Adjustment disorder (usually less severe stressor and different symptoms)

Acute stress disorder (if less than 1 month has elapsed since trauma)

Dissociative disorders (if prominent dissociative symptoms)

Factitious disorders or malingering (especially if there could be apparent secondary gain)

---

### Organic Mental Disorders

Mild concussions may leave no immediate apparent neurological signs but may have residual long-term effects on mood and concentration. Malnutrition may occur during prolonged stressful periods and may also lead to organic brain syndromes. Other causes of organic mental disorder may occasionally mimic PTSD if anxiety, depression, personality changes, or abnormal behaviors are present.

### Mood and Anxiety Disorders

**Major depression.**  There is much overlap between PTSD and major mood disorders. Symptoms such as psychic numbing, irritability, sleep disturbance, fatigue, anhedonia, impairments in family and social relationships, anger, concern with physical health, and pessimistic outlook may occur in both disorders. Major depression is a frequent complication of PTSD; when it occurs, it must be treated aggressively because comorbidity carries an increased risk of suicide. If major depression develops secondary to PTSD, both disorders should be diagnosed.

**Phobic disorders.**  Following a traumatic event, patients may be aversively conditioned to the surroundings of the trauma and develop a phobia of objects, surroundings, or situations that remind them of the trauma itself. Phobic patients experience anxiety in the feared situation, whereas avoidance is accompanied by anxiety reduction that reinforces the avoidant behavior.

**Generalized anxiety disorder.**  The symptoms of GAD, such as motor tension, autonomic hyperactivity, apprehensive expectation, and vigilance and scanning, are also present in PTSD. However, the onset and course of the illness differ: GAD has an insidious or a gradual onset and a course that fluctuates with environmental stressors, whereas PTSD has an acute onset often followed by a chronic course.

**Panic disorder.**  Patients with PTSD also may experience panic attacks. In some patients, panic attacks predate the PTSD or do not occur exclusively in the context of stimuli reminiscent of the traumatic event. In some patients, however, panic attacks develop after the PTSD and are cued solely by traumatic stimuli.

**Adjustment disorder.** Adjustment disorders are maladaptive reactions to identifiable psychosocial pressures. If symptoms are of sufficient severity to meet other Axis I criteria, then the diagnosis of adjustment disorder is not made. Adjustment disorder differs from PTSD in that the stressor is usually less severe and within the range of common experience, and the characteristic symptoms of PTSD, such as reexperiencing the trauma, are absent.

**Compensation neurosis (factitious disorder and malingering).** Both factitious disorder and malingering involve conscious deception and feigning of illness, although the motivation for each condition differs. Factitious disorder may present with physical or psychological symptoms; the feigning of symptoms is under voluntary control, and the motivation is to assume the "patient" role. Chronic factitious disorder with physical symptoms (i.e., Munchausen syndrome) involves frequent doctor visits and surgical interventions.

Malingering involves the conscious fabrication of an illness for the purpose of achieving a definite goal such as money or compensation. Malingerers often reveal an inconsistent history, unexpected symptom clusters, a history of antisocial behavior and substance abuse, and a chaotic lifestyle, and there is often a discrepancy between history, claimed distress, and objective data.

**Postconcussion syndrome.** Psychological symptoms are extremely common after mild closed head injuries, even without loss of consciousness. The so-called postconcussion syndrome comprises the symptoms of headache, dizziness, irritability, and emotional lability after a head injury with concussion.

## Treatment

### Pharmacotherapy

A variety of different psychopharmacological agents have been used in the treatment of PTSD by clinicians and reported in the literature as case reports, open clinic trials, and controlled studies. The findings for these medications are summarized in the following sections (Table 19–34).

**Serotonin reuptake inhibitors.** SSRIs have become established as first-line medications for PTSD treatment (D.J. Stein et al. 2006). Several initial open trials of fluoxetine reported marked improvement in PTSD symptoms at a wide range of dosages (Davidson et al. 1991; McDougle et al. 1991; Shay 1992). Currently, sertraline is FDA approved for the treatment of PTSD.

**TABLE 19–34.   Pharmacotherapy for posttraumatic stress disorder (PTSD)**

**Selective serotonin reuptake inhibitors (SSRIs)**

*General indications:*   First-line treatment; well tolerated; once-a-day dosing; documented efficacy

*Sertraline:*   U.S. Food and Drug Administration–approved; large controlled trials

*Other SSRIs:*   similar efficacy

*Venlafaxine, mirtazapine*

**Other antidepressants**

*Tricyclic antidepressants:*   overall modest results when tested in double-blind fashion

*Monoamine oxidase inhibitors:*   may be superior to tricyclics, especially for intrusive symptoms

**Other medications**

*General indications:*   When response to first-line options not adequate; additional treatment of specific PTSD symptoms or comorbid disorders.

*Prazosin:*   nightmares and daytime intrusions

*Atypical antipsychotics:*   several studies documenting some benefit

*Clonidine:*   some efficacy in open treatment

*Lithium:*   improvement in intrusive symptoms and irritability in open trial

*Anticonvulsants (carbamazepine, valproate, lamotrigine, tiagabine, topiramate, levetiracetam, phenytoin):*   mostly open trials showing some efficacy

*Buspirone:*   efficacy in an open trial

*Triiodothyronine:*   improvement in small open trial, possibly antidepressant response

*Trazodone, benzodiazepines, diphenhydramine:*   sleep disturbance

A controlled comparison of venlafaxine extended-release (mean dosage=225 mg/day), sertraline (150 mg/day), and placebo reported modest benefits, with response rates of 30%, 24%, and 20%, respectively (Davidson et al. 2006). A randomized comparison of mirtazapine (mean dosage=34 mg/day) and sertraline (100 mg/day) reported comparable outcomes at 6 weeks, with large reductions in PTSD symptoms (Chung et al. 2004). A small double-blind trial of mirtazapine monotherapy, at dosages up to 45 mg/day, reported a responder rate of 65%, significantly higher than the 20% placebo responder rate (Davidson et al. 2003).

**Tricyclic antidepressants.**  A positive effect of imipramine on posttraumatic night terrors was reported by Marshall (1975). Controlled studies of TCAs in PTSD have not overall reported much success in decreasing posttraumatic symptoms.

**Monoamine oxidase inhibitors.**  Positive effects of phenelzine on intrusive posttraumatic symptoms have been reported in subsequent small open trials (Davidson et al. 1987; van der Kolk 1983). Subsequently, an 8-week randomized, double-blind trial compared phenelzine (71 mg), imipramine (240 mg), and placebo in 34 veterans with PTSD (Frank et al. 1988) and found that phenelzine tended to be superior to imipramine.

**Adrenergic blockers.**  Kolb et al. (1984) treated 12 Vietnam veterans with PTSD in an open trial of the β-blocker propranolol over a 6-month period. Dosage ranged from 120 to 160 mg daily. Eleven patients reported a positive change in self-assessment at the end of the 6-month period, with less explosiveness, fewer nightmares, improved sleep, and a decrease in intrusive thoughts, hyperalertness, and startle. Another open pilot study by this group (Kolb et al. 1984) using clonidine, a noradrenergic $\alpha_2$-agonist, was conducted with nine Vietnam veterans with PTSD. Dosages of 0.2–0.4 mg/day of clonidine were administered over a 6-month period. Eight patients reported improvements in their capacity to control their emotions and lessened explosiveness, and a majority reported improvements in sleep and nightmares, as well as psychosocial improvement, and lowered startle, hyperalertness, and intrusive thinking.

Recently, the $\alpha_1$-adrenergic antagonist prazosin has emerged as a very promising agent in the treatment of PTSD. Evidence supporting its use is mostly available for bedtime administration, but benefits can also occur for daytime symptoms. In an initial 6-week trial of prazosin in five patients given 1–4 mg/day, all showed moderate to marked improvement in PTSD, with at least moderate improvement of nightmares (Taylor and Raskind 2002).

**Mood stabilizers and anticonvulsants.**  In a small open trial of lithium for treating PTSD, van der Kolk (1983) reported improvement in intrusive recollections and irritability in more than half of the patients treated. However, there have been no controlled trials. In an open trial of carbamazepine in 10 patients with PTSD, Lipper et al. (1986) reported moderate to great improvement in intrusive symptoms in 7 patients. Wolf et al. (1988) reported decreased impulsivity and angry outbursts in 10 veterans who were also taking carbamazepine; all patients had normal electroencephalogram findings. An open trial of 16 patients treated openly with valproate for 8 weeks reported a significant decrease in hyperarousal and intrusion but not numbing (Clark et al. 1999b), whereas another 8-week open trial of valproate monotherapy reported no benefits (Otte et al. 2004).

In a very small placebo-controlled trial of lamotrigine at dosages up to 500 mg/day, more patients appeared to respond to lamotrigine (Hertzberg et al. 1999); this finding warrants larger studies of lamotrigine. Tiagabine was also reported effective in a 12-week acute treatment trial, with increasing likelihood of remission during continuation treatment (Connor et al. 2006), as well as in a case series at a mean dosage of 8 mg/day (Taylor 2003). Levetiracetam was reported to be an effective augmentation, with a 56% responder rate in a retrospective analysis of patients with treatment-resistant PTSD (Kinrys et al. 2006). Topiramate also looked promising in treating PTSD in one open trial of 33 civilians with chronic nonhallucinatory PTSD; at a median dosage of 50 mg/day, about three-fourths of the patients were rated as responders after 4 weeks, with a rapid median response interval of 9 days (Berlant 2004).

**Other medications.**  A small open trial of buspirone reported that seven of eight patients experienced a significant reduction in PTSD symptoms (Duffy and Malloy 1994). In a small open trial, triiodothyronine was reported to result in significant clinical improvement in four of five PTSD patients whose symptoms had only partial responses to SSRIs (Agid et al. 2001). Cyproheptadine has been reported to greatly decrease the nightmares characteristic of PTSD (Clark et al. 1999a; Gupta et al. 1998). An open trial of bupropion in PTSD reported global improvement secondary to decreased depression, but PTSD symptoms remained mostly unchanged (Canive et al. 1998).

An open trial with risperidone, 2–4 mg/day, in veterans with psychotic PTSD led to an overall improvement of both PTSD and psychotic symptoms (Kozaric-Kovacic et al. 2005). A small 8-week placebo-controlled risperidone trial in women with PTSD related to childhood abuse reported a significant improvement in intrusive and arousal symptoms. An open quetiapine augmentation trial, using a mean dosage of 100 mg/day, resulted in an approximately 25% decline in PTSD symptom severity (Hamner et al. 2003). Quetiapine may be helpful in improving the sleep disturbance associated with the disorder (Robert et al. 2005).

## Psychotherapy

**General principles.**   The "phase-oriented" treatment model suggested by Horowitz (1976) strikes a balance between initial supportive interventions to minimize the traumatic state and increasingly aggressive working through at later stages of treatment. Establishment of a safe and communicative relationship, reappraisal of the traumatic event, revision of the patient's inner model of self and world, and planning for termination with a reexperiencing of loss are all important therapeutic issues in the treatment of PTSD. Herman et al. (1989) emphasized the importance of validating the patient's traumatic experiences as a precondition for reparation of damaged self-identity.

Embry (1990) outlined seven major parameters for effective psychotherapy in war veterans with chronic PTSD: 1) initial rapport building, 2) limit setting and supportive confrontation, 3) affective modeling, 4) defocusing on stress and focusing on current life events, 5) sensitivity to transference/countertransference issues, 6) understanding of secondary gain, and 7) therapist's maintenance of a positive treatment attitude.

**Cognitive and behavioral therapies.**   A variety of cognitive and behavioral techniques have gained increasing popularity and validation in the treatment of PTSD (Table 19–35).

People involved in traumatic events such as accidents frequently develop phobias or phobic anxiety related to or associated with these situations. When a phobia or phobic anxiety is associated with PTSD, systematic desensitization or graded exposure has been found to be effective. This is based on the principle that when patients are gradually exposed to a phobic or anxiety-provoking stimulus, they will become habituated or deconditioned to the stimulus. Variations of this treatment include using imaginal techniques (i.e., imaginal desensitization) and exposure to real-life situations (i.e., in vivo desensitization). Prolonged exposure, a form of extended repeat exposure

**TABLE 19–35.   Cognitive and behavioral approaches to treating posttraumatic stress disorder**

Graded exposure (imaginal and/or in vivo)

Prolonged exposure

Virtual reality exposure

Cognitive reprocessing

Stress inoculation training

Hypnosis

Affect management

Eye movement desensitization and reprocessing

to the same traumatic memory over a series of sessions, if tolerated, is an effective technique first reported to be successful in the treatment of Vietnam veterans (Fairbank and Keane 1982) and has become established as a first-line treatment of PTSD (Foa et al. 2000). Virtual reality exposure is another computer-based exposure technique that has been piloted in Vietnam veterans and appears promising (Rothbaum et al. 2001).

Relaxation techniques produce the beneficial physiological result of reducing motor tension and lowering the activity of the autonomic nervous system, effects that may be particularly efficacious in PTSD. Progressive muscle relaxation involves contracting and relaxing various muscle groups to induce the relaxation response. This is useful for symptoms of autonomic arousal such as somatic symptoms, anxiety, and insomnia. Hypnosis also has been used to induce the relaxation response with success in PTSD. Relaxation, combined with elements of distraction, thought-stopping, and self-guided dialogue, is a technique known as stress inoculation training.

Cognitive therapy, also referred to as cognitive reprocessing or restructuring, involves various cognitive formulations and corrections of patients' traumatic recollections—that is, identifying distorted and maladaptive cognitions and replacing them with more realistic ones (Resick et al. 2002). Cognitive processing therapy was shown to be more efficacious than wait-list control in a study of women with childhood sexual abuse (Chard 2005).

# Key Points: Anxiety Disorders

• Anxiety disorders are prevalent in the general population, with lifetime prevalence ranging from about 2%–3% for panic disorder and OCD to 15% for social anxiety disorder.

• Anxiety disorders are highly treatable: medication and CBT constitute first-line treatments for all these disorders.

• The "neurocircuitry of fear" has been implicated in all anxiety disorders except for OCD, in which there is evidence of a hyperactive orbitofrontal-limbic-basal ganglia-thalamic circuitry.

• Serotonin reuptake inhibitors are the first-line treatment for all anxiety disorders.

• Exposure, relaxation, and cognitive restructuring are the main types of psychotherapies helpful in treating the anxiety disorders.

# References

Abelson JL, Glitz D, Cameron OG, et al: Blunted growth hormone response to clonidine in patients with generalized anxiety disorder. Arch Gen Psychiatry 48:157–162, 1991

Agid O, Shalev AY, Lerer B: Triiodothyronine augmentation of selective serotonin reuptake inhibitors in posttraumatic stress disorder. J Clin Psychiatry 62:169–173, 2001

Akhtar S, Wig NN, Varma VK, et al: A phenomenological analysis of symptoms in obsessive-compulsive neurosis. Br J Psychiatry 127:342–348, 1975

Allgulander C, Dahl AA, Austin C, et al: Efficacy of sertraline in a 12-week trial for generalized anxiety disorder. Am J Psychiatry 161:1642–1649, 2004

American Psychiatric Association: Diagnostic and Statistical Manual of Mental Disorders, 3rd Edition. Washington, DC, American Psychiatric Association, 1980

American Psychiatric Association: Diagnostic and Statistical Manual of Mental Disorders, 3rd Edition, Revised. Washington, DC, American Psychiatric Association, 1987

American Psychiatric Association: Diagnostic and Statistical Manual of Mental Disorders, 4th Edition. Washington, DC, American Psychiatric Association, 1994

American Psychiatric Association: Diagnostic and Statistical Manual of Mental Disorders, 4th Edition, Text Revision. Washington, DC, American Psychiatric Association, 2000

Arntz A: Cognitive therapy versus applied relaxation as treatment of generalized anxiety disorder. Behav Res Ther 41:633–646, 2003

Bakker A, van Balkom AJ, Spinhoven P: SSRIs vs. TCAs in the treatment of panic disorder: a meta-analysis. Acta Psychiatr Scand 106:163–167, 2002

Baldwin D, Bobes J, Stein DJ, et al: Paroxetine in social phobia/social anxiety disorder. Randomised, double-blind, placebo-controlled study. Br J Psychiatry 175:120–126, 1999

Ball SG, Kuhn A, Wall D, et al: Selective serotonin reuptake inhibitor treatment for generalized anxiety disorder: a double-blind, prospective comparison between paroxetine and sertraline. J Clin Psychiatry 66:94–99, 2005

Bandelow B, Spath C, Tichauer GA, et al: Early traumatic life events, parental attitudes, family history, and birth risk factors in patients with panic disorder. Compr Psychiatry 43:269–278, 2002

Bandelow B, Behnke K, Lenoir S, et al: Sertraline versus paroxetine in the treatment of panic disorder: an acute, double-blind noninferiority comparison. J Clin Psychiatry 65:405–413, 2004

Banerjee SO, Bhandari RP, Rosenberg DR: Use of low dose selective serotonin reuptake inhibitors for severe, refractory choking phobia in childhood. J Dev Behav Pediatr 26:123–127, 2005

Barlow DH: Anxiety and Its Disorders: The Nature and Treatment of Anxiety and Panic. New York, Guilford, 1988

Barlow DH, Rapee RM, Brown TA: Behavioral treatment of generalized anxiety disorder. Behav Ther 23:551–570, 1992

Bellew KM, McCafferty JP, Iyengar M, et al: Paroxetine treatment of GAD: a double-blind, placebo-controlled trial. Presentation at the 153rd annual meeting of the American Psychiatric Association, Chicago, IL, May 13–18, 2000

Benjamin J, Ben-Zion IZ, Karbofsky E, et al: Double-blind, placebo-controlled study of paroxetine for specific phobia. Psychopharmacology (Berl) 149:194–196, 2000

Berlant JL: Prospective open-label study of add-on and monotherapy topiramate in civilians with chronic nonhallucinatory posttraumatic stress disorder. BMC Psychiatry 4:24, 2004

Black A: The natural history of obsessional neurosis, in Obsessional States. Edited by Beech HK. London, England, Methuen, 1974, pp 19–54

Black DW, Noyes R, Goldstein RB, et al: A family study of obsessive-compulsive disorder. Arch Gen Psychiatry 49:362–368, 1992

Borkovec TD, Costello E: Efficacy of applied relaxation and cognitive-behavioral therapy in the treatment of generalized anxiety disorder. J Consult Clin Psychol 61:611–619, 1993

Bouwer C, Stein DJ: Use of the selective serotonin reuptake inhibitor citalopram in the treatment of generalized social phobia. J Affect Disord 49:79–82, 1998

Bradwejn J, Ahokas A, Stein DJ, et al: Venlafaxine extended-release capsules in panic disorder: flexible-dose, double-blind, placebo-controlled study. Br J Psychiatry 187:352–359, 2005

Bremner JD, Licinio J, Darnell A, et al: Elevated CSF corticotropin-releasing factor concentrations in posttraumatic stress disorder. Am J Psychiatry 154:624–629, 1997

Breslau N, Davis GC, Andreski P, et al: Traumatic events and posttraumatic stress disorder in an urban population of young adults. Arch Gen Psychiatry 48:216–222, 1991

Breslau N, Davis GC, Andreski P, et al: Sex differences in posttraumatic stress disorder. Arch Gen Psychiatry 54:1044–1048, 1997

Breslau N, Kessler RC, Chilcoat HD, et al: Trauma and posttraumatic stress disorder in the community: the 1996 Detroit Area Survey of Trauma. Arch Gen Psychiatry 55:626–632, 1998

Breslau N, Davis GC, Peterson EL, et al: A second look at comorbidity in victims of trauma: the posttraumatic stress disorder–major depression connection. Biol Psychiatry 48:902–909, 2000

Butler G, Fennell M, Robson P, et al: Comparison of behavior therapy and cognitive behavior therapy in the treatment of generalized anxiety disorder. J Consult Clin Psychol 59:167–175, 1991

Canive JM, Clark RD, Calais LA, et al: Bupropion treatment in veterans with posttraumatic stress disorder: an open study. J Clin Psychopharmacol 18:379–383, 1998

Carey G, Gottesman II: Twin and family studies of anxiety, phobic, and obsessive disorders, in Anxiety: New Research and Changing Concepts. Edited by Klein DF, Rabkin J. New York, Raven, 1981, pp 117–136

Carter RM, Wittchen HU, Pfister H, et al: One-year prevalence of subthreshold and threshold DSM-IV generalized anxiety disorder in a nationally representative sample. Depress Anxiety 13:78–88, 2001

Cassidy J: Attachment and generalized anxiety disorder, in Rochester Symposium on Developmental Psychopathology, Vol 6: Emotion, Cognition and Representation. Edited by Cicchetti D, Toth S. New York, University of Rochester Press, 1995, pp 343–370

Chambless DL, Gillis MM: Cognitive therapy of anxiety disorders. J Consult Clin Psychol 61:248–260, 1993

Chard KM: An evaluation of cognitive processing therapy for the treatment of posttraumatic stress disorder related to childhood sexual abuse. J Consult Clin Psychol 73:965–971, 2005

Charney DS, Heninger GR, Breier A: Noradrenergic function in panic anxiety: effects of yohimbine in healthy subjects and patients with agoraphobia and panic disorder. Arch Gen Psychiatry 41:751–763, 1984

Chung MY, Min KH, Jun YJ, et al: Efficacy and tolerability of mirtazapine and sertraline in Korean veterans with posttraumatic stress disorder: a randomized open label trial. Hum Psychopharmacol 19:489–494, 2004

Clark RD, Canive JM, Calais LA, et al: Cyproheptadine treatment of nightmares associated with posttraumatic stress disorder. J Clin Psychopharmacol 19:486–487, 1999a

Clark RD, Canive JM, Calais LA, et al: Divalproex in posttraumatic stress disorder: an open-label clinical trial. J Trauma Stress 12:395–401, 1999b

Clomipramine Collaborative Study Group: Clomipramine in the treatment of patients with obsessive-compulsive disorder. Arch Gen Psychiatry 48:730–738, 1991

Connor KM, Davidson JR, Weisler RH, et al: Tiagabine for posttraumatic stress disorder: effects of open label and double blind discontinuation treatment. Psychopharmacology (Berl) 184:21–25, 2006

Cooper AM: Will neurobiology influence psychoanalysis? Am J Psychiatry 142:1395–1402, 1985

Cottraux J, Note I, Albuisson E, et al: Cognitive behavior therapy versus supportive therapy in social phobia: a randomized controlled trial. Psychother Psychosom 69:137–146, 2000

Cottraux J, Note I, Yao SN, et al: A randomized controlled trial of cognitive therapy versus intensive behavior therapy in obsessive compulsive disorder. Psychother Psychosom 70:288–297, 2001

Crowe RR, Noyes R, Pauls DL, et al: A family study of panic disorder. Arch Gen Psychiatry 40:1065–1069, 1983

Dahl AA, Ravindran A, Allgulander C, et al: Sertraline in generalized anxiety disorder: efficacy in treating the psychic and somatic anxiety factors. Acta Psychiatr Scand 111:429–435, 2005

Dale RC, Heyman I, Giovannoni G, et al: Incidence of antibrain antibodies in children with obsessive compulsive disorder. Br J Psychiatry 187:314–319, 2005

Davidson J, Walker JI, Kilts C: A pilot study of phenelzine in the treatment of post-traumatic stress disorder. Br J Psychiatry 150:252–255, 1987

Davidson J, Roth S, Newman E: Fluoxetine in post-traumatic stress disorder. J Trauma Stress 4:419–423, 1991

Davidson J, Potts N, Richichi E, et al: Treatment of social phobia with clonazepam and placebo. J Clin Psychopharmacol 13:423–428, 1993

Davidson JR, DuPont RL, Hedges D, et al: Efficacy, safety, and tolerability of venlafaxine extended release and buspirone in outpatients with generalized anxiety disorder. J Clin Psychiatry 60:528–535, 1999

Davidson JR, Rothbaum BO, van der Kolk BA, et al: Multicenter, double blind comparison of sertraline and placebo in the treatment of posttraumatic stress disorder. Arch Gen Psychiatry 58:485–492, 2001

Davidson JR, Weisler RH, Butterfield MI, et al: Mirtazapine vs placebo in posttraumatic stress disorder: a pilot trial. Biol Psychiatry 53:188–191, 2003

Davidson JR, Foa E, Huppert JD, et al: Fluoxetine, comprehensive cognitive behavioral therapy, and placebo in generalized social phobia. Arch Gen Psychiatry 61:1005–1013, 2004

Davidson JR, Rothbaum BO, Tucker P, et al: Venlafaxine extended release in posttraumatic stress disorder: a sertraline and placebo controlled study. J Clin Psychopharmacol 26:259–267, 2006

Duffy JD, Malloy PF: Efficacy of buspirone in the treatment of posttraumatic stress disorder: an open trial. Ann Clin Psychiatry 6:33–37, 1994

Durham RC, Murphy R, Allan T, et al: Cognitive therapy, analytic psychotherapy and anxiety management training for generalised anxiety disorder. Br J Psychiatry 165:315–323, 1994

Ehlers A, Clark DM: A cognitive model of posttraumatic stress disorder. Behav Res Ther 38:319–345, 2000

Embry CK: Psychotherapeutic interventions in chronic posttraumatic stress disorder, in Posttraumatic Stress Disorder: Etiology, Phenomenology, and Treatment. Edited by Wolf ME, Mosnaim AD. Washington, DC, American Psychiatric Press, 1990, pp 226–236

Emmanuel NP, Lydiard BR, Ballenger JC: Treatment of social phobia with bupropion. J Clin Psychopharmacol 1:276–277, 1991

Fairbank TA, Keane TM: Flooding for combat-related stress disorders: assessment of anxiety reduction across traumatic memories. Behav Ther 13:499–510, 1982

Fava GA, Ruini C, Rafanelli C, et al: Well-being therapy of generalized anxiety disorder. Psychother Psychosom 74:26–30, 2005

Ferrarese C, Appollonio I, Frigo M, et al: Decreased density of benzodiazepine receptors in lymphocytes of anxious patients: reversal after chronic diazepam treatment. Acta Psychiatr Scand 82:169–173, 1990

Flint AJ: Epidemiology and comorbidity of anxiety disorders in the elderly. Am J Psychiatry 151:640–649, 1994

Foa EB, Keane TM, Friedman MJ: Effective Treatments for PTSD: Practice Guidelines From the International Society for Traumatic Stress Studies. New York, Guilford, 2000

Frank JB, Kosten TR, Giller EL Jr, et al: A randomized clinical trial of phenelzine and imipramine for posttraumatic stress disorder. Am J Psychiatry 145:1289–1291, 1988

Freud S: On the grounds for detaching a particular syndrome from neurasthenia under the description "anxiety neurosis" (1895[1894]), in The Standard Edition of the Complete Psychological Works of Sigmund Freud, Vol 3. Translated and edited by Strachey J. London, England, Hogarth, 1962, pp 85–117

Freud S: Analysis of a phobia in a five-year-old boy (1909), in The Standard Edition of the Complete Psychological Works of Sigmund Freud, Vol 10. Translated and edited by Strachey J. London, England, Hogarth, 1955, pp 1–149

Freud S: The disposition to obsessional neurosis: a contribution to the problem of choice of neurosis (1913), in The Standard Edition of the Complete Psychological Works of Sigmund Freud, Vol 12. Translated and edited by Strachey J. London, Hogarth, 1958, pp 311–326

Freud S: Inhibitions, symptoms and anxiety (1926), in The Standard Edition of the Complete Psychological Works of Sigmund Freud, Vol 20. Translated and edited by Strachey J. London, England, Hogarth, 1959, pp 75–175

Furukawa TA, Watanabe N, Churchill R: Psychotherapy plus antidepressant for panic disorder with and without agoraphobia: systematic review. Br J Psychiatry 188:305–312, 2006

Gabbard GO: Psychodynamic Psychiatry in Clinical Practice. Washington, DC, American Psychiatric Press, 1990

Gelenberg AJ, Lydiard RB, Rudolph RL, et al: Efficacy of venlafaxine extended-release capsules in nondepressed outpatients with generalized anxiety disorder: a 6-month randomized controlled trial. JAMA 283:3082–3088, 2000

Geracioti TD Jr, Baker DG, Ekhator NN, et al: CSF norepinephrine concentrations in posttraumatic stress disorder. Am J Psychiatry 158:1227–1230, 2001

Germine M, Goddard AW, Woods SW, et al: Anger and anxiety responses to m-chlorophenylpiperazine in generalized anxiety disorder. Biol Psychiatry 32:457–461, 1992

Giedd JN, Rapoport JL, Garvey MA, et al: MRI assessment of children with obsessive-compulsive disorder or tics associated with streptococcal infection. Am J Psychiatry 157:281–283, 2000

Goodman WK, Bose A, Wang Q: Treatment of generalized anxiety disorder with escitalopram: pooled results from double-blind, placebo-controlled trials. J Affect Disord 87:161–167, 2005

Goodwin RD, Fergusson DM, Horwood LJ: Childhood abuse and familial violence and the risk of panic attacks and panic disorder in young adulthood. Psychol Med 35:881–890, 2005

Gorman JM, Askanazi J, Liebowitz MR, et al: Response to hyperventilation in a group of patients with panic disorder. Am J Psychiatry 141:857–861, 1984

Gorman JM, Kent JM, Sullivan GM, et al: Neuroanatomical hypothesis of panic disorder, revised. Am J Psychiatry 157:493–505, 2000

Grady TA, Pigott TA, L'Heureux F, et al: Double-blind study of adjuvant buspirone for fluoxetine-treated patients with obsessive-compulsive disorder. Am J Psychiatry 150:819–821, 1993

Grant BF, Hasin DS, Blanco C, et al: The epidemiology of social anxiety disorder in the United States: results from the National Epidemiologic Survey on Alcohol and Related Conditions. J Clin Psychiatry 66:1351–1361, 2005a

Grant BF, Hasin DS, Stinson FS, et al: Prevalence, correlates, comorbidity, and comparative disability of DSM-IV generalized anxiety disorder in the USA: results from the National Epidemiologic Survey on Alcohol and Related Conditions. Psychol Med 35:1747–1759, 2005b

Grant BF, Hasin DS, Stinson FS, et al: The epidemiology of DSM-IV panic disorder and agoraphobia in the United States: results from the National Epidemiologic Survey on Alcohol and Related Conditions. J Clin Psychiatry 67:363–374, 2006

370

Greist JH, Chouinard G, DuBoff E, et al: Double-blind parallel comparison of three dosages of sertraline and placebo in outpatients with obsessive-compulsive disorder. Arch Gen Psychiatry 52:289–295, 1995a

Greist JH, Jefferson JW, Kobak KA, et al: A 1-year double-blind placebo-controlled fixed dose study of sertraline in the treatment of obsessive-compulsive disorder. Int Clin Psychopharmacol 10:57–65, 1995b

Gupta S, Popli A, Bathurst E, et al: Efficacy of cyproheptadine for nightmares associated with posttraumatic stress disorder. Compr Psychiatry 39:160–164, 1998

Hamner MB, Deitsch SE, Brodrick PS, et al: Quetiapine treatment in patients with posttraumatic stress disorder: an open trial of adjunctive therapy. J Clin Psychopharmacol 23:15–20, 2003

Heimberg RG, Dodge CS, Hope DA, et al: Cognitive behavioral group treatment for social phobia: comparison with a credible placebo control. Cognit Ther Res 14:1–23, 1990

Heimberg RG, Liebowitz MR, Hope DA, et al: Cognitive behavioral group therapy vs phenelzine therapy for social phobia: a 12-week outcome. Arch Gen Psychiatry 55:1133–1141, 1998

Herman JL, Perry JC, van der Kolk BA: Childhood trauma in borderline personality disorder. Am J Psychiatry 146:490–495, 1989

Hertzberg MA, Butterfield MI, Feldman ME, et al: A preliminary study of lamotrigine for the treatment of posttraumatic stress disorder. Biol Psychiatry 45:1226–1229, 1999

Hettema JM, Prescott CA, Kendler KS: Genetic and environmental sources of covariation between generalized anxiety disorder and neuroticism. Am J Psychiatry 161:1581–1587, 2004

Hewlett WA, Vinogradov S, Agras WS: Clomipramine, clonazepam, and clonidine treatment of obsessive-compulsive disorder. J Clin Psychopharmacol 12:420–430, 1992

Hoehn-Saric R, McLeod DR, Zimmerli WD: Differential effects of alprazolam and imipramine in generalized anxiety disorder: somatic versus psychic symptoms. J Clin Psychiatry 49:293–301, 1988

Hoehn-Saric R, Hazlett RL, McLeod DR: Generalized anxiety disorder with early and late onset of anxiety symptoms. Compr Psychiatry 34:291–298, 1993

Hofmann SG, Moscovitch DA, Kim HJ, et al: Changes in self perception during treatment of social phobia. J Consult Clin Psychol 72:588–596, 2004

Hollander E, Friedberg J, Wasserman D, et al: Venlafaxine in treatment resistant obsessive compulsive disorder. J Clin Psychiatry 64:546–550, 2003a

Hollander E, Koran LM, Goodman WK, et al: A double blind, placebo controlled study of the efficacy and safety of controlled release fluvoxamine in patients with obsessive compulsive disorder. J Clin Psychiatry 64:640–647, 2003b

Hollifield M, Thompson PM, Ruiz JE, et al: Potential effectiveness and safety of olanzapine in refractory panic disorder. Depress Anxiety 21:33–40, 2005

Hornig CD, McNally RJ: Panic disorder and suicide attempt: a reanalysis of data from the Epidemiologic Catchment Area study. Br J Psychiatry 167:76–79, 1995

Horowitz MJ: Stress-Response Syndromes. New York, Jason Aronson, 1976

Horowitz MJ, Wilner N, Kaltreider N, et al: Signs and symptoms of posttraumatic stress disorder. Arch Gen Psychiatry 37:88–92, 1980

Hudson J, Rapee R: The origins of social phobia. Behav Modif 24:102–129, 2000

Janet P: Les obsessions et la psychasthénie, 2nd Edition. Paris, France, Baillière, 1908

Jenike MA, Hyman S, Baer L, et al: A controlled trial of fluvoxamine in obsessive-compulsive disorder: implications for a serotonergic theory. Am J Psychiatry 147:1209–1215, 1990

Johnson J, Weissman MM, Klerman GL: Panic disorder, comorbidity, and suicide attempts. Arch Gen Psychiatry 47:805–808, 1990

Kasper S, Stein DJ, Loft H, et al: Escitalopram in the treatment of social anxiety disorder: randomised, placebo controlled, flexible-dosage study. Br J Psychiatry 186:222–226, 2005

Katzelnick DJ, Kobak KA, Greist JH, et al: Sertraline for social phobia: a double-blind, placebo-controlled crossover study. Am J Psychiatry 152:1368–1371, 1995

Keck PE Jr, Taylor VE, Tugrul KC, et al: Valproate treatment of panic disorder and lactate-induced panic attacks. Biol Psychiatry 33:542–546, 1993

Kendler KS, Neale MC, Kessler RC, et al: Generalized anxiety disorder in women: a population-based twin study. Arch Gen Psychiatry 49:267–272, 1992

Kessler RC, McGonagle KA, Zhao S, et al: Lifetime and 12-month prevalence of DSM-III-R psychiatric disorders in the United States: results from the National Comorbidity Survey. Arch Gen Psychiatry 51:8–19, 1994

Kessler RC, Sonnega A, Bromet E, et al: Posttraumatic stress disorder in the National Comorbidity Survey. Arch Gen Psychiatry 52:1048–1060, 1995

Kessler RC, Stang P, Wittchen HU, et al: Lifetime comorbidities between social phobia and mood disorders in the US National Comorbidity Survey. Psychol Med 29:555–567, 1999

Kinrys G, Wygant LE, Pardo TB, et al: Levetiracetam for treatment-refractory posttraumatic stress disorder. J Clin Psychiatry 67:211–214, 2006

Kolb LC: A neuropsychological hypothesis explaining posttraumatic stress disorders. Am J Psychiatry 144:989–995, 1987

Kolb LC, Burris BC, Griffiths S: Propranolol and clonidine in treatment of the chronic post-traumatic stress disorders of war, in Post-Traumatic Stress Disorder: Psychological and Biological Sequelae. Edited by van der Kolk BA. Washington, DC, American Psychiatric Press, 1984, pp 97–105

Koran LM, Gamel NN, Choung HW, et al: Mirtazapine for obsessive compulsive disorder: an open trial followed by double blind discontinuation. J Clin Psychiatry 66:515–520, 2005

Kozaric-Kovacic D, Pivac N, Muck Seler D, et al: Risperidone in psychotic combat related posttraumatic stress disorder: an open label trial. J Clin Psychiatry 66:922–927, 2005

Kronig MH, Apter J, Asnis G, et al: Placebo-controlled, multicenter study of sertraline treatment for obsessive-compulsive disorder. J Clin Psychopharmacol 19:172–176, 1999

Leskin GA, Sheikh JI: Lifetime trauma history and panic disorder: findings from the National Comorbidity Survey. J Anxiety Disord 16:599–603, 2002

Liebowitz MR, Schneier F, Campeas R, et al: Phenelzine vs atenolol in social phobia: a placebo-controlled comparison. Arch Gen Psychiatry 49:290–300, 1992

Lipper S, Davidson JRT, Grady TA, et al: Preliminary study of carbamazepine in post-traumatic stress disorder. Psychosomatics 27:849–854, 1986

Lipschitz DS, Mayes LM, Rasmussen AM, et al: Baseline and modulated acoustic startle responses in adolescent girls with posttraumatic stress disorder. J Am Acad Child Adolesc Psychiatry 44:807–814, 2005

Lipsitz JD, Mannuzza S, Klein DF, et al: Specific phobia 10–16 years after treatment. Depress Anxiety 10:105–111, 1999

Magee WJ, Eaton WW, Wittchen HU, et al: Agoraphobia, simple phobia, and social phobia in the National Comorbidity Survey. Arch Gen Psychiatry 53:159–168, 1996

Mannuzza S, Schneier FR, Chapman TF, et al: Generalized social phobia: reliability and validity. Arch Gen Psychiatry 52:230–237, 1995

Marshall JR: The treatment of night terrors associated with the posttraumatic syndrome. Am J Psychiatry 132:293–295, 1975

Mason JW, Giller EL, Kosten TR, et al: Urinary free-cortisol levels in posttraumatic stress disorder patients. J Nerv Ment Dis 174:145–149, 1986

Mason JW, Giller EL, Kosten TR, et al: Elevation of urinary norepinephrine/cortisol ratio in posttraumatic stress disorder. J Nerv Ment Dis 176:498–502, 1988

Massion AO, Dyck IR, Shea MT, et al: Personality disorders and time to remission in generalized anxiety disorder, social phobia, and panic disorder. Arch Gen Psychiatry 59:434–440, 2002

Mathew RJ, Ho BT, Kralik P, et al: Catecholamines and monoamine oxidase activity in anxiety. Acta Psychiatr Scand 63:245–252, 1981

Mavissakalian M, Perel JM: Imipramine dose-response relationship in panic disorder with agoraphobia: preliminary findings. Arch Gen Psychiatry 46:127–131, 1989

Mavissakalian M, Perel JM: Clinical experiments in maintenance and discontinuation of imipramine therapy in panic disorder with agoraphobia. Arch Gen Psychiatry 49:318–323, 1992

McDougle CJ, Goodman WK, Price LH, et al: Neuroleptic addition in fluvoxamine-refractory obsessive-compulsive disorder. Am J Psychiatry 147:652–654, 1990

McDougle CJ, Southwick SM, Charney DS, et al: An open trial of fluoxetine in the treatment of posttraumatic stress disorder. J Clin Psychopharmacol 11:325–327, 1991

McDougle CJ, Goodman WK, Leckman JF, et al: The efficacy of fluvoxamine in obsessive-compulsive disorder: effects of comorbid chronic tic disorder. J Clin Psychopharmacol 13:354–358, 1993a

McDougle CJ, Goodman WK, Leckman JF, et al: Limited therapeutic effect of addition of buspirone in fluvoxamine-refractory obsessive-compulsive disorder. Am J Psychiatry 150:647–649, 1993b

McDougle CJ, Goodman WK, Leckman JF, et al: Haloperidol addition in fluvoxamine-refractory obsessive-compulsive disorder: a double-blind, placebo-controlled study in patients with and without tics. Arch Gen Psychiatry 51:302–308, 1994

Mindus, Jenike MA: Neurosurgical treatment of malignant obsessive-compulsive disorder. Psychiatr Clin North Am 15:921–938, 1992

Mitte K: Meta-analysis of cognitive-behavioral treatments for generalized anxiety disorder: a comparison with pharmacotherapy. Psychol Bull 131:785–795, 2005

Montgomery SA, McIntyre A, Osterheider M, et al: A double-blind, placebo-controlled study of fluoxetine in patients with DSM-III-R obsessive-compulsive disorder. The Lilly European OCD Study Group. Eur Neuropsychopharmacol 3:143–152, 1993

Mowrer OH: A stimulus-response analysis of anxiety and its role as a reinforcing agent. Psychol Rev 46:553–565, 1939

Muehlbacher M, Nickel MK, Nickel C, et al: Mirtazapine treatment of social phobia in women: a randomized, double-blind, placebo-controlled study. J Clin Psychopharmacol 25:580–583, 2005

Murphy TK, Goodman WK, Fudge MW, et al: B lymphocyte antigen D8/17: a peripheral marker for childhood-onset obsessive-compulsive disorder and Tourette's syndrome? Am J Psychiatry 154:402–407, 1997

Nee LE, Caine ED, Polinsky RJ, et al: Gilles de la Tourette syndrome: clinical and family study of 50 cases. Ann Neurol 7:41–49, 1982

Neziroglu F, Anemone R, Yaryura-Tobias JA: Onset of obsessive-compulsive disorder in pregnancy. Am J Psychiatry 149:947–950, 1992

Ninan PT, Koran LM, Kiev A, et al: High-dose sertraline strategy for nonresponders to acute treatment for obsessive-compulsive disorder: a multicenter double-blind trial. J Clin Psychiatry 67:15–22, 2006

Orr SP, Metzger LJ, Lasko NB, et al: De novo conditioning in trauma-exposed individuals with and without posttraumatic stress disorder. J Abnorm Psychol 109:290–298, 2000

Ost LG, Breitholtz E: Applied relaxation versus cognitive therapy in the treatment of generalized anxiety disorder. Behav Res Ther 38:777–790, 2000

Otte C, Wiedemann K, Yassouridis A, et al: Valproate monotherapy in the treatment of civilian patients with non combat related posttraumatic stress disorder: an open label study. J Clin Psychopharmacol 24:106–108, 2004

Otto MW, Pollack MH, Gould RA, et al: A comparison of the efficacy of clonazepam and cognitive-behavioral group therapy for the treatment of social phobia. J Anxiety Disord 14:345–358, 2000

Pande AC, Pollack MH, Crockatt J, et al: Placebo-controlled study of gabapentin treatment of panic disorder. J Clin Psychopharmacol 20:467–471, 2000

Pato MT, Pigott TA, Hill JL, et al: Controlled comparison of buspirone and clomipramine in obsessive-compulsive disorder. Am J Psychiatry 148:127–129, 1991

Pauls DL, Towbin KE, Leckman JF, et al: Gilles de la Tourette's syndrome and obsessive-compulsive disorder: evidence supporting a genetic relationship. Arch Gen Psychiatry 43:1180–1182, 1986

Pecknold JC, Swinson RP, Kuch K, et al: Alprazolam in panic disorder and agoraphobia: results from a multicenter trial, III: discontinuation effects. Arch Gen Psychiatry 45:429–436, 1988

Peri T, Ben Shakhar G, Orr SP, et al: Psychophysiological assessment of aversive conditioning in posttraumatic stress disorder. Biol Psychiatry 47:512–519, 2000

Perry BD, Giller EL Jr, Southwick SM: Altered plasma alpha$_2$-adrenergic binding sites in posttraumatic stress disorder (letter). Am J Psychiatry 144:1511–1512, 1987

Pigott TA, L'Heureux F, Hill JL, et al: A double-blind study of adjuvant buspirone hydrochloride in clomipramine-treated patients with obsessive-compulsive disorder. J Clin Psychopharmacol 12:11–18, 1992

Pitman RK, Orr SP, Forgue DF, et al: Psychophysiological assessment of post-traumatic stress disorder imagery in Vietnam combat veterans. Arch Gen Psychiatry 44:970–975, 1987

Pollack MH, Zaninelli R, Goddard A, et al: Paroxetine in the treatment of generalized anxiety disorder: results of a placebo-controlled, flexible-dosage trial. J Clin Psychiatry 62:350–357, 2001

Quitkin F, Babkin J: Hidden psychiatric diagnosis in the alcoholic, in Alcoholism and Clinical Psychiatry. Edited by Solomon J. New York, Plenum, 1982, pp 129–140

Rachman SJ, Hodgson RJ: Obsessions and Compulsions. Englewood Cliffs, NJ, Prentice-Hall, 1980

Ralevski E, Sanislow CA, Grilo CM, et al: Avoidant personality disorder and social phobia: distinct enough to be separate disorders? Acta Psychiatr Scand 112:208–214, 2005

Regier DA, Boyd JH, Burke JD Jr, et al: One-month prevalence of mental disorders in the United States, based on five Epidemiologic Catchment Area sites. Arch Gen Psychiatry 45:977–986, 1988

Resick PA, Nishith P, Weaver TL, et al: A comparison of cognitive processing therapy with prolonged exposure and a waiting condition for the treatment of chronic posttraumatic stress disorder in female rape victims. J Consult Clin Psychol 70:867–879, 2002

Ressler KJ, Rothbaum BO, Tannenbaum L, et al: Cognitive enhancers as adjuncts to psychotherapy: use of D-cycloserine in phobic individuals to facilitate extinction of fear. Arch Gen Psychiatry 61:1136–1144, 2004

Rettew DC: Avoidant personality disorder, generalized social phobia, and shyness: putting the personality back into personality disorders. Harv Rev Psychiatry 8:283–297, 2000

Rickels K, Schweizer E, Csanalosi I, et al: Long-term treatment of anxiety and risk of withdrawal: prospective comparison of clorazepate and buspirone. Arch Gen Psychiatry 45:444–450, 1988

Rickels K, Downing R, Schweizer E, et al: Antidepressants for the treatment of generalized anxiety disorder: a placebo-controlled comparison of imipramine, trazodone, and diazepam. Arch Gen Psychiatry 50:884–895, 1993

Rickels K, DeMartinis N, Garcìa-España F, et al: Imipramine and buspirone in treatment of patients with generalized anxiety disorder who are discontinuing long-term benzodiazepine therapy. Am J Psychiatry 157:1973–1979, 2000

Rickels K, Zaninelli R, McCafferty J: Paroxetine treatment of generalized anxiety disorder: a double-blind, placebo-controlled study. Am J Psychiatry 160:749–756, 2003

Rickels K, Mangano R, Khan A: A double blind placebo controlled study of a flexible dose of venlafaxine ER in adult outpatients with generalized social anxiety disorder. J Clin Psychopharmacol 24:488–496, 2004

Robert S, Hamner MB, Kose S, et al: Quetiapine improves sleep disturbances in combat veterans with PTSD: sleep data from a prospective, open label study. J Clin Psychopharmacol 25:387–388, 2005

Rocca P, Beoni AM, Eva C, et al: Peripheral benzodiazepine receptor messenger RNA is decreased in lymphocytes of generalized anxiety disorder patients. Biol Psychiatry 43:767–773, 1998

Romach M, Busto U, Somer G, et al: Clinical aspects of chronic use of alprazolam and lorazepam. Am J Psychiatry 152:1161–1167, 1995

Rosenbaum JF, Moroz G, Bowden CL: Clonazepam in the treatment of panic disorder with or without agoraphobia: a dose–response study of efficacy, safety, and discontinuance. Clonazepam Panic Disorder Dose-Response Study Group. J Clin Psychopharmacol 17:390–400, 1997

Rothbaum BO, Hodges LF, Ready D, et al: Virtual reality exposure therapy for Vietnam veterans with posttraumatic stress disorder. J Clin Psychiatry 62:617–622, 2001

Sarchiapone M, Armore M, De Risio S, et al: Mirtazapine in the treatment of panic disorder: an open-label trial. Int Clin Psychopharmacol 18:35–38, 2003

Scrignar CB: Post-traumatic Stress Disorder: Diagnosis, Treatment, and Legal Issues. New York, Praeger, 1984

Senkowski D, Linden M, Zubragel D, et al: Evidence for disturbed cortical signal processing and altered serotonergic neurotransmission in generalized anxiety disorder. Biol Psychiatry 53:304–314, 2003

Sepede G, Mancini E, Salerno RM, et al: Olanzapine augmentation in treatment-resistant panic disorder: a 12-week, fixed-dose, open-label trial. J Clin Psychopharmacol 26:45–49, 2006

Sevy S, Papadimitriou GN, Surmont DW, et al: Noradrenergic function in generalized anxiety disorder, major depressive disorder, and healthy subjects. Biol Psychiatry 15:141–152, 1989

Shay J: Fluoxetine reduces explosiveness and elevates mood of Vietnam combat vets with PTSD. J Trauma Stress 5:97–101, 1992

Simon NM, Emmanuel N, Ballenger J, et al: Bupropion sustained release for panic disorder. Psychopharmacol Bull 37:66–72, 2003

Simpson HB, Gorfinkle KS, Liebowitz MR: Cognitive-behavioral therapy as an adjunct to serotonin reuptake inhibitors in obsessive-compulsive disorder: an open trial. J Clin Psychiatry 60:584–590, 1999

Smith MA, Davidson J, Ritchie JC, et al: The corticotropin releasing hormone test in patients with posttraumatic stress disorder. Biol Psychiatry 26:349–355, 1989

Southwick SM, Krystal JH, Bremner JD, et al: Noradrenergic and serotonergic function in posttraumatic stress disorder. Arch Gen Psychiatry 54:749–758, 1997

Spivak B, Vered Y, Graff E, et al: Low platelet-poor plasma concentrations of serotonin in patients with combat-related posttraumatic stress disorder. Biol Psychiatry 45:840–845, 1999

Stein DJ, Ipser JC, Seedat S: Pharmacotherapy for post traumatic stress disorder. Cochrane Database Syst Rev (1): CD002795, 2006

Stein MB, Walker JR, Anderson G, et al: Childhood physical and sexual abuse in patients with anxiety disorders and in a community sample. Am J Psychiatry 153:275–277, 1996

Stein MB, Liebowitz MR, Lydiard B, et al: Paroxetine treatment of generalized social phobia (social anxiety disorder): a randomized controlled trial. JAMA 280:708–713, 1998

Stein MB, Fyer AJ, Davidson JRT, et al: Fluvoxamine treatment of social phobia (social anxiety disorder): a double-blind, placebo-controlled study. Am J Psychiatry 156:756–760, 1999

Stemberger RT, Turner SM, Beidel DC, et al: Social phobia: an analysis of possible developmental factors. J Abnorm Psychol 104:526–531, 1995

Swedo SE, Rapoport JL, Cheslow DL, et al: Increased incidence of obsessive-compulsive symptoms in patients with Sydenham's chorea. Am J Psychiatry 146:246–249, 1989a

Swedo SE, Rapoport JL, Leonard H, et al: Obsessive-compulsive disorder in children and adolescents: clinical phenomenology of 70 consecutive cases. Arch Gen Psychiatry 46:335–341, 1989b

Tancer ME, Stein MB, Uhde TW: Growth hormone response to intravenous clonidine in social phobia: comparison to patients with panic disorder and healthy volunteers. Biol Psychiatry 34:591–595, 1993

Tancer ME, Mailman RB, Stein MB, et al: Neuroendocrine responsivity to monoaminergic system probes in generalized social phobia. Anxiety 1:216–223, 1994

Taylor FB: Tiagabine for posttraumatic stress disorder: a case series of 7 women. J Clin Psychiatry 64:1421–1425, 2003

Taylor FB, Raskind MA: The alpha1-adrenergic antagonist prazosin improves sleep and nightmares in civilian trauma posttraumatic stress disorder. J Clin Psychopharmacol 22:82–85, 2002

Tolin DF, Maltby N, Diefenbach GJ, et al: Cognitive behavioral therapy for medication nonresponders with obsessive compulsive disorder: a wait list controlled open trial. J Clin Psychiatry 65:922–931, 2004

Tollefson GD, Rampey AH, Potvin JH, et al: A multicenter investigation of fixed-dose fluoxetine in the treatment of obsessive-compulsive disorder. Arch Gen Psychiatry 51:559–567, 1994

Torgersen S: Genetic factors in anxiety disorders. Arch Gen Psychiatry 40:1085–1089, 1983

True WR, Rice J, Eisen SA, et al: A twin study of genetic and environmental contributions to liability for posttraumatic stress symptoms. Arch Gen Psychiatry 50:257–264, 1993

Van Ameringen M, Mancini C, Streiner DL: Fluoxetine efficacy in social phobia. J Clin Psychiatry 54:27–32, 1993

Van Den Hout M, Tenney N, Huygens K, et al: Preconscious processing bias in specific phobia. Behav Res Ther 35:29–34, 1997

van der Kolk BA: Psychopharmacological issues in posttraumatic stress disorder. Hosp Community Psychiatry 34:683–691, 1983

van der Kolk BA: The compulsion to repeat the trauma: reenactment, revictimization, and masochism. Psychiatr Clin North Am 12:389–411, 1989

van der Kolk BA, Saporta J: The biological response to psychic trauma: mechanisms and treatment of intrusion and numbing. Anxiety Res 4:199–212, 1991

van Oppen P, de Haan E, van Balkom AJ, et al: Cognitive therapy and exposure in vivo in the treatment of obsessive compulsive disorder. Behav Res Ther 33:379–390, 1995

van Vliet IM, den Boer JA, Westenberg HG: Psychopharmacological treatment of social phobia: a double blind placebo controlled study with fluvoxamine. Psychopharmacology (Berl) 115:128–134, 1994

Versiani M, Mundim FD, Nardi AE, et al: Tranylcypromine in social phobia. J Clin Psychopharmacol 8:279–283, 1988

Vickers K, McNally RJ: Panic disorder and suicide attempt in the National Comorbidity Survey. J Abnorm Psychol 113:582–591, 2004

Warshaw MG, Dolan RT, Keller MB: Suicidal behavior in patients with current or past panic disorder: five years of prospective data from the Harvard/Brown Anxiety Research Program. Am J Psychiatry 157:1876–1878, 2000

Whittal ML, Thordarson DS, McLean PD, et al: Treatment of obsessive compulsive disorder: cognitive behavior therapy vs. exposure and response prevention. Behav Res Ther 43:1559–1576, 2005

Wittchen HU, Zhao S, Kessler RC, et al: DSM-III-R generalized anxiety disorder in the National Comorbidity Survey. Arch Gen Psychiatry 51:355–364, 1994

Wittchen HU, Carter RM, Pfister H, et al: Disabilities and quality of life in pure and comorbid generalized anxiety disorder and major depression in a national survey. Int Clin Psychopharmacol 15:319–328, 2000

Wlazlo Z, Schroeder-Hartwig K, Hand I, et al: Exposure in vivo vs social skills training for social phobia: long-term outcome and differential effects. Behav Res Ther 28:181–193, 1990

Wolf ME, Alavi A, Mosnaim AD: Posttraumatic stress disorder in Vietnam veterans, clinical and EEG findings: possible therapeutic effects of carbamazepine. Biol Psychiatry 23:642–644, 1988

Woodman CL, Noyes R: Panic disorder: treatment with valproate. J Clin Psychiatry 55:134–136, 1994

Woody SR, Chambless DL, Glass CR: Self-focused attention in the treatment of social phobia. Behav Res Ther 35:117–129, 1997

# 20

# Somatoform Disorders

SEAN H. YUTZY, M.D.

BROOKE S. PARISH, M.D.

In DSM-IV-TR (American Psychiatric Association 2000), the disorders included under the somatoform rubric are somatization disorder, undifferentiated somatoform disorder, conversion disorder, pain disorder, hypochondriasis, body dysmorphic disorder, and the residual category somatoform disorder not otherwise specified (NOS).

## Somatization Disorder

### Definition and Clinical Description

Somatization disorder is the most pervasive somatoform disorder. By definition, somatization disorder is a polysymptomatic disorder affecting multiple body systems. Symptoms of other specific somatoform disorders (e.g., conversion disorder and pain disorder) are included in the diagnostic criteria for somatization disorder (Table 20–1).

### Diagnosis

#### Differential Diagnosis

According to Cloninger (1994), three features are useful in discriminating between somatization disorder and physical illness: 1) involvement of multiple organ systems, 2) early onset and chronic course without development of physical signs of structural abnormalities, and 3) absence of characteristic laboratory abnormalities of the suggested

physical disorder (Table 20–2). These features should be considered in cases for which careful analysis leaves the etiology unclear. The clinician also should be aware that several medical disorders may be confused with somatization disorder (Table 20–3).

According to Cloninger (1994), three psychiatric disorders must be carefully considered in the differential diagnosis of somatization disorder: anxiety disorders (in particular, panic disorder), mood disorders, and schizophrenia. The most troublesome distinction is between anxiety disorders and somatization disorder. Individuals with generalized anxiety disorder may have a multitude of physical complaints that are also frequently found in patients with somatization disorder. Individuals with anxiety disorders also may have disease concerns and hypochondriacal complaints common to somatization disorder. Similarly, patients with somatization disorder often report panic (anxiety) attacks. The presence of histrionic personality traits, conversion and dissociative symptoms, sexual and menstrual problems, and social impairment supports a diagnosis of somatization disorder (Cloninger 1994). In addition, gender should be considered because men are much more likely to have anxiety disorders than somatization disorder.

Patients with mood disorders, especially depression, may have somatic complaints. However, such symptoms resolve with successful treatment of the mood disorder, whereas in somatization disorder, the physical complaints continue. Patients with somatization disorder frequently

**TABLE 20–1.  DSM-IV-TR diagnostic criteria for somatization disorder**

A.  A history of many physical complaints beginning before age 30 years that occur over a period of several years and result in treatment being sought or significant impairment in social, occupational, or other important areas of functioning.

B.  Each of the following criteria must have been met, with individual symptoms occurring at any time during the course of the disturbance:

  (1)  *four pain symptoms:*  a history of pain related to at least four different sites or functions (e.g., head, abdomen, back, joints, extremities, chest, rectum, during menstruation, during sexual intercourse, or during urination)

  (2)  *two gastrointestinal symptoms:*  a history of at least two gastrointestinal symptoms other than pain (e.g., nausea, bloating, vomiting other than during pregnancy, diarrhea, or intolerance of several different foods)

  (3)  *one sexual symptom:*  a history of at least one sexual or reproductive symptom other than pain (e.g., sexual indifference, erectile or ejaculatory dysfunction, irregular menses, excessive menstrual bleeding, vomiting throughout pregnancy)

  (4)  *one pseudoneurological symptom:*  a history of at least one symptom or deficit suggesting a neurological condition not limited to pain (conversion symptoms such as impaired coordination or balance, paralysis or localized weakness, difficulty swallowing or lump in throat, aphonia, urinary retention, hallucinations, loss of touch or pain sensation, double vision, blindness, deafness, seizures; dissociative symptoms such as amnesia; or loss of consciousness other than fainting)

C.  Either (1) or (2):

  (1)  after appropriate investigation, each of the symptoms in Criterion B cannot be fully explained by a known general medical condition or the direct effects of a substance (e.g., a drug of abuse, a medication)

  (2)  when there is a related general medical condition, the physical complaints or resulting social or occupational impairment are in excess of what would be expected from the history, physical examination, or laboratory findings

D.  The symptoms are not intentionally produced or feigned (as in factitious disorder or malingering).

**TABLE 20–2.  Features useful in discriminating between somatization disorder and general medical conditions**

Involvement of multiple organ systems

Early onset and chronic course without development of physical signs of structural abnormalities

Absence of characteristic laboratory abnormalities of the suggested physical disorder

**TABLE 20–3.  General medical conditions that may be confused with somatization disorder**

Multiple sclerosis

Systemic lupus erythematosus

Acute intermittent porphyria

Hemochromatosis

complain of depression and often fulfill the criteria for major depression (DeSouza et al. 1988).

Patients with schizophrenia may have unexplained somatic complaints. Careful evaluation often identifies delusions, hallucinations, and/or a formal thought disorder. As described in the section on conversion disorder later in this chapter, reports of hallucinations are common among women with somatization disorder (R.L. Martin, unpublished observations, 1998).

Individuals with antisocial, borderline, and/or histrionic personality disorder may have an associated somatization disorder (Cloninger et al. 1997; Hudziak et al. 1996; Stern et al. 1993). Antisocial personality disorder has been shown to cluster both within individuals and within families (Cloninger and Guze 1970; Cloninger et al. 1975) and may have a common etiology in many cases.

Patients with somatization disorder often complain of psychological or interpersonal problems in addition to somatic symptoms. Wetzel et al. (1994) summarized these as "psychoform symptoms." In this study, Minnesota Multiphasic Personality Inventory (Hathaway and McKinley 1943) profiles of somatization disorder patients mimicked multiple psychiatric disorders.

## Natural History

Somatization disorder is a chronic illness with fluctuations in the frequency and diversity of symptoms, but it rarely, if ever, totally remits (Guze and Perley 1963; Guze et al. 1986). The most active symptomatic phase is usually early adulthood, but aging does not lead to total remission (Goodwin and Guze 1996). Longitudinal prospective studies have confirmed that 80%–90% of the patients diagnosed with somatization disorder maintain a consistent clinical syndrome and retain the same diagnosis over many years (Cloninger et al. 1986; Guze et al. 1986; Perley and Guze 1962).

Avoiding the prescribing of habit-forming or addictive substances for persistent or recurrent complaints of pain should be paramount in the mind of the treating physician. Suicide attempts are common, but completed suicide is not (Martin et al. 1985; Murphy and Wetzel 1982).

## Epidemiology

The lifetime risk for somatization disorder was estimated at about 2% in women when age at onset and method of assessment were taken into account (Cloninger et al. 1975). However, the Epidemiologic Catchment Area (ECA) study (Robins et al. 1984), using nonphysician interviewers, found a lifetime risk of somatization disorder of only 0.2%–0.3% for women. In a study by Robins et al. (1981), nonphysicians, when compared with psychiatrists, showed high (i.e., 97%–99%) diagnostic specificity for somatization disorder. However, diagnostic sensitivity for nonphysicians was low (55% for Feighner-defined hysteria and 41% for DSM-III-defined [American Psychiatric Association 1980] somatization disorder). Somatization disorder is diagnosed predominantly in women and rarely in men.

## Etiology

The etiology of somatization disorder is unknown, but it is clearly a familial disorder. In several studies, approximately 20% of the female first-degree relatives of patients with somatization disorder also met criteria for the disorder (Cloninger and Guze 1970; Guze et al. 1986; Woerner and Guze 1968). Overall, these findings suggest that somatization disorder in women shares a common etiology

with antisocial personality disorder, whereas somatization disorder in men may be related more to anxiety disorders (Cloninger et al. 1984, 1986).

A relation between somatization disorder and certain personality disorders has been posited. Hudziak et al. (1996) and Cloninger et al. (1997) identified similarities and even overlap between somatization disorder and borderline personality disorder, as did Stern et al. (1993) with personality disorders broadly.

## Treatment

An eclectic approach accords well with the general principles of treatment recommended by Quill (1985), Cloninger (1994), and Smith et al. (1986). Three important suggestions emerge from review of these reports: 1) establish a firm therapeutic alliance with the patient, 2) educate the patient about the manifestations of somatization disorder, and 3) provide consistent reassurance (Table 20–4). Implementation of these principles, as described in more detail in the following paragraphs, may greatly facilitate clinical management of somatization disorder and prevent potentially serious complications, including the effects of unnecessary diagnostic and therapeutic procedures.

**TABLE 20–4. Main treatment principles in approaching a patient with somatization disorder**

1. Establish a firm therapeutic alliance at the outset.
2. Provide education about the illness.
3. Offer consistent reassurance.

Generally, multiple physicians already have been consulted in an attempt to discover a physical explanation for the symptoms offered. The patient usually has received the message (overtly or covertly) that the difficulty is "mental," "psychological," or "psychiatric," and the physician is not particularly interested in continuing to provide care to him or her. That message promotes a pattern of "doctor shopping," which may lead to unnecessary diagnostic procedures and treatments. The first step in establishing a firm therapeutic alliance is for the physician to acknowledge the patient's pain and suffering. This acknowledgment communicates to the patient that the physician is caring, compassionate, and interested in providing assistance. The physician should then conduct an exhaustive review of the patient's medical history, including careful examination of medical records. After the diagnosis of somatization disorder is firmly established, elaborate diagnostic evaluations should be conducted based on objective evidence and not just subjective complaints.

Education is the second general principle. Cloninger (1994) favors informing the patient of the diagnosis and describing the various facets of somatization disorder in a positive light. The patient should be advised that he or she is not "crazy" but has a medically recognized illness. The clinician should be careful to strike a balance between painting a positive picture of the disorder and conducting a realistic discussion of prognosis, goals, and treatment.

The third principle is consistent reassurance. Patients with somatization disorder often become concerned that the physician is not performing a sufficiently thorough evaluation and may threaten to seek care from a different physician. The patient should be reassured that there is no evidence of a physical cause for the complaint but that there may be a link with stress. A thorough review of complaints commonly identifies a temporal association of symptoms with interpersonal, social, or occupational problems. In patients for whom introspection is difficult, modification of behavior by using simple behavioral management techniques may be useful.

Because patients with somatization disorder also frequently complain of anxiety and depressive symptoms, prescription medications for these complaints should be held to a minimum and carefully monitored. Although chlordiazepoxide was recommended for reasons of safety, patient preference, and effectiveness in symptom relief, the best results were obtained by optimistic physicians using low dosages of anxiolytic medications, regardless of which drug was given (Wheatley 1965).

# Undifferentiated Somatoform Disorder

## Definition and Clinical Description

The essential aspect of undifferentiated somatoform disorder is the presence of one or more clinically significant, medically unexplained somatic symptoms with a duration of 6 months or more that are not better accounted for by another mental disorder (Table 20–5).

## Differential Diagnosis

Principal considerations in the differential diagnosis include the question of whether, with follow-up, criteria for somatization disorder will be met.

---

**TABLE 20–5.  DSM-IV-TR diagnostic criteria for undifferentiated somatoform disorder**

A.  One or more physical complaints (e.g., fatigue, loss of appetite, gastrointestinal or urinary complaints).

B.  Either (1) or (2):

(1)  after appropriate investigation, the symptoms cannot be fully explained by a known general medical condition or the direct effects of a substance (e.g., a drug of abuse, a medication)

(2)  when there is a related general medical condition, the physical complaints or resulting social or occupational impairment is in excess of what would be expected from the history, physical examination, or laboratory findings

C.  The symptoms cause clinically significant distress or impairment in social, occupational, or other important areas of functioning.

D.  The duration of the disturbance is at least 6 months.

E.  The disturbance is not better accounted for by another mental disorder (e.g., another somatoform disorder, sexual dysfunction, mood disorder, anxiety disorder, sleep disorder, or psychotic disorder).

F.  The symptom is not intentionally produced or feigned (as in factitious disorder or malingering).

---

## Epidemiology

Some investigators have argued that undifferentiated somatoform disorder is the most common somatoform disorder.

## Etiology

If undifferentiated somatoform disorder is simply an abridged form of somatization disorder, etiological theories reviewed under that diagnosis should also apply to undifferentiated somatoform disorder.

## Treatment

Several studies suggested that improvement is accelerated with psychotherapy of a supportive, rather than nondirective, type. However, a substantial proportion of patients improve or recover with no formal psychotherapy. Judicious use of pharmacotherapy appears to be beneficial, with trials of antidepressant medications indicated for patients with depressive symptoms and trials of buspirone, benzodiazepines, and propranolol for patients with anxiety symptoms.

# Conversion Disorder

## Definition and Clinical Description

The essential features of conversion disorder are the nonintentionally produced symptoms or deficits affecting voluntary motor or sensory function that suggest but are not fully explained by a neurological or general medical condition, by the direct effects of a substance, or by a culturally sanctioned behavior or experience. Specific symptoms mentioned as examples in DSM-IV-TR include motor symptoms such as impaired coordination or balance, paralysis or localized weakness, difficulty swallowing or lump in throat (e.g., "globus hystericus"), aphonia, and urinary retention; sensory symptoms, including hallucinations, loss of touch or pain sensation, double vision, blindness, and deafness; and seizures or convulsions with voluntary motor or sensory components. Psychological factors generally appear to be involved because symptoms often occur in the context of a conflictual situation that may in some way be resolved with the development of the symptom.

## Diagnosis

### DSM-IV-TR Criteria

As defined in DSM-IV-TR, nonintentional "symptoms or deficits affecting voluntary motor or sensory function" (American Psychiatric Association 2000, p. 498) are central to conversion disorder (Table 20–6). The majority of such symptoms will suggest a neurological condition (i.e., are pseudoneurological), but other general medical conditions may be suggested as well. Pseudoneurological symptoms remain the classic symptomatology. By definition, symptoms limited to pain or disturbance in sexual functioning are not included.

In conversion disorder, as in the other somatoform disorders, the symptom cannot be fully explained by a known physical disorder.

### Differential Diagnosis

Neurologists are frequently consulted by primary care physicians for such symptoms because most suggest neurological disease. It has been estimated that 1% of the patients admitted to the hospital for neurological problems have conversion symptoms (Marsden 1986), and up to one-third of new neurology clinic patients have medically unexplained symptoms (Carson et al. 2003; Stone et al. 2003).

---

**TABLE 20–6. DSM-IV-TR diagnostic criteria for conversion disorder**

A. One or more symptoms or deficits affecting voluntary motor or sensory function that suggest a neurological or other general medical condition.

B. Psychological factors are judged to be associated with the symptom or deficit because the initiation or exacerbation of the symptom or deficit is preceded by conflicts or other stressors.

C. The symptom or deficit is not intentionally produced or feigned (as in factitious disorder or malingering).

D. The symptom or deficit cannot, after appropriate investigation, be fully explained by a general medical condition, or by the direct effects of a substance, or as a culturally sanctioned behavior or experience.

E. The symptom or deficit causes clinically significant distress or impairment in social, occupational, or other important areas of functioning or warrants medical evaluation.

F. The symptom or deficit is not limited to pain or sexual dysfunction, does not occur exclusively during the course of somatization disorder, and is not better accounted for by another mental disorder.

*Specify* type of symptom or deficit:

**With motor symptom or deficit**

**With sensory symptom or deficit**

**With seizures or convulsions**

**With mixed presentation**

---

Symptoms of various neurological illnesses may seem to be inconsistent with known neurophysiology or neuropathology and may suggest conversion. Diseases to be considered include multiple sclerosis, myasthenia gravis, periodic paralysis, myoglobinuric myopathy, polymyositis, other acquired myopathies, and Guillain-Barré syndrome (Cloninger 1994).

Longitudinal studies show the factor that most reliably predicts that a patient with apparent conversion symptoms will not later be shown to have a physical disorder is a history of conversion or other unexplained symptoms (Cloninger 1994). Patients with somatization disorder will manifest multiple symptoms in multiple organ systems, including the voluntary motor and sensory nervous systems. Although conversion symptoms may occur at any age, vulnerability for conversion symptoms is first manifested most often in late adolescence or early adulthood (Cloninger 1994).

*Natural History*

Onset of conversion disorder is generally from late childhood to early adulthood. Conversion disorder is rare before age 10 years (Maloney 1980) and seldom first presents after age 35 years.

Onset of conversion disorder is generally acute, but it may be characterized by gradually increasing symptomatology. The typical course of individual conversion symptoms is generally short; half (Folks et al. 1984) to nearly all (Carter 1949) patients show a disappearance of symptoms by the time of hospital discharge. However, 20%–25% will relapse within 1 year. Factors traditionally associated with good prognosis include acute onset, presence of clearly identifiable stress at the time of onset, short interval between onset and institution of treatment, and good intelligence (Toone 1990). Generally, individual conversion symptoms are self-limited and do not lead to physical changes or disabilities.

## Epidemiology

Lifetime prevalence rates of treated conversion symptoms in general populations have ranged from 11 in 100,000 to 500 in 100,000 (Ford and Folks 1985; Toone 1990). A marked excess of women compared with men develop conversion symptoms. Approximately 5%–24% of psychiatric outpatients, 5%–14% of general hospital patients, and 1%–3% of outpatient psychiatric referrals have a history of conversion symptoms (Cloninger 1994; Ford 1983; Toone 1990). Conversion is associated with lower socioeconomic status, lower education, lack of psychological sophistication, and a rural setting (Folks et al. 1984; Guze and Perley 1963; Lazare 1981; Stefansson et al. 1976; Weinstein et al. 1969). Consistent with this finding, much higher rates (nearly 10%) of outpatient psychiatric referrals in developing countries are for conversion symptoms.

## Etiology

An etiological hypothesis is implicit in the term *conversion*. Several psychological factors have been implicated in the pathogenesis, or at least pathophysiology, of conversion disorder (see Table 20–7 for definitions).

In primary gain, anxiety is theoretically reduced by keeping an internal conflict or need out of awareness by symbolic expression of an unconscious wish as a conversion symptom. However, individuals with active conversion symptoms often continue to show marked anxiety, especially on psychological tests (Lader and Sartorius

**TABLE 20–7. Key terms**

**Conversion:** Hypothesized conversion of a psychological conflict into a somatic complaint.

**Primary gain:** Anxiety is theoretically reduced by keeping an internal conflict or need out of conscious awareness through production of a symptom; the symptom is involuntarily produced and not under conscious control.

**Secondary gain:** The symptom is voluntarily produced and under conscious control; production is for the purpose of a goal, such as avoiding work, obtaining money (i.e., malingering).

*La belle indifférence:* The individual seems indifferent to or disinterested in personal medical issues that should concern anyone.

1968; Meares and Horvath 1972). Symbolism is infrequently evident, and its evaluation involves highly inferential and unreliable judgments (Raskin et al. 1966). Interpretation of symbolism in persons with occult medical disorder has been noted to contribute to misdiagnosis. Secondary gain, whereby conversion symptoms allow avoidance of noxious activities or the obtaining of otherwise unavailable support, also may occur in persons who have medical conditions, who often take advantage of such benefits (Raskin et al. 1966; Watson and Buranen 1979).

Individuals with conversion disorder may show a lack of concern, in keeping with the nature or implications of the symptom (the so-called *belle indifférence*). Conversion symptoms may be revealed in a dramatic or histrionic fashion. A minority of individuals with conversion disorder fulfill criteria for histrionic personality disorder. Patients with conversion disorder may have a history of disturbed sexuality (Lewis 1974), with many (one-third) reporting a history of sexual abuse, especially incestuous. (Thus, two-thirds do not report such a history.)

## Treatment

Generally, the initial aim in treating conversion disorder is removal of the symptom. The pressure behind accomplishing this goal depends on the distress and disability associated with the symptom (Merskey 1989). In any situation, direct confrontation is not recommended. A conservative approach of reassurance and relaxation is effective. Reassurance need not come from a psychiatrist but can be performed effectively by the primary physician. After physical illness is excluded, prognosis for conversion symptoms is good.

If symptoms do not resolve with a conservative approach and there is an immediate need for symptom resolution, several techniques, including narcoanalysis (e.g., amobarbital interview), hypnosis, and behavior therapy, may be tried (Merskey 1989).

# Hypochondriasis

## Definition and Clinical Description

The essential feature in hypochondriasis is preoccupation not with the symptoms themselves but rather with the fear or idea of having a serious disease, based on the misinterpretation of bodily signs and sensations. The preoccupation persists despite evidence to the contrary and reassurance from physicians.

## Diagnosis

### *DSM-IV-TR Criteria*

Specific criteria for the diagnosis of hypochondriasis are presented in Table 20–8.

### *Differential Diagnosis*

If, after appropriate assessment, the probability of physical illness appears low, the condition should be considered relative to other psychiatric disorders. Patients with hypochondriasis as a primary disorder, although extremely preoccupied, are generally able to acknowledge the possibility that their concerns are unfounded. Delusional patients, on the other hand, are not. Somatic delusions of serious illness are seen in some cases of major depressive disorder and in schizophrenia. A useful discriminator is the presence of other psychiatric symptoms.

### *Natural History*

Traditionally, limited data suggested that approximately one-fourth of the patients with a diagnosis of hypochondriasis do poorly, two-thirds show a chronic but fluctuating course, and one-tenth recover.

## Epidemiology

The ECA study (Robins et al. 1984) did not assess for hypochondriasis. More recent studies suggest a prevalence in general medical practice of 3%–9% (Barsky et al. 1990; Escobar et al. 1998; Kellner et al. 1983/1984).

**TABLE 20–8.** **DSM-IV-TR diagnostic criteria for hypochondriasis**

A. Preoccupation with fears of having, or the idea that one has, a serious disease based on the person's misinterpretation of bodily symptoms.

B. The preoccupation persists despite appropriate medical evaluation and reassurance.

C. The belief in Criterion A is not of delusional intensity (as in delusional disorder, somatic type) and is not restricted to a circumscribed concern about appearance (as in body dysmorphic disorder).

D. The preoccupation causes clinically significant distress or impairment in social, occupational, or other important areas of functioning.

E. The duration of the disturbance is at least 6 months.

F. The preoccupation is not better accounted for by generalized anxiety disorder, obsessive-compulsive disorder, panic disorder, a major depressive episode, separation anxiety, or another somatoform disorder.

*Specify* if:

**With poor insight:** if, for most of the time during the current episode, the person does not recognize that the concern about having a serious illness is excessive or unreasonable

## Etiology

In considering hypochondriasis as an aspect of depression or anxiety disorders, it has been posited that these conditions create a state of hypervigilance to insult, including overperception of physical problems (Barsky and Klerman 1983).

## Treatment

Patients referred early for psychiatric evaluation and treatment of hypochondriasis appear to have a better prognosis than do those continuing with only medical evaluations and treatments (Kellner 1983). Psychiatric referral should be performed with sensitivity. Perhaps the best guideline to follow is for the referring physician to stress that the patient's distress is serious and that psychiatric evaluation will be a supplement to, not a replacement for, continued medical care.

Hypochondriacal symptoms secondary to depressive and anxiety disorders may improve with successful treatment of the primary disorder. However, until recently, hypochondriasis as a primary condition was not considered to be responsive to known psychopharmacological medications. Early results of placebo-controlled, double-blind studies are pending, but anecdotal case reports, open-label trials, and review of preliminary data show some promise for the selective serotonin reuptake inhibitors (Fallon et al. 1996). Stoudemire (1988) suggested an approach that includes consistent treatment, generally by the same primary physician, with supportive, regularly scheduled office visits not based on the evaluation of symptoms. Hospitalization, medical tests, and medications with addictive potential are to be avoided if possible. Focus during the office visits gradually should be shifted from symptoms to social or interpersonal problems. Psychotherapeutic approaches may be enhanced greatly by the promising potential of effective pharmacotherapy. Of note, cognitive-behavioral therapy (CBT) recently has been found to be effective in one study, in which 57% of CBT-treated patients at 12-month follow-up had a lessening of hypochondriacal beliefs (Barsky and Ahern 2004).

# Body Dysmorphic Disorder

## Definition and Clinical Description

The essential feature of body dysmorphic disorder is a preoccupation with some imagined defect in appearance or markedly excessive concern with a minor physical anomaly (Table 20–9). Such preoccupation persists even after reassurance. Common complaints include a diversity of imagined flaws of the face or head, such as various defects in the hair (too much or too little), skin, shape of the face, or facial features. It is not surprising, then, that patients with body dysmorphic disorder are found most commonly among persons seeking cosmetic surgery.

---

TABLE 20–9.    **DSM-IV-TR diagnostic criteria for body dysmorphic disorder**

A.    Preoccupation with an imagined defect in appearance. If a slight physical anomaly is present, the person's concern is markedly excessive.

B.    The preoccupation causes clinically significant distress or impairment in social, occupational, or other important areas of functioning.

C.    The preoccupation is not better accounted for by another mental disorder (e.g., dissatisfaction with body shape and size in anorexia nervosa).

---

## Diagnosis

### Differential Diagnosis

Anorexia nervosa, in which there is dissatisfaction with body shape and size, is specifically mentioned in the criteria as an example of an exclusion. Diagnostic problems may develop when a patient has the mood-congruent ruminations of major depression. However, such concerns generally lack the focus on a particular body part that is seen in body dysmorphic disorder. Somatic obsessions and even grooming or cleaning rituals in obsessive-compulsive disorder (OCD) may suggest body dysmorphic disorder; however, in such cases, other obsessions and compulsions are seen as well. In body dysmorphic disorder, the preoccupations are limited to concerns with appearance.

### Natural History

Onset of body dysmorphic disorder is usually in adolescence or early adulthood (Phillips 1991). The disorder is generally a chronic condition, with a waxing and waning of intensity but rarely full remission (Phillips et al. 1993). Over a lifetime, multiple preoccupations are typical. (In their study, Phillips et al. [1993] found an average of four preoccupations.)

Recent studies of special populations have reported varying findings regarding outcomes, with one study finding that at 4-year follow-up, 58% of patients were in full remission and 84% were in partial remission (Phillips et al. 2005). A second study found that only 9% experienced full remission, with 21% experiencing partial remission (Phillips et al. 2006). Body dysmorphic disorder is highly incapacitating. Almost all persons with this disorder show marked impairment in social and occupational activities. Superimposed depressive episodes are common, as are suicidal ideation and suicide attempts. The estimated lifetime risk of depression is 76% (Gunstad and Phillips 2003). The lifetime suicide attempt rate has been estimated at 22%–24% (Phillips and Diaz 1997; Veale et al. 1996).

## Epidemiology

Studies have reported prevalences varying from 0.7% to 5% in special populations (Bohne et al. 2002; Otto et al. 2001; Rief et al. 2006). Although body dysmorphic disorder is seldom reported in psychiatric settings, Andreasen and Bardach (1977) estimated that 2% of the patients seeking corrective cosmetic surgery have this disorder. The male-to-female ratio is about 1:1 (Phillips 1995).

## Etiology

Although the etiology of body dysmorphic disorder remains elusive, there has been significant nosological debate recently in several areas. First, the possibility that the label represents a spectrum of disorders as opposed to simply psychotic versus nonpsychotic variants has been raised. The second issue is whether body dysmorphic disorder should be classified as an anxiety disorder, particularly a variant of OCD. Phillips and Stout (2005) found that only 10% of patients had resolution of their body dysmorphic symptoms after their OCD symptoms resolved.

## Treatment

Simply recognizing that a complaint derives from body dysmorphic disorder may have therapeutic benefit by interrupting an unending procession of repeated evaluations by physicians and eliminating the possibility of needless surgery. There is a long history of anecdotal reports suggesting the value of diverse treatments, including behavior therapy, dynamic psychotherapy, and pharmacotherapy.

Recommended medications include neuroleptics and antidepressants (De Leon et al. 1989). Delusional syndromes, in general, may respond to neuroleptics, whereas in body dysmorphic disorder, even when the bodily preoccupations are psychotic, there is less likelihood of success.

# Somatoform Disorder Not Otherwise Specified

## Definition and Clinical Description

Somatoform disorder NOS is the true residual category for the somatoform disorders. By definition, conditions included under this category are characterized by somatoform symptoms that do not meet the criteria for any of the specified somatoform disorders. DSM-IV-TR gives several examples, but syndromes potentially included under this category are not limited to those examples (see Table 20–10).

Unlike undifferentiated somatoform disorder, no minimum duration is required. In fact, some disorders may be relegated to the NOS category because they do not meet the time requirements for a specified somatoform disorder.

**TABLE 20–10.　DSM-IV-TR somatoform disorder not otherwise specified**

This category includes disorders with somatoform symptoms that do not meet the criteria for any specific somatoform disorder. Examples include

1. Pseudocyesis: a false belief of being pregnant that is associated with objective signs of pregnancy, which may include abdominal enlargement (although the umbilicus does not become everted), reduced menstrual flow, amenorrhea, subjective sensation of fetal movement, nausea, breast engorgement and secretions, and labor pains at the expected date of delivery. Endocrine changes may be present, but the syndrome cannot be explained by a general medical condition that causes endocrine changes (e.g., a hormone-secreting tumor).

2. A disorder involving nonpsychotic hypochondriacal symptoms of less than 6 months' duration.

3. A disorder involving unexplained physical complaints (e.g., fatigue or body weakness) of less than 6 months' duration that are not due to another mental disorder.

## Diagnosis

### *DSM-IV-TR Criteria*

The basic DSM-IV-TR requirement for a diagnosis of somatoform disorder NOS is that a disorder with somatoform symptoms does not meet criteria for a specified somatoform disorder (Table 20–10). The first example of such a disorder listed in DSM-IV-TR is pseudocyesis.

### *Differential Diagnosis*

Pseudocyesis deserves further attention. Its presumed mechanism was ambivalence about pregnancy, with the resulting conflict expressed somatically, leading to resolution (primary gain) and unconsciously needed environmental support (secondary gain). Pseudocyesis could have been subsumed under the heading "Psychological Factors Affecting Medical Condition." An argument can be made for its inclusion as a medical condition because, based on a literature review (Martin 1995), in most if not all cases, it appears that a neuroendocrine change accompanies, and at times may antedate, the false belief of pregnancy. However, in most instances, a discrete general medical condition (such as a hormone-secreting tumor) cannot be identified. It might have been included as a specified somatoform disorder except for its rarity; Whelan and Stewart (1990) reported six cases in 20 years of consulting to a unit delivering 2,500 women per year.

## Epidemiology, Etiology, and Treatment

Discussion of epidemiology, etiology, and treatment for a residual category such as somatoform disorder NOS would not be meaningful because it represents a grouping of diverse disorders. Conditions that would warrant diagnosis of a specified somatoform disorder except for their insufficient duration (less than 6 months) are probably best considered to be in the spectrum of the resembled disorder. Thus, the epidemiological, etiological, and treatment considerations pertaining to the specified disorder should be reviewed because these may apply, at least in part, to the shorter-duration syndromes.

## Key Points: Somatoform Disorders

- The somatoform disorders are grouped because they suggest a physical disorder for which there are no organic findings or known physiological mechanism or there is a strong presumption that the symptoms are linked to psychological issues.

- Somatization disorder is uncommon, but it is considered one of very few valid and reliable mental illnesses.

- Conversion disorder is a diagnosis that should be applied only after significant effort has been expended to eliminate any possible treatable organic disorder.

- Hypochondriasis is a rather uncommon disorder that usually follows a fluctuating course.

- Body dysmorphic disorder is a diagnosis in evolution, with conflicting data regarding amenability to treatment.

## References

American Psychiatric Association: Diagnostic and Statistical Manual of Mental Disorders, 3rd Edition. Washington, DC, American Psychiatric Association, 1980

American Psychiatric Association: Diagnostic and Statistical Manual of Mental Disorders, 4th Edition, Text Revision. Washington, DC, American Psychiatric Association, 2000

Andreasen NC, Bardach J: Dysmorphophobia: symptom or disease? Am J Psychiatry 134:673–676, 1977

Barsky AJ, Ahern DK: Cognitive behavior therapy for hypochondriasis. JAMA 291:1464–1470, 2004

Barsky AJ, Klerman GL: Overview: hypochondriasis, bodily complaints, and somatic styles. Am J Psychiatry 140:273–283, 1983

Barsky AJ, Wyshak G, Klerman GL, et al: The prevalence of hypochondriasis in medical outpatients. Soc Psychiatry Psychiatr Epidemiol 25:89–94, 1990

Bohne A, Wilhelm S, Keuthen N, et al: Prevalence of body dysmorphic disorder in a German college student sample. Psychiatry Res 109:101–104, 2002

Carson A, Best S, Postma K, et al: The outcome of neurology patients with medically unexplained symptoms: a prospective study. J Neurol Neurosurg Psychiatry 74:897–900, 2003

Carter AB: The prognosis of certain hysterical symptoms. Br Med J 1:1076–1079, 1949

Cloninger CR: Somatoform and dissociative disorders, in The Medical Basis of Psychiatry, 2nd Edition. Edited by Winokur G, Clayton P. Philadelphia, PA, WB Saunders, 1994, pp 169–192

Cloninger CR, Guze SB: Psychiatric illness and female criminality: the role of sociopathy and hysteria in the antisocial woman. Am J Psychiatry 127:303–311, 1970

Cloninger CR, Reich T, Guze SB: The multifactorial model of disease transmission, III: familial relationship between sociopathy and hysteria (Briquet's syndrome). Br J Psychiatry 127:23–32, 1975

Cloninger CR, Sigvardsson S, von Knorring A-L, et al: An adoption study of somatoform disorders, II: identification of two discrete somatoform disorders. Arch Gen Psychiatry 41:863–871, 1984

Cloninger CR, Martin RL, Guze SB, et al: A prospective follow-up and family study of somatization in men and women. Am J Psychiatry 143:873–878, 1986

Cloninger CR, Bayon C, Przybeck TR: Epidemiology and Axis I comorbidity of antisocial personality, in Handbook of Antisocial Behavior. Edited by Stoff DM, Breiling J, Maser JD. New York, Wiley, 1997, pp 12–21

De Leon J, Bott A, Simpson GM: Dysmorphophobia: body dysmorphic disorder or delusional disorder, somatic subtype? Compr Psychiatry 30:457–472, 1989

DeSouza C, Othmer E, Gabrielli W Jr, et al: Major depression and somatization disorder: the overlooked differential diagnosis. Psychiatr Ann 18:340–348, 1988

Escobar JL, Gara MA, Waitzkins H, et al: DSM-IV hypochondriasis in primary care. Gen Hosp Psychiatry 20:155–159, 1998

Fallon BA, Schneier FR, Marshall R, et al: The pharmacotherapy of hypochondriasis. Psychopharmacol Bull 32:607–611, 1996

Folks DG, Ford CV, Regan WM: Conversion symptoms in a general hospital. Psychosomatics 25:285–295, 1984

Ford CV: The Somatizing Disorders: Illness as a Way of Life. New York, Elsevier, 1983

Ford CV, Folks DG: Conversion disorders: an overview. Psychosomatics 26:371–383, 1985

Goodwin DW, Guze SB: Psychiatric Diagnosis, 5th Edition. New York, Oxford University Press, 1996

Gunstad J, Phillips KA: Axis I comorbidity in body dysmorphic disorder. Compr Psychiatry 44:270–276, 2003

Guze SB, Perley MJ: Observations on the natural history of hysteria. Am J Psychiatry 119:960–965, 1963

Guze SB, Cloninger CR, Martin RL, et al: A follow-up and family study of Briquet's syndrome. Br J Psychiatry 149:17–23, 1986

Hathaway SR, McKinley JC: The Minnesota Multiphasic Personality Inventory. Minneapolis, University of Minnesota Press, 1943

Hudziak JJ, Boffeli TJ, Kreisman JJ, et al: Clinical study of the relation of borderline personality disorder to Briquet's syndrome (hysteria), somatization disorder, antisocial personality disorder, and substance abuse disorders. Am J Psychiatry 153:1598–1606, 1996

Kellner R: The prognosis of treated hypochondriasis: a clinical study. Acta Psychiatr Scand 67:69–79, 1983

Kellner R, Abbott P, Pathak D, et al: Hypochondriacal beliefs and attitudes in family practice and psychiatric patients. Int J Psychiatry Med 13:127–139, 1983/1984

Lader M, Sartorius N: Anxiety in patients with hysterical conversion symptoms. J Neurol Neurosurg Psychiatry 31:490–495, 1968

Lazare A: Conversion symptoms. N Engl J Med 305:745–748, 1981

Lewis WC: Hysteria: the consultant's dilemma: twentieth century demonology, pejorative epithet, or useful diagnosis? Arch Gen Psychiatry 30:145–151, 1974

Maloney MJ: Diagnosing hysterical conversion disorders in children. J Pediatr 97:1016–1020, 1980

Marsden CD: Hysteria: a neurologist's view. Psychol Med 16:277–288, 1986

Martin RL: DSM-IV changes in the somatoform disorders. Psychiatr Ann 25:29–39, 1995

Martin RL, Cloninger CR, Guze SB, et al: Mortality in a follow-up of 500 psychiatric outpatients, II: cause-specific mortality. Arch Gen Psychiatry 42:58–66, 1985

Meares R, Horvath TB: "Acute" and "chronic" hysteria. Br J Psychiatry 121:653–657, 1972

Merskey H: Conversion disorder, in Treatments of Psychiatric Disorders: A Task Force Report of the American Psychiatric Association, Vol 3. Washington, DC, American Psychiatric Association, 1989, pp 2152–2159

Murphy GE, Wetzel RD: Family history of suicidal behavior among suicide attempters. J Nerv Ment Dis 170:86–90, 1982

Otto M, Wilhelm S, Cohen L, et al: Prevalence of body dysmorphic disorder in a community sample of women. Am J Psychiatry 158:2061–2063, 2001

Perley M, Guze SB: Hysteria: the stability and usefulness of clinical criteria: a quantitative study based upon a 6- to 8-year follow-up of 39 patients. N Engl J Med 266:421–426, 1962

Phillips KA: Body dysmorphic disorder: the distress of imagined ugliness. Am J Psychiatry 148:1138–1149, 1991

Phillips KA: Body dysmorphic disorder: clinical features and drug treatment. CNS Drugs 3:30–40, 1995

Phillips KA, Diaz SF: Gender differences in body dysmorphic disorder. J Nerv Ment Dis 185:570–577, 1997

Phillips KA, Stout RL: Associations in the longitudinal course of body dysmorphic disorder with major depression, obsessive-compulsive disorder and social phobia. J Psychiatr Res 40:360–369, 2005

Phillips KA, McElroy SL, Keck PE Jr, et al: Body dysmorphic disorder: 30 cases of imagined ugliness. Am J Psychiatry 150:302–308, 1993

Phillips KA, Grant JE, Siniscalchi JM, et al: A retrospective follow-up study of body dysmorphic disorder. Compr Psychiatry 46:315–321, 2005

Phillips KA, Pagano ME, Menard W, et al: A 12-month follow-up study of the course of body dysmorphic disorder. Am J Psychiatry 163:907–912, 2006

Quill TE: Somatization disorder: one of medicine's blind spots. JAMA 254:3075–3079, 1985

Raskin M, Talbott JA, Meyerson AT: Diagnosis of conversion reactions: predictive value of psychiatric criteria. JAMA 197:530–534, 1966

Rief W, Buhlmann U, Wilhelm A, et al: The prevalence of body dysmorphic disorder in a population based survey. Psychol Med 36:877–885, 2006

Robins LN, Helzer JE, Croughan J, et al: National Institute of Mental Health Diagnostic Interview Schedule: its history, characteristics, and validity. Arch Gen Psychiatry 38:381–389, 1981

Robins LN, Helzer JE, Weissman MM, et al: Lifetime prevalence of specific psychiatric disorders in three sites. Arch Gen Psychiatry 41:949–958, 1984

Smith GR Jr, Monson RA, Ray DC: Psychiatric consultation in somatization disorder: a randomized controlled study. N Engl J Med 314:1407–1413, 1986

Stefansson JH, Messina JA, Meyerowitz S: Hysterical neurosis, conversion type: clinical and epidemiological considerations. Acta Psychiatr Scand 59:119–138, 1976

Stern J, Murphy M, Bass C: Personality disorders in patients with somatization disorder: a controlled study. Br J Psychiatry 163:785–789, 1993

Stone J, Sharpe M, Rothwell PM, et al: The 12 year prognosis of unilateral functional weakness and sensory disturbance. J Neurol Neurosurg Psychiatry 74:591–596, 2003

Stoudemire GA: Somatoform disorders, factitious disorders, and malingering, in The American Psychiatric Press Textbook of Psychiatry. Edited by Talbott JA, Hales RE, Yudofsky SC. Washington, DC, American Psychiatric Press, 1988, pp 533–556

Toone BK: Disorders of hysterical conversion, in Physical Symptoms and Psychological Illness. Edited by Bass C. London, England, Blackwell Scientific, 1990, pp 207–234

Veale D, Boocock A, Gournay K, et al: Body dysmorphic disorder: a survey of fifty cases. Br J Psychiatry 169:196–201, 1996

Watson CG, Buranen C: The frequency and identification of false positive conversion reactions. J Nerv Ment Dis 167:243–247, 1979

Weinstein EA, Eck RA, Lyerly OG: Conversion hysteria in Appalachia. Psychiatry 32:334–341, 1969

Wetzel RD, Guze SB, Cloninger CR, et al: Briquet's syndrome (hysteria) is both a somatoform and a "psychoform" illness: an MMPI study. Psychosom Med 56:564–569, 1994

Wheatley D: General practitioner clinical trials: chlordiazepoxide in anxiety states, II: long-term study. Practitioner 195:692–695, 1965

Whelan CI, Stewart DE: Pseudocyesis: a review and report of six cases. Int J Psychiatry Med 20:97–108, 1990

Woerner PI, Guze SB: A family and marital study of hysteria. Br J Psychiatry 114:161–168, 1968

21

# Factitious Disorder and Malingering

BARBARA E. McDERMOTT, Ph.D.

MARTIN H. LEAMON, M.D.

MARC D. FELDMAN, M.D.

CHARLES L. SCOTT, M.D.

## Factitious Disorder

Factitious disorder is characterized by a person intentionally fabricating or inducing signs or symptoms of other illnesses solely to become identified as "ill" or as a patient. The concept became firmly established in modern medical thinking in 1951 when Asher (1951) described what has since been classified as a subtype of factitious disorder known as Munchausen syndrome. Factitious disorder causes significant morbidity and mortality (Baker and Major 1994; Folks 1995), consumes an astonishing amount of medical resources (Feldman 1994), and produces significant emotional distress in the patients themselves, in their caregivers, and in their close relationships (Feldman and Smith 1996).

In recent years, the medical literature about factitious disorders has continued to expand, with the publication of lay and professional books on the topic (Feldman 2004; Feldman and Eisendrath 1996; Feldman et al. 1994) and the establishment of a factitious disorder Web site (http://munchausen.com) and discussion group (http://health.groups.yahoo.com/group/cravin4care/).

## Classification

DSM-IV-TR (American Psychiatric Association 2000) requires three criteria for the diagnosis of factitious disorder (Table 21–1). The first, the intentional production or feigning of physical or psychological signs or symptoms, distinguishes factitious disorder from the somatoform disorders, in which physical symptoms are viewed as unconsciously produced. The second and third criteria, that the motivation for the behavior is to assume the sick role and that external incentives for the behavior are absent, distinguish factitious disorder from malingering. DSM-IV-TR classifies the disorder based on the predominant type of factitious symptoms presented, whether physical or psychological (Table 21–1). The fourth subtype is factitious disorder not otherwise specified (Table 21–2).

Nadelson (1979) distinguished between factitious disorders of the Munchausen and the non-Munchausen type. Munchausen syndrome comprises about 10% of patients with factitious disorders (Eisendrath 1994). In this subtype of factitious disorder, multiple hospitalizations with dramatic and often life-threatening presentations, wandering from hospital to hospital (peregrination), and pathological lying (*pseudologia fantastica*, the telling of dramatic tales that merge truth and falsehood and that the listener initially finds intriguing) are prominent.

---

**TABLE 21–1.   DSM-IV-TR diagnostic criteria for factitious disorder**

A. Intentional production or feigning of physical or psychological signs or symptoms.

B. The motivation for the behavior is to assume the sick role.

C. External incentives for the behavior (such as economic gain, avoiding legal responsibility, or improving physical well-being, as in malingering) are absent.

*Code* based on type:

**300.16   with predominantly psychological signs and symptoms:** if psychological signs and symptoms predominate in the clinical presentation

**300.19   with predominantly physical signs and symptoms:** if physical signs and symptoms predominate in the clinical presentation

**300.19   with combined psychological and physical signs and symptoms:** if both psychological and physical signs and symptoms are present but neither predominates in the clinical presentation

---

**TABLE 21–2.   DSM-IV-TR diagnostic criteria for factitious disorder not otherwise specified**

This category includes disorders with factitious symptoms that do not meet the criteria for factitious disorder. An example is factitious disorder by proxy: the intentional production or feigning of physical or psychological signs or symptoms in another person who is under the individual's care for the purpose of indirectly assuming the sick role.

---

As described, the vast majority of factitious disorders are of the non-Munchausen type. Patients with these factitious disorders are mostly young women with conforming lifestyles and more family support and involvement compared with Munchausen patients. These patients have been described as passive and immature, and a significant proportion have health-related jobs or training. Most are not wanderers, have single-system complaints, and generate fewer hospitalizations than do Munchausen patients, but the overall severity and morbidity of their illness may be just as great (Sutherland and Rodin 1990).

## Diagnosis

Many factors can suggest a diagnosis of factitious disorder (Freyberger et al. 1994; Popli et al. 1992). There can be discrepancies between objective findings, such as pronounced differences between oral, rectal, axillary, and urine temperatures or involuntary contractions measured in "paralyzed" limbs (Ziv et al. 1998). Objective findings might be inconsistent with clinical history or symptoms, such as when mixed bowel flora is isolated from "spontaneous" skin lesions. The illness course could be markedly atypical, or the condition can fail to respond as expected to usual therapies, as indicated by erratic blood sugars or failure of wounds to heal. A patient may be unusually acquiescent to invasive diagnostic studies or may be unusually quarrelsome and argumentative with staff, particularly when it comes to trying to obtain old records to confirm history. A patient who describes a flamboyant, fascinating life with connections to well-known people may nevertheless have no visitors or callers. Unexplained medical paraphernalia or medications may be found in the patient's hospital room.

These indicators notwithstanding, verification of the first criterion requires that the patient be feigning or intentionally producing illness. The physician becomes a detective, working against the patient's overt desires, trying to discover the ruse. The dilemma is especially complex when patients have combinations of feigned and actual illness (Nordmeyer 1994; Sutherland and Rodin 1990) or develop an actual illness in the attempt to simulate one. Additionally, some general medical conditions may be difficult to diagnose initially, leading to an erroneous clinical impression of fabricated symptoms (Baddley et al. 1998; Koo et al. 1996). Other illnesses, such as multiple sclerosis or systemic lupus erythematosus, may have fluctuating courses or in themselves produce inconsistent findings suggestive of factitious disorder (Liebson et al. 1996).

Furthermore, the patient's specific motivation must be "to assume the sick role" (American Psychiatric Association 2000). Yet such patients often are unaware of their motivations, despite being aware of their role in producing their illness (Eisendrath 1996). Patients can be extremely resistant to psychological inquiry or may prematurely leave the hospital (Bauer and Boegner 1996), rendering psychological motivational assessment incomplete (Baker and Major 1994; Topazian and Binder 1994). Motivations may be multiple and mixed (Rogers et al. 1989), with clear secondary gains coexisting with less conscious or more subtle ones (Khan et al. 2000; Lawrie et al. 1993).

Another factor complicating the diagnosis is the high prevalence of comorbid disorders (Sutherland and Rodin 1990). Substance use disorders (Bauer and Boegner 1996; Parker 1993; Popli et al. 1992), personality disorders (particularly borderline and antisocial) (Bauer and Boegner 1996; Nadelson 1979; Overholser 1990), malingering (Gorman and Winograd 1988; Harrington et al. 1990), dissociative disorders (Toth and Baggaley 1991), eating disorders (Mizuta et al. 2000), suicidality, and mood disorders (Gielder 1994; Sutherland and Rodin 1990) may coexist.

## Epidemiology

Sutherland and Rodin (1990) diagnosed factitious disorder in 0.8% of all psychiatric consultation-liaison service referrals of medical or surgical inpatients. Bhugra (1988) found 0.5% of psychiatric admissions to have Munchausen syndrome. Bauer and Boegner (1996) diagnosed factitious disorders in 0.3% of neurological admissions. Others (Eisendrath 1996) have reported rates between approximately 2% and 10%, with the higher rates in case series of fevers of unknown origin. Most reported cases have been in patients in their 20s–40s (Angus et al. 2007; Libow 2000; Zimmerman et al. 1991).

## Etiology

Many authors have noted the apparent prevalence of histories of early childhood physical or sexual abuse, with disturbed parental relationships and emotional deprivation. Histories of early illness or extended hospitalizations also have been noted. Nadelson (1979) conceptualized factitious disorder as a manifestation of borderline character pathology rather than as an isolated clinical syndrome. Projection of hostility and worthlessness onto the caregiver occurs as he or she is both desired and rejected.

## Treatment

Once the diagnosis is suspected, it is essential to examine the treatment system for countertransference reactions (Crawford et al. 2005). Plassmann (1994) saw the patient's ability to induce a countertransference identification in the physician as a core of the disorder, and several authors (Freyberger et al. 1994; Kalivas 1996) viewed the physician's countertransference feelings as partially diagnostic for the disorder. In general medical settings, the risk of nontherapeutic countertransference reactions usually calls for obtaining psychiatric consultation (Stotland 1989)

that then often involves working with the entire treatment team of physicians, nurses, ethics and risk management committees, and others (Eisendrath and Feder 1996). As Feldman and Feldman (1995) described, countertransference can lead to several adverse consequences. Anger and aversion can rupture any therapeutic alliance, undermine the unity of a treatment team, or lead to punitive acting-out against the patient. Genuine comorbid or concomitant illness may be overlooked. Nonemergent breaches of confidentiality may ensue in the diagnostic hunt or in the supposed effort to "warn" colleagues.

As discussed previously, the diagnosis must be confirmed. The patient then must be informed of a change in treatment plan, and an attempt must be made to enlist him or her in that plan. The literature generally refers to this process (perhaps alluding to countertransference aspects) as containing an element of "confrontation." There is now general agreement that treatment begins at this point and that it is best done indirectly, with minimal expectation that the patient "confess" or acknowledge the deception.

# Factitious Disorder by Proxy

In 1977, the British pediatrician Roy Meadow described another scenario involving factitious illness. He presented his observations on a number of cases, in each of which a mother had intentionally induced illness in her infant, not in herself. Concealing the deception, the mother then presented the child for medical care, resulting in extensive, often invasive, evaluations and examinations of the child. Despite the outward appearance of being concerned and caring, the mother continued to fabricate illness in her child. Meadow employed the term *Munchausen syndrome by proxy* to describe such scenarios. The children in these situations may be subject to considerable and prolonged morbidity, with a mortality rate of 6%–10% (Rosenberg 1987; Schreier and Libow 1993; Sheridan 2003).

## Classification

DSM-IV-TR provides research criteria for factitious disorder by proxy in Appendix B, "Criteria Sets and Axes Provided for Further Study" (American Psychiatric Association 2000). The criteria are similar to those for factitious disorder, with the addition of the "by proxy" specification (Table 21–3). Much of the literature, however, retains the use of the eponym *Munchausen syndrome by*

---

**TABLE 21–3. DSM-IV-TR research criteria for factitious disorder by proxy**

A. Intentional production or feigning of physical or psychological signs or symptoms in another person who is under the individual's care.

B. The motivation for the perpetrator's behavior is to assume the sick role by proxy.

C. External incentives for the behavior (such as economic gain) are absent.

D. The behavior is not better accounted for by another mental disorder.

---

*proxy*, and there is considerable debate about how best to use that term and the term *factitious disorder by proxy* (Fisher and Mitchell 1995; Meadow 1995).

The debate revolves around four questions:

1. Does the syndrome require legally defined child abuse and/or neglect to have occurred?
2. Does the syndrome pertain to the diagnosis of an individual (implying some degree of homogeneous individual psychopathology), or does it pertain to a situation (without homogeneous psychopathology in the fabricator)?
3. Does the syndrome require an attribution or determination of the fabricator's primary motivation, and if so, what is the nature of that motivation?
4. Does the conferring of a psychiatric diagnosis mitigate the fabricator's responsibility for egregious behavior?

## Diagnosis

The mother's principal motivation must be determined (Kahan and Yorker 1991; Morley 1995), and any motivation other than attaining the sick role by proxy must be ruled out (Bools 1996; Meadow 1995). Also required is the determination that the mother is intentionally fabricating or inducing the child's illness. Because child abuse is a crime, proving the fabrication becomes a forensic process rather than a clinical medical investigation (Yorker 1996). Various techniques have been used, including covert video surveillance in the hospital (Samuels et al. 1992), searching of rooms and belongings (Ford 1996), and special handling of laboratory specimens (Kahan and Yorker 1991).

## Epidemiology

The prevalence of factitious disorder by proxy is unknown, but one study that made the diagnosis very conservatively estimated 2.8 cases per 100,000 children age 1 year or younger or 0.5 cases per 100,000 children age 16 years or younger (McClure et al. 1996). Among select populations, such as in cases of fevers of unknown origin (Aduan et al. 1979), discharges against medical advice (Jani et al. 1992), or pediatric specialty registers (Schreier and Libow 1993), the rates may be substantially higher. The child typically is 2–5 years old at diagnosis (Sheridan 2003; Yorker and Kahan 1990). Length of time from onset of symptoms in the child to diagnosis can vary widely, averaging 15 months (±14 months) in one series (Rosenberg 1987) to years in another (Libow 1995). Methods are legion, but smothering, poisoning, and fabricated history of seizures or fever are most commonly reported (McClure et al. 1996).

## Etiology

Although perpetrators rarely make themselves available for psychiatric or psychological study, most authors postulate that the maternal pathology arises from childhood roots, characterized by "quietly traumatic" emotional neglect and abandonment. Adshead and Bluglass (2005) found unresolved trauma or loss reactions in the majority of their sample. They concluded that insecure attachment is a risk factor.

## Treatment and Prognosis

The first stage of treatment in factitious disorder by proxy usually begins with the involvement of child protection authorities, the initiation of legal proceedings against the parent, and the removal of the child from the home. Management of factitious disorder by proxy requires coordinated multidisciplinary, multiagency involvement (Coombe 1995; Parnell and Day 1998). Individual treatment includes long-term psychotherapy (group, individual, or combined) and focuses on helping the perpetrator express feelings and needs for support and recognition more directly, with less use of projection and with the development of empathic capacity (Coombe 1995). As with the treatment of factitious disorder, the factitious behavior is rarely the primary focus. Pharmacotherapy is used only to treat comorbid conditions.

# Malingering

## Classification

DSM-IV-TR classifies malingering under "Additional Conditions That May Be a Focus of Clinical Attention." Malingering in this nomenclature is not considered to be a diagnosis, as by definition it is "the intentional production of false or grossly exaggerated physical or psychological symptoms, motivated by external incentives" (American Psychiatric Association 2000). External incentives that may motivate a person to malinger symptoms include avoiding work, evading criminal prosecution, obtaining drugs, receiving financial compensation, avoiding military duty, and escaping other intolerable situations. Table 21–4 provides the DSM-IV-TR guidelines for when to suspect malingering.

---

**TABLE 21–4.** **DSM-IV-TR warning signs for malingering**

The individual's evaluation occurs in a medicolegal context, such as referral from an attorney.

A marked discrepancy exists between the person's claims and objective findings.

The individual is uncooperative during the diagnostic evaluation and in complying with the prescribed treatment regimen.

Antisocial personality disorder is present.

---

Diagnostic confusion between malingering and other mental disorders, particularly factitious disorder, can be traced to Asher's (1951) original description of Munchausen syndrome. He attributed several possible motives to Munchausen syndrome, including "a desire to escape from the police" and "a desire to get free board and lodgings for the night" (p. 339), motives that would now clearly classify feigned illness behavior as malingering. The tendency to include malingering within the factitious disorder spectrum was further reinforced by Spiro (1968), who recommended that in individuals with Munchausen syndrome, "malingering should only be diagnosed in the absence of psychiatric illness and the presence of behavior appropriately adaptive to a clear-cut long-term goal" (p. 569). There are, however, many examples of patients with factitious disorder who also malinger (see "Diagnosis" subsection of "Factitious Disorder" section earlier in this chapter). Other disorders to consider in the differential diagnosis of malingering include conversion disorder and other somatoform disorders. Although all of these diagnoses may involve physical symptoms, none involve the production of symptoms for external incentives. The individual with conversion disorder or another somatoform disorder experiences symptoms that cannot be fully explained by a medical condition and are often connected to psychological reasons of which the person is unaware. Finally, individuals who confabulate should be distinguished from malingerers because they are unintentionally filling in information that they believed to have happened, when, in fact, it did not happen at all (Newmark et al. 1999; Resnick 2000).

## Detection ("Diagnosis")

The detection of malingering in the forensic arena is particularly crucial because the avoidance of criminal prosecution is a strong motivation (Resnick 1984). The detection of malingered psychosis in particular is especially important because psychotic symptoms often are offered as the basis for an insanity defense (Cornell and Hawk 1989). However, erroneously concluding that a defendant is malingering can have rather serious negative consequences. In addition to delaying potentially appropriate treatment, such mislabeling may lead to the inappropriate conviction of truly mentally ill individuals. Thus, the detection of malingered psychosis, and distinguishing such from true psychosis, is of paramount importance.

Cornell and Hawk (1989) contrasted the clinical presentations of two groups of criminal defendants: those diagnosed as genuinely psychotic and those diagnosed as malingering. Interestingly, they found the incidence of malingering to be relatively low: 8%, or 25 cases out of 314 evaluations. They found that defendants diagnosed as malingering presented with visual hallucinations, exaggerated behavior, and symptoms that typically do not cluster together (such as psychomotor retardation and hallucinations). In contrast, genuinely psychotic patients evidenced disturbed affect and formal thought disorders (see Table 21–5). The authors concluded that malingerers may overlook more subtle, but more common, symptoms of psychosis such as thought disorder and disturbances of affect.

Consistent with this research, Resnick (2000) noted that the better clinicians understand characteristics of a true illness, the more likely it is they will be able to detect feigned symptoms. Malingering is "so easy to define but so difficult to diagnose" (Resnick 1997, p. 48). When a clinician suspects that a symptom may be fabricated or exaggerated, he or she should be on alert for various incon-

**TABLE 21–5.  Clinical decision model for the assessment of malingering of psychosis**

The evaluee's presentation meets the following criteria:

A.  Understandable motive to malinger

B.  Marked variability of presentation as observed in at least one of the following:
  1.  Marked discrepancies in interview and noninterview behavior
  2.  Gross inconsistencies in reported psychotic symptoms
  3.  Blatant contradictions between reported prior episodes and documented psychiatric history

C.  Improbable psychiatric symptoms as evidenced by one or more of the following:
  1.  Reporting elaborate psychotic symptoms that lack common paranoid, grandiose, or religious themes
  2.  Sudden emergence of purported psychotic symptoms to explain antisocial behavior
  3.  Atypical hallucinations or delusions (see Table 21–6)

D.  Confirmation of malingered psychosis by either
  1.  Admission of malingering following confrontation
  2.  Presence of strong corroborative information, such as psychometric data or history of malingering

*Source.*  Resnick 1997.

sistencies that may appear in the individual's evaluation. First, the individual may present inconsistencies in what he or she actually reports. For example, a person may report that he or she is currently unable to talk, despite speaking eloquently throughout the interview. Second, a malingerer's observed behavior may differ significantly from the symptoms he or she reports. The person who describes active, continuous, disturbing hallucinations during the interview but shows no evidence of distraction illustrates this type of inconsistency, suggestive of malingering. Third, malingerers may behave in a dramatically different way depending on who they believe is observing them. This disparity in presentation is illustrated by a person who acts in a confused, disoriented manner in the clinician's office and shortly after leaving is observed by ward staff winning a brilliant game of chess. Fourth, psycholog-

ical test data may be inconsistent with the history provided by malingerers. Finally, malingerers often report symptoms that are inconsistent with how genuine symptoms normally manifest.

Table 21–5 provides a suggested clinical decision model for the assessment of malingered psychosis (Resnick 1997). In determining whether reported hallucinations or delusions are fabricated or exaggerated, the factors outlined in Table 21–6 also may prove helpful (Resnick 1997). Note that a bona fide diagnosis of a past psychotic disorder does not necessarily exclude a presentation of manufactured psychotic symptoms (Tyrer et al. 2001).

**TABLE 21–6.  Threshold model for the assessment of hallucinations and delusions**

Malingering should be suspected if any combination of the following is observed:

**Hallucinations**

Continuous rather than intermittent hallucinations

Vague or inaudible hallucinations

Hallucinations not associated with delusions

Stilted language reported in hallucinations

Inability to state strategies to diminish voices

Self-report that all command hallucinations were obeyed

Visual hallucinations in black and white

**Delusions**

Abrupt onset or termination

Eagerness to call attention to delusions

Conduct markedly inconsistent with delusions

Bizarre content without disordered thinking

*Source.*  Resnick 1997.

Psychological testing is often used in malingering assessments and may include structured interviews to evaluate psychotic symptoms (Rogers et al. 1992), various personality inventories, and neuropsychological testing to assess cognitive deficits (Liebson et al. 1996). Witztum et al. (1996) described several military inductees who received erroneous diagnoses of malingering; diagnoses of severe psychiatric disorders were missed because of assessment problems. They also noted, as did DuAlba and Scott (1993), the important role of cross-cultural issues in the assessment of malingering.

## Structured Assessments of Malingering

Although suggestions have been outlined for the clinical assessment of malingering (Cornell and Hawk 1989; Resnick 1997), structured assessments recently have been developed to aid in the detection of malingering. Prior to the development of these specialized assessments, subscales of standard psychological tests were used as an indicator of assessment attitudes, both for malingering and for other dissimulation. Perhaps the most common and extensively researched of these is the Minnesota Multiphasic Personality Inventory (MMPI) and its revision, the MMPI-2 (Butcher et al. 1989). In two meta-analyses of the validity scales of the MMPI (Berry et al. 1991) and the MMPI-2 (Rogers et al. 1994), the F scale (Infrequency) and the F–K index (Dissimulation) were shown to be superior to other indices of malingering. Because these indices can be elevated in individuals with true psychiatric disorders, other scales have been developed in an effort to aid in this distinction. For example, Arbisi and Ben-Porath (1995) developed the Infrequency-Psychopathology scale [F(p)] using items endorsed infrequently even by psychiatric inpatients. However, recent research suggests that this scale does not improve the detection of malingerers over the F scale when used alone (Kucharski et al. 2004).

## Epidemiology

The reported incidence of malingering varies depending on the population in question. In a study of malingered mental illness in a metropolitan emergency department, 13% of the patients were strongly suspected or considered to be malingering. Reasons identified for malingering included seeking hospitalization for food and shelter, attempting to gain medication, attempting to avoid incarceration, and seeking financial gain (Yates et al. 1996).

## Treatment

Depending on the situation, the clinician may elect to confront the individual with the assessment. Pankratz and Erickson (1990) emphasized the importance of permitting the malingerer to save face. Possible verbal interventions include statements such as "You haven't told me the whole truth" or "The type of symptoms that you are reporting are not consistent with known mental illness" (Inbau and Reid 1967). The clinician should be prepared for some individuals to react defensively and to refuse to accept this diagnosis, even when faced with strong evidence that they are faking symptoms. In contrast, when other individuals are confronted, they admit that their symptoms are faked and give up the charade. Han (1997) described a method of intervention based on cognitive-behavioral techniques that effectively reduced the likelihood of the recurrence of malingering. This intervention, termed *comprehensive management of prisoners*, included family, educational, and occupational interventions designed to reduce the motivation to malinger. The management of malingering must first be based on an understanding of the motivations for symptom production (Adetunji et al. 2006).

# Key Points: Factitious Disorder and Malingering

- Distinction between factitious disorder and malingering lies in underlying motivation for symptom production.
- The motivation for factitious disorder is to assume the sick role and is often presumed to be unconscious.
- The motivation for malingering involves the attainment of a tangible reward.
- Factors suggestive of factitious disorder include discrepancies between objective findings, inconsistencies between objective findings and clinical history or symptoms, an atypical illness course, and conditions that fail to respond to usual therapies.
- Factors suggestive of malingering include inconsistencies between reported versus observed behavior and the reporting of improbable or absurd symptoms in the presence of an understandable motive to malinger.
- The treatment/management of both factitious disorder and malingering involves "delicate" confrontation with minimal expectations of confessions.
- The treatment for factitious disorder involves focusing on the underlying motivation for the behavior, which often can be psychodynamic in nature.
- The management of malingering involves understanding the secondary gains associated with the production of symptoms in order to address these expectations.
- Factitious disorder by proxy involves maltreatment and, when suspected, must be reported to child protection authorities.

# References

Adetunji BA, Basil B, Mathews M, et al: Detection and management of malingering in a clinical setting. Prim Psychiatry 13:61–69, 2006

Adshead G, Bluglass K: Attachment representations in mothers with abnormal illness behavior by proxy. Br J Psychiatry 187:328–333, 2005

Aduan RP, Fauci AS, Dale DC, et al: Factitious fever and self-induced infection: a report of 32 cases and review of the literature. Ann Intern Med 90:230–242, 1979

American Psychiatric Association: Diagnostic and Statistical Manual of Mental Disorders, 4th Edition, Text Revision. Washington, DC, American Psychiatric Association, 2000

Angus J, Affleck AG, Croft JC, et al: Dermatitis artefacta in a 12-year-old girl mimicking cutaneous T-cell lymphoma. Pediatr Dermatol 24:327–329, 2007

Arbisi PA, Ben-Porath YS: An MMPI-2 infrequent response scale for use with psychopathological populations: the Infrequency-Psychopathology Scale, F(p). Psychol Assess 7:424–431, 1995

Asher R: Munchausen's syndrome. Lancet 1(6):339–341, 1951

Baddley J, Daberkow D, Hilton C: Insulinoma masquerading as factitious hypoglycemia. South Med J 91:1067–1069, 1998

Baker CE, Major E: Munchausen's syndrome: a case presenting as asthma requiring ventilation. Anaesthesia 49:1050–1051, 1994

Bauer M, Boegner F: Neurological syndromes in factitious disorder. J Nerv Ment Dis 184:281–288, 1996

Berry DTR, Baer RA, Harris MJ: Detection of malingering on the MMPI: a meta-analytic review. Clin Psychol Rev 11:585–598, 1991

Bhugra D: Psychiatric Munchausen's syndrome: literature review with case reports. Acta Psychiatr Scand 77:497–503, 1988

Bools C: Factitious illness by proxy: Munchausen syndrome by proxy. Br J Psychiatry 169:268–275, 1996

Butcher JN, Dahlstrom WG, Graham JR, et al: MMPI-2: Manual for Administration and Scoring. Minneapolis, University of Minnesota Press, 1989

Coombe P: The inpatient psychotherapy of a mother and child at the Cassel Hospital: a case of Munchausen's syndrome by proxy. Br J Psychother 12:195–207, 1995

Cornell DG, Hawk GL: Clinical presentation of malingerers diagnosed by experienced forensic psychologists. Law Hum Behav 13:375–383, 1989

Crawford SM, Jeyasanger G, Wright M: A visitor with Munchausen's syndrome. Clin Med 5:400–401, 2005

DuAlba L, Scott RL: Somatization and malingering for workers' compensation applicants: a cross-cultural MMPI study. J Clin Psychol 49:913–917, 1993

Eisendrath SJ: Factitious physical disorders. West J Med 160:177–179, 1994

Eisendrath SJ: Current overview of factitious physical disorders, in The Spectrum of Factitious Disorders. Edited by Feldman MD, Eisendrath SJ. Washington, DC, American Psychiatric Press, 1996, pp 21–36

Eisendrath SJ, Feder A: Management of factitious disorders, in The Spectrum of Factitious Disorders. Edited by Feldman MD, Eisendrath SJ. Washington, DC, American Psychiatric Press, 1996, pp 195–213

Feldman MD: The costs of factitious disorders. Psychosomatics 35:506–507, 1994

Feldman MD: Playing Sick? Untangling the Web of Munchausen syndrome, Munchausen by Proxy, Malingering and Factitious Disorder. New York, Brunner-Routledge, 2004

Feldman MD, Eisendrath SJ (eds): The Spectrum of Factitious Disorders. Washington, DC, American Psychiatric Press, 1996

Feldman MD, Feldman JM: Tangled in the web: countertransference in the therapy of factitious disorders. Int J Psychiatry Med 25:389–399, 1995

Feldman MD, Smith R: Personal and interpersonal toll of factitious disorders, in The Spectrum of Factitious Disorders. Edited by Feldman MD, Eisendrath SJ. Washington, DC, American Psychiatric Press, 1996, pp 175–194

Feldman MD, Ford CV, Reinhold T: Patient or Pretender: Inside the Strange World of Factitious Disorders. New York, Wiley, 1994

Fisher GC, Mitchell I: Is Munchausen syndrome by proxy really a syndrome? Arch Dis Child 72:530–534, 1995

Folks DG: Munchausen's syndrome and other factitious disorders. Neurol Clin 13:267–281, 1995

Ford CV: Ethical and legal issues in factitious disorders: an overview, in The Spectrum of Factitious Disorders. Edited by Feldman MD, Eisendrath SJ. Washington, DC, American Psychiatric Press, 1996, pp 51–63

Freyberger H, Nordmeyer JP, Freyberger HJ, et al: Patients suffering from factitious disorders in the clinico-psychosomatic consultation liaison service: psychodynamic processes, psychotherapeutic initial care and clinico-interdisciplinary cooperation. Psychother Psychosom 62:108–122, 1994

Gielder U: Factitious disease in the field of dermatology. Psychother Psychosom 62:48–55, 1994

Gorman WF, Winograd M: Crossing the border from Munchausen to malingering. J Fla Med Assoc 75:147–150, 1988

Han S: Social rehabilitation of ex-malingerers from prison. Int Med J 4:73–75, 1997

Harrington WZ, Jackimczyk KC, Seligson RA: Thiopental-facilitated interview in respiratory Munchausen's syndrome. Ann Emerg Med 19:941–942, 1990

Inbau FE, Reid JE: Criminal Interrogation and Confessions. Baltimore, MD, Williams & Wilkins, 1967

Jani S, White M, Rosenberg LA, et al: Munchausen syndrome by proxy. Int J Psychiatry Med 22:343–349, 1992

Kahan B, Yorker BC: Munchausen syndrome by proxy: clinical review and legal issues. Behav Sci Law 9:73–83, 1991

Kalivas J: Malingering versus factitious disorder (letter). Am J Psychiatry 153:1108, 1996

Khan I, Fayaz I, Ridgley J, et al: Factitious clock drawing and constructional apraxia. J Neurol Neurosurg Psychiatry 68:106–107, 2000

Koo J, Gambla C, Fried R: Pseudopsychodermatological disease. Dermatol Clin 14:525–530, 1996

Kucharski LT, Johnsen D, Procell S: The utility of the MMPI-2 Infrequency Psychopathology F(p) and the revised infrequency psychopathology scales in the detection of malingering. Am J Forensic Psychol 22:33–40, 2004

Lawrie SM, Goodwin G, Masterton G: Munchausen's syndrome and organic brain disorder. Br J Psychiatry 162:545–549, 1993

Libow J: Munchausen by proxy victims in adulthood: a first look. Child Abuse Negl 19:1131–1142, 1995

Libow J: Child and adolescent illness falsification. Pediatrics 105:336–342, 2000

Liebson E, White R, Albert M: Cognitive inconsistencies in abnormal illness behavior and neurologic disease. J Nerv Ment Dis 184:122–125, 1996

McClure RJ, Davis PM, Meadow SR, et al: Epidemiology of Munchausen syndrome by proxy, nonaccidental poisoning, and nonaccidental suffocation. Arch Dis Child 75:57–61, 1996

Meadow R: What is, and what is not, "Munchausen syndrome by proxy"? Arch Dis Child 72:534–538, 1995

Mizuta I, Fukunaga T, Sato H, et al: A case report of comorbid eating disorder and factitious disorder. Psychiatry Clin Neurosci 54:603–606, 2000

Morley CJ: Practical concerns about the diagnosis of Munchausen syndrome by proxy. Arch Dis Child 72:528–529, 1995

Nadelson T: The Munchausen spectrum: borderline character features. Gen Hosp Psychiatry 1:11–17, 1979

Newmark N, Adityanjee, Kay J: Pseudologia fantastica and factitious disorder: review of the literature and a case report. Compr Psychiatry 40:89–95, 1999

Nordmeyer JP: An internist's view of patients with factitious disorders and factitious clinical symptomatology. Psychother Psychosom 62:30–40, 1994

Overholser JC: Differential diagnosis of malingering and factitious disorder with physical symptoms. Special issue: malingering and deception—an update. Behav Sci Law 8:55–65, 1990

Pankratz L, Erickson RC: Two views of malingering. Clin Neuropsychol 4:379–389, 1990

Parker PE: A case report of Munchausen syndrome with mixed psychological features. Psychosomatics 34:360–364, 1993

Parnell TF, Day DO: Munchausen by Proxy Syndrome: Misunderstood Child Abuse. Thousand Oaks, CA, Sage, 1998

Plassmann R: Münchausen syndromes and factitious diseases. Psychother Psychosom 62:7–26, 1994

Popli AP, Masand PS, Dewan MJ: Factitious disorders with psychological symptoms. J Clin Psychiatry 53:315–318, 1992

Resnick PJ: The detection of malingered mental illness. Behav Sci Law 2:20–38, 1984

Resnick PJ: Malingered psychosis, in Clinical Assessment of Malingering and Deception, 2nd Edition. Edited by Rogers R. New York, Guilford, 1997, pp 47–67

Resnick PJ: The clinical assessment of malingered mental illness, in Annual Board Review Course Syllabus. Bloomfield, CT, American Academy of Psychiatry and the Law, 2000, pp 842–866

Rogers R, Bagby RM, Rector N: Diagnostic legitimacy of factitious disorder with psychological symptoms. Am J Psychiatry 146:1312–1314, 1989

Rogers R, Bagby RM, Dickens SE: Structured Interview of Reported Symptoms (SIRS) and Professional Manual. Odessa, FL, Psychological Assessment Resources, 1992

Rogers R, Sewell KW, Salekin RT: A meta-analysis of malingering on the MMPI-2. Assessment 1:227–237, 1994

Rosenberg DA: Web of deceit: a literature review of Munchausen syndrome by proxy. Child Abuse Negl 11:547–563, 1987

Samuels MP, McClaughlin W, Jacobson RR, et al: Fourteen cases of imposed upper airway obstruction. Arch Dis Child 67:162–170, 1992

Schreier HA, Libow JA: Munchausen syndrome by proxy: diagnosis and prevalence. Am J Orthopsychiatry 63:318–321, 1993

Sheridan MS: The deceit continues: an updated literature review of Munchausen syndrome by proxy. Child Abuse Negl 27:431–451, 2003

Spiro HR: Chronic factitious illness: Munchausen's syndrome. Arch Gen Psychiatry 18:569–579, 1968

Stotland NL: Munchausen syndrome. JAMA 261:447, 1989

Sutherland AJ, Rodin GM: Factitious disorders in a general hospital setting: clinical features and a review of the literature. Psychosomatics 31:392–399, 1990

Topazian M, Binder HJ: Factitious diarrhea detected by measurement of stool osmolality. N Engl J Med 330:1418–1419, 1994

Toth EL, Baggaley A: Coexistence of Munchausen's syndrome and multiple personality disorder: detailed report of a case and theoretical discussion. Psychiatry 54:176–186, 1991

Tyrer P, Babidge N, Emmanuel J, et al: Instrumental psychosis: the Good Soldier Svejk syndrome. J R Soc Med 94:22–25, 2001

Witztum E, Grinshpoon A, Margolin J, et al: The erroneous diagnosis of malingering in a military setting. Mil Med 161:225–229, 1996

Yates BD, Nordquist CR, Schultz-Ross RA: Feigned psychiatric symptoms in the emergency room. Psychiatr Serv 47:998–1000, 1996

Yorker BC: Legal issues in factitious disorder by proxy, in The Spectrum of Factitious Disorders. Edited by Feldman MD, Eisendrath SJ. Washington, DC, American Psychiatric Press, 1996, pp 135–156

Yorker BC, Kahan BB: Munchausen's syndrome by proxy as a form of child abuse. Arch Psychiatr Nurs 4:313–318, 1990

Zimmerman JG, Hussian RA, Tintner R, et al: Factitious disorder in a geriatric patient. Clin Gerontol 11:3–11, 1991

Ziv I, Djaldetti R, Zoldan Y, et al: Diagnosis of "nonorganic" limb paresis by a novel objective motor assessment: the quantitative Hoover's test. J Neurol 245:797–802, 1998

# 22

# Dissociative Disorders

JOSÉ R. MALDONADO, M.D., F.A.P.M., F.A.C.F.E.

DAVID SPIEGEL, M.D.

The dissociative disorders involve a disturbance in the integrated organization of identity, memory, perception, or consciousness. When memories are poorly integrated, the resulting disorder is *dissociative amnesia*. Fragmentation of identity results in *dissociative fugue* or *dissociative identity disorder* (DID; formerly multiple personality disorder). Disordered perception yields *depersonalization disorder*. Dissociation of aspects of consciousness produces *acute stress disorder* and various dissociative trance and possession states (Table 22–1).

Repression as a general model for keeping information out of conscious awareness differs from dissociation in six important ways (Table 22–2).

## Acute Stress Disorder

Although acute stress disorder is classified among the anxiety disorders in DSM-IV-TR (American Psychiatric Association 2000), mention is made of it in this chapter because half of the symptoms of this disorder are dissociative in nature (Table 22–3). These symptoms are strongly predictive of later development of posttraumatic stress disorder (PTSD) in some studies. Similarly, the occurrence of PTSD is predicted by intrusion, avoidance, and hyperarousal symptoms in the immediate aftermath of rape (Rothbaum and Foa 1993) and combat trauma (Blank 1993; Solomon and Mikulincer 1988).

Dissociation may work well at the time of trauma, but if the defense persists too long, it interferes with the working through (in Lindemann's terms, the "grief work" [Lindemann 1944/1994; D. Spiegel 1981]) necessary to

| TABLE 22–1. | DSM-IV-TR dissociative disorders |
|---|---|

Dissociative amnesia (300.12)

Dissociative fugue (300.13)

Dissociative identity disorder (300.14; formerly multiple personality disorder)

Depersonalization disorder (300.6)

Dissociative disorder not otherwise specified (300.15)

Related disorders

    Dissociative trance disorder

    Acute stress disorder (308.3)

put traumatic experience into perspective and reduce the likelihood of later PTSD or other symptomatology. Therefore, psychotherapy aimed at helping individuals acknowledge, bear, and put into perspective traumatic experience shortly after the trauma should be helpful in reducing the incidence of later PTSD.

## Dissociative Amnesia

The hallmark of dissociative amnesia is the inability to recall important personal information, usually of a traumatic or stressful nature, that cannot be explained by ordinary forgetfulness (American Psychiatric Association 2000) (Table 22–4). Dissociative amnesia is considered the most common of all dissociative disorders (Putnam 1985). Amnesia is a symptom commonly found in several other dissociative and anxiety disorders, including acute stress

TABLE 22–2.    Differences between dissociation and repression

|  | Dissociation | Repression |
|---|---|---|
| Organizational structure | Horizontal | Vertical |
| Barriers | Amnesia | Dynamic conflict |
| Etiology | Trauma | Developmental conflict over unacceptable wishes |
| Contents | Untransformed: traumatic memories | Disguised primary process: dreams, slips |
| Means of access | Hypnosis | Interpretation |
| Psychotherapy | Access, control, and work through traumatic memories | Interpretation, transference |

disorder, PTSD, somatization disorder, dissociative fugue, and DID (American Psychiatric Association 2000). A higher incidence of dissociative amnesia has been described in the context of war and natural and other disasters (Maldonado et al. 2000). There appears to be a direct relation between the severity of the exposure to trauma and the incidence of amnesia (G.R. Brown and Anderson 1991; Chu and Dill 1990; Putnam 1985, 1993).

Dissociative amnesia is the classical functional disorder of memory and involves difficulty in retrieving discrete components of episodic memory. Because the amnesia primarily involves difficulties in retrieval rather than encoding or storage, the memory deficits usually are reversible. Dissociative amnesia has three primary characteristics:

1.  The memory loss is episodic. The first-person recollection of certain events is lost, rather than knowledge of procedures.
2.  The memory loss is for a discrete period of time, ranging from minutes to years. It is not vagueness or inefficient retrieval of memories, but rather a dense unavailability of memories that were clearly accessible. Unlike in the amnestic disorders, there is usually no difficulty in learning *new* episodic information.
3.  The memory loss is generally for events of a traumatic or stressful nature.

Dissociative amnesia is most common in the third and fourth decades of life (Coons and Milstein 1986). It usually involves one episode, but multiple periods of lost memory are not uncommon (Coons and Milstein 1986). Comorbidity with conversion disorder, bulimia, alcohol abuse, and depression is common, and Axis II diagnoses of histrionic, dependent, and borderline personality disorders occur in a substantial minority of such patients (Coons and Milstein 1986). Legal difficulties, such as

driving under the influence of alcohol, also accompany dissociative amnesia in a minority of cases. In a recent study of community adults, the prevalence of dissociative amnesia was 1.8% (Johnson et al. 2006).

Individuals with such a disorder lose the ability to recall what happened during a specific time. They demonstrate not vagueness or spotty memory but rather a loss of any episodic memory for a finite period. Such individuals initially may not be aware of the memory loss—that is, they may not remember that they do not remember. However, they may find, for example, new purchases in their homes but have no memory of having obtained them. They report being told that they have done or said things that they cannot remember.

Dissociative amnesia most frequently occurs after an episode of trauma, and the onset may be sudden or gradual. Some individuals do experience episodes of selective amnesia, usually for specific traumatic incidents, that may be more interwoven with periods of intact memory. In these cases, the amnesia is for a type of material remembered rather than for a discrete period of time.

Despite the fact that certain information is kept out of consciousness in dissociative amnesia, such information may exert an influence on consciousness. For example, a rape victim with no conscious recollection of the assault will nonetheless behave like someone who has been sexually victimized. Such individuals often show detachment and demoralization, are unable to enjoy intimate relationships, and show hyperarousal to stimuli reminiscent of the trauma.

Individuals with dissociative amnesia generally do not have disturbances of identity, except to the extent that their identity is influenced by the warded-off memory. It is not uncommon for such individuals to develop depressive symptoms as well, especially when the amnesia is in the wake of a traumatic episode.

---

**TABLE 22–3.** DSM-IV-TR diagnostic criteria for acute stress disorder

A. The person has been exposed to a traumatic event in which both of the following were present:
  (1) the person experienced, witnessed, or was confronted with an event or events that involved actual or threatened death or serious injury, or a threat to the physical integrity of self or others
  (2) the person's response involved intense fear, helplessness, or horror

B. Either while experiencing or after experiencing the distressing event, the individual has three (or more) of the following dissociative symptoms:
  (1) a subjective sense of numbing, detachment, or absence of emotional responsiveness
  (2) a reduction in awareness of his or her surroundings (e.g., "being in a daze")
  (3) derealization
  (4) depersonalization
  (5) dissociative amnesia (i.e., inability to recall an important aspect of the trauma)

C. The traumatic event is persistently reexperienced in at least one of the following ways: recurrent images, thoughts, dreams, illusions, flashback episodes, or a sense of reliving the experience; or distress on exposure to reminders of the traumatic event.

D. Marked avoidance of stimuli that arouse recollections of the trauma (e.g., thoughts, feelings, conversations, activities, places, people).

E. Marked symptoms of anxiety or increased arousal (e.g., difficulty sleeping, irritability, poor concentration, hypervigilance, exaggerated startle response, motor restlessness).

F. The disturbance causes clinically significant distress or impairment in social, occupational, or other important areas of functioning or impairs the individual's ability to pursue some necessary task, such as obtaining necessary assistance or mobilizing personal resources by telling family members about the traumatic experience.

G. The disturbance lasts for a minimum of 2 days and a maximum of 4 weeks and occurs within 4 weeks of the traumatic event.

H. The disturbance is not due to the direct physiological effects of a substance (e.g., a drug of abuse, a medication) or a general medical condition, is not better accounted for by brief psychotic disorder, and is not merely an exacerbation of a preexisting Axis I or Axis II disorder.

---

**TABLE 22–4.** DSM-IV-TR diagnostic criteria for dissociative amnesia

A. The predominant disturbance is one or more episodes of inability to recall important personal information, usually of a traumatic or stressful nature, that is too extensive to be explained by ordinary forgetfulness.

B. The disturbance does not occur exclusively during the course of dissociative identity disorder, dissociative fugue, posttraumatic stress disorder, acute stress disorder, or somatization disorder and is not due to the direct physiological effects of a substance (e.g., a drug of abuse, a medication) or a neurological or other general medical condition (e.g., amnestic disorder due to head trauma).

C. The symptoms cause clinically significant distress or impairment in social, occupational, or other important areas of functioning.

---

## Treatment

No established pharmacological treatments are available, except for the use of benzodiazepines or barbiturates for drug-assisted interviews (Maldonado et al. 2000). Most cases of dissociative amnesia revert spontaneously, especially when the individuals are removed from stressful or threatening situations, when they feel physically and psychologically safe, and/or when they are exposed to cues from the past (e.g., family members) (W. Brown 1918; Kardiner and Spiegel 1947; Loewenstein 1991; Maldonado et al. 2000; Reither and Stoudemire 1988). When a safe environment is not enough to restore normal memory functioning, the amnesia sometimes can be breached using techniques such as pharmacologically mediated interviews (i.e., barbiturates and benzodiazepines) (Baron and Nagy 1988; Naples and Hackett 1978; Perry and Jacobs 1982; Wettstein and Fauman 1979).

On the other hand, most patients with dissociative disorder are highly hypnotizable on formal testing and therefore are easily able to make use of hypnotic techniques such as age regression (H. Spiegel and Spiegel 2004). Patients are hypnotized and instructed to experience a time before the onset of the amnesia as though it were the present. Then the patients are reoriented in hypnosis to experience events during the amnesic period. Hypnosis can enable such patients to reorient temporally and therefore to achieve access to otherwise dissociated memories.

One technique that can help bring such memories into consciousness while modulating the affective response to them is the split-screen technique (D. Spiegel 1981). In this approach, patients are taught, by using hypnosis, to relive the traumatic event as if they were watching it on an imaginary movie or television screen. This technique is often helpful for individuals who are unable to relive the event as if it were occurring in the present tense, either because that process is too emotionally taxing or because they are not sufficiently hypnotizable to be able to engage in hypnotic age regression. The screen technique also can be used to provide dissociation between the psychological and the somatic aspects of the memory retrieval. Individuals can be put into self-hypnosis and instructed to get their bodies into a state of floating comfort and safety. They are reminded that no matter what they see on the screen, their bodies will be safe and comfortable.

Psychotherapy for dissociative amnesia involves accessing the dissociated memories, working through affectively loaded aspects of these memories, and supporting the patient through the process of integrating these memories into consciousness.

# Dissociative Fugue

Dissociative fugue combines failure of integration of certain aspects of personal memory with loss of customary identity and automatisms of motor behavior (Table 22–5). Patients appear "normal," usually showing no signs of psychopathology or cognitive deficit. Fugue involves one or more episodes of sudden, unexpected, purposeful travel away from home, coupled with an inability to recall portions or all of one's past, and a loss of identity or the assumption of a new identity. In contrast to patients who have DID, if patients with dissociative fugue develop a new identity, the old and new identities do not alternate. The onset is usually sudden, and it frequently occurs after a traumatic experience or bereavement. A single episode is not uncommon, and spontaneous remission of symptoms can occur without treatment.

Hypnosis can be helpful in accessing otherwise unavailable components of memory and identity. The approach used is similar to that for dissociative amnesia. Hypnotic age regression can be used as the framework for accessing information available at a previous time. Demonstrating to patients that such information can be made available to consciousness enhances their sense of control over the material and facilitates the therapeutic working through of its emotionally laden aspects.

Once reorientation is established and the overt aspects of the fugue have been resolved, it is important to work

**TABLE 22–5. DSM-IV-TR diagnostic criteria for dissociative fugue**

A. The predominant disturbance is sudden, unexpected travel away from home or one's customary place of work, with inability to recall one's past.

B. Confusion about personal identity or assumption of a new identity (partial or complete).

C. The disturbance does not occur exclusively during the course of dissociative identity disorder and is not due to the direct physiological effects of a substance (e.g., a drug of abuse, a medication) or a general medical condition (e.g., temporal lobe epilepsy).

D. The symptoms cause clinically significant distress or impairment in social, occupational, or other important areas of functioning.

through interpersonal or intrapsychic issues that underlie the dissociative defenses. Individuals with dissociative fugue are often relatively unaware of their reactions to stress because they so effectively can dissociate them (H. Spiegel 1974). Thus, effective psychotherapy is also anticipatory, in that it helps patients to recognize and modify their tendency to set aside their own feelings in favor of those of others.

Patients with dissociative fugue may be helped with a psychotherapeutic approach that facilitates conscious integration of dissociated memories and motivations for behavior previously experienced as automatic and unwilled. It is often helpful to address current psychosocial stressors, such as marital conflict, with the involved individuals. To the extent that current psychosocial stress triggers fugue, resolution of that stress can help resolve the fugue state and reduce the likelihood of recurrence. Highly hypnotizable individuals prone to these extreme dissociative symptoms (D. Spiegel et al. 1988; H. Spiegel 1974; H. Spiegel and Spiegel 2004) often have great difficulty in asserting their own point of view in a personal relationship. Rather, they interact with others as though they were undergoing a spontaneous trance experience. One such individual described herself as a "disciple in search of a teacher." Psychotherapy can be effective in helping such individuals recognize and modify their tendency toward unthinking compliance with others and toward extreme sensitivity to rejection and disapproval.

In the past, sodium amobarbital or other short-acting sedatives were used to reverse dissociative amnesia or fugue. More recently, Ilechukwu and Henry (2006) described the use of intravenous lorazepam for the same purpose. However, such techniques offer no advantage over hypnosis and are not especially effective (Perry and Jacobs 1982).

# Depersonalization Disorder

The essential feature of depersonalization disorder is the occurrence of persistent feelings of unreality, detachment, or estrangement from oneself or one's body, usually with the feeling that one is an outside observer of one's own mental processes (Steinberg 1991). Thus, depersonalization disorder is primarily a disturbance in the integration of perceptual experience (Table 22–6). Individuals who have depersonalization disorder are distressed by it. Different from those with delusional disorders and other psychotic processes, those with depersonalization disorder have intact reality testing. Patients are aware of some distortion in their perceptual experience and therefore are not delusional. The symptom is often transient and may co-occur with a variety of other symptoms, especially anxiety, panic, or phobic symptoms. Derealization frequently co-occurs with depersonalization disorder, in which affected individuals notice an altered perception of their surroundings, resulting in the world seeming unreal or dreamlike. Affected individuals often will ruminate about this alteration and be preoccupied with their own somatic and mental functioning.

---

**TABLE 22–6.  DSM-IV-TR diagnostic criteria for depersonalization disorder**

A. Persistent or recurrent experiences of feeling detached from, and as if one is an outside observer of, one's mental processes or body (e.g., feeling like one is in a dream).

B. During the depersonalization experience, reality testing remains intact.

C. The depersonalization causes clinically significant distress or impairment in social, occupational, or other important areas of functioning.

D. The depersonalization experience does not occur exclusively during the course of another mental disorder, such as schizophrenia, panic disorder, acute stress disorder, or another dissociative disorder, and is not due to the direct physiological effects of a substance (e.g., a drug of abuse, a medication) or a general medical condition (e.g., temporal lobe epilepsy).

---

Hunter et al. (2004) conducted a study using computerized databases and citation searches to assess the prevalence of symptoms of depersonalization and derealization in both clinical and nonclinical settings. They found that transient symptoms of depersonalization/derealization are common in the general population, with a lifetime prevalence rate between 26% and 74% and a current prevalence rate between 31% and 66% at the time of a traumatic event. Community surveys employing standardized diagnostic interviews found rates of between 1.2% and 1.7% for 1-month prevalence of symptoms of depersonalization/derealization in a U.K. sample and a 2.4% current prevalence rate in a Canadian sample. Current prevalence rates between 1% and 16% were reported in samples of consecutive inpatient admissions, although these rates were considered to be underestimates. Prevalence rates in clinical samples of specific psychiatric disorders varied between 30% (for war veterans with PTSD) and 60% (for those with unipolar depression). There was a high prevalence of depersonalization/derealization symptoms within panic disorder samples, with rates varying from 7.8% to 82.6%.

## Treatment

Depersonalization is most often transient and may remit without formal treatment. Recurrent or persistent depersonalization should be thought of both as a symptom in and of itself and as a component of other syndromes requiring treatment, such as anxiety disorders and schizophrenia.

The symptom itself may respond to self-hypnosis training. Often, hypnotic induction will induce transient depersonalization symptoms in patients. This is a useful exercise because by having a structure for inducing the symptoms, one provides patients with a context for understanding and controlling them. The symptoms are presented as a spontaneous form of hypnotic dissociation that can be modified. Individuals for whom this approach is effective can be taught to induce a pleasant sense of floating lightness or heaviness in place of the anxiety-related somatic detachment. Often, the use of an imaginary screen to picture problems in a way that detaches them from the typical somatic response is also helpful (H. Spiegel and Spiegel 2004).

Other treatment modalities used (Maldonado et al. 2000) include behavioral techniques such as paradoxical intention, record keeping, positive reward, flooding, psychotherapy (especially psychodynamic), cognitive-behavioral therapy, and psychoeducation. Hunter et al.

(2005) reported on an open study in which 21 patients with depersonalization disorder were treated individually with cognitive-behavioral therapy. The authors reported significant improvements in patient-defined measures of depersonalization/derealization severity as well as in standardized measures of dissociation, depression, anxiety, and general functioning at the end of treatment and at 6-month follow-up.

Virtually all types of psychotropic medications, including psychostimulants, antidepressants, antipsychotics, anticonvulsants, and benzodiazepines, have been tried with modest success. Appropriate treatment of comorbid disorders is an important part of treatment.

# Dissociative Identity Disorder (Multiple Personality Disorder)

## Prevalence

There are no convincing studies of the absolute prevalence of DID. The initial systematic report on the epidemiology of DID estimated a prevalence in the general population of 0.01% (Coons 1984). The estimated prevalence is approximately 3% of psychiatric inpatients (Ross 1991; Ross et al. 1991). Studies conducted in the general population suggest a prevalence higher than initially reported by Coons (1984) but lower (about 1%) than the one described in psychiatric settings and specialized treatment units (Ross 1991; Vanderlinden et al. 1991). Loewenstein (1994) reported that the prevalence in North America is about 1%, compared with a prevalence of 10% for all dissociative disorders as a group. Loewenstein's findings were replicated by Rifkin et al. (1998), who studied 100 randomly selected women, ages 16–50 years, who had been admitted to an acute psychiatric hospital and found that 1% of the subjects had DID. There is evidence that dissociative disorders are often underdiagnosed (D. Spiegel 2006). Foote et al. (2006) carefully assessed 231 consecutive admissions to an inner-city mental health clinic and interviewed 82 of those willing to cooperate with the study. Twenty-nine percent of this sample met DSM-IV (American Psychiatric Association 1994) criteria for a dissociative disorder (8 with dissociative amnesia, 7 with dissociative disorder not otherwise specified, 5 with DID, and 4 with depersonalization disorder). Only 5% of this sample had previously been diagnosed with a dissociative disorder. Furthermore, the study provided additional evidence linking both physical and sexual abuse to dissociative symptoms, determining an odds ratio of 5.86 for

physical abuse and 7.87 for sexual abuse. In a recent study of community adults, the prevalence of DID was 1.5% (Johnson et al. 2006).

The number of reported DID cases has risen considerably in recent years. Factors that account for this increase include a more general awareness of the diagnosis among mental health professionals; the availability, starting with DSM-III (American Psychiatric Association 1980), of specific diagnostic criteria (Table 22–7); and reduced misdiagnosis of DID as schizophrenia or borderline personality disorder.

---

**TABLE 22–7.    DSM-IV-TR diagnostic criteria for dissociative identity disorder**

A.  The presence of two or more distinct identities or personality states (each with its own relatively enduring pattern of perceiving, relating to, and thinking about the environment and self).

B.  At least two of these identities or personality states recurrently take control of the person's behavior.

C.  Inability to recall important personal information that is too extensive to be explained by ordinary forgetfulness.

D.  The disturbance is not due to the direct physiological effects of a substance (e.g., blackouts or chaotic behavior during alcohol intoxication) or a general medical condition (e.g., complex partial seizures). **Note:** In children, the symptoms are not attributable to imaginary playmates or other fantasy play.

---

## Course

DID is diagnosed in childhood with increasing frequency (Kluft 1984a, 1984b) but typically emerges between adolescence and the third decade of life; it rarely presents as a new disorder after an individual reaches age 40 years, but there is often considerable delay between initial symptom presentation and diagnosis (American Psychiatric Association 2000; Putnam et al. 1986). The female-to-male sex ratio of DID is 5 to 4 in children and adolescents and 9 to 1 in adults (Hocke and Schmidtke 1998; Sno and Schalken 1999).

Untreated, DID is a chronic and recurrent disorder. The dissociation itself hampers self-monitoring and accurate reporting of symptoms. Many patients with the disorder are not fully aware of the extent of their dissociative symptomatology. They may be reluctant to bring up symptoms because of having encountered frequent skepticism.

Furthermore, because most patients with DID report histories of sexual and physical abuse (Coons and Milstein 1992; Coons et al. 1988; Kluft 1985b, 1988, 1991; Putnam 1988; Putnam et al. 1986; Ross 1989; Ross et al. 1990; Schultz et al. 1989; D. Spiegel 1984), the shame associated with that experience, as well as fear of retribution, may inhibit reporting of symptoms.

## Comorbidity

To find comorbid Axis I or II disorders in patients diagnosed with DID is the norm (Maldonado and Spiegel 2005). The major comorbid psychiatric illnesses of DID are the depressive disorders (Putnam et al. 1986; Ross and Norton 1989; Ross et al. 1989; Sar et al. 2007; Yargic et al. 1998), substance use disorders (Anderson et al. 1993; Dunn et al. 1995; Ellason et al. 1996; Karadag et al. 2005; Putnam et al. 1986; Rivera 1991), and borderline personality disorder (Anderson et al. 1993; Brodsky et al. 1995; Ross 2007; Sar et al. 2007; Shearer 1994; Yargic et al. 1998). Sexual (Brenner 1996; van der Kolk et al. 1994), eating (Berger et al. 1994; Valdiserri and Kihlstrom 1995; van der Kolk et al. 1994), somatoform (Spitzer et al. 1999; Yargic et al. 1998), and sleep (Putnam et al. 1986) disorders occur less commonly. Patients with DID frequently engage in self-mutilative behavior (Gainer and Torem 1993; Putnam et al. 1986; Ross and Norton 1989; Zweig-Frank et al. 1994), impulsiveness, and overvaluing and devaluing of relationships, and approximately a third of DID patients fit the criteria for borderline personality disorder as well.

In a study attempting to identify the risk factors associated with the dissociative symptomatology of borderline personality disorder patients, four risk factors were found to be significantly associated with the level of dissociation reported: 1) inconsistent treatment by a caregiver, 2) sexual abuse by a caregiver, 3) witnessing sexual violence as a child, and 4) adult rape history (Zanarini et al. 2000). A recent study by Watson et al. (2006) suggested that patients with borderline personality disorder show levels of dissociation that increase with levels of childhood trauma, supporting the hypothesis that traumatic childhood experiences engender dissociative symptoms later in life. Their study findings also suggested that emotional abuse and neglect may be at least as important as physical and sexual abuse in the development of dissociative symptoms.

Comorbidity is complex in that patients with concurrent diagnoses of DID and borderline personality disorder (approximately one-third) also are more likely to meet the criteria for major depressive disorder. In addition, they frequently meet the criteria for PTSD, with intrusive flashbacks, recurring dreams of physical and sexual abuse, avoidance of and loss of pleasure from usually pleasurable activities, and symptoms of hyperarousal, especially when exposed to reminders of childhood trauma (Kluft 1985a, 1991; Putnam 1993; D. Spiegel 1990; van der Kolk and Fisler 1995; van der Kolk et al. 1994, 1996). Ross (2007) studied a group of 93 inpatient subjects who met criteria for borderline personality disorder and compared them with a group (*n*=108) who did not. The two groups were then compared on dissociative symptoms and disorders. The subjects with borderline personality disorder reported significantly more dissociative symptoms and disorders on all measures. He found that 59% of the borderline patients met criteria for a dissociative disorder on the Dissociative Disorders Interview Schedule, compared with 22% of the nonborderline patients. Furthermore, in a sample of 1,301 college students in Turkey, Sar et al. (2006) found that 8.5% met diagnostic criteria for borderline personality disorder (as measured by the Structured Clinical Interview for DSM-IV Axis II Personality Disorders). A significant majority (72.5%) of the borderline personality disorder group had a comorbid dissociative disorder, compared with only 18.0% for the comparison group of students without borderline personality disorder ($P<0.001$).

Individuals with DID report an average of 15 somatic or conversion symptoms (Anderson et al. 1993; Bowman 1993; Bowman and Markand 1996; Kaplan et al. 1995; Ross et al. 1989, 1990) and other psychosomatic symptoms such as migraine headaches (Frances and Spiegel 1987). Studies show that approximately one-third of these patients have complex partial seizures (Schenk and Bear 1981), although more recent studies have not found seizure rates to be that high and do not show substantial elevations in Dissociative Experiences Scale scores in patients with complex partial seizures compared with scores in other neurological patients (Loewenstein and Putnam 1988). There is sufficient comorbidity that patients receiving recent diagnoses of DID should be evaluated for the possibility of a seizure disorder.

## Psychological Testing

The diagnosis of DID can be facilitated by psychological testing (Scroppo et al. 1998). Form level on the Rorschach test usually is within the normal range, but emotionally dramatic responses are common, often involving mutilation, especially on the color cards (such responses are often seen in patients with histrionic personality disorder as well). Good form level is useful in distinguishing DID patients from schizophrenic patients, who have poor form level. Leavitt and Labott (1998) replicated these findings. Their results indicated that Rorschach signs for the Labott, Barach, and Wagner Rorschach markers were significantly better than chance at classifying patients as having DID or as not having DID. The Labott system, which performed the best, was able to accurately classify 92% of the sample. The fact that two relatively rare sets of signs (DID and Rorschach) converged in the same small sector of the psychiatric population represents evidence of linkage that is clinically meaningful and not explainable on the basis of artificial creation. That the Rorschach signs operate independent of external bias, yet correspond to the diagnoses obtained through psychiatric evaluation in an inpatient setting, argues for the validity of the DID diagnosis. Also, unlike individuals with schizophrenia, those with DID score far higher than healthy individuals on standard measures of hypnotizability, whereas patients with schizophrenia tend to show lower than normal or an absence of high hypnotizability (Lavoie and Sabourin 1980; Pettinati et al. 1990; D. Spiegel and Fink 1979; D. Spiegel et al. 1982; van der Hart and Spiegel 1993). Thus, there is comparatively little overlap in the hypnotizability scores of schizophrenic patients and those of DID patients.

## Treatment

### *Psychotherapy*

**Therapeutic direction.** Maldonado (2000) described a series of "rules of engagement" (Table 22–8) to be used in the treatment of DID. These rules were designed to facilitate the therapist–patient contract by establishing clear lines of communication, delineating therapeutic boundaries, eliminating splitting, and enhancing control over dissociative experiences. The rules call for free access to all pertinent old records and permission to discuss all past and current pertinent information with previous therapists; cooperation in the completion of a full organic/neurological workup; a contract for safety; the establishment of a hierarchical pattern of communication and a hierarchical pattern of responsibility; agreement for a limited exploration followed by therapeutic condensation of memories—that is, an "all details are not needed" policy rather than an endless fishing exploration; a "no secrets" policy; an increased level of communication and cooperation between patient and therapist and among alters; detailed rules regarding therapist–patient contact during

**TABLE 22–8.** "Rules of engagement" in the treatment of dissociative identity disorder

1. Free access to all pertinent records
2. Review of all available and pertinent records
3. Freedom to discuss all past and current pertinent information with previous therapists
4. Complete organic/neurological workup
5. Contract for safety
6. Increased communication and cooperation among alters
7. "No secrets" policy
8. Establishment of hierarchical pattern of communication
9. Establishment of hierarchical pattern of responsibility
10. Limited exploration followed by therapeutic condensation of memories
11. "All details are not needed" policy
12. Rules regarding contact during hospitalizations and continued therapy after discharge
13. Videotaping
14. Ultimate goal: "full integration"
15. "One day you will make me obsolete" principle

hospitalization and continued therapy after discharge; need for videotaping; and, finally, clear understanding of the ultimate treatment goal: "full integration."

**Hypnosis.** Hypnosis can be helpful in therapy as well as in diagnosis (Kluft 1982, 1985a, 1985c, 1992, 1999; Maldonado and Spiegel 1995, 1998; Maldonado et al. 2000; Smith 1993; H. Spiegel and Spiegel 2004).

First, the simple structure of hypnotic induction may elicit dissociative phenomena. Most of these patients have the experience of being unable to stop dissociative symptoms but are often intrigued by the possibility of starting them. This carries with it the potential for changing or stopping the symptoms as well.

Hypnosis can be helpful in facilitating access to dissociated personalities. The personalities may simply occur spontaneously during hypnotic induction. An alternative strategy is to hypnotize the patient and use age regression to help the patient reorient to a time when a different personality state was manifest. An instruction later to change times back to the present tense usually elicits a return to the other personality state. This then becomes an alternative means of teaching the patient control over the dissociation.

Alternatively, entering the state of hypnosis may make it possible to simply "call up" different identities or personality states. Patients can be taught a simple self-hypnosis exercise. For example, the patient can be told to count to himself or herself from 1 to 3: On 1, do one thing: look up. On 2, do two things: slowly close your eyes, and take a deep breath. On 3, do three things: let the breath out, let your eyes relax but keep them closed, and let your body float. Then let one hand float up into the air like a balloon. Develop a pleasant sense of floating throughout your body. After some formal exercises such as this, it is often possible to simply ask to speak with a given alter personality, without the formal use of hypnosis.

**Memory retrieval.** Because loss of memory in DID is complex and chronic, its retrieval is likewise a more extended and integral part of the psychotherapeutic process. The therapy becomes an integrating experience of information sharing among disparate personality elements. In conceptualizing DID as a chronic PTSD, the psychotherapeutic strategy involves a focus on working through traumatic memories in addition to controlling the dissociation.

Controlled access to memories greatly facilitates psychotherapy. As in the treatment of dissociative amnesia, a variety of strategies can be used to help DID patients break down amnesic barriers. Use of hypnosis to go to that place in imagination and ask one or more such parts of the self to interact can be helpful.

Once these memories of earlier traumatic experiences have been brought into consciousness, it is crucial to help the patient work through the painful affect, inappropriate self-blame, and other reactions to these memories. A model of grief work is helpful, enabling the patient to acknowledge and bear the import of such memories (Lindemann 1944/1994; D. Spiegel 1981). It may be useful to have the patient visualize the memories rather than relive them, as a way of making their intensity more manageable. It also can be useful to have the patient divide the memories onto two sides of an imaginary screen—for example, on one side, picturing something an abuser did to him or her, and on the other side, picturing how the patient tried to protect himself or herself from the abuse.

This technique and similar approaches can help these individuals work through traumatic memories, enabling them to bear the memories in consciousness and therefore reducing the need for dissociation as a means of keeping such memories out of consciousness. Although these techniques can be helpful and often result in reduced fragmentation and integration (Kluft 1985a, 1985c, 1986, 1992; Maldonado and Spiegel 1995, 1998; D. Spiegel

1984, 1986a), several complications can occur in the psychotherapy of these patients as well.

The information retrieved from memory in these ways should be reviewed, traumatic memories put into perspective, and emotional expression encouraged and worked through, with the goal of sharing the information as widely as possible among various parts of the patient's personality structure. Instructing other alter personalities to "listen" while a given alter is talking, and reviewing previously dissociated material uncovered, can be helpful. The therapist conveys his or her desire to disseminate the information, without accepting responsibility for transmitting it across all personality boundaries.

**The "rule of thirds."** Psychotherapy with a DID patient can be a time-consuming and emotionally taxing process. The "rule of thirds" (Kluft 1988, 1991) is a helpful guideline. The therapist should spend the first third of the psychotherapy session assessing the patient's current mental state and life problems and defining a problem area that might benefit from retrieval into conscious memory and working through. The therapist should spend the second third of the session accessing and working through this memory. The therapist should allow a final third for helping the patient assimilate the information, regulate and modulate emotional responses, and discuss any responses to the therapist and plans for the immediate future.

Given the intensity of the material that often emerges, involving memories of sexual and physical abuse, and the sudden shifts in mental state accompanied by amnesia, the therapist is called on to take a clear and structured role in managing the psychotherapy. Appropriate limits must be set about self-destructive or threatening behavior and agreements made regarding physical safety and treatment compliance, and other matters must be presented to the patient in such a way that dissociative ignorance is not an acceptable explanation for failure to live up to agreements.

**Traumatic transference.** Transference applies with special meaning in patients who have been physically and sexually abused. These patients have had presumed caregivers who acted instead in an exploitative and sometimes sadistic fashion. These patients thus expect the same from their therapists. Although their reality testing is good enough that they can perceive genuine caring, they expect therapists either to exploit them, with the patients viewing the working through of traumatic memories as a re-inflicting of the trauma and the therapists' taking sadistic pleasure in the patients' suffering, or to be excessively passive, with the patients identifying the therapists with some uncaring family figure who knew abuse was occurring but did little or nothing to stop it. It is important in managing the therapy to keep these issues in mind and make them frequent topics of discussion. Attention to these issues can diffuse, but not eliminate, such traumatic transference distortions of the therapeutic relationship (Maldonado and Spiegel 1995, 1998; D. Spiegel 1988).

**Integration.**    The ultimate goal of psychotherapy for patients with DID is integration of the disparate states. There can be considerable resistance to this process. Early in therapy, the patient views the dissociation as tremendous protection: "I knew my father could get some of me, but he couldn't get all of me." Indeed, he or she may experience efforts of integration as an attempt on the part of the therapist to "kill" personalities. These fears must be worked through and the patient shown how to control the degree of integration, a process that will give the patient a sense of gradually being able to control his or her dissociative processes in the service of working through traumatic memories. The process of the psychotherapy, in emphasizing control, must alter rather than reinforce the content, which involves reexperiencing of helplessness, a symbolic reenactment of trauma (D. Spiegel 1986b).

### Cognitive-Behavioral Approaches

Fine (1999) summarized the tactical-integration model for the treatment of dissociative disorders. This consists of structured cognitive-behavioral–based treatments that foster symptom relief, followed by integration of the personalities and/or ego states into one mainstream of consciousness. This approach promotes proficiency in control over posttraumatic and dissociative symptoms, is collaborative and exploratory, and conveys a consistent message of empowerment to the patient.

    In addition, both cognitive analytic therapy (CAT; Kellett 2005; Ryle and Fawkes 2007) and dialectical behavioral therapy (Braakmann et al. 2007) have been found to be helpful as adjunctive or primary treatment of DID. In CAT, multiplicity is understood in terms of a range of self–other patterns (i.e., reciprocal role relationships) originating in childhood. These patterns alternate in determining experience and action according to the situation (i.e., contextual multiplicity). They may be restricted by adverse childhood experiences (i.e., diminished multiplicity), and severe deprivation or abuse may result in a structural dissociation of self-processes (i.e., pathological multiplicity). In CAT practice (Ryle and Fawkes 2007), descriptions of

dysfunctional relationship patterns and of transitions between them are worked out by therapist and patient at the start of therapy and are used by both throughout its course.

### Psychopharmacology

To date, no good evidence shows that medication of any type has a direct therapeutic effect on the dissociative process manifested by patients with DID (Loewenstein 1991; Markowitz and Gill 1996; Putnam 1989). Antidepressants are the most useful class of psychotropic agents for patients with DID. Such patients frequently have dysthymic disorder or major depression as well, and when these disorders are present, especially with somatic signs and suicidal ideation, antidepressant medication can be helpful. At least two studies report on the successful use of antidepressant medications (Barkin et al. 1986; Kluft 1984a, 1985b). The use of antidepressants should be limited to the treatment of DID patients who experience symptoms of major depression (Barkin et al. 1986). The selective serotonin reuptake inhibitors are effective at reducing comorbid depressive symptoms and have the advantage of far less lethality in overdose compared with tricyclics and monoamine oxidase inhibitors. Medication compliance is a problem with such patients because dissociated personality states may interfere with the taking of medication, with the patients "hiding" or hoarding pills or possibly taking an overdose.

# Dissociative Trance Disorder

## Cultural Context

Dissociative phenomena are ubiquitous around the world, occurring in virtually every culture (Castillo 1994a, 1994b; Kirmayer 1993; Lewis-Fernandez 1993). These phenomena seem to be more prevalent in the less heavily industrialized second and third world countries.

    Most scholars agree that the most common clinical features of trance states are amnesia, emotional disturbances, and loss of identity (Li and Spiegel 1992). In a study comparing the characteristic features of the possession trance in three different ethnic groups of Chinese, Malayans, and Indians, Kua et al. (1986) found a set of similarities, including alteration in the level of consciousness, amnesia for the period of the trance, stereotyped behavior characteristic of a deity, duration of less than 1 hour, fatigue at the termination of the trance, normal behavior in the interval between trances, onset before age 25 years, low socioeconomic status, low educational attainment, and prior witnessing of a trance.

The DSM-IV-TR research criteria for dissociative trance disorder are shown in Table 22–9. The major purposes served by possession and trance states include the need to gain power, prestige, and status and the desire to express aggressive and sexual impulses (Shirali et al. 1986), especially given the cultural overdetermination of women's selfhood (Boddy 1988). Spirit possession rituals may mystify the source of women's suppression and absolve women of any responsibility for an otherwise unacceptable challenge to patriarchal control (Sered 1994). They also may provide the subject with a sense of social association and ultimately attempt to make something socially useful from feelings such as aggression that were previously socially destructive (Tantam 1993), may provide a release from normative structural constraints, and may facilitate role reversal and role enhancement (McLellan 1991). Dissociative trance disorders, especially possession disorder, are probably more common than is usually thought. Ferracuti et al. (1996) reported on 10 patients undergoing exorcisms for devil trance possession state. Subjects were studied with the Dissociative Disorders Interview Schedule and the Rorschach test. Subjects were found to have many traits in common with patients with DID. Despite claiming possession by a demon and various paranormal phenomena, most of them managed to maintain normal social functioning.

The trance and possession categories of dissociative trance disorder constitute by far the most common kinds of dissociative disorders around the world. Cultural and biological factors may account for the different content and form of dissociative symptoms. Nonetheless, the underlying dissociative mechanism inhibiting integration of perception, memory, and identity makes these syndromes an important class of dissociative disorders.

These dissociative episodes usually are understood as an idiom of distress, yet they are not viewed as normal. That is, they are not a generally accepted part of cultural and religious practice that may often involve normal trance phenomena, such as trance dancing in the Balinese Hindu culture. Trance dancers in that culture are remarkable for being the only portion of this socially stable society able to elevate their social status. This elevation of social status is done through developing an ability to enter trance states. The dancers are able within the social ceremony to induce an altered state of consciousness in which they dance over hot coals, hold a sword at their throat, or in other ways show exceptional powers of concentration and physical prowess. They are frequently watched by other dancers to make sure that they retain control and do not hurt themselves. This form of trance is con-

---

**TABLE 22–9. DSM-IV-TR research criteria for dissociative trance disorder**

A. Either (1) or (2):

   (1) trance, i.e., temporary marked alteration in the state of consciousness or loss of customary sense of personal identity without replacement by an alternate identity, associated with at least one of the following:

      (a) narrowing of awareness of immediate surroundings, or unusually narrow and selective focusing on environmental stimuli

      (b) stereotyped behaviors or movements that are experienced as being beyond one's control

   (2) possession trance, a single or episodic alteration in the state of consciousness characterized by the replacement of customary sense of personal identity by a new identity. This is attributed to the influence of a spirit, power, deity, or other person, as evidenced by one (or more) of the following:

      (a) stereotyped and culturally determined behaviors or movements that are experienced as being controlled by the possessing agent

      (b) full or partial amnesia for the event

B. The trance or possession trance state is not accepted as a normal part of a collective cultural or religious practice.

C. The trance or possession trance state causes clinically significant distress or impairment in social, occupational, or other important areas of functioning.

D. The trance or possession trance state does not occur exclusively during the course of a psychotic disorder (including mood disorder with psychotic features and brief psychotic disorder) or dissociative identity disorder and is not due to the direct physiological effects of a substance or a general medical condition.

---

sidered socially normal and even exalted. By contrast, trance and possession disorder is viewed by the local community as a common but aberrant form of behavior that requires intervention. Although trance and possession disorder is clearly an idiom of distress (e.g., discomfort in a new family environment), most individuals use an array of alternative strategies for coping with such distress. Thus, cultural informants make it clear that persons with trance and possession trance disorders are acting abnormally, if recognizably.

**TABLE 22–10.  Comparison of Western and Eastern types of dissociative syndromes**

| Dissociative phenomena | Western | Eastern |
|---|---|---|
| Identity | Dissociative identity disorder: multiple internal identities<br>Dissociative fugue | Possession trance: control by external identities |
| Memory | Dissociative amnesia | Secondary in dissociative trance, more common in possession trance |
| Perception | Depersonalization disorder | Dissociative trance (e.g., *latah*, *ataque de nervios*) |
| Consciousness | Acute stress disorder | Dissociative trance |

## Classification

Dissociative trance disorder has been divided into two broad categories: dissociative trance and possession trance (Table 22–10).

### Dissociative Trance

Dissociative trance phenomena are characterized by a sudden alteration in consciousness not accompanied by distinct alternative identities. In this form, the dissociative symptom involves consciousness rather than identity. Also, in dissociative trance, the activities performed are rather simple, usually involving sudden collapse, immobilization, dizziness, shrieking, screaming, or crying. Memory is rarely affected, and amnesia, if any, is fragmented.

### Possession Trance

In contrast to dissociative trance, possession trance involves the assumption of a distinct alternative identity, usually that of a deity, an ancestor, or a spirit. The person in this trance often engages in rather complex activities,

which may take the form of expressing otherwise forbidden thoughts or needs, negotiating for change in family or social status, or engaging in aggressive behavior. Possession usually involves amnesia for a large portion of the episode during which the alternative identity was in control of the person's behavior.

## Treatment

Treatment of these disorders varies from culture to culture. Most syndromes occur within the context of acute social stress and thus serve the purpose of recruiting help from the family and other support systems or removing the subject from the immediate danger or threat. Ceremonies to remove or appease the invading spirit are commonly used (Piñeros et al. 1998). The role of psychiatry should be focused on ruling out any possible organic cause for the symptoms shown, treating comorbid psychiatric conditions (if any are present), avoiding excess medication, understanding the social context and role of the syndrome, and facilitating a favorable outcome.

# Key Points: Dissociative Disorders

- Dissociative disorders are underdiagnosed.
- Dissociation is a common component of acute response to trauma, and dissociative fugue, amnesia, and identity disorders often have a traumatic etiology.
- Dissociation represents a failure of integration of identity, memory, perception, and consciousness.
- The primary treatments for dissociative disorders involve various psychotherapies, including hypnosis, trauma-related psychotherapies, and cognitive therapies.
- Common comorbid condiions requiring treatment include depression, substance use disorders, and borderline personality disorder.
- Dissociative symptoms are ubiquitous around the world, but the content of the dissociative symptoms varies, involving "possession" by external entities more often in the East, and fragmentation of individual identity in the West.

# References

American Psychiatric Association: Diagnostic and Statistical Manual of Mental Disorders, 3rd Edition. Washington, DC, American Psychiatric Association, 1980

American Psychiatric Association: Diagnostic and Statistical Manual of Mental Disorders, 4th Edition. Washington, DC, American Psychiatric Association, 1994

American Psychiatric Association: Diagnostic and Statistical Manual of Mental Disorders, 4th Edition, Text Revision. Washington, DC, American Psychiatric Association, 2000

Anderson G, Yasenik L, Ross CA: Dissociative experiences and disorders among women who identify themselves as sexual abuse survivors. Child Abuse Negl 17:677–686, 1993

Barkin R, Braun BG, Kluft RP: The dilemma of drug therapy for multiple personality disorder, in Treatment of Multiple Personality Disorder. Edited by Braun BG. Washington, DC, American Psychiatric Press, 1986, pp 107–132

Baron DA, Nagy R: The amobarbital interview in a general hospital setting, friend or foe: a case report. Gen Hosp Psychiatry 10:220–222, 1988

Berger D, Saito S, Ono Y, et al: Dissociation and child abuse histories in an eating disorder cohort in Japan. Acta Psychiatr Scand 90:274–280, 1994

Blank AS Jr: The longitudinal course of posttraumatic stress disorder, in Posttraumatic Stress Disorder: DSM-IV and Beyond. Edited by Davidson JRT, Foa EB. Washington, DC, American Psychiatric Press, 1993, pp 3–22

Boddy J: Spirits and selves in Northern Sudan: the cultural therapeutics of possession and trance. American Ethnologist 15:4–27, 1988

Bowman ES: Etiology and clinical course of pseudoseizures: relationship to trauma, depression, and dissociation. Psychosomatics 34:333–342, 1993

Bowman ES, Markand ON: Psychodynamics and psychiatric diagnoses of pseudoseizure subjects. Am J Psychiatry 153:57–63, 1996

Braakmann D, Ludewig S, Milde J, et al: Dissociative symptoms during treatment of borderline personality disorder. Psychother Psychosom Med Psychol 57(3–4):154–160, 2007

Brenner I: On trauma, perversion, and "multiple personality." J Am Psychoanal Assoc 44:785–814, 1996

Brodsky BS, Cloitre M, Dulit RA: Relationship of dissociation to self-mutilation and childhood abuse in borderline personality disorder. Am J Psychiatry 152:1788–1792, 1995

Brown GR, Anderson B: Psychiatric morbidity in adult inpatients with childhood histories of sexual and physical abuse. Am J Psychiatry 148:55–61, 1991

Brown W: The treatment of cases of shell shock in an advanced neurological centre. Lancet 2:197–200, 1918

Castillo RJ: Spirit possession in South Asia, dissociation or hysteria? I: theoretical background. Cult Med Psychiatry 18:1–21, 1994a

Castillo RJ: Spirit possession in South Asia, dissociation or hysteria? II: case histories. Cult Med Psychiatry 18:141–162, 1994b

Chu JA, Dill DL: Dissociative symptoms in relation to childhood physical and sexual abuse. Am J Psychiatry 147:887–892, 1990

Coons PM: The differential diagnosis of multiple personality: a comprehensive review. Psychiatr Clin North Am 7:51–65, 1984

Coons PM, Milstein V: Psychosexual disturbances in multiple personality: characteristics, etiology, and treatment. J Clin Psychiatry 47:106–110, 1986

Coons PM, Milstein V: Psychogenic amnesia: a clinical investigation of 25 cases. Dissociation 5:73–79, 1992

Coons PM, Bowman ES, Milstein V: Multiple personality disorder: a clinical investigation of 50 cases. J Nerv Ment Dis 17:519–527, 1988

Dunn GE, Ryan JJ, Paolo AM, et al: Comorbidity of dissociative disorders among patients with substance use disorders. Psychiatr Serv 46:153–156, 1995

Ellason JW, Ross CA, Sainton K, et al: Axis I and II comorbidity and childhood trauma history in chemical dependency. Bull Menninger Clin 60:39–51, 1996

Ferracuti S, Sacco R, Lazzari R: Dissociative trance disorder: clinical and Rorschach findings in 10 persons reporting demon possession and treated by exorcism. J Pers Assess 66:525–539, 1996

Fine CG: The tactical-integration model for the treatment of dissociative identity disorder and allied dissociative disorders. Am J Psychother 53:361–376, 1999

Foote B, Smolin Y, Kaplan M, et al: Prevalence of dissociative disorders in psychiatric outpatients. Am J Psychiatry 163:623–629, 2006

Frances A, Spiegel D: Chronic pain masks depression, multiple personality disorder. Hosp Community Psychiatry 38:933–935, 1987

Gainer MJ, Torem MS: Ego-state therapy for self-injurious behavior. Am J Clin Hypn 35:257–266, 1993

Hocke V, Schmidtke A: "Multiple personality disorder" in childhood and adolescence. Z Kinder Jugendpsychiatr Psychother 26:273–284, 1998

Hunter EC, Sierra M, David AS: The epidemiology of depersonalisation and derealisation: a systematic review. Soc Psychiatry Psychiatr Epidemiol 39:9–18, 2004

Hunter EC, Baker D, Phillips ML, et al: Cognitive-behavioural therapy for depersonalisation disorder: an open study. Behav Res Ther 43:1121–1130, 2005

Ilechukwu ST, Henry T: Amytal interview using intravenous lorazepam in a patient with dissociative fugue. Gen Hosp Psychiatry 28:544–545, 2006

Johnson JG, Cohen P, Kasen S, et al: Dissociative disorders among adults in the community, impaired functioning, and Axis I and II comorbidity. J Psychiatr Res 40:131–140, 2006

Kaplan ML, Asnis GM, Lipschitz DS, et al: Suicidal behavior and abuse in psychiatric outpatients. Compr Psychiatry 36:229–235, 1995

Karadag F, Sar V, Tamar-Gurol D, et al: Dissociative disorders among inpatients with drug or alcohol dependency. J Clin Psychiatry 66:1247–1253, 2005

Kardiner A, Spiegel H: War, Stress and Neurotic Illness. New York, Hoeber, 1947

Kellett S: The treatment of dissociative identity disorder with cognitive analytic therapy: experimental evidence of sudden gains. J Trauma Dissociation 6:55–81, 2005

Kirmayer LJ: Pacing the void: social and cultural dimensions of dissociation, in Dissociation: Culture, Mind, and Body. Edited by Spiegel D. Washington, DC, American Psychiatric Press, 1993, pp 91–122

Kluft RP: Varieties of hypnotic intervention in the treatment of multiple personality. Am J Clin Hypn 24:230–240, 1982

Kluft RP: An introduction to multiple personality disorder. Psychiatr Ann 14:19–24, 1984a

Kluft RP: Multiple personality in childhood. Psychiatr Clin North Am 7:121–134, 1984b

Kluft RP: Hypnotherapy of childhood multiple personality disorder. Am J Clin Hypn 27:201–210, 1985a

Kluft RP: The natural history of multiple personality disorder, in Childhood Antecedents of Multiple Personality. Edited by Kluft RP. Washington, DC, American Psychiatric Press, 1985b, pp 197–238

Kluft RP: Using hypnotic inquiry protocols to monitor treatment progress and stability in multiple personality disorder. Am J Clin Hypn 28:63–75, 1985c

Kluft RP: Personality unification in multiple personality disorder: a follow-up study, in Treatment of Multiple Personality Disorder. Edited by Braun BG. Washington, DC, American Psychiatric Press, 1986, pp 29–60

Kluft RP: The dissociative disorders, in The American Psychiatric Press Textbook of Psychiatry. Edited by Talbott JA, Hales RE, Yudofsky SC. Washington, DC, American Psychiatric Press, 1988, pp 557–585

Kluft RP: Multiple personality disorder, in American Psychiatric Press Review of Psychiatry, Vol 10. Edited by Tasman A, Goldfinger SM. Washington, DC, American Psychiatric Press, 1991, pp 161–188

Kluft RP: The use of hypnosis with dissociative disorders. Psychiatr Med 10:31–46, 1992

Kluft RP: An overview of the psychotherapy of dissociative identity disorder. Am J Psychother 53:289–319, 1999

Kua EH, Sim LP, Chee KT: A cross-cultural study of the possession-trance in Singapore. Aust N Z J Psychiatry 20:361–364, 1986

Lavoie G, Sabourin M: Hypnosis and schizophrenia: a review of experimental and clinical studies, in Handbook of Hypnosis and Psychosomatic Medicine. Edited by Burrows GD, Dennerstein L. New York, Elsevier, 1980

Leavitt F, Labott SM: Rorschach indicators of dissociative identity disorders: clinical utility and theoretical implications. J Clin Psychol 54:803–810, 1998

Lewis-Fernandez R: Culture and dissociation: a comparison of ataque de nervios among Puerto Ricans and "possession syndrome" in India, in Dissociation: Culture, Mind, and Body. Edited by Spiegel D. Washington, DC, American Psychiatric Press, 1993, pp 123–167

Li D, Spiegel D: A neural network model of dissociative disorders. Psychiatr Ann 22:144–147, 1992

Lindemann E: Symptomatology and management of acute grief. 1944. Am J Psychiatry 151 (6 suppl):155–160, 1994

Loewenstein RJ: Psychogenic amnesia and psychogenic fugue: a comprehensive review, in American Psychiatric Press Review of Psychiatry, Vol 10. Edited by Tasman A, Goldfinger SM. Washington, DC, American Psychiatric Press, 1991, pp 189–222

Loewenstein RJ: Diagnosis, epidemiology, clinical course, treatment, and cost effectiveness of treatment of dissociative disorders and MPD: report submitted to the Clinton Administration Task Force on Health Care Financing Reform. Dissociation 7:3–11, 1994

Loewenstein RJ, Putnam FW: A comparative study of dissociative symptoms in patients with complex partial seizures, multiple personality disorder and posttraumatic stress disorder. Dissociation 1:17–23, 1988

Maldonado JR: Diagnosis and treatment of dissociative disorders, in Manual for the Course "Advanced Hypnosis: The Use of Hypnosis in Medicine and Psychiatry," at the 153rd annual meeting of the American Psychiatric Association, Chicago, IL, May 13–18, 2000

Maldonado JR, Spiegel D: Using hypnosis, in Treating Women Molested in Childhood. Edited by Classen C. San Francisco, CA, Jossey-Bass, 1995, pp 163–186

Maldonado JR, Spiegel D: Trauma, dissociation, and hypnotizability, in Trauma, Memory, and Dissociation. Edited by Marmar CR, Bremner JD. Washington, DC, American Psychiatric Press, 1998, pp 57–106

Maldonado JR, Spiegel D: Dissociative states in personality disorders, in The American Psychiatric Publishing Textbook of Personality Disorders. Edited by Oldham JM, Skodol AE, Bender DS. Washington, DC, American Psychiatric Publishing, 2005, pp 493–521

Maldonado JR, Butler LD, Spiegel D: Treatment of dissociative disorders, in Treatments That Work. Edited by Nathan P, Gorman JM. New York, Oxford University Press, 2000, pp 463–493

Markowitz JS, Gill HS: Pharmacotherapy of dissociative identity disorder. Ann Pharmacother 30:1498–1499, 1996

McLellan S: Deviant spirits in West Malaysian factories. Anthropologica 33:145–160, 1991

Naples M, Hackett T: The Amytal interview: history and current uses. Psychosomatics 19:98–105, 1978

Perry JC, Jacobs D: Overview: clinical applications of the Amytal interview in psychiatric emergency settings. Am J Psychiatry 139:552–559, 1982

Pettinati HM, Kogan LG, Evans FJ, et al: Hypnotizability of psychiatric inpatients according to two different scales. Am J Psychiatry 147:69–75, 1990

Piñeros M, Rosselli D, Calderon C: An epidemic of collective conversion and dissociation disorder in an indigenous group of Colombia: its relation to cultural change. Soc Sci Med 46:1425–1428, 1998

Putnam FW: Dissociation as a response to extreme trauma, in Childhood Antecedents of Multiple Personality. Edited by Kluft RP. Washington, DC, American Psychiatric Press, 1985, pp 65–97

Putnam FW: The disturbance of "self" in victims of childhood sexual abuse, in Incest-Related Syndromes of Adult Psychopathology. Edited by Kluft RP. Washington, DC, American Psychiatric Press, 1988, pp 113–132

Putnam FW: Diagnosis and Treatment of Multiple Personality Disorder. New York, Guilford, 1989

Putnam FW: Dissociative disorders in children: behavioral profiles and problems. Child Abuse Negl 17:39–45, 1993

Putnam FW, Guroff JJ, Silberman EK, et al: The clinical phenomenology of multiple personality disorder: review of 100 recent cases. J Clin Psychiatry 47:285–293, 1986

Reither AM, Stoudemire A: Psychogenic fugue states: a review. South Med J 81:568–571, 1988

Rifkin A, Ghisalbert D, Dimatou S, et al: Dissociative identity disorder in psychiatric inpatients. Am J Psychiatry 155:844–845, 1998

Rivera M: Multiple personality disorder and the social systems: 185 cases. Dissociation 4:79–82, 1991

Ross CA: Multiple Personality Disorder: Diagnosis, Clinical Features, and Treatment. New York, Wiley, 1989

Ross CA: Epidemiology of multiple personality disorder and dissociation. Psychiatr Clin North Am 14:503–518, 1991

Ross CA: Borderline personality disorder and dissociation. J Trauma Dissociation 8:71–80, 2007

Ross CA, Norton GR: Suicide and parasuicide in multiple personality disorder. Psychiatry 52:365–371, 1989

Ross CA, Norton GR, Wozney K: Multiple personality disorder: an analysis of 236 cases. Can J Psychiatry 34:413–418, 1989

Ross CA, Miller SD, Reagor P, et al: Structured interview data on 102 cases of multiple personality disorder from four centers. Am J Psychiatry 147:596–601, 1990

Ross CA, Anderson G, Fleischer WP, et al: The frequency of multiple personality disorder among psychiatric inpatients. Am J Psychiatry 148:1717–1720, 1991

Rothbaum BO, Foa EB: Subtypes of posttraumatic stress disorder and duration of symptoms, in Posttraumatic Stress Disorder: DSM-IV and Beyond. Edited by Davidson JRT, Foa EB. Washington, DC, American Psychiatric Press, 1993, pp 23–35

Ryle A, Fawkes L: Multiplicity of selves and others: cognitive analytic therapy. J Clin Psychol 63:165–174, 2007

Sar V, Akyuz G, Kugu N, et al: Axis I dissociative disorder comorbidity in borderline personality disorder and reports of childhood trauma. J Clin Psychiatry 67:1583–1590, 2006

Sar V, Koyuncu A, Ozturk E, et al: Dissociative disorders in the psychiatric emergency ward. Gen Hosp Psychiatry 29:45–50, 2007

Schenk L, Bear D: Multiple personality and related dissociative phenomena in patients with temporal lobe epilepsy. Am J Psychiatry 138:1311–1316, 1981

Schultz R, Braun BG, Kluft RP: Multiple personality disorder: phenomenology of selected variables in comparison to major depression. Dissociation 2:45–51, 1989

Scroppo JC, Drob SL, Weinberger JL, et al: Identifying dissociative identity disorder: a self-report and projective study. J Abnorm Psychol 107:272–284, 1998

Sered SS: Ideology, autonomy, and sisterhood: an analysis of the secular consequences of women's religions. Gend Soc 8:486–506, 1994

Shearer SL: Dissociative phenomena in women with borderline personality disorder. Am J Psychiatry 151:1324–1328, 1994

Shirali P, Kishwar A, Bharti SP: Life stress, demographic variables and personality (TAT) in eleven cases of possession (trance-medium) in Shimla Tehsil. Personality Study and Group Behaviour 6:73–81, 1986

Smith WH: Incorporating hypnosis into the psychotherapy of patients with multiple personality disorder. Bull Menninger Clin 57:344–354, 1993

Sno HN, Schalken HF: Dissociative identity disorder: diagnosis and treatment in the Netherlands. Eur Psychiatry 14:270–277, 1999

Solomon Z, Mikulincer M: Psychological sequelae of war: a 2-year follow-up study of Israeli combat stress reaction casualties. J Nerv Ment Dis 176:264–269, 1988

Spiegel D: Vietnam grief work using hypnosis. Am J Clin Hypn 24:33–40, 1981

Spiegel D: Multiple personality as a post-traumatic stress disorder. Psychiatr Clin North Am 7:101–110, 1984

Spiegel D: Dissociating damage. Am J Clin Hypn 29:123–131, 1986a

Spiegel D: Dissociation, double binds, and posttraumatic stress in multiple personality disorder, in Treatment of Multiple Personality Disorder. Edited by Braun BG. Washington, DC, American Psychiatric Press, 1986b, pp 61–77

Spiegel D: Dissociation and hypnosis in posttraumatic stress disorders. J Trauma Stress 1:17–33, 1988

Spiegel D: Trauma, dissociation, and hypnosis, in Incest-Related Syndromes of Adult Psychopathology. Edited by Kluft RL. Washington, DC, American Psychiatric Press, 1990, pp 247–261

Spiegel D: Recognizing traumatic dissociation. Am J Psychiatry 163:566–568, 2006

Spiegel D, Fink R: Hysterical psychosis and hypnotizability. Am J Psychiatry 136:777–781, 1979

Spiegel D, Detrick D, Frischholz E: Hypnotizability and psychopathology. Am J Psychiatry 139:431–437, 1982

Spiegel D, Hunt T, Dondershine HE: Dissociation and hypnotizability in posttraumatic stress disorder. Am J Psychiatry 145:301–305, 1988

Spiegel H: The grade 5 syndrome: the highly hypnotizable person. Int J Clin Exp Hypn 22:303–319, 1974

Spiegel H, Spiegel D: Trance and Treatment: Clinical Uses of Hypnosis, 2nd Edition. Washington, DC, American Psychiatric Publishing, 2004

Spitzer C, Spelsberg B, Grabe HJ, et al: Dissociative experiences and psychopathology in conversion disorders. J Psychosom Res 46:291–294, 1999

Steinberg M: The spectrum of depersonalization: assessment and treatment, in American Psychiatric Press Review of Psychiatry, Vol 10. Edited by Tasman A, Goldfinger SM. Washington, DC, American Psychiatric Press, 1991, pp 223–247

Tantam D: An exorcism in Zanzibar: insights into groups from another culture. Group Analysis 26:251–260, 1993

Valdiserri S, Kihlstrom JF: Abnormal eating and dissociative experiences. Int J Eat Disord 17:373–380, 1995

van der Hart O, Spiegel D: Hypnotic assessment and treatment of trauma-induced psychoses: the early psychotherapy of H. Breukink and modern views. Int J Clin Exp Hypn 41:191–209, 1993

van der Kolk BA, Fisler R: Dissociation and the fragmentary nature of traumatic memories: overview and exploratory study. J Trauma Stress 8:505–525, 1995

van der Kolk BA, Hostetler A, Herron N, et al: Trauma and the development of borderline personality disorder. Psychiatr Clin North Am 17:715–730, 1994

van der Kolk BA, Pelcovitz D, Roth S, et al: Dissociation, somatization, and affect dysregulation: the complexity of adaptation of trauma. Am J Psychiatry 153 (suppl 7):83–93, 1996

Vanderlinden J, Van Dyck R, Vandereycken W, et al: Dissociative experiences in the general population of the Netherlands and Belgium: a study with the Dissociative Questionnaire (DIS-Q). Dissociation 4:180–184, 1991

Watson S, Chilton R, Fairchild H, et al: Association between childhood trauma and dissociation among patients with borderline personality disorder. Aust N Z J Psychiatry 40:478–481, 2006

Wettstein RM, Fauman BJ: The amobarbital interview. JACEP 8:272–274, 1979

Yargic LI, Sar V, Tutkun H, et al: Comparison of dissociative identity disorder with other diagnostic groups using a structured interview in Turkey. Compr Psychiatry 39:345–351, 1998

Zanarini MC, Ruser TF, Frankenburg FR, et al: Risk factors associated with the dissociative experiences of borderline patients. J Nerv Ment Dis 188:26–30, 2000

Zweig-Frank H, Paris J, Guzder J: Psychological risk factors for dissociation and self-mutilation in female patients with borderline personality disorder. Can J Psychiatry 39:259–264, 1994

# 23

# Sexual Disorders

JUDITH V. BECKER, Ph.D.

JILL D. STINSON, Ph.D.

The classifications of sexual dysfunctions discussed in this chapter are found in DSM-IV-TR (American Psychiatric Association 2000) and are listed in Table 23–1.

## Sexual Dysfunctions

### Male and Female Physiology

It is readily apparent that normal sexual functioning and processes require intact neural and vascular connections to the genitals along with normal endocrine functioning. Any illness that interferes with these systems can lead to sexual dysfunction: neurological diseases (e.g., multiple sclerosis, lumbar or sacral spinal cord trauma, herniated disks), thrombosis of the arteries or veins of the penis, diabetes mellitus (which causes both neurological and vascular damage), endocrine disorders (e.g., hyperprolactinemia), liver disease (which leads to a buildup of estrogen), and so forth.

Similarly, drugs that affect these systems also can impair sexual functioning (see Table 23–2). Thus, antihypertensives, because of their antiadrenergic effects, can impair erectile function in men and vaginal lubrication in women. Antipsychotics, tricyclic antidepressants, and monoamine oxidase inhibitors can inhibit these same functions through their anticholinergic effects. Antipsychotics can impair arousal and orgasm because of their dopamine-blocking effects, whereas serotonin reuptake inhibitors (e.g., fluoxetine, sertraline, paroxetine, fluvoxamine, citalopram) can inhibit arousal and orgasm through their

**TABLE 23–1.** DSM-IV-TR classifications of sexual dysfunctions

**Sexual desire disorders**

Hypoactive sexual desire disorder

Sexual aversion disorder

**Sexual arousal disorders**

Female sexual arousal disorder

Male erectile disorder

**Orgasmic disorders**

Female orgasmic disorder

Male orgasmic disorder

Premature ejaculation

**Sexual pain disorders**

Dyspareunia (not due to a general medical condition)

Vaginismus (not due to a general medical condition)

**Others**

Sexual dysfunction due to a general medical condition

Substance-induced sexual dysfunction

Sexual dysfunction not otherwise specified

serotonergic effects. Spironolactone, steroids, and estrogens can decrease sexual desire through their antiandrogenic effects.

The sexual response cycle of men and women consists of four stages: excitement, plateau, orgasm, and resolution (Masters and Johnson 1966, 1970) (Table 23–3; Figure 23–1).

**TABLE 23–2.     Commonly used medications that may interfere with sexual functioning**

| Abused drugs | Antihypertensives | Antipsychotics | Antidepressants | Others |
|---|---|---|---|---|
| Alcohol | Diuretics | Thioridazine | Tricyclic antidepressants | Cimetidine |
| Marijuana | Methyldopa | Thiothixene | Mirtazapine (rare) | Estrogens |
| Opiates | Clonidine | Chlorpromazine | MAOIs | Steroids |
| Cocaine | Beta-blockers | Perphenazine | Nefazodone (rare) | |
| Amphetamines | Guanethidine | Fluphenazine | Serotonin reuptake inhibitors | |
| MDMA ("Ecstasy") | ACE inhibitors | Risperidone | Trazodone (priapism) | |
| | | Olanzapine | Venlafaxine | |

ACE=angiotensin-converting enzyme; MAOI=monoamine oxidase inhibitor; MDMA=methylenedioxymethamphetamine.

**TABLE 23–3.     Four stages of the sexual response cycle**

## Excitement

Initiated by physical or psychological erotic stimulation

Increases in heart rate, breathing, and blood pressure; vasocongestion in the skin becomes apparent

In males, increased blood flow to the penis and partial erection

In females, increased blood flow to the genitals, vaginal lubrication, and nipples become stiff and erect

## Plateau

Further increases in heart rate, blood flow, and muscle tension

Increase of sexual pleasure with additional stimulation

In males, penis becomes more fully erect and begins to secrete seminal fluid

In females, increased blood flow to and some swelling of the genitals; further lubrication of the vagina

## Orgasm

Both males and females experience quick muscular contractions in pelvic muscles (as well as uterine and vaginal muscles in females) and an associated euphoric sensation; males ejaculate approximately 2–5 mL of semen

## Resolution

Occurs following orgasm; relaxation of muscles and activity of parasympathetic nervous system

Some may return to plateau phase here and experience multiple orgasms, whereas others may not respond to sexual stimulation while in this phase

## Epidemiology

The estimated prevalence of various sexual disorders for men and women is shown in Table 23–4.

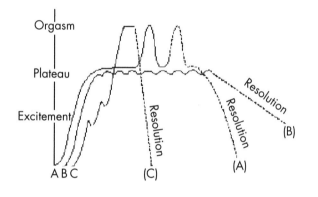

**FIGURE 23–1.     The human sexual response cycle, as seen in three different patients.**

*Source.* Masters and Johnson 1966.

## Etiology

Kaplan (1974) argued for a multicausal theory of sexual dysfunctions, combining intrapsychic, interpersonal, and behavioral characteristics into four factors that play a role in the development of these disorders (Table 23–5).

Other factors may lead to the development of a sexual dysfunction. One such etiological consideration is an unacknowledged homosexual orientation, with attempts to function sexually with a person of the opposite sex. This could lead to decreased sexual desire or arousal as well as difficulties with orgasm. Another factor to consider is the presence of other sexual dysfunctions. Some sexual dysfunctions can lead to secondary sexual problems; for example, a person who does not have erections or cannot achieve orgasm may develop a lack of sexual desire secondary to not experiencing any positive gratification from the sexual interaction. Many sexual problems may be related to sexual trauma. For example, a history of incest,

TABLE 23–4. Prevalence estimates for male and female sexual dysfunctions

**TABLE 23–4.** Prevalence estimates for male and female sexual dysfunctions

| Male sexual dysfunction | % | Female sexual dysfunction | % |
|---|---|---|---|
| Premature ejaculation | 27 | Female hypoactive sexual desire | 33 |
| Male orgasmic disorder | 10 | Female orgasmic disorder | 25 |
| Erectile dysfunction | 10 | Female arousal disorder | 20 |
| Male dyspareunia | 3 | Female dyspareunia | 15 |

*Source.* American Psychiatric Association 2000.

child sexual abuse, or rape may place an individual at risk for developing sexual problems later (Becker et al. 1986; Leonard and Follette 2002). Sexual dysfunctions can occur as secondary to major psychiatric disorders such as schizophrenia, depression, and severe personality disorders. As previously discussed, physical, neurological, and physiological problems can lead to sexual dysfunction. The use of a single medication, or of multiple medications, is one of the most common causes of sexual dysfunction. Medications that may affect sexual functioning are discussed later in this chapter.

## Differential Diagnosis

A number of physiological assessments are also available to supplement the information reported by the patient. Psychophysiological procedures have been developed to assess patients' erections. During rapid eye movement (REM) sleep, men experience penile erections defined as nocturnal penile tumescence (NPT). Although NPT measures can be equivocal, they can be of help in discriminating potential organic factors in a patient with self-reported erectile problems.

**TABLE 23–5.** Multicausal theory of sexual dysfunctions

1. Misinformation or ignorance regarding sexual and social interaction
2. Unconscious guilt and anxiety concerning sex
3. Performance anxiety, as the most common cause of erectile and orgasmic dysfunctions
4. Partners' failure to communicate to each other their sexual feelings and those behaviors in which they want to engage

**TABLE 23–6.** DSM-IV-TR diagnostic criteria for hypoactive sexual desire disorder

A. Persistently or recurrently deficient (or absent) sexual fantasies and desire for sexual activity. The judgment of deficiency or absence is made by the clinician, taking into account factors that affect sexual functioning, such as age and the context of the person's life.

B. The disturbance causes marked distress or interpersonal difficulty.

C. The sexual dysfunction is not better accounted for by another Axis I disorder (except another sexual dysfunction) and is not due exclusively to the direct physiological effects of a substance (e.g., a drug of abuse, a medication) or a general medical condition.

*Specify* type:
   **Lifelong type**
   **Acquired type**
*Specify* type:
   **Situational type**
   **Generalized type**
*Specify*:
   **Due to psychological factors**
   **Due to combined factors**

Typical physiological measures of arousal in females evaluate vaginal blood volume and vaginal pulse amplitude. Vaginal photoplethysmography is perhaps the most commonly used physiological measurement in both research and clinical samples (Hoon et al. 1976; Laan et al. 1995; Sintchak and Geer 1975).

# Descriptions and Treatments of Sexual Dysfunctions

## Sexual Desire Disorders

### Hypoactive Sexual Desire Disorder

The DSM-IV-TR diagnostic criteria for hypoactive sexual desire disorder (also known as inhibited sexual desire) are shown in Table 23–6.

It is also important to determine whether hypoactive sexual desire is the primary problem or the consequence of another underlying sexual problem. Frequently, a male or female who is experiencing either inhibited sexual excitement or an orgasmic problem may develop hypoactive sexual desire because sexual activity is not found to be reinforcing. It is also important to differentiate this disorder, in which there is an absence of sexual desire and fantasies, from sexual aversion, in which there is avoidance of sexual activity because of extreme anxiety. As with the other dysfunctions, this disorder may be lifelong, may occur after a period of good sexual appetite, or may occur only in a certain context (e.g., with the individual's current partner). It is important to assess whether the desire disorder is substance-induced (i.e., due to the effects of drugs or medications). The assessment of individuals with hypoactive sexual desire disorder requires a medical workup, psychological evaluation, and assessment of the relationship.

Hypoactive sexual desire disorder is perhaps the most common sexual complaint among females, but until recently, there was no validated instrument to assess its severity. The Female Sexual Function Index (Rosen et al. 2000), the Sexual Interest and Desire Inventory—Female (Sills et al. 2005), and the Sexual Desire Inventory (Spector et al. 1996) are all measures designed to assess the nature and severity of sexual dysfunction in women who have hypoactive sexual desire.

Hypoactive sexual desire disorder has been the most difficult of all the dysfunctions to treat. Testosterone has been used for both males and females to treat inhibited sexual desire; however, masculinizing side effects make its use problematic in women.

Bupropion sustained-release has also been used in the treatment of hypoactive sexual desire disorder in women. Results from an empirical study evaluating its effectiveness in nondepressed women indicated that 29% of the evaluable participants responded to the treatment (Segraves et al. 2001).

The most effective treatments involve a combination of cognitive therapy to deal with maladaptive beliefs (e.g., that partners must always want sex at the same time), behavioral treatment (e.g., exercises to enhance sexual pleasure and communication), and marital therapy (e.g., to deal with the individual's use of sex to control the relationship). When the problem is secondary to prescription medication, one could consider waiting for the patient to accommodate to the drug, lowering the dose, giving drug holidays, changing to another drug within the same therapeutic class, changing to a new therapeutic class, or adding a pharmacological antidote (although none is currently approved by the U.S. Food and Drug Administration for this purpose) (Finger 2001).

### Sexual Aversion Disorder

The DSM-IV-TR diagnostic criteria for sexual aversion disorder are shown in Table 23–7.

---

**TABLE 23–7. DSM-IV-TR diagnostic criteria for sexual aversion disorder**

A. Persistent or recurrent extreme aversion to, and avoidance of, all (or almost all) genital sexual contact with a sexual partner.

B. The disturbance causes marked distress or interpersonal difficulty.

C. The sexual dysfunction is not better accounted for by another Axis I disorder (except another sexual dysfunction).

*Specify* type:
**Lifelong type**
**Acquired type**

*Specify* type:
**Situational type**
**Generalized type**

*Specify*:
**Due to psychological factors**
**Due to combined factors**

---

The major goal of treatment is to reduce the patient's fear and avoidance of sexual activity. This goal can be accomplished via systematic desensitization. The patient is gradually exposed to sexual scenarios in his or her imagination and then progressively moves toward in vivo exposure to the actual sexual situations that generate anxiety. The successful treatment of sexual phobias using tricyclic antidepressants as well as sex therapy has also been reported (Carey 1998; Kaplan et al. 1982).

## Sexual Arousal Disorders

### Female Sexual Arousal Disorder

The DSM-IV-TR diagnostic criteria for female sexual arousal disorder are shown in Table 23–8.

Treatment of impairment of sexual arousal in women often involves the reduction of anxiety associated with sexual activity. Thus, behavioral techniques such as those involving sensate focus are most often effective (Kaplan 1974). Sensate focus exercises (Masters and Johnson 1970) are techniques in which the patient engages in nongenital,

| TABLE 23–8. DSM-IV-TR diagnostic criteria for female sexual arousal disorder |
| --- |

A. Persistent or recurrent inability to attain, or to maintain until completion of the sexual activity, an adequate lubrication-swelling response of sexual excitement.

B. The disturbance causes marked distress or interpersonal difficulty.

C. The sexual dysfunction is not better accounted for by another Axis I disorder (except another sexual dysfunction) and is not due exclusively to the direct physiological effects of a substance (e.g., a drug of abuse, a medication) or a general medical condition.

*Specify* type:

**Lifelong type**

**Acquired type**

*Specify* type:

**Situational type**

**Generalized type**

*Specify*:

**Due to psychological factors**

**Due to combined factors**

| TABLE 23–9. DSM-IV-TR diagnostic criteria for male erectile disorder |
| --- |

A. Persistent or recurrent inability to attain, or to maintain until completion of the sexual activity, an adequate erection.

B. The disturbance causes marked distress or interpersonal difficulty.

C. The erectile dysfunction is not better accounted for by another Axis I disorder (other than a sexual dysfunction) and is not due exclusively to the direct physiological effects of a substance (e.g., a drug of abuse, a medication) or a general medical condition.

*Specify* type:

**Lifelong type**

**Acquired type**

*Specify* type:

**Situational type**

**Generalized type**

*Specify*:

**Due to psychological factors**

**Due to combined factors**

nondemand caressing with a partner and concentrates on pleasurable feelings. Gradually, the patient engages in pleasurable genital sexual activities (e.g., touch, oral contact), with no penetration permitted until anxiety has been decreased sufficiently.

The pharmacological agent sildenafil also has been described as being successful in the treatment of psychotropic-induced sexual dysfunctions in females. Use of topical alprostadil cream applied to the genital area may also serve as a viable treatment method (Islam et al. 2001; Padma-Nathan et al. 2003).

## Male Erectile Disorder

The DSM-IV-TR diagnostic criteria for male erectile disorder are shown in Table 23–9.

The treatment of erectile problems is generally easier if the patient has a willing sexual partner to participate in therapy. However, treatment is possible without a partner's attendance. Initially, the clinician should inform the patient with male erectile dysfunction that he is not alone in this problem and that, in fact, most men are unable to generate an erection at some time in their lives. Epidemiology research suggests that approximately one-third of

men experience erectile dysfunction, affecting 20%–25% of males younger than 40 years and more than 50% of men age 60 years or older (Heruti et al. 2004; Jackson et al. 2006). Until recently, the most frequently used interventions have been behavioral. However, with the introduction of new pharmacological agents such as sildenafil citrate, tadalafil, and vardenafil—all phosphodiesterase 5 inhibitors that relax smooth muscles in the penis and thereby allow for increased blood flow and engorgement of penile tissues—many patients are opting for a convenient medication as treatment.

A successful treatment for arousal and erectile disorders in patients with partners has been the use of behavioral assignments to gradually decrease performance anxiety. Sensate focus exercises, described earlier, are used to reduce anxiety and increase erectile functioning and show moderate success in decreasing experiences of erectile dysfunction. Group therapy, hypnotherapy, and systematic desensitization also have been used successfully in cases of erectile difficulties. Although psychoanalysis is not indicated in the treatment of simple erectile dysfunction, psychodynamic interventions may be helpful in alleviating intrapsychic conflicts contributing to performance anxiety. Couples therapy also is often helpful in treating these patients (Leiblum and Rosen 1991). Recent comparisons of behavioral and pharmacological treatments suggest that these nonmedical interventions are equally successful at reducing rates of erectile dysfunction in those patients with psychogenic causes of the disorder (Melnik and Abdo 2005).

Various somatic treatments also can be used for erectile disorders, even when these disorders are primarily due to nonorganic factors. Testosterone is often used by nonpsychiatric physicians to treat impotence; however, there is no indication for its use except when erectile problems are due to hypogonadism (O'Carroll and Bancroft 1984; Shabsigh 2005). Vasoactive injections into the corpora cavernosa also can be used to treat erectile disorders and may produce erections lasting up to several hours. Most injections consist of a combination of papaverine (a smooth-muscle relaxant) and phentolamine (an α-adrenergic blocker), although other agents (e.g., prostaglandin E₁) also can be used. Success rates for this treatment are high (about 85%) (Althof et al. 1991). The combination of traditional sex therapy techniques and these injections may be helpful even in those men with purely psychogenic erectile dysfunction (Weiss et al. 1991). However, side effects of the injections, including priapism (i.e., a prolonged, painful erection), fibrotic nodules in the penis, and mild alteration in liver function test results, as well as pain at the site of the injection and limitations on frequent use, often prevent men from using this treatment (Cooper 1991; Levine et al. 1989). Topical medications also may play a role in the treatment of erectile dysfunction by directly relaxing arterial smooth muscle in the penis. Nitroglycerin patches have been found to improve erectile function in about 40% of patients (Meyhoff et al. 1992); the most common side effect is headache.

Early oral medications included the α-adrenergic antagonist yohimbine (Witt 1998) and dopamine agonists such as bromocriptine (Lal et al. 1991), which were beneficial in treating erectile dysfunction. However, the more recent introduction of phosphodiesterase 5 inhibitors such as sildenafil sulfate, tadalafil, and vardenafil has greatly changed the way in which this dysfunction is now treated. These medications operate by releasing nitric oxide into the corpus cavernosum, which then activates the enzyme guanylate cyclase and results in increased levels of cyclic guanosine monophosphate (cGMP). This produces smooth-muscle relaxation in the corpus cavernosum and allows the inflow of blood during sexual stimulation.

A major noninvasive, nonpharmacological treatment for erectile dysfunction is an external vacuum device. The device consists of a plastic cylinder with one end open and the other end connected to a vacuum pump. A vacuum is created that draws blood into the penis. A tension ring is then slipped from the cylinder to the base of the penis for up to 30 minutes.

For men with pure organic or combination organic-psychogenic impotence who do not respond to other treatment measures, penile prostheses can be implanted. Two types are currently available: a bendable silicone implant and an inflatable implant.

## Orgasmic Disorders

### Female Orgasmic Disorder

The DSM-IV-TR diagnostic criteria for female orgasmic disorder are shown in Table 23–10.

TABLE 23–10.    DSM-IV-TR diagnostic criteria for female orgasmic disorder

A. Persistent or recurrent delay in, or absence of, orgasm following a normal sexual excitement phase. Women exhibit wide variability in the type or intensity of stimulation that triggers orgasm. The diagnosis of female orgasmic disorder should be based on the clinician's judgment that the woman's orgasmic capacity is less than would be reasonable for her age, sexual experience, and the adequacy of sexual stimulation she receives.

B. The disturbance causes marked distress or interpersonal difficulty.

C. The orgasmic dysfunction is not better accounted for by another Axis I disorder (except another sexual dysfunction) and is not due exclusively to the direct physiological effects of a substance (e.g., a drug of abuse, a medication) or a general medical condition.

*Specify* type:
   **Lifelong type**
   **Acquired type**
*Specify* type:
   **Situational type**
   **Generalized type**
*Specify*:
   **Due to psychological factors**
   **Due to combined factors**

The most likely way for a woman with general anorgasmia (i.e., never having had an orgasm) to become orgasmic is through a program of directed masturbation (LoPiccolo and Stock 1986). Any discomfort that the patient may feel about exploring her own body should be discussed. Next, the patient should be instructed in a systematic program for exercising the pubococcygeal muscle, a muscle involved in orgasms. Once the patient has mastered these exercises, she should be placed on a masturbatory program that begins with a gradual visual and tactile exploration of her body and moves toward focused genital touching. Use of sexual fantasies combined with stimulation is also taught. The clinician may recommend use of a vibrator if the woman is unable to have an orgasm when engaging in focused genital touching. Once the woman is able to have an orgasm through self-stimulation, she then teaches her sexual partner (using sensate focus exercises) the type of genital stimulation she requires to have an orgasm.

For a woman with anorgasmia, it is imperative to explore the relationship and involve her partner in treatment. Couples therapy, if indicated, and graduated exposure exercises also can be used in treatment. Treatments that focus on communication and relationship skills have been found to have high success rates (Milan et al. 1988).

Communication is vital in the process of assisting anorgasmic women to become orgasmic (Kelly et al. 2006). A recent study assessed communication patterns in heterosexual couples in which the woman was experiencing female orgasmic disorder and compared them with the communication patterns of two groups of control couples. Results indicated that the sexually dysfunctional couples experienced poorer communication, greater blame, and less openness than did the control groups while discussing sexual topics.

The most frequent complaint of women experiencing an orgasmic problem is that they are not orgasmic through penile–vaginal intercourse. When becoming orgasmic through intercourse is a patient's treatment goal, the clinician should ensure that she and her partner are aware that adequate stimulation both before and during intercourse is necessary. In addition, the clinician may suggest various sexual positions that allow stimulation of the clitoris by the patient or her partner during intercourse. For women who are fearful of "letting go" during intercourse, systematic desensitization is often helpful. The therapist may wish to explore with the patient any religious concerns or personal beliefs regarding intercourse and sexual pleasure. Finally, the patient should be told not to expect to have an orgasm every time she has intercourse, given that only a minority of women are regularly orgasmic during intercourse.

Some medications have also been useful in increasing orgasmic responding in women. Sildenafil has been used for the treatment of low arousal and anorgasmia, with 67% of women in two studies reporting an increasing ability to achieve orgasm (Berman et al. 2001; Salerian et al. 2000). Other medications used to treat different sexual dysfunctions also may be useful in increasing orgasmic response in women (Dobkin et al. 2006).

### Male Orgasmic Disorder

The DSM-IV-TR diagnostic criteria for male orgasmic disorder are shown in Table 23–11.

---

**TABLE 23–11.  DSM-IV-TR diagnostic criteria for male orgasmic disorder**

A.  Persistent or recurrent delay in, or absence of, orgasm following a normal sexual excitement phase during sexual activity that the clinician, taking into account the person's age, judges to be adequate in focus, intensity, and duration.

B.  The disturbance causes marked distress or interpersonal difficulty.

C.  The orgasmic dysfunction is not better accounted for by another Axis I disorder (except another sexual dysfunction) and is not due exclusively to the direct physiological effects of a substance (e.g., a drug of abuse, a medication) or a general medical condition.

*Specify* type:
   **Lifelong type**
   **Acquired type**

*Specify* type:
   **Situational type**
   **Generalized type**

*Specify*:
   **Due to psychological factors**
   **Due to combined factors**

---

The treatment of male orgasmic disorder is similar to that of female orgasmic disorder. The patient should be told that when he masturbates, he should masturbate as quickly as possible to ejaculation while fantasizing that his penis is inside his partner's vagina and ejaculating. A second technique is to teach the patient and his partner sensate focus exercises. If the patient is able to masturbate in the presence of his partner, he is instructed to place his partner's hand over his so that she can see how much touching he requires. He should then place his hand over hers while she masturbates him to ejaculation. Finally, she should sit astride him and stimulate him, eventually putting his penis in her vagina when he reaches the point of ejaculatory inevitability. If a man is uncomfortable ejaculating in the presence of his partner, systematic desensitization is used to help him become more comfortable in her presence.

Much like females with orgasmic disorder or other sexual dysfunctions, males with psychotropically induced orgasmic disorder also show improvement after taking sildenafil (Salerian et al. 2000), with approximately 77% reporting increased orgasmic functioning. Imipramine also has shown success in treating psychotropically induced orgasmic dysfunction in male patients (Aizenburg et al. 1996).

### Premature Ejaculation

The DSM-IV-TR diagnostic criteria for premature ejaculation are shown in Table 23–12.

---

**TABLE 23–12.    DSM-IV-TR diagnostic criteria for premature ejaculation**

A. Persistent or recurrent ejaculation with minimal sexual stimulation before, on, or shortly after penetration and before the person wishes it. The clinician must take into account factors that affect duration of the excitement phase, such as age, novelty of the sexual partner or situation, and recent frequency of sexual activity.

B. The disturbance causes marked distress or interpersonal difficulty.

C. The premature ejaculation is not due exclusively to the direct effects of a substance (e.g., withdrawal from opioids).

*Specify* type:
   **Lifelong type**
   **Acquired type**

*Specify* type:
   **Situational type**
   **Generalized type**

*Specify*:
   **Due to psychological factors**
   **Due to combined factors**

---

Premature ejaculation is the most prevalent of all male sexual problems. The treatment of premature ejaculation can involve training the individual to tolerate high levels of excitement without ejaculating, and reducing anxiety associated with sexual arousal. One successful intervention is the start–stop technique (Semans 1956). This procedure involves having the patient lie on his back while his partner strokes his penis. The patient then focuses on the pleasurable feelings resulting from the penile stimulation and the sensations that precede his urge to ejaculate. When he feels that he is about to ejaculate, he signals his partner to stop stimulation. The patient should start and stop at least four times before he allows himself to ejaculate.

A second procedure, the "squeeze" technique (Masters and Johnson 1970), can be done in conjunction with the start–stop technique. In the squeeze technique, the patient's partner is taught to place her thumb on the frenulum of the penis and her first and second fingers on the opposite sides of the head of the penis. When the patient feels that he is going to ejaculate, the partner squeezes for up to 5 seconds and then releases the penis for up to 30 seconds. This technique is continued until the individual is no longer on the verge of ejaculating, at which time the patient's partner then resumes penile stimulation.

Several subtypes of biogenic and psychogenic premature ejaculation have been identified (Metz and Pryor 2000). Biogenic types include 1) neurological constitution, 2) physical illness, 3) physical injury, and 4) pharmacological side effects. Medical conditions that can contribute to premature ejaculation include arteriosclerosis, benign prostatic hyperplasia, cardiovascular disease, diabetes, injury to the sympathetic nervous system, pelvic injuries, prostate cancer, prostatitis, urethritis, urinary incontinence, polycythemia, and polyneuritis (Baum and Spieler 2001). Psychogenic types consist of 1) psychological constitution or chronic psychological disorders, 2) psychological distress, and 3) psychosexual skills deficit. A fourth psychogenic subtype is concomitant with another sexual dysfunction. Specific treatments for this disorder should be determined following a comprehensive assessment of the relevant subtype (Metz and Pryor 2000).

A new functional–sexological treatment for premature ejaculation has been recently introduced (de Carufel and Trudel 2006) and involves the modulation of sexual excitement through several techniques. Men are instructed in specific ways of altering their typical bodily movements and positioning during sexual intercourse, the use of positions that require less muscular tension, variations in the speed and intensity of pelvic movements, and breathing involving the diaphragm, and are provided education regarding sensuality and the sexual responses of men and women. When compared with traditional behavioral treatments, including the squeeze and start–stop techniques, this functional–sexological treatment shows similar effectiveness in improving subjective duration of intercourse, sexual satisfaction, and satisfaction with overall treatment results.

Somatic treatments for premature ejaculation have included intracavernous injection of papaverine and phentolamine (Fein 1990) and the use of oral medications such as the tricyclic antidepressant clomipramine (Richardson and Goldmeier 2005; Segraves et al. 1993; Strassberg et al. 1999) and selective serotonin reuptake inhibitors (Baum and Spieler 2001; Richardson and Goldmeier 2005; Waldinger et al. 2003), which can decrease libido and delay orgasm, as well as oral analgesics such as tramadol (Safarinejad and Hosseini 2006), which reduce penile sensation. Other potential somatic interventions include topical agents such as SS-cream, which can cause mild penile burning or pain, or anesthetic creams, which may cause penile numbness (Baum and Spieler 2001; Richardson and Goldmeier 2005). Chloraseptic mouthwash may also retard sexual stimulation and result in increased ejaculation latency (Baum and Spieler 2001). However, many of these medications and somatic interventions may lead to negative side effects that should be discussed with the patient (Althof 1995; de Carufel and Trudel 2006).

## Sexual Pain Disorders

### *Dyspareunia*

The DSM-IV-TR diagnostic criteria for dyspareunia are shown in Table 23–13.

It is imperative that a comprehensive physical and gynecological or urological examination be conducted. In the absence of organic pathology, the patient's fear and anxiety underlying sexual functioning should be investigated. Systematic desensitization has been found to be successful in the treatment of this disorder in some women. Physiotherapy also has been recommended as a potential treatment for dyspareunia and involves several techniques designed to decrease pelvic and vulvar pain and increase circulation and muscular mobility and flexibility in these regions (Graziottin and Brotto 2004; Rosenbaum 2005). A diagnosis incorporating medical as well as psychosexual factors is a crucial step in the effective treatment of this disorder (Graziottin 2001). Therefore, in addition to the physiological interventions described earlier, therapy related to the individual's or couple's psychosexual issues also may be beneficial.

---

**TABLE 23–13. DSM-IV-TR diagnostic criteria for dyspareunia**

A. Recurrent or persistent genital pain associated with sexual intercourse in either a male or a female.

B. The disturbance causes marked distress or interpersonal difficulty.

C. The disturbance is not caused exclusively by vaginismus or lack of lubrication, is not better accounted for by another Axis I disorder (except another sexual dysfunction), and is not due exclusively to the direct physiological effects of a substance (e.g., a drug of abuse, a medication) or a general medical condition.

*Specify* type:
   **Lifelong type**
   **Acquired type**

*Specify* type:
   **Situational type**
   **Generalized type**

*Specify*:
   **Due to psychological factors**
   **Due to combined factors**

---

### *Vaginismus*

The DSM-IV-TR diagnostic criteria for vaginismus are shown in Table 23–14.

Vaginismus can be diagnosed with certainty only through a gynecological examination. Some women who are anxious about sex may experience muscular tightening and some pain during penetration, but these women do not have vaginismus. It is important to rule out other Axis I disorders (e.g., somatization disorder), substance-induced disorders, or a general medical condition.

Systematic desensitization has been the most effective treatment method for vaginismus. A useful procedure involves the systematic insertion of dilators of graduated sizes, either in the physician's office or in the privacy of the patient's home. Some clinicians have the patient or her partner gradually insert a tampon or fingers until penile penetration can be effected (Kaplan 1974). The clinician may suggest that the patient gently stroke her genitals, including her clitoris, during the insertion procedure. Additionally, penile penetration should be effected with the partner lying on his back and the patient controlling the actual insertion and subsequent movement during intercourse. Follow-up studies have reported maintenance

---

**TABLE 23–14.   DSM-IV-TR diagnostic criteria for vaginismus**

A. Recurrent or persistent involuntary spasm of the musculature of the outer third of the vagina that interferes with sexual intercourse.

B. The disturbance causes marked distress or interpersonal difficulty.

C. The disturbance is not better accounted for by another Axis I disorder (e.g., somatization disorder) and is not due exclusively to the direct physiological effects of a general medical condition.

*Specify* type:
   **Lifelong type**
   **Acquired type**

*Specify* type:
   **Situational type**
   **Generalized type**

*Specify*:
   **Due to psychological factors**
   **Due to combined factors**

---

of treatment gains over time for most women (Scholl 1988). As described earlier in the chapter, physiotherapy with targeted relaxation and desensitization procedures also may be useful in the treatment of this disorder (Rosenbaum 2005).

## Sexual Dysfunction Due to a General Medical Condition

The diagnosis of sexual dysfunction due to a general medical condition is made if there is evidence from the history, physical examination, or laboratory findings of a general medical condition judged to be etiologically related to the sexual dysfunction (e.g., male erectile disorder due to a general medical condition, dyspareunia due to a general medical condition). Several examples of medical conditions associated with sexual dysfunction were listed in the beginning of this chapter, including those that interfere with circulation and normative endocrine functioning.

## Substance-Induced Sexual Dysfunction

A number of substances have shown an adverse effect on sexual functioning (see Table 23–2). Alcohol, psychomotor stimulants such as cocaine or amphetamines, opiates, antipsychotic medications, antidepressants, sedatives, and marijuana may reduce sexual arousal in both males and females when used at high doses or over a long period of time. Chronic use of cocaine or amphetamines, as well as typical use of some antipsychotic medications, can impair the ejaculatory response in males.

These drugs of abuse can impair sexual functioning through various mechanisms, which were briefly discussed at the beginning of this chapter. Cocaine may impair sexual functioning because of its ability to deplete dopamine stores with chronic use. Chronic opiate and alcohol use also may interfere with endogenous dopamine and serotonin functioning, leading to impaired sexual functioning. Long-term opiate use also may reduce testosterone levels in the body, thereby decreasing normal sexual arousal. A similar but temporary effect may be seen after marijuana use. Evidence also suggests that the negative effects of methylenedioxymethamphetamine (MDMA; "Ecstasy") on the brain's serotonergic systems can lead to significant sexual dysfunction in heavy or chronic users (Parrott 2006).

# Key Points: Sexual Disorders

- Sexual dysfunctions are divided into four primary categories: sexual desire disorders, sexual arousal disorders, orgasmic disorders, and sexual pain disorders. DSM-IV-TR diagnostic criteria for each of these categories are outlined in this chapter.

- Sexual dysfunctions are relatively common disorders in both males and females, affecting up to 20%–30% of the population at some point in their lives. Improvements in assessment and diagnosis have increased our understanding of sexual dysfunction and its variation across the life span.

- Causes of sexual dysfunction are numerous and varied, with external influences such as disease, medication, or substance use and internal influences such as anxiety, other psychological disorders, or lack of communication regarding sexual interests or desires all playing a role.

- Treatments for sexual dysfunctions often involve a combination of psychological and behavioral interventions. Recent advances in pharmacological agents designed to affect sexual performance have also helped in the treatment of sexual dysfunctions, particularly male orgasmic disorders. Successful treatment may require addressing both psychogenic and physiological etiologies of the dysfunction.

# References

Aizenburg D, Shiloh R, Zemishlany Z, et al: Low-dose imipramine for thioridazine-induced male orgasmic disorder. J Sex Marital Ther 22:225–229, 1996

Althof SE: Pharmacological treatment for rapid ejaculation: preliminary strategies, concerns, and questions. Sex Marital Ther 10:247–251, 1995

Althof SE, Turner LA, Levine SB, et al: Sexual, psychological, and marital impact of self-injection of papaverine and phentolamine: a long-term prospective study. J Sex Marital Ther 17:101–112, 1991

American Psychiatric Association: Diagnostic and Statistical Manual of Mental Disorders, 4th Edition, Text Revision. Washington, DC, American Psychiatric Association, 2000

Baum N, Spieler B: Medical management of premature ejaculation. Med Aspects Hum Sex 1:15–25, 2001

Becker JV, Skinner LJ, Abel GG, et al: Level of postassault sexual functioning in rape and incest victims. Arch Sex Behav 15:37–49, 1986

Berman JR, Berman LA, Lin H, et al: Effect of sildenafil on subjective and physiologic parameters of the female sexual response in women with sexual arousal disorder. J Sex Marital Ther 27:411–420, 2001

Carey MP: Cognitive-behavioral treatment of sexual dysfunctions, in International Handbook of Cognitive and Behavioural Treatments for Psychological Disorders. Edited by Caballo VE. Oxford, England, Pergamon/Elsevier Science, 1998, pp 251–280

Cooper AJ: Evaluation of I-C papaverine in patients with psychogenic and organic impotence. Can J Psychiatry 36:574–578, 1991

de Carufel F, Trudel G: Effects of a new functional-sexological treatment for premature ejaculation. J Sex Marital Ther 32:97–114, 2006

Dobkin RD, Menza M, Marin H, et al: Bupropion improves sexual functioning in depressed minority women: an open-label switch study. J Clin Psychopharmacol 26:21–26, 2006

Fein RL: Intracavernous medication for treatment of premature ejaculation. Urology 35:301–303, 1990

Finger WW: Antidepressants and sexual dysfunction: managing common treatment pitfalls. Med Aspects Hum Sex 1:12–18, 2001

Graziottin A: Clinical approaches to dyspareunia. J Sex Marital Ther 27:489–501, 2001

Graziottin A, Brotto LA: Vulvar vestibulitis syndrome: a clinical approach. J Sex Marital Ther 30:125–139, 2004

Heruti R, Shochat T, Tekes-Manova D, et al: Prevalence of erectile dysfunction among young adults: results of a large-scale survey. J Sex Med 1:284–291, 2004

Hoon PW, Wincze JP, Hoon EF: Physiological assessment of sexual arousal in women. Psychophysiology 13:196–204, 1976

Islam A, Mitchel J, Rosen R, et al: Topical alprostadil in the treatment of female sexual arousal disorder: a pilot study. J Sex Marital Ther 27:531–540, 2001

Jackson G, Rosen RC, Kloner RA, et al: The second Princeton consensus on sexual dysfunction and cardiac risk: new guidelines for sexual medicine. J Sex Med 3:28–36, 2006

Kaplan HS: The New Sex Therapy: Active Treatment of Sexual Dysfunctions. New York, Brunner/Mazel, 1974

Kaplan HS, Fyer AJ, Novick A: The treatment of sexual phobias: the combined use of antipanic medication and sex therapy. J Sex Marital Ther 8:3–28, 1982

Kelly MP, Strassberg DS, Turner CM: Behavioral assessment of couples' communication in female orgasmic disorder. J Sex Marital Ther 32:81–95, 2006

Laan E, Everaerd W, Evers A: Assessment of female sexual arousal: response specificity and construct validity. Psychophysiology 32:476–485, 1995

Lal S, Kiely ME, Thavundayil JX, et al: Effect of bromocriptine in patients with apomorphine-responsive erectile impotence: an open study. J Psychiatry Neurosci 16:262–266, 1991

Leiblum SR, Rosen RC: Couples therapy for erectile disorders: conceptual and clinical considerations. J Sex Marital Ther 17:147–159, 1991

Leonard LM, Follette VM: Sexual functioning in women reporting a history of child sexual abuse: review of the empirical literature and clinical implications. Annu Rev Sex Res 13:346–388, 2002

Levine SB, Althof SE, Turner LA, et al: Side effects of self-administration of intracavernous papaverine and phentolamine for the treatment of impotence. J Urol 141:54–57, 1989

LoPiccolo J, Stock WE: Treatment of sexual dysfunction. J Consult Clin Psychol 54:158–167, 1986

Masters WH, Johnson VE: Human Sexual Response. Boston, MA, Little, Brown, 1966

Masters WH, Johnson VE: Human Sexual Inadequacy. Boston, MA, Little, Brown, 1970

Melnik T, Abdo CHN: Psychogenic erectile dysfunction: comparative study of three therapeutic approaches. J Sex Marital Ther 31:243–255, 2005

Metz ME, Pryor JL: Premature ejaculation: a psychophysiological approach for assessment and management. J Sex Marital Ther 26:293–320, 2000

Meyhoff HH, Rosenkilde P, Bodker A: Non-invasive management of impotence with transcutaneous nitroglycerin. Br J Urol 69:88–90, 1992

Milan RJ Jr, Kilmann PR, Boland JP: Treatment outcome of secondary orgasmic dysfunction: a two- to six-year follow-up. Arch Sex Behav 17:463–480, 1988

O'Carroll R, Bancroft J: Testosterone therapy for low sexual interest and erectile dysfunctions in men: a controlled study. Br J Psychiatry 145:146–151, 1984

Padma-Nathan H, Brown C, Fendl J, et al: Efficacy and safety of topical alprostadil cream for the treatment of female sexual arousal disorder (FSAD): a double-blind, multicenter, randomized, and placebo-controlled clinical trial. J Sex Marital Ther 29:329–344, 2003

Parrott AC: MDMA in humans: factors which affect the neuropsychobiological profiles of recreational ecstasy users, the integrative role of bioenergetic stress. J Psychopharmacol 20:147–163, 2006

Richardson D, Goldmeier D: Pharmacological treatment for premature ejaculation. Int J STD AIDS 16:709–711, 2005

Rosen R, Brown C, Heiman J, et al: The Female Sexual Function Index (FSFI): a multidimensional self-report instrument for the assessment of female sexual function. J Sex Marital Ther 26:191–208, 2000

Rosenbaum TY: Physiotherapy treatment of sexual pain disorders. J Sex Marital Ther 31:329–340, 2005

Safarinejad MR, Hosseini SY: Pharmacotherapy for premature ejaculation. Current Drug Therapy 1:37–46, 2006

Salerian AJ, Vittone BJ, Geyer SP, et al: Sildenafil for psychotropic-induced sexual dysfunction in 31 women and 61 men. J Sex Marital Ther 26:133–140, 2000

Scholl GM: Prognostic variables in treating vaginismus. Obstet Gynecol 72:231–235, 1988

Segraves RT, Saran A, Segraves K, et al: Clomipramine versus placebo in the treatment of premature ejaculation: a pilot study. J Sex Marital Ther 19:198–200, 1993

Segraves RT, Croft H, Kavoussi R, et al: Bupropion sustained release (SR) for the treatment of hypoactive sexual desire disorder (HSDD) in nondepressed women. J Sex Marital Ther 27:303–316, 2001

Semans JH: Premature ejaculation: a new approach. South Med J 9:353–357, 1956

Shabsigh R: Testosterone therapy in erectile dysfunction and hypogonadism. J Sex Med 2:785–792, 2005

Sills T, Wunderlich G, Pyke R, et al: The Sexual Interest and Desire Inventory—Female (SIDI-F): item response analyses of data from women diagnosed with hypoactive sexual desire disorder. J Sex Med 2:801–818, 2005

Sintchak G, Geer JH: A vaginal plethysmograph system. Psychophysiology 12:113–115, 1975

Spector IP, Carey MP, Steinberg L: The Sexual Desire Inventory: development, factor structure, and evidence of reliability. J Sex Marital Ther 22:175–190, 1996

Strassberg DS, de Gouveia Brazao CA, Rowland DL, et al: Clomipramine in the treatment of rapid (premature) ejaculation. J Sex Marital Ther 25:89–101, 1999

Waldinger MD, Zwinderman AH, Olivier B: Antidepressants and ejaculation: a double-blind, randomized, fixed-dose study with mirtazapine and paroxetine. J Clin Psychopharmacol 23:467–470, 2003

Weiss JN, Ravalli R, Badlani GH: Intracavernous pharmacotherapy in psychogenic impotence. Urology 37:441–443, 1991

Witt DK: Yohimbine for erectile dysfunction. J Fam Pract 46:282–283, 1998

# 24

# Gender Identity Disorders and Paraphilias

JUDITH V. BECKER, Ph.D.

BRADLEY R. JOHNSON, M.D.

## Gender Identity Disorders

### Criteria for Diagnosing Gender Identity Disorder

Currently, it is accepted that there are two necessary components of gender identity disorder: a strong and persistent cross-gender identification (not merely a desire for any perceived cultural advantages of being the other sex) and a persistent discomfort with one's sex or sense of inappropriateness in the gender role of that sex (Table 24–1). The diagnosis is not given if the person has a concurrent physical condition such as partial androgen insensitivity syndrome or congenital adrenal hyperplasia, and as with many other diagnoses in DSM-IV-TR, there must be evidence of clinically significant distress or impairment (American Psychiatric Association 2000).

### Gender Identity Disorder of Adulthood

#### Epidemiology

Gender identity disorder of adulthood is thought to be rare, with prior estimates of 30,000 cases worldwide (Lothstein 1980). Approximately 1 per 30,000 adult men and 1 per 100,000 women seek sex reassignment surgery (American Psychiatric Association 2000). Transsexual individuals most commonly request *sex reassignment*—that is, change in their physical appearance (usually by hor-

monal and surgical means) to correspond with their self-perceived gender. However, it is important to remember that not all those who seek sex reassignment are transsexual; cross-gender wishes may occur in transvestism (i.e., wearing opposite-gender clothes for erotic purposes) or effeminate homosexuality in men.

#### Comorbidity

Among those adults who are diagnosed as having gender identity disorder, there is a high degree of concomitant psychiatric disorder, most commonly borderline, antisocial, or narcissistic personality disorder; substance abuse; and suicidal or self-destructive behavior (J.K. Meyer 1982).

#### Etiology

Gender identity appears to be established and influenced by psychosocial factors during the first few years of life. However, many authors have argued that biological factors, if not causative, may predispose an individual to a gender identity disorder.

#### Diagnosis and Evaluation

Individuals who request sex reassignment require careful evaluation by a psychiatrist or psychologist with experience in the management of gender identity disorders. They should undergo a complete psychosexual evaluation, in addition to a thorough psychiatric or psychological exam-

---

**TABLE 24–1.    DSM-IV-TR diagnostic criteria for gender identity disorder**

---

A.  A strong and persistent cross-gender identification (not merely a desire for any perceived cultural advantages of being the other sex).

    In children, the disturbance is manifested by four (or more) of the following:

    (1)  repeatedly stated desire to be, or insistence that he or she is, the other sex

    (2)  in boys, preference for cross-dressing or simulating female attire; in girls, insistence on wearing only stereotypical masculine clothing

    (3)  strong and persistent preferences for cross-sex roles in make-believe play or persistent fantasies of being the other sex

    (4)  intense desire to participate in the stereotypical games and pastimes of the other sex

    (5)  strong preference for playmates of the other sex

    In adolescents and adults, the disturbance is manifested by symptoms such as a stated desire to be the other sex, frequent passing as the other sex, desire to live or be treated as the other sex, or the conviction that he or she has the typical feelings and reactions of the other sex.

B.  Persistent discomfort with his or her sex or sense of inappropriateness in the gender role of that sex.

    In children, the disturbance is manifested by any of the following: in boys, assertion that his penis or testes are disgusting or will disappear or assertion that it would be better not to have a penis, or aversion toward rough-and-tumble play and rejection of male stereotypical toys, games, and activities; in girls, rejection of urinating in a sitting position, assertion that she has or will grow a penis, or assertion that she does not want to grow breasts or menstruate, or marked aversion toward normative feminine clothing.

    In adolescents and adults, the disturbance is manifested by symptoms such as preoccupation with getting rid of primary and secondary sex characteristics (e.g., request for hormones, surgery, or other procedures to physically alter sexual characteristics to simulate the other sex) or belief that he or she was born the wrong sex.

C.  The disturbance is not concurrent with a physical intersex condition.

D.  The disturbance causes clinically significant distress or impairment in social, occupational, or other important areas of functioning.

*Code* based on current age:

    **302.6    Gender identity disorder in children**

    **302.85  Gender identity disorder in adolescents or adults**

*Specify* if (for sexually mature individuals):

    **Sexually attracted to males**

    **Sexually attracted to females**

    **Sexually attracted to both**

    **Sexually attracted to neither**

---

ination. Patients with other primary psychiatric diagnoses may present as transsexuals. Psychotic patients may have delusions centered around their genitalia (e.g., that someone has substituted the incorrect genitals, that God is telling them to change their sex). When the psychosis is treated, the cross-gender wishes usually resolve. Individuals with severe personality disorders, especially borderline, can have transient wishes to change gender as part of their overall identity diffusion during times of stress. Effeminate homosexual men may desire to change sex in order to be more attractive to men; usually this desire fluctuates with time. Transvestites (described in the "Paraphilias" section later in this chapter) are heterosexual men aroused by wearing female garments. To increase their arousal, they may progress to actually wishing to become a woman; again, however, this wish is usually not continuous over a long period, and their gender identity is male. Adolescents sometimes become gender dysphoric because of developing homosexual feelings that need to be resolved.

## Treatment

Because most gender dysphoric individuals have adamant requests for sex reassignment (many often are already taking opposite-sex hormones supplied by other physicians), it is extremely difficult to engage these patients in treatment with anything other than surgical sex reassignment as the goal. However, because surgery is irreversible, it is important to engage these patients in psychotherapy, even if surgery is indicated. The therapist should be careful to base the goals of therapy on what is desired by the patient. These goals should be identified at the beginning of therapy, including a discussion on informed consent as to the possible outcomes and complications that could arise secondary to the use of psychotherapy.

Supportive psychotherapy can serve various purposes in transsexual individuals. First, there have been reports, albeit few, of reversal of patients' gender identity disorders. Second, a trial of psychotherapy is often useful in cases in which the diagnosis is not clear. Third, dealing with patients' fears of homosexuality may sometimes change their wishes for surgical reassignments. Fourth, psychotherapy plays an important role in patients' adjustment to the process of sex reassignment. Finally, therapy is often helpful in the postsurgical adjustment of patients with gender identity disorder.

Sexual reassignment to the opposite sex has been the most widely used and studied treatment modality for adults with gender identity disorder. Early reports of outcome were extremely positive, with dramatic changes in social functioning and satisfaction. Hormonal treatment and surgery have become more readily available for adults with gender identity disorder, often with little preparation other than a brief consultation with a psychiatrist. This approach led to an increase in the reports of poor results and realization that sex reassignment is not a panacea. Clinicians who are considering providing services to gender dysphoric patients should familiarize themselves with *The Standards of Care for Gender Identity Disorders* (M. Meyer et al. 2001), which is published by the Harry Benjamin International Gender Dysphoria Association.

Sex reassignment is a long process that must be carefully monitored. Patients with other primary psychiatric diagnoses and secondary transsexuals should be screened out and given other appropriate treatment. If the patient is considered appropriate for sex reassignment, psychotherapy should be started to prepare the patient for the cross-gender role. The patient should then go out into the world and live in the cross-gender role before surgical reassignment. After 1–2 years, if these measures have been successful and the patient still wishes reassignment, hor-

mone treatment is begun. After 1–2 years of hormone therapy, the patient may be considered for surgical reassignment if such a procedure is still desired. In the male-to-female patient, this consists of bilateral orchiectomy, penile amputation, and creation of an artificial vagina. Female-to-male patients undergo bilateral mastectomy and optional hysterectomy with removal of ovaries. Efforts to create an artificial penis have met with mixed results thus far; at this point, it is better to counsel the patient to focus on mutual body caressing, oral-genital stimulation, and other forms of sexual pleasuring that do not necessarily involve having a penis sufficient for vaginal penetration. Overall cosmetic and functional results from surgery have been variable in both male and female transsexuals. *The Standards of Care for Gender Identity Disorders* states, "benefit from psychotherapy may be attained at every stage of gender evolution" including "the postsurgical period when the anatomic obstacles to gender comfort have been removed and the person continues to feel a lack of genuine comfort and skill in living in the new gender role" (M. Meyer et al. 2001).

## Gender Identity Disorder of Childhood

### Prevalence and Etiology

One study looking at children referred to a specificity clinic for gender identity disorder from the period 1978–1995 found a boy-to-girl sex ratio of 6.6:1 (Zucker et al. 1997). As with adult gender dysphoria, the etiology of childhood gender identity disorder is unclear.

### Physical Appearance

It is interesting to note that several studies have associated gender identity disorder with greater physical attractiveness in boys when compared with the physical attractiveness of clinical control subjects who did not have the disorder (Green 1987; Zucker et al. 1993). Fridell et al. (1996) concluded that girls with gender identity disorder often were seen as less attractive than those in a control group.

### Course

Retrospective studies of transsexuals (Green 1974) have shown a high incidence of childhood cross-gender behavior. There appear to be two main pathways to adult gender identity disorder, one that involves childhood gender identity disorder and one that develops in early to middle adulthood, sometimes concurrent with transvestic fetishism (American Psychiatric Association 2000). Longitudinal research with boys who have gender identity disorder and a comparison group found that a large proportion of the boys with gender identity disorder (about 68%) were bisexually or homosexually oriented, whereas none of a demographically matched comparison sample reported a bisexual or homosexual orientation (Green 1985). According to the American Psychiatric Association (2000, p. 580), "only a very small number of children with GID [gender identity disorder] will continue to have symptoms that meet criteria in adolescence or adulthood" and "by late adolescence or adulthood, about three-quarters of boys who had a childhood history of Gender Identity Disorder report a homosexual or bisexual orientation, but without concurrent Gender Identity Disorder." The proportion of female children with gender identity disorder who report bisexual or homosexual orientation in adolescence and adulthood is unknown.

### Treatment

A comprehensive assessment is required to provide appropriate services to a child with gender identity disorder. Hormonal or surgical therapies should not be considered for this age group. M. Meyer et al. (2001) recommend that

1. The professional recognize and accept the gender identity problem.
2. The assessment explore the nature and characteristics of the child's or adolescent's gender identity.
3. Therapy focus on ameliorating any comorbid problems in the child's life and on reducing distress the child experiences from his or her gender identity problem and other difficulties.

Not all children with childhood gender identity disorder will develop the adult disorder. Consequently, when a child presents with gender identity disorder, the clinician should assess what is in the best interest of the child, considering parental concerns and the child's wishes. Unfortunately, such children can be subject to social ostracism; therefore, support needs to be provided to the child, and parents may be given information as to how best to protect their child from harassment. Zucker and Bradley (1995) stated that treatment has three goals: increasing peer support and acceptance, treating co-occurring mental health concerns, and reducing the likelihood of transsexualism in adulthood (Zucker and Bradley 1995). Behavior therapy has been used in the past to modify specific cross-gender behaviors in a manner similar to that described for adults as well as to enhance contingency management (e.g.,

reinforcing behaviors consistent with the child's phenotype sex). Analytically oriented treatment has dealt with the family dynamics (e.g., a powerful, masculine-devaluing mother; an ineffective, emotionally absent father) and individual dynamics (e.g., castration anxiety following surgery) of the child.

In treating adolescents with gender identity disorder, clinicians should take a conservative approach, given that a hallmark of adolescence involves identity issues. As with young children, therapy may involve individual and family therapy. The adolescents also need to learn coping skills to deal with any harassment or ostracism they may experience. M. Meyer et al. (2001) indicated that adolescents may be eligible for fully and partially reversible physical interventions.

## Paraphilias

The paraphilias (Table 24–2) are characterized by experiencing, over a period of at least 6 months, "recurrent, intense sexually arousing fantasies, sexual urges, or behaviors" (American Psychiatric Association 2000, p. 566) generally involving nonhuman objects or nonconsenting partners.

## Types of Paraphilias

### Exhibitionism

*Exhibitionism* is defined as the exposure of one's genitals to an unsuspecting person or stranger. It may involve masturbation during the exposure, and in some cases the individual tries to surprise or shock the observer. The individual may hope or desire that the observer will become sexually aroused or join in the sexual activity. It is generally thought to be a disorder of males, sometimes has an early onset (before age 18 years), and is directed primarily at females (Murphy 1997). As with many types of paraphilias, there are no good personality profiles for exhibitionists (Blair and Lanyon 1981). Few arrests occur in offenders older than 40, suggesting that the condition may become less common after about 40 years of age (American Psychiatric Association 2000).

### Fetishism

*Fetishism* is sexual arousal involving the use of nonliving objects such as women's underpants, bras, stockings, shoes, boots, or other apparel (American Psychiatric Association 2000). Masturbation may accompany the person holding, rubbing, or smelling the item. In general, the person may

**TABLE 24–2.  Paraphilias**

| | |
|---|---|
| Exhibitionism | Exposure of genitals to an unsuspecting stranger |
| Fetishism | Arousal to nonliving objects |
| Frotteurism | Touching and rubbing against a nonconsenting person |
| Pedophilia | Urges and fantasies involving prepubescent children |
| Sexual masochism | Deriving sexual excitement from being humiliated, beaten, bound, or otherwise made to suffer |
| Sexual sadism | Urges and fantasies of acts in which psychological and/or physical suffering of the victim is sexually exciting |
| Transvestic fetishism | Urges and fantasies involving cross-dressing |
| Voyeurism | Observing an unsuspecting person naked, disrobing, or engaged in sex |
| Necrophilia | Contact with corpses |
| Urophilia | Urine |
| Zoophilia | Animals |
| Klismaphilia | Enemas |
| Telephone scatologia | Obscene telephone calls |
| Partialism | Exclusive focus on one part of body |

have difficulty in getting sexually aroused in the absence of the item. Mason (1997) concluded that this paraphilia appears to be more common in males than females.

## Frotteurism

*Frotteurism* involves touching and rubbing against another nonconsenting person (American Psychiatric Association 2000). It frequently takes place in crowded places such as on a bus or subway, in a crowded hall, or on a busy sidewalk. Although there are many different ways that a person can engage in frotteuristic activity, it is not uncommon that a male would rub his genitals against the unsuspecting victim; however, the behavior may include touching or rubbing the genitals or sexual organs of victims without their being aware that they have been offended.

## Pedophilia

*Pedophilia* is defined as sexual attraction to, or sexual behavior involving, a prepubescent boy or girl, generally age 13 or younger. By definition, in order for a diagnosis of pedophilia to be made, the individual must be at least 16 years old and at least 5 years older than the child. It is not uncommon for an individual with pedophilia to have a certain age range of child to which he or she is sexually attracted, and the attraction can be gender specific or to both male and female children. There are specifiers listed in DSM-IV-TR (American Psychiatric Association 2000), including being limited to incest, exclusive type (attracted only to children), and nonexclusive type.

## Sexual Masochism

The diagnostic criteria for *sexual masochism* are intense sexually arousing fantasies, urges, or behaviors involving the act, whether real or simulated, of "being humiliated, beaten, bound, or otherwise made to suffer" (American Psychiatric Association 2000, p. 573). Such acts may include restraint, blindfolding, paddling, spanking, whipping, beating, electrical shocks, cutting, piercing, and humiliating acts such as being urinated on or defecated on. *Hypoxyphilia* is a dangerous and potentially life-threatening form of sexual masochism that involves sexual arousal by oxygen deprivation through a number of possible means.

## Sexual Sadism

*Sexual sadism* involves real acts (not simulated) in which sexual arousal is achieved from the psychological or physical suffering of the victim (American Psychiatric Association 2000). Although it may involve a consenting partner who has sexual masochistic desires, it often involves nonconsenting victims. The sadistic acts may involve things such as controlling or dominating the victim but also may include things such as restraint, blindfolding, paddling, spanking, whipping, pinching, beating, burning, electrical shocks, rape, cutting, stabbing, strangulation, torture, mutilation, or even killing. Such fantasies may have begun in childhood but are usually present in these patients by early adulthood. Hucker (1997) discussed that sexual sadism may include several subcategories of paraphilia, including necrophilia (sexual attraction or behavior with a corpse), sadistic and lust murders (sexual arousal from killing), and sadistic rape.

### Transvestic Fetishism

Identified separate from the general concept of fetishism, *transvestic fetishism* involves cross-dressing by a male in women's attire, in most cases producing sexual arousal (American Psychiatric Association 2000). The disorder has only been described in heterosexual males and is not diagnosed if it occurs exclusively in the case of gender identity disorder. It may begin in childhood or may start in adulthood, may be temporary or chronic, and may lead to gender dysphoria in some cases.

### Voyeurism

*Voyeurism* is commonly seen as the act of becoming sexually aroused while viewing nudity or sexual activity by others when they do not realize they are being watched or have not given permission. The act of looking while another unsuspecting person is naked, is disrobing, or is engaging in sexual activity leads to sexual excitement, but generally there is no sexual activity between the voyeur and the victim. The person is usually masturbating while watching, or shortly thereafter, and in some cases, the voyeuristic behavior may be the sole form of sexual activity for the person. This type of behavior often starts in adolescence and can become chronic (American Psychiatric Association 2000).

## Epidemiology

The paraphilias rarely cause personal distress, and individuals with these disorders usually come for treatment because of pressure from their partners or the authorities. Thus, there are few data on the prevalence or course of many of these disorders. Historically, information on those paraphilias involving victims (pedophilia, exhibitionism) has been obtained from studies of incarcerated sex offenders.

In contrast, studies of nonincarcerated pedophiles have been enlightening regarding what has been learned about paraphilias in general. Abel et al. (1987) gathered data through structured clinical interviews of 561 men with paraphilias regarding demographic characteristics, frequency and variety of deviant sexual acts, and number and characteristics of victims. Most of their participants (all of whom who gave information under a Certificate of Confidentiality) were well educated; half had formed a significant relationship with an adult partner; and 67% fell into the age range of 20–39 years. The authors reported an average number of crimes and victims that was substantially higher than had been realized before and reported that their subjects molested young boys five times more often than they did young girls. The vast majority of individuals with these disorders are men.

## Etiology

Various theories have been put forth to explain the development of paraphilias. As with the gender identity disorders, biological factors have been postulated. Destruction of parts of the limbic system in animals causes hypersexual behavior (Klüver-Bucy syndrome), and temporal lobe diseases such as psychomotor seizures or temporal lobe tumors have been implicated in some persons with paraphilias. It also has been suggested that abnormal levels of androgens may contribute to inappropriate sexual arousal. Most studies, however, have dealt only with violent sex offenders and have yielded inconclusive results (Bradford and McLean 1984).

Psychoanalytic theories have postulated that severe castration anxiety during the oedipal phase of development leads to the substitution of a symbolic object (inanimate object or an anatomical part) for the mother, as in fetishism and transvestism. Similarly, anxiety over arousal to the mother can lead to the choice of "safe," inappropriate sexual partners, as in pedophilia or zoophilia, or safe sexual behaviors in which there is no sexual contact, as in exhibitionism and voyeurism. Some psychoanalytic theories have suggested that a paraphilia represents an attempt by an individual to re-create and master early childhood punishment or humiliation (Stoller 1975a, 1975b).

According to learning theory, sexual arousal develops when an individual engages in a sexual behavior that is subsequently reinforced through sexual fantasies and masturbation. It is thought that there are certain vulnerable periods (e.g., puberty) when the development of sexual arousal can occur.

Finkelhor (1984) hypothesized that there were four underlying factors involved in child molestation. Specifically, sex offenders of children experienced emotional congruence; that is, they found sex with children to be emotionally satisfying. They also found the behavior to be sexually arousing. A third factor related to having sex with children is that these men were unable to meet their needs in a sexually and socially appropriate way (blockage). Finally, child molesters experienced disinhibition in that they are able to behave in ways contrary to social norms.

Hall and Hirschman (1992) proposed a quadripartite model of child molestation. The four components include physiological sexual arousal, cognitive distortions that justify sex with children, personality problems, and affective dyscontrol. Marshall and Barbaree (1990) proposed that individuals who engage in sexual activity with children during their own childhood experience developmentally adverse events. As those children enter adolescence, their sexual fantasies may involve sexual scripts that involve aggression and sex. These youths might lack self-regulation skills, may be lacking in social skills, and may experience negative states that increase the probability that they will engage in inappropriate sexual behavior.

## Diagnosis

It is important to distinguish between paraphilias such as fetishism and transvestism and normal variations of sexual behavior. Some couples occasionally augment their usual sexual activities with activities such as bondage or cross-dressing. Transvestism, however, would be diagnosed only if a heterosexual male, over a period of at least 6 months, had recurrent, intense sexual urges and sexually arousing fantasies involving cross-dressing and if the person is distressed by the urges or has acted on them. Only when these activities are the exclusive or preferred means of achieving sexual excitement and orgasm, or when the sexual behavior is not consensual, is the paraphilia diagnosed. Obviously, nonconsensual sexual activities such as sexual contact with children or exhibitionism never can be appropriate; children never can give consent for sexual activity with an adult.

## Clinical Evaluation

Table 24–3 lists information that is important to collect during a clinical psychosexual interview, which may then be confirmed with collateral sources. Table 24–4 lists specific details that may be covered in the sexual history portion of the evaluation.

## Therapeutic Treatment of Paraphilias

A variety of behavior therapies have been used to treat paraphilias. Various aversive conditioning methods (e.g., noxious odors) and covert sensitization have been used to decrease deviant sexual behavior. (In the latter approach, the individual pairs his or her inappropriate sexual fantasies with aversive, anxiety-provoking scenes, under the guidance of a therapist.) *Satiation* is a technique in which the individual uses his or her deviant fantasies postorgasm in a

**TABLE 24–3. Psychosexual assessment**

A history of present and past psychiatric illness and treatments

A family psychiatric history

A social history

A medical history, including things such as past surgical procedures, chronic medical illnesses, acute traumatic injury, head trauma, history of seizures, and history of loss of consciousness

A history of current and past medications and other medical treatments

A developmental history, learning things such as whether the child was the product of a planned pregnancy; whether the mother was exposed to alcohol, drugs, or abuse during the pregnancy; and whether there were any complications with the delivery

Information about the temperament of the youth as he or she was a developing infant and toddler

A history of interactions with other children and adults while growing up

A history of educational development, including whether he or she was referred for special education services or has learning disabilities

An employment history

Family history and functioning

Future plans for employment, education, and family

Emotional, physical, and sexual abuse history

The current living arrangements and social and financial support

A history of legal problems

A history of gang involvement

A history of violent behaviors

Alcohol and substance use history

A detailed sexual history

repetitive manner to the point of satiating himself or herself with the deviant stimuli, in essence making the fantasies and behavior boring (Marshall and Barbaree 1978).

Skills training and cognitive restructuring to change the individual's maladaptive beliefs are also used in behavioral treatments. Marshall et al. (1991), in a comprehensive review of the literature of treatment outcome studies for a variety of sex offenders, concluded that treatment programs that use comprehensive cognitive-behavioral interventions, as well as those that use antiandrogens in combination with psychological treatment, are the most effective.

---

**TABLE 24–4.    Sexual history**

When puberty began

When the person as an adolescent first became aware of his or her own sexuality (for a male, when he became aware of obtaining erections and when the erections correlated with sexual stimuli or fantasies)

Personal beliefs about sex

How the person's sexual relationships developed (such as when the person experienced his or her first crush and romantic kiss and how the person first learned about sex)

The nature of his or her first type of sexual contact (such as prolonged kissing, touching, oral sexual contact, anal sexual contact, and actual intercourse)

Number of sexual contacts

Age range of sexual fantasies and contacts

Gender of sexual fantasies and contacts

Exposure to sexually stimulating materials (such as magazines, videos, books, Internet Web sites, sexual toll telephone calls, adult bookstores, strip clubs)

Personal feelings about his or her body and sexual organs and any sexual dysfunctions

Fantasies and behaviors regarding common as well as serious sexual paraphilias and related topics (such as exhibitionism, voyeurism, frotteurism, pedophilia, sexual masochism, sexual sadism, transvestism, zoophilia, necrophilia, rape, killing, torture, control)

History of gender identity concerns or disorder

Any other pertinent sexual issue not covered previously

---

Psychoanalysis and psychodynamic therapy have been used in treating paraphilias. Identification and resolution of early conflicts, trauma, and humiliation are thought to remove the individual's anxiety toward appropriate partners and enable him or her to give up the paraphilic fantasies. Although psychodynamic psychotherapy has been useful in the treatment of some individuals, there has been disappointment with the results of this therapy as the sole form of treatment in cases of deviant sexual arousal (Crawford 1981).

Most work conducted to date is focused on static risk factors, including criminal history, personality traits, and demographic characteristics, as long-term predictors of recidivism. Only recently has the focus been on dynamic risk factors, when, in fact, dynamic risk factors are probably the more appropriate target of treatment, given their amenability to change. Researchers need to determine the mechanisms of change that produce reductions in sexual

recidivism. Given the heterogeneity among sex offender populations, it is important to identify moderating variables. Treatment should be tailored to specific subtypes of offenders. Much of current treatment is geared toward establishing goals that involve the avoidance of behaviors, and less attention is paid to creating positive goals such as striving toward engaging in prosocial behaviors. Very little research has been directed toward what factors are related to treatment dropout and to motivation for treatment. We conclude that sex offender theory and treatment should be guided by empirical evidence, and targeted research in the field will lead to development of more optimal treatment programs.

## Biological and Pharmacological Treatments of Paraphilias

### Hormonal Treatments

Biological treatments traditionally have been reserved for individuals with pedophilia, sexual sadism, or exhibitionism, although occasionally individuals with other paraphilias receive treatment with medications (Bradford and Kaye 1999).

Hormonal treatments have been attempted for a number of years in the paraphilic population, with the initial treatments focusing on blocking or decreasing the level of circulating androgens. Surgical castration has been used widely in Europe with incarcerated sex offenders. However, some have suggested that surgical castration is not always an effective means of eliminating deviant sexual behavior and that almost one-third of castrated men can still engage in intercourse. Many view surgical castration not only as highly intrusive but also as cruel and unusual punishment. The results from this procedure are variable, unpredictable, and irreversible (Heim 1981; Wille and Beier 1989).

Interestingly, Weinberger et al. (2005) recently reviewed the relation of surgical castration and sexual recidivism in a sexually violent predator/sexually dangerous person population, concluding that surgically castrated sex offenders have a very low incidence of sexual recidivism. However, they also pointed out that whereas orchiectomy can reduce sexual desire, it does not completely eliminate the ability to obtain an erection in response to sexually stimulating material, and the effects can be reversed by testosterone replacement. Berlin (2005) responded by saying that from a treatment standpoint, if lowering testosterone can provide a decrease in sexual appetite in this population, there seems to be little reason to use surgical castration, because the same effects can be achieved with testosterone-lowering medications.

Antiandrogenic medications have been used throughout the world since the late 1960s to treat sex offenders. As early as the 1940s, estrogens were used to treat sex offenders, but by the 1960s this practice had been discontinued because of serious side effects (Neuman and Kalmus 1991). Next, a progestin derivative, cyproterone acetate, was introduced in Europe and Canada, but it has never been made available in the United States. Medroxyprogesterone acetate is available in the United States, and now gonadotropin-releasing hormone agonists are being used, including leuprolide acetate. Each of these medications works because of its effect on sexual libido by ultimately (albeit by different mechanisms) lowering testosterone levels. For example, medroxyprogesterone acetate appears to act by blocking testosterone synthesis, whereas cyproterone acetate acts primarily by blocking central and peripheral androgen receptors. Both may be given orally or via long-acting intramuscular depot injection (to improve compliance). They do not appear to influence the direction of sexual drive toward appropriate adult partners; rather, they act to decrease libido and thus break the individual's pattern of compulsive deviant sexual behavior. These agents thus work best in those paraphilic persons with a high sexual drive and less well in those with a low sexual drive or an antisocial personality (Cooper 1986). Leuprolide acetate works by stimulating follicle-stimulating hormone and luteinizing hormone secretion initially, and then downregulating luteinizing hormone–releasing hormone receptors on follicle-stimulating hormone– and luteinizing hormone–secreting cells in the pituitary. This, in turn, decreases testosterone production.

### Other Pharmacological Treatments

Another promising focus of research has been on the use of other forms of pharmacological treatment for paraphilias. There have now been a number of case reports and open-label studies in which the selective serotonin reuptake inhibitors (SSRIs) were used to treat paraphilias and nonparaphilic sexual disorders (Bradford 1996; Kafka 2000; Saleh 2004). Although sexual libido may decrease as a side effect of an SSRI, one has to keep in mind that there may be multiple reasons as to these agents' possible effectiveness. SSRIs have been approved for disorders such as major depression, generalized anxiety disorder, panic disorder, and obsessive-compulsive disorder. However, there have been studies to show their benefit in off-label uses such as aggression, self-injurious behavior, and impulsivity. Hollander et al. (1996, 2000) proposed that sexual compulsions may overlap with impulsive disorders and obsessive-compulsive disorders. Is it possible that serotonergic agents may help improve mood, decrease impulsivity, decrease sexual obsessions, and lead to sexual dysfunction (Rothschild 2000), which in combination decrease the chance of recidivism in men with paraphilias?

## Risk Assessment of Sex Offenders

A question that mental health professionals who evaluate or treat individuals with paraphilias that involve victims are often asked to address is whether the individual is at risk to reoffend. This is also important in those states that have sexually violent predators legislation and where individuals may be petitioned for civil commitment. Sixteen states at present have relevant statutes that allow for the civil commitment of individuals who have committed sexual offenses and remain a risk to society. Although the terminology of the statutes may vary from state to state, in general the commitment criteria involve an individual who has been convicted of a sexually violent offense or adjudicated insane and currently has a mental disorder, paraphilia, personality disorder, or conduct disorder that predisposes the person to commit sexual acts such as to render him or her a danger to the health and safety of others.

Historically, individuals have used clinical judgment in determining whether a person poses a risk of either violent or sexually violent behavior. Doren (2002) noted that different methods have been used to conduct risk assessments, including unguided clinical judgment, guided clinical judgment, clinical judgment based on an amnestic approach, research-guided clinical judgment, a clinically adjusted actuarial approach, and a purely actuarial approach. The field of risk assessment now has available a number of actuarial risk assessment instruments for use. Doren (2002) noted that when selecting what instrument to use, the following issues need to be addressed: statistical demonstration of reliability and validity; degree of concordance between what the instrument was designed to measure and the legally defined risk; availability of information required to use the instrument; and availability of interpretive information. Actuarial assessment instruments include the STATIC-99, the Sex Offender Risk Appraisal Guide, the Violence Risk Appraisal Guide, the Rapid Risk Assessment for Sex Offense Recidivism, and the Minnesota Sex Offender Screening Tool—Revised. When conducting a risk assessment, it is important that the assessment be comprehensive and include a review of official court documents and interview of the offender, use of a risk assessment instrument, and assessment of dynamic risk factors. See Doren (2002) for information on risk assessment instruments as well as information on report writing and court testimony.

## Key Points: Gender Identity Disorders and Paraphilias

- Whereas the genetic sex of an individual is determined at conception, gender identity develops during the early years of life.

- Gender identity disorder requires a strong and persistent cross-gender identification and a persistent discomfort with one's sex or sense of inappropriateness in the gender role of that sex.

- Approximately 1 in 30,000 adult men and 1 in 100,000 women seek sex reassignment surgery. After surgery, patients report few problems and marked improvement in their sexuality.

- The paraphilias are characterized by experiencing, over a period of at least 6 months, recurrent, intense sexually arousing fantasies, sexual urges, or behaviors, generally involving nonhuman objects or nonconsenting partners.

- The most common paraphilias are exhibitionism, fetishism, frotteurism, pedophilia, sexual masochism, sexual sadism, transvestic fetishism, and voyeurism.

- A variety of behavior therapies, hormonal treatments, and psychopharmacological treatments have been used to manage paraphilias.

# References

Abel GG, Becker JV, Mittelman M, et al: Self-reported sex crimes of nonincarcerated paraphiliacs. J Interpers Violence 2:3–25, 1987

American Psychiatric Association: Diagnostic and Statistical Manual of Mental Disorders, 4th Edition, Text Revision. Washington, DC, American Psychiatric Association, 2000

Berlin FS: Commentary: the impact of surgical castration on sexual recidivism risk among civilly committed sexual offenders. J Am Acad Psychiatry Law 33:37–41, 2005

Blair CD, Lanyon RI: Exhibitionism: etiology and treatment. Psychol Bull 89:439–463, 1981

Bradford J: The role of serotonin in the future of forensic psychiatry. Bull Am Acad Psychiatry Law 24:57–72, 1996

Bradford J, Kaye NS: Pharmacological treatment of sexual offenders. Newsl Am Acad Psychiatry Law 24:16–17, 1999

Bradford J, McLean D: Sexual offenders, violence, and testosterone: a clinical study. Can J Psychiatry 29:335–343, 1984

Cooper AJ: Progestogens in the treatment of male sex offenders: a review. Can J Psychiatry 31:73–79, 1986

Crawford D: Treatment approaches with pedophiles, in Adult Sexual Interest in Children. Edited by Cook M, Howells K. New York, Academic Press, 1981, pp 181–217

Doren DM: Evaluating Sex Offenders: A Manual for Civil Commitment and Beyond. Thousand Oaks, CA, Sage, 2002

Finkelhor D: Child Abuse: New Theory and Research. New York, Free Press, 1984

Fridell SR, Zucker KJ, Bradley SJ, et al: Physical attractiveness of girls with gender identity disorder. Arch Sex Behav 25:17–31, 1996

Green R: Sexual Identity Conflict in Children and Adults. New York, Basic Books, 1974

Green R: Gender identity in childhood and later sexual orientation: follow-up of 78 males. Am J Psychiatry 142:339–341, 1985

Green R: The Sissy Boys Syndrome and the Development of Homosexuality. New Haven, CT, Yale University Press, 1987

Hall G, Hirschman R: Sexual aggression against children: a conceptual perspective of etiology. Crim Justice Behav 19:8–23, 1992

Heim N: Sexual behavior of castrated sex offenders. Arch Sex Behav 10:11–19, 1981

Hollander E, Kwon JH, Stein DJ, et al: Obsessive-compulsive and spectrum disorders: overview and quality of life issues. J Clin Psychiatry 57(suppl):3–6, 1996

Hollander E, Twersky R, Bienstock C: The obsessive compulsive spectrum: a survey of 800 practitioners. CNS Spectr 5:61–63, 2000

Hucker SJ: Sexual sadism, in Sexual Deviance. Edited by Laws DR, O'Donohue W. New York, Guilford, 1997, pp 194–209

Kafka MP: Psychopharmacological treatments for nonparaphilic compulsive sexual behaviors. CNS Spectr 5:49–59, 2000

Lothstein L: The postsurgical transsexual: empirical and theoretical considerations. Arch Sex Behav 9:547–564, 1980

Marshall WL, Barbaree HE: The reduction of deviant arousal: satiation treatment for sexual aggressors. Crim Justice Behav 5:294–303, 1978

Marshall WL, Barbaree HE: An integrated theory of etiology of sexual offending, in Handbook of Sexual Assault: Issues, Theories and Treatment of the Offender. Edited by Marshall WL, Laws DR, Barbaree HE. New York, Plenum, 1990, pp 257–275

Marshall WL, Jones R, Ward T, et al: Treatment outcome with sex offenders. Clin Psychol Rev 11:465–485, 1991

Mason FL: Fetishism: psychopathology and theory, in Sexual Deviance. Edited by Laws DR, O'Donohue W. New York, Guilford, 1997, pp 75–91

Meyer JK: The theory of gender identity disorders. J Am Psychoanal Assoc 30:381–418, 1982

Meyer M III, Bockting WO, Cohen-Kettenis P, et al: Harry Benjamin International Gender Dysphoria Association's The Standards of Care for Gender Identity Disorders, 6th Version. Minneapolis, MN, Harry Benjamin International Gender Dysphoria Association, 2001. Available at: http://www.symposion.com/ijt/soc_2001/index.htm. Accessed October 15, 2007.

Murphy WD: Exhibitionism: psychopathology and theory, in Sexual Deviance. Edited by Laws DR, O'Donohue W. New York, Guilford, 1997, pp 22–39

Neuman F, Kalmus J: Hormonal treatment of sexual deviations. Arch Gen Psychiatry 57:1012–1032, 1991

Rothschild AJ: Sexual side effects of antidepressants. J Clin Psychiatry 61(suppl):28–36, 2000

Saleh FM: Serotonin reuptake inhibitors and the paraphilias. Newsl Am Acad Psychiatry Law 29:12–13, 2004

Stoller RJ: Perversion: The Erotic Form of Hatred. New York, Pantheon, 1975a

Stoller RJ: Sex and Gender, Vol 2: The Transsexual Experiment. London, England, Hogarth, 1975b

Weinberger LE, Sreenivasan S, Garrick T, et al: The impact of surgical castration on sexual recidivism risk among sexually violent predatory offenders. J Am Acad Psychiatry Law 33:16–36, 2005

Wille R, Beier K: Castration in Germany. Annals of Sex Research 2:103–133, 1989

Zucker KJ, Bradley SJ: Gender Identity Disorder and Psychosexual Problems in Children and Adolescents. New York, Guilford, 1995

Zucker KJ, Bradley SJ, Lowry Sullivan CB, et al: A gender identity interview for children. J Pers Assess 61:443–456, 1993

Zucker KJ, Bradley SJ, Sanikhani M: Sex differences in referral rates of children with gender identity disorder: some hypotheses. J Abnorm Child Psychol 25:217–227, 1997

# 25

# Eating Disorders

## KATHERINE A. HALMI, M.D.

## Anorexia Nervosa

### Definition

Anorexia nervosa is a disorder characterized by preoccupation with body weight and food, behavior directed toward losing weight, peculiar patterns of handling food, weight loss, intense fear of gaining weight, disturbance of body image, and amenorrhea. DSM-IV-TR (American Psychiatric Association 2000a) criteria for anorexia nervosa are included in Table 25–1.

### Clinical Features

Individuals with anorexia nervosa typically express an intense fear of gaining weight, tend to be preoccupied with thoughts of food, and worry irrationally about fatness. Denial of their own clearly observable symptoms is characteristic of anorexic patients. They frequently look in mirrors to make sure they are thin, and they incessantly express concern about looking fat and feeling flabby. Collecting recipes and preparing elaborate meals for their families are other behaviors that reflect their preoccupation with food. Peculiar handling of food is frequent in individuals with anorexia. They will hide carbohydrate-rich foods and hoard large quantities of candies, carrying them in their pockets and purses. Often, they will try to dispose of their food surreptitiously to avoid eating. Anorexic persons will spend a great deal of time cutting food into small pieces and rearranging the food on the plate.

Anorexic patients' fear that they are gaining weight exists even in the face of increasing cachexia, and they characteristically show disinterest in and even resistance

**TABLE 25–1.  DSM-IV-TR diagnostic criteria for anorexia nervosa**

A.  Refusal to maintain body weight at or above a minimally normal weight for age and height (e.g., weight loss leading to maintenance of body weight less than 85% of that expected; or failure to make expected weight gain during period of growth, leading to body weight less than 85% of that expected).

B.  Intense fear of gaining weight or becoming fat, even though underweight.

C.  Disturbance in the way in which one's body weight or shape is experienced, undue influence of body weight or shape on self-evaluation, or denial of the seriousness of the current low body weight.

D.  In postmenarcheal females, amenorrhea, i.e., the absence of at least three consecutive menstrual cycles. (A woman is considered to have amenorrhea if her periods occur only following hormone, e.g., estrogen, administration.)

*Specify* type:

**Restricting type:**   during the current episode of anorexia nervosa, the person has not regularly engaged in binge-eating or purging behavior (i.e., self-induced vomiting or the misuse of laxatives, diuretics, or enemas)

**Binge-eating/purging type:**   during the current episode of anorexia nervosa, the person has regularly engaged in binge-eating or purging behavior (i.e., self-induced vomiting or the misuse of laxatives, diuretics, or enemas) to treatment. Persons with this disorder lose weight by drastically reducing their total food intake and disproportionately decreasing the intake of high-carbohydrate and fatty foods. Some individuals with anorexia will develop rigorous exercise programs, and others simply will be as active as possible at all times. Self-induced vomiting and laxative and diuretic abuse are other purging behaviors by which anorexic persons attempt to lose weight. Weight loss and a refusal to maintain body weight over a minimal normal weight for age and height are the most characteristic features of this disorder. Anorexic individuals have a disturbance in the way in which they experience their body weight and shape. They often fail to recognize that their degree of emaciation is dangerous. Their cognition is so distorted that they judge their self-worth predominantly by body shape and weight.

Obsessive-compulsive behavior often develops after the onset of anorexia nervosa. An obsession with cleanliness, an increase in housecleaning activities, and a more compulsive approach to studying are not uncommonly observed in these patients.

Amenorrhea can appear before noticeable weight loss has occurred. Poor sexual adjustment is frequently present in patients with anorexia. Many adolescent patients with anorexia have delayed psychosocial sexual development, and adults often have a markedly decreased interest in sex with the onset of anorexia nervosa.

Patients with anorexia nervosa can be divided into two groups: those who binge eat and purge and those who merely restrict food intake to lose weight. There is a relatively frequent association with impulsive behavior such as suicide attempts, self-mutilation, stealing, and substance abuse (including alcohol abuse) among bulimic individuals with anorexia, who are also less likely to be regressed in their sexual activity and may in fact be promiscuous. Also, bulimic anorexic patients are more likely to have discrete personality disorder diagnoses (Halmi 1987).

## Medical Complications

Most of the physiological and metabolic changes in anorexia nervosa are secondary to the starvation state or purging behavior and are reversed with nutritional rehabilitation (Table 25–2).

## Epidemiology, Course, and Prognosis

The incidence of anorexia nervosa has increased since the mid–twentieth century, both in the United States and in Western Europe. The lifetime prevalence of anorexia nervosa is 0.6% (Lewinsohn et al. 2000). Only 4%–6% of the anorexic population is male (Halmi 1974).

The course of anorexia nervosa varies from a single episode with weight and psychological recovery, to nutritional rehabilitation with relapses, to an unremitting course resulting in death. Two of the most methodologically satisfying long-term follow-up studies have shown a mortality rate of 6.6% at 10 years after a well-defined treatment program (Halmi et al. 1991) and a mortality rate of 18% at 30-year follow-up (Theander 1985).

These studies, in addition to a follow-up study by Hsu et al. (1979), found that many patients with anorexia may show considerable improvement in their medical condition but most still had the characteristic psychological set of the illness. Fewer than one-fourth of these patients could be considered to have made a good psychological adjustment when they were followed up to ages 20–50 years. At the end of his 30-year follow-up study, Theander (1985) found that 75% of his patients could be classified as being in a psychologically stable state. This was not true at the time of earlier follow-up examinations. Generally speaking, poor outcome in the studies mentioned earlier was associated with longer duration of illness, older age at onset, previous admissions to psychiatric hospitals, poor childhood social adjustment, premorbid personality difficulties, and disturbed relationships between patients and other family members.

## Etiology and Pathogenesis

A specific etiology and pathogenesis leading to development of anorexia nervosa are unknown. Anorexia nervosa begins after a period of severe food deprivation (Table 25–3). In addition, several neurotransmitters and neuropeptides are involved in eating behavior (Table 25–4).

## Treatment

A multifaceted treatment endeavor with medical management and behavioral, individual, cognitive, and family therapy is necessary to treat anorexia nervosa (Table 23–5). The first step in treatment is to obtain the anorexic patient's cooperation in a treatment program. Most patients with anorexia nervosa are disinterested and even resistant to treatment and are brought to the therapist's office unwillingly by relatives or friends. For these patients, it is important to emphasize the benefits of treatment and to reassure them that treatment can bring about a relief of insomnia and depressive symptoms, a decrease in the ob-

**TABLE 25–2.**   **Medical complications of anorexia nervosa**

**Cardiovascular**
Bradycardia
Orthostatic hypotension
Arrhythmias
Electrocardiogram changes—QTc prolongation
ST–T wave abnormalities

**Central nervous system**
Peripheral neuropathy
Enlarged ventricles
Decreased gray and white matter
Cognitive impairment

**Endocrine/metabolic**
Hypothermia
Amenorrhea
Hypokalemia
Electrolyte abnormalities
Hypercholesterolemia

**Gastrointestinal**
Vomiting
Constipation
Diarrhea
Parotid hyperplasia
Increased serum amylase
Abnormal liver function tests

**Renal**
Hypokalemic nephropathy

**Hematological**
Anemia
Leukopenia with relative lymphocytosis

**Integument**
Lanugo
Carotenoderma

**Muscular**
Muscle wasting
Creatine kinase abnormalities

**Pulmonary**
Decreased pulmonary capacity

**Reproductive**
Amenorrhea, secondary or primary
Decreased serum estrogen in females
Decreased serum testosterone in males
Loss of libido

**Skeletal**
Osteopenia
Osteoporosis
Pathological stress fractures

**TABLE 25–3.**   **Common reasons for severe food deprivation**

Willful dieting for the purpose of being more attractive

Willful dieting for the purpose of being more professionally competent (e.g., ballet dancers, gymnasts, jockeys)

Food restriction secondary to severe stress

Food restriction secondary to severe illness and/or surgery

Involuntary starvation

sessive thoughts about food and body weight that interfere with the ability to concentrate on other matters, an increase in physical well-being and energy, and an improvement in peer relationships.

The immediate aim of treatment should be to restore the patient's nutritional state to normal. Mere emaciation or the state of being mildly underweight (15%–25% below normal weight) can cause irritability, depression, preoccupation with food, and sleep disturbance. It is exceedingly difficult to achieve behavior change with psychotherapy in a patient who is experiencing the psychological effects of emaciation. Outpatient therapy as an initial approach has the best chance for success in patients with anorexia who 1) have had the illness for less than 6 months, 2) are not bingeing and vomiting, and 3) have parents who are likely to cooperate and effectively participate in family therapy.

The more severely ill patient with anorexia may present an extremely difficult medical-management challenge and should be hospitalized and undergo daily monitoring of weight, food and calorie intake, and urine output. In the patient who is vomiting, frequent assessment of serum electrolytes is necessary. Behavior therapy is most effective in the medical management and nutritional rehabilitation of the patient with anorexia, although there are times when other target behaviors can be changed with this approach. Behavior therapy can be used in both outpatient and inpatient settings.

The operant conditioning paradigm has been the most effective form of behavior therapy for the treatment of anorexia nervosa. This can be used both in the context of a structured ward setting and in an individualized treatment program set up after a behavioral analysis of the patient has been completed. Positive reinforcements are used and consist of increased physical activity, visiting privileges, and social activities contingent on weight gain.

**TABLE 25–4.   Neurotransmitters and neuropeptides in anorexia nervosa**

| Hormone | Effect on eating behavior | Functional status in anorexia nervosa | Clinical manifestations |
|---|---|---|---|
| Norepinephrine | Inhibits the CRF-inhibiting feeding effect | ↓ | Decreased food intake |
| Serotonin | Facilitates satiety | ↑ | Feeling full after a minimal intake of food |
| Dopamine | Mediates rewarding effects of food | ↓ | ? |
| Corticotropin-releasing factor (CRF) | Inhibits feeding; stimulates motor activity | ↑ | Decreased food intake; increased motor activity |
| Neuropeptide Y | Increases food intake | ↑ | Should stimulate feeding, but ineffective in anorexia nervosa |
| Cholecystokinin | Attenuates feeding | ↑ | Decreased meal size |

*Note.*   This table is, of course, oversimplified; actual phenomena are more complex.

An individual behavioral analysis may show other positive reinforcements to be more clinically relevant in the particular cases. The timing of reinforcement is important in behavior therapy. An adolescent patient needs at least a daily reinforcement for weight increase, which should be approximately 0.5 lb or 0.2 kg per day. Making positive reinforcements contingent only on weight gain is helpful in reducing the staff–patient arguments and stressful interactions concerning how and what the patient is eating, because weight is an objective measure. In addition to being used to induce weight gain, behavior therapy can be used to stop vomiting. A response-prevention technique is used when bingeing and purging patients are required to stay in an observed dayroom area for 2–3 hours after every meal. Very few patients vomit in front of other people, and thus the emesis response is prevented and, eventually, stopped completely.

Cognitive therapy techniques for treating anorexia nervosa were developed by Garner and Bemis (1982). The assessment of cognition is a first step in cognitive therapy. Patients are asked to write down their thoughts on an assessment form so that cognitions can be examined for systematic distortions in the processing and interpretation of events. Cognitive techniques include operationalizing beliefs, decentering, using the "what if" technique, evaluating autonomic thoughts, testing prospective hypotheses, reinterpreting body image misperception, examining underlying assumptions, and modifying basic assumptions.

Cognitive-behavioral therapy (CBT) for prevention of relapse of anorexia nervosa was further developed by Klei-field et al. (1996), who created an easy-to-use treatment manual. CBT is based on two core assumptions about the disorder. The first assumption is that anorexia nervosa has a significant positive function in the patient's life and develops as a way of coping with adverse experiences often associated with developmental transitions and distressing life events. The anorexic patient's deficient coping abilities produce anxiety and fear, and the patient is distracted from these anxieties by an overwhelming preoccupation with food and weight. The anorexic condition is also a reinforcing one in that the patient experiences a surge of confidence and a sense of competence and control after being successful in dieting. The second assumption is that food restriction and ritualistic food avoidance behaviors become independent of the events or issues provoking them. The anorexic patient's extreme anxiety about gaining weight and becoming fat is alleviated by not eating. The relief of anxiety about gaining weight—the anxiety being alleviated through avoidance of food—is another strong reinforcement and thus a key factor in the persistence with which these patients pursue food restriction.

On the basis of the aforementioned assumptions, two separate pathways are taken in treatment. First, the dietary restriction is regarded as a food phobia, and change in eating behavior is a primary objective. Behavioral methods such as monitoring food intake and the details surrounding food intake, along with techniques such as increasing exposure, are used to increase the patient's food intake gradually. Then, cognitive-behavioral methods are used to reduce the anxiety associated with behavior change.

TABLE 25–5.  **Treatment of anorexia nervosa**

| Type of treatment | Key elements | Measurements | Indications |
|---|---|---|---|
| Medical management | Weight restoration | Weight (outpatient—weekly; inpatient—daily) | Below normal weight for age and height by ≥10% |
| | Rehydration and correction of serum electrolytes | Serum electrolytes | History of vomiting, laxative abuse, severe restriction of food and fluids |
| Behavior therapy | Positive reinforcements for weight gain | Weight (outpatient—weekly; inpatient—daily) | Underweight |
| | Response prevention for binge eating and purging | Serum electrolytes and serum amylase | Weakness, puffy cheeks—parotid enlargement, scars on dorsum of hands, fainting spells |
| Cognitive therapy | Operationalizing beliefs, evaluating automatic thoughts, prospective hypothesis testing, examination of underlying assumptions | Assessment of distorted cognitions (e.g., all-or-none/black-or-white thinking), feeling fat, self-worth measured solely by body image, pervasive sense of ineffectiveness except in losing weight | Disturbance in way one's body weight or shape is experienced; denial of seriousness of low body weight; relentless pursuit of thinness for control of environment |
| Family therapy | Family counseling or therapy format based on needs of specific family | Analysis of family functioning, roles, and interactions | If patient is living with family, some type of family counseling or therapy is essential |
| Pharmacotherapy | | | |
| Chlorpromazine | Liquid form, start low doses, such as 10 mg three times a day, and gradually increase | Complete blood count, lying and standing blood pressure | Severely delusional, overactive, hospitalized patients |
| Cyproheptadine | Liquid form, start 4 mg twice a day and increase to 8 mg three times a day if necessary | Complete blood count with platelets | Severely overactive anorexic patient who does not binge and purge |
| Fluoxetine | Preferable to use after weight restoration because of tendency to induce arousal | Complete blood count, observation of total sleep and activity | Severely obsessive-compulsive behaviors related or unrelated to eating disorders, severe depression |
| Clomipramine | Necessary to start in very low doses because of hypotension side effects; preferable to use after weight restoration | Complete blood count, lying and standing blood pressure, electrocardiogram | Severely obsessive-compulsive behaviors |
| Tricyclic antidepressants | Necessary to start in very low doses because of hypotension side effects; preferable to use after weight restoration | Complete blood count, lying and standing blood pressure, electrocardiogram | Severe depression |

Cognitive techniques such as cognitive restructuring and problem solving help the patient deal with distorted and overvalued beliefs about food and thinness and cope with life's stresses.

A family analysis should be done on all patients with anorexia who are living with their families. On the basis of this analysis, a clinical judgment should be made regarding what type of family therapy or counseling is clinically advisable. In some cases, family therapy will not be possible. However, in those cases, issues of family relationships must be dealt with in individual therapy and, in some cases, in brief counseling sessions with immediate family members.

Drugs can be useful adjuncts in the treatment of anorexia nervosa. The first drug used in treating anorexia was chlorpromazine. This medication is especially effective in patients with anorexia who are severely obsessive-compulsive. More recently, atypical antipsychotics have been studied in acutely ill anorexia nervosa patients.

Another category of drugs frequently used in the treatment of anorexia nervosa is the antidepressants. A double-blind study in which 72 patients with anorexia were randomly assigned to amitriptyline, cyproheptadine (an antihistaminic drug), or placebo therapy showed that both cyproheptadine and amitriptyline had a marginal effect in decreasing the number of days necessary to achieve a normal weight. Cyproheptadine had an unexpected antidepressant effect, indicated by a significant decrease in scores on the Hamilton Rating Scale for Depression (Halmi et al. 1986). In the bulimic subgroups of patients with anorexia, cyproheptadine had a negative effect compared with both placebo and amitriptyline. This differential effect within the bulimic anorexic subgroups indicates a real medical distinction and appears to justify this subgrouping. Cyproheptadine has the advantage of not having the tricyclic antidepressant side effects of reducing blood pressure and increasing heart rate.

The results of small studies exploring the efficacy of fluoxetine and clomipramine suggest that both of these medications warrant further study (Crisp et al. 1987; Gwirtsman et al. 1990). These medications may be effective in preventing relapse in anorexia nervosa. Because of certain side effects (anorexia and hyperactivity in fluoxetine therapy; hypotension and tachycardia in clomipramine therapy), special caution is necessary when these medications are given to underweight anorexic patients. At a 6- to 18-month follow-up of 31 patients who had been taking fluoxetine after inpatient weight restoration, 29 patients were found to have maintained their weight at or above 85% of average body weight (Kaye et al. 2001). In this study, restricting anorexic patients responded significantly better than did bulimic and purging-type anorexic patients. The authors judged the overall response to be good in 10 patients, partial in 17 patients, and poor in 4 patients.

In a study of 122 anorexia nervosa patients randomized to CBT, fluoxetine, or their combination for a 1-year treatment, the overall dropout rate was 46%. Treatment acceptance defined as staying in treatment for at least 5 weeks occurred in 73% of the randomized cases. Of the 41 patients assigned to medication alone, acceptance occurred in 56%, and in the other two groups the acceptance rate was 81%. This study showed that anorexia nervosa patients will not accept medication unless it is combined with psychotherapy. Among patients who accepted treatment, those with high self-esteem were more likely than those with low self-esteem to complete treatment (Halmi et al. 2005).

A multifaceted treatment approach is necessary for effective care of patients with anorexia nervosa. As medical rehabilitation proceeds, an associated improvement in psychological state occurs. Behavioral contingencies are useful for inducing weight gain and changing the medical condition of the patient. Cyproheptadine may be helpful in facilitating weight gain and decreasing depressive symptomatology in the restricting anorexic patient. If an anorexic patient has a predominance of depressive symptoms and is within 80% of a normal weight range, fluoxetine should be useful for treating the depression.

Severely obsessive-compulsive, anxious, and agitated anorexic patients are likely to require chlorpromazine or an atypical antipsychotic medication such as risperidone or olanzapine. All patients need individual cognitive psychotherapy. The more severely ill patients need hospitalization initially, followed by a well-planned continued outpatient treatment program (Garner and Garfinkel 1985). Prevention of relapse is a major part of the treatment of anorexia nervosa. Family therapy is essential for children younger than 18 years of age and is equally effective in conjoint or separated format. Effectively treating adolescents before age 18 years is the best way to prevent chronic anorexia nervosa.

It is obvious that treating chronic anorexia nervosa involves high rates of morbidity and mortality. Preventing the chronicity of anorexia nervosa should be a major aim. Focusing on early diagnosis and adequate treatment of the younger anorexic patient would be the best strategy to prevent chronic anorexia nervosa.

# Bulimia Nervosa

## Definition

Bulimia nervosa is a disorder in which bulimia or binge eating is the predominant behavior (Table 25–6).

*Binge eating* is defined as an episodic, uncontrolled, rapid ingestion of large quantities of food over a short period. Abdominal pain or discomfort, self-induced vomiting, sleep, or social interruption terminates the bulimic episode. Feelings of guilt, depression, or self-disgust follow. Bulimic patients often use cathartics for weight control and have an eating pattern of alternate binges and fasts. Bulimic patients have a fear of not being able to stop eating voluntarily. The food consumed during a binge usually has a highly dense calorie content and a texture that facilitates rapid eating. Frequent weight fluctuations occur, but without the severity of weight loss present in anorexia nervosa.

## Clinical Features

Bulimia nervosa usually begins after a period of dieting of a few weeks to a year or longer. Most binge-eating episodes are followed by self-induced vomiting. Episodes are less frequently followed by use of laxatives. A minority of bulimic patients use diuretics for weight control. The average length of a bingeing episode is about 1 hour. Most patients learn to vomit by sticking their fingers down their throat, and after a short time they learn to vomit on a reflex basis. Some patients have abrasions and scars on the backs of their hands (called *Russell's sign*) from their persistent efforts to induce vomiting. Most bulimic patients do not eat regular meals and have difficulty feeling satiety at the end of a normal meal. Bulimic patients usually prefer to eat alone and at their homes. Approximately one-third to one-fifth of bulimic patients will choose a weight within a normal weight range as their ideal body weight. About one-fourth to one-third of the patients with bulimia nervosa have had a history of anorexia nervosa.

Most bulimic patients have depressive signs and symptoms. They have problems with interpersonal relationships, self-concept, and impulsive behaviors and show high levels of anxiety and compulsivity. Chemical dependency is not unusual in this disorder, alcohol abuse being the most common. Bulimic persons will abuse amphetamines to reduce their appetite and to lose weight. Impulsive stealing usually occurs after the onset of binge eating; however, about one-fourth of patients actually begin stealing before the onset of bulimia.

**TABLE 25–6. DSM-IV-TR diagnostic criteria for bulimia nervosa**

A. Recurrent episodes of binge eating. An episode of binge eating is characterized by both of the following:

(1) eating, in a discrete period of time (e.g., within any 2-hour period), an amount of food that is definitely larger than most people would eat during a similar period of time and under similar circumstances

(2) a sense of lack of control over eating during the episode (e.g., a feeling that one cannot stop eating or control what or how much one is eating)

B. Recurrent inappropriate compensatory behavior in order to prevent weight gain, such as self-induced vomiting; misuse of laxatives, diuretics, enemas, or other medications; fasting; or excessive exercise.

C. The binge eating and inappropriate compensatory behaviors both occur, on average, at least twice a week for 3 months.

D. Self-evaluation is unduly influenced by body shape and weight.

E. The disturbance does not occur exclusively during episodes of anorexia nervosa.

*Specify* type:

**Purging type:** during the current episode of bulimia nervosa, the person has regularly engaged in self-induced vomiting or the misuse of laxatives, diuretics, or enemas

**Nonpurging type:** during the current episode of bulimia nervosa, the person has used other inappropriate compensatory behaviors, such as fasting or excessive exercise, but has not regularly engaged in self-induced vomiting or the misuse of laxatives, diuretics, or enemas

## Medical Complications

Patients with bulimia nervosa who engage in self-induced vomiting and abuse purgatives or diuretics are susceptible to hypokalemic alkalosis. These patients have electrolyte abnormalities, including elevated serum bicarbonate levels, hypochloremia, hypokalemia, and, in a few cases, low serum bicarbonate levels indicating a metabolic acidosis. The latter is particularly true among individuals who abuse laxatives. It is important to remember that fasting can promote dehydration, which results in volume depletion. This can promote generation of aldosterone, which promotes further potassium excretion from the kidneys. Thus, there can be an indirect renal loss of potassium as well as a direct loss through self-induced vomiting. Patients with electrolyte disturbances have physical symptoms of weakness and lethargy and at times have cardiac arrhythmias. The latter, of course, can lead to a sudden cardiac arrest. Patients with bulimia nervosa can have severe attrition and erosion of the teeth, causing an irritating sensitivity, pathological pulp exposures, loss of integrity of the dental arches, diminished masticatory ability, and an unaesthetic appearance.

Parotid gland enlargement associated with elevated serum amylase levels is commonly observed in patients who binge and vomit. In fact, the serum amylase level is an excellent way to follow reduction of vomiting in patients with eating disorders who deny purging episodes. Acute dilatation of the stomach is a rare emergency condition for patients who binge. Esophageal tears also can occur through the process of self-induced vomiting. A complication of shock can result subsequent to the esophageal tear and should be treated by experienced medical and surgical personnel. Severe abdominal pain in the patient with bulimia nervosa should alert the physician to a diagnosis of gastric dilatation and the need for nasogastric suction, X rays, and surgical consultation.

Cardiac failure caused by cardiomyopathy from ipecac intoxication is a medical emergency that is being reported more frequently and that usually results in death. Symptoms of precordial pain, dyspnea, and generalized muscle weakness associated with hypotension, tachycardia, and abnormalities on the electrocardiogram should alert one to possible ipecac intoxication. Other laboratory findings may include elevated liver enzymes and an increased erythrocyte sedimentation rate. An echocardiogram will show a cardiomyopathy contraction pattern associated with congestive heart failure.

A summary of medical complications of bulimia nervosa is presented in Table 25–7.

## Epidemiology, Course, and Prognosis

Soundy et al. (1995) screened all medical records of health care providers, general practitioners, and specialists in Rochester, Minnesota, over the period 1980–1990 for a clinical diagnosis of bulimia nervosa and found an annual incidence of 3.5 cases per 100,000 population. Hoek et al. (1995), using DSM-III-R (American Psychiatric Association 1987) criteria, examined a large general practice study representative of the population covering the period

**TABLE 25–7. Medical complications of bulimia nervosa**

| Behavioral and physical aberrations | Physiological disturbances |
|---|---|
| Binge eating | Acute dilatation of stomach—shock |
| Self-induced vomiting | Esophageal tears—shock; dehydration |
| | Metabolic alkalosis—hypochloremia, hypokalemia, weakness, lethargy |
| | Cardiac arrhythmias—cardiac arrest |
| | Erosion of dental enamel—caries, exposure of pulp |
| Parotid gland enlargement (self-induced vomiting or excessive gum chewing) | Elevated serum amylase |
| Ipecac use | Hypotension, tachycardia, electrocardiographic abnormalities, elevated liver enzymes |

1985–1989 in the Netherlands and found an annual incidence of 11.5 cases per 100,000 population. Turnbull et al. (1996) screened the United Kingdom General Practice Research Database covering a large representative sample of the English and Welsh population for bulimia nervosa in 1993 and found an annual incidence of 12.2 cases per 100,000 population. Studies that used strict criteria found prevalence rates between 1 and 3.8 per 100 females (Hart and Ollendick 1985; Schotte and Stunkard 1987). In a study combining surveys and interviews of women in the first year of college, Kurth et al. (1995) found the prevalence of bulimia nervosa to be 2%. In a Canadian community sample in which a structured interview was used, prevalence rates of this disorder were 1% (Garfinkel et al. 1995). Hoek (1991) found a 1-year prevalence rate of bulimia nervosa of 0.17% among adolescent girls and young women 15–29 years old in a primary care health delivery system. The prevalence of males in the bulimia nervosa population varies between 10% and 15%. In most studies, the average age at onset of bulimia nervosa is 18 years (range=12–35 years). These studies have shown a much higher representation of social classes IV and V (include workers with low personal incomes and no college degrees and persons who drift in and out of poverty) in patients with bulimia nervosa compared with patients with anorexia nervosa.

Combining the results of meta-analyses by Keel and Mitchell (1997) and Nielsen (2001) yields a corrected mortality rate for bulimia nervosa of 0.4% (11 deaths in 2,692 patients), which indicates that persons with bulimia nervosa have an increased risk of mortality of 1.5.

## Etiology and Pathogenesis

Fairburn and Cooper (1984) found that a rigid diet was the most commonly reported precipitant of binge-eating behavior and that a gross bingeing bout was the most common precipitant for vomiting behavior. This finding may shed some light on the physiological mechanisms involved in binge eating and purging. For example, the period of strict dieting may influence peptide and neurotransmitter secretion, which may in turn affect appetite and satiety mechanisms. Studies of satiety responses in patients with eating disorders have shown that the perceptions of hunger and satiety are disturbed in patients who binge and purge (Halmi and Sunday 1991). Another study showed distinct differences in taste preferences for sweetness and "fattiness" in restricting anorexic patients, bulimic anorexic patients, normal-weight bulimic patients, and control subjects (Sunday and Halmi 1990).

## Treatment

Specific therapy techniques such as behavior therapy, cognitive therapy, psychodynamic therapy, and "psychoeducation therapy" have been conducted in both individual and group formats (Table 25–8). Multiple controlled drug treatment studies also have been conducted in the past decade. Often a variety of therapy techniques such as cognitive therapy, behavior therapy, and drug treatment may be used together in either individual or group therapy. The American Psychiatric Association (2000b) revised practice guideline for the treatment of patients with eating disorders has a helpful section on developing a treatment plan for the individual patient. Factors that need to be considered are level of care (outpatient, intensive outpatient, partial hospitalization, residential treatment center, or inpatient hospitalization), site of treatment (availability of medical care), and family assessment and treatment.

### *Psychodynamic Therapy*

Lacey (1983) described the use of psychodynamic therapy with cognitive and behavioral techniques in both individual and group therapy formats. Common themes that need

to be dealt with are poor self-esteem, dependency problems, and a sense of ineffectiveness.

### *Cognitive-Behavioral Therapy*

Fourteen published controlled studies have examined the efficacy of CBT in bulimia nervosa. One of the first and best descriptions of CBT was by Fairburn (1981). All of the subjects in these 14 studies were outpatients, with the exception of one study of the effectiveness of CBT in individual therapy that involved inpatients. Nearly all of the studies used a psychoeducational component that included information on the social-cultural emphasis on thinness; set point theory; the physical effects and medical complications of bingeing, purging, and abuse of laxatives and diuretics; and how dieting and fasting precipitate binge–purge cycles. Self-monitoring was an important part of all of these studies and usually consisted of a daily record of the times and durations of meals and a record of binge-eating and purging episodes as well as descriptions of moods and circumstances surrounding binge–purge episodes. The studies stressed the importance of eating regular meals.

Cognitive restructuring is the basis of all the CBT programs. The first step in cognitive therapy is the assessment of cognition. Patients are asked to write their thoughts on an assessment form so that cognitions can be examined for systematic distortions in the processing and interpretation of events. Two reviews of controlled studies of CBT for bulimia nervosa concluded that CBT benefits most patients (Fairburn et al. 1992a; Gotestam and Agras 1989). CBT was more effective than treatment with antidepressants alone, self-monitoring plus supportive psychotherapy, and behavioral treatment without the cognitive treatment component. One-year follow-up studies with CBT have shown a good maintenance of change, superior to that following treatment with antidepressants.

Behavior therapy is used specifically to stop the binge-eating/purging behaviors. Behavioral approaches include restricting exposure to cues that trigger a binge–purge episode, developing a strategy of alternative behaviors, and delaying the vomiting response to eating. Response prevention is a technique used specifically to prevent vomiting. After eating, a patient is placed in a situation in which it is very difficult for him or her comfortably to vomit. Adding exposure (i.e., requiring the patient to binge) did not seem to enhance the effects of response prevention (Rosen 1982).

The combined effects of CBT and antidepressant medication for bulimia nervosa were examined in three studies. Mitchell et al. (1990) found that group CBT was

**TABLE 25–8.    Treatment of bulimia nervosa**

| Type of treatment | Indications | Measurements | Key elements |
|---|---|---|---|
| Cognitive-behavioral therapy (CBT) | | | |
| Group | Outpatients—young adults | Psychiatric and medical evaluations before entering therapy | Psychoeducational component on all aspects of the bulimic disorder |
| Individual | Inpatients; outpatients— adolescents and adults with severe character disorders | Self-recording of medical consultations available throughout treatment | Self-monitoring, cognitive restructuring |
| Behavior therapy | Usually used in conjunction with computed tomography | Same as for CBT | Restricting exposure to cues, developing alternative behaviors, response prevention to stop vomiting |
| Interpersonal therapy | Outpatients—young adults | Psychiatric and medical evaluations before entering therapy and consultation available during treatment | Focuses on interpersonal relationships |
| Pharmacotherapy | | | |
| Antidepressants Fluoxetine Desipramine Imipramine Nortriptyline | Binge-eating behavior, depression, unwillingness to enter CBT | Initial evaluation: complete blood count, serum electrolytes and amylase, electrocardiogram, blood pressure; repeat above after 1 week and then as often as clinically indicated | Antidepressant drugs affect catecholamine and indoleamine function, which modulates eating behavior |

superior to imipramine therapy for decreasing binge eating and purging, and the combined treatment showed no additive effects compared with treatment with group CBT alone. Agras et al. (1992) had similar results comparing individual CBT, desipramine therapy, and the combination at 16 weeks. However, at 32 weeks, only the combined treatment given for 24 weeks was superior to medication given for 16 weeks. In a third study, CBT plus medication (desipramine, followed by fluoxetine in nonresponders) was superior to medication alone, but supportive psychotherapy plus medication was not. CBT plus medication was superior to CBT alone.

A study of interpersonal therapy (IPT), which targets interpersonal functioning, showed that IPT was equivalent to CBT in reducing bulimic symptoms and psychopathology; at follow-up, it was actually superior to CBT (Fairburn et al. 1992b). This was the first study to show that bulimia nervosa may be treated successfully without focusing directly on the patient's eating habits and attitudes toward shape and weight. In a multisite study comparing CBT with IPT, bulimic patients had 19 sessions of treatment over a 20-week period and were evaluated for 1 year after treatment. CBT was significantly superior to IPT at the end of treatment for the number of participants recovered (29% vs. 6%). At a 1-year follow-up, no significant difference was found between the two treatments. However, CBT was significantly more rapid in initiating improvement in patients with bulimia nervosa compared with IPT. Therefore, the authors suggested that CBT should be considered the preferred psychotherapeutic treatment for bulimia nervosa (Agras et al. 2000).

A multicenter treatment study that used a sequential design, which more realistically represents the practice of treating bulimia nervosa by primary care physicians, showed that those patients who failed to respond to CBT and were randomized to either IPT or fluoxetine improved equally in both treatments. However, only 20% of these patients in each form of treatment became abstinent, which is not a very impressive figure (Mitchell et al. 2002). One study showed that individuals with bulimia nervosa who did not respond to or had relapsed following CBT or IPT had a significantly better response to fluoxetine compared with placebo (Walsh et al. 2000). In the next 3–4 years, these studies will yield some very useful data to aid in the decisions about what kind of therapy should be given to which patients.

*Drug Therapy*

Studies of antidepressant medications have consistently shown some efficacy in the treatment of bulimia nervosa. Since 1980, more than a dozen double-blind, placebo-controlled trials of various antidepressants have been conducted in normal-weight outpatients with bulimia nervosa. (For a review of these studies, see Fairburn et al. 1992a.) All of these trials found a significantly greater reduction in binge eating when antidepressant medication was administered than when placebo was given. Antidepressants improved mood and reduced psychopathological symptoms such as preoccupation with shape and weight. These studies provide evidence for the short-term efficacy of antidepressant medication, but long-term efficacy remains unknown. The average rate of abstinence from bingeing and purging in these studies was 22%, indicating that most patients remain symptomatic at the end of treatment with antidepressants. Both of the systematic studies conducted to evaluate maintenance of change in bulimic symptomatology yielded disappointing results: most subjects did not maintain improvement (Pyle et al. 1990; Walsh et al. 1991). The dosage of antidepressant medication to treat bulimia nervosa was similar to that used in the treatment of depression. The antidepressants used in the controlled-treatment studies of bulimia nervosa included desipramine, imipramine, amitriptyline, nortriptyline, phenelzine, and fluoxetine. It should be noted that bulimic patients are impulsive and cannot follow diets; therefore, the drug phenelzine should not be used to treat binge eating in bulimia nervosa patients. Topiramate, an antiepileptic agent, was shown in a placebo-controlled, double-blind trial to be effective in reducing binge–purge behavior in binge-eating disorder (McElroy et al. 2003), and more recently studies have been under way with topiramate in treating bulimia nervosa.

## Key Points: Eating Disorders

- Chronic anorexia nervosa is best prevented by early diagnosis and early intensive treatment.
- Adolescents with anorexia nervosa are most effectively treated with family therapy, either conjoint or with separate parental counseling.
- CBT specific for bulimia is the most effective treatment for bulimia nervosa.
- Serotonin reuptake inhibitors are effective in reducing bingeing episodes and have a more benign side-effect profile compared with tricyclic antidepressants.

# References

Agras WS, Rossiter EM, Arnow B, et al: Pharmacological and cognitive-behavioral treatment for bulimia nervosa: a controlled comparison. Am J Psychiatry 149:82–87, 1992

Agras WS, Walsh BT, Fairburn CG: A multicenter comparison of cognitive-behavioral therapy and interpersonal psychotherapy for bulimia nervosa. Arch Gen Psychiatry 57:459–466, 2000

American Psychiatric Association: Diagnostic and Statistical Manual of Mental Disorders, 3rd Edition, Revised. Washington, DC, American Psychiatric Association, 1987

American Psychiatric Association: Diagnostic and Statistical Manual of Mental Disorders, 4th Edition, Text Revision. Washington, DC, American Psychiatric Association, 2000a

American Psychiatric Association: Practice guideline for the treatment of patients with eating disorders (revision). Am J Psychiatry 157(suppl):1–39, 2000b

Crisp AH, Lacey JH, Crutchfield M: Clomipramine and "drive" in people with anorexia nervosa: an inpatient study. Br J Psychiatry 150:355–358, 1987

Fairburn C: A cognitive behavioral approach to the treatment of bulimia. Psychol Med 11:707–711, 1981

Fairburn CG, Cooper PJ: The clinical features of bulimia nervosa. Br J Psychiatry 144:238–246, 1984

Fairburn CG, Agra WS, Wilson GT: The research on the treatment of bulimia nervosa: practical and theoretical implications, in Biology of Feast and Famine: Relevance to Eating Disorders. Edited by Anderson GH, Kennedy SH. New York, Academic Press, 1992a, pp 318–340

Fairburn CG, Jones R, Pevelar RC, et al: Three psychological treatments for bulimia nervosa: a comparative trial. Arch Gen Psychiatry 48:463–469, 1992b

Garfinkel PE, Lin E, Goering P, et al: Bulimia nervosa in a Canadian community sample: prevalence and comparison of subgroups. Am J Psychiatry 152:1052–1058, 1995

Garner DM, Bemis KM: A cognitive-behavioral approach to anorexia nervosa. Cognit Ther Res 6:1223–1250, 1982

Garner DM, Garfinkel PE: Handbook of Psychotherapy for Anorexia Nervosa. New York, Guilford, 1985

Gotestam KA, Agras WS: Bulimia nervosa: pharmacological and psychological approaches to treatment. Nord Psykiatr Tidsskr 43:543–551, 1989

Gwirtsman HE, Guze BH, Yager J, et al: Fluoxetine treatment of anorexia nervosa: an open trial. J Clin Psychiatry 51:378–382, 1990

Halmi KA: Anorexia nervosa: demographic and clinical features in 94 cases. Psychosom Med 36:18–26, 1974

Halmi KA: Anorexia nervosa and bulimia, in Handbook of Adolescent Psychology. Edited by Hersen M, Van Hasselt T. New York, Pergamon, 1987, pp 265–287

Halmi KA, Sunday SR: Temporal patterns of hunger and satiety ratings and related cognitions in anorexia and bulimia. Appetite 16:219–237, 1991

Halmi KA, Eckert E, LaDu T, et al: Anorexia nervosa: treatment efficacy of cyproheptadine and amitriptyline. Arch Gen Psychiatry 43:177–181, 1986

Halmi KA, Eckert E, Marchi P, et al: Comorbidity of psychiatric diagnoses in anorexia nervosa. Arch Gen Psychiatry 48:712–718, 1991

Halmi KA, Agras S, Crow S, et al: Predictors of treatment acceptance and completion in anorexia nervosa. Arch Gen Psychiatry 62:1–6, 2005

Hart K, Ollendick TH: Prevalence of bulimia in working and university women. Am J Psychiatry 142:851–854, 1985

Hoek H: The incidence and prevalence of anorexia nervosa and bulimia nervosa in primary care. Psychol Med 21:455–460, 1991

Hoek HW, Bartelds A, Bosveld J, et al: Impact of urbanization on detection rates of eating disorders. Am J Psychiatry 152:1272–1278, 1995

Hsu LK, Crisp AH, Harding B: Outcome of anorexia nervosa. Lancet 1(8107):61–65, 1979

Kaye WH, Nagata T, Weltzin TE, et al: Double-blind placebo-controlled administration of fluoxetine in restricting- and restricting-purging-type anorexia nervosa. Biol Psychiatry 49:644–652, 2001

Keel PK, Mitchell JE: Outcome in bulimia nervosa. Am J Psychiatry 154:313–321, 1997

Kleifield E, Wagner S, Halmi K: Cognitive-behavioral treatment of anorexia nervosa. Psychiatr Clin North Am 19:715–734, 1996

Kurth C, Krahn D, Nairn K, et al: The severity of dieting and bingeing behaviors in college women: interview validation of survey data. J Psychiatry Res 29:211–225, 1995

Lacey JH: An outpatient treatment program for bulimia nervosa. Int J Eat Disord 2:209–241, 1983

Lewinsohn PM, Striegel-Moore RH, Seeley JR: Epidemiology and natural course of eating disorders in young women from adolescence to young adulthood. J Am Acad Child Adolesc Psychiatry 39:1284–1292, 2000

McElroy SL, Arnold LM, Shapira N: Topiramate in the treatment of binge eating disorder associated with obesity: a randomized, placebo-controlled trial. Am J Psychiatry 160:255–261, 2003

Mitchell JE, Pyle RL, Eckert ED, et al: A comparison study of antidepressants and structured intensive group therapy in the treatment of bulimia nervosa. Arch Gen Psychiatry 47:149–157, 1990

Mitchell JE, Halmi K, Wilson GT, et al: A randomized secondary treatment study of women with bulimia nervosa who failed to respond to CBT. Int J Eat Disord 32:271–278, 2002

Nielsen S: Epidemiology and mortality of eating disorders. Psychiatr Clin North Am 24:201–214, 2001

Pyle RL, Mitchell JE, Eckert ED, et al: Maintenance treatment and 6 month outcome for bulimia patients who respond to initial treatment. Am J Psychiatry 147:871–875, 1990

Rosen J: Bulimia nervosa: treatment with exposure and response prevention. Behav Ther 13:117–124, 1982

Schotte D, Stunkard A: Bulimia vs. bulimic behaviors on a college campus. JAMA 9:1213–1215, 1987

Soundy TJ, Lucas AR, Suman VJ: Bulimia nervosa in Rochester, Minnesota from 1980 to 1990. Psychol Med 25:1065–1071, 1995

Sunday SR, Halmi KA: Taste perceptions and hedonics in eating disorders. Physiol Behav 48:587–594, 1990

Theander S: Outcome and prognosis in anorexia nervosa and bulimia, in Anorexia Nervosa and Bulimic Disorders. Edited by Szmukler GI, Slade PD, Harris P, et al. London, Pergamon, 1985, pp 493–508

Turnbull S, Ward A, Treasure J, et al: The demand for eating disorder care: an epidemiological study using the General Practice Research Database. Br J Psychiatry 169:705–712, 1996

Walsh BT, Hadigan CM, Devlin MJ, et al: Long-term outcome of antidepressant treatment for bulimia nervosa. Am J Psychiatry 148:1206–1212, 1991

Walsh BT, Agras WS, Devlin MJ, et al: Fluoxetine in bulimia nervosa following poor response to psychotherapy. Am J Psychiatry 157:1332–1334, 2000

# Sleep Disorders

DANIEL J. BUYSSE, M.D.

JED E. BLACK, M.D.

PHYLLIS G. ZEE, M.D., Ph.D.

JOHN W. WINKELMAN, M.D., Ph.D.

In humans, the electrophysiological characteristics of sleep can be characterized by polysomnography, an adaptation of electroencephalography. Patterns of electroencephalographic activity, eye movements, and muscle tone show clear differences between wakefulness and sleep, which is further divided into two states, rapid eye movement (REM) sleep and non–rapid eye movement (NREM) sleep (Carskadon and Rechtschaffen 2005). These three states are distinguished by characteristic patterns of environmental responsiveness, general physiology, electroencephalographic waveforms, muscle tone, and mental activity (Table 26–1).

NREM sleep is subdivided into four stages of increasing "depth," which correlate with decreasing arousability. NREM and REM sleep cycle periodically across the night. Most Stage 3–4 NREM sleep ("deep" or "delta" sleep) occurs in the first half of the night. NREM and REM sleep alternate approximately every 90–100 minutes during the sleep period. REM sleep episodes become longer and more intense toward the morning hours, as measured by the number of eye movements and complexity of dream mentation (Figure 26–1).

Sleep stages are affected by a number of individual and environmental factors. Age is the most important of these (Ohayon et al. 2004). Newborns spend nearly 50% of sleep in a form of sleep resembling REM, but this decreases rapidly in the first year of life. Sleep duration also dramatically decreases from infancy through childhood and then increases slightly in adolescence. Across the adult life span, Stage 3–4 sleep gradually diminishes from its peak in late adolescence. In later adulthood, the number and duration of awakenings and the amount of Stage 1 sleep increase, but Stage 2 NREM and REM sleep are relatively consistent. In addition, the entire sleep period tends to phase delay during adolescence and then phase advance during later adulthood.

Physiologically, human sleep is regulated by two processes, a homeostatic factor and a circadian factor (Figure 26–2). The homeostatic factor represents an increase in sleep "drive" as a function of prior wakefulness and can be measured in the time course of electroencephalographic slow-wave activity across a sleep period. Homeostatic sleep drive builds up during waking hours and then decreases during subsequent sleep. The second regulatory factor is the circadian rhythm of sleep and wakefulness. In humans, the circadian drive for sleep is highest in the second half of the usual sleep period. Homeostatic and circadian sleep factors typically function interactively. Homeostatic sleep drive builds up near the approaching usual sleep time at night and ensures rapid entry into deep NREM sleep. As homeostatic sleep drive weakens during the middle of the night, circadian sleep drive increases, maintaining sleep for the second half of the sleep period.

**TABLE 26–1.    Physiological characteristics of sleep–wake states**

|  | Wake | NREM | REM |
|---|---|---|---|
| Electroencephalogram | Fast, low voltage | Slow, high voltage | Fast, low voltage |
| Eye movement | Vision-related | Slow, irregular | Rapid |
| Muscle tone | ++ | + | 0 |
| Neuronal activity in LDT/PPT | + | 0 | ++ |
| Neuronal activity in LC/DR/TMN | ++ | + | 0 |
| Neuronal activity in VLPO (cluster) | 0 | ++ | +? |
| Neuronal activity in VLPO (extended) | 0 | +? | ++ |
| Neuronal activity in hypocretin neurons | ++ | 0? | 0? |
| Heart rate, blood pressure, respiratory rate | Variable | Slow/low, regular | Variable, higher than NREM |
| Responses to hypoxia and hypercarbia | Active | Reduced responsiveness | Lowest responsiveness |
| Thermoregulation | Behavioral and physiological regulation | Physiological regulation only | Reduced physiological regulation |
| Mental activity | Full | None or limited | Story-like dreams |

*Note.*  +, ++=activity level; 0=inactive; DR=dorsal raphe; LC=locus coeruleus; LDT=laterodorsal pontine tegmentum; NREM= non–rapid eye movement sleep; PPT=pedunculopontine tegmentum; REM=rapid eye movement sleep; TMN = tuberomammillary nucleus; VLPO (cluster)=central portion of ventrolateral preoptic nucleus; VLPO (extended)=peripheral portion of ventrolateral preoptic nucleus.
*Source.*   Adapted from Saper et al. 2001.

# Clinical Assessment of Sleep and Sleep Disorders

The diagnosis and management of patients with sleep complaints rest on an accurate clinical history. Important elements of the history include the nature, severity, and frequency of the symptoms; duration of the complaint; associated impairments; and exacerbating and alleviating factors. The following aspects of the clinical evaluation are particularly relevant to sleep and circadian rhythm disorders:

- *24-hour history.* Because sleep affects wakefulness and vice versa, it is important to assess both nighttime and daytime symptoms. Following the chronology of a "typical" night and day is essential for assessing sleep problems and daytime sleepiness.
- *Regularity of sleep–wake patterns.* Many patients with sleep disorders develop highly irregular schedules, seeking to "catch" sleep whenever they can. This pattern can itself contribute to further sleep difficulties.

- *Bed partner history.* Certain symptoms, including snoring and sleep-related behaviors, may not be evident to the person with the disorder itself.
- *Medical, neurological, and psychiatric disorders.* Sleep problems are associated with a wide variety of other disorders that may exacerbate symptoms (Table 26–2).
- *Medications and substances.* All drugs affecting control of nervous system function, and many used for medical disorders, can affect sleep (Table 26–3).
- *Physical examination.* Although most sleep disorders have no specific physical findings, sleep apnea syndromes often do. Thus it is useful to evaluate the following minimal features in patients presenting with sleep–wake complaints: height, weight, and body mass index; neck circumference; patency or oral and nasal airways; and craniofacial abnormalities, including retrognathia. Cardiopulmonary and neurological examinations can identify associated heart failure in sleep apnea or neuropathies that may contribute to restless legs syndrome (RLS).
- *Questionnaires.* Sleep–wake diaries may give a more complete picture of the individual's sleep patterns and

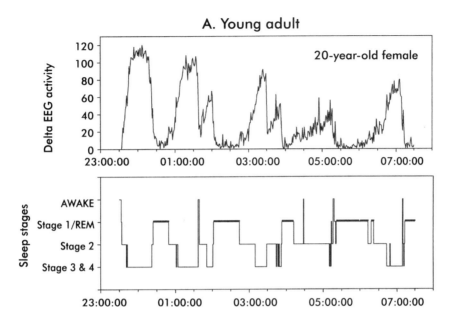

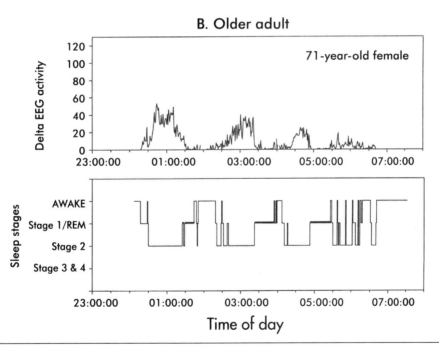

FIGURE 26–1.  **Hypnograms of sleep stages in healthy subjects.**

Each 20- to 30-second epoch of sleep for an entire night is assigned a sleep stage by a human "scorer." These epoch scores can then be displayed graphically in a "hypnogram," to display the progression of sleep stages across the night. (*A*) Hypnogram for an entire night of sleep in a healthy young adult. Sleep stages are indicated by increasing "depth" on the vertical axis, with rapid eye movement (REM) sleep represented by heavy horizontal lines. Time is indicated on the horizontal axis. Note that most Stage 3–4 non-REM (NREM) sleep occurs in the early part of the night, and REM periods get longer toward the end of the night. (*B*) Hypnogram for an older adult. Note the absence of Stage 3–4 NREM sleep and the greater amount of wakefulness during the sleep period. EEG=electroencephalogram.

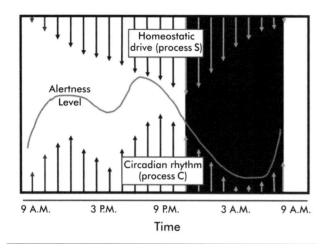

FIGURE 26–2.  **The two-process model.**

Alertness level is determined by the interaction between two processes. The sleep homeostatic drive (Process S) promotes sleep and builds up during wake, reaching a maximum in the late evening (near the usual sleep time). The circadian rhythm system (Process C) promotes wakefulness during the day. It is biphasic and tends to dip in the midafternoon. Process C also reaches its peak in the evening to counterbalance the accumulation of homeostatic drive that has built up throughout the day and it begins to fall just before the usual bedtime. This system promotes wakefulness during the day and consolidates sleep at night.

*Source.*   Reprinted from Buysse DJ (ed.): *Sleep Disorders and Psychiatry* (Review of Psychiatry Series, Vol. 24, No. 2; Oldham JM and Riba MB, series eds.). Washington, DC, American Psychiatric Publishing, 2005, p. 191. Copyright 2005, American Psychiatric Publishing. Used with permission.

day-to-day variability and may even help the individual identify patterns that are contributing to sleep problems. The Epworth Sleepiness Scale (Johns 1991) assesses daytime sleepiness by asking about the likelihood of falling asleep in specific behavioral situations. Scores range from 0 (no sleepiness) to 24 (extreme sleepiness). The Pittsburgh Sleep Quality Index is a 19-item self-rated scale that assesses global sleep quality, with scores ranging from 0 (good sleep quality) to 21 (poor sleep quality) (Buysse et al. 1989). A score greater than 5 is associated with significant sleep problems.

• *Actigraphy.* Actigraphy measures body movement patterns during sleep through a small accelerometer worn on the wrist. Patterns of motor activity correspond reasonably well to sleep and wakefulness and may be useful for assessing sleep–wake patterns over time.

**TABLE 26–2.  Medical and psychiatric disorders and conditions associated with insomnia**

| System | Examples |
| --- | --- |
| Cardiovascular | Congestive heart failure |
| Pulmonary | Chronic obstructive pulmonary disease, asthma |
| Renal and genitourinary | Chronic renal failure, prostatic hypertrophy |
| Gastrointestinal | Gastroesophageal reflux disease |
| Musculoskeletal | Fibromyalgia, osteoarthritis, rheumatoid arthritis |
| Endocrine | Hyperthyroidism, diabetes |
| Neurological | Parkinson's disease, cerebrovascular disease |
| Other | Menopause |
| Mood disorders | Major depression, dysthymic disorder, bipolar affective disorder |
| Anxiety disorders | Generalized anxiety disorder, panic disorder, posttraumatic stress disorder |
| Psychotic disorders | Schizophrenia |
| Substance use disorders | Alcohol, sedatives |

• *Polysomnography.* In addition to electroencephalography, electro-oculography, and electromyography, clinical polysomnography typically includes measurements of nasal–oral airflow, nasal pressure, and chest and abdominal movements to assess breathing; oximetry to measure desaturation events; electrocardiography; and anterior tibialis electromyography to assess leg movements during sleep.

## Insomnia Disorders

### Definition and Description

*Insomnia* refers to the complaint of difficulty falling asleep, frequent or prolonged awakenings, inadequate sleep quality, or short overall sleep duration in an individual who has adequate time available for sleep. Insomnia is not defined by polysomnography or a specific sleep duration. Because insomnia occurs only when there is adequate opportunity for sleep, it must be distinguished from sleep

**TABLE 26–3. Medications and substances associated with insomnia**

Alcohol (acute use, withdrawal)

Caffeine

Nicotine

Antidepressants (selective serotonin reuptake inhibitor, serotonin-norepinephrine reuptake inhibitor)

Corticosteroids

Decongestants (phenylpropanolamine, pseudoephedrine)

Beta-agonists, theophylline derivatives

Beta-antagonists

Statins

Stimulants

Dopamine agonists

deprivation, in which the individual has relatively normal sleep ability but inadequate opportunity for sleep.

## Epidemiology and Consequences

The 1-year prevalence of insomnia symptoms is approximately 30%–40% in the general population and up to 66% in primary care and psychiatric settings. The prevalence of primary insomnia as a specific disorder is in the range of 5%–10% of the general population (Ohayon 2002). Established risk factors for insomnia include advancing age, female sex, being divorced or separated, unemployment, and comorbid medical and psychiatric illness. Factors that commonly initiate or maintain insomnia include psychosocial stresses such as moves, relationship difficulties, occupational and financial problems, and caregiving responsibilities.

## Pathophysiology and Etiology

Insomnia is often thought to result from increased arousal. *Arousal* refers to the individual's state of central nervous system (CNS) activity and reactivity, ranging from sleep to wakefulness with excitement or panic. *Hyperarousal* is characterized by a high level of alertness either tonically or in response to specific situations such as the sleep environment. Hyperarousal in insomnia is suggested by psychophysiological, metabolic, electrophysiological, neuroendocrine, and functional neuroanatomical evidence (reviewed in Perlis et al. 2005). Functional imaging studies

demonstrate increased glucose metabolic rates during wakefulness and sleep and attenuation of the usual NREM sleep–related decline in metabolism in brain-stem arousal centers in subjects with insomnia compared with healthy control subjects. Self-reported wakefulness during sleep is related to increased metabolic activity in the same regions (Nofzinger 2006; Nofzinger et al. 2004).

Psychological and behavioral theories also may help to explain the development and persistence of insomnia. In Spielman et al.'s (1987) behavioral model (Figure 26–3), individual predisposing factors such as heightened physiological or cognitive arousal interact with external precipitating factors or stressors to produce acute insomnia. Perpetuating factors—that is, maladaptive coping strategies such as spending more time in bed—maintain and reinforce insomnia even after the original precipitants recede. In Morin's (1993) model, cognitive hyperarousal is indicated by sleep-focused, ruminative thoughts, particularly around bedtime. A vicious cycle of cognitive arousal, physiological arousal, sleep disturbance, and daytime consequences ensues, leading to the adoption of maladaptive coping strategies. Perlis et al. (1997) proposed a neurocognitive model of insomnia emphasizing the central role of cortical arousal. This model suggests that cortical arousal, as measured by beta electroencephalographic activity, leads to both physiological and cognitive arousal. Harvey (2002) proposed that cognitive strategies used by people with insomnia maintain sleep disturbances by producing selective attention and monitoring toward autonomic symptoms and environmental cues associated with sleeplessness. Psychological and behavioral theories of insomnia are important not only for their heuristic value but also for the interventions they have generated.

## Assessment and Diagnosis

The assessment of patients with insomnia rests on a detailed clinical history focusing on specific symptoms, chronology, exacerbating and alleviating factors, and response to previous treatments. The insomnia history should cover the patient's usual sleep and wake periods, specifically considering behaviors, cognitions, and environmental factors related to bedtime and sleep and variability of sleep from day to day. Symptoms of RLS, snoring or breathing problems, and pain or limitations to mobility during sleep also should be assessed. Other important elements of the history include exercise routines, regularity of work and daytime activities, limitations in these activities, and daytime sleepiness and napping.

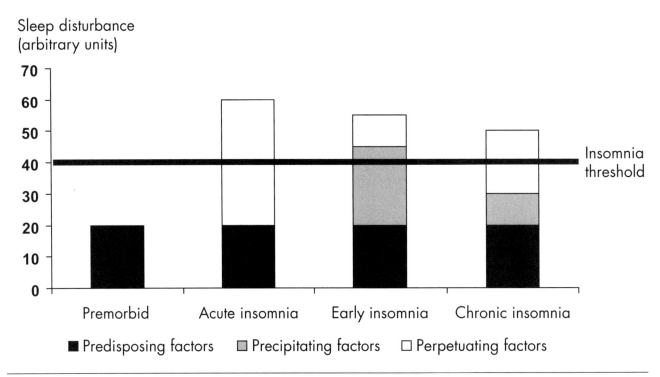

Sleep disturbance
(arbitrary units)

FIGURE 26–3.   **Heuristic model of the development of insomnia.**

This behavioral model of insomnia proposes that individuals have varying predispositions for insomnia and that specific precipitating factors will lead vulnerable individuals to cross the insomnia "threshold." Behavioral factors lead to perpetuation of the insomnia after the original precipitants have receded. The y axis indicates sleep disturbance (higher numbers=worse), and the x axis represents successive stages of insomnia.

*Source.*   Adapted from Spielman 1986.

## Behavioral and Psychological Treatment

Behavioral and psychological treatments aim to reduce sleep latency and improve sleep consolidation by changing behaviors, habits, and cognitions that interfere with sleep. Table 26–4 summarizes the major components of behavioral and psychological treatments for insomnia, which can be administered in individual or group format.

## Pharmacological Treatment

### *Benzodiazepine Receptor Agonists*

Benzodiazepine receptor agonists (BzRAs) are indicated for the treatment of acute insomnia and chronic primary insomnia. They are useful as adjunctive therapies for secondary insomnia related to certain medical conditions, psychiatric disorders, and other primary sleep disorders such as RLS and circadian rhythm sleep disorders (CRSDs). These agents bind at specific recognition sites on the γ-aminobutyric acid type A (GABA$_A$) receptor.

GABA$_A$ receptors are widely distributed in the CNS, including the cortex, basal ganglia, and cerebellum. The GABA$_A$ receptor comprises five protein subunits; BzRAs bind at the interface of α and γ subunits (Bateson 2004). Some of these drugs, such as zolpidem and zaleplon, bind relatively selectively at GABA$_A$ receptors containing α$_1$ subunits. The clinical significance of this selectivity is not clear, although such agents may be relatively more specific for hypnotic effects and have lower abuse liability. GABA$_A$ receptors with α$_1$ subunits mediate the sedative, amnestic, and anticonvulsant effects of BzRAs, whereas those containing α$_2$ and α$_3$ subunits mediate anxiolytic and myorelaxant effects (Mohler et al. 2002).

The BzRAs have different clinical effects primarily as a result of their different pharmacokinetic properties, including rate of absorption, extent of distribution, and terminal elimination half-life (Table 26–5).

As a class, BzRAs decrease sleep latency; those with longer duration of action also decrease the number and duration of awakenings from sleep and increase sleep duration. Most decrease Stage 3–4 NREM sleep and REM

**TABLE 26–4.** Cognitive-behavioral interventions for insomnia

| Intervention | General description | Specific techniques |
|---|---|---|
| Stimulus control | A set of behaviors that promote associative conditioning between the sleep environment and sleepiness | Go to bed only when feeling sleepy and intending to fall asleep.<br>If unable to fall asleep within 10–20 minutes (without watching the clock, 10–20 minutes is equivalent to repositioning yourself twice to try to fall asleep), leave the bed and the bedroom. Return only when feeling sleepy again.<br>Use the bed and bedroom for sleep only. Do not read, watch television, talk on the telephone, worry, or plan activities in the bedroom.<br>Set the alarm, and wake up at a regular time every day.<br>Do not snooze or nap during the day. |
| Sleep restriction therapy | Sleep practices that increase sleep "drive" and facilitate the ability to sleep | Restrict time awake in bed by setting strict bedtime and rising schedules limited to the average number of hours of actual sleep reported in one night.<br>Increase time in bed by advancing bedtime by 15–30 minutes when the time spent asleep is at least 85% of the allowed time in bed.<br>Keep a fixed wakeup time, regardless of actual sleep duration.<br>If after 10 days sleep efficiency is lower than 85%, delay bedtime by 15–30 minutes. |
| Relaxation training | Training in techniques that decrease waking arousal and facilitate sleep at night (muscular tension and cognitive arousal are incompatible with sleep). | Practice muscle relaxation daily, using progressive relaxation training.<br>Use guided imagery to decrease rumination at bedtime by replacing arousing mental content with soothing images and deliberately avoiding intrusive thoughts. |
| Cognitive restructuring of irrational sleep-related beliefs | Identification, challenge, and replacement of dysfunctional beliefs and attitudes regarding sleep and sleep loss. These beliefs increase arousal and tension, which in turn impede sleep and reinforce the dysfunctional beliefs. | Address irrational beliefs and fears about sleep, including<br>Overestimation of numbers of hours of sleep necessary to be rested.<br>Overall apprehensive expectation that sleep cannot be controlled.<br>Fear of getting out of bed when awake for fear of the time when sleep will come. |
| Sleep hygiene | Promote behaviors that improve sleep; limit behaviors that harm sleep. | Avoid naps.<br>Get regular exercise, at least 6 hours before sleep.<br>Maintain a regular sleep schedule 7 nights a week.<br>Avoid stimulants (caffeine, nicotine).<br>Limit alcohol intake.<br>Do not look at the clock when awake in bed. |

**TABLE 26–5.   Benzodiazepine receptor agonists: pharmacokinetics**

| Drug | Onset of action (min) | Elimination half-life (h) | Typical adult dosage (mg) |
|---|---|---|---|
| Zaleplon | 10–20 | 1.0 | 5–20 |
| Zolpidem | 10–20 | 1.5–2.4 | 5–10 (IR) |
| | | | 5–10 (MR) |
| Eszopiclone | 10–30 | 5–6 | 1–3 |
| Triazolam | 10–20 | 1.5–5 | 0.125–0.25 |
| Temazepam | 45–60 | 8–20 | 7.5–30 |
| Estazolam[a] | 15–30 | 20–30 | 0.5–2 |
| Quazepam[a] | 15–30 | 15–120 | 7.5–15 |
| Flurazepam[a] | 15–30 | 36–120 | 15–30 |

*Note.*   IR=immediate release; MR=modified release. [a]Has active metabolite.

sleep by small amounts, but the clinical significance of these changes is unclear. Meta-analyses have found these agents to be efficacious in the treatment of chronic insomnia (Holbrook et al. 2000; Nowell et al. 1997; Soldatos et al. 1999) on self-reported outcomes of sleep latency, sleep duration, number of awakenings, and sleep quality.

Although tolerance has long been a concern with BzRAs, evidence presented here shows no general loss of efficacy with nightly or intermittent treatment. Epidemiological studies show that up to two-thirds of patients taking hypnotics chronically report substantial ongoing benefit (Ohayon and Guilleminault 1999). In many placebo-controlled BzRA trials, placebo-treated groups show gradual improvements over time, which may also account for some of the apparent loss of efficacy with BzRA treatment. Discontinuance effects include *rebound insomnia*, defined as an increase in sleep problems to a level greater than the baseline level on discontinuation of the drug. A meta-analysis suggests that rebound insomnia is a short-lived, dosage-dependent phenomenon (Soldatos et al. 1999). Nevertheless, abrupt discontinuation of BzRAs does lead to worsening of symptoms compared with the treatment period. BzRAs have a marginal tendency for self-administration in animals—this is often used as a model of abuse potential in humans (Woods and Winger 1995)—and they are rarely the drug of choice in humans who abuse drugs. Individuals with a history of substance abuse, particularly of sedatives or alcohol, should be treated cautiously (Griffiths and Weerts 1997).

### Melatonin and Melatonin Receptor Agonists

Melatonin is a pineal hormone secreted exclusively at night in a strong circadian rhythm. Exogenous melatonin has been studied as a hypnotic. It is rapidly absorbed, with peak levels occurring in 20–30 minutes, and has an elimination half-life of 40–60 minutes. Studies of subjective effects in healthy young adults given melatonin during the daytime, when activity of the suprachiasmatic nucleus is greatest, support its hypnotic efficacy (Cajochen et al. 2003). When given at night, melatonin can decrease subjective sleep latency, although other effects are less consistent (Brzezinski et al. 2005), and its efficacy on polysomnographic measures is not well documented. Ramelteon is a synthetic agonist of melatonin $MT_1$ and $MT_2$ receptors, with much higher affinity than endogenous melatonin. Controlled clinical trials have indicated its efficacy for reducing sleep latency, but with variable effects on sleep duration (Buysse et al. 2005a; Erman et al. 2006).

### Other Agents

Other drugs and compounds are often used to treat insomnia, despite the lack of a U.S. Food and Drug Administration indication and the small amount of efficacy and safety data supporting their use (reviewed in Buysse et al. 2005b). The use of sedating antidepressants may be related to their lack of abuse potential as well as the perception that they may help subsyndromal depression. Small placebo-controlled clinical trials in primary insomnia support the efficacy of trazodone, doxepin, and trimipramine. Mirtazapine has been evaluated in small studies of healthy adults and patients with depression that documented improvements in sleep latency, awakenings, Stage 1 NREM sleep, and Stage 3–4 NREM sleep (Winokur et al. 2000). Effects of sedating antidepressants are summarized in Table 26–6.

**TABLE 26–6. Summary of other drugs used to treat insomnia[a]**

| Drug | Sleep latency | Sleep continuity[b] | Stage 3/4 NREM sleep amount (%) | REM sleep | Other |
|---|---|---|---|---|---|
| Trazodone | ↓ | ↔ to ↑ | ↑ | ↔ Amount, % (↓ to ↑ in individual studies) | Infrequent side effect of priapism |
| Doxepin | ↓ | ↑ | ↔ | ↓ Amount, % of REM; ↑ phasic eye movements (REM density) | ↓ Sleep apnea (minor effect); ↔ or ↑ periodic limb movements; ↑ restless legs symptoms; may induce eye movements during NREM sleep; anticholinergic effects |
| Amitriptyline | ↓ | ↑ | ↔ | ↓Amount, % of REM; ↑ phasic eye movements (REM density) | |
| Trimipramine | ↓ | ↑ | ↔ | ↔ Amount, % | |
| Mirtazapine | ↓ | ↑ | ↔ | ↔ | May cause weight gain |
| Melatonin | ↓ | ↔ to ↑ | ↔ | ↔ | |
| Diphenhydramine | ↓ | ↔ to ↑ | ↔ to ↑ | ↓ | Anticholinergic effects |
| Valerian | ↓ | ↔ to ↑ | ↔ to ↑ | ↔ to ↑ | Inconsistent effects on sleep continuity, Stage 3/4 |
| Gabapentin | ↔ | ↔ to ↑ | ↑ | ↔ | ↓ Periodic limb movements |
| Tiagabine | ↔ | ↑ | ↑ | ↔ | Infrequent side effect of seizures |
| Olanzapine, quetiapine | ↔ to ↓ | ↑ | ↑ | ↔ to ↓ | Reports of increased periodic limb movements, sleep-related eating |
| γ-Hydroxybutyrate | ↔ to ↓ | ↑ | ↑ | ↔ to ↓ | Side effects of sleepwalking, enuresis; abuse potential |
| Chloral hydrate | ↓ | ↑ | ↔ | ↔ to ↓ | Rapid tolerance; hepatotoxicity |

*Note.* NREM=non–rapid eye movement sleep; REM=rapid eye movement sleep.

[a]Reported effects are based on preponderance of evidence from published studies (see text for details). Many effects are inconsistent between individual studies. ↑ indicates increase from pretreatment baseline; ↓ indicates decrease from pretreatment baseline; ↔ indicates no change from pretreatment baseline.

[b]*Sleep continuity* refers to the proportion of sleep relative to wakefulness after sleep onset as reflected by measures such as sleep efficiency. Other indicators of sleep continuity, such as wakefulness after sleep onset or number of awakenings, would have opposite signs. Thus, ↑ indicates improvement in overall sleep continuity.

**TABLE 26–7.    Comorbidities and consequences associated with obstructive sleep apnea syndrome**

| Cardiovascular complications | Metabolic complications | Neurocognitive complications |
|---|---|---|
| Nocturnal dysrhythmias | Leptin resistance | Daytime sleepiness |
| Bradydysrhythmias | Insulin resistance | Motor vehicle accidents |
| Atrial fibrillation | | Work-related accidents |
| Nocturnal hypertension | | Impaired neuropsychological function |
| Diurnal hypertension | | Impaired quality of life |
| Pulmonary hypertension | | |
| Congestive heart failure | | |
| Myocardial infarction | | |
| Stroke | | |

# Sleep-Related Breathing Disorders

## Obstructive Sleep Apnea

### Definition and Description

Obstructive sleep apnea (OSA) is characterized by repetitive episodes of complete (apnea) or partial (hypopnea) upper airway obstruction during sleep that often result in oxygen desaturation and terminate with brief arousals. By definition, apnea and hypopnea events last for 10 seconds or longer and are accompanied by continued efforts to breathe. Obstructive hypopneas are typically defined by a decrease in airflow of 30% or more with desaturation of 4% or more (Strollo and Rogers 1996).

### Epidemiology and Consequences

In predominantly white middle-aged cohorts, the prevalence of the OSA defined as an apnea–hypopnea index (AHI) of 10 or greater with daytime sleepiness and/or hypertension is approximately 5% (Young et al. 2002). In a longitudinal family study, the 5-year incidence of mild OSA (AHI=10–15) and moderate to severe OSA (AHI≥15) was 7.5% and 16%, respectively (Tishler et al. 2003). Clinical studies indicate an increased risk in men, with a male-to-female prevalence ratio of 3.3 to 1 (Bixler et al. 2001; Young et al. 1993). Increasing weight and advancing age also increase the risk of OSA (Young et al. 2002), although the age effect plateaus after age 65 years (Young et al. 1993).

OSA is associated with significant cardiovascular, metabolic, and neurocognitive consequences (see Table 26–7).

### Pathophysiology

The human upper airway lacks rigid support from bone or cartilage in the retropalatal and retrolingual airway.

During inspiration, negative intrathoracic pressure results in a suction force applied to this small, compliant upper airway, and narrowing (hypopnea) or closure (apnea) may occur. Vibration of these structures produces snoring. Thus, the primary cause for apnea is small functional airway diameter.

Craniofacial structure and function and obesity are the major determinants of small airway diameter in adults. During the transition from wakefulness to sleep, muscle tone decreases and snoring and airway narrowing occur in vulnerable individuals. Arousal from sleep, precipitated by increased airway resistance, hypopnea, or apnea, stimulates resumption of breathing (Gleeson et al. 1990).

### Assessment and Diagnosis

The history and physical examination can identify patients at high risk for OSA, which is then confirmed with polysomnography. Nightly loud snoring, breathing pauses during sleep, snorting, choking, and subjective daytime sleepiness all suggest the diagnosis of OSA. Obesity (particularly upper-body obesity) and systemic hypertension are often present. In some individuals, craniofacial abnormalities (retrognathia or micrognathia) and/or soft tissue abnormalities, such as enlarged tonsils, lateral narrowing of the airway, or an elongated soft palate, place the patient at risk for OSA (Schellenberg et al. 2000; Zonato et al. 2003).

### Treatment

Behavioral treatments play a minor role in treatment of OSA. Because obesity is a major risk factor for OSA, weight loss improves both sleep and breathing (Peppard et al. 2000). Sleep deprivation increases the severity of daytime sleepiness and decreases upper airway muscle tone and should therefore be avoided. Alcohol and BzRA hypnotics also reduce upper airway muscle tone. If the patient clearly has positional OSA (typically worse in the supine position), the lateral sleep position or elevation of the head of the bed may be helpful.

Positive pressure delivered via nasal or nasal–oral mask reliably treats airway closure during sleep and is the first-line treatment for OSA. Positive pressure therapy works by pneumatically "splinting" the airway open during sleep. The treatment effect is virtually immediate when proper positive pressure titration is performed. Positive pressure can be applied as continuous positive airway pressure (CPAP) or as bilevel positive airway pressure (BPAP). With BPAP, the pressure setting is higher during inspiration than expiration, accounting for normal variation in pressure during the respiratory cycle.

Oral appliance therapy modifies the position of the mandible and tongue to increase the upper airway size and reduce collapsibility. Oral appliance therapy is regarded as second-line therapy for OSA because it requires multiple adjustments over weeks to months, it is not 100% effective, and objective adherence is difficult to measure.

Surgical therapy has a small but important role in the management of adult OSA and can be broadly divided into two categories: tracheostomy (bypass of the upper airway) and reconstruction of the upper airway, which can involve multiple sites from the nasopharynx to the epiglottis. Tracheostomy was the original treatment for severe OSA but is now reserved for the small group of patients with severe and potentially life-threatening OSA who are intolerant of CPAP/BPAP. There are few well-designed studies to definitively evaluate the effect of simple reconstructive upper airway surgery on OSA (Bridgman and Dunn 2000). The most common procedure is uvulopalatopharyngoplasty, which involves altering the size and the stiffness of the soft palate. This procedure is highly effective in treating loud snoring, but its effect on OSA is less certain, with reported success ranging from 7% to 60% (Sher 1995).

Modafinil is an efficacious adjunctive therapy for OSA patients with residual daytime sleepiness despite adequate treatment with CPAP (Pack et al. 2001). Insomnia also can be encountered in OSA, although its true prevalence is unknown. Some reports have suggested improvement of insomnia with positive pressure treatment (Guilleminault et al. 2002a, 2002b).

BzRAs generally should be avoided in patients with OSA or suspected OSA unless they have been diagnosed and treated.

# Hypersomnias of Central Origin

## Narcolepsy

### Definition and Description

Narcolepsy is a syndrome characterized by profound excessive daytime sleepiness (EDS), which often occurs in association with cataplexy, hypnagogic or hypnopompic hallucinations, sleep paralysis, automatic behavior, and disrupted nocturnal sleep (American Academy of Sleep Medicine 2005). It is subdivided into two types: narcolepsy with cataplexy and narcolepsy without cataplexy. EDS is manifest as an increased propensity to fall asleep in relaxed or sedentary situations or a struggle to avoid sleeping in these situations. EDS may be so severe as to be irresistible, leading to sleep in inappropriate or dangerous situations. Brief naps temporarily relieve the sleepiness in many patients. EDS can lead to related symptoms, including automatic behavior (behavior that the individual does not recall), irritability, and poor memory, concentration, and attention. The overall amount of sleep per 24 hours is not increased in narcolepsy. In fact, many patients report fragmented nocturnal sleep, suggesting that the underlying disorder is an inability to maintain any stable sleep–wake state (Guilleminault and Fromherz 2005).

*Cataplexy* is the partial or complete loss of bilateral voluntary muscle tone in response to strong emotion and occurs in 60%–100% of patients with narcolepsy. The atonia may be minimal, occurring in a few muscle groups and causing subtle symptoms (ptosis, head drooping, slurred speech, dropping objects) or severe, resulting in complete collapse. Cataplectic episodes usually last from a few seconds to a minute or two (Honda 1988). The patient is awake and oriented during these episodes, a feature that distinguishes cataplexy from sleep episodes. Cataplexy is most often triggered by positive emotional experiences, such as laughter, but can be triggered by other strong emotions (Gelb et al. 1994). It is exacerbated by stress, fatigue, or sleepiness. The onset of cataplexy typically occurs within a few months of the onset of EDS but may be delayed by years (Honda 1988). *Hypnagogic* and *hypnopompic hallucinations* are visual, tactile, auditory, or multisensory events lasting up to a few minutes during the transition from wakefulness to sleep (hypnagogic) or from sleep to wakefulness (hypnopompic). Hallucinations may combine elements of dream sleep and consciousness and are often bizarre or disturbing to patients. *Sleep paralysis* is the inability to move for a few seconds to a few minutes during wake–sleep or sleep–wake transitions. Sleep paralysis can be frightening, particularly when accompanied by hallucinations or the sensation of being unable to breathe. Hypnagogic hallucinations, sleep paralysis, and automatic behavior are not specific to narcolepsy and may occur in other sleep disorders as well as in healthy individuals. However, their co-occurrence with EDS strongly suggests narcolepsy.

### Epidemiology

EDS occurring 3 or more days per week and interfering with daily activities has been reported in approximately 15% of the adult population in Western countries (Ohayon et al. 2002). The prevalence of narcolepsy in the United States, Western Europe, the Middle East, and Japan is approximately 0.05%, with a range of 0.002%–0.160% (Mignot 1998).

### Pathophysiology

Narcolepsy results from dysfunction of the hypothalamic peptide neuromodulator hypocretin (orexin). Although mutations in hypocretin-related genes are extremely rare in humans, the majority (85%–90%) of patients with narcolepsy–cataplexy have low or undetectable levels of hypocretin 1 in their cerebrospinal fluid (Nishino et al. 2000), a finding specific for this disorder (Mignot 2005).

### Assessment and Diagnosis

Clinical assessment of individuals presenting with EDS should focus on the severity, frequency, and situations in which sleepiness occurs. The relation between EDS and nighttime sleep is also important; individuals with narcolepsy frequently report no strong relation, which distinguishes narcolepsy from sleep deprivation. A clinical history of severe EDS coupled with cataplexy and/or sleep-related hallucinations or sleep paralysis is virtually diagnostic of narcolepsy. Polysomnography is also an important part of the evaluation and differential diagnosis. It can identify OSA, periodic limb movement disorder, and REM sleep behavior disorder that may contribute to EDS and nocturnal sleep disruption (Overeem et al. 2001). Individuals with narcolepsy also may have sleep-onset REM periods during nocturnal polysomnography testing. The multiple sleep latency test (MSLT) identifies reduced sleep latency (≤8 minutes) coupled with two or more sleep-onset REM periods. *Sleep-onset REM periods* are not specific for narcolepsy and may be due to sleep deprivation, rebound from REM-suppressing medication, altered sleep schedules, OSA, or delayed sleep phase

disorder. However, when these conditions are ruled out, these periods are highly suggestive of narcolepsy (Guilleminault and Fromherz 2005).

### Treatment

The effective treatment of EDS requires regular, structured nocturnal sleep and planned daytime naps. A nocturnal sleep period of 8 hours or more should be encouraged, with consistent bedtimes and awakening times. Shift work in any form is usually problematic for individuals with narcolepsy. Scheduling two or more brief naps at regular times during the day is almost always necessary to further enhance daytime function in patients with narcolepsy.

Stimulants are indicated for the treatment of EDS in narcolepsy (Guilleminault and Fromherz 2005; Mitler et al. 1994; Table 26–8). These drugs produce substantial improvement but do not restore daytime alertness to normal levels. Traditional stimulants include methylphenidate, dextroamphetamine, and methamphetamine. Dosages of 20–80 mg/day are typical for most stimulants (10–40 mg for methamphetamine). Modafinil is a wake-promoting agent that is somewhat less potent than traditional agents, but with greater tolerability. The mechanism of action of modafinil appears to be mediated through inhibition of the dopamine transporter (Wisor and Eriksson 2005). The duration of effect of modafinil is relatively long as a result of its half-life of 12–15 hours. The efficacy of modafinil has been evaluated extensively in EDS due to narcolepsy, idiopathic hypersomnia, and sleep apnea (U.S. Modafinil in Narcolepsy Multicenter Study Group 1998). An agent unrelated to the traditional stimulants that also enhances alertness in narcolepsy is sodium oxybate (γ-hydroxybutyrate) (Mamelak et al. 2004). Sodium oxybate has similar efficacy as other agents, and its effect may be additive with that of other stimulants (U.S. Xyrem Multicenter Study Group 2002) (see Table 26–8).

## Circadian Rhythm Sleep Disorders

Alterations in the regulation of the circadian timing system, or a misalignment between the endogenous circadian rhythm and the external physical or social environment, can affect the timing or duration of sleep and give rise to CRSD (Reid and Zee 2005). Several distinct subtypes of CRSD have been described (Figure 26–4). The approach to assessment and diagnosis is described first because this is similar across all subtypes.

**TABLE 26–8.** Common alerting agents for the treatment of excessive daytime sleepiness

| Agent | Receptor | Elimination half-life (h) | Time to maximal plasma concentration (h) | Usual dosage | Side effects |
|---|---|---|---|---|---|
| Modafinil | Unknown | 15 | 2–4 | 100–400 mg + once daily or divided | Headache, nausea, anxiety, irritability |
| Amphetamines | Dopamine agonist | 10 (SR: 15+) | 2 (SR: 8–10) | 5–60 mg divided | Both amphetamines and methylphenidate: headache, anxiety/irritability, increased blood pressure, palpitation, appetite suppression, tremor, insomnia |
| Methylphenidate | Dopamine agonist | 4 (SR: 8–10) | 2 (SR: 5) | 5–60 mg divided | |
| Pemoline[a] | Dopamine agonist | 12 | 2–4 | 18.75–112.5 mg daily or divided | As above, but milder |
| γ-Hydroxybutyrate | Inadequately characterized | 2 | 1 | 6–9 g + liquid solution divided nightly | Sedation, nausea, confusional arousals, sleepwalking |

*Note.* SR=sustained-release.
[a]Potentially hepatotoxic—frequent liver function monitoring required; withdrawn from the U.S. market in 2007.

## Assessment and Diagnosis

The diagnosis of CRSD rests on clinical history. CRSDs are distinguished from subclinical symptoms or circadian preferences by impairment in social, occupational, or other areas of functioning. Sleep–wake diaries are useful for confirming abnormalities of sleep–wake timing, and actigraphy provides objective verification of rest–activity patterns. Sleep diaries and actigraphy should be obtained for 1–2 weeks in order to capture the individual's typical schedule variations, such as work and nonwork days. Physiological markers of circadian phase, such as melatonin or core body temperature rhythms, can confirm abnormal circadian phase but are rarely used in clinical practice.

Although polysomnography is not required for the diagnosis of CRSD, it may be useful to exclude other sleep disorders such as OSA or RLS. Polysomnographic findings in individuals with CRSD may vary depending on the time of the sleep recording in relation to the individual's usual sleep–wake schedule.

When objective evaluation of sleepiness is needed, such as in shift work disorder when safety is of significant concern, the MSLT should be conducted during usual work hours.

Medical history is an important aspect of assessment in CRSD. Shift work disorder is associated with increased prevalence of medical disorders such as cardiovascular and gastrointestinal disorders, sleep apnea, obesity, and miscarriage (Scott 2000; Wagner 1996). Neurological disorders affecting the structure of the circadian pacemaker, its afferents, or its efferents (e.g., visual impairment, tumors, dementia, stroke) should be considered in individuals with irregular sleep–wake pattern and nonentrained type.

Evaluation of CRSD should routinely include screening for psychiatric disorders and psychoactive medications. The prevalence of affective and personality disorders is high in patients with CRSDs such as delayed sleep phase disorder and irregular sleep–wake pattern (Dagan 2002). Mood and personality disorders may contribute to social withdrawal, which can lead to a decrease in light exposure, physical activity, and social cues, thereby perpetuating abnormal sleep timing. Because depressed patients often complain of early-morning awakening, it is important to distinguish advanced sleep phase disorder from major depression and other mood disorders (Wagner 1996). Individuals with CRSD may use alcohol, sedative-hypnotics, and stimulants to alleviate symptoms, which may lead to substance dependence.

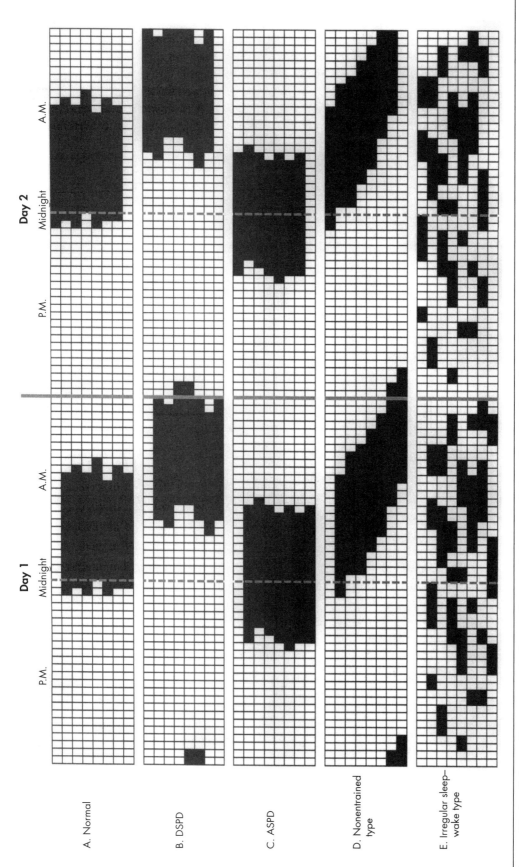

FIGURE 26–4.  Schematic representations of normal sleep and circadian rhythm sleep disorders.

Data are shown for 7 days and nights for each condition. *Black bars:* sleep; *open rectangles:* wakefulness. For each hypothetical condition, sleep–wake data are "double plotted" (i.e., each day's data are shown both to the right of and below the previous day) to facilitate viewing the pattern across days. Each *horizontal line* shows 2 days; the *heavy vertical line* separates successive days. The *dashed vertical line* indicates midnight. For comparative purposes, each condition is shown with a total sleep time of approximately 8 hours. **(A)** Normal sleep. Sleep hours across successive days fall at about midnight to 7:00 A.M. **(B)** Delayed sleep phase disorder (DSPD). Sleep hours are consistently delayed, with average sleep times of approximately 4:00 A.M. to noon. **(C)** Advanced sleep phase disorder (ASPD). Sleep hours are consistently advanced, with average sleep times of approximately 8:00 P.M. to 4:00 A.M. **(D)** Nonentrained type. Sleep hours are progressively later each day, following an underlying circadian rhythm period closer to 25 hours than 24. **(E)** Irregular sleep–wake type. Sleep–wake hours occur irregularly over the 24-hour day, with no discernible circadian pattern.

**TABLE 26–9.  Overview of parasomnias**

| | NREM parasomnias | | | REM parasomnias | |
|---|---|---|---|---|---|
| | **Confusional arousals** | **Sleepwalking** | **Sleep terrors** | **REM sleep behavior disorder** | **Nightmare disorder** |
| Stage of arousal | NREM 2–4 | NREM 3–4 | NREM 3–4 | REM | REM |
| Time of night | Anytime | First 2 hours | First 2 hours | Anytime | Anytime |
| EEG with event | NA | Mixed | Mixed | Characteristic of REM | NA |
| EMG with event | Low | Low | Low | High, variable | NA |
| Relative unresponsiveness during event | Yes | Yes | Yes | Yes | Yes |
| Autonomic activity | Low | Low | High | High | High |
| Amnesia | Yes | Yes | Yes | No | No |
| Confusion following episode | Yes | Yes | Yes | No | No |
| Family history of parasomnias | Yes | Yes | Yes | No | No |

*Note.*   EEG=electroencephalogram; EMG=electromyogram; NA=not available; NREM=non–rapid eye movement; REM = rapid eye movement.

The role of voluntary behavior often poses a problem in the evaluation of CRSD. For instance, some adolescents and young adults prefer delayed sleep–wake schedules and are not strongly motivated to change this pattern; socially withdrawn or cognitively impaired individuals may not see an irregular sleep–wake pattern as undesirable. In such cases, altered timing of light exposure can lead to a self-perpetuating cycle of sleep–wake disturbance.

# Parasomnias

The term *parasomnia* derives from the Latin *para* (next to) and *somnus* (sleep). Parasomnias are defined as undesirable physical or experiential events that accompany sleep (American Academy of Sleep Medicine 2005) and are generally divided into those arising from NREM sleep and those arising from REM sleep. These types of parasomnias can often be distinguished by their clinical features, time of occurrence, and associated autonomic activation (Table 26–9).

## NREM Parasomnias

### Clinical Features, Epidemiology, Pathophysiology

Arousal from sleep is not an all-or-none phenomenon, but rather a continuum of reestablishing alertness, judgment,

and control over behavior (Mahowald and Schenck 2001). Behaviors or mood states can be expressed during such partial arousals, which may be partially or completely divorced from awareness. Most commonly, such behaviors involve dissociated motor activities (walking, eating, sexual activity) or emotional responses (fear, anger, sexual excitement) (Schenck and Mahowald 2000). They are distinguished from waking behavior by the absence of complex mentation and sound judgment and by reduced response to environmental feedback. The relation between sleep-related behaviors and emotional states and waking motivations, psychological states, or psychopathology is unclear. NREM parasomnias show clear familial aggregation (Mahowald and Cramer Bornemann 2005). Specific NREM parasomnias share many features that may provide insight into their pathophysiology.

*Confusional arousals* are brief, simple motor behaviors that usually occur without strong affective expression during partial arousals from NREM sleep. Confusional arousals may occur during daytime naps. Mental confusion with automatic behavior, indistinct speech, and relative unresponsiveness to the environment are hallmarks (Mahowald and Cramer Bornemann 2005). Amnesia for events is dense; without an observer's report, they may go unnoticed. Individuals do not report dreams on achieving full alertness, but rather simple mentation. Electroencephalographic recordings at the time of confusional arousals may show delta waves (characteristic of slow-wave sleep), theta or alpha activity, or alternation between sleep and waking activity (Gaudreau et al. 2000). Epidemiological information is unreliable, but approximately 10%–20% of children and 2%–5% of adults report a history of confusional arousals (Ohayon et al. 1999). The expression of confusional arousals depends on a genetic predisposition combined with a precipitating event, which may be endogenous (e.g., OSA, pain, leg movements) or exogenous (e.g., forced awakening or environmental disruption) (Hublin et al. 2001). In predisposed individuals, sleep deprivation, medications, sleep disorders, stress, and circadian misalignment may aggravate or precipitate NREM parasomnia.

*Sleepwalking* also occurs within the first 1 or 2 hours of sleep without substantial affective activity, but it involves more elaborate behavior than in confusional arousals. Actions are typically simple, such as attempts to use the bathroom, go to the kitchen, or leave the home. Although the sleepwalker's eyes are open, behavior is often clumsy (Crisp 1996). Dreaming is usually not present or consists of only simple mentation (e.g., "had to find my ring"). If the episode is interrupted, responses may be absent, incomplete, or inappropriate. If left alone, sleepwalkers usually return to sleep, at times in unusual places; if attempts are made to arouse them, they may take a prolonged period of time to become fully alert. Individuals may become violent or agitated if sleepwalking episodes are interrupted. As in other NREM parasomnias, full or partial amnesia is typical.

Sleepwalking occurs in 10%–20% of children and 1%–4% of adults (Ohayon et al. 1999). It is most common in children between ages 5 and 10 years and becomes less and less prevalent with increasing age. There are no gender or racial differences in prevalence. Genetic factors appear to play an important role in sleepwalking, as evidenced by epidemiological and twin studies (Hublin et al. 2001). Risk of sleepwalking roughly doubles when one parent has a positive history and triples when both parents have a history. Genetic factors account for approximately 60%–80% of the variance in sleepwalking.

Approximately 80% of adults with sleepwalking report a continuous history from childhood, although many will not come to medical attention until their 20s or 30s as a result of bed-partner concerns. The frequency of sleepwalking is quite variable, but it usually occurs infrequently—that is, once or twice a month.

*Sleep terrors* share many features with sleepwalking but are characterized by more intense motor, autonomic, and affective activity and experience. Sleepwalking and sleep terrors may occur in the same individual. In children, sleep terrors are heralded by a piercing scream, with apparent extreme fear, crying, and inconsolability (Mahowald and Cramer Bornemann 2005). In adults, agitation is common, with the perception of an imminent threat requiring escape or defense (Schenck et al. 1997). For this reason, persons with sleep terrors may cause injury to themselves, others, or property. Dreams are usually not reported, but simple thoughts are sometimes present ("The room is on fire," or "I am being attacked") that can be difficult to dispel, even after awakening. The individual may incorporate bed partners or family members into the threatening scenario, potentially harming them. For this reason, individuals having a sleep terror should be gently redirected. Recollection of the event afterward is limited.

Sleep terrors are less common than sleepwalking, with about 5% of children and 1%–2% of adults reporting a history of such events (Ohayon et al. 1999). As with sleepwalking, genetic factors appear to increase susceptibility to sleep terrors, and precipitating factors can be either endogenous or exogenous. Polysomnography may not capture episodes, although multiple brief arousals from slow-wave sleep with heightened autonomic activity may be observed (Gaudreau et al. 2000).

## Assessment and Diagnosis

The differential diagnosis of patients with abnormal sleep-related motor or affective behaviors includes nocturnal panic attacks, nocturnal dissociative episodes, frontal lobe seizures, delirium associated with medical or neurological disorders, and REM sleep behavior disorder. A daytime history of behaviors similar to the nocturnal behaviors (e.g., panic or dissociative episode) suggests a diagnosis other than NREM parasomnia. Similarly, overnight polysomnographic monitoring may confirm REM sleep behavior disorder or a seizure disorder.

## Treatment

The decision to treat NREM parasomnias is based on the frequency of events, risk of injury to self or others, and distress the behaviors cause the patient or family members (Schenck and Mahowald 2000). Parasomnias typically occur infrequently but unpredictably, raising the question of whether chronic treatment of episodic events is warranted.

For most children, parasomnias do not require treatment because there is little risk of harm and the child is unaware of the events. Regulating the sleep–wake schedule and avoiding sleep deprivation can reduce the frequency of events. For sleepwalking, the sleeping environment must be made safe by locking doors and windows and keeping hallways and stairs well lit.

Treatment of sleepwalking or sleep terrors in adults involves three steps: modification of predisposing and precipitating factors; enhancing safety of the sleeping environment; and, when these are not successful, pharmacotherapy. Sleep disorders, medical disorders (pain, nocturia, dyspnea), and sleep-disrupting medications should be addressed when possible. If the parasomnia occurs within the first half of the sleep period, short-acting BzRAs such as triazolam (0.125–0.25 mg at bedtime) or zolpidem (5–10 mg at bedtime) are recommended. Clonazepam (0.5–1.0 mg at bedtime) is the most commonly used BzRA for parasomnias and has been used successfully for extended periods without the development of tolerance (Schenck and Mahowald 1996). These medications may suppress arousals or decrease slow-wave sleep. However, no controlled efficacy trials have been performed for NREM parasomnias.

## REM-Related Parasomnias

### REM Sleep Behavior Disorder

In REM sleep behavior disorder, the usual atonia of REM sleep is absent, allowing the sleeper to enact dreams that, when agitated or violent, can result in injury to the sleeper or bed partner (Mahowald and Schenck 2005). During such episodes, the sleeper has his or her eyes closed and is completely unresponsive to the environment until awakened, at which point he or she will achieve rapid and full alertness and report a dream that usually corresponds to the exhibited behavior. Fully expressed episodes of the disorder are intermittent, but talking, shouting, and fragmentary motor activity often occur between such events.

REM sleep behavior disorder is chronic and usually observed in men older than 50 years. It is strongly associated with neurological disorders characterized by accumulation of α-synuclein protein (Parkinson's disease, dementia with Lewy bodies, and multiple system atrophy) and may serve as an early marker of these disorders (Boeve et al. 2003). Up to two-thirds of patients followed up for 10 years developed Parkinson's disease (Schenck et al. 1996). REM-suppressing antidepressants, including selective serotonin reuptake inhibitors and monoamine oxidase inhibitors, are an important risk factor for REM sleep behavior disorder (Mahowald and Schenck 2005). Acute and chronic administration of serotonergic antidepressants can produce subclinical illness, in which motor tone is disinhibited during REM sleep (Winkelman and James 2004).

The diagnosis of REM sleep behavior disorder is made by polysomnography, which shows elevated muscle tone or excessive phasic muscle activity during REM sleep (American Academy of Sleep Medicine 2005). Large body movements and REM-related behaviors also may appear during the polysomnogram. Periodic limb movements of sleep may be observed during both REM and NREM sleep.

First-line treatment consists of BzRAs. The most commonly used agent is clonazepam (0.5–1.0 mg), which decreases the number and extent of pathological dream-enacting behaviors (Mahowald and Schenck 2005). Although clonazepam is generally well tolerated, its long half-life and the age of most patients with the disorder may lead to daytime sleepiness and/or cognitive impairment. In this case, shorter-acting benzodiazepines (e.g., lorazepam 1–2 mg) may be preferable. Melatonin (3–15 mg at bedtime) and pramipexole (0.5–1.0 mg at bedtime) also have been used with some success. Discontinuing medications such as antidepressants should be attempted if clinically possible. As with the NREM parasomnias, ensuring the safety of the sleeping environment for both the patient and the bed partner is essential (Mahowald and Schenck 2005).

### Nightmare Disorder

Nightmare disorder is characterized by recurrent distressing dreams that usually arise from REM sleep and are followed by an awakening, with full recall. The dominant emotion is usually fear, although anger, sadness, and embarrassment also may be present. Nightmares may occur at any time of night but are more common in the final third of the night, when REM is most prominent (American Academy of Sleep Medicine 2005; Nielsen and Zadra 2005). In distinction to sleep terrors, return to sleep after a nightmare is usually delayed, and frequent nightmares may lead to a fear of going to sleep. Nightmares are not associated with complex acting out of dreams as in REM sleep behavior disorder.

Nightmare treatment includes pharmacological and behavioral/psychological approaches. Prazosin (4–12 mg at bedtime; Raskind et al. 2003), cyproheptadine (Gupta et al. 1998), anticonvulsants (Berlant and Van Kammen 2002), and antipsychotic medications (Labbate and Douglas 2000) all have been efficacious in placebo-controlled trials and/or uncontrolled case series. Imagery rehearsal, in which new versions (with better outcomes) of nightmares are rehearsed during the day, has shown consistent benefit for trauma-related and non-trauma-related nightmares (Krakow et al. 2001).

## Key Points: Sleep Disorders

- Human sleep is regulated physiologically by the interaction of homeostatic sleep drive and the circadian timing system. Dysregulation of these factors can contribute to insomnia, hypersomnia, and circadian rhythm sleep disorders. Behavioral treatments of sleep disorders work in part by reinforcing the activity of these regulatory processes.

- Insomnia is a complaint of poor sleep and impaired daytime function in an individual with adequate sleep opportunity. Efficacy has been well demonstrated for behavioral treatments and BzRAs.

- OSA should be suspected in overweight patients with daytime sleepiness, loud snoring, and neurocognitive symptoms including depression. Continuous positive pressure applied via nasal mask is an efficacious first-line treatment.

- Narcolepsy, a disorder characterized by extreme sleepiness, cataplexy, and sleep-related hallucinations and paralysis, is caused by dysfunction of hypocretin-containing neurons in the hypothalamus. Treatment includes stimulants for improving daytime sleepiness and agents such as antidepressants or sodium oxybate to control cataplexy.

- CRSDs result from misalignment of the individual's circadian timing system with the light–dark cycle of the work, social, or physical environment. Behavioral interventions, appropriately timed exposure to light and darkness, and exogenous melatonin may all improve circadian alignment.

- RLS is characterized by unpleasant feelings in the legs and an urge to move, which are temporarily relieved by movement. Efficacious treatments include dopamine receptor agonists, BzRAs, antiepileptic drugs, and opiate analgesics.

- Parasomnias are abnormal behavioral or affective events that occur in association with sleep or arousals from sleep. Distinctive clinical features characterize those occurring in association with NREM sleep and those occurring in association with REM sleep.

## References

American Academy of Sleep Medicine: The International Classification of Sleep Disorders, 2nd Edition (ICSD-2): Diagnostic and Coding Manual. Westchester, IL, American Academy of Sleep Medicine, 2005

Bateson AN: The benzodiazepine site of the GABA$_A$ receptor: an old target with new potential? Sleep Med 5 (suppl 1):S9–S15, 2004

Berlant J, Van Kammen DP: Open-label topiramate as primary or adjunctive therapy in chronic civilian posttraumatic stress disorder: a preliminary report. J Clin Psychiatry 63:15–20, 2002

Bixler EO, Vgontzas AN, Lin HM, et al: Prevalence of sleep-disordered breathing in women: effects of gender. Am J Respir Crit Care Med 163:608–613, 2001

Boeve BF, Silber MH, Parisi JE, et al: Synucleinopathy pathology and REM sleep behavior disorder plus dementia or parkinsonism. Neurology 61:40–45, 2003

Bridgman SA, Dunn KM: Surgery for obstructive sleep apnea. Cochrane Database Syst Rev (2):CD001004, 2000

Brzezinski A, Vangel MG, Wurtman RJ, et al: Effects of exogenous melatonin on sleep: a meta-analysis. Sleep Med Rev 9:41–50, 2005

Buysse DJ, Reynolds CF, Monk TH, et al: The Pittsburgh Sleep Quality Index: a new instrument for psychiatric practice and research. Psychiatry Res 28:193–213, 1989

Buysse D, Bate G, Kirkpatrick P: Fresh from the pipeline: ramelteon. Nat Rev Drug Discov 4:881–882, 2005a

Buysse DJ, Schweitzer PK, Moul DE: Clinical pharmacology of other drugs used as hypnotics, in Principles and Practice of Sleep Medicine, 4th Edition. Edited by Kryger MH, Roth T, Dement WC. Philadelphia, PA, Elsevier, 2005b, pp 452–467

Cajochen C, Kräuchi K, Wirz-Justice A: Role of melatonin in the regulation of human circadian rhythms and sleep. J Neuroendocrinol 15:432–437, 2003

Carskadon MA, Rechtschaffen A: Monitoring and staging human sleep, in Principles and Practice of Sleep Medicine, 4th Edition. Edited by Kryger MH, Roth T, Dement WC. Philadelphia, PA, Elsevier, 2005, pp 1359–1377

Crisp AH: The sleepwalking/night terrors syndrome in adults. Postgrad Med J 72:599–604, 1996

Dagan Y: Circadian rhythm sleep disorders (CRSD). Sleep Med Rev 6:45–54, 2002

Erman M, Seiden D, Zammit G, et al: An efficacy, safety, and dose-response study of ramelteon in patients with chronic primary insomnia. Sleep Med 7:17–24, 2006

Gaudreau H, Joncas S, Zadra A, et al: Dynamics of slow-wave activity during the NREM sleep of sleepwalkers and control subjects. Sleep 23:755–760, 2000

Gelb M, Guilleminault C, Kraemer H, et al: Stability of cataplexy over several months: information for the design of therapeutic trials. Sleep 17:265–273, 1994

Gleeson K, Zwillich CW, White DP: The influence of increasing ventilatory effort on arousal from sleep. Am Rev Respir Dis 142:295–300, 1990

Griffiths RR, Weerts EM: Benzodiazepine self-administration in humans and laboratory animals: implications for problems of long-term use and abuse. Psychopharmacology (Berl) 134:1–37, 1997

Guilleminault C, Fromherz S: Narcolepsy: diagnosis and management, in Principles and Practice of Sleep Medicine, 4th Edition. Edited by Kryger MH, Roth T, Dement WC. Philadelphia, PA, Elsevier, 2005, pp 780–790

Guilleminault C, Palombini L, Poyares D, et al: Chronic insomnia, premenopausal women and sleep disordered breathing: part 1. J Psychosom Res 53:611–615, 2002a

Guilleminault C, Palombini L, Poyares D, et al: Chronic insomnia, premenopausal women and sleep disordered breathing: part 2. J Psychosom Res 53:617–623, 2002b

Gupta S, Popli A, Bathurst E, et al: Efficacy of cyproheptadine for nightmares associated with posttraumatic stress disorder. Compr Psychiatry 39:160–164, 1998

Harvey AG: A cognitive model of insomnia. Behav Res Ther 40:869–893, 2002

Holbrook AM, Crowther R, Lotter A, et al: Meta-analysis of benzodiazepine use in the treatment of insomnia. CMAJ 162:225–233, 2000

Honda Y: Clinical features of narcolepsy: Japanese experiences, in HLA in Narcolepsy. Edited by Honda Y, Juti T. Berlin, Germany, Springer-Verlag, 1988, pp 24–57

Hublin C, Kaprio J, Partinen M, et al: Parasomnias: co-occurrence and genetics. Psychiatr Genet 11:65–70, 2001

Johns MW: A new method for measuring daytime sleepiness: the Epworth Sleepiness Scale. Sleep 14:540–545, 1991

Krakow B, Hollifield M, Johnston L, et al: Imagery rehearsal therapy for chronic nightmares in sexual assault survivors with posttraumatic stress disorder: a randomized controlled trial. JAMA 286:537–545, 2001

Labbate LA, Douglas S: Olanzapine for nightmares and sleep disturbance in posttraumatic stress disorder (PTSD). Can J Psychiatry 45:667–668, 2000

Mahowald MW, Cramer Bornemann MA: NREM sleep-arousal parasomnias, in Principles and Practice of Sleep Medicine, 4th Edition. Edited by Kryger MH, Roth T, Dement WC. Philadelphia, PA, Elsevier, 2005, pp 889–896

Mahowald MW, Schenck CH: Evolving concepts of human state dissociation. Arch Ital Biol 139:269–300, 2001

Mahowald MW, Schenck CH: REM sleep parasomnias, in Principles and Practice of Sleep Medicine, 4th Edition. Edited by Kryger MH, Roth T, Dement WC. Philadelphia, PA, Elsevier, 2005, pp 897–916

Mamelak M, Black J, Montplaisir J, et al: A pilot study on the effects of sodium oxybate on sleep architecture and daytime alertness in narcolepsy. Sleep 27:1327–1334, 2004

Mignot E: Genetic and familial aspects of narcolepsy. Neurology 50:S16–S22, 1998

Mignot E: Narcolepsy: pharmacology, pathophysiology, and genetics, in Principles and Practice of Sleep Medicine, 4th Edition. Edited by Kryger MH, Roth T, Dement WC. Philadelphia, PA, Elsevier, 2005, pp 761–779

Mitler MM, Aldrich MS, Koob GF, et al: Narcolepsy and its treatment with stimulants: ASDA standards of practice. Sleep 17:352–371, 1994

Mohler H, Fritschy J, Rudolph U: A new benzodiazepine pharmacology. J Pharmacol Exp Ther 300:2–8, 2002

Morin CM: Insomnia: Psychological Assessment and Management, 17th Edition. New York, Guilford, 1993

Nielsen TA, Zadra A: Nightmares and other common dream disturbances, in Principles and Practice of Sleep Medicine, 4th Edition. Edited by Kryger MH, Roth T, Dement WC. Philadelphia, PA, Elsevier, 2005, pp 926–935

Nishino S, Ripley B, Overeem S, et al: Hypocretin (orexin) deficiency in human narcolepsy. Lancet 355:39–40, 2000

Nofzinger EA: Neuroimaging of sleep and sleep disorders. Curr Neurol Neurosci Rep 6:149–155, 2006

Nofzinger EA, Buysse DJ, Germain A, et al: Functional neuroimaging evidence for hyperarousal in insomnia. Am J Psychiatry 161:2126–2131, 2004

Nowell PD, Mazumdar S, Buysse DJ, et al: Benzodiazepines and zolpidem for chronic insomnia: a meta-analysis of treatment efficacy. JAMA 278:2170–2177, 1997

Ohayon MM: Epidemiology of insomnia: what we know and what we still need to learn. Sleep Med Rev 6:97–111, 2002

Ohayon MM, Guilleminault C: Epidemiology of sleep disorders, in Sleep Disorders Medicine: Basic Science, Technical Considerations and Clinical Aspects. Edited by Chokroverty S. Boston, MA, Butterworth-Heinemann, 1999, pp 301–316

Ohayon MM, Guilleminault C, Priest RG: Night terrors, sleepwalking, and confusional arousals in the general population: their frequency and relationship to other sleep and mental disorders. J Clin Psychiatry 60:268–276, 1999

Ohayon MM, Priest RG, Zulley J, et al: Prevalence of narcolepsy symptomatology and diagnosis in the European general population. Neurology 58:1826–1833, 2002

Ohayon MM, Carskadon MA, Guilleminault C, et al: Meta-analysis of quantitative sleep parameters from childhood to old age in healthy individuals: developing normative sleep values across the human life span. Sleep 27:1255–1273, 2004

Overeem S, Mignot E, van Dijk JG, et al: Narcolepsy: clinical features, new pathophysiologic insights, and future perspectives. J Clin Neurophysiol 18:78–105, 2001

Pack AI, Black JE, Schwartz JR, et al: Modafinil as adjunct therapy for daytime sleepiness in obstructive sleep apnea. Am J Respir Crit Care Med 164:1675–1681, 2001

Peppard PE, Young T, Palta M, et al: Longitudinal study of moderate weight change and sleep-disordered breathing. JAMA 284:3015–3021, 2000

Perlis ML, Giles DE, Mendelson WB, et al: Psychophysiological insomnia: the behavioural model and a neurocognitive perspective. J Sleep Res 6:179–188, 1997

Perlis ML, Smith MT, Pigeon WR: Etiology and pathophysiology of insomnia, in Principles and Practice of Sleep Medicine, 4th Edition. Edited by Kryger MH, Roth T, Dement WC. Philadelphia, PA, Elsevier, 2005, pp 714–725

Raskind MA, Peskind ER, Kanter ED, et al: Reduction of nightmares and other PTSD symptoms in combat veterans by prazosin: a placebo-controlled study. Am J Psychiatry 160:371–373, 2003

Reid KJ, Zee PC: Circadian disorders of the sleep–wake cycle, in Principles and Practices of Sleep Medicine, 4th Edition. Edited by Kryger MH, Roth T, Dement WC. Philadelphia, PA, Elsevier, 2005, pp 691–701

Saper CB, Chou TC, Scammel TE: The sleep switch: hypothalamic control of sleep and wakefulness. Trends Neurosci 24:726–731, 2001

Schellenberg JB, Maislin G, Schwab RJ: Physical findings and the risk for obstructive sleep apnea: the importance of oropharyngeal structures. Am J Respir Crit Care Med 162:740–748, 2000

Schenck CH, Mahowald MW: Long-term, nightly benzodiazepine treatment of injurious parasomnias and other disorders of disrupted nocturnal sleep in 170 adults. Am J Med 100:333–337, 1996

Schenck CH, Mahowald MW: Parasomnias: managing bizarre sleep-related behavior disorders. Postgrad Med 107:145–156, 2000

Schenck CH, Bundlie SR, Mahowald MW: Delayed emergence of a parkinsonian disorder in 38% of 29 older men initially diagnosed with idiopathic rapid eye movement sleep behaviour disorder. Neurology 46:388–393, 1996

Schenck CH, Boyd JL, Mahowald MW: A parasomnia overlap disorder involving sleepwalking, sleep terrors, and REM sleep behavior disorder in 33 polysomnographically confirmed cases. Sleep 20:972–981, 1997

Scott AJ: Shift work and health. Prim Care 27:1057–1079, 2000

Sher AE: Update on upper airway surgery for obstructive sleep apnea. Curr Opin Pulm Med 1:504–511, 1995

Soldatos CR, Dikeos DG, Whitehead A: Tolerance and rebound insomnia with rapidly eliminated hypnotics: a meta-analysis of sleep laboratory studies. Int Clin Psychopharmacol 14:287–303, 1999

Spielman AJ: Assessment of insomnia. Clin Psychol Rev 6:11–25, 1986

Spielman AJ, Caruso LS, Glovinsky PB: A behavioral perspective on insomnia treatment. Psychiatr Clin North Am 10:541–553, 1987

Strollo PJ, Rogers RM: Obstructive sleep apnea. N Engl J Med 334:99–104, 1996

Tishler PV, Larkin EK, Schluchter MD, et al: Incidence of sleep-disordered breathing in an urban adult population: the relative importance of risk factors in the development of sleep-disordered breathing. JAMA 289:2230–2237, 2003

U.S. Modafinil in Narcolepsy Multicenter Study Group: Randomized trial of modafinil for the treatment of pathological somnolence in narcolepsy. Ann Neurol 43:88–97, 1998

U.S. Xyrem Multicenter Study Group: A randomized, double-blind, placebo-controlled multicenter trial comparing effects of three doses of orally administered sodium oxybate with placebo for the treatment of narcolepsy. Sleep 25:42–49, 2002

Wagner DR: Disorders of the circadian sleep–wake cycle. Neurol Clin 14:651–670, 1996

Winkelman JW, James L: Serotonergic antidepressants are associated with REM sleep without atonia. Sleep 27:317–321, 2004

Winokur A, Sateia MJ, Hayes JB, et al: Acute effects of mirtazapine on sleep continuity and sleep architecture in depressed patients: a pilot study. Biol Psychiatry 48:75–78, 2000

Wisor JP, Eriksson KS: Dopaminergic-adrenergic interactions in the wake-promoting mechanism of modafinil. Neuroscience 132:1027–1034, 2005

Woods J, Winger G: Current benzodiazepine issues. Psychopharmacology (Berl) 118:107–115; discussion 118, 1995

Young T, Palta M, Dempsey J, et al: The occurrence of sleep-disordered breathing among middle-aged adults. N Engl J Med 328:1230–1235, 1993

Young T, Peppard PE, Gottlieb DJ: Epidemiology of obstructive sleep apnea: a population health perspective. Am J Respir Crit Care Med 165:1217–1239, 2002

Zonato AI, Bittencourt LR, Martinho FL, et al: Association of systematic head and neck physical examination with severity of obstructive sleep apnea-hypopnea syndrome. Laryngoscope 113:973–980, 2003

27

# Impulse-Control Disorders Not Elsewhere Classified

ERIC HOLLANDER, M.D.

HEATHER A. BERLIN, D.Phil., M.P.H.

DAN J. STEIN, M.D., Ph.D.

Whereas impulse-control disorders (ICDs) were once conceptualized as either addictive or compulsive behaviors, they are now classified within the DSM-IV-TR (American Psychiatric Association 2000) ICD category. These include intermittent explosive disorder (IED; failure to resist aggressive impulses), kleptomania (failure to resist urges to steal items), pyromania (failure to resist urges to set fires), pathological gambling (failure to resist urges to gamble), and trichotillomania (failure to resist urges to pull one's hair) (Table 27–1).

In DSM-IV-TR, ICDs are characterized by five stages of symptomatic behavior (Table 27–2). First is the increased sense of tension or arousal, followed by the failure to resist the urge to act. Third, there is a heightened sense of arousal. Once the act has been completed, there is a sense of relief from the urge. Finally, the patient experiences guilt and remorse at having committed the act.

## Intermittent Explosive Disorder

### Definition and Diagnostic Criteria

IED is a DSM diagnosis used to describe people with pathological impulsive aggression. Many clinicians and researchers rarely consider this diagnosis, although impulsive aggressive behavior is relatively common. In community surveys, 12%–25% of men and women in the United States reported engaging in physical fights as adults, a frequent manifestation of impulsive aggression (Robins and Regier 1991). Impulsive aggressive behavior usually is pathological and causes substantial psychosocial distress or dysfunction (McElroy et al. 1998) (see Table 27–3).

### Epidemiology

Several studies have looked at clinical populations, and one community survey has been done to determine the prevalence of IED. Numbers range between 1.1% and 6.3%. Most of the limited published data on gender differences suggest that males outnumber females with IED. However, more recent data suggest that the male-to-female ratio is approximately 1:1 (Coccaro et al. 2005).

### Comorbidity

Subjects with IED most frequently have other Axis I and II disorders. The most frequent Axis I diagnoses comorbid with IED are mood, anxiety, substance, eating, and other ICDs, with lifetime rates ranging from 7% to 89% (Coccaro et al. 1998a; McElroy et al. 1998).

**TABLE 27–1.   DSM-IV-TR impulse-control disorders**

**Impulse-control disorders not elsewhere classified**

Intermittent explosive disorder

Kleptomania

Pyromania

Pathological gambling

Trichotillomania

**Impulse-control disorders not otherwise specified**

Impulsive-compulsive sexual disorder

Impulsive-compulsive self-injurious disorder

Impulsive-compulsive Internet usage disorder

Impulsive-compulsive buying disorder

**Other disorders with impulsivity**

Childhood conduct disorders

Binge-eating disorder

Bulimia nervosa

Paraphilias

    Exhibitionism

    Fetishism

    Frotteurism

    Pedophilia

    Sexual masochism

    Sexual sadism

    Transvestic fetishism

    Voyeurism

    Paraphilia not otherwise specified

Bipolar disorder

Attention-deficit/hyperactivity disorder

Substance use disorders

Cluster B personality disorders

Neurological disorder with disinhibition

*Source.* American Psychiatric Association 2000.

**TABLE 27–2.   Core features of impulse-control disorders**

| | |
|---|---|
| Essential features | Failure to resist an impulse, drive, or temptation to perform an act that is harmful to the person or to others |
| Before the act | The individual feels an increasing sense of tension or arousal |
| At the time of committing the act | The individual experiences pleasure, gratification, or relief |
| After the act | The individual experiences a sense of relief from the urge |
| | The individual may or may not feel regret, self-reproach, or guilt |

*Source.* American Psychiatric Association 2000.

**TABLE 27–3.   DSM-IV-TR diagnostic criteria for intermittent explosive disorder**

A. Several discrete episodes of failure to resist aggressive impulses that result in serious assaultive acts or destruction of property.

B. The degree of aggressiveness expressed during the episodes is grossly out of proportion to any precipitating psychosocial stressors.

C. The aggressive episodes are not better accounted for by another mental disorder (e.g., antisocial personality disorder, borderline personality disorder, a psychotic disorder, a manic episode, conduct disorder, or attention-deficit/hyperactivity disorder) and are not due to the direct physiological effects of a substance (e.g., a drug of abuse, a medication) or a general medical condition (e.g., head trauma, Alzheimer's disease).

## Bipolar Disorder

McElroy et al. (1998) reported that the aggressive episodes observed in their subjects resembled "microdysphoric" manic episodes. Symptoms in common with both manic and IED episodes included irritability (79%–92%), increased energy (83%–96%), racing thoughts (62%–67%), anxiety (21%–42%), and depressed (dysphoric) mood (17%–33%). However, this finding may not be surprising because 56% of the subjects in question had a comorbid bipolar diagnosis of some type (bipolar I, 33%; bipolar II, 11%; bipolar not otherwise specified or cyclothymia, 11%).

Regardless, clinicians should fully evaluate for bipolar disorder prior to determining treatment for IED because mood stabilizers, rather than selective serotonin reuptake inhibitors (SSRIs), would be the first-line treatment for IED comorbid with bipolar disorder.

## Other Impulse-Control Disorders

McElroy et al. (1998) reported that up to 44% of their IED subjects had another ICD, such as compulsive buying (37%) or kleptomania (19%).

### Borderline and Antisocial Personality Disorders

Coccaro et al. (1998a) reported the rate of borderline personality disorder (BPD) and/or antisocial personality disorder in IED subjects to be 38%. However, higher rates of IED have been noted in BPD subjects (78%) and in subjects with antisocial personality disorder (58%) (Coccaro et al. 1998a). Regardless, BPD and antisocial personality disorder subjects with a comorbid diagnosis of IED do appear to have higher scores for aggression and lower scores for general psychosocial function than do BPD and antisocial personality disorder subjects without IED (Coccaro et al. 2005).

## Pathogenesis

### Family and Twin Studies

Clinical observation and family history data suggest that IED is familial. Familial aggregation of temper outbursts and IED has been reported in psychiatric patients with "temper problems" (Mattes and Fink 1987), and McElroy et al. (1998) reported that nearly a third of first-degree relatives of IED probands had IED.

### Biological Correlates

Measures examining central (as well as peripheral) serotonin function correlate inversely with life history, questionnaire, and laboratory measures of aggression. The type of aggression associated with reduced central serotonin function appears to be *impulsive*, as opposed to *nonimpulsive*, aggression (Linnoila et al. 1983; Virkkunen et al. 1994).

Evidence also supports the role of other nonserotonergic brain systems and modulators in impulsive aggression. These findings suggest a facilitating role for dopamine (DePue et al. 1994), norepinephrine (Coccaro et al. 1991), vasopressin (Coccaro et al. 1998b), brain-derived neurotrophic factor (Lyons et al. 1991), opiates (Post et al. 1984), and testosterone (Giammanco et al. 2005; Virkkunen et al. 1994) and an inhibitory interaction between neuronal nitric oxide synthase and testosterone in rodents (Kriegsfeld et al. 1997).

## Course

Limited research is available concerning the age at onset and natural course of IED. However, according to DSM-IV-TR, the onset appears to be from childhood to the early 20s. The age at onset and course of IED distinguish it as separate from its comorbid diagnoses. The course of IED is variable, with an episodic course in some and a more chronic course in others.

## Treatment

### Pharmacotherapy

Several medications have been used to treat impulsive aggression, such as tricyclic antidepressants, benzodiazepines, mood stabilizers, and neuroleptics. Recently, pharmacotherapy studies of aggression have turned to SSRIs and mood stabilizers as first-line treatments. Fluoxetine and other SSRIs have been studied in impulsive aggressive subjects and IED patients. In a treatment trial of subjects meeting Integrated Research Criteria for intermittent explosive disorder, impulsive aggressive behavior did respond to fluoxetine (Coccaro and Kavoussi 1997), but non-serotonin-specific antidepressants had little benefit for impulsive aggression and many side effects in treatment studies. Soloff et al. (1986a) found that affective symptoms improved with amitriptyline in some BPD and schizotypal personality disorder inpatients, but impulsivity and aggression worsened in a set of patients, perhaps because of the noradrenergic effects of tricyclic antidepressants (Links et al. 1990). Thus, clinicians should be cautious when using the new dual-action antidepressants in these patients.

Monoamine oxidase inhibitors such as tranylcypromine and phenelzine also have been studied in impulsively aggressive subjects. In a double-blind study, Soloff et al. (1993) found that compared with placebo and haloperidol, phenelzine produced a moderate reduction in anger and hostility in BPD patients. Yet in a 16-week continuation phase, the subjects had experienced only minor benefits in depression and irritability and remained substantially impaired after the treatment phase (Cornelius et al. 1993; Soloff et al. 1993). In a double-blind crossover trial (Cowdry and Gardner 1988), treatment-resistant BPD patients with a history of impulsive aggression showed improvement with tranylcypromine, carbamazepine (decreased severity of behavioral dyscontrol), and trifluoperazine but had an increase in the severity and frequency of the episodes of serious dyscontrol with alprazolam. Benzodiazepine treatment might have released the subjects' control or inhibition of these episodes.

Mood stabilizers also have been used to treat aggression. Links et al. (1990) found that objective ratings of anger and suicidality in BPD outpatients improved the most on lithium compared with desipramine and placebo, but subjects and their clinicians did not report any improvement in mood. Sheard et al. (1976) found an improvement with lithium compared with placebo in chronically aggressive prisoners. Again, however, only objective findings supported this result; no improvement was reported subjectively. Barratt et al. (1997) also reported a reduction in aggression with phenytoin in impulsive aggressive prisoners.

The other mood stabilizers studied for impulsive aggression are carbamazepine and divalproex. In the Cowdry and Gardner (1988) study, carbamazepine lessened episodes of impulsive aggression in BPD subjects, but 18% of the subjects had a worsening of mood that improved once carbamazepine was stopped. Kavoussi and Coccaro (1998) and Hollander et al. (2003) reported an antiaggressive effect of divalproex sodium in IED subjects with a Cluster B personality disorder. Given the relative adverse event profiles for SSRIs versus mood stabilizers, it is likely that clinical treatment of IED should start with SSRIs unless the subject is extremely aggressive or has a history of a bipolar disorder, in which case treatment with a mood stabilizer would be more appropriate.

The neuroleptics haloperidol, trifluoperazine, and depot flupenthixol have all been studied in BPD patients. Cowdry and Gardner's (1988) subjects showed significant improvement in depression and anxiety objective ratings with trifluoperazine, but subjective ratings did not support this. Trifluoperazine was seen as less useful than tranylcypromine (a monoamine oxidase inhibitor) and carbamazepine in improving behavior and affect among subjects. Soloff et al. (1986b, 1989) found that BPD inpatients improved on hostility and global function measurements with haloperidol, but considerable depression remained. Montgomery and Montgomery (1982) found that suicidal and parasuicidal behavior, in subjects with a history of such behaviors, decreased in a depot flupenthixol treatment group compared with a placebo group. Zanarini and Frankenburg (2001) compared the atypical antipsychotic olanzapine with placebo in outpatients with BPD. The treatment improved anger, hostility, and other symptoms but did not improve depression, and patients remained quite ill.

*Psychotherapy*

Anger treatment studies focus on treatment of anger as a component of other psychiatric illnesses, such as substance abuse, posttraumatic stress disorder, and depression; in forensic and mentally impaired populations; and in the context of domestic violence. Therapy for anger and aggression focuses on cognitive-behavioral group therapy. In a few rare cases, anger is addressed as the primary or only problem, and a limited number of treatments have been described. Imaginal exposure therapy, used frequently in anxiety disorders, was studied in a noncontrolled pilot study of anger treatment (Grodnitzky

and Tafrate 2000). Subjects habituated to anger-provoking scenarios, and the treatment was believed to be useful.

Other versions of cognitive-behavioral therapy (CBT), such as dialectical behavior therapy, have been studied in BPD patients. One study showed improvement in anger, social adjustment, and global functioning compared with a treatment-as-usual condition (Linehan et al. 1994). Improvement in anger and impulsivity has been shown with dialectical behavior therapy across many disorders. There are no published double-blind, placebo-controlled studies on IED subjects in therapy, but studies of therapy for IED subjects are ongoing.

# Kleptomania

## Definition and Diagnostic Criteria

Kleptomania was officially designated a psychiatric disorder in 1980 in DSM-III (American Psychiatric Association 1980), and in DSM-III-R (American Psychiatric Association 1987) it was grouped under the category "disorders of impulse control not elsewhere classified." Kleptomania is currently classified in DSM-IV-TR as an ICD, but it is still poorly understood and has received very little empirical study. The DSM-IV-TR criteria for kleptomania are listed in Table 27–4.

**TABLE 27–4.  DSM-IV-TR diagnostic criteria for kleptomania**

A. Recurrent failure to resist impulses to steal objects that are not needed for personal use or for their monetary value.

B. Increasing sense of tension immediately before committing the theft.

C. Pleasure, gratification, or relief at the time of committing the theft.

D. The stealing is not committed to express anger or vengeance and is not in response to a delusion or a hallucination.

E. The stealing is not better accounted for by conduct disorder, a manic episode, or antisocial personality disorder.

Patients with kleptomania often report amnesia surrounding the act of shoplifting (Goldman 1991; Grant 2004) and deny feelings of tension or arousal prior to shoplifting and feelings of pleasure or relief after the thefts. They often recall entering and leaving a store but have no memory of events in the store, including the theft (Grant 2004). Other patients, who are not amnestic for the thefts, describe shoplifting as "automatic" or "a habit" and also may deny feelings of tension prior to a theft or pleasure after the act (DSM-IV-TR Criterion B or C), although they report an inability to control their shoplifting (Criterion A).

## Epidemiology

A recent study in the United States of 204 adult psychiatric inpatients with multiple disorders reported that kleptomania may in fact be fairly common. The study found that 7.8% (*n*=16) endorsed current symptoms consistent with a diagnosis of kleptomania and 9.3% (*n*=19) had a lifetime diagnosis of kleptomania (Grant et al. 2005). Kleptomania appeared equally common in patients with mood, anxiety, substance use, or psychotic disorders.

The literature clearly suggests that most patients with kleptomania are women (e.g., Grant and Kim 2002b; McElroy et al. 1991b; Presta et al. 2002). The severity of kleptomania symptoms and the clinical presentation of symptoms do not appear to differ based on gender (Grant and Kim 2002b).

## Comorbidity

Rates of lifetime comorbid affective disorders range from 59% (Grant and Kim 2002b) to 100% (McElroy et al. 1991b). The rate of lifetime comorbid bipolar disorder has been reported as ranging from 9% (Grant and Kim 2002b) to 27% (Bayle et al. 2003) to 60% (McElroy et al. 1991b). Studies also have found high lifetime rates of comorbid anxiety disorders (60%–80%; McElroy et al. 1991b, 1992), ICDs (20%–46%; Grant and Kim 2003), substance use disorders (23%–50%; Grant and Kim 2002b; McElroy et al. 1991b), and eating disorders (60%; McElroy et al. 1991b). Personality disorders have been found in 43%–55% of patients with kleptomania, the most common being paranoid personality disorder and histrionic personality disorder (Bayle et al. 2003; Grant 2004).

## Pathogenesis

### Biological Theories

**Serotonin and inhibition.** The most well-studied inhibitory pathways involve serotonin and the prefrontal cortex (Chambers et al. 2003). Decreased measures of serotonin have long been associated with a variety of adult risk-taking behaviors, including alcoholism, fire setting, and pathological gambling (Moreno et al. 1991; Virkkunen et al. 1994). Blunted serotonergic responses in the ventromedial prefrontal cortex have been seen in people with impulsive aggression (New et al. 2002), and this region also has been implicated in poor decision making (Bechara 2003), as seen in those with kleptomania.

**Dopamine and reward deficiency.** Dopaminergic systems influencing rewarding and reinforcing behaviors also have been implicated in ICDs and may play a role in the pathogenesis of kleptomania. Alterations in dopaminergic pathways have been proposed as underlying the seeking of rewards (e.g., shoplifting) that trigger the release of dopamine and produce feelings of pleasure (Blum et al. 2000). Furthermore, dopamine release into the nucleus accumbens has been implicated in the translation of motivated drive into action, serving as a "go" signal (Chambers et al. 2003). Dopamine release into the nucleus accumbens seems maximal when reward probability is most uncertain, suggesting that it plays a central role in guiding behavior during risk-taking situations (Fiorillo et al. 2003). The structure and function of dopamine neurons within the nucleus accumbens, in conjunction with glutamatergic afferent and intrinsic γ-aminobutyric acid (GABA)–ergic activities, appear to change in response to experiences that influence the function of the nucleus accumbens.

**Opioid system, cravings, and pleasure.** The μ-opioid system is thought to underlie urge regulation by processing reward, pleasure, and pain at least in part via modulation of dopamine neurons in the mesolimbic pathway through GABA interneurons (Potenza and Hollander 2002). Studies of naltrexone, a μ-opioid antagonist, have shown its efficacy in reducing urges in those with kleptomania and other ICDs (Dannon et al. 1999; Grant and Kim 2002c; Kim et al. 2001).

### Psychological Theories

Kleptomania may result from an attempt to relieve feelings of depression through stimulation (Goldman 1991; McElroy et al. 1991a). Risk-taking behavior may produce an antidepressant effect for some patients (Fishbain 1987; Goldman 1991). Shoplifting may distract depressed patients from stressors and unpleasant cognitions. Ironically, problems resulting directly from shoplifting (e.g., embarrassment and shame from getting caught) may lead to even more shoplifting as a misguided means of symptom management (Goldman 1991).

Behavioral models also provide clues as to the pathogenesis of kleptomania. From an operant viewpoint, the positive reinforcer in kleptomania is the acquisition of items for nothing, and the intermittent reinforcement (e.g., not always being able to shoplift because of store security) of kleptomanic behavior may therefore be particularly resistant to extinction. Physiological arousal related to shoplifting (Goldman 1991) may be another reinforcer that initiates and perpetuates the behavior.

## Course

Kleptomania may begin in childhood, adolescence, or adulthood and sometimes in late adulthood. However, most patients have an onset of symptoms before age 21 years (i.e., by late adolescence; Goldman 1991; Grant and Kim 2002b; McElroy et al. 1991a, 1991b; Presta et al. 2002).

## Treatment

### Pharmacotherapy

Various medications—tricyclic antidepressants, SSRIs (Lepkifker et al. 1999), mood stabilizers, and opioid antagonists—have been examined for the treatment of kleptomania (Grant and Kim 2002c; McElroy et al. 1989). McElroy et al. (1991b) reported treatment response in 10 of 20 patients with the following single agents: fluoxetine, nortriptyline, trazodone, clonazepam, valproate, and lithium. Other agents used successfully as monotherapy for kleptomania include fluvoxamine (Chong and Low 1996) and paroxetine (Kraus 1999). Combinations of medications also have been effective in case reports: lithium plus fluoxetine (Burstein 1992), fluvoxamine plus buspirone (Durst et al. 1997), fluoxetine plus lithium, fluoxetine plus imipramine (McElroy et al. 1991b), and fluvoxamine plus valproate (Kmetz et al. 1997).

In the only open-label medication trial for kleptomania, naltrexone (mean effective dosage=145 mg/day) resulted in a significant decline in the intensity of urges to steal, stealing thoughts, and stealing behavior (Grant and Kim 2002c). A lower dosage, possibly 50 mg/day, may be effective in younger people with kleptomania (Grant and Kim 2002a).

### Psychotherapy

Imaginal desensitization uses the idea of imagining the steps of stealing while maintaining a relaxed state. The patient then imagines the potential scene of stealing but also imagines his or her ability to not steal in that context.

# Pyromania

## Definition and Diagnostic Criteria

The essential feature of pyromania is multiple deliberate and purposeful (rather than accidental) fire setting (Table 27–5).

---

**TABLE 27–5.    DSM-IV-TR diagnostic criteria for pyromania**

A. Deliberate and purposeful fire setting on more than one occasion.

B. Tension or affective arousal before the act.

C. Fascination with, interest in, curiosity about, or attraction to fire and its situational contexts (e.g., paraphernalia, uses, consequences).

D. Pleasure, gratification, or relief when setting fires, or when witnessing or participating in their aftermath.

E. The fire setting is not done for monetary gain, as an expression of sociopolitical ideology, to conceal criminal activity, to express anger or vengeance, to improve one's living circumstances, in response to a delusion or hallucination, or as a result of impaired judgment (e.g., in dementia, mental retardation, substance intoxication).

F. The fire setting is not better accounted for by conduct disorder, a manic episode, or antisocial personality disorder.

---

Another important clinical feature of pyromania is the fascination with fire. People with pyromania are prone to being "watchers" at fires in their neighborhoods, setting off false fire alarms, or working or volunteering as firefighters.

## Epidemiology

Lewis and Yarnell (1951), in their classic study *Pathological Firesetting (Pyromania)*, found that of those arrested for firesetting, 39% did not have a profit motive and were diagnosed with pyromania.

## Comorbidity

Comorbid conditions often include substance use disorders, mental retardation, conduct disorder, mania, schizophrenia, and antisocial personality disorder.

TABLE 27–6. Pyromania: treatment summary

| Authors | Treatment | Description |
| --- | --- | --- |
| McGrath and Marshall 1979 | Behavioral therapy | Child fire setter ($N=1$); successful |
| Koles and Jenson 1985 | Behavioral therapy | Child fire setter ($N=1$); successful |
| Bumpass et al. 1983 | Technique that sequentially correlates external stress, behavior, and feelings on graph paper to help patients become aware of the cause–effect relation between feelings and behavior so as to substitute an acceptable behavior | Child fire setters ($N=29$); after treatment (average follow-up, 2.5 years), only 2 of the 29 children continued to set fires |
| Franklin et al. 2002 | Trauma Burn Outreach Prevention Program (TBOPP), 1-day interactive program focusing on the medical, financial, legal, and societal impact of fire setting, emphasizing individual accountability and responsibility | 132 juveniles (66 arsonists, 66 fire setters) in the TBOPP group; 102 juveniles (33 arsonists and 66 fire setters) in the no-TBOPP group; TBOPP participants had essentially no recidivism compared with the no-TBOPP group |

## Pathogenesis

### *Biological Markers*

Virkkunen et al. (1987, 1994) suggested that pyromania may be associated with reactive hypoglycemia and/or lower concentrations of 3-methoxy-4-hydroxyphenylglycol (MHPG) and cerebrospinal fluid 5-hydroxyindoleacetic acid.

## Course

In individuals with pyromania, fire-setting incidents are episodic and may wax and wane in frequency. Studies indicate that the recidivism rate for fire setters ranges from 4.5% (Mavromatis and Lion 1977) to 28% (Lewis and Yarnell 1951).

## Treatment

The treatment of pyromania is summarized in Table 27–6.

# Pathological Gambling

## Definition and Diagnostic Criteria

DSM-IV-TR currently classifies pathological gambling as an ICD not elsewhere classified. The essential feature of pathological gambling is recurrent gambling behavior that is maladaptive (e.g., loss of judgment, excessive gam-

bling) and in which personal, family, or vocational endeavors are disrupted (Table 27–7).

## Epidemiology

A meta-analysis of 120 published studies indicated that the lifetime prevalence of serious gambling (meeting DSM criteria for pathological gambling) among adults is 1.6% (Shaffer et al. 1999).

## Comorbidity

The literature to date strongly suggests that three Axis I disorders frequently co-occur with pathological gambling: substance abuse or dependence, bipolar spectrum disorders, and attention-deficit/hyperactivity disorder.

## Pathogenesis

### *Neurobiology*

There is evidence of serotonergic, noradrenergic, and dopaminergic dysfunction in the pathogenesis of pathological gambling (Table 27–8).

### *Genetics*

At present, the main source of evidence for the genetic influence in the etiology of pathological gambling derives from a study of 3,359 male twin pairs from the Vietnam Era Twin Registry cohort (Eisen et al. 1998, 2001; Slutske et al. 2000). These data suggest that gambling problems

## TABLE 27–7. DSM-IV-TR diagnostic criteria for pathological gambling

A. Persistent and recurrent maladaptive gambling behavior as indicated by five (or more) of the following:

(1) is preoccupied with gambling (e.g., preoccupied with reliving past gambling experiences, handicapping or planning the next venture, or thinking of ways to get money with which to gamble)

(2) needs to gamble with increasing amounts of money in order to achieve the desired excitement

(3) has repeated unsuccessful efforts to control, cut back, or stop gambling

(4) is restless or irritable when attempting to cut down or stop gambling

(5) gambles as a way of escaping from problems or of relieving a dysphoric mood (e.g., feelings of helplessness, guilt, anxiety, depression)

(6) after losing money gambling, often returns another day to get even ("chasing" one's losses)

(7) lies to family members, therapist, or others to conceal the extent of involvement with gambling

(8) has committed illegal acts such as forgery, fraud, theft, or embezzlement to finance gambling

(9) has jeopardized or lost a significant relationship, job, or educational or career opportunity because of gambling

(10) relies on others to provide money to relieve a desperate financial situation caused by gambling

B. The gambling behavior is not better accounted for by a manic episode.

## TABLE 27–8. Developmental and neurobiological model of pathological gambling

### Vulnerable state
Primed genetically/neurobiologically

Repeated environmental exposure

### Gambling cycle: behavioral mechanisms

Stimulation readiness → norepinephrine

Behavioral initiation → serotonin

Reward/reinforcement → dopamine

Behavioral disinhibition → serotonin

*Source.* Reprinted from Pallanti S, Baldini Rossi N, Hollander E: "Pathological Gambling," in *Clinical Manual of Impulse-Control Disorders*. Edited by Hollander E, Stein DJ. Washington, DC, American Psychiatric Publishing, 2006, p. 262. Used with permission.

Chronicity is usually associated with increases in the frequency of gambling and the amount gambled. Gambling may increase during periods of increased stress. Gambling behavior frequently leads to severe personal, familial, financial, social, and occupational impairment.

Psychiatric disorders such as major depression and alcohol or substance abuse and dependence may develop from or be exacerbated by pathological gambling. There is also a mortality risk associated with pathological gambling. Estimates of suicide attempts in pathological gamblers range from 17% to 24% (Ciarrochi and Richardson 1989; Hollander et al. 2000a).

In males, the disorder usually begins in adolescence (Hollander et al. 2000a) and may remain undiagnosed for years; male pathological gamblers often present with a 20- to 30-year gambling history, with gradual development of dependence. In contrast, onset of pathological gambling in females is more likely to occur later in life. Prior to their seeking treatment, the duration of pathological gambling in women is approximately 3 years.

## Treatment

### *Pharmacotherapy*

Pharmacological treatment studies of pathological gambling have had some promising results with the use of serotonin reuptake inhibitors (de la Gandara 1999; Hollander et al. 1992, 1998, 2000b; Kim et al. 2002; Zimmerman et al. 2002), serotonin antagonists (Pallanti et al. 2002a), mood stabilizers (Haller and Hinterhuber 1994; Hollander et al. 2002; Pallanti et al. 2002b), opiate antag-

of increasing severity represent a single continuum of vulnerability rather than distinct entities (Eisen et al. 1998, 2001), indicate genetic susceptibility in pathological gambling (Eisen et al. 1998), and suggest a common genetic vulnerability for pathological gambling and alcohol dependence in men (Slutske et al. 2000).

## Course

The course of pathological gambling tends to be chronic, but the pattern of gambling may be regular or episodic.

onists (Kim et al. 2001), and atypical antipsychotics (Potenza and Chambers 2001).

### Psychotherapy

The most popular intervention for problem gambling is Gamblers Anonymous (GA), which is similar to Alcoholics Anonymous and Narcotics Anonymous. However, evidence suggests that GA may not be very effective when used without other treatment modalities (Petry and Armentano 1999). Retrospective studies show a dropout rate of up to 70% within the first year (Stewart and Brown 1988), and overall dropout rates range from 75% to 90% (Moody 1990). Only 8% of GA members report total abstinence at 1-year follow-up and 7% at 2-year follow-up (Brown 1985).

Inpatient programs for pathological gambling have included various combinations of individual and group psychotherapy and substance use treatment (Taber 1981), and most strongly encouraged or required attendance at GA meetings. Many patients improved in all programs, and outcome studies have shown 55% of patients reporting abstinence at 1-year follow-up (Russo et al. 1984; Taber et al. 1987).

Behavioral, cognitive, and combined cognitive-behavioral methods have been used in treating pathological gambling. Aversive therapy has been used to reach the goal of total abstinence of gambling, as have behavior monitoring, contingency management, contingency contracting, covert sensitization, systematic desensitization, imaginal desensitization, in vivo exposure, imaginal relaxation, psychoeducation, cognitive restructuring, problem-solving skills training, social skills training, and relapse prevention (Ladouceur 1990).

# Trichotillomania

## Definition and Diagnostic Criteria

Trichotillomania is a chronic ICD characterized by repetitive pulling out of one's own hair, resulting in noticeable hair loss. The DSM-IV-TR criteria for trichotillomania are listed in Table 27–9.

## Epidemiology

In studies involving college samples, 10%–13% of students reported hair pulling, with the prevalence of clinically significant pulling ranging between 1% and 3.5% (Christenson et al. 1991c; Rothbaum et al. 1993).

**TABLE 27–9. DSM-IV-TR diagnostic criteria for trichotillomania**

A. Recurrent pulling out of one's hair resulting in noticeable hair loss.

B. An increasing sense of tension immediately before pulling out the hair or when attempting to resist the behavior.

C. Pleasure, gratification, or relief when pulling out the hair.

D. The disturbance is not better accounted for by another mental disorder and is not due to a general medical condition (e.g., a dermatological condition).

E. The disturbance causes clinically significant distress or impairment in social, occupational, or other important areas of functioning.

## Comorbidity

Christenson et al. (1991a) found that approximately 82% of an adult sample with trichotillomania met criteria for a past or current comorbid Axis I disorder, the most common being mood, anxiety, and addictive disorders. Of the patients with comorbid disorders, there was a lifetime prevalence rate of 65% for mood disorders, 57% for anxiety disorders, 22% for substance abuse disorders, 20% for eating disorders, and 42% for personality disorders. The most frequently cited comorbid personality disorders are histrionic, borderline, and obsessive-compulsive (Christenson et al. 1992; Schlosser et al. 1994; Swedo and Leonard 1992).

A key debate in the field is whether trichotillomania should be conceptualized as an ICD or a variant of obsessive-compulsive disorder (OCD). In support of the classification as an obsessive-compulsive spectrum disorder is the apparent similarity between compulsions and the repetitive and perceived uncontrollable nature of hair pulling and accompanying anxiety relief (Swedo 1993; Swedo and Leonard 1992), the possible selective responsiveness of trichotillomania to serotonin reuptake inhibitors, and the elevated rates of OCD in patients with trichotillomania (Christenson et al. 1991a).

## Pathogenesis

### Biological Vulnerability

Familial research suggests that trichotillomania may be associated with increased rates of OCD or other excessive habits among first-degree relatives (Bienvenu et al. 2000; King et al. 1995).

### Hair-Pulling Cues

The behavioral model of hair pulling suggests that pulling begins as a normal response to stress but eventually becomes associated with a variety of internal and external cues through conditioning (Mansueto et al. 1997).

### Reinforcement

Hair pulling is often preceded by negative internal states such as unpleasant emotions, aversive physiological sensations, or dysregulated arousal. Hair pulling appears to result in a decrease of these states. Over time, hair-pulling urges that are reinforced by pulling lead to stronger urges to pull, which perpetuates the behavioral cycle. Trichotillomania patients report retrospectively that pulling leads to reduced feelings of tension, boredom, and anxiety, and nonclinical hair pullers also report reductions in sadness and anger (Stanley et al. 1995).

## Course

Age at onset usually ranges from early childhood to young adulthood. Initial onset after young adulthood is uncommon.

Trichotillomania in adolescents and adults typically follows a chronic course, involves multiple hair sites, and is associated with high rates of psychiatric comorbidity (Christenson et al. 1991a).

## Treatment

### Pharmacotherapy

Of the six randomized controlled trials evaluating the efficacy of pharmacotherapy conducted to date, five involved serotonin reuptake inhibitors. In summary, results from these controlled studies of serotonin reuptake inhibitors are equivocal at best, although in view of the small sample sizes, more controlled research should be conducted to determine the efficacy of these medications more definitively (Christenson et al. 1991b; Ninan et al. 2000; Streichenwein and Thornby 1995; Swedo et al. 1989, 1993; van Minnen et al. 2003). However, several case studies indicated that augmentation of SSRIs with atypical antipsychotics may be beneficial (Epperson et al. 1999).

### Psychotherapy

With respect to behavioral approaches and CBT, a variety of specific techniques have been applied, including awareness training, self-monitoring, aversion, covert sensitization, negative practice, relaxation training, habit reversal, competing response training, stimulus control, and overcorrection. Although the state of the CBT literature justifies only cautious recommendations, habit reversal, awareness training, and stimulus control are generally purported as the core efficacious interventions for trichotillomania.

## Key Points: Impulse-Control Disorders

- Pathological impulsivity is a useful construct in understanding a broad range of psychiatric symptoms and disorders, including the ICDs not otherwise specified.

- ICDs are highly prevalent and associated with significant disability and costs but receive disproportionately little attention from clinicians and researchers.

- There are now structured diagnostic instruments and standardized rating scales that allow reliable diagnosis and assessment of the ICDs.

- There have been significant advances in our understanding of the neuronal circuitry that mediates impulsivity, as well as in the delineating of the contributing genes and proteins in this circuitry.

- Ultimately, a better understanding of the psychobiological underpinnings of impulsivity, behavior addiction, and other related constructs may lead to changes in our classification of these disorders.

- Although no medication is registered for the treatment of ICDs, a number of randomized, controlled trials have demonstrated the potential value of pharmacotherapy.

- Current clinical practice also emphasizes the need for a comprehensive approach to management that includes psychotherapy and family intervention. Additional work is needed to improve efficacy.

# References

American Psychiatric Association: Diagnostic and Statistical Manual of Mental Disorders, 3rd Edition. Washington, DC, American Psychiatric Association, 1980

American Psychiatric Association: Diagnostic and Statistical Manual of Mental Disorders, 3rd Edition, Revised. Washington, DC, American Psychiatric Association, 1987

American Psychiatric Association: Diagnostic and Statistical Manual of Mental Disorders, 4th Edition, Text Revision. Washington, DC, American Psychiatric Association, 2000

Barratt ES, Stanford MS, Felthous AR, et al: The effects of phenytoin on impulsive and premeditated aggression: a controlled study. J Clin Psychopharmacol 17:341–349, 1997

Bayle FJ, Caci H, Millet B, et al: Psychopathology and comorbidity of psychiatric disorders in patients with kleptomania. Am J Psychiatry 160:1509–1513, 2003

Bechara A: Risky business: emotion, decision-making, and addiction. J Gambl Stud 19:23–51, 2003

Bienvenu OJ, Samuels JF, Riddle MA, et al: The relationship of obsessive-compulsive disorder to possible spectrum disorders: results from a family study. Biol Psychiatry 48:287–293, 2000

Blum K, Braverman ER, Holder JM, et al: Reward deficiency syndrome: a biogenetic model for the diagnosis and treatment of impulsive, addictive, and compulsive behaviors. J Psychoactive Drugs 32(suppl):1–68, 2000

Brown RI: The effectiveness of Gamblers Anonymous, in The Gambling Studies: Proceedings of the 6th National Conference on Gambling and Risk-Taking. Edited by Eadington WR. Reno, University of Nevada, 1985

Bumpass ER, Fagelman FD, Brix RJ: Intervention with children who set fires. Am J Psychother 37:328–345, 1983

Burstein A: Fluoxetine-lithium treatment for kleptomania. J Clin Psychiatry 53:28–29, 1992

Chambers RA, Taylor JR, Potenza MN: Developmental neurocircuitry of motivation in adolescence: a critical period of addiction vulnerability. Am J Psychiatry 160:1041–1052, 2003

Chong SA, Low BL: Treatment of kleptomania with fluvoxamine. Acta Psychiatr Scand 93:314–315, 1996

Christenson GA, Mackenzie TB, Mitchell JE: Characteristics of 60 adult chronic hair pullers. Am J Psychiatry 148:365–370, 1991a

Christenson GA, Mackenzie TB, Mitchell JE, et al: A placebo-controlled, double-blind crossover study of fluoxetine in trichotillomania. Am J Psychiatry 148:1566–1571, 1991b

Christenson GA, Pyle RL, Mitchell JE: Estimated lifetime prevalence of trichotillomania in college students. J Clin Psychol 52:415–417, 1991c

Christenson GA, Chernoff-Clementz E, Clementz BA: Personality and clinical characteristics in patients with trichotillomania. J Clin Psychiatry 53:407–413, 1992

Ciarrochi J, Richardson R: Profile of compulsive gamblers in treatment: update and comparisons. Journal of Gambling Behavior 5:53–65, 1989

Coccaro EF, Kavoussi RJ: Fluoxetine and impulsive aggressive behavior in personality disordered subjects. Arch Gen Psychiatry 54:1081–1088, 1997

Coccaro EF, Lawrence T, Trestman R, et al: Growth hormone responses to intravenous clonidine challenge correlate with behavioral irritability in psychiatric patients and healthy volunteers. Psychiatry Res 39:129–139, 1991

Coccaro EF, Kavoussi RJ, Berman ME, et al: Intermittent explosive disorder—revised: development, reliability, and validity of research criteria. Compr Psychiatry 39:368–376, 1998a

Coccaro EF, Kavoussi RJ, Hauger RL, et al: Cerebrospinal fluid vasopressin levels: correlates with aggression and serotonin function in personality-disordered subjects. Arch Gen Psychiatry 55:708–714, 1998b

Coccaro EF, Posternak MA, Zimmerman M: Prevalence and features of intermittent explosive disorder in a clinical setting. J Clin Psychiatry 66:1221–1227, 2005

Cornelius JR, Soloff P, Perel JM, et al: Continuation pharmacotherapy of borderline personality disorder with haloperidol and phenelzine. Arch Gen Psychiatry 150:1843–1848, 1993

Cowdry RW, Gardner DL: Pharmacotherapy of borderline personality disorder: alprazolam, carbamazepine, trifluoperazine, and tranylcypromine. Arch Gen Psychiatry 45:111–119, 1988

Dannon PN, Iancu I, Grunhaus L: Naltrexone treatment in kleptomanic patients. Hum Psychopharmacol 14:583–585, 1999

de la Gandara JJ: Fluoxetine: open-trial in pathological gambling. Paper presented at the 152nd annual meeting of the American Psychiatric Association, Washington, DC, May 1999

DePue RA, Luciana M, Arbisi P, et al: Dopamine and the structure of personality: relation of agonist-induced dopamine activity to positive emotionality. J Pers Soc Psychol 67:485–498, 1994

Durst R, Katz G, Knobler HY: Buspirone augmentation of fluvoxamine in the treatment of kleptomania. J Nerv Ment Dis 185:586–588, 1997

Eisen SA, Lin N, Lyons MJ, et al: Familial influences on gambling behavior: an analysis of 3359 twin pairs. Addiction 93:1375–1384, 1998

Eisen SA, Slutske WS, Lyons MJ, et al: The genetics of pathological gambling. Semin Clin Neuropsychiatry 6:195–204, 2001

Epperson NC, Fasula D, Wasylink S, et al: Risperidone addition in serotonin reuptake inhibitor–resistant trichotillomania: three cases. J Child Adolesc Psychopharmacol 9:43–49, 1999

Fiorillo CD, Tobler PN, Schultz W: Discrete coding of reward probability and uncertainty by dopamine neurons. Science 299:1898–1902, 2003

Fishbain DA: Kleptomania as risk-taking behavior in response to depression. Am J Psychother 41:598–603, 1987

Franklin GA, Pucci PS, Arbabi S, et al: Decreased juvenile arson and firesetting recidivism after implementation of a multidisciplinary prevention program. J Trauma 53:260–266, 2002

Giammanco M, Tabacchi G, Giammanco S, et al: Testosterone and aggressiveness. Med Sci Monit 11:RA136–RA145, 2005

Goldman MJ: Kleptomania: making sense of the nonsensical. Am J Psychiatry 148:986–996, 1991

Grant JE: Co-occurrence of personality disorders in persons with kleptomania: a preliminary investigation. J Am Acad Law Psychiatry 34:395–398, 2004

Grant JE, Kim SW: Adolescent kleptomania treated with naltrexone: a case report. Eur Child Adolesc Psychiatry 11:92–95, 2002a

Grant JE, Kim SW: Clinical characteristics and associated psychopathology of 22 patients with kleptomania. Compr Psychiatry 43:378–384, 2002b

Grant JE, Kim SW: An open label study of naltrexone in the treatment of kleptomania. J Clin Psychiatry 63:349–356, 2002c

Grant JE, Kim SW: Comorbidity of impulse-control disorders among pathological gamblers. Acta Psychiatr Scand 108:207–213, 2003

Grant JE, Levine L, Kim D, et al: Impulse-control disorders in adult psychiatric inpatients. Am J Psychiatry 162:2184–2188, 2005

Grodnitzky GR, Tafrate RC: Imaginal exposure for anger reduction in adult outpatients: a pilot study. J Behav Ther Exp Psychiatry 31:259–279, 2000

Haller R, Hinterhuber H: Treatment of pathological gambling with carbamazepine. Pharmacopsychiatry 27:129, 1994

Hollander E, Frenkel M, DeCaria C, et al: Treatment of pathological gambling with clomipramine (letter). Am J Psychiatry 149:710–711, 1992

Hollander E, DeCaria CM, Mari E, et al: Short-term single-blind fluvoxamine treatment of pathological gambling. Am J Psychiatry 155:1781–1783, 1998

Hollander E, Buchalter AJ, DeCaria CM: Pathological gambling. Psychiatr Clin North Am 23:629–642, 2000a

Hollander E, DeCaria CM, Finkell JN, et al: A randomized double-blind fluvoxamine/placebo crossover trial in pathological gambling. Biol Psychiatry 47:813–817, 2000b

Hollander E, Pallanti S, Baldini Rossi N, et al: Sustained release lithium/placebo treatment response in bipolar spectrum pathological gamblers. Paper presented at the New Clinical Drug Evaluation (NCDEU) Annual Meeting, Boca Raton, FL, June 2002

Hollander E, Tracy KA, Swann AC, et al: Divalproex in the treatment of impulsive aggression: efficacy in cluster B personality disorders. Neuropsychopharmacology 28:1186–1197, 2003

Kavoussi RK, Coccaro EF: Divalproex sodium for impulsive aggressive behavior in patients with personality disorder. J Clin Psychiatry 59:676–680, 1998

Kim SW, Grant JE, Adson DE, et al: Double-blind naltrexone and placebo comparison study in the treatment of pathological gambling. Biol Psychiatry 49:914–921, 2001

Kim SW, Grant JE, Adson DE, et al: A double-blind placebo-controlled study of the efficacy and safety of paroxetine in the treatment of pathological gambling. J Clin Psychiatry 63:501–507, 2002

King RA, Scahill L, Vitulano LA, et al: Childhood trichotillomania: clinical phenomenology, comorbidity, and family genetics. J Am Acad Child Adolesc Psychiatry 34:1451–1459, 1995

Kmetz GF, McElroy SL, Collins DJ: Response of kleptomania and mixed mania to valproate. Am J Psychiatry 154:580–581, 1997

Koles MR, Jenson WR: Comprehensive treatment of chronic fire setting in a severely disordered boy. J Behav Ther Exp Psychiatry 16:81–85, 1985

Kraus JE: Treatment of kleptomania with paroxetine (letter). J Clin Psychiatry 60:793, 1999

Kriegsfeld LJ, Dawson TM, Dawson VL, et al: Aggressive behavior in male mice lacking the gene for neuronal nitric oxide synthase requires testosterone. Brain Res 769:66–70, 1997

Ladouceur R: Cognitive activities among gamblers. Paper presented at the Association for Advancement of Behavior Therapy (AABT) Convention, San Francisco, CA, November 1990

Lepkifker E, Dannon PN, Ziv R, et al: The treatment of kleptomania with serotonin reuptake inhibitors. Clin Neuropharmacol 22:40–43, 1999

Lewis NDC, Yarnell H: Pathological Firesetting (Pyromania) (Nervous and Mental Disease Monographs, No 82). New York, Coolidge Foundation, 1951

Linehan MM, Tutek DA, Heard HL, et al: Interpersonal outcome of cognitive behavioral treatment for chronically suicidal borderline patients. Am J Psychiatry 151:1771–1776, 1994

Links PS, Steiner M, Boiago I, et al: Lithium therapy for borderline patients: preliminary findings. J Personal Disord 4:173–181, 1990

Linnoila M, Virkkunen M, Scheinin M, et al: Low cerebrospinal fluid 5-hydroxyindoleacetic acid concentration differentiates impulsive from nonimpulsive violent behavior. Life Sci 33:2609–2614, 1983

Lyons WE, Mamounas LA, Ricaurte GA: Brain-derived neurotrophic factor–deficient mice develop aggressiveness and hyperphagia in conjunction with brain serotonergic abnormalities. Proc Natl Acad Sci U S A 96:15239–15244, 1991

Mansueto CS, Stemberger RMT, Thomas AM, et al: Trichotillomania: a comprehensive behavioral model. Clin Psychol Rev 17:567–577, 1997

Mattes JA, Fink M: A family study of patients with temper outbursts. J Psychiatr Res 21:249–255, 1987

Mavromatis M, Lion JR: A primer on pyromania. Dis Nerv Syst 38:954–955, 1977

McElroy SL, Keck PE Jr, Pope HG Jr, et al: Pharmacological treatment of kleptomania and bulimia nervosa. J Clin Psychopharmacol 9:358–360, 1989

McElroy SL, Hudson JI, Pope HG Jr, et al: Kleptomania: clinical characteristics and associated psychopathology. Psychol Med 21:93–108, 1991a

McElroy SL, Pope HG Jr, Hudson JI, et al: Kleptomania: a report of 20 cases. Am J Psychiatry 148:652–657, 1991b

McElroy SL, Hudson JI, Pope HG Jr, et al: The DSM-III-R impulse-control disorders not elsewhere classified: clinical characteristics and relationship to other psychiatric disorders. Am J Psychiatry 149:318–327, 1992

McElroy SL, Soutullo CA, Beckman DA, et al: DSM-IV intermittent explosive disorder: a report of 27 cases. J Clin Psychiatry 59:203–210, 1998

McGrath P, Marshall PG: A comprehensive treatment program for a fire-setting child. J Behav Ther Exp Psychiatry 10:69–72, 1979

Montgomery SA, Montgomery D: Pharmacological prevention of suicidal behavior. J Affect Disord 4:291–298, 1982

Moody G: Quit Compulsive Gambling. London, Thorsons, 1990

Moreno I, Saiz-Ruiz J, Lopez-Ibor JJ: Serotonin and gambling dependence. Hum Psychopharmacol 6:9–12, 1991

New AS, Hazlett EA, Buchsbaum MS: Blunted prefrontal cortical [18]fluorodeoxyglucose positron emission tomography response to meta-chlorophenylpiperazine in impulsive aggression. Arch Gen Psychiatry 59:621–629, 2002

Ninan PT, Rothbaum BO, Marsteller FA, et al: A placebo-controlled trial of cognitive-behavioral therapy and clomipramine in trichotillomania. J Clin Psychiatry 61:47–50, 2000

Pallanti S, Baldini Rossi N, Sood E, et al: Nefazodone treatment of pathological gambling: a prospective open-label controlled trial. J Clin Psychiatry 63:1034–1039, 2002a

Pallanti S, Quercioli L, Sood E, et al: Lithium and valproate treatment of pathological gambling: a randomized single-blind study. J Clin Psychiatry 63:559–564, 2002b

Petry NM, Armentano C: Prevalence, assessment, and treatment of pathological gambling: a review. Psychiatr Serv 50:1021–1027, 1999

Post RM, Pickar D, Ballenger JC, et al: Endogenous opiates in cerebrospinal fluid: relationship to mood and anxiety, in Neurobiology of Mood Disorders. Edited by Post RM, Ballenger JC. Baltimore, MD, Williams & Wilkins, 1984, pp 356–368

Potenza MN, Chambers RA: Schizophrenia and pathological gambling. Am J Psychiatry 158:497–498, 2001

Potenza MN, Hollander E: Pathological gambling and impulse-control disorders, in Neuropsychopharmacology: The Fifth Generation of Progress. Edited by Coyle JT, Nemeroff C, Charney D, et al. Baltimore, MD, Lippincott Williams & Wilkins, 2002, pp 1725–1741

Presta S, Marazziti D, Dell'Osso L, et al: Kleptomania: clinical features and comorbidity in an Italian sample. Compr Psychiatry 43:7–12, 2002

Robins LN, Regier DA: Psychiatric Disorders in America. New York, Free Press, 1991

Rothbaum BO, Shaw L, Morris R, et al: Prevalence of trichotillomania in a college freshman population (letter). J Clin Psychiatry 54:72, 1993

Russo AM, Taber JI, McCormick RA, et al: An outcome study of an inpatient treatment program for pathological gambling. Hosp Community Psychiatry 35:823–827, 1984

Schlosser S, Black DW, Blum N, et al: The demography, phenomenology, and family history of 22 persons with compulsive hair pulling. Ann Clin Psychiatry 6:147–152, 1994

Shaffer HJ, Hall MN, Vanderbilt J: Estimating the prevalence of disordered gambling behavior in United States and Canada: a research synthesis. Am J Public Health 89:1369–1376, 1999

Sheard M, Manini J, Bridges C, et al: The effect of lithium on impulsive aggressive behavior in man. Am J Psychiatry 133:1409–1413, 1976

Slutske WS, Eisen S, True WR, et al: Common genetic vulnerability for pathological gambling and alcohol dependence in men. Arch Gen Psychiatry 57:666–673, 2000

Soloff PH, George A, Nathan RS, et al: Paradoxical effects of amitriptyline in borderline patients. Am J Psychiatry 143:1603–1605, 1986a

Soloff PH, George A, Nathan RS, et al: Progress in pharmacotherapy of borderline disorders. Arch Gen Psychiatry 43:691–697, 1986b

Soloff PH, George A, Nathan RS, et al: Amitriptyline versus haloperidol in borderlines: final outcomes and predictors of response. J Clin Psychopharmacol 9:238–246, 1989

Soloff PH, Cornelius J, George A, et al: Efficacy of phenelzine and haloperidol in borderline personality disorder. Arch Gen Psychiatry 50:377–385, 1993

Stanley MA, Borden JW, Mouton SG, et al: Nonclinical hair-pulling: affective correlates and comparison with clinical samples. Behav Res Ther 33:179–186, 1995

Stewart RM, Brown RIF: An outcome study of Gamblers Anonymous. Br J Psychiatry 152:284–288, 1988

Streichenwein SM, Thornby JI: A long-term, double-blind, placebo-controlled crossover trial of the efficacy of fluoxetine for trichotillomania. Am J Psychiatry 152:1192–1196, 1995

Swedo SE: Trichotillomania. Psychiatr Ann 23:402–407, 1993

Swedo SE, Leonard HL: Trichotillomania: an obsessive compulsive spectrum disorder? Psychiatr Clin North Am 15:777–790, 1992

Swedo SE, Leonard HL, Rapoport JL, et al: A double-blind comparison of clomipramine and desipramine in the treatment of trichotillomania (hair pulling). N Engl J Med 321:497–501, 1989

Swedo SE, Lenane MC, Leonard HL: Long-term treatment of trichotillomania (hair pulling) (letter). N Engl J Med 329:141–142, 1993

Taber JI: Group psychotherapy with pathological gamblers. Paper presented at the 5th National Conference on Gambling and Risk-Taking, South Lake Tahoe, NV, October 1981

Taber JI, McCormick RA, Russo AM, et al: Follow-up of pathological gamblers after treatment. Am J Psychiatry 144:757–761, 1987

van Minnen A, Hoogduin KA, Keijsers GP, et al: Treatment of trichotillomania with behavioral therapy or fluoxetine. Arch Gen Psychiatry 60:517–522, 2003

Virkkunen M, Nuutila A, Goodwin FK: Cerebrospinal fluid monoamine metabolite levels in male arsonists. Arch Gen Psychiatry 44:241–247, 1987

Virkkunen M, Rawlings, Tokola R: CSF biochemistries, glucose metabolism, and diurnal activity rhythms in alcoholic, violent offenders, fire setters, and healthy volunteers. Arch Gen Psychiatry 51:20–27, 1994

Zanarini MC, Frankenburg FR: Olanzapine treatment of female borderline personality disorder patients: a double-blind, placebo-controlled pilot study. J Clin Psychiatry 62:849–854, 2001

Zimmerman M, Breen RB, Posternak MA: An open-label study of citalopram in the treatment of pathological gambling. J Clin Psychiatry 63:44–48, 2002

# 28

# Adjustment Disorders

JAMES J. STRAIN, M.D.

KIMBERLY G. KLIPSTEIN, M.D.

JEFFREY H. NEWCORN, M.D.

No symptom inventory or checklist has been constructed or easily emanates from the DSM-IV-TR (American Psychiatric Association 2000) diagnostic criteria (see Table 28–1).

According to DSM-IV (American Psychiatric Association 1994), "[t]he essential feature of an adjustment disorder is the development of clinically significant emotional or behavioral symptoms in response to an identifiable psychosocial stressor or stressors" (p. 623). In the recent DSM-IV text revision (DSM-IV-TR; American Psychiatric Association 2000), the term *psychosocial stressor* was changed to the broader concept of *stressor*.

In DSM-IV-TR, the section on "Prevalence" has been altered to include rates in children, adolescents, and the elderly (with the rate of adjustment disorder being 2%–8% in community samples). Adjustment disorder "has been diagnosed in up to 12% of general hospital inpatients who are referred for a mental health consultation, in 10%–30% of those in mental health outpatient settings, and in as many as 50% in special populations that have experienced a specific stressor (e.g., following cardiac surgery)" (American Psychiatric Association 2000, p. 681). Those populations with increased stressors (e.g., indigent pa-

tients, medically ill patients) are at higher risk for developing adjustment disorder.

Adjustment disorder is a stress-related phenomenon in which the stressor has precipitated maladaptation and symptoms (within 3 months of the occurrence of the stressor) that are time limited until the stressor is removed or a new state of adaptation has occurred (see Table 28–1).

## Definition

In reviewing the diagnosis of adjustment disorder for DSM-IV, two issues emerged as fundamental. First, the effect of the imprecision of this diagnosis on reliability and validity because of the lack of behavioral or operational criteria must be determined. One study (Aoki et al. 1995) found three psychological tests—Zung's Self-Rating Anxiety Scale (Zung 1971), Zung's Self-Rating Depression Scale (Zung 1965), and Profile of Mood States (McNair et al. 1971)—to be useful tools for the diagnosis of adjustment disorder among physical rehabilitation patients. Although Aoki et al. (1995) succeeded in

This work was funded by The Malcolm Gibbs Foundation, Inc., New York, New York.

**TABLE 28–1.    DSM-IV-TR diagnostic criteria for adjustment disorders**

A.  The development of emotional or behavioral symptoms in response to an identifiable stressor(s) occurring within 3 months of the onset of the stressor(s).

B.  These symptoms or behaviors are clinically significant as evidenced by either of the following:

(1)  marked distress that is in excess of what would be expected from exposure to the stressor

(2)  significant impairment in social or occupational (academic) functioning

C.  The stress-related disturbance does not meet the criteria for another specific Axis I disorder and is not merely an exacerbation of a preexisting Axis I or Axis II disorder.

D.  The symptoms do not represent bereavement.

E.  Once the stressor (or its consequences) has terminated, the symptoms do not persist for more than an additional 6 months.

*Specify* if:

**Acute:**  if the disturbance lasts less than 6 months

**Chronic:**  if the disturbance lasts for 6 months or longer

Adjustment disorders are coded based on the subtype, which is selected according to the predominant symptoms. The specific stressor(s) can be specified on Axis IV.

309.0   **With depressed mood**

309.24  **With anxiety**

309.28  **With mixed anxiety and depressed mood**

309.3   **With disturbance of conduct**

309.4   **With mixed disturbance of emotions and conduct**

309.9   **Unspecified**

reliably differentiating patients with adjustment disorder from healthy patients, they did not distinguish them from patients with major depression or posttraumatic stress disorder.

Second, the classification of syndromes that do not fulfill the criteria for a major mental illness but indicate serious (or incipient) symptomatology that requires intervention and/or treatment, by default, may be viewed as "subthreshold" and afforded a subthreshold interest by health care workers and third-party payers. Thus, the con-

struct of adjustment disorder is designed as a means for classifying psychiatric conditions having a symptom profile that is as yet insufficient to meet the more specifically operationalized criteria for the major syndromes but that is 1) clinically significant and deemed to be in excess of a normal reaction to the stressor in question (taking culture into account), 2) associated with impaired vocational or interpersonal functioning, and 3) not solely the result of a psychosocial problem (V code) requiring medical attention (e.g., noncompliance, phase-of-life problem).

With the lack of specificity that characterizes the adjustment disorder diagnoses, however, it is often difficult to truly distinguish them from other psychiatric syndromes. Spalletta et al. (1996) observed that assessment of suicidal behavior is an important tool in differentiating major depression, dysthymia, and adjustment disorder. Furthermore, patients with adjustment disorder were observed to be among the most common recipients of a deliberate self-harm diagnosis, with the majority involving self-poisoning (Vlachos et al. 1994). Thus, deliberate self-harm is more common in these patients (Vlachos et al. 1994), whereas the percentage of suicidal behavior was found to be higher in depressed patients (Spalletta et al. 1996). In a more recent study, Casey et al. (2006) examined variables that might distinguish adjustment disorder from other depressive episodes. The patients were screened for depression severity with the Beck Depression Inventory (BDI) and then interviewed with the Schedule for Clinical Assessment in Neuropsychiatry, which includes questions assessing the presence of adjustment disorder. The authors were unable to find any independent variables that distinguished adjustment disorder from other depressive episodes, including the severity of the BDI score at the outset.

## Epidemiology

Andreasen and Wasek (1980) reported that 5% of an inpatient and outpatient sample were labeled as having adjustment disorder. Fabrega et al. (1987) observed that 2.3% of a sample of patients at a walk-in clinic (diagnostic and evaluation center) met criteria for adjustment disorder, with no other diagnoses on Axis I or Axis II; 20% had the diagnosis of adjustment disorder when patients with other Axis I diagnoses (i.e., Axis I comorbidities) also were included. In general hospital psychiatric consultation populations, adjustment disorder was diagnosed in 21.5% (Popkin et al. 1990), 18.5% (Foster and Oxman 1994), and 11.5% (Snyder and Strain 1989).

Strain et al. (1998) examined the consultation-liaison data from seven university teaching hospitals in the United States, Canada, and Australia. The sites had all used a common computerized clinical database to examine 1,039 consecutive referrals—the MICRO-CARES software system (Strain et al. 1998). Adjustment disorder was diagnosed in 125 patients (12.0%); it was the sole diagnosis in 81 (7.8%) and comorbid with other Axis I and II diagnoses in 44 (4.2%). It had been considered as a "rule-out" diagnosis in an additional 110 (10.6%). Adjustment disorder with depressed mood, with anxious mood, and with mixed emotions were the most common subcategories used. Adjustment disorder was diagnosed comorbidly most frequently with personality disorder and organic mental disorder. Sixty-seven subjects (6.4%) were assigned a V-code diagnosis only. Patients with adjustment disorder were referred significantly more often for problems of anxiety, coping, and depression; had less past psychiatric illness; and were rated as functioning better than those patients with major mental disorders—all consistent with the construct of adjustment disorder as a maladaptation to a psychosocial stressor. Interventions used for this general hospital inpatient cohort were similar to those for other Axis I and II diagnoses—in particular, the prescription of antidepressant medications.

## Etiology

Cohen (1981) argued that 1) acute stresses are different from chronic ones in both psychological and physiological terms, 2) the meaning of the stress is affected by "modifiers" (e.g., ego strengths, support systems, prior mastery), and 3) the manifest and latent meanings of the stressor(s) must be differentiated (e.g., loss of job may be a relief or a catastrophe). Adjustment disorder with maladaptive denial of pregnancy, for example, can be a consequence of a stressor such as separation from a partner (Brezinka et al. 1994). An objectively overwhelming stress may have little effect on one individual, whereas a minor one could be regarded as cataclysmic by another.

Several recent studies of young male soldiers with adjustment disorder secondary to conscription found that stress at a young age, such as abusive and overprotective parenting or adverse early family events, is a risk factor for the later development of adjustment disorder (For-Wey et al. 2002; Hansen-Schwartz et al. 2005). In a similar cohort, a history of childhood separation anxiety was found to be correlated with the later development of adjustment disorder (Giotakos and Konstantakopoulos 2002).

## Clinical Features

In DSM-IV-TR, adjustment disorder was reduced to six types that are classified according to their clinical features: with depressed mood, with anxiety, with mixed anxiety and depressed mood, with disturbance of conduct, with mixed disturbance of emotions and conduct, and unspecified (Table 28–2).

## Treatment

### Psychotherapy

Treatment of adjustment disorder rests primarily on psychotherapeutic measures that enable reduction of the stressor, enhanced coping with the stressor that cannot be reduced or removed, and establishment of a support system to maximize adaptation. The first goal is to note significant dysfunction secondary to a stressor and to help the patient moderate this imbalance. Many stressors may be avoided or minimized. Other stressors may elicit an overreaction on the part of the patient. The patient may attempt suicide or become reclusive, damaging his or her source of income. In this situation, the therapist would attempt to help the patient put his or her rage and other feelings into words rather than into destructive actions and assist with more optimal adaptation and mastery of the trauma–stressor. The role of verbalization cannot be overestimated in an attempt to reduce the pressure of the stressor and enhance coping. The therapist also needs to clarify and interpret the meaning of the stressor for the patient. For example, a mastectomy may have devastated a patient's feelings about her body and herself. It is necessary to clarify that the patient is still a woman, capable of having a fulfilling relationship, including a sexual one, and that the patient can have the cancer removed or treated and not have a recurrence. Otherwise, the patient's pernicious fantasies—"all is lost"—may take over in response to the stressor (i.e., the mastectomy) and make her dysfunctional in work and/or sex and precipitate a painful disturbance of mood that is incapacitating.

Many types of therapeutic modalities have a place in the treatment of adjustment disorders. Wise (1988), drawing from military psychiatry, emphasized the treatment variables of Brevity, Immediacy, Centrality, Expectance, Proximity, and Simplicity (BICEPS principles). The treatment approach is brief, usually no more than 72 hours (True and Benway 1992). Such treatment would be similar to that prescribed for an acute stress disorder—

**TABLE 28–2.    Types of DSM-IV-TR adjustment disorder**

| | |
|---|---|
| With depressed mood | The predominant symptoms are those of a minor depression. For example, the symptoms might be depressed mood, tearfulness, and hopelessness. |
| With anxiety | This type of adjustment disorder is diagnosed when anxiety symptoms are predominant, such as nervousness, worry, and jitteriness. The differential diagnosis would include anxiety disorders. |
| With mixed anxiety and depressed mood | This category should be used when the predominant symptoms are a combination of depression and anxiety or other emotions. An example would be an adolescent who, after moving away from home and parental supervision, reacts with ambivalence, depression, anger, and signs of increased dependence. |
| With disturbance of conduct | The symptomatic manifestations are those of behavioral misconduct that violate societal norms or the rights of others. Examples are fighting, truancy, vandalism, and reckless driving. |
| With mixed disturbance of emotions and conduct | This diagnosis is made when the disturbance combines affective and behavioral features of adjustment disorder with mixed emotional features and adjustment disorder with disturbance of conduct. |
| Unspecified | This is a residual diagnosis within the diagnostic category. This diagnosis can be used when a maladaptive reaction that is not classified under other adjustment disorders occurs in response to stress. An example would be a patient who, when given a diagnosis of cancer, denies the diagnosis of malignancy and is noncompliant with treatment recommendations. |

the new diagnosis proposed by Spiegel and included in DSM-IV and DSM-IV-TR. The implication that maladaptation secondary to stressors requires immediate amelioration is important for the adjustment disorders, to avoid losses and dysfunction at work, in school, or with relationships.

## Pharmacotherapy

Reynolds (1992), reviewing randomized controlled trials, stated that bereavement-related syndromal depression also appears to respond to antidepressant medication. By definition, however, bereavement is considered not as an adjustment disorder but rather as a stress-related response disorder and as such is classified as a V code—a problem-level diagnosis—warranting the attention of a mental health professional. Ordinarily, medication is not prescribed for problem-level diagnoses; rather, counseling, psychotherapy, support, and so forth are the interventions of choice. If medication is prescribed for minor disorders (including subthreshold disorders), the predominant mood that accompanies the (adjustment) disorder is an important consideration.

Schatzberg (1990) recommended that therapists consider both psychotherapy and pharmacotherapy in adjust-

ment disorders with anxious mood and that anxiolytics should be part of psychiatrists' armamentarium. Nguyen et al. (2006), using a double-blind, randomized controlled trial, compared the efficacies of etifoxine, a nonbenzodiazepine anxiolytic drug, and lorazepam, a benzodiazepine, in the treatment of adjustment disorder with anxiety in a primary care setting. Efficacy was evaluated on days 7 and 28 with the Hamilton Rating Scale for Anxiety. The two drugs were found to be equivalent in anxiolytic efficacy on day 28. However, overall, more etifoxine recipients responded to the treatment. Moreover, 1 week after stopping treatment, fewer patients taking etifoxine experienced rebound anxiety compared with lorazepam patients.

Whether psychotherapy or pharmacotherapy is used alone or in combination, a significant aspect of treatment is for the physician to keep alert to the fact that the diagnosis of adjustment disorder may indicate a patient who is in the early phase of a major mental disorder that has not yet evolved to full-blown symptoms. Therefore, if a patient continues to worsen, becomes more symptomatic, and does not respond to treatment, it is critical to review the patient's symptoms and the diagnosis for the presence of a major mental disorder.

## Course and Prognosis

DSM-IV-TR Criterion E for adjustment disorder implies a good long-term outcome by stating "once the stressor (or its consequences) has terminated, the symptoms do not persist for more than an additional 6 months" (American Psychiatric Association 2000, p. 683). Andreasen and Hoenk's (1982) landmark study confirmed this by showing that prognosis is favorable for adults but that in adolescents, many major psychiatric illnesses eventually occur. At 5-year follow-up, 71% of the adults were completely well, 8% had an intervening problem, and 21% had developed a major depressive disorder or alcoholism. In adolescents at 5-year follow-up, only 44% were without a psychiatric diagnosis, 13% had an intervening psychiatric illness, and 43% had gone on to develop major psychiatric morbidity (e.g., schizophrenia, schizoaffective disorder, major depression, bipolar disorder, substance abuse, personality disorders). In contrast to the predictors for major pathology in adults, the chronicity of the illness and the presence of behavioral symptoms in the adolescents were the strongest predictors for major pathology at the 5-year follow-up. The number and type of symptoms were less useful than the length of treatment and chronicity of symptoms as predictors of future outcome.

Although most studies do point to a more benign prognosis for the adjustment disorders, it is important to realize that the risk of serious morbidity and mortality still exists. Many studies investigating the association between suicide and adjustment disorder underscore the importance of monitoring patients closely for suicidality. Runeson et al. (1996) observed from psychological autopsy methods that the median interval between first suicidal communication and suicide was very short in the patients with adjustment disorder (<1 month) compared with patients who had major depression (3 months), borderline personality disorder (30 months), or schizophrenia (47 months). Portzky et al. (2005) conducted psychological autopsies on adolescents with adjustment disorder who had committed suicide and found that suicidal thinking in these patients was brief and evolved rapidly and without warning.

A slightly different profile was found in two other studies that looked at suicide attempters with a diagnosis of adjustment disorder. These patients were more likely to have poor overall psychosocial functioning, prior psychiatric treatment, personality disorders, substance abuse histories, and a current "mixed" symptom profile of depressed mood and behavioral disturbances (Kryzhanovskaya and Canterbury 2001; Pelkonen et al. 2005).

A study of the neurochemical variables of adjustment disorder patients of all ages who had attempted suicide reported biological correlates consistent with the more major psychiatric disorders. Attempters were found to have lower platelet monoamine oxidase activity, higher 3-methoxy-4-hydroxyphenylglycol (MHPG) activity, and higher cortisol levels than control subjects had. Although these findings differ from the lower MHPG and cortisol levels found in patients with major depression and suicidality, they are similar to findings in other major stress-related conditions.

## Key Points: Adjustment Disorders

- Adjustment disorders are of two forms: acute (6 months or less) and chronic (greater than 6 months).

- In children, adjustment disorders are predictive of more serious mental illnesses for late adolescence and adulthood.

- An adjustment disorder diagnosis can be used concurrently with another Axis I diagnosis.

- The adjustment disorders have a clear threshold for when they are supplanted by another Axis I diagnosis, because the other diagnoses have established thresholds and symptom guidelines. The point at which the patient crosses the threshold between normal behavior and an adjustment disorder is less clear, however, because the symptom guidelines for entry are less specific.

- It has been suggested that adjustment disorders could be placed with other diagnoses identified by the mood and behavior; for example, adjustment disorder with depressed mood could be positioned as an affective disorder.

# References

American Psychiatric Association: Diagnostic and Statistical Manual of Mental Disorders, 4th Edition. Washington, DC, American Psychiatric Association, 1994

American Psychiatric Association: Diagnostic and Statistical Manual of Mental Disorders, 4th Edition, Text Revision. Washington, DC, American Psychiatric Association, 2000

Andreasen NC, Hoenk PR: The predictive value of adjustment disorders: a follow-up study. Am J Psychiatry 139:584–590, 1982

Andreasen NC, Wasek P: Adjustment disorders in adolescents and adults. Arch Gen Psychiatry 37:1166–1170, 1980

Aoki T, Hosaka T, Ishida A: Psychiatric evaluation of physical rehabilitation patients. Gen Hosp Psychiatry 17:440–443, 1995

Brezinka C, Huter O, Biebl W, et al: Denial of pregnancy: obstetrical aspects. J Psychosom Obstet Gynaecol 15:1–8, 1994

Casey P, Maracy M, Kelly BD, et al: Can adjustment disorder and depressive episode be distinguished? J Affect Disord 92:291–297, 2006

Cohen F: Stress and bodily illness. Psychiatr Clin North Am 4:269–286, 1981

Fabrega H Jr, Mezzich JE, Mezzich AC: Adjustment disorder as a marginal or transitional illness category in DSM-III. Arch Gen Psychiatry 44:567–572, 1987

For-Wey L, Fei-Yin L, Bih-Ching S: The relationship between life adjustment and parental bonding in military personnel with adjustment disorder in Taiwan. Mil Med 167:678–682, 2002

Foster P, Oxman T: A descriptive study of adjustment disorder diagnoses in general hospital patients. Ir J Psychol Med 11:153–157, 1994

Giotakos O, Konstantakopoulos G: Parenting received in childhood and early separation anxiety in male conscripts with adjustment disorder. Mil Med 167:28–33, 2002

Hansen-Schwartz J, Kijne B, Johnsen A, et al: The course of adjustment disorder in Danish male conscripts. Nord J Psychiatry 59:193–196, 2005

Kryzhanovskaya L, Canterbury R: Suicidal behavior in patients with adjustment disorders. Crisis 22:125–131, 2001

McNair DM, Lorr M, Doppelman LF (eds): Manual for the Profile of Mood States. San Diego, CA, Educational and Industrial Testing Service, 1971

Nguyen N, Fakra E, Pradel V, et al: Efficacy of etifoxine compared to lorazepam monotherapy in the treatment of patients with adjustment disorders with anxiety: a double-blind controlled study in general practice. Hum Psychopharmacol 21:139–149, 2006

Pelkonen M, Marttunen M, Henriksson M, et al: Suicidality in adjustment disorder—clinical characteristics of adolescent outpatients. Eur Child Adolesc Psychiatry 14:174–180, 2005

Popkin MK, Callies AL, Colon EA, et al: Adjustment disorders in medically ill patients referred for consultation in a university hospital. Psychosomatics 31:410–414, 1990

Portzky G, Audenaert K, van Heeringen K: Adjustment disorder and the course of the suicidal process in adolescents. J Affect Disord 87:265–270, 2005

Reynolds CF 3rd: Treatment of depression in special populations. J Clin Psychiatry 53 (9, suppl):45–53, 1992

Runeson BS, Beskow J, Waern M: The suicidal process in suicides among young people. Acta Psychiatr Scand 93:35–42, 1996

Schatzberg AF: Anxiety and adjustment disorder: a treatment approach. J Clin Psychiatry 51(suppl):20–24, 1990

Snyder S, Strain JJ: Differentiation of major depression and adjustment disorder with depressed mood in the medical setting. Gen Hosp Psychiatry 12:159–165, 1989

Spalletta G, Troisi A, Saracco M, et al: Symptom profile: Axis II comorbidity and suicidal behavior in young males with DSM-III-R depressive illnesses. J Affect Disord 39:141–148, 1996

Strain JJ, Smith GC, Hammer JS, et al: Adjustment disorder: a multisite study of its utilization and interventions in the consultation-liaison psychiatry setting. Gen Hosp Psychiatry 20:139–149, 1998

True PK, Benway MW: Treatment of stress reaction prior to combat using the "BICEPS" model. Mil Med 157:380–381, 1992

Vlachos IO, Bouras N, Watson JP, et al: Deliberate self-harm referrals. Eur Psychiatry 8:25–28, 1994

Wise MG: Adjustment disorders and impulse disorders not otherwise classified, in American Psychiatric Press Textbook of Psychiatry. Edited by Talbot JA, Hales RE, Yudofsky SC. Washington, DC, American Psychiatric Press, 1988, pp 605–620

Zung W: A self-rating depression scale. Arch Gen Psychiatry 12:63–70, 1965

Zung W: A rating instrument for anxiety disorders. Psychosomatics 12:371–379, 1971

# 29

# Personality Disorders

ANDREW E. SKODOL, M.D.

JOHN G. GUNDERSON, M.D.

## General Considerations

### What Is a Personality Disorder?

According to DSM-IV-TR (American Psychiatric Association 2000), personality disorders are patterns of inflexible and maladaptive personality traits and behaviors that cause subjective distress, significant impairment in social or occupational functioning, or both. These patterns deviate markedly from the culturally expected and accepted range and are manifest in two or more of the following areas: cognition, affectivity, control over impulses and need gratification, and ways of relating to others. The maladaptive traits and behaviors are pervasive—that is, they are expressed across a broad range of contexts and situations rather than in only one specific triggering situation or in response to a particular stimulus or person. Finally, the patterns must have been stably present and enduring since adolescence or early adulthood.

### Classification Issues

Since DSM-III (American Psychiatric Association 1980), the personality disorders have been grouped into three clusters: the *odd or eccentric Cluster A* (paranoid, schizoid, and schizotypal); the *dramatic, emotional, or erratic Cluster B* (borderline, histrionic, narcissistic, and antisocial); and the *anxious or fearful Cluster C* (avoidant, dependent, and obsessive-compulsive) (Table 29–1).

The most widely used dimensional approaches describe personality according to a number of broad factors and more narrow trait dimensions and assess the degree to which traits are present for a given patient. These may more comprehensively cover both normal and pathological personality traits. Indeed, one of the recent large-scale efforts in personality research has been to describe DSM personality disorder types in terms of dimensions of general personality functioning (Widiger 2000). Of special significance are the widely heralded "Big Five" dimensions of the Five-Factor Model of Personality: neuroticism, extraversion, openness, agreeableness, and conscientiousness (Costa and McCrae 1990). Cloninger's seven-dimension psychobiological model of temperament and character (Table 29–2; Cloninger et al. 1993), which was theoretically linked to abnormalities in specific neurotransmitter systems, has generated a large body of research, but the data generally have not supported these neurobiological hypotheses (Paris 2005b).

### Comprehensiveness of Evaluation

A skilled clinical interview is the mainstay of personality disorder diagnosis and requires the clinician to be familiar with DSM criteria, take a longitudinal view, and use multiple sources of information. A psychodynamic perspective may contribute depth to the assessment through its attention to defenses, attitudes, and development. However, because an open-ended approach may provide insufficient information to assess all Axis II disorders, a self-

**TABLE 29–1.    DSM-IV-TR personality clusters, specific types, and their defining clinical features**

| Cluster | Type | Characteristic features |
|---|---|---|
| A (odd or eccentric) | Paranoid | Pervasive distrust and suspiciousness of others such that their motives are interpreted as malevolent |
| | Schizoid | Pervasive pattern of detachment from social relationships and restricted range of expression of emotions in interpersonal settings |
| | Schizotypal | Pervasive pattern of social and interpersonal deficits marked by acute discomfort with, and reduced capacity for, close relationships as well as by cognitive or perceptual distortions and eccentricities of behavior |
| B (dramatic, emotional, or erratic) | Antisocial | History of conduct disorder before age 15 years; pervasive pattern of disregard for and violation of the rights of others; current age at least 18 years |
| | Borderline | Pervasive pattern of instability of interpersonal relationships, self-image, and affects and marked impulsivity |
| | Histrionic | Pervasive pattern of excessive emotionality and attention seeking |
| | Narcissistic | Pervasive pattern of grandiosity (in fantasy or behavior), need for admiration, and lack of empathy |
| C (anxious or fearful) | Avoidant | Pervasive pattern of social inhibition, feelings of inadequacy, and hypersensitivity to negative evaluation |
| | Dependent | Pervasive and excessive need to be taken care of that leads to submissive and clinging behavior and fears of separation |
| | Obsessive-compulsive | Pervasive pattern of preoccupation with orderliness, perfectionism, and mental and interpersonal control at the expense of flexibility, openness, and efficiency |

*Source.*   Adapted from American Psychiatric Association 2000.

report or semistructured (i.e., interviewer-administered) personality disorder assessment instrument may be used to augment a clinical interview (Table 29–3) (Kaye and Shea 2000; McDermut and Zimmerman 2005). Such instruments systematically assess each personality disorder criterion with standard questions or probes. Although self-report instruments have the advantage of saving interviewer time and being free of interviewer bias, they often yield false-positive diagnoses and allow contamination of Axis II traits by Axis I states. Semistructured interviews—which require the interviewer to use certain questions, but allow further probing—facilitate accurate diagnosis in several ways: they ensure coverage of relevant domains of personality psychopathology, allow the interviewer to attempt to differentiate Axis II traits from Axis I states, encourage clarification of contradictions or ambiguities in the patient's response, and provide the opportunity to determine that traits are pervasive (i.e., by eliciting multiple examples of trait expression) rather than limited to a specific situation.

## Clinical Significance of Personality Disorders

Several studies have compared patients with personality disorders with patients with no personality disorder or with Axis I disorders and have found that patients with personality disorders were more likely to be separated, divorced, or never married and to have had more unemployment, frequent job changes, or periods of disability. Patients with personality disorders only rarely have been found to be less well educated, however. Studies that have examined quality of functioning have found poorer social functioning or interpersonal relationships and poorer work functioning or occupational achievement and satisfaction. Among patients with different personality disorders, those with severe types, such as schizotypal and borderline, have been found to have significantly more impairment at work, in social relationships, and at leisure than patients with less severe types, such as obsessive-compulsive disorder, or with an impairing Axis I disorder, such as major depressive disorder in the absence of personality disorder. Even the less impaired patients with

TABLE 29–2. The seven-factor model of personality: temperament and character inventory

| Temperament | Descriptors of extreme variants | | Character | Descriptors of extreme variants | |
|---|---|---|---|---|---|
| | High | Low | | High | Low |
| Harm avoidance | Pessimistic | Optimistic | Self-directedness | Responsible | Blaming |
| | Fearful | Daring | | Purposeful | Aimless |
| | Shy | Outgoing | | Resourceful | Inept |
| | Fatigable | Energetic | | Self-accepting | Vain |
| | | | | Disciplined | Undisciplined |
| Novelty seeking | Exploratory | Reserved | Cooperative | Tender-hearted | Intolerant |
| | Impulsive | Rigid | | Empathic | Insensitive |
| | Extravagant | Frugal | | Helpful | Hostile |
| | Irritable | Stoic | | Compassionate | Revengeful |
| | | | | Principled | Opportunistic |
| Reward dependence | Sentimental | Critical | Self-transcendent | Self-forgetful | Unimaginative |
| | Open | Aloof | | Transpersonal | Controlling |
| | Warm | Detached | | Spiritual | Materialistic |
| | Sympathetic | Independent | | Enlightened | Possessive |
| | | | | Idealistic | Practical |
| Persistence | Industrious | Lazy | | | |
| | Determined | Spoiled | | | |
| | Ambitious | Underachieving | | | |
| | Perfectionistic | Pragmatic | | | |

*Source.* Adapted from Cloninger CR: "The Genetics and Psychobiology of the Seven-Factor Model of Personality," in *Biology of Personality Disorders.* Edited by Silk KR. Washington, DC, American Psychiatric Press, 1998, pp. 63–92. Copyright 1998, American Psychiatric Press. Used with permission.

personality disorders (e.g., obsessive-compulsive), however, have moderate to severe impairment in at least one area of functioning (or a Global Assessment of Functioning rating of 60 or less) (Skodol et al. 2002). Thus, patients with specific personality disorders differ from one another not only in the degree of associated functional impairment but also in the breadth of impairment across functional domains.

Impairment in functioning in patients with personality disorders tends to be persistent even beyond apparent improvement in personality disorder psychopathology itself (Seivewright et al. 2004; Skodol et al. 2005). The persistence of impairment is understandable because personality disorder psychopathology has usually been relatively long-standing and therefore has disrupted a person's work and social development over a period of time (Roberts et al. 2003). The "scars" or residua of personality

disorder pathology may take time to heal or be overcome. With time (and treatment), however, improvements in functioning can occur.

Personality disorders also often cause problems for others and are costly to society. They are associated with elevated rates of separation, divorce, conflict with family members and romantic partners, child custody proceedings, homelessness, high-risk sexual behavior, and perpetration of child abuse. Those with personality disorders also have increased rates of accidents; police contacts; emergency department visits; medical hospitalization and treatment utilization; violence and criminal behavior, including homicide; self-injurious behavior; attempted suicide; and completed suicide. A high percentage of individuals with criminal convictions (70%–85% in some studies), 60%–70% of individuals with alcoholism, and 70%–90% of persons who abuse drugs have a personality disorder.

**TABLE 29–3. Features of interviews and self-report instruments for the assessment of personality disorders**

| Interview or instrument | Author | Type | Special features |
|---|---|---|---|
| Structured Interview for DSM-IV Personality (SIDP-IV) | Pfohl et al. 1997 | Interview | Patient and informant questions |
| International Personality Disorder Examination (IPDE) | Loranger 1999 | Interview | Detailed instruction manual; translated into several languages |
| Structured Clinical Interview for DSM-IV Axis II Personality Disorders (SCID-II) | First et al. 1997 | Interview | Axis I section; Axis II screening questionnaire |
| Diagnostic Interview for DSM-IV Personality Disorders (DIPD-IV) | Zanarini et al. 1996 | Interview | Good test–retest reliability |
| Personality Disorder Interview–IV (PDI-IV) | Widiger et al. 1995 | Interview | Detailed instruction manual; categorical and dimensional assessments |
| Personality Diagnostic Questionnaire–4 (PDQ-4) | Hyler 1994 | Self-report | Face-valid items; useful for screening |
| Millon Clinical Multiaxial Inventory–III (MCMI-III) | Millon et al. 1997 | Self-report | Dimensions of Axis I and Axis II psychopathology |
| Wisconsin Personality Inventory–IV (WPI-IV) | Klein 1993 | Self-report | Integrated structural analysis of social behavior model[a] |
| Schedule for Nonadaptive and Adaptive Personality (SNAP) | Clark 1993 | Self-report | Normal and abnormal personality trait measures; DSM-IV diagnoses |

*Note.* All instruments listed assess the full range of personality disorders. Other instruments are available to assess certain individual personality disorders.
[a]See Benjamin 1974.
*Source.* Adapted from Skodol and Oldham 1991.

Personality disorders often need to be a focus of treatment or, at the very least, need to be taken into account when comorbid Axis I disorders are treated, because their presence often affects an Axis I disorder's prognosis and treatment response. As most clinicians are well aware, the characteristics of patients with personality disorders are likely to be manifested in the treatment relationship regardless of whether the personality disorder is the focus of treatment. Although individuals with personality disorders tend to use psychiatric services extensively (Bender et al. 2001), they are more likely to be dissatisfied with the treatment they receive (Kent et al. 1995).

## Etiology and Pathogenesis

All available data suggest that personality disorders (as well as normal personality traits) result from a complex combination of, and interaction between, temperament (genetic and other biological factors) and psychological (develop-mental or environmental) factors (Paris 2005a). Although the degree to which genetic and environmental factors contribute to etiology may vary for different personality disorders, the first major twin study indicates that both factors are important in all of these disorders (Torgersen et al. 2000). Of relevance, too, are studies showing that approximately half the observed variance in personality traits such as neuroticism, introversion, and submissiveness can be traced to genetic variation (Carey and DiLalla 1994).

Increasing numbers of studies of environmental antecedents of personality disorders, such as family environment and sexual and physical abuse, are substantiating a likely role for such factors in the development of certain disorders, particularly borderline personality disorder (BPD) (Zanarini 1997). In addition, defense mechanisms appear to play an important role in the expression of personality disorders, which are characterized by less mature defense mechanisms such as projection and acting-out

(Perry and Bond 2005). Research in these areas is expected to continue to increase rapidly. In addition to providing information about the origins of the personality disorders, such findings are expected to open new avenues for treating these often difficult-to-treat patients.

## Treatment

Psychoanalysts pioneered the notion that persons with personality disorders could respond to treatment (Gabbard 2005). The original conception of neurosis as a specific set of symptoms related to a discrete developmental phase or to discrete conflicts was gradually replaced by the idea that more enduring defensive styles and identification processes were the building blocks of character traits. From this perspective, Wilhelm Reich (1949) and others developed the concepts of *character analysis* and *defense analysis.* These processes refer to an analyst's efforts to address the ways in which a person resists learning and the confrontations by which the analyst draws attention to the maladaptive effects of the patient's character traits. A parallel development in technique evolved from group therapy experience. Maxwell Jones (1953) identified the value of confrontations delivered within group settings in which peer pressure made it difficult for patients to ignore feedback or to leave the group (Piper and Ogrodniczuk 2005).

Reviews of psychotherapy outcome studies, including psychodynamic/interpersonal, cognitive-behavioral, mixed, and supportive therapies, have found that psychotherapy was associated with a significantly faster rate of recovery compared with the natural course of personality disorders (Leichsenring and Leibing 2003; Perry et al. 1999).

A significant development has been the application of cognitive-behavioral strategies to personality disorders. These strategies generally are more focused and struc-

tured than psychodynamic therapies. Cognitive strategies involve identifying specific internal mental schemes by which patients typically misunderstand certain situations or misrepresent themselves and then learning how to modify those internal schemes (Beck et al. 2004). Cognitive therapy for personality disorders is more complicated than for most Axis I disorders because of the unique challenges (e.g., cognitive and affective avoidance, lack of psychological flexibility, pervasiveness of problems, and ambivalence about having problems and getting treatment for them) that character pathology presents. Behavioral strategies involve efforts to diminish traits such as impulsivity or to increase assertiveness by using relaxation techniques, role-playing exercises, and other behavioral techniques. A specific type of cognitive-behavioral therapy called dialectical behavior therapy (Linehan 1993), developed for suicidal and self-injuring patients with BPD, has recently come into broad use (Stanley and Brodsky 2005).

Although psychotherapy remains the mainstay of the treatment of personality disorders, in the past two decades the use of pharmacotherapy has begun to be explored as biological dimensions of personality psychopathology that may respond to different medication classes have been identified. For example, research has increasingly suggested that impulsivity and aggression may respond to serotonergic medications; mood instability and lability may respond to serotonergic medications, other antidepressants, and mood stabilizers; and psychotic-like experiences may respond to antipsychotics (Soloff 2005). These principles have been incorporated into the "Practice Guideline for the Treatment of Patients With Borderline Personality Disorder" (American Psychiatric Association 2001).

An overview of our knowledge about the potential usefulness of the three major types of psychiatric treatment is provided in Table 29–4.

**TABLE 29–4.** **Evidence of treatment effectiveness for personality disorders**

|  | ST | SZ | P | B | AS | H | N | OC | D | AV |
|---|---|---|---|---|---|---|---|---|---|---|
| Psychotherapies | – | + | – | ++ | – | + | ++ | ++ | ++ | ++ |
| Sociotherapies[a] | ± | + | – | ++ | + | – | – | – | + | + |
| Pharmacotherapies | + | – | ± | + | – | – | – | – | – | ± |

*Note.* –=no support; ±=uncertain support; +=modestly helpful; ++=significantly helpful. AS=antisocial; AV=avoidant; B = borderline; D=dependent; H=histrionic; N=narcissistic; OC=obsessive-compulsive; P=paranoid; ST=schizotypal; SZ=schizoid.
[a]Includes group, family, and milieu therapies.

# Specific Personality Disorders

## Paranoid Personality Disorder

### *Epidemiology*

Paranoid personality disorder is estimated to occur in 1.25%–1.5% of the general population (Torgersen 2005). It has been found to be more common among men than women (Zimmerman and Coryell 1990).

### *Clinical Features*

Persons with paranoid personality disorder have a pervasive, persistent, and inappropriate mistrust of others (Table 29–5). They are suspicious of others' motives and assume that others intend to exploit, harm, or deceive them. Thus, they may question, without justification, the loyalty or trustworthiness of friends or romantic partners, and they are reluctant to confide in others for fear the information will be used against them. Persons with paranoid personality disorder appear guarded, tense, and hypervigilant, and they frequently scan their environments for clues of possible attack, deception, or betrayal. They often find "evidence" of such malevolence by misinterpreting benign events (such as a glance in their direction) as demeaning or threatening. In response to perceived or actual insults or betrayals, these individuals overreact quickly, becoming excessively angry and responding with counterattacking behavior. They are unable to forgive or forget such incidents and instead bear long-term grudges against their supposed betrayers; some persons with paranoid personality disorder are extremely litigious. Whereas individuals with this disorder can appear quietly and tensely aloof and hostile, others are overtly angry and combative. Persons with this disorder are usually socially isolated and, because of their paranoia, often have difficulties with bosses and coworkers.

### *Differential Diagnosis*

Unlike paranoid personality disorder, the Axis I disorders *paranoid schizophrenia* and *delusional disorder, persecutory type*, are both characterized by prominent and persistent paranoid delusions of psychotic proportions; paranoid schizophrenia is also accompanied by hallucinations and other core symptoms of schizophrenia. Although paranoid and schizotypal personality disorders both involve suspiciousness, paranoid personality disorder does not include magical thinking, perceptual distortions, or odd thinking or speech. People who are extremely self-conscious may fear that others are watching them or have negative or critical thoughts about them. They are pro-

**TABLE 29–5.**   **DSM-IV-TR diagnostic criteria for paranoid personality disorder**

A.  A pervasive distrust and suspiciousness of others such that their motives are interpreted as malevolent, beginning by early adulthood and present in a variety of contexts, as indicated by four (or more) of the following:

   (1)  suspects, without sufficient basis, that others are exploiting, harming, or deceiving him or her

   (2)  is preoccupied with unjustified doubts about the loyalty or trustworthiness of friends or associates

   (3)  is reluctant to confide in others because of unwarranted fear that the information will be used maliciously against him or her

   (4)  reads hidden demeaning or threatening meanings into benign remarks or events

   (5)  persistently bears grudges, i.e., is unforgiving of insults, injuries, or slights

   (6)  perceives attacks on his or her character or reputation that are not apparent to others and is quick to react angrily or to counterattack

   (7)  has recurrent suspicions, without justification, regarding fidelity of spouse or sexual partner

B.  Does not occur exclusively during the course of schizophrenia, a mood disorder with psychotic features, or another psychotic disorder and is not due to the direct physiological effects of a general medical condition.

**Note:**   If criteria are met prior to the onset of schizophrenia, add "premorbid," e.g., "paranoid personality disorder (premorbid)."

---

jecting their negative ideas about themselves onto others, whereas paranoid people project malevolent thoughts and feelings onto others.

### *Etiology*

Some psychological theories suggest that paranoid personality disorder originates from having been the object of excessive parental rage or from having been repeatedly humiliated by others. Either type of experience could lead to feelings of inadequacy and vulnerability, followed by projection onto others of hostility and rage, as well as a tendency to blame others for one's shortcomings and problems. The defense mechanism of projection is generally assumed to be involved in the expression of this disorder's features.

## Treatment

Because they mistrust others, persons with paranoid personality disorder usually avoid psychiatric treatment. If they do seek treatment, the therapist immediately encounters the challenge of engaging them and keeping them in treatment. This can best be accomplished by maintaining an unusually respectful, straightforward, and unintrusive style aimed at building trust. If a rupture develops in the treatment relationship—for example, the patient accuses the therapist of some fault—it is best simply to offer a straightforward apology, if warranted, rather than to respond evasively or defensively. It is also best to avoid an overly warm style because excessive warmth and expression of interest can intensify the patient's thoughts about the therapist's motives (Appelbaum 2005). A supportive individual psychotherapy that incorporates such approaches may be the best treatment for these patients (Gabbard 2000).

Although seldom studied, antipsychotic medications may be sometimes useful in the treatment of paranoid personality disorder. Patients may view such treatment with mistrust; however, these medications are more clearly indicated in the treatment of the overtly psychotic decompensations that these patients sometimes experience.

## Schizoid Personality Disorder

### Epidemiology

Schizoid personality disorder is one of the rarest personality disorders, occurring in less than 1% of the general population (Torgersen 2005). Like paranoid personality disorder, schizoid personality disorder is more common among men than women (Torgersen et al. 2001; Zimmerman and Coryell 1990).

### Clinical Features

Schizoid personality disorder is characterized by a profound defect in the ability to relate to others in a meaningful way (Table 29–6). Persons with this disorder have little or no desire for relationships with others and, as a result, are extremely socially isolated. They prefer to engage in solitary, often intellectual, activities, such as computer games or puzzles, and they often create an elaborate fantasy world that they retreat into and that substitutes for relationships with real people. As a result of their lack of interest in relationships, they have few or no close friends or confidants. They date infrequently, seldom marry, and have little interest in sex, and they often work at jobs requiring little interpersonal interaction (e.g., as a night watchman). These individuals are also notable for

their lack of emotional expression or affect. They usually appear cold, detached, aloof, and constricted, and they have particular discomfort with warm feelings. Few, if any, activities or experiences give them pleasure, resulting in chronic anhedonia.

---

**TABLE 29–6.** **DSM-IV-TR diagnostic criteria for schizoid personality disorder**

A. A pervasive pattern of detachment from social relationships and a restricted range of expression of emotions in interpersonal settings, beginning by early adulthood and present in a variety of contexts, as indicated by four (or more) of the following:

   (1) neither desires nor enjoys close relationships, including being part of a family

   (2) almost always chooses solitary activities

   (3) has little, if any, interest in having sexual experiences with another person

   (4) takes pleasure in few, if any, activities

   (5) lacks close friends or confidants other than first-degree relatives

   (6) appears indifferent to the praise or criticism of others

   (7) shows emotional coldness, detachment, or flattened affectivity

B. Does not occur exclusively during the course of schizophrenia, a mood disorder with psychotic features, another psychotic disorder, or a pervasive developmental disorder and is not due to the direct physiological effects of a general medical condition.

**Note:** If criteria are met prior to the onset of schizophrenia, add "premorbid," e.g., "schizoid personality disorder (premorbid)."

---

### Differential Diagnosis

Schizoid personality disorder shares the features of social isolation and restricted emotional expression with schizotypal personality disorder, but it lacks the latter disorder's characteristic cognitive and perceptual distortions. Unlike individuals with avoidant personality disorder, who intensely desire relationships but avoid them because of exaggerated fears of rejection, persons with schizoid personality disorder have little or no apparent interest in developing relationships with others. Schizoid individuals can be distinguished from those with paranoid personality disorder by the lack of suspiciousness and mistrust. They can be differentiated from milder forms of autistic disorder or Asperger's disorder by the more severely impaired social interactions and stereotyped behavior and interests seen in the latter.

### Etiology

Clinicians have noted that schizoid personality disorder occurs in adults who experienced cold, neglectful, and ungratifying relationships in early childhood, which presumably led these persons to assume that relationships are not valuable or worth pursuing. There is reason to believe that constitutional factors contribute to the childhood pattern of shyness that often precedes the disorder. Introversion (intimacy problems, inhibition), which characterizes schizoid (as well as avoidant and schizotypal) personality disorder, appears to be substantially heritable (DiLalla et al. 1996).

### Treatment

Persons with schizoid personality disorder, like those with paranoid personality disorder, rarely seek treatment. They do not perceive the formation of any relationship—including a therapeutic relationship—as potentially valuable or beneficial. They may, however, occasionally seek treatment for an associated problem, such as depression, or they may be brought for treatment by others. Whereas some patients can tolerate only a supportive therapy or treatment aimed at the resolution of a crisis or associated Axis I disorder, others may actually do well with insight-oriented psychotherapy aimed at effecting a basic shift in their comfort with intimacy and affects. Although many patients may be unwilling to participate in a group, group therapy may also facilitate the development of social skills and relationships (Piper and Ogrodniczuk 2005) (Table 29–7).

---

TABLE 29–7. **Treatment of schizoid personality disorder**

Supportive individual psychotherapy
Psychodynamic individual psychotherapy
Cognitive-behavioral psychotherapy
Group psychotherapy

---

## Schizotypal Personality Disorder

### Epidemiology

Schizotypal personality disorder occurs in 0.7%–1.2% of the general population (Torgersen 2005). Unlike the other two Cluster A personality disorders, no gender difference in prevalence has been found for this disorder (Torgersen et al. 2001; Zimmerman and Coryell 1990).

### Clinical Features

Schizotypal personality disorder, like schizophrenia, is characterized by positive, psychotic-like symptoms and negative, deficit-like symptoms (Table 29–8). Persons with schizotypal personality disorder experience cognitive or perceptual distortions (positive), behave in an eccentric manner, and are socially withdrawn and anxious (negative). Common cognitive and perceptual distortions include ideas of reference, bodily illusions, and unusual telepathic and clairvoyant experiences. These distortions, which are inconsistent with subcultural norms, occur frequently and are an important and pervasive component of the person's experience. They help explain the odd and eccentric behavior characteristic of this disorder. Individuals with schizotypal personality disorder may, for example, talk to themselves in public, gesture for no apparent reason, or dress in a peculiar or unkempt fashion. Their speech is often odd and idiosyncratic—for example, unusually circumstantial, metaphorical, or vague—and their affect is constricted or inappropriate. Such a person may, for example, laugh inappropriately when discussing his or her problems.

### Differential Diagnosis

Schizotypal personality disorder shares the feature of suspiciousness with paranoid personality disorder and that of social isolation with schizoid personality disorder, but the latter two disorders lack the markedly peculiar behavior and significant cognitive and perceptual distortions typical of schizotypal personality disorder. The symptoms of schizotypal personality disorder appear to be attenuated versions of the symptoms of schizophrenia, but enduring periods of overt psychosis and social deterioration over time are not characteristic.

### Etiology

Schizotypal personality disorder is considered a schizophrenia spectrum disorder—that is, related to Axis I schizophrenia (Siever and Davis 2004). Phenomenological as well as genetic, biological, treatment, and outcome data support this link. In addition, at least some forms of schizotypal personality disorder involve abnormalities of brain structure, physiology, chemistry, and functioning characteristic of schizophrenia—for example, increased cerebrospinal fluid and reduced cortical vol-

## TABLE 29–8. DSM-IV-TR diagnostic criteria for schizotypal personality disorder

A. A pervasive pattern of social and interpersonal deficits marked by acute discomfort with, and reduced capacity for, close relationships as well as by cognitive or perceptual distortions and eccentricities of behavior, beginning by early adulthood and present in a variety of contexts, as indicated by five (or more) of the following:

(1) ideas of reference (excluding delusions of reference)

(2) odd beliefs or magical thinking that influences behavior and is inconsistent with subcultural norms (e.g., superstitiousness, belief in clairvoyance, telepathy, or "sixth sense"; in children and adolescents, bizarre fantasies or preoccupations)

(3) unusual perceptual experiences, including bodily illusions

(4) odd thinking and speech (e.g., vague, circumstantial, metaphorical, overelaborate, or stereotyped)

(5) suspiciousness or paranoid ideation

(6) inappropriate or constricted affect

(7) behavior or appearance that is odd, eccentric, or peculiar

(8) lack of close friends or confidants other than first-degree relatives

(9) excessive social anxiety that does not diminish with familiarity and tends to be associated with paranoid fears rather than negative judgments about self

B. Does not occur exclusively during the course of schizophrenia, a mood disorder with psychotic features, another psychotic disorder, or a pervasive developmental disorder.

**Note:** If criteria are met prior to the onset of schizophrenia, add "premorbid," e.g., "schizotypal personality disorder (premorbid)."

ume; temporal lobe volume reductions and dysfunctions; and abnormalities of brain physiological functions that modulate attention and inhibit sensory input, such as P50 suppression, prepulse inhibition, impaired smooth-pursuit eye movements, and poor performance on the continuous performance task.

### Treatment

Because they are socially anxious and somewhat paranoid, persons with schizotypal personality disorder usually avoid psychiatric treatment. They may, however, seek such treatment—or be brought for treatment by concerned family members—when they become depressed or overtly psychotic. As with patients with paranoid personality disorder, it is difficult to establish an alliance with schizotypal patients, and they are unlikely to tolerate exploratory techniques that emphasize interpretation or confrontation. A supportive relationship that counters cognitive distortions and ego-boundary problems may be useful (Stone 1985). This may involve an educational approach that fosters the development of social skills or encourages risk-taking behavior in social situations or, if these efforts fail, encourages the development of activities with less social involvement. If the patient is willing to participate, cognitive-behavioral therapy and highly structured educational groups with a social skills focus also may be helpful.

Several studies support the usefulness of low-dosage antipsychotic medications in the treatment of schizotypal personality disorder. These agents include atypical antipsychotics such as risperidone (double-blind, placebo-controlled study; Koenigsberg et al. 2003) and olanzapine (Keshavan et al. 2004). These medications may ameliorate the anxiety and psychotic-like features associated with this disorder, and they are particularly indicated in the treatment of the more overt psychotic decompensations that patients with this disorder can experience (Table 29–9).

## TABLE 29–9. Treatment of schizotypal personality disorder

Supportive individual psychotherapy

Cognitive-behavioral psychotherapy

Psychoeducational, social skills group therapy

Low-dosage antipsychotic medications

## Antisocial Personality Disorder

### Epidemiology

Antisocial personality disorder occurs in about 1.7% of the general population (Torgersen 2005). It is much more common among men than women (Torgersen et al. 2001; Zimmerman and Coryell 1989).

## Clinical Features

The central feature of antisocial personality disorder is a long-standing pattern of socially irresponsible behaviors that reflects a disregard for the rights of others (Table 29–10). Many persons with this disorder engage in repeated unlawful acts. The more prevailing personality characteristics include a lack of interest in or concern for the feelings of others, deceitfulness, and, most notably, a lack of remorse for the harm they may cause others. These characteristics generally make antisocial individuals fail in roles requiring fidelity (e.g., as a spouse), honesty (e.g., as an employee), or reliability (e.g., as a parent). Some antisocial persons possess a glibness and charm that can be used to seduce, outwit, and exploit others. Although most antisocial persons are indifferent to their effects on others, a notable subgroup takes sadistic pleasure in doing harm (Stone 2005). Recent research has shown that psychopathy is multidimensional and that each dimension may have distinct developmental trajectories (Edens et al. 2006) and may be variants of normal personality traits and behaviors (Hare and Neumann 2005). Antisocial personality syndromes are associated with high rates of substance abuse (Compton et al. 2005), which may contribute to the persistence of antisocial behavior over time (Malone et al. 2004).

## Differential Diagnosis

The primary differential diagnostic issue involves narcissistic personality disorder. Indeed, these two disorders may be variants of the same basic type of psychopathology (Hare et al. 1991). However, the antisocial person, unlike the narcissistic person, is likely to be reckless and impulsive. In addition, narcissistic individuals' exploitiveness and disregard for others are attributable to their sense of uniqueness and superiority rather than to a desire for materialistic gains.

## Etiology

Twin and adoption studies indicate that genetic factors predispose to the development of antisocial personality disorder (Grove et al. 1990; Lyons et al. 1995). Nonetheless, it is unclear how much variance is accounted for by genetic factors and whether the nature of the predisposition is relatively specific or is best conceptualized in terms of relatively nonspecific traits such as impulsivity, excitability, or hostility. Conduct problems (56%), stimulus seeking (40%), and callousness (56%) are antisocial traits that have substantial heritability (Jang et al. 1996). Psychopathic traits of fearless dominance and impulsive anti-

---

**TABLE 29–10.   DSM-IV-TR diagnostic criteria for antisocial personality disorder**

A.  There is a pervasive pattern of disregard for and violation of the rights of others occurring since age 15 years, as indicated by three (or more) of the following:

   (1)  failure to conform to social norms with respect to lawful behaviors as indicated by repeatedly performing acts that are grounds for arrest

   (2)  deceitfulness, as indicated by repeated lying, use of aliases, or conning others for personal profit or pleasure

   (3)  impulsivity or failure to plan ahead

   (4)  irritability and aggressiveness, as indicated by repeated physical fights or assaults

   (5)  reckless disregard for safety of self or others

   (6)  consistent irresponsibility, as indicated by repeated failure to sustain consistent work behavior or honor financial obligations

   (7)  lack of remorse, as indicated by being indifferent to or rationalizing having hurt, mistreated, or stolen from another

B.  The individual is at least age 18 years.

C.  There is evidence of conduct disorder (see DSM-IV-TR p. 98) with onset before age 15 years.

D.  The occurrence of antisocial behavior is not exclusively during the course of schizophrenia or a manic episode.

---

sociality also show significant genetic influences (Blonigen et al. 2005). Growing evidence indicates that the impulsive and aggressive behaviors may be mediated by abnormal serotonin transporter functioning in the brain (Coccaro et al. 1996).

In addition to biological factors, it is also clear that the early family lives of these persons often pose severe environmental handicaps in the form of absent, inconsistent, or abusive parenting. Indeed, many family members also have significant action-oriented psychopathology, such as substance abuse or antisocial personality disorder itself. Modern behavioral genetic research is focusing on interactions between genes and the environment to explain the genesis of antisocial behavior (Moffitt 2005; Reiss et al. 1995).

## Treatment

It is clinically important to recognize antisocial personality disorder because an uncritical acceptance of these individuals' glib or shallow statements of good intentions and collaboration can permit them to have disruptive influences on treatment teams and other patients. However, there is little evidence to suggest that this disorder can be successfully treated by usual psychiatric interventions. Of interest, nonetheless, are reports suggesting that in confined settings, such as the military or prisons, depressive and introspective concerns may surface. Under these circumstances, confrontation by peers may bring about changes in the antisocial person's social behaviors. It is also notable that some antisocial patients have an ability to form a therapeutic alliance with psychotherapists, which augurs well for these patients' future course (Woody et al. 1985). These findings contrast with the clinical tradition that emphasizes such persons' inability to learn from harmful consequences. Yet longitudinal follow-up studies have shown that the prevalence of this disorder diminishes with age as these individuals become more aware of the social and interpersonal maladaptiveness of their most harmful social behaviors.

## Borderline Personality Disorder

### *Epidemiology*

BPD occurs in 1%–1.5% of the general population (Torgersen 2005). Although it has been shown to be more common among women than men in clinical settings (Morey et al. 2005), this difference may be largely the result of sampling bias (i.e., more women seek treatment) because no gender difference in prevalence has been found in community-based studies (Torgersen et al. 2001; Zimmerman and Coryell 1990).

### *Clinical Features*

BPD is characterized by instability and dysfunction in affective, behavioral, and interpersonal domains. Central to the psychopathology of this disorder are a severely impaired capacity for attachment (Levy et al. 2005) and predictably maladaptive behavior patterns related to separation (Gunderson 1996). When borderline patients feel cared for, held on to, and supported, depressive features (notably, loneliness and emptiness) are most evident (Table 29–11). When the threat of losing such a sustaining relationship arises, the idealized image of a beneficent caregiver is replaced by a devalued image of a cruel persecutor. This shift between idealization and devaluation is called *splitting*. An impending separation also evokes intense abandonment fears. To minimize these fears and to prevent the separation, rageful accusations of mistreatment and cruelty and angry self-destructive behaviors

may occur. These behaviors often elicit a guilty or fearful protective response from others.

---

**TABLE 29–11. DSM-IV-TR diagnostic criteria for borderline personality disorder**

A pervasive pattern of instability of interpersonal relationships, self-image, and affects, and marked impulsivity beginning by early adulthood and present in a variety of contexts, as indicated by five (or more) of the following:

(1) frantic efforts to avoid real or imagined abandonment. **Note:** Do not include suicidal or self-mutilating behavior covered in Criterion 5.

(2) a pattern of unstable and intense interpersonal relationships characterized by alternating between extremes of idealization and devaluation

(3) identity disturbance: markedly and persistently unstable self-image or sense of self

(4) impulsivity in at least two areas that are potentially self-damaging (e.g., spending, sex, substance abuse, reckless driving, binge eating). **Note:** Do not include suicidal or self-mutilating behavior covered in Criterion 5.

(5) recurrent suicidal behavior, gestures, or threats, or self-mutilating behavior

(6) affective instability due to a marked reactivity of mood (e.g., intense episodic dysphoria, irritability, or anxiety usually lasting a few hours and only rarely more than a few days)

(7) chronic feelings of emptiness

(8) inappropriate, intense anger or difficulty controlling anger (e.g., frequent displays of temper, constant anger, recurrent physical fights)

(9) transient, stress-related paranoid ideation or severe dissociative symptoms

---

Another central feature of this disorder is extreme affective instability that often leads to impulsive and self-destructive behaviors. These episodes are usually brief and reactive and involve extreme alternations between angry and depressed states. The experience and expression of anger can be particularly difficult for the borderline patient. During periods of unusual stress, dissociative experiences, ideas of reference, or desperate impulsive acts (including substance abuse and promiscuity) commonly occur.

## Differential Diagnosis

The most common differential diagnosis involves the interface of BPD with bipolar disorder—particularly bipolar II. The major distinctions are that bipolar patients have periods of elation, and borderline patients have abandonment fears and repeated episodes of self-harm when alone.

Borderline patients' intense feelings of being bad or evil are distinctly different from the idealized self-image of narcissistic persons. Patients with BPD differ from those with antisocial personality disorder in that the impulsive behaviors of borderline patients are primarily interpersonally oriented and aimed toward obtaining support rather than materialistic gains. Paranoid ideas may also occur in patients with schizotypal or paranoid personality disorder, but these symptoms are more transient, interpersonally reactive, and responsive to external structuring in borderline patients. Patients with dependent personality disorder (DPD) are characterized by fear of abandonment, but they react to such threats by efforts at appeasement and submissiveness rather than with feelings of emptiness and rage.

## Etiology

Psychoanalytic theories have emphasized the importance of early parent–child relationships in the etiology of BPD. These theories have emphasized 1) maternal mismanagement of the 2- to 3-year-old child's efforts to become autonomous (Masterson 1972), 2) exaggerated maternal frustration that aggravates the child's anger (Kernberg 1975), or 3) inattention to the child's emotions and attitudes (Adler 1985). A considerable body of empirical research has embellished these theories by documenting a high frequency of traumatic early abandonment, physical abuse, and sexual abuse (Johnson et al. 2005). These traumatic experiences appear to occur within a context of sustained neglect, from which the preborderline child develops enduring rage and self-hatred. The lack of reliably involved attachment to caregivers during development is a source of borderline patients' inability to maintain stable senses of themselves or of others without ongoing contact (i.e., their defects of object constancy or lack of stable introjects) (Gunderson 1996).

Zanarini and Frankenburg (1997) proposed a tripartite causative model of BPD consisting of a traumatic childhood, a vulnerable temperament, and triggering events. Linehan's biosocial theory suggests that a biological disposition toward emotional vulnerability, exposure to invalidating environments, and deficits in emotion-regulation skills are key etiological factors (Linehan 1993). Joyce et al. (2003) proposed a distinctive combination of risk factors consisting of a temperament characterized by high novelty seeking and high harm avoidance, childhood abuse and/or neglect, and childhood or adolescent psychopathology in the affective, conduct, and substance abuse domains.

## Treatment

Borderline patients are high utilizers of psychiatric outpatient, inpatient, and psychopharmacological treatment (Table 29–12). The extensive literature on the treatment of BPD universally notes the extreme difficulties that clinicians encounter with these patients. These problems derive from the patients' appeal to their treaters' nurturing qualities and their rageful accusations in response to their treaters' perceived failures. Often therapists develop intense countertransference reactions that lead them to attempt to re-parent or, conversely, to reject borderline patients. As a consequence, regardless of the treatment approach used, personal maturity and considerable clinical experience are important assets.

TABLE 29–12. **Treatment of borderline personality disorder**

Psychodynamic individual psychotherapy

Supportive individual psychotherapy

Cognitive-behavioral or schema-focused psychotherapy

Dialectical behavior therapy

Interpersonal psychotherapy

Family psychoeducation

Selective serotonin reuptake inhibitor antidepressant medications

Atypical antipsychotic medications

Anticonvulsant medications

Much of the early treatment literature focused on the value of intensive exploratory psychotherapies directed at modifying borderline patients' basic character structure. However, this literature has increasingly suggested that improvement may be related not to the acquisition of insight but to the corrective experience of developing a stable, trusting relationship with a therapist who fails to retaliate in response to these patients' angry and disruptive behaviors. Paralleling this development has been the suggestion that supportive psychotherapies or group ther-

**TABLE 29–13.** Medication efficacy in borderline personality disorder

| Medication | Affective dysregulation | Impulsivity | Psychotic-like features |
| --- | --- | --- | --- |
| Monoamine oxidase inhibitors | + | + | ? |
| Serotonin reuptake inhibitors[a] | ++ | ++ | ? |
| Tricyclic antidepressants | ± | ± | ± |
| Typical antipsychotics | + | + | ++ |
| Atypical antipsychotics | + | + | ++ |
| Mood stabilizers | + | + | + |
| Benzodiazepines | ± | − | ? |

*Note.* ++=clear improvement; +=modest improvement; ±=variable improvement or worsening; −=some worsening. The information in this table should be considered tentative; some medications have received relatively little investigation, many medication trials have been small and open, and few of the medications listed have been directly compared with one another.
[a]Most published studies of serotonin reuptake inhibitors have used fluoxetine.

apies may bring about similar changes (Appelbaum 2005; Piper and Ogrodniczuk 2005). Evidence has provided support for the effectiveness of an 18-month psychoanalytic treatment called "mentalization-based treatment" that took place in a partial hospital setting (Bateman and Fonagy 1999). In addition, a long-term phased model of psychodynamic therapy that combined hospital-based and community-based strategies was reported to be more effective than hospital-based treatment alone (Chiesa and Fonagy 2000).

At present, treatment of BPD typically includes cognitive-behavioral and pharmacological interventions (American Psychiatric Association 2001). Linehan et al. (2006) have shown that behavioral treatment consisting of a once-weekly individual and twice-weekly group regimen can effectively diminish the self-destructive behaviors and hospitalizations of borderline patients. The success and cost benefits of this treatment, called *dialectical behavior therapy*, have led to its widespread adoption and to modifications that can be used in a variety of settings. *Schema-focused therapy* is a newer cognitive therapy that also has been shown to be efficacious (Giesen-Bloo et al. 2006).

Although no one medication has been found to have dramatic or predictable effects, studies indicate that many medications may diminish specific problems such as impulsivity, affective lability, or intermittent cognitive and perceptual disturbances (Table 29–13), as well as irritability and aggressive behavior (Soloff 2005). Most recently, studies have shown efficacy for atypical antipsychotics for dysphoria and aggression (Soler et al. 2005) and anticonvulsants for anger and aggression (Hollander et al. 2005). In general, the profusion of treatment modalities and the introduction of empiricism

point toward the increasing use of more focused treatment strategies.

## Histrionic Personality Disorder

### *Epidemiology*

Histrionic personality disorder is one of the most frequently occurring personality disorders; it occurs in almost 2% of the general population (Torgersen 2005). Those with histrionic personality disorder are more often women (Torgersen et al. 2001; Zimmerman and Coryell 1990).

### *Clinical Features*

Central to histrionic personality disorder is an overconcern with attention and appearance (Table 29–14). Persons with this disorder spend an excessive amount of time seeking attention and making themselves attractive. The desire to be found attractive may lead to inappropriately seductive or provocative dress and flirtatious behavior, and the desire for attention may lead to other flamboyant acts or self-dramatizing behavior. All of these features reflect these persons' underlying insecurity about their value as anything other than fetching companions. Persons with histrionic personality disorder also have an effusive, but labile and shallow, range of feelings. They are often overly impressionistic and given to hyperbolic descriptions of others. More generally, these persons do not attend to detail or facts, and they are reluctant or unable to make reasoned critical analyses of problems or situations. Persons with this disorder often present with complaints of depression, somatic problems of unclear origin, and a history of disappointing romantic relationships.

---

**TABLE 29–14.    DSM-IV-TR diagnostic criteria for histrionic personality disorder**

A pervasive pattern of excessive emotionality and attention seeking, beginning by early adulthood and present in a variety of contexts, as indicated by five (or more) of the following:

(1)  is uncomfortable in situations in which he or she is not the center of attention

(2)  interaction with others is often characterized by inappropriate sexually seductive or provocative behavior

(3)  displays rapidly shifting and shallow expression of emotions

(4)  consistently uses physical appearance to draw attention to self

(5)  has a style of speech that is excessively impressionistic and lacking in detail

(6)  shows self-dramatization, theatricality, and exaggerated expression of emotion

(7)  is suggestible, i.e., easily influenced by others or circumstances

(8)  considers relationships to be more intimate than they actually are

---

## Differential Diagnosis

Histrionic personality disorder can be confused with dependent, borderline, and narcissistic personality disorders. Histrionic individuals are often willing, even eager, to have others make decisions and organize their activities for them. However, unlike persons with DPD, histrionic persons are uninhibited and lively companions who willfully forgo appearing autonomous because they believe that this attracts others. Unlike persons with BPD, those with histrionic personality do not perceive themselves as bad, and they lack ongoing problems with rage or willful self-destructiveness. Persons with narcissistic personality disorder also seek attention to sustain their self-esteem but differ in that their self-esteem is characterized by grandiosity, and the attention they crave must be admiring.

## Etiology

Psychoanalytic theory proposes that histrionic personality disorder originates in the oedipal phase of development (i.e., age 3–5 years), when an overly eroticized relationship with the opposite-sex parent is unduly encouraged and the child fears that the consequences of this excitement will be the loss of, or retaliation by, the

same-sex parent. This conflict results in lasting character formations of exaggerated fantasy and exhibitionistic promise with inhibited factual analysis and diminished actual productivity. Research suggests that qualities such as emotional expressiveness (Jang et al. 1996) and egocentricity (Torgersen et al. 1993) are heritable temperaments. From this perspective, histrionic personality disorder would consist of extreme variants of temperamental dispositions, the environmental contributions of which may be less specific than those of the aforementioned theories.

## Treatment

Individual psychodynamic psychotherapy, including psychoanalysis, remains the cornerstone of most treatment for persons with histrionic personality disorder (Gabbard 2005). This treatment is directed at increasing patients' awareness of 1) how their self-esteem is maladaptively tied to their ability to attract attention at the expense of developing other skills and 2) how their shallow relationships and emotional experience reflect unconscious fears of real commitments. Much of this increase in awareness occurs through analysis of the here-and-now doctor–patient relationship rather than through the reconstruction of childhood experiences. Therapists should be aware that the typical idealization and eroticization that such patients bring into treatment are the material for exploration, and thus therapists should be aware of countertransferential gratification.

# Narcissistic Personality Disorder

## Epidemiology

Narcissistic personality disorder is among the rarest disorders found in community studies, with a prevalence of only about 0.5% (Torgersen 2005). It appears to be more common among men (Torgersen et al. 2001; Zimmerman and Coryell 1990).

## Clinical Features

Because persons with narcissistic personality disorder have grandiose self-esteem, fantasies of unlimited potential, a sense of entitlement, and needs for admiration, they are vulnerable to intense reactions when their self-image is damaged (Table 29–15). They respond with strong feelings of hurt or anger to even small slights, rejections, defeats, or criticisms. As a result, persons with narcissistic personality disorder usually go to great lengths to avoid exposure to such experiences, and when that fails, they react by becoming devaluative or rageful. Serious depression can ensue, which is the usual precipitant for their seeking clinical help. In relationships, narcissistic persons are often quite distant and try to sustain "an illusion of self-sufficiency" (Modell 1975). They lack empathy for others, are often envious, and may exploit others for self-serving ends. They are likely to feel that those with whom they associate need to be special and unique because they see themselves in these terms; thus, they usually wish to be associated only with persons, institutions, or possessions that will confirm their sense of superiority.

---

**TABLE 29–15. DSM-IV-TR diagnostic criteria for narcissistic personality disorder**

A pervasive pattern of grandiosity (in fantasy or behavior), need for admiration, and lack of empathy, beginning by early adulthood and present in a variety of contexts, as indicated by five (or more) of the following:

(1) has a grandiose sense of self-importance (e.g., exaggerates achievements and talents, expects to be recognized as superior without commensurate achievements)

(2) is preoccupied with fantasies of unlimited success, power, brilliance, beauty, or ideal love

(3) believes that he or she is "special" and unique and can only be understood by, or should associate with, other special or high-status people (or institutions)

(4) requires excessive admiration

(5) has a sense of entitlement, i.e., unreasonable expectations of especially favorable treatment or automatic compliance with his or her expectations

(6) is interpersonally exploitative, i.e., takes advantage of others to achieve his or her own ends

(7) lacks empathy: is unwilling to recognize or identify with the feelings and needs of others

(8) is often envious of others or believes that others are envious of him or her

(9) shows arrogant, haughty behaviors or attitudes

---

## Differential Diagnosis

Narcissistic personality disorder can be most readily confused with antisocial and histrionic personality disorders. Like persons with antisocial personality disorder, those with narcissistic personality disorder are capable of exploiting others, but narcissistic persons usually rationalize their behavior on the basis of the specialness of their goals or their personal virtue. In contrast, antisocial persons'

goals are materialistic, and their rationalizations, if offered, are based on a view that others would do the same to them. The narcissistic person's excessive pride in achievements, relative constraint in expression of feelings, and disregard for other people's rights and sensitivities help distinguish him or her from persons with histrionic personality disorder. Perhaps the most difficult differential diagnostic problem is whether a person who meets criteria for narcissistic personality disorder has a stable personality disorder or is in an episode of an Axis I disorder, such as an adjustment reaction. If the emergence of narcissistic traits has been defensively triggered by experiences of failure or rejection, these traits may diminish radically and self-esteem may be restored when new relationships or successes occur. When manic, patients with bipolar disorder can appear quite similar to those with narcissistic personality disorder.

## Etiology

Little scientific evidence is available about the pathogenesis of narcissistic personality disorder. Reconstructions based on developmental history and observations in psychoanalytic treatment indicate that this disorder develops in persons who have had their fears, failures, or dependency responded to with criticism, disdain, or neglect during their childhood years. Such experiences leave them contemptuous of such reactions in themselves and others and inexperienced in viewing others as sources of comfort and support. They develop a veneer of invulnerability and self-sufficiency that masks their underlying emptiness and constricts their capacity to feel deeply.

## Treatment

Individual psychodynamic psychotherapy, including psychoanalysis, is the cornerstone of treatment for persons with narcissistic personality disorder (Gabbard 2005). Following Kohut's lead, some therapists believe that the vulnerability to narcissistic injury indicates that intervention should be directed at conveying empathy for the patient's sensitivities and disappointments. This approach, in theory, allows a positive idealized transference to develop that will then be gradually disillusioned by the inevitable frustrations encountered in therapy—disillusionment that will clarify the excessive nature of the patient's reactions to frustrations and disappointments. An alternative view, explicated by Kernberg (1975), is that the vulnerability should be addressed earlier and more directly by interpretations and confrontations through which these persons will come to recognize their grandiosity and its maladaptive consequences. With either approach, the psychotherapeutic process usually requires a relatively intensive schedule over a period of years in which the narcissistic patient's hypersensitivity to slights and tendency to treat the therapist almost exclusively as an object for gratifying his or her needs must be foremost in the therapist's mind and interventions.

## Avoidant Personality Disorder

### *Epidemiology*

Estimates of the prevalence of avoidant personality disorder based on epidemiological studies vary widely, resulting in a mean prevalence of 1.35% but a pooled prevalence of almost 3% (Torgersen 2005). This is in part due to the frequency with which it was found in a Scandinavian study (Torgersen et al. 2001), which illustrates how culture may contribute to the form a personality disorder takes. Avoidant personality disorder may be more common among women (Zimmerman and Coryell 1989, 1990).

### *Clinical Features*

Persons with avoidant personality disorder experience excessive and pervasive anxiety and discomfort in social situations and in intimate relationships (Table 29–16). Although strongly desiring relationships, they avoid them because they fear being ridiculed, criticized, rejected, or humiliated. These fears reflect their low self-esteem and hypersensitivity to negative evaluation by others. When they do enter into social situations or relationships, they feel inept and are self-conscious, shy, awkward, and preoccupied with being criticized or rejected. Their lives are constricted in that they tend to avoid not only relationships but also any new activities because they fear that they will embarrass or humiliate themselves. Patients with avoidant personality disorder may engage in deliberate self-harm (Klonsky et al. 2003) and experience disability in social, educational, and physical realms (Kessler 2003).

### *Differential Diagnosis*

Schizoid personality disorder also involves social isolation, but the schizoid person does not desire relationships, whereas the avoidant person desires them but avoids them because of anxiety and fears of humiliation and rejection. Whereas avoidant personality disorder is characterized by avoidance of situations and relationships involving possible rejection, disappointment, ridicule, or shame, Axis I social phobia usually consists of specific fears related to

---

**TABLE 29–16.    DSM-IV-TR diagnostic criteria for avoidant personality disorder**

A pervasive pattern of social inhibition, feelings of inadequacy, and hypersensitivity to negative evaluation, beginning by early adulthood and present in a variety of contexts, as indicated by four (or more) of the following:

(1) avoids occupational activities that involve significant interpersonal contact, because of fears of criticism, disapproval, or rejection

(2) is unwilling to get involved with people unless certain of being liked

(3) shows restraint within intimate relationships because of the fear of being shamed or ridiculed

(4) is preoccupied with being criticized or rejected in social situations

(5) is inhibited in new interpersonal situations because of feelings of inadequacy

(6) views self as socially inept, personally unappealing, or inferior to others

(7) is unusually reluctant to take personal risks or to engage in any new activities because they may prove embarrassing

---

social performance (e.g., a fear of saying something inappropriate or of being unable to answer questions in front of other people). Furthermore, patterns of avoidance in persons with avoidant personality disorder often extend beyond social situations to include emotional and novelty avoidance (Taylor et al. 2004). Some avoidant persons are actually vulnerable subtypes of narcissistic character styles (Dickinson and Pincus 2003).

### *Etiology*

Millon (1981) suggested that avoidant personality disorder develops from parental rejection and censure, which may be reinforced by rejecting peers. Psychodynamic theory suggests that avoidant behavior may derive from early life experiences that lead to an exaggerated desire for acceptance or an intolerance of criticism. Research on childhood experiences of avoidant persons identifies negative childhood memories (e.g., of isolation, rejection) (Meyer and Carver 2000); poorer athletic performance, less involvement in hobbies, and less popularity (Rettew et al. 2003); and parental neglect (Joyce et al. 2003). Research in the biological sphere has implicated the importance of inborn temperament in the development of avoidant behavior. Kagan (1989) found that some children as young as 21 months manifest increased physiological arousal and avoidant traits in social situations (e.g., retreat from the unfamiliar and avoidance of interaction with strangers) and that this social inhibition tends to persist for many years. Family studies have found elevated rates of trait and social anxiety, as well as personality traits such as harm avoidance, in the first-degree relatives of patients with generalized social phobia, suggesting that social anxiety lies on a continuum that may be influenced by familial factors (Stein et al. 2001).

### Treatment

Because of their excessive fear of rejection and criticism and their reluctance to form relationships, persons with avoidant personality disorder may be difficult to engage in treatment. Engagement in psychotherapy may be facilitated by the therapist's use of supportive techniques, sensitivity to the patient's hypersensitivity, and gentle interpretation of the defensive use of avoidance. Although early in treatment these patients may tolerate only supportive techniques, they may eventually respond well to all kinds of psychotherapy (Gabbard 2005). Clinicians should be aware of the potential for countertransference reactions such as overprotectiveness, hesitancy to adequately challenge the patient, or excessive expectations for change.

Although few data exist, it seems likely that assertiveness and social skills training may increase patients' confidence and willingness to take risks in social situations. Cognitive techniques that gently challenge patients' pathological assumptions about their sense of ineptness also may be useful (Beck et al. 2004). Group experiences—perhaps, in particular, homogeneous supportive groups that emphasize the development of social skills—may prove useful for avoidant patients (Piper and Ogrodniczuk 2005).

Promising preliminary data suggest that avoidant personality disorder may improve with treatment with monoamine oxidase inhibitors or serotonin reuptake inhibitors. Anxiolytics sometimes help patients better manage anxiety (especially severe anxiety) caused by facing previously avoided situations or trying new behaviors (Table 29–17).

## Dependent Personality Disorder

### Epidemiology

DPD occurs in about 1.25% of the general population (Torgersen 2005) and is much more common among women (Torgersen et al. 2001; Zimmerman and Coryell 1989, 1990).

**TABLE 29–17. Treatment of avoidant personality disorder**

Supportive individual psychotherapy

Psychodynamic individual psychotherapy

Cognitive-behavioral psychotherapy

Assertiveness and social skills training

Group psychotherapy

Monoamine oxidase inhibitor and selective serotonin reuptake inhibitor antidepressant medications

Antianxiety medications

### Clinical Features

Dependent personality is characterized by an excessive need to be cared for by others, which leads to submissive and clinging behavior and excessive fears of separation (Table 29–18). Although these individuals are able to care for themselves, they doubt their abilities and judgment, and they view others as much stronger and more capable than they are. These persons excessively rely on "powerful" others to initiate and do things for them, make their decisions, assume responsibility for their actions, and guide them through life. Low self-esteem and doubts about their effectiveness lead them to avoid positions of responsibility. Because they feel unable to function without excessive guidance, they go to great lengths to maintain dependent relationships. They may, for example, always agree with those on whom they depend, and they tend to be excessively passive and self-sacrificing. Because they feel incapable of caring for themselves when relationships end, these individuals feel helpless and fearful. They may indiscriminately begin another relationship so that they can be provided with direction and nurturance—an unfulfilling or even abusive relationship may seem better than being on their own.

### Differential Diagnosis

Although persons with BPD also dread being alone and need ongoing support, dependent persons want others to assume a controlling function that would frighten the borderline patient. Moreover, persons with DPD become appeasing rather than rageful or self-destructive when threatened with separation. Although both avoidant and dependent personality disorders are characterized by low self-esteem, rejection sensitivity, and an excessive need for reassurance, persons with DPD seek out rather than avoid relationships, and they quickly and indiscriminately replace ended relationships instead of further withdrawing from others.

---

**TABLE 29–18.   DSM-IV-TR diagnostic criteria for dependent personality disorder**

A pervasive and excessive need to be taken care of that leads to submissive and clinging behavior and fears of separation, beginning by early adulthood and present in a variety of contexts, as indicated by five (or more) of the following:

(1)  has difficulty making everyday decisions without an excessive amount of advice and reassurance from others

(2)  needs others to assume responsibility for most major areas of his or her life

(3)  has difficulty expressing disagreement with others because of fear of loss of support or approval.
    **Note:** Do not include realistic fears of retribution.

(4)  has difficulty initiating projects or doing things on his or her own (because of a lack of self-confidence in judgment or abilities rather than a lack of motivation or energy)

(5)  goes to excessive lengths to obtain nurturance and support from others, to the point of volunteering to do things that are unpleasant

(6)  feels uncomfortable or helpless when alone because of exaggerated fears of being unable to care for himself or herself

(7)  urgently seeks another relationship as a source of care and support when a close relationship ends

(8)  is unrealistically preoccupied with fears of being left to take care of himself or herself

---

### Etiology

Abraham (1927) suggested that the dependent character derives from either overindulgence or underindulgence during the oral phase of development (i.e., birth to age 2 years). Subsequent empirical data have given more support to the underindulgence hypothesis. However, studies of adults have not supported a specific association between feeding or other oral habits in childhood and dependency in adulthood. Caretaking patterns unrelated to the oral phase, per se—for example, in the care of a child with chronic physical illness or parenting that punishes independent behaviors—are probably more important to this disorder's development.

Genetic or constitutional factors, such as innate submissiveness, also may contribute to this disorder's etiology; a twin study found heritability of 45% on a scale measuring submissiveness (Jang et al. 1996).

### Treatment

Patients with DPD often enter therapy with complaints of depression or anxiety that may be precipitated by the threatened or actual loss of a dependent relationship. They often respond well to various types of individual psychotherapy. Treatment may be particularly helpful if it explores the patients' fears of independence; uses the transference to explore their dependency; and is directed toward increasing patients' self-esteem, sense of effectiveness, assertiveness, and independent functioning. These patients often seek an excessively dependent relationship with the therapist, which can lead to countertransference problems that may actually reinforce their dependence.

Group therapy (Piper and Ogrodniczuk 2005) and cognitive-behavioral therapy (Beck et al. 2004) aimed at increasing independent functioning, including assertiveness and social skills training, may be useful for some patients. If the patient is in a relationship that is maintaining and reinforcing his or her excessive dependence, couples or family therapy may be helpful (Table 29–19).

---

**TABLE 29–19.   Treatment of dependent personality disorder**

Psychodynamic individual psychotherapy

Cognitive-behavioral psychotherapy

Group psychotherapy

Assertiveness and social skills training

Couples therapy

Family therapy

---

## Obsessive-Compulsive Personality Disorder

### Epidemiology

Obsessive-compulsive personality disorder (OCPD), like histrionic personality disorder, is one of the most common in the general population, with a prevalence of about 2% (Torgersen 2005). Unlike histrionic personality, however, OCPD is more common in men than in women (Torgersen et al. 2001; Zimmerman and Coryell 1989, 1990).

### Clinical Features

As Freud noted, and as DSM-IV-TR criteria reflect, persons with OCPD are excessively orderly (Table 29–20). They are neat, punctual, overly organized, and overly conscientious. Although these traits might be considered virtues, especially in cultures that subscribe to the Puritan

---

**TABLE 29–20. DSM-IV-TR diagnostic criteria for obsessive-compulsive personality disorder**

A pervasive pattern of preoccupation with orderliness, perfectionism, and mental and interpersonal control, at the expense of flexibility, openness, and efficiency, beginning by early adulthood and present in a variety of contexts, as indicated by four (or more) of the following:

(1) is preoccupied with details, rules, lists, order, organization, or schedules to the extent that the major point of the activity is lost

(2) shows perfectionism that interferes with task completion (e.g., is unable to complete a project because his or her own overly strict standards are not met)

(3) is excessively devoted to work and productivity to the exclusion of leisure activities and friendships (not accounted for by obvious economic necessity)

(4) is overconscientious, scrupulous, and inflexible about matters of morality, ethics, or values (not accounted for by cultural or religious identification)

(5) is unable to discard worn-out or worthless objects even when they have no sentimental value

(6) is reluctant to delegate tasks or to work with others unless they submit to exactly his or her way of doing things

(7) adopts a miserly spending style toward both self and others; money is viewed as something to be hoarded for future catastrophes

(8) shows rigidity and stubbornness

---

work ethic, to qualify as OCPD the traits must be so extreme that they cause significant distress or impairment in functioning. As Abraham (1923) noted, these individuals' perseverance is unproductive. Although these individuals tend to work extremely hard, they do so at the expense of leisure activities and relationships.

These individuals also tend to be overly concerned with control—not only over the details of their own lives but also over their emotions and other people. They have difficulty expressing warm and tender feelings, often using stilted, distant phrasing that reveals little of their inner experience. They may be obstinate and reluctant to delegate tasks or to work with others unless others submit exactly to their ways of doing things, which reflects their needs for interpersonal control as well as their fears of making mistakes. Their tendency to doubt and worry also manifests itself in their inability to discard worn-out or worthless objects that might be needed in the future, and as

Freud and Jones noted, persons with OCPD are miserly toward themselves and others.

## Differential Diagnosis

OCPD differs from Axis I obsessive-compulsive disorder in that the latter disorder is characterized by specific repetitive thoughts and ritualistic behaviors rather than the personality traits of orderliness, perfectionism, and control. In addition, the symptoms of obsessive-compulsive disorder have traditionally been considered ego-dystonic, whereas the traits and behaviors of OCPD have been considered ego-syntonic. These two disorders are sometimes, but not often, comorbid.

## Etiology

Freud's view that OCPD derives from difficulties occurring during the anal stage of psychosexual development (age 2–4 years) was echoed and elaborated on by subsequent psychoanalytic thinkers such as Karl Abraham and Wilhelm Reich (Reich 1933). According to this theory, children's infantile anal–erotic libidinal impulses conflict with parental attempts to socialize them—in particular, to toilet train them. Although these theories emphasize the importance of children's perceptions of parental disapproval during toilet training, and of ensuing parent–child control struggles—what Rado (1959) referred to as "the battle of the chamber pot"—these factors are not currently considered central to this disorder's etiology. It may be, however, that conflicts arising during toilet training— such as those characteristic of Erikson's (1950) stage of autonomy versus shame—and continuing during other developmental stages do play a role. In particular, excessive parental control, criticism, and shaming may result in an insecurity that is defended against with perfectionism, orderliness, and an attempt to maintain self-control.

## Treatment

Persons with OCPD may seem difficult to treat because of their excessive intellectualization and difficulty expressing emotion. However, these patients often respond well to psychoanalytic psychotherapy or psychoanalysis (Gabbard 2005). Therapists usually need to be relatively active in treatment. They should also avoid being drawn into interesting but affectless discussions that are unlikely to have therapeutic benefit. In other words, rather than intellectualizing with patients, therapists should focus on the feelings these patients usually avoid. Other defenses common in this disorder, such as rationalization, isolation, undoing, and reaction formation, also should be identified and clarified. Power struggles that may occur in treatment offer opportunities to address the patient's excessive need for control.

Cognitive techniques also may be used to diminish the patient's excessive need for control and perfection (Beck et al. 2004). Although patients may resist group treatment because of their need for control, dynamically oriented groups that focus on feelings may provide insight and increase patients' comfort with exploring and expressing new affects (Table 29–21).

**TABLE 29–21.   Treatment of obsessive-compulsive personality disorder**

Psychodynamic individual psychotherapy

Psychoanalysis

Cognitive-behavioral therapy

Psychodynamic group psychotherapy

## Key Points: Personality Disorders

Personality disorders

- Are common in clinical settings and in the community.

- Can be challenging to diagnose.

- Cause significant problems for those who have them and for others and are costly to society.

- Often complicate the treatment of other mental disorders.

- Result from an interaction between temperamental (genetic/biological) and psychological (developmental/ environmental) factors.

## References

Abraham K: Contributions to the theory of the anal character. Int J Psychoanal 4:400–418, 1923

Abraham K: The influence of oral eroticism on character formation, in Selected Papers on Psychoanalysis. Edited by Jones E. London, England, Hogarth Press, 1927, pp 393–406

Adler G: Borderline Psychopathology and Its Treatment. New York, Jason Aronson, 1985

American Psychiatric Association: Diagnostic and Statistical Manual of Mental Disorders, 3rd Edition. Washington, DC, American Psychiatric Association, 1980

American Psychiatric Association: Diagnostic and Statistical Manual of Mental Disorders, 4th Edition, Text Revision. Washington, DC, American Psychiatric Association, 2000

American Psychiatric Association: Practice guideline for the treatment of patients with borderline personality disorder. Am J Psychiatry 158(suppl):1–52, 2001

Appelbaum AH: Supportive therapy, in The American Psychiatric Publishing Textbook of Personality Disorders. Edited by Oldham JM, Skodol AE, Bender DS. Washington, DC, American Psychiatric Publishing, 2005, pp 335–346

Bateman A, Fonagy P: Effectiveness of partial hospitalization in the treatment of borderline personality disorder: a randomized controlled trial. Am J Psychiatry 156:1563–1569, 1999

Beck AT, Freeman A, Davis DD, et al: Cognitive Therapy of Personality Disorders, 2nd Edition. New York, Guilford, 2004

Bender DS, Dolan RT, Skodol AE, et al: Treatment utilization by patients with personality disorders. Am J Psychiatry 158:295–302, 2001

Benjamin LS: Structural analysis of social behavior. Psychol Rev 81:392–425, 1974

Blonigen DM, Hicks BM, Krueger RF, et al: Psychopathic personality traits: heritability and genetic overlap with internalizing and externalizing psychopathology. Psychol Med 35:637–648, 2005

Carey G, DiLalla DL: Personality and psychopathology: genetic perspectives. J Abnorm Psychol 103:32–43, 1994

Chiesa M, Fonagy P: Cassel Personality Disorder Study. Br J Psychiatry 176:485–491, 2000

Clark LA: Schedule for Nonadaptive and Adaptive Personality (SNAP). Minneapolis, University of Minnesota Press, 1993

Cloninger CR, Svrakic DM, Przybeck TR: A psychobiological model of temperament and character. Arch Gen Psychiatry 50:975–990, 1993

Coccaro EF, Kavoussi RJ, Sheline YI, et al: Impulsive aggression in personality disorder correlates with tritiated paroxetine binding in the platelet. Arch Gen Psychiatry 53:531–536, 1996

Compton WM, Conway KP, Stinson FS, et al: Prevalence, correlates, and comorbidity of DSM-IV antisocial personality syndromes and alcohol and specific drug use disorders in the United States: results from the National Epidemiologic Study on Alcohol and Related Conditions. J Clin Psychiatry 66:677–685, 2005

Costa P, McCrae R: Personality disorders and the five-factor model of personality. J Personal Disord 4:362–371, 1990

Dickinson KA, Pincus AL: Interpersonal analysis of grandiose and vulnerable narcissism. J Personal Disord 17:188–207, 2003

DiLalla DL, Carey G, Gottesman II, et al: Heritability of MMPI personality indicators of psychopathology in twins reared apart. J Abnorm Psychol 105:491–499, 1996

Edens JF, Marcus DK, Lillienfeld SO, et al: Psychopathic, not psychopath: taxometric evidence for the dimensional structure of psychopathy. J Abnorm Psychol 115:131–144, 2006

Erikson EH: Childhood and Society. New York, WW Norton, 1950

First MB, Gibbon M, Spitzer RL, et al: Structured Clinical Interview for DSM-IV Axis II Personality Disorders (SCID-II). Washington, DC, American Psychiatric Press, 1997

Gabbard GO: Psychodynamic Psychiatry in Clinical Practice, 3rd Edition. Washington, DC, American Psychiatric Publishing, 2000

Gabbard GO: Psychoanalysis, in The American Psychiatric Publishing Textbook of Personality Disorders. Edited by Oldham JM, Skodol AE, Bender DS. Washington, DC, American Psychiatric Publishing, 2005, pp 257–273

Giesen-Bloo J, van Dyck R, Spinhoven P, et al: Outpatient psychotherapy for borderline personality disorder: randomized trial of schema-focused therapy vs. transference-focused psychotherapy. Arch Gen Psychiatry 63:649–658, 2006

Grove WM, Eckert ED, Heston L, et al: Heritability of substance abuse and antisocial behavior: a study of monozygotic twins reared apart. Biol Psychiatry 27:1293–1304, 1990

Gunderson JG: The borderline patient's intolerance of aloneness: insecure attachment and therapist availability. Am J Psychiatry 153:752–758, 1996

Hare RD, Neumann CS: Structural models of psychopathy. Curr Psychiatry Rep 7:57–64, 2005

Hare RD, Hart SD, Harpur TJ: Psychopathy and the DSM-IV criteria for antisocial personality disorder. J Abnorm Psychol 100:391–398, 1991

Hollander E, Swann AC, Coccaro EF, et al: Impact of trait impulsivity and state aggression on divalproex versus placebo response in borderline personality disorder. Am J Psychiatry 162:621–624, 2005

Hyler SE: Personality Diagnostic Questionnaire–4 (PDQ-4). New York, New York State Psychiatric Institute, 1994

Jang KL, Livesley WJ, Vernon PA, et al: Heritability of personality disorder traits: a twin study. Acta Psychiatr Scand 94:438–444, 1996

Johnson JG, Bromley E, McGeoch PG: Role of childhood experiences in the development of maladaptive and adaptive personality traits, in The American Psychiatric Publishing Textbook of Personality Disorders. Edited by Oldham JM, Skodol AE, Bender DS. Washington, DC, American Psychiatric Publishing, 2005, pp 209–221

Jones M: The Therapeutic Community: A New Treatment in Psychiatry. New York, Basic Books, 1953

Joyce PR, McKenzie JM, Luty SE, et al: Temperament, childhood environment and psychopathology as risk factors for avoidant and borderline personality disorders. Aust N Z J Psychiatry 37:756–764, 2003

Kagan J: Temperamental influences on the preservation of styles of social behavior. McLean Hospital Journal 14:23–34, 1989

Kaye AL, Shea MT: Personality disorders, personality traits, and defense mechanisms measures, in Handbook of Psychiatric Measures. Washington, DC, American Psychiatric Association, 2000, pp 713–749

Kent S, Fogarty M, Yellowlees P: A review of studies of heavy users of psychiatric services. Psychiatr Serv 46:1247–1253, 1995

Kernberg OF: Borderline Conditions and Pathological Narcissism. New York, Jason Aronson, 1975

Keshavan M, Shad M, Soloff P, et al: Efficacy and tolerability of olanzapine in the treatment of schizotypal personality disorder. Schizophr Res 71:97–101, 2004

Kessler RC: The impairments caused by social phobia in the general population: implications for intervention. Acta Psychiatr Scand Suppl (417):19–27, 2003

Klein M: Wisconsin Personality Inventory–IV (WPI-IV). Madison, University of Wisconsin, 1993

Klonsky ED, Oltmanns TF, Turkheimer E: Deliberate self-harm in a nonclinical population: prevalence and psychological correlates. Am J Psychiatry 160:1501–1508, 2003

Koenigsberg HW, Reynolds D, Goodman M, et al: Risperidone in the treatment of schizotypal personality disorder. J Clin Psychiatry 64:628–634, 2003

Leichsenring F, Leibing E: The effectiveness of psychodynamic therapy and cognitive behavior therapy in the treatment of personality disorders: a meta-analysis. Am J Psychiatry 160:1223–1232, 2003

Levy KN, Meehan KB, Weber M, et al: Attachment and borderline personality disorder: implications for psychotherapy. Psychopathology 38:64–74, 2005

Linehan MM: Cognitive-Behavioral Treatment of Borderline Personality Disorder. New York, Guilford, 1993

Linehan MM, Comtois KA, Murray AM, et al: Two-year randomized controlled trial and follow-up of dialectical behavior therapy vs. therapy by experts for suicidal behaviors and borderline personality disorder. Arch Gen Psychiatry 63:757–766, 2006

Loranger AW: International Personality Disorder Examination (IPDE) Manual. Odessa, FL, Psychological Assessment Resources, 1999

Lyons MJ, True WR, Eisen SA, et al: Differential heritability of adult and juvenile antisocial traits. Arch Gen Psychiatry 52:906–915, 1995

Malone SM, Taylor J, Marmorstein NR, et al: Genetic and environmental influences on antisocial behavior and alcohol dependence from adolescence to early adulthood. Dev Psychopathol 16:943–966, 2004

Masterson JF: Treatment of the Borderline Adolescent: A Developmental Approach. New York, Wiley-Interscience, 1972

McDermut W, Zimmerman M: Assessment instruments and standardized evaluation, in The American Psychiatric Publishing Textbook of Personality Disorders. Edited by Oldham JM, Skodol AE, Bender DS. Washington, DC, American Psychiatric Publishing, 2005, pp 89–101

Meyer B, Carver CS: Negative childhood accounts, sensitivity, and pessimism: a study of avoidant personality disorder features in college students. J Personal Disord 14:233–248, 2000

Millon T: Disorders of Personality: DSM-III, Axis II. New York, Wiley, 1981

Millon T, Davis R, Millon C: Manual for the MCMI-III. Minneapolis, MN, National Computer Systems, 1997

Modell AH: A narcissistic defense against affects and the illusion of self-sufficiency. Int J Psychoanal 56:275–282, 1975

Moffitt TE: The new look of behavioral genetics in developmental psychopathology: gene-environment interplay in antisocial behaviors. Psychol Bull 131:533–554, 2005

Morey LC, Alexander GM, Boggs C: Gender, in The American Psychiatric Publishing Textbook of Personality Disorders. Edited by Oldham JM, Skodol AE, Bender DS. Washington, DC, American Psychiatric Publishing, 2005, pp 541–559

Paris J: A current integrative perspective on personality disorders, in The American Psychiatric Publishing Textbook of Personality Disorders. Edited by Oldham JM, Skodol AE, Bender DS. Washington, DC, American Psychiatric Publishing, 2005a, pp 119–128

Paris J: Neurobiological dimensional models of personality: a review of the models of Cloninger, Depue, and Siever. J Personal Disord 19:156–170, 2005b

Perry JC, Bond M: Defensive functioning, in The American Psychiatric Publishing Textbook of Personality Disorders. Edited by Oldham JM, Skodol AE, Bender DS. Washington, DC, American Psychiatric Publishing, 2005, pp 523–540

Perry JC, Banon E, Ianni F: Effectiveness of psychotherapy for personality disorders. Am J Psychiatry 156:1312–1321, 1999

Pfohl B, Blum N, Zimmerman M: Structured Interview for DSM-IV Personality. Washington, DC, American Psychiatric Press, 1997

Piper WE, Ogrodniczuk JS: Group treatment, in The American Psychiatric Publishing Textbook of Personality Disorders. Edited by Oldham JM, Skodol AE, Bender DS. Washington, DC, American Psychiatric Publishing, 2005, pp 347–357

Rado S: Obsessive behavior, in American Handbook of Psychiatry, Vol 1. Edited by Arieti S. New York, Basic Books, 1959, pp 324–344

Reich W: Charakteranalyse: Technik und Grundlagen für studierende und praktizierende Analytiker. Leipzig, Germany, IM Selbstverlage des Verfassers, 1933

Reich W: On the technique of character analysis, in Character Analysis, 3rd Edition. New York, Simon & Schuster, 1949, pp 39–113

Reiss D, Hetherington EM, Plomin R, et al: Genetic questions for environmental studies: differential parenting and psychopathology in adolescence. Arch Gen Psychiatry 52:925–936, 1995

Rettew DC, Zanarini MC, Yen S, et al: Childhood antecedents of avoidant personality disorder: a retrospective study. J Am Acad Child Adolesc Psychiatry 42:1122–1130, 2003

Roberts BW, Caspi A, Moffitt TE: Work experiences and personality development in young adulthood. J Pers Soc Psychol 84:582–593, 2003

Seivewright H, Tyrer P, Johnson T: Persistent social dysfunction in anxious and depressed patients with personality disorder. Acta Psychiatr Scand 109:104–109, 2004

Siever LJ, Davis KL: The pathophysiology of schizophrenia disorders: perspectives from the spectrum. Am J Psychiatry 161:398–413, 2004

Skodol AE, Oldham JM: Assessment and diagnosis of borderline personality disorder. Hosp Community Psychiatry 42:1021–1028, 1991

Skodol AE, Gunderson JG, McGlashan TH, et al: Functional impairment in patients with schizotypal, borderline, avoidant, or obsessive-compulsive personality disorder. Am J Psychiatry 159:276–283, 2002

Skodol AE, Pagano MP, Bender DS, et al: Stability of functional impairment in patients with schizotypal, borderline, avoidant, or obsessive-compulsive personality disorder over two years. Psychol Med 35:443–451, 2005

Soler J, Pascual JC, Carlos J, et al: Double-blind, placebo-controlled study of dialectical behavior therapy plus olanzapine for borderline personality disorder. Am J Psychiatry 162:1221–1224, 2005

Soloff PH: Somatic treatments, in The American Psychiatric Publishing Textbook of Personality Disorders. Edited by Oldham JM, Skodol AE, Bender DS. Washington, DC, American Psychiatric Publishing, 2005, pp 387–403

Stanley B, Brodsky BS: Dialectical behavior therapy, in The American Psychiatric Publishing Textbook of Personality Disorders. Edited by Oldham JM, Skodol AE, Bender DS. Washington, DC, American Psychiatric Publishing, 2005, pp 307–320

Stein MB, Chartier MJ, Lizak MV, et al: Familial aggregation of anxiety-related quantitative traits in generalized social phobia: clues to understanding "disorder" heritability? Am J Med Genet 105:79–83, 2001

Stone M: Schizotypal personality: psychotherapeutic aspects. Schizophr Bull 11:576–589, 1985

Stone M: Violence, in The American Psychiatric Publishing Textbook of Personality Disorders. Edited by Oldham JM, Skodol AE, Bender DS. Washington, DC, American Psychiatric Publishing, 2005, pp 477–491

Taylor CT, Laposa JM, Alden LE: Is avoidant personality disorder more than just social avoidance? J Personal Disord 18:571–594, 2004

Torgersen S: Epidemiology, in The American Psychiatric Publishing Textbook of Personality Disorders. Edited by Oldham JM, Skodol AE, Bender DS. Washington, DC, American Psychiatric Publishing, 2005, pp 129–141

Torgersen S, Onstad S, Skre I, et al: "True" schizotypal personality disorder: a study of co-twins and relatives of schizophrenic probands. Am J Psychiatry 150:1661–1667, 1993

Torgersen S, Lygren S, Øien PA, et al: A twin study of personality disorders. Compr Psychiatry 41:416–425, 2000

Torgersen S, Kringlen E, Cramer V: The prevalence of personality disorders in a community sample. Arch Gen Psychiatry 58:590–596, 2001

Widiger TA: Personality disorders in the 21st century. J Personal Disord 14:3–16, 2000

Widiger TA, Mangine S, Corbitt EM, et al: Personality Disorder Interview–IV (PDI-IV): A Semi-Structured Interview for the Assessment of Personality Disorders. Professional Manual. Odessa, FL, Psychological Assessment Resources, 1995

Woody GE, McLellan AT, Luborsky L, et al: Sociopathy and psychotherapy outcome. Arch Gen Psychiatry 42:1081–1086, 1985

Zanarini M: Role of Sexual Abuse in the Etiology of Borderline Personality Disorder. Washington, DC, American Psychiatric Press, 1997

Zanarini M, Frankenburg FR: Pathways to the development of borderline personality disorder. J Personal Disord 11:93–104, 1997

Zanarini MC, Frankenburg FR, Chauncey DL, et al: The Diagnostic Interview for DSM-IV Personality Disorders. Belmont, MA, McLean Hospital, Laboratory for the Study of Adult Development, 1996

Zimmerman M, Coryell W: DSM-III personality disorder diagnoses in a nonpatient sample: demographic correlates and comorbidity. Arch Gen Psychiatry 46:682–689, 1989

Zimmerman M, Coryell W: Diagnosing personality disorders in the community: a comparison of self-report and interview measures. Arch Gen Psychiatry 47:527–531, 1990

# Section III

# Treatments and Special Topics

# 30

# Psychopharmacology

MELISSA MARTINEZ, M.D.

LAUREN B. MARANGELL, M.D.

JAMES M. MARTINEZ, M.D.

## General Principles

### Medication Selection

Because so many medication options exist, a clinician must consider numerous factors when selecting a specific psychotropic medication for a given patient. These factors include the presence of comorbid medical conditions (which may preclude the use of certain medications); the presence of comorbid psychiatric disorders (which may be exacerbated by certain medications but effectively treated by others); the use of concomitant psychotropic and nonpsychotropic medications (which may pose a risk for significant drug–drug interactions); history of response and tolerability to medication; family history of medication responses; patient-specific life circumstances that may be affected by particular side effects; patient concerns regarding the avoidance of particular side effects; and treatment costs.

### Generic Substitution

Generic drugs are less expensive alternatives to original proprietary (brand-name) formulations. Some patients may favor the use of a generic medication, if available, so that they may benefit from the cost savings. However, some caution is warranted with respect to generic drugs because generic "equivalents" are not always truly equivalent. The current U.S. Food and Drug Administration (FDA) requirements center around the concept of *bioequivalence*. Products are bioequivalent if they have no significant difference in the rate at which or extent to which the active ingredient becomes available at the site of action, given the same dose and conditions. In some cases, even small differences between a proprietary formulation and a generic preparation may have clinically meaningful consequences.

### Drug Interactions

The three main types of drug interactions are *pharmacokinetic interactions*, *pharmacodynamic interactions*, and *idiosyncratic interactions*. Pharmacokinetic interactions occur when one medication alters the pharmacokinetics (absorption, distribution, metabolism, or excretion) of another drug. Pharmacodynamic interactions occur when the action of a drug changes at a receptor or biologically active

The text and tables in this chapter were derived, in part, from Marangell LB, Martinez JM: *Concise Guide to Psychopharmacology*, 2nd Edition, which had its genesis in our chapter in the fourth edition of *The American Psychiatric Publishing Textbook of Psychiatry*.

The authors wish to express sincere gratitude and acknowledgment to Stuart C. Yudofsky, M.D., Donald C. Goff, M.D., and Jonathan M. Silver, M.D., who were coauthors on the previous version of this chapter, and to Dr. Yudofsky and Dr. Silver, who also were coauthors on the first edition of the *Concise Guide to Psychopharmacology*. The "Drug Interactions" sections contain material developed over many years by Lauren B. Marangell, M.D., in collaboration with Ann Callahan, M.D., and Terence Ketter, M.D.

site, which alters the pharmacological effect of a given plasma concentration of the drug. Idiosyncratic interactions occur unpredictably in a small number of patients; they are unexpected given the known pharmacological actions of the individual drugs.

### Cytochrome P450 Enzymes

Most psychotropic medications, except for lithium, are metabolized by cytochrome P450 enzymes. These enzymes are classified by families and subfamilies on the basis of similarities in amino acid sequence. Enzymes within subfamilies have relatively specific affinities for various drugs and other substances. The enzymes primarily involved in drug metabolism include CYP1A2, CYP2C9, CYP2C10, CYP2C19, CYP2D6, CYP3A3, and CYP3A4.

One important drug interaction that may involve cytochrome P450 enzymes is *enzyme inhibition*. Some medications, including several psychotropic medications, can cause clinically meaningful inhibition of one or more cytochrome P450 enzymes. If a cytochrome P450 enzyme is inhibited by a medication, then the plasma levels of concurrently administered drugs that rely on that enzyme for metabolism may increase. For example, CYP2D6 is essential for the usual metabolism of tricyclic antidepressants (TCAs). If a patient is taking a TCA and a medication that inhibits the CYP2D6 enzyme is introduced, or vice versa, plasma TCA levels increase, which may result in increased TCA-related side effects or TCA toxicity. A clinician who is aware of the potential for this reaction might choose to use a lower dose of the TCA. This example illustrates a key clinical principle of prescribing enzyme inhibitors: in many cases, the concomitant administration of an enzyme inhibitor and a medication that is a substrate for that enzyme is not contraindicated, but the patient should be monitored for signs and symptoms related to increased substrate levels, and the substrate dose should be decreased if necessary.

With regard to many medications, the specific cytochrome P450 enzymes responsible for metabolism are not yet known, but information about the role of cytochrome P450 enzymes in drug metabolism is rapidly accumulating. A partial list of clinically important substrates for and inhibitors of the cytochrome P450 enzymes most commonly involved in drug metabolism is presented in Table 30–1.

The effects of inhibitors occur relatively rapidly (in minutes to hours) and are reversible within a time frame that depends on the half-life of the inhibitor. Additionally, there is a large amount of interindividual variation in drug metabolism and the propensity for enzyme inhibition to alter metabolism. Part of this variation is the result of genetic polymorphism, which is a heritable alteration of the enzyme. Persons who have a genetic polymorphism that causes a large reduction in the amount of active enzyme are referred to as *poor metabolizers* and are at risk for increased drug levels, which may lead to toxicity. In contrast, some people have increased amounts of an enzyme. These individuals, referred to as *ultrarapid metabolizers,* may have reduced levels of drugs that are metabolized by the enzyme, resulting in decreased efficacy.

Another important interaction that may occur with cytochrome P450 enzymes is *enzyme induction*. Induction occurs when the liver produces a greater amount of the enzyme. This increase in enzyme availability can increase elimination and reduce plasma levels of a drug (or metabolite) that is a substrate for that enzyme. One risk inherent with this interaction is a potential loss of efficacy for drugs metabolized by the induced enzyme. Indeed, if a drug's clinical effectiveness is diminished as a result of this interaction, the dose of the affected drug should be increased to achieve the same serum concentration that was previously therapeutically effective.

### Protein Binding

Another potential drug–drug interaction may occur when drugs compete for protein-binding sites. In short, medications are distributed to their various sites of action through the circulatory system. In the bloodstream, most psychotropic medications (except lithium) are bound to plasma proteins to different degrees. For drugs that are protein bound, the unbound fraction of the drug is pharmacologically active, whereas the bound fraction is not. When two drugs that bind to plasma proteins are present in plasma simultaneously, competition for protein-binding sites occurs. This competition for protein-binding sites can cause displacement of a previously protein-bound drug, which in the free state becomes pharmacologically active. These interactions are often referred to as *protein-binding interactions*. This type of interaction may be clinically significant if the drugs involved are highly protein bound (which results in a large change in plasma concentration of free drug from a small amount of drug displacement) and have a low therapeutic index or narrow therapeutic window (in which case small changes in plasma levels can result in toxicity or loss of efficacy) (Callahan et al. 1996).

**TABLE 30–1.** Partial list of cytochrome P450 (CYP) substrates and inhibitors

| | CYP1A2 | CYP2D6 | CYP3A3/4 |
|---|---|---|---|
| Substrates[a] | Aminophylline | Most antipsychotics | Acetaminophen |
| | Amitriptyline | Amphetamine | Alprazolam |
| | Caffeine | Codeine | Amiodarone |
| | Clozapine (in part) | Donepezil | Antiarrhythmics |
| | Cyclobenzaprine | Encainide | Calcium channel blockers |
| | Flutamide | Flecainide | Carbamazepine |
| | Imipramine | Galantamine | Cyclosporine |
| | Riluzole | Lipophilic β-blockers | Donepezil |
| | Ramelteon | Mexiletine | Eszopiclone |
| | Theophylline | Oxycodone | Ethosuximide |
| | | Tricyclic antidepressants[b] | Galantamine |
| | | Tramadol | HMG-CoA reductase inhibitors |
| | | Trazodone | Lamotrigine |
| | | Type Ic antiarrhythmics | Lidocaine |
| | | Venlafaxine | Midazolam |
| | | | Most antineoplastics |
| | | | Oral contraceptives |
| | | | Oxcarbazepine |
| | | | Phosphodiesterase inhibitors |
| | | | Pimozide |
| | | | Propafenone |
| | | | Protease inhibitors |
| | | | Quinidine |
| | | | Steroids |
| | | | Zaleplon |
| | | | Zolpidem |

| | CYP1A2 | CYP2D6 | CYP3A3/4 |
|---|---|---|---|
| Inhibitors[c] | Cimetidine | Bupropion | Diltiazem |
| | Ciprofloxacin | Cimetidine | Fluvoxamine |
| | Enoxacin | Duloxetine | Grapefruit juice |
| | Flutamide | Fluoxetine | Imidazole antifungal agents |
| | Fluvoxamine | Paroxetine | Some macrolides |
| | Grapefruit juice | Quinidine | Nefazodone |
| | Ketoconazole | Ritonavir | Protease inhibitors |
| | Lomefloxacin | Sertraline | Verapamil |
| | Norfloxacin | | |

*Note.* HMG-CoA=3-hydroxy-3-methylglutaryl coenzyme A.
[a]Medications and substances metabolized by a given enzyme.
[b]The 2D6 enzyme is the final common pathway for the metabolism of tricyclic antidepressants.
[c]May increase levels of substrates.
*Source.* Callahan et al. 1996; Cozza et al. 2003; Greenblatt et al. 1998, 1999; Michalets 1998. Adapted from Marangell LB, Martinez JM: *Concise Guide to Psychopharmacology*, 2nd Edition. Washington, DC, American Psychiatric Publishing, 2006. Used with permission.

### Absorption and Excretion

Changes in plasma levels as a result of alterations in absorption or excretion are less common with psychiatric medications. Changes in plasma concentrations as a result of changes in excretion are most frequent with lithium, which is dependent on renal excretion (see "Mood Stabilizers" section later in this chapter).

### Pharmacodynamic Interactions

In pharmacodynamic interactions, the pharmacological effect of a drug is changed by the action of a second drug at a common receptor or bioactive site. To avoid these interactions to the extent possible, the clinician must be aware of all medications that a patient is taking, including over-the-counter medications, and be knowledgeable about each medication's various mechanisms of action and receptor effects.

## Antidepressant Medications

## Mechanisms of Action

All currently available antidepressant drugs affect serotonergic and/or noradrenergic neurotransmission. The effects of antidepressants on monoamine availability are immediate, but the clinical response is typically delayed for several weeks. Downregulation of receptors more closely parallels the time course of clinical response. This downregulation can be conceptualized as a marker of antidepressant-induced neuronal adaptation.

## Indications and Efficacy

All antidepressants are effective in the treatment of major depression. Additionally, some antidepressants are effective in obsessive-compulsive disorder (OCD; selective serotonin reuptake inhibitors [SSRIs] and clomipramine), panic disorder (TCAs and SSRIs), generalized anxiety disorder (venlafaxine and SSRIs), bulimia (TCAs, SSRIs, and monoamine oxidase inhibitors [MAOIs]), dysthymia (SSRIs), bipolar depression (with treatment with a mood stabilizer), social phobia (SSRIs, venlafaxine, MAOIs), posttraumatic stress disorder (SSRIs), irritable bowel syndrome (TCAs), enuresis (TCAs), neuropathic pain (TCAs, duloxetine), migraine headaches (TCAs), attention-deficit/hyperactivity disorder (bupropion), autism (SSRIs), late luteal phase dysphoric disorder (SSRIs), borderline personality disorder (SSRIs), and smoking cessation (bupropion).

## Clinical Use

In the following subsections, clinically relevant information is presented for each commonly used class of antidepressant individually. The pharmacological treatment of depression is also discussed. Information on doses and half-lives is summarized in Table 30–2, and a list of key features and side effects is presented in Table 30–3. The antidepressants currently available are classified according to their effects on neurotransmitter receptors or catabolic enzymes. The choice of a specific antidepressant medication is based on several factors, including the patient's psychiatric symptoms, history of previous treatment response and tolerability, family members' history of response, medication side-effect profiles, drug–drug interaction potentials, and the presence of comorbid disorders that may respond to (or preclude the use of) specific antidepressants.

## Antidepressants and Suicide

Long-term pharmacological treatment is associated with a decreased suicide rate (Angst et al. 2002), but the acute phases of treatment with antidepressants have been associated with increased risks of suicidal thoughts and behaviors. This is of particular concern in children and adolescents.

At this time, warnings apply to all antidepressant medications. Although data from adult placebo-controlled trials have not been evaluated in the same systematic manner, some adult patients might be at risk for suicide in the initial weeks of treatment. Thus, it is imperative that clinicians monitor all patients, including adults, for the emergence or worsening of suicidal thoughts or behavior during treatment with antidepressants. These warnings also underscore the need for thoughtful patient education.

## Selective Serotonin Reuptake Inhibitors

### Background

SSRIs inhibit serotonin reuptake and are largely devoid of four other major pharmacological properties inherent to other antidepressants (e.g., TCAs)—namely, muscarinic receptor blockade, histamine type 1 ($H_1$) receptor blockade, $\alpha_1$-adrenergic receptor blockade, and norepinephrine reuptake inhibition. This pharmacological selectivity has several advantages, including a reduction in dangerous side effects. SSRIs are unlikely to affect the seizure threshold or cardiac conduction, and are relatively safe in overdose. Despite their highly selective pharmacological activity,

TABLE 30–2. Antidepressant medications: dosing and half-life information

| Generic drug name | Proprietary drug name | Usual starting dose (mg)[a] | Usual daily dose (mg) | Available oral doses (mg) | Mean half-life, hours (active metabolites)[b] |
|---|---|---|---|---|---|
| **Monoamine oxidase inhibitors** | | | | | |
| *Irreversible, nonselective monoamine oxidase inhibitors* | | | | | |
| Isocarboxazid | Marplan | 10 | 20–60 | 10 | 2 |
| Phenelzine | Nardil | 15 | 15–90 | 15 | 2 |
| Tranylcypromine | Parnate | 10 | 30–60 | 10 | 2 |
| *Transdermal monoamine oxidase inhibitors* | | | | | |
| Transdermal selegiline | EMSAM | 6 | 6 | None Transdermal doses: 6 mg/24 hours 9 mg/24 hours 12 mg/24 hours | 18–25 |
| *Reversible inhibitors of monoamine oxidase A* | | | | | |
| Moclobemide[c] | Aurorix, Manerix | 150 | 300–600 | 100, 150 | 2 |
| **Tricyclic antidepressants** | | | | | |
| *Tertiary-amine tricyclic antidepressants* | | | | | |
| Amitriptyline | Elavil | 25–50 | 100–300 | 10, 25, 50, 75, 100, 150 | 16 (27) |
| Clomipramine | Anafranil | 25 | 100–250 | 25, 50, 75 | 32 (69) |
| Doxepin | Sinequan | 25–50 | 100–300 | 10, 25, 50, 75, 100, 150, L | 17 |
| Imipramine | Tofranil | 25–50 | 100–300 | 10, 25, 50, 75, 100, 125, 150 | 8 (17) |
| Trimipramine | Surmontil | 25–50 | 100–300 | 25, 50, 100 | 24 |
| *Secondary-amine tricyclic antidepressants* | | | | | |
| Desipramine | Norpramin | 25–50 | 100–300 | 10, 25, 50, 75, 100, 150 | 17 |
| Nortriptyline | Pamelor, Aventyl | 25 | 50–150 | 10, 25, 50, 75, L | 27 |
| Protriptyline | Vivactil | 10 | 15–60 | 5, 10 | 79 |
| **Tetracyclic antidepressants** | | | | | |
| Amoxapine | Asendin | 50 | 100–400 | 25, 50, 100, 150 | 8 |
| Maprotiline | Ludiomil | 50 | 100–225 | 25, 50, 75 | 43 |
| **Selective serotonin reuptake inhibitors** | | | | | |
| Citalopram | Celexa | 20 | 20–40[d] | 10, 20, 40, L | 35 |
| Escitalopram | Lexapro | 10 | 10–20 | 5, 10, 20, L | 27–32 |
| Fluoxetine | Prozac | 20 | 20–60[d] | 10, 20, 40, L | 72 (216) |
| Fluoxetine Weekly | Prozac Weekly | 90 | NA | 90 | — |
| Fluvoxamine[e] | Luvox | 50 | 50–300[d] | 25, 50, 100 | 15 |
| Paroxetine | Paxil | 20 | 20–60[d] | 10, 20, 30, 40, L | 20 |
| Paroxetine CR | Paxil CR | 25 | 25–62.5 | 12.5, 25, 37.5 | 15–20 |
| Sertraline | Zoloft | 50 | 50–200[d] | 25, 50, 100 | 26 (66) |

**TABLE 30–2.**    Antidepressant medications: dosing and half-life information *(continued)*

| Generic drug name | Proprietary drug name | Usual starting dose (mg)[a] | Usual daily dose (mg) | Available oral doses (mg) | Mean half-life, hours (active metabolites)[b] |
|---|---|---|---|---|---|
| **Serotonin-norepinephrine reuptake inhibitors** | | | | | |
| Duloxetine | Cymbalta | 30 | 60–90 | 20, 30, 60 | 12 |
| Venlafaxine | Effexor | 37.5 | 75–225 | 25, 37.5, 50, 75, 100 | 5 (11) |
| Venlafaxine XR | Effexor XR | 37.5 | 75–225 | 37.5, 75, 150 | 5 (11) |
| **Serotonin modulators** | | | | | |
| Nefazodone[e] | Serzone | 50 | 150–300 | 100, 150, 200, 250 | 4 |
| Trazodone | Desyrel | 50 | 75–300 | 50, 100, 150, 300 | 7 |
| **Norepinephrine-serotonin modulators** | | | | | |
| Mirtazapine | Remeron | 15 | 15–45 | 7.5, 15, 30, 45, SolTab | 20 |
| **Norepinephrine-dopamine reuptake inhibitors** | | | | | |
| Bupropion | Wellbutrin | 150 | 300 | 75, 100 | 14 |
| Bupropion SR | Wellbutrin SR | 150 | 300 | 100, 150 | 21 |
| Bupropion XL | Wellbutrin XL | 300 | 300 | 100, 150 | 21 |

*Note.*    CR=controlled release; L=liquid; NA=not applicable; SolTab=orally disintegrating tablets; SR=sustained release; XL or XR=extended release.
[a]Lower starting doses are recommended for elderly patients and patients with panic disorder, significant anxiety, or hepatic disease.
[b]Mean half-lives of active metabolites are given in parentheses.
[c]Not available in the United States.
[d]Dose varies with diagnosis. See text for specific guidelines.
[e]Generic only.
*Source.*    Dosing information from American Psychiatric Association 2000. Half-life data from Physicians' Desk Reference 2005. Dosing and half-life information for transdermal selegiline system from EMSAM 2006. Adapted from Marangell LB, Martinez JM: *Concise Guide to Psychopharmacology*, 2nd Edition. Washington, DC, American Psychiatric Publishing, 2006, pp. 13–16. Used with permission.

SSRIs have a broad spectrum of action. They are efficacious in the treatment of depression and of many other psychiatric disorders, including many major anxiety disorders.

All the SSRIs have similar spectrums of efficacy and similar side-effect profiles. However, they are structurally and, in some instances, clinically distinct. Importantly, SSRIs also have distinct pharmacokinetic properties, including differences in half-life (see Table 30–2) and drug–drug interaction potential (see Table 30–1).

## *Clinical Use*

Although all patients with depression should undergo a thorough medical evaluation, no specific tests are required

before SSRI therapy is initiated. The usual starting doses of SSRIs are summarized in Table 30–2. These standard doses generally should be decreased by 50% in patients with hepatic disease and in elderly persons. In addition, patients with significant anxiety symptoms, or those who are generally sensitive to medication side effects, may experience better tolerability if lower initial doses are used; however, it is important to titrate the dose to a potentially effective dose once tolerability is achieved.

In patients with depression, SSRIs have a flat dose–response curve, meaning that higher doses tend not to be more effective than standard doses, although some patients may respond better to higher doses. Premature escalation of the SSRI dose may result in increased side

**TABLE 30–3.** Key side effects of major antidepressant drugs

| Medications | Sedation | Weight gain | Sexual dysfunction | Other key side effects |
|---|---|---|---|---|
| Tricyclic antidepressants (TCAs) | Most, yes | Yes | Yes | Anticholinergic effects, orthostasis, quinidine-like effects on cardiac conduction; lethal in overdose |
| Selective serotonin reuptake inhibitors (SSRIs) | Minimal | Rare | Yes | Initial: nausea, loose bowel movements, headache, insomnia |
| Bupropion XL | Rare | Rare | Rare | Initial: nausea, headache, insomnia, anxiety or agitation; seizure risk |
| Venlafaxine XR | Minimal | Rare | Yes | Similar to SSRI side effects; dose-dependent hypertension |
| Duloxetine | Minimal | Rare | Some | Initial: nausea; similar to SSRI side effects; avoid in patients with substantial alcohol use, hepatic insufficiency, chronic liver disease, or severe renal impairment |
| Trazodone | Yes | Rare | Rare | Sedation, priapism, dizziness, orthostasis |
| Mirtazapine | Yes | Yes | Rare | Anticholinergic effects; may increase serum lipid levels; rare: orthostasis, hypertension, peripheral edema, agranulocytosis |
| Monoamine oxidase inhibitors (MAOIs) | Rare | Yes | Yes | Orthostatic hypotension, insomnia, peripheral edema; avoid in patients with CHF; avoid phenelzine in patients with hepatic impairment; potentially life-threatening drug interactions; dietary restrictions |

*Note.* CHF=congestive heart failure; XL or XR=extended release.
*Source.* Adapted from Marangell LB, Martinez JM: *Concise Guide to Psychopharmacology*, 2nd Edition. Washington, DC, American Psychiatric Publishing, 2006, pp. 18–20. Used with permission.

effects without necessarily improving antidepressant efficacy. Therefore, we recommend maintaining the usual therapeutic dose for at least 4 weeks. If no improvement is seen after 4 weeks, a trial of a higher dose may be warranted. If a partial response is evident after 4 weeks of therapy, the dose should remain constant for an additional 2 weeks because further improvement at the initial dose may occur.

Treatment of OCD requires a longer duration and higher doses to assess efficacy. A therapeutic trial for OCD should last 8–12 weeks.

Late luteal phase dysphoric disorder is more responsive to serotonergic agents than to noradrenergic agents. Interestingly, late luteal phase dysphoric disorder can be treated with medication administered only during the symptomatic period before menses or on a continuous basis (Pearlstein et al. 2000; Wikander et al. 1998; Yonkers et al. 1997).

## Risks, Side Effects, and Their Management

**Common side effects.** Nausea, loose bowel movements, anxiety, headache, insomnia, and increased sweating are frequent initial side effects of SSRIs. They are usually dose related and may be minimized with low initial dosing and gradual titration. These early adverse effects almost always attenuate after the first few weeks of treatment. Sexual dysfunction (see "Sexual Dysfunction" subsection later in this section) is a common long-term side effect of SSRIs.

**Gastrointestinal symptoms.** Nausea is a common early, and typically transient, side effect of SSRIs. Some patients report less nausea if they take the medication with food.

**Sexual dysfunction.** Decreased libido, anorgasmia, and delayed ejaculation are common side effects of SSRIs. When significant sexual dysfunction persists despite a positive response to treatment, a reduction in the dose may be considered. However, the clinician must balance efficacy and tolerability; for some patients, a lower dose may improve tolerability without compromising the therapeutic benefits, whereas others may not have an adequate therapeutic response to the medication at lower doses. Importantly, some patients may experience sexual side effects throughout the medication dose range. If sexual side effects remain problematic, two main strategies are available: the antidepressant can be replaced with an alternative, or other drugs can be prescribed concomitantly to counteract the side effects. Antidepressants that do not commonly cause sexual dysfunction include bupropion and mirtazapine. Several medications have been suggested as antidotes for the sexual side effects associated with antidepressant therapy. Bupropion, 75 or 150 mg/day, has been added to an SSRI regimen with some success in terms of improving libido (Labbate and Pollack 1994). Sildenafil has been used on an as-needed basis before sexual activity (Fava et al. 1998).

**Stimulation and insomnia.** Some patients taking an SSRI may experience jitteriness, restlessness, muscle tension, and disturbed sleep, particularly during the early course of treatment. Patients should be informed of the possibility of the emergence of these side effects and be reassured that if they develop, they tend to be transient. In patients with prominent anxiety, SSRI therapy should be started at low doses, with subsequent titration as tolerated. Additionally, the short-term use of a benzodiazepine (if otherwise safe) may help the patient cope with overstimulation in the early stages of treatment. Despite these transient stimulating effects, SSRIs are effective in patients with anxiety or agitated depression. Similarly, insomnia may occur early in treatment, and short-term, symptomatic treatment with a hypnotic at bedtime is reasonable if necessary.

**Sedation.** SSRIs may induce sedation in some patients. Altering the time of administration often is not successful.

**Vivid dreams.** Reports of vivid dreams (not nightmares) are common with SSRI therapy.

**Bleeding.** SSRIs affect serotonin systems throughout the body, including serotonin in platelets. Because platelets cannot synthesize serotonin, this effect tends to decrease platelet aggregation, which may lead to abnormal bleeding.

**Neurological effects.** Headaches are common early in treatment and usually can be managed with over-the-counter pain relief preparations. SSRIs may initially worsen migraine headaches but are often effective in reducing the severity and frequency of these headaches.

Tremor and akathisia also may occur, and they can be managed with dose reduction or the addition of a β-blocker such as propranolol (10–40 mg). There are isolated case reports of SSRI-related dystonia and increasing reports of SSRI-related exacerbation of Parkinson's disease (Di Rocco et al. 1998; Linazasoro 2000).

**Weight change.** All SSRIs have the potential to cause weight gain in some individuals.

**Rash.** As with other medications, some patients taking an SSRI may experience a rash during the course of treatment.

**Syndrome of inappropriate secretion of antidiuretic hormone.** Some patients taking SSRIs may develop the syndrome of inappropriate antidiuretic hormone secretion (SIADH). Symptoms include lethargy, headache, hyponatremia, increased urinary sodium excretion, and hyperosmotic urine. Acute treatment of this syndrome should consist of discontinuation of the drug as well as restriction of fluid intake. Patients experiencing severe confusion, convulsions, or coma should receive intravenous sodium chloride.

**Apathy syndrome.** We and others have noted an apathy syndrome in some patients after months or years of successful treatment with SSRIs. The syndrome is characterized by a loss of motivation, increased passivity, and feelings of lethargy and "flatness." The apathy syndrome appears to be dose dependent and reversible.

**Serotonin syndrome.** The serotonin syndrome results from excess serotonergic stimulation and can range in severity from mild to life threatening. The most common symptoms are confusion, flushing, diaphoresis, tremor, and myoclonic jerks. The patient may have symptoms of the serotonin syndrome in the context of monotherapy with a serotonergic medication, but this scenario is less common than symptoms resulting from use of two or more serotonergic drugs simultaneously. Discontinuation of the serotonergic medications is the first step in treatment, followed by emergency medical treatment. The serotonin type 2A (5-HT$_{2A}$) receptor antagonist cyproheptadine can be used if further treatment is warranted, beginning with an oral dose of 12 mg and then administration of 2 mg every 2 hours. However, efficacy for this presumed antidote has not been established.

**Discontinuation syndrome.** Some patients may experience a series of symptoms after discontinuation or dose reduction of serotonergic antidepressant medications, including dizziness, headache, paresthesia, nausea, diarrhea, insomnia, and irritability. These symptoms also may be seen when a patient misses doses of a serotonergic antidepressant. To avoid a discontinuation syndrome, clinicians should slowly taper antidepressant medications on discontinuation of the drug, particularly medications with short half-lives.

### Teratogenicity

Managing major depression, or any psychiatric disorder, in the context of pregnancy is challenging. Although minimizing the risk to the fetus is a clear goal, many patients, families, and even some practitioners need to be reminded that the illness of depression can have adverse effects on the fetus and neonate. Each woman who is facing pregnancy and related psychiatric treatment decisions needs to be approached and advised in the context of her unique circumstances. Some data indicate that the incidence of congenital abnormalities associated with the SSRIs is comparable to that associated with placebo, but other reports note an increased risk of congenital abnormalities, including septal heart defects, with first-trimester exposure and that this risk may be greater with paroxetine and clomipramine (Källén and Otterblad Olausson 2006). These data have resulted in a new FDA Category D pregnancy classification for paroxetine. Other data indicate that antidepressants may increase the risk of pulmonary hypertension by about sixfold with exposure after week 20 (Chambers et al. 2006).

### Drug Interactions

Several deaths have been reported among patients taking a combination of serotonergic antidepressants and MAOIs (Hodgman et al. 1997; Kolecki 1997). Because of the potential lethality of this interaction, a patient who needs to switch from an SSRI to an MAOI must not begin taking the MAOI until the SSRI has been fully eliminated from his or her body. Thus, a period equivalent to at least five times the half-life of the SSRI is required after stopping the SSRI before an MAOI can be initiated. A 2-week waiting period is required after stopping an MAOI before an SSRI can be initiated, to allow resynthesis of the monoamine oxidase enzyme in the absence of the MAOI.

The concurrent use of SSRIs and triptans (e.g., sumatriptan) has been reported to result in symptoms consistent with mild to moderate serotonin syndrome, but most patients tolerate this combination. Medications within the SSRI class also may inhibit one or more cytochrome P450 enzymes, and the SSRIs vary with regard to inhibition of specific enzymes (see Table 30–1 and extensive review in Cozza et al. 2003).

## Serotonin-Norepinephrine Reuptake Inhibitors

### Background

Serotonin-norepinephrine reuptake inhibitors (SNRIs) are dual reuptake inhibitors that affect serotonin and norepinephrine but have little effect on muscarinic, $H_1$, or $\alpha_1$-adrenergic receptors. Thus, these medications share many of the tolerability and safety benefits of the SSRIs but add an additional pharmacological action compared with SSRIs—namely, norepinephrine reuptake inhibition. Two SNRIs are currently available in the United States: venlafaxine and duloxetine.

### Venlafaxine

**Background.** Venlafaxine is a dual reuptake inhibitor for both serotonin and norepinephrine; serotonin reuptake inhibition is prominent at lower doses, whereas norepinephrine reuptake inhibition becomes more significant at higher doses.

**Clinical use.** The recommended dosage range of venlafaxine is 75–225 mg/day. The extended-release (XL) preparation, which allows for once-daily dosing in most patients, is preferred over the short-acting preparation. The usual starting dosage is 37.5–75 mg/day. Dosages up to 375 mg/day have been used in patients who were otherwise nonresponsive to treatment. Blood pressure monitoring during therapy is recommended because of a dose-dependent risk of increases in mean diastolic blood pressure in some patients.

Unlike SSRIs, venlafaxine shows a positive dose–response relation: patients with mild depression may respond to lower doses, whereas patients with more severe or recurrent depression may respond better to higher doses.

**Risks, side effects, and their management.** The side-effect profile of venlafaxine is similar to that of SSRIs and includes gastrointestinal symptoms, sexual dysfunction, and transient discontinuation symptoms. Like the SSRIs, venlafaxine does not affect cardiac conduction or lower the seizure threshold. In most patients, venlafaxine is not associated with sedation or weight gain. Side effects that differ from those of SSRIs are hypothesized to be related to the increased noradrenergic activity of this drug at higher doses; these side effects include dose-dependent anxiety (in some patients) and dose-dependent hypertension.

Dose-dependent increases in blood pressure may occur with venlafaxine treatment. A meta-analysis found that the magnitude of change in blood pressure associated with venlafaxine use is statistically significant but is unlikely to be of clinical significance at dosages less than 300 mg/day. However, the incidence of hypertension is 13% at dosages greater than 300 mg/day.

**Overdose.**   Few data are available regarding venlafaxine in overdose, but the drug's pharmacological profile suggests that it is safer than TCAs. In other cases, somnolence, mild sinus tachycardia, and generalized convulsions were noted. Recommended treatment includes general supportive and symptomatic measures. In severe cases, dialysis should be considered.

**Drug interactions.**   Venlafaxine does not appear to inhibit cytochrome P450 enzymes significantly and is not highly protein bound; thus, venlafaxine is less likely to contribute to protein-binding interactions than most other antidepressants. However, venlafaxine should not be combined with MAOIs because of the risk for serotonin syndrome.

### Duloxetine

**Background.**   Duloxetine hydrochloride is an SNRI that is approved by the FDA for the treatment of both major depression and the pain associated with diabetic peripheral neuropathy. Its half-life is approximately 12 hours, and it is highly protein bound. The most frequent side effect is early nausea, which is dose dependent and typically transient. Like venlafaxine, duloxetine typically is not associated with significant changes in weight.

**Clinical use.**   The recommended dosage for the treatment of major depression is 60 mg/day, whereas in diabetic neuropathy, a dosage of up to 120 mg/day is recommended. Nausea in the early phases of treatment is dose dependent, so treatment-naive patients might benefit from starting at 30 mg/day for the first week and then increasing to the target dose of 60 mg. At present, duloxetine is not recommended for use in patients with end-stage renal disease, severe renal impairment, or any hepatic insufficiency (Cymbalta 2006).

**Risks, side effects, and their management.**   The side-effect profile of duloxetine is similar to that of SSRIs. In most patients, duloxetine is not associated with sedation. Nausea may occur during treatment initiation, but it is generally transient.

Duloxetine has been associated with increases in serum transaminase levels. In controlled trials in major depressive disorder, elevations of alanine transaminase (ALT) to greater than three times the upper limit of normal occurred in 0.9% (8 of 930) of the duloxetine-treated patients and in 0.3% (2 of 652) of the placebo-treated patients (Cymbalta 2006). Additionally, postmarketing reports have indicated occurrences of hepatitis, hepatomegaly with liver enzyme elevation, severe hepatic enzyme elevation, and cholestatic jaundice (see Cymbalta 2006). Current labeling advises that duloxetine should not be prescribed to patients with significant alcohol use (because duloxetine may interact with alcohol to produce liver injury) or evidence of chronic liver disease (Cymbalta 2006).

As with SSRIs and venlafaxine, males who received duloxetine experienced more difficulty with ability to reach orgasm than did males who received placebo. However, females taking duloxetine did not experience more sexual dysfunction than did those taking placebo (Cymbalta 2006).

**Overdose.**   Few data are available regarding duloxetine in overdose. Recommended treatment includes general supportive and symptomatic measures. Dialysis is not recommended because the drug is highly protein bound.

**Drug interactions.**   Duloxetine is a moderate inhibitor of the CYP2D6 enzyme and may increase the levels of other medications that use this enzyme. Because of the risk of serotonin syndrome, duloxetine should not be combined with MAOIs. Because duloxetine is highly bound to plasma protein, combination with another drug that is highly protein bound may cause increased free concentrations of the other drug, potentially resulting in adverse events.

### Bupropion

**Background.**   Bupropion facilitates dopamine transmission; thus, many clinicians preferentially use this agent for depressed patients with Parkinson's disease. The fact that dopamine is integrally related to the brain's reward mechanisms, which are stimulated by nicotine and other addictive substances, has provided the theoretical underpinning for recent research indicating that bupropion is an effective aid in smoking cessation. Placebo-controlled trials involving nondepressed, chronic cigarette smokers found a dose-dependent increase in the percentage of patients able to achieve abstinence. Individuals receiving 300 mg/day of bupropion were able to sustain abstinence longer than those receiving 150 mg/day, and results achieved by patients given bupropion were superior to those achieved in the placebo groups (Zyban 2005).

Overall, bupropion has a favorable side-effect profile. The drug is associated with little or no weight gain, has few effects on cardiac conduction, and has minimal sexual side effects. Disadvantages include an increased risk of medication-induced seizures at higher-than-recommended doses.

**Clinical use.** Use of the XL preparation is preferred because of increased tolerability, decreased seizure risk, and the convenience of once-daily dosing. Treatment with the sustained-release (SR) or XL preparation is initiated at a dose of 150 mg, preferably taken in the morning. After 4 days, the dosage may be increased to 150 mg twice a day (SR) or 300 mg once daily in the morning (XL).

**Contraindications.** Patients with seizure disorders should not take bupropion. Similarly, an alternative treatment should be considered in patients with a history of significant head trauma, a central nervous system (CNS) tumor, or an active eating disorder.

**Risks, side effects, and their management.** The most common side effects of bupropion are initial headache, anxiety, insomnia, increased sweating, and gastrointestinal upset. Tremor and akathisia also may occur. Management is the same as for SSRI side effects. Bupropion is not associated with anticholinergic side effects, orthostatic hypotension, weight gain, or cardiac conduction changes.

*Seizures.* The incidence of seizures with the immediate-release preparation is 0.4% at doses less than 450 mg/day, provided no single dose of the short-acting preparation exceeds 150 mg. The incidence increases to 5% at dosages between 450 and 600 mg/day. The SR preparation is associated with seizure incidences of 0.1% at dosages less than 300 mg/day and 0.4% at dosages between 300 and 400 mg/day. Higher doses of the SR preparation have not been evaluated. No single dose of greater than 200 mg is recommended for the SR preparation, whereas up to 450 mg in a single dose may be given with the XL preparation. Bupropion should be used with caution in patients who are taking concomitant medications that lower the seizure threshold.

*Psychosis.* Reports of delusions, hallucinations, and paranoia are consistent with bupropion-mediated increases in central dopamine.

**Overdose.** Reported reactions to overdose with the immediate-release form include seizures, hallucinations, loss of consciousness, and sinus tachycardia. Treatment of overdose should include induction of vomiting, administration of activated charcoal, and electrocardiographic and electroencephalographic monitoring. For seizures, an intravenous benzodiazepine preparation is recommended.

**Drug interactions.** The combination of bupropion with an MAOI is potentially dangerous but less so than the combination of serotonergic drugs and MAOIs.

Data to date suggest that bupropion is metabolized by CYP2B6 (Faucette et al. 2000). Bupropion inhibits CYP2D6. Because of the risk of dose-dependent seizures, caution is warranted when bupropion is combined with other medications that might inhibit its metabolism.

### Trazodone

**Background.** Trazodone is an antidepressant that is associated with significant sedation. Currently, trazodone is not recommended as a first-line antidepressant because of an increased risk of orthostatic hypotension, arrhythmias, and priapism. However, trazodone may be useful in some patients with insomnia.

**Clinical use.** The recommended dose range for trazodone is 200–400 mg/day in divided doses. Initial dosing should begin at 50 mg/day. For many patients, even low doses of trazodone may be associated with significant sedation; thus, most of the daily dose should be administered at night.

**Risks, side effects, and their management.** Excessive sedation is the most commonly encountered side effect of trazodone. Although trazodone has virtually no anticholinergic side effects, dry mouth and blurred vision occur more frequently with trazodone treatment than with placebo.

Trazodone can cause orthostatic hypotension and dizziness. Additionally, there have been reports of increased ventricular irritability among patients with conduction defects and preexisting ventricular arrhythmias (Aronson and Hafez 1986; Jankowsky et al. 1983; Vitullo et al. 1990).

Trazodone has been associated with priapism (Scher et al. 1983), which may be irreversible and require surgical intervention.

**Overdose.** Trazodone overdose carries a risk of myocardial irritation in patients with preexisting ventricular conduction abnormalities.

## Mirtazapine

**Background.** Mirtazapine has been shown to reduce anxiety symptoms and sleep disturbances associated with depression as early as 1 week after the start of treatment. Other advantages are minimal sexual dysfunction, minimal nausea, and once-daily dosing. In addition, mirtazapine is unlikely to be associated with cytochrome P450–mediated drug interactions.

**Mechanism of action.** Mirtazapine facilitates central serotonergic and noradrenergic transmission by antagonizing $\alpha_2$-noradrenergic autoreceptors and heteroreceptors (De Boer 1996). In addition, mirtazapine antagonizes postsynaptic 5-HT$_{2A}$, 5-HT$_3$, and H$_1$ receptors and has moderate activity at $\alpha_1$-adrenergic and muscarinic receptors.

**Clinical use.** Mirtazapine treatment is initiated at a dosage of 15 mg at bedtime. The maximum recommended daily dose is 45 mg. Elderly patients and individuals with renal or hepatic disease may require lower doses.

**Risks, side effects, and their management.**

*Common side effects.* The most common side effects associated with mirtazapine are sedation, weight gain, and dizziness. Somnolence occurs in more than 50% of the patients taking mirtazapine (Bremner 1995; Smith et al. 1990).

*Agranulocytosis.* In preliminary clinical trials, 2 of 2,796 mirtazapine-treated patients developed agranulocytosis, and 1 developed severe neutropenia. All 3 patients recovered after medication discontinuation, and other possible etiologies were present in at least 1 of these individuals. Thirteen patients with pretreatment neutropenia did develop more severe neutropenia or agranulocytosis.

*Anticholinergic effects.* Mirtazapine is associated with modest anticholinergic side effects, including dry mouth and constipation.

*Cardiovascular effects.* Hypertension, orthostatic hypotension, dizziness, and vasodilation with peripheral edema may occur with mirtazapine treatment.

**Overdose.** Warning signs include drowsiness, impaired memory, and tachycardia. Recommended treatment includes gastric lavage, cardiac monitoring, and supportive measures.

**Drug interactions.** Mirtazapine does not significantly inhibit hepatic cytochrome P450 enzymes. Additive effects may occur when mirtazapine is combined with other drugs with sedative or vascular effects. Mirtazapine should not be used in combination with an MAOI or within 14 days of discontinuing treatment with an MAOI. When mirtazapine is combined with fluvoxamine, a potent inhibitor of P450 enzymes—including 1A2, 2D6, and 3A4—that metabolizes mirtazapine, the plasma concentration of mirtazapine may be increased up to fourfold.

## Tricyclic and Heterocyclic Antidepressants

### Background

Imipramine, amitriptyline, clomipramine, trimipramine, and doxepin are tertiary-amine TCAs. Desipramine, nortriptyline, and protriptyline are secondary-amine TCAs. Tertiary-amine tricyclics have more potent serotonin reuptake inhibition, and secondary-amine tricyclics have more potent noradrenergic reuptake inhibition. Tertiary-amine TCAs tend to have more side effects than do secondary-amine TCAs. Desipramine and protriptyline tend to be activating. Among the TCAs, nortriptyline is the least likely to produce orthostatic hypotension. Because amoxapine has an active metabolite that antagonizes dopamine type 2 (D$_2$) receptors, it can cause treatment-emergent extrapyramidal side effects (EPS).

### Mechanism of Action

TCAs inhibit norepinephrine, serotonin, and (to a lesser degree) dopamine reuptake. They also exert inhibitory effects on H$_1$, muscarinic, and $\alpha_1$-adrenergic receptors.

### Clinical Use

Because of potential cardiovascular effects and risks associated with TCAs, the clinician should obtain a cardiovascular history before initiating TCA therapy. In patients with preexisting heart disease and patients older than 40 years, an electrocardiogram (ECG) should be obtained before TCA treatment. TCAs should not be used in patients with bundle branch block unless all other options have failed. Additionally, other treatment options should be considered for patients with ischemic heart disease. Because orthostatic hypotension can occur with TCA treatment, other potential risk factors for hypotension should be explored.

Imipramine, amitriptyline, doxepin, desipramine, clomipramine, and trimipramine therapy can be initiated at 25–50 mg/day. Divided dosing may be used at first to minimize side effects, but eventually the entire dose can be given at bedtime. The dosage can be increased to 150 mg/day the second week, 225 mg/day the third week, and 300 mg/day the fourth week. The clomipramine dosage should not exceed 250 mg/day because of an increased risk of seizures at higher doses.

Nortriptyline therapy should be initiated at 25 mg/day, and the dosage should be increased to 75 mg/day over 1–2 weeks depending on tolerability and clinical response. Some patients require dosages of up to 150 mg/day. Amoxapine should be started at 50 mg/day, and the dosage should be titrated to 400 mg/day. Amoxapine has a short half-life and should be given in divided doses. Treatment with protriptyline can be started at 10 mg/day, and the dosage can be increased to 60 mg/day. Maprotiline therapy should be started at 50 mg/day, and that dosage should be maintained for 2 weeks; the risk of seizure increases if the dosage is raised too quickly. The dosage can be increased over 4 weeks to 225 mg/day.

### TCA Plasma Levels and Therapeutic Monitoring

Clinically meaningful plasma levels are available for imipramine, desipramine, and nortriptyline. For imipramine, the sum of the plasma levels of imipramine and the desmethyl metabolite (desipramine) should be greater than 200 ng/mL. Desipramine levels should be greater than 125 ng/mL. A therapeutic window has been noted for nortriptyline, with optimal response between 50 and 150 ng/mL. These therapeutic levels are based on steady-state concentrations, which are reached after 5–7 days of administration of these medications. Blood should be drawn approximately 10–14 hours after the last dose of medication.

### Risks, Side Effects, and Their Management

**Anticholinergic effects.** Common anticholinergic side effects include dry mouth, constipation, urinary retention, blurred vision, and tachycardia. Additionally, anticholinergic medications may cause cognitive impairment and confusion. Because the tertiary-amine TCAs and protriptyline have a particularly high affinity for muscarinic receptors, these medications are more likely than others within the TCA class to have anticholinergic side effects.

One must proceed with great caution when using antidepressants with anticholinergic side effects in treating patients with prostatic hypertrophy, narrow-angle glaucoma, or cognitive impairment.

**Sedation.** The sedative properties of TCAs appear to parallel their respective histamine receptor binding affinities.

**Cardiovascular effects.** Cardiovascular effects include orthostatic hypotension, tachycardia, and cardiac conduction delays. Although TCAs at toxic levels can cause life-threatening arrhythmias, TCAs are potent antiarrhythmic agents, possessing quinidine-like properties. Because prolongation of PR and QRS intervals can occur with TCA use, these drugs should not be used in patients with preexisting heart block (especially right bundle branch block and left bundle branch block).

**Weight gain.** Weight gain is a common side effect of TCA treatment.

**Seizures.** A dose-related risk of seizures has been found with clomipramine, which has led to the recommendation that the total daily dose of this drug not exceed 250 mg. Overdoses of TCAs, particularly amoxapine and desipramine, also are associated with seizures.

**Extrapyramidal side effects (amoxapine only).** Amoxapine, which has a mild neuroleptic effect, can cause EPS, akathisia, and even tardive dyskinesias.

### Overdose

Complications of TCA overdose may include neuropsychiatric impairment, hypotension, cardiac arrhythmias, and seizures. Anticholinergic delirium may occur, as well as other complications of anticholinergic overdose, including agitation, supraventricular arrhythmias, hallucinations, severe hypertension, and seizures.

Hypotension, which may result from norepinephrine depletion or have other causes related to peripheral and central effects of TCAs, should be treated with vigorous fluid replacement. Seizures and cardiac complications also may occur with TCA overdose. When the QRS interval is less than 0.10 second, the likelihood of seizures or ventricular arrhythmias decreases. Ventricular arrhythmias that occur secondary to overdose are typical of arrhythmias resulting from high doses of quinidine-like agents and begin within the first 24 hours after hospital admission.

### Drug Interactions

Drugs that induce hepatic microsomal enzymes or inhibit hepatic enzymes (particularly CYP2D6 inhibitors) may

TABLE 30–4.    Monoamine oxidase inhibitor reversibility and selectivity

| Generic drug (proprietary names) | Monoamine oxidase enzyme inhibition | |
| | Inhibition type | Enzyme selectivity |
| --- | --- | --- |
| Isocarboxazid (Marplan) | Irreversible | MAO-A+B |
| Phenelzine (Nardil) | Irreversible | MAO-A+B |
| Tranylcypromine (Parnate) | Irreversible | MAO-A+B |
| Selegiline (Eldepryl; EMSAM) | Irreversible | MAO-B[a] |
| Moclobemide[b] (Aurorix; Manerix) | Reversible | MAO-A |

*Note.*    MAO=monoamine oxidase.
[a]Selective at lower doses, nonselective at higher doses. Transdermal selegiline system allows for selegiline inhibition of both MAO-A and MAO-B. Oral selegiline is not indicated for the treatment of depression.
[b]Not available in the United States.
*Source.*    Adapted from Marangell LB, Martinez JM: *Concise Guide to Psychopharmacology*, 2nd Edition. Washington, DC, American Psychiatric Publishing, 2006, p. 47. Used with permission.

alter plasma tricyclic levels. The coadministration of a TCA and a potent CYP2D6 inhibitor may result in dangerously high levels of the TCA.

Although several medications may affect TCA levels, TCAs rarely affect the metabolism of other drugs. A notable exception is valproate sodium, levels of which may decrease when a TCA is administered concurrently (Preskorn and Burke 1992).

## Monoamine Oxidase Inhibitors

### *Background*

Patients with atypical depression, characterized by oversleeping and overeating, show a preferential response to MAOI therapy (Quitkin et al. 1979). Recently, a patch containing the MAOI selegiline has become available.

### *Mechanism of Action*

The enzyme monoamine oxidase A (MAO-A) acts selectively on norepinephrine and serotonin, whereas monoamine oxidase B (MAO-B) preferentially affects phenylethylamine. Both MAO-A and MAO-B oxidize dopamine and tyramine. MAO-A inhibition appears to be most relevant to the antidepressant effects of these drugs. Drugs that inhibit both MAO-A and MAO-B are called nonselective. Because tyramine can be metabolized by either MAO-A or MAO-B, drugs that selectively inhibit one of these enzymes but not the other do not require dietary restrictions. MAO-A–selective drugs, such as moclobemide, are available in other countries for the treatment of depression. MAO-B–selective drugs, such as pargyline,

are marketed for other indications. Selegiline is an irreversible MAOI that is selective for MAO-B at lower doses—namely, those doses typically used in the treatment of Parkinson's disease, but selegiline inhibits both MAO-A and MAO-B at antidepressant doses.

In addition to potential selectivity for MAO-A or MAO-B, MAOIs may produce either reversible or irreversible enzyme inhibition. An *irreversible inhibitor* permanently disables the enzyme, and the enzyme must be resynthesized in the absence of the drug before the activity of the enzyme can be reestablished. MAO enzyme resynthesis may take up to 2 weeks in the absence of an MAOI; thus, an interval of approximately 14 days is required after discontinuing an irreversible MAOI before instituting treatment with other antidepressants, permitting the use of contraindicated drugs, or permitting the consumption of contraindicated foods. On the other hand, a *reversible inhibitor* can move away from the active site of the enzyme, making the enzyme available to metabolize other substances. The reversibility and selectivity of the currently available MAOIs are summarized in Table 30–4.

### *Clinical Use*

The physician should discuss the risks associated with MAOI use with the patient and should review and discuss the need to adhere to the appropriate dietary restrictions and avoid medications that may lead to potentially dangerous interactions (Table 30–5). The patient should also be given written instructions that include a list of restricted foods and drugs, a list of safe concomitant medications, common side effects and precautions, signs and symptoms of potentially serious adverse events and instructions for action if they occur, and the importance of letting other health care providers, including dentists, know that he or she is taking an MAOI before any other treatments are prescribed or used, including anesthetic agents. Additionally, patients should be advised not to start any new medications without first informing their physician.

Phenelzine therapy is initiated at a dose of 15 mg in the morning, and the dose is increased by 15 mg every other day until a total daily dose of 60 mg is reached. If no response occurs within 2 weeks, the dose may be increased in 15-mg increments to a usual maximum of 90 mg/day. Higher doses are sometimes used, if tolerated, in patients with severe refractory depression. Treatment with tranylcypromine is initiated at a dose of 10 mg, and the dose is then increased every other day to 30 mg/day. As with phenelzine, higher doses may be necessary when the condition is refractory to treatment (Amsterdam and Berwish 1989). After tolerance to the hypotensive side effects has developed, usually after 1 or 2 weeks, the patient may take the medication in a single daily dose in the morning. Morning dosing is preferred because these medications tend to be activating; this is especially true of tranylcypromine, which is related to amphetamine.

Selegiline is an irreversible MAOI that is selective for MAO-B at lower doses and, when administered orally, undergoes extensive first-pass metabolism to amphetamine and methamphetamine metabolites (Karoum et al. 1982). Transdermal selegiline (EMSAM), which allows selegiline to be absorbed directly into the bloodstream, avoids first-pass metabolism (Rohatagi et al. 1997) and selectively targets MAO-A and MAO-B enzymes in the brain relative to those in the gastrointestinal tract (Wecker et al. 2003). Transdermal selegiline has been shown to be effective in the short-term treatment of depression in controlled trials (Amsterdam 2003; Bodkin and Amsterdam 2002). Transdermal selegiline is applied to dry skin on the upper torso, upper thigh, or outer surface of the upper arm once every 24 hours and not applied to the same site on consecutive days (EMSAM 2006). Patients should be advised to wash their hands after applying the transdermal system and also to avoid exposing the transdermal selegiline patch to external sources of heat.

Currently, transdermal selegiline is available in three dosages: 6 mg/24 hours (20 mg/20 cm²), 9 mg/24 hours (30 mg/30 cm²), and 12 mg/24 hours (40 mg/40 cm²). The recommended starting and target dose is 6 mg/24 hours, and dose increases in increments of 3 mg/24 hours should occur at intervals of at least 2 weeks. The maximum recom-

mended daily dosage is 12 mg/24 hours. At present, no dose adjustment is required for mild to moderate renal or hepatic impairment. Additionally, current product labeling does not require dietary restrictions for the 6-mg/24-hour dosing but does require dietary restrictions for the 9-mg/24-hour and 12-mg/24-hour dosings (EMSAM 2006). However, the concomitant medication warnings and restrictions apply across all transdermal selegiline dosages. A medication guide with safety information, dietary restrictions, drug interaction information, and instructions for use is available for patients.

### Risks, Side Effects, and Their Management

The following side effects apply to the irreversible, nonselective MAOI antidepressants (phenelzine and tranylcypromine). The most common side effects are orthostatic hypotension, headache, insomnia, weight gain, sexual dysfunction, peripheral edema, and afternoon somnolence. Although MAOIs do not have significant affinity for muscarinic receptors, anticholinergic-like side effects are present at the beginning of treatment. Dry mouth is common but not as marked as in TCA therapy. Fortunately, the more serious side effects, such as hypertensive crisis and serotonin syndrome, are not common.

Transdermal selegiline was generally well tolerated in controlled trials; common adverse events included headache, insomnia, diarrhea, dry mouth, dyspepsia, and rash (EMSAM 2006). The most commonly reported treatment-emergent adverse event was application site reaction, which was generally mild to moderate in most cases. The rates of most adverse events were similar between transdermal selegiline and placebo, with a local skin site reaction occurring significantly more frequently with the transdermal selegiline compared with placebo (Bodkin and Amsterdam 2002).

**Hypertensive crisis.** Inactivation of intestinal MAO impairs the metabolism of tyramine. Tyramine can act as a false transmitter and displace norepinephrine from presynaptic storage granules. Therefore, large amounts of dietary tyramine can result in a hypertensive crisis in patients taking MAOIs, because increased amounts of norepinephrine are displaced from adrenergic terminals, resulting in profound α-adrenergic activation. This reaction has also been called the "cheese reaction" because tyramine is present in relatively high concentrations in aged cheeses.

**TABLE 30–5.  Dietary and medication restrictions for patients taking nonselective monoamine oxidase inhibitors (MAOIs)**

## Foods to avoid while taking an MAOI and for 2 weeks after discontinuing the medication[a]

| | |
|---|---|
| Aged cheeses | Sauerkraut |
| Aged or fermented meats (e.g., sausage, salami, pepperoni) | Soy sauce |
| All foods that may be spoiled | Tap beer, including nonalcoholic tap beer |
| Fava beans and broad bean pods | Yeast extracts (e.g., Marmite) |
| Meat extracts (e.g., Bovril) | |

## Safe foods

| | |
|---|---|
| Alcohol (but not tap beer), in moderation | Fresh yogurt |
| Fresh cheeses (e.g., cream cheese, cottage cheese, ricotta cheese, American cheese, moderate amounts of mozzarella) | Smoked salmon and whitefish |
| | Yeast and baked goods containing yeast |

## Drugs to avoid while taking an MAOI and for 2 weeks after discontinuing the medication

*All sympathomimetic and stimulant drugs*

| | |
|---|---|
| Amphetamines | Local anesthetic drugs containing epinephrine or cocaine |
| Buspirone | Meperidine |
| Diet medications | Methylphenidate |
| Ephedrine | Other antidepressant medications |
| Fenfluramine and dexfenfluramine | Phenylephrine |
| Isoproterenol | Phenylpropanolamine |
| Levodopa and dopamine | |

*Over-the-counter nasal decongestants; cold, sinus, and allergy medications containing pseudoephedrine, phenylephrine, or phenylpropanolamine; and supplements*

| | |
|---|---|
| Actifed | NyQuil |
| Alka-Seltzer Plus | Robitussin PE, DM, CF, Night Relief |
| Allerest | Sine-Aid |
| Contac | Sine-Off |
| Coricidin D | Sinex |
| CoTylenol | St. John's wort |
| Dristan | Triaminic |
| L-Tryptophan | Tylenol (other than plain) |
| Neo-Synephrine | Vicks 44M, 44D |

*Other medications*

| | |
|---|---|
| Carbamazepine | Oxcarbazepine |

## Safe cold and allergy medications

| | |
|---|---|
| Alka-Seltzer (plain) | Robitussin (plain) |
| Chlor-Trimeton Allergy (without decongestant) | Tylenol (plain) |

## Other safe medications

| | |
|---|---|
| Antibiotics | Local anesthetics without epinephrine or cocaine |
| Codeine | Morphine |
| Laxatives and stool softeners | Nonsteroidal anti-inflammatory drugs |

[a]Food restrictions based on tyramine content data from Walker et al. 1996.
[b]It is strongly advised that the reader consult the current *Physicians' Desk Reference* before prescribing any medication in combination with an MAOI.
*Source.*  EMSAM 2006; Feinberg and Holzer 1997, 2000; Gardner et al. 1996; Physicians' Desk Reference 2006; Shulman and Walker 1999, 2000; Shulman et al. 1997; Walker et al. 1996, 1997; Wing and Chen 1997. Adapted from Marangell LB, Martinez JM: *Concise Guide to Psychopharmacology,* 2nd Edition. Washington, DC, American Psychiatric Publishing, 2006, pp. 48–50. Used with permission.

Tyramine is formed in foods by the decarboxylation of tyrosine during the aging, ripening, or decaying process of foods. Patients receiving MAOIs should be instructed to avoid the foods listed in Table 30–5. Fresh unaged cheeses (such as cottage cheese, ricotta, and cream cheese) are safe. Several foods that were formerly considered dangerous are no longer on the list of prohibited substances. For example, domestic bottled or canned beer is now considered safe when consumed in moderation (Gardner et al. 1996). However, tap beer, including nonalcoholic tap beer, continues to be considered dangerous. Most wines and liquors are also considered safe when drunk in moderation. Caffeine and chocolate are of concern when consumed in large amounts.

Some drugs with sympathomimetic activity, including certain decongestants and cough syrups, should be avoided because they may precipitate a hypertensive crisis (see Table 30–5). However, pure antihistaminic drugs, such as diphenhydramine, and pure expectorants without dextromethorphan, such as guaifenesin, are permissible.

A patient with a mild reaction may complain of sweating, palpitations, and a slight headache. The most severe reaction manifests as a hypertensive crisis, with severe headache, increased blood pressure, and possible intracerebral hemorrhage. If a patient taking an MAOI experiences a severe headache, he or she should seek immediate medical evaluation.

Patients taking MAOIs are advised to carry identification cards that indicate that they are taking MAOIs. Before accepting any medication or anesthetic, patients should notify their physicians that they are taking MAOIs. When patients undergo dental procedures, local anesthetics without vasoconstrictors (e.g., epinephrine) must be used.

**Serotonin syndrome.**  The combination of serotonergic drugs, such as SSRIs, with MAOIs can result in a potentially fatal hypermetabolic reaction, often referred to as the *serotonin syndrome*. Affected individuals may experience lethargy, restlessness, confusion, flushing, diaphoresis, tremor, and myoclonic jerks. As the condition progresses, hyperthermia, hypertonicity, myoclonus, and death may occur. The syndrome must be identified as rapidly as possible. Discontinuation of the serotonergic medications is the first step in treatment, followed by emergency medical treatment as required.

The combination of MAOIs with meperidine, and perhaps with other phenylpiperidine analgesics, also has been implicated in fatal reactions attributed to the serotonin syndrome. Aspirin, nonsteroidal anti-inflammatory drugs, and acetaminophen should be used for mild to moderate pain. Of the narcotic agents, codeine and morphine are safe in combination with MAOIs, although doses may need to be lower than usual.

**Cardiovascular effects.**  The MAOIs cause significant hypotension, which is often their dose-limiting side effect. Expansion of intravascular volume through administration of salt tablets or fludrocortisone may be an effective treatment.

**Weight gain.**  MAOIs are associated with a risk of significant weight gain during treatment.

**Sexual dysfunction.**  MAOIs are commonly associated with treatment-emergent sexual dysfunction, including decreased libido, delayed ejaculation, anorgasmia, and impotence.

**CNS effects.**  Headache and insomnia are common initial side effects that usually disappear after the first few weeks of treatment.

### Overdose

Most complications related to MAOI overdose arise from the drugs' stimulation of the sympathetic nervous system. MAOIs are most dangerous when patients experience hypertensive crises as the result of ingesting foods with high tyramine content.

### Drug Interactions

Inhibition of MAO can cause severe interactions with other drugs, as detailed in the "Hypertensive Crisis" and "Serotonin Syndrome" subsections earlier in this section. A list of some drugs that interact with the nonselective MAOIs is provided in Table 30–5.

## Discontinuation of Antidepressants

Discontinuation of antidepressant medication should be concordant with the guidelines for treatment duration. It is advisable to taper the dose while monitoring for signs and symptoms of relapse. Abrupt discontinuation is also more likely to lead to antidepressant discontinuation symptoms, often referred to as *withdrawal symptoms*. The occurrence of these symptoms after medication discontinuation does not imply that antidepressants are addictive.

Discontinuation symptoms appear to occur most commonly after discontinuation of short-half-life serotonergic drugs (Coupland et al. 1996), such as fluvoxamine, paroxetine, and venlafaxine. Patients describe symptoms as "flulike," including nausea, diarrhea, insomnia, malaise, muscle aches, anxiety, irritability, dizziness, vertigo, and vivid dreams (Coupland et al. 1996). Patients also may experience transient "electric shock" sensations. This unique symptom is diagnostically useful and strongly suggests to the clinician that the patient is experiencing antidepressant discontinuation symptoms, because the symptom rarely occurs in other conditions or as a side effect of a new medication.

Discontinuation symptoms usually occur within 1–2 days after abrupt discontinuation of a medication and subside within 7–10 days. In some instances, symptoms also may occur during tapering and dose reduction, and they may persist for up to 3 weeks. Restarting treatment with the medication and then tapering more slowly may be necessary, although it is often possible to attenuate withdrawal symptoms produced by short-half-life SSRIs by administering one dose of fluoxetine (which has a longer half-life).

## Antidepressant Switching

Particular care must be exercised when switching from an MAOI to other antidepressant classes. In patients who have completed an MAOI trial without achieving a therapeutic response, treatment with other antidepressants should not be started until 14 days after discontinuation of the original MAOI. Equal care is required when switching from most other antidepressants to an MAOI. An interval equal to five times the half-life of the drug, including active metabolites, is required between stopping treatment with other antidepressant medications and starting MAOI therapy. A 2-week interval is also recommended when switching from phenelzine to tranylcypromine because tranylcypromine is an amphetamine derivative.

Switching from one SSRI or SNRI to another can be accomplished by a direct switch from one medication to the next. Although abrupt discontinuation of SSRIs or SNRIs, particularly those with short half-lives, may be associated with discontinuation effects (Rosenbaum et al. 1998), such effects generally are not seen if another medication is substituted that also inhibits the serotonin reuptake pump. Although both agents will be present until a time equal to five times the half-life of the first medication, this is not usually a problem in practice. Similarly, higher levels of either medication may occur if one or both medications inhibit cytochrome P450 enzymes

(e.g., paroxetine or fluoxetine). This may lead to transient side effects, but it is not usually a safety issue. In most cases, a direct switch from one medication to another is better tolerated than a washing out of the first agent. Although cross-tapering may be useful when medications with different receptor effects are used (e.g., an SSRI and bupropion or mirtazapine), this strategy is not useful when both medications are SSRIs.

# Anxiolytics, Sedatives, and Hypnotics

## Overview

Anxiety and insomnia are prevalent symptoms with multiple etiologies. Effective treatments are available, but they vary by diagnosis. In most instances, the best course of action is to treat the underlying disorder rather than reflexively instituting treatment with a nonspecific anxiolytic.

In some cases, anxiolytics serve a transitional purpose. For example, for a patient with acute-onset panic disorder, severe anticipatory anxiety, and a family history of depression, administration of an antidepressant medication that also has antipanic effects may be the optimal treatment, but this will not help the patient for several weeks, during which time there is a risk of progression to agoraphobia. For this patient, starting antidepressant therapy and also attempting to obtain acute symptom relief with a benzodiazepine may be helpful. After 4 weeks, the benzodiazepine dose should be slowly tapered so that the patient's condition is controlled with the antidepressant alone.

In this section, we review the pharmacology of medications that are primarily classified as anxiolytic, sedative, or hypnotic agents. Diagnosis-specific treatment guidelines are outlined in Table 30–6. Common anxiolytics and hypnotics are shown in Table 30–7.

## Benzodiazepines

### Mechanisms of Action

Benzodiazepines facilitate inhibition by γ-aminobutyric acid (GABA), a major inhibitory neurotransmitter in the brain (reviewed by Tallman et al. 1980). The benzodiazepine receptor is a subtype of the $GABA_A$ receptor. Activation of the benzodiazepine receptor facilitates the action of endogenous GABA, which results in the opening of chloride ion channels and a decrease in neuronal excitability.

**TABLE 30–6. Medications for the treatment of major anxiety disorders**

| Anxiety disorder | Medication options |
| --- | --- |
| Generalized anxiety disorder | Buspirone, benzodiazepines, venlafaxine, SSRIs[a] |
| Obsessive-compulsive disorder | Clomipramine, SSRIs[b] |
| Panic disorder | SSRIs,[c] TCAs, MAOIs, benzodiazepines |
| Performance anxiety | β-Blockers, benzodiazepines |
| Social phobia | SSRIs,[d] venlafaxine, MAOIs, benzodiazepines, buspirone |

*Note.* MAOIs=monoamine oxidase inhibitors; SSRIs=selective serotonin reuptake inhibitors; TCAs=tricyclic antidepressants.
[a]SSRIs currently approved by the U.S. Food and Drug Administration (FDA) for the treatment of generalized anxiety disorder include paroxetine and escitalopram.
[b]SSRIs currently approved by the FDA for the treatment of obsessive-compulsive disorder include paroxetine, sertraline, and fluoxetine.
[c]SSRIs currently approved by the FDA for the treatment of panic disorder include paroxetine, sertraline, and fluoxetine.
[d]SSRIs currently approved by the FDA for the treatment of social phobia include paroxetine and sertraline.
*Source.* Adapted from Marangell LB, Martinez JM: *Concise Guide to Psychopharmacology*, 2nd Edition. Washington, DC, American Psychiatric Publishing, 2006, p. 70. Used with permission.

## Indications and Efficacy

Benzodiazepines are highly effective anxiolytics and sedatives. They also have muscle relaxant, amnestic, and anticonvulsant properties. Benzodiazepines effectively treat acute and chronic generalized anxiety and panic disorder. The high-potency benzodiazepines alprazolam and clonazepam have received more attention as antipanic agents, but double-blind studies also have confirmed the efficacy of diazepam and lorazepam in the treatment of panic disorder. Although only a few benzodiazepines are specifically approved by the FDA for the treatment of insomnia, almost all benzodiazepines may be used for this purpose. Benzodiazepines are most clearly valuable as hypnotics in the hospital setting, where high levels of sensory stimulation, pain, and acute stress may interfere with sleep. The safe, effective, and time-limited use of benzodiazepine hypnotics may, in fact, prevent chronic sleep difficulties (NIMH/NIH Consensus Development Conference Statement 1985). Benzodiazepines are also used to treat akathisia and catatonia and as adjuncts in the treatment of acute mania.

Because alcohol and barbiturates also act, in part, via the $GABA_A$ receptor–mediated chloride ion channel, benzodiazepines show cross-tolerance with these substances. Thus, benzodiazepines are used frequently for treating alcohol or barbiturate withdrawal and detoxification. Alcohol and barbiturates are more dangerous than benzodiazepines because they can act directly at the chloride ion channel at higher doses. In contrast, benzodiazepines have no direct effect on the ion channel; the effects of benzodiazepines are limited by the amount of endogenous GABA.

## Benzodiazepine Selection

At equipotent doses, all benzodiazepines have similar effects. The choice of benzodiazepine is generally based on half-life, rapidity of onset, metabolism, and potency. In patients with moderate to severe hepatic dysfunction, it may be useful to avoid benzodiazepines. All benzodiazepines are metabolized at various levels by the liver, which leads to an increased risk of sedation and confusion in patients with hepatic failure. If it is necessary to prescribe this class of medication, lorazepam and oxazepam are reasonable choices because their elimination will not be significantly affected (Abernethy et al. 1984).

## Risks, Side Effects, and Their Management

**Sedation and impairment of performance.** Benzodiazepine-induced sedation may be considered either a therapeutic action or a side effect. When a patient takes a benzodiazepine at night, particularly an agent with a long half-life, residual sedation may be present on awakening. Additionally, any benzodiazepine has the potential to cause sedation.

**Dependence, withdrawal, and rebound effects.** Most benzodiazepines have a low abuse potential when they are properly prescribed and their use is supervised (American Psychiatric Association 1990). However, physical dependence often occurs when benzodiazepines are taken at higher-than-usual doses or for prolonged periods.

If benzodiazepines are discontinued precipitously, withdrawal effects (including hyperpyrexia, seizures, psychosis, and even death) may occur. Signs and symptoms of with-

TABLE 30–7.    Commonly used anxiolytic and hypnotic agents

| Generic drug | Proprietary name | Dose equivalence (mg) | Typical starting dose in adults[a] (mg) | Typical daily dosage range in adults[a] (mg/day) |
|---|---|---|---|---|
| **Anxiolytic medications** | | | | |
| *Benzodiazepines used as anxiolytics* | | | | |
| Alprazolam | Xanax | 0.5 | 0.25–0.5 tid (0.5 tid for panic) | 0.75–4 (divided) (1–6 for panic) |
| Alprazolam extended-release | Xanax XR | NA | 0.5–1 | 3–6 |
| Chlordiazepoxide | Librium | 10 | 5–25 tid or qid | 15–100 (divided tid or qid) |
| Clonazepam | Klonopin | 0.25 | 0.25 bid | 1–4 |
| Clorazepate | Tranxene | 7.5 | 15 (T-tab) | T-tab: 15–60 (divided) SD: 22.5 qd to replace T-tab 7.5 tid |
| Diazepam | Valium | 5 | 2–10 bid–qid | 4–40 (divided) |
| Lorazepam | Ativan | 1 | 0.5–2 tid–qid | 2–4 (divided) |
| Oxazepam | Serax | 15 | 10–30 tid–qid | 30–120 (divided) |
| *Nonbenzodiazepines used as anxiolytics* | | | | |
| Buspirone | BuSpar | NA | 10–30 (divided) | 30–60 (divided) |
| **Hypnotic medications** | | | | |
| *Benzodiazepines used as anxiolytics* | | | | |
| Estazolam | ProSom | — | 1 | 1–2 |
| Flurazepam | Dalmane | — | 15–30 | 15–30 |
| Quazepam | Doral | — | 7.5–15 | 7.5–15 |
| Temazepam | Restoril | — | 15 | 15–30 |
| Triazolam | Halcion | — | 0.125 | 0.125–0.25 |
| *Nonbenzodiazepine GABA–benzodiazepine receptor agonists used as hypnotics* | | | | |
| Eszopiclone | Lunesta | NA | 2 | 2–3 |
| Zaleplon | Sonata | NA | 5–10 | 5–10 |
| Zolpidem | Ambien | NA | 5–10 | 5–10 |
| Zolpidem extended-release | Ambien CR | NA | 12.5 | 6.25–12.5 |
| *Nonbenzodiazepine melatonin $MT_1$ and $MT_2$ receptor agonists used as hypnotics* | | | | |
| Ramelteon | Rozerem | NA | 8 | 8 |

*Note.*    bid=twice-daily dosing; qd=once-daily dosing; qid=four-times-per-day dosing; tid=three-times-per-day dosing; CR=extended release; GABA=γ-aminobutyric acid; NA=not applicable; SD=single dose; T-tab=T-shaped tablet.
[a]The typical starting doses are for healthy adults. Special populations, such as the elderly, debilitated, or hepatically or renally impaired, may require lower doses or may preclude the use of certain agents.
*Source.*    Drug Facts and Comparisons 2002; Fuller and Sajatovic 2004, p. 1420; Jenkins et al. 2001; Nishino et al. 2004; Physicians' Desk Reference 2006; Pies 1998; Shader and Greenblatt 2003.

drawal may include tachycardia, increased blood pressure, muscle cramps, anxiety, insomnia, panic attacks, impairment of memory and concentration, perceptual disturbances, and delirium. In addition, withdrawal-related derealization, hallucinations, and other psychotic symptoms may occur. These withdrawal symptoms may begin as early as the day after discontinuation of the benzodiazepine, and they may continue for weeks to months. Evidence indicates that withdrawal reactions associated with shorter-half-life benzodiazepines peak more rapidly and more intensely. These withdrawal symptoms may be alleviated by reintroducing the withdrawn benzodiazepine.

Rebound anxiety and insomnia also may occur when benzodiazepines are abruptly discontinued. As a general rule, most psychoactive medications should be discontinued gradually, not abruptly. For patients who have been taking benzodiazepines for longer than 2–3 months, the benzodiazepine dose should be decreased by approximately 10% per week. Therefore, in the case of a patient receiving alprazolam 4 mg/day, the dose should be tapered by 0.5 mg/week for 8 weeks.

**Memory impairment.** Benzodiazepines are associated with anterograde amnesia, especially when they are administered intravenously and in high doses (Dixon et al. 1984; Lucki et al. 1986; Reitan et al. 1986).

**Disinhibition and dyscontrol.** Anecdotal reports suggest that benzodiazepines may occasionally cause paradoxical anger and behavioral disinhibition (see review by Rothschild 1992). A history of hostility, impulsivity, or borderline or antisocial personality disorder is a potential predictor of this reaction.

### Overdose

Benzodiazepines are remarkably safe in overdose when taken alone. Dangerous effects occur when the overdose includes several sedative drugs, especially alcohol, because of synergistic effects at the chloride ion site and resultant membrane hyperpolarization. In an emergency setting, the benzodiazepine antagonist flumazenil may be given intravenously to reverse the effects of a potential overdose of a benzodiazepine.

### Drug Interactions

Most sedative drugs, including narcotics and alcohol, potentiate the sedative effects of benzodiazepines. In addition, medications that inhibit hepatic CYP3A3/4 increase blood levels and hence side effects of clonazepam, alpraz-

olam, midazolam, and triazolam. Lorazepam, oxazepam, and temazepam are not dependent on hepatic enzymes for metabolism; thus, cytochrome P450 enzyme inhibition should not significantly affect these particular benzodiazepines.

### Use in Pregnancy

Anxiolytics, like most medications, should be avoided during pregnancy and breast-feeding when possible. There have been concerns that benzodiazepines, when administered during the first trimester of pregnancy, may increase the risk of malformations, particularly cleft palate. Pooled data from cohort studies do not support an increased risk, but data from case-control studies do suggest a risk (Rosenberg et al. 1983). Until further data are available, a high-quality ultrasound should be considered for women who have used benzodiazepines in the first trimester (Dolovich et al. 1998).

## Buspirone

### Background

Buspirone is a partial agonist at 5-HT$_{1A}$ receptors. It is important to note that buspirone does not interact with the GABA receptor or chloride ion channels. Therefore, it does not produce sedation, interact with alcohol, impair psychomotor performance, or pose a risk of abuse. Like the antidepressants, buspirone has a relatively slow onset of action.

### Indications and Efficacy

Buspirone is effective in the treatment of generalized anxiety. Although the onset of therapeutic action is less rapid, buspirone's efficacy is not statistically different from that of benzodiazepines (Cohn and Wilcox 1986; Goldberg and Finnerty 1979). Despite its success in the treatment of generalized anxiety disorder, buspirone does not appear to be effective against panic disorder (Sheehan et al. 1990). Buspirone is also used as an augmenting agent in the treatment of OCD (Harvey and Balon 1995; Laird 1996) and depression (Sramek et al. 1996; Trivedi et al. 2006), and some evidence suggests that buspirone therapy may be an effective treatment for social phobia (Munjack et al. 1991; Schneier et al. 1992).

### Clinical Use

The usual initial dosage is 7.5 mg twice a day, increased after 1 week to 15 mg twice a day. The dose may then be increased as needed to achieve optimal therapeutic re-sponse. The usual recommended maximum daily dose is 60 mg. Because buspirone is metabolized by the liver and excreted by the kidneys, it should not be administered to patients with severe hepatic or renal impairment.

### Side Effects

The side effects that are more common with buspirone therapy than with benzodiazepine therapy are nausea, headache, nervousness, insomnia, dizziness, and light-headedness (Rakel 1990). Restlessness also has been reported.

### Overdose

No fatal outcomes of buspirone overdose have been reported. However, overdose of buspirone with other drugs may result in more serious outcomes.

### Drug Interactions

Buspirone is metabolized by CYP3A3/4. Therefore, the initial dose should be lower in patients who are also taking medications known to inhibit this enzyme. Additionally, buspirone should not be administered in combination with an MAOI.

## Zolpidem and Zaleplon

Zolpidem and zaleplon are hypnotics that act at the omega-1 receptor of the central $GABA_A$ receptor com-plex. This selectivity is hypothesized to be associated with a lower risk of dependence. Unlike benzodiazepines, zolpidem and zaleplon do not appear to have significant anxiolytic, muscle relaxant, or anticonvulsant properties. However, amnestic effects may occur.

### Indications and Efficacy

Zolpidem is a short-acting hypnotic with established effi-cacy in inducing and maintaining sleep. Because of the short half-life of this drug, most patients taking zolpidem report minimal daytime sedation. Zaleplon is an ultra-short-acting hypnotic; minimal residual sedative effects are seen 4 hours after administration.

### Clinical Use

Both zolpidem and zaleplon are available in 5- and 10-mg tablets for oral administration. The maximum recom-mended dosages for adults are 10 mg/day and 20 mg/day,

respectively, administered at night. The initial dose for elderly persons should not exceed 5 mg. Caution is ad-vised in patients with hepatic dysfunction. In general, hypnotics should be limited to short-term use, with re-evaluation for more extended therapy. Zolpidem XL is available in 6.25- and 12.5-mg tablets. The recommended dose for adults is 12.5 mg before sleep (6.25 mg for eld-erly patients).

### Side Effects

In general, side effects of zolpidem and zaleplon are sim-ilar to those of short-acting benzodiazepines. These agents should not be considered free of abuse potential.

### Overdose

Both zolpidem and zaleplon appear to be nonfatal in overdose. However, overdoses in combination with other CNS depressant agents pose a greater risk. Recommended treatment consists of general symptomatic and supportive measures, including gastric lavage. Use of flumazenil may be helpful.

### Drug Interactions

Research on drug interactions is limited, but any drug with CNS depressant effects could potentially enhance the CNS depressant effects of zolpidem and zaleplon through pharmacodynamic interactions. In addition, zolpidem is primarily metabolized by CYP3A3/4, and zaleplon is par-tially metabolized by CYP3A3/4. Thus, inhibitors of these enzymes may increase blood levels and the toxicity of zolpidem.

## Ramelteon

Ramelteon is a hypnotic medication with melatonin receptor agonist activity targeting melatonin $MT_1$ and $MT_2$ receptors. It has not been proven to induce depen-dence. No appreciable activity on serotonin, dopamine, GABA, or acetylcholine occurs with the parent com-pound, but in vitro studies report that ramelteon's pri-mary metabolite, M-II, has weak $5\text{-}HT_{2B}$ receptor ago-nist activity.

### Indications and Efficacy

Ramelteon is indicated for the treatment of insomnia. Because its half-life is 1–2.6 hours, this medication is not thought to be associated with daytime sedation.

## Clinical Use

Ramelteon is available in 8-mg tablets for oral administration. The current maximum dosage is 8 mg administered at night. Ramelteon should be used with caution in elderly patients because plasma levels were twice those in healthy adults in clinical trials. Ramelteon should not be used by patients with severe hepatic impairment.

## Side Effects

Common side effects include somnolence, dizziness, and fatigue. Additionally, ramelteon has been associated with decreased testosterone levels and increased prolactin levels. To date, trials of ramelteon have not indicated high abuse potential with this medication.

## Overdose

Supportive measures are recommended if overdose occurs. Gastric lavage also should be considered.

## Drug Interactions

Ramelteon is metabolized by hepatic metabolism; CYP1A2 is the major isoenzyme involved. Caution is recommended with other inhibitory agents such as fluvoxamine. Ramelteon is also metabolized, to a lesser extent, by CYP2C9 and CYP3A4; thus, additional caution is warranted with medications that affect these cytochrome P450 enzymes.

## Eszopiclone

Eszopiclone is a hypnotic agent that is thought to act on GABA receptor complexes close to benzodiazepine receptors.

### Indications and Efficacy

Eszopiclone has a half-life of approximately 6 hours and is indicated for the treatment of insomnia.

### Clinical Use

Eszopiclone is available in 1-, 2-, and 3-mg tablets for oral administration. The maximum recommended dose is 3 mg/night. In the elderly, this dose is reduced to a maximum of 2 mg. No evidence of tolerance or dependence has been reported, but long-term use should be approached with caution. In addition, eszopiclone should be used cautiously in patients with substance abuse because clinical trials have shown euphoric effects at high doses.

### Side Effects

Dizziness, headache, and unpleasant taste were the most commonly reported side effects in patients taking eszopiclone in clinical trials (Lunesta 2005).

### Overdose

No fatalities have been reported with up to 36 mg being taken in overdose. Overdose symptoms include impairment in consciousness, including somnolence or coma. Treatment is symptom-driven and supportive. Flumazenil may be beneficial.

### Drug Interactions

Eszopiclone is metabolized in the liver by CYP3A4. Eszopiclone should not be used in patients with severe hepatic impairment. Dose adjustment and caution are recommended when prescribing eszopiclone to patients taking enzyme inhibitors such as ketoconazole, ciprofloxacin, erythromycin, isoniazid, or nefazodone. The use of other sedative-hypnotics is not recommended with administration of this medication.

# Antipsychotic Medications

## Background

Antipsychotic medications, previously referred to as *major tranquilizers* or *neuroleptics,* are effective for the treatment of a variety of psychotic symptoms. Antipsychotics can be classified in several ways. One classification system is based on chemical structure; for example, phenothiazines and butyrophenones make up two chemical classes. We use the term *conventional* to signify older or first-generation antipsychotic drugs—to differentiate them from newer *atypical* or second-generation antipsychotics. Among the conventional antipsychotics, we distinguish between high- and low-potency agents because the level of potency predicts side effects. Although the term *atypical antipsychotic* lacks a single consistent definition, it generally refers to the newer antipsychotic medications that affect both 5-HT$_2$ and D$_2$ receptors. Atypical antipsychotics available in the United States include clozapine, olanzapine, risperidone, quetiapine, ziprasidone, and aripiprazole.

The favorable neurological side-effect profile of atypical antipsychotics led to their use as first-line agents for the treatment of psychosis. Additionally, atypical antipsychotics as a class were often considered to be more effective than conventional antipsychotics. As discussed later in this section, superior efficacy has clearly been documented for clozapine but not necessarily for all agents in the class (Lieberman et al. 2005). Although neurological side effects are less frequent with atypical antipsychotics compared with conventional agents, atypical antipsychotics may place some patients at risk for medical morbidity resulting from weight gain and adverse metabolic effects.

## Mechanisms of Action

All available antipsychotics antagonize $D_2$ receptors in vitro. However, the theory that psychosis results from hyperdopaminergia is overly simplistic. Underactivity of dopamine in mesocortical pathways, specifically those projecting to the frontal lobes, may account for the negative symptoms of schizophrenia (e.g., anergia, apathy, lack of spontaneity) (Davis et al. 1991; Goff and Evins 1998). In addition, this underactivity in the frontal lobes may serve to disinhibit mesolimbic dopamine activity via a corticolimbic feedback loop. Overactivity of mesolimbic dopamine is the result, which manifests as the positive symptoms of schizophrenia (e.g., hallucinations, delusions).

The atypical antipsychotics have other physiological properties as well, some of which appear to relate to antagonism of the 5-$HT_2$ receptor, which may modify dopamine activity in a regionally specific manner. This dual 5-$HT_2$/$D_2$ antagonism is believed to account, at least in part, for the unique properties of this group of medications. An additional hypothesis is that the atypical antipsychotic medications have a lower liability for EPS because they have looser binding to the $D_2$ receptor (Kapur and Seeman 2001).

## Indications and Efficacy

The most common indications for antipsychotic drugs are the treatment of acute psychosis and the maintenance of psychotic symptom remission in patients with schizophrenia. All conventional antipsychotics have comparable efficacy in schizophrenia when given in equivalent doses (Table 30–8) but differ somewhat in their propensity for some side effects. The atypical antipsychotics appear to be at least as effective as the conventional antipsychotics in the treatment of schizophrenia (Glick and Marder 2005; Goff et al. 1998), but they differ with respect to their tolerability profiles. Clozapine has shown efficacy in patients with schizophrenia after nonresponse to one or more

antipsychotic medication trials, including other atypical antipsychotics (Kane 1996; Lewis et al. 2006; McEvoy et al. 2006).

Atypical antipsychotics also have become a key part of the pharmacological armamentarium to treat bipolar disorder. Indeed, all atypical antipsychotics (except clozapine) are approved by the FDA for the treatment of acute mania. Additionally, olanzapine and aripiprazole are approved as maintenance treatments for bipolar disorder. As of September 2007, olanzapine/fluoxetine combination therapy (marketed in the United States under the trade name Symbyax) and quetiapine are the only medications approved by the FDA specifically for the treatment of acute bipolar depressive episodes.

Antipsychotic drugs also effectively target psychotic symptoms associated with drug intoxications, delusional disorders, and nonspecific agitation, although the data supporting their use in these conditions are limited. In addition, low doses of antipsychotics may be effective in some patients with borderline or schizotypal personality disorders, particularly when psychotic ideation is targeted (Oldham 2005). In patients with severe OCD, antipsychotics have been used to augment treatment with antiobsessional agents. Antipsychotics and other drugs with dopamine receptor–blocking action (e.g., metoclopramide) are also used for their antiemetic effect. Gilles de la Tourette's syndrome also may be controlled with antipsychotic agents.

## Clinical Use

### Medication Selection

The choice of antipsychotic medication is often determined, in part, by its safety and tolerability profiles. The prescribing clinician should engage the patient in a discussion of available treatment options and their potential for both short- and long-term side effects. Clozapine is generally reserved for patients with refractory illness, particularly for patients whose symptoms have failed to respond to two or more antipsychotic medication trials (Lewis et al. 2006), because of the risk of agranulocytosis.

A useful construct for conceptualizing differences in side-effect profiles for the conventional antipsychotics is the concept of "high potency" versus "low potency." *Drug potency* refers to the milligram equivalence of drugs. For example, although haloperidol is more potent than chlorpromazine (haloperidol 2 mg=chlorpromazine 100 mg), therapeutically equivalent doses are equally effective (haloperidol 12 mg=chlorpromazine 600 mg). As a rule, for conventional antipsychotics only, the high-potency antipsychotic drugs

**TABLE 30–8.** Commonly used atypical and conventional antipsychotic drugs

| Generic drug name | Trade name | Usual adult daily dose (mg) | Formulations for administration | Available oral doses (mg) | Approximate oral dose equivalents (mg) |
|---|---|---|---|---|---|
| **Atypical antipsychotics** | | | | | |
| Aripiprazole | Abilify | 15–30 | po, L, ODT | 5, 10, 15, 20, 30; 1 mg/mL | 4 |
| Clozapine | Clozaril | 250–500 | po, ODT | 25, 100 | 100 |
| Olanzapine | Zyprexa | 10–20 | po, ODT, im | 2.5, 5, 7.5, 10, 15, 20 | 4 |
| Paliperidone | Invega | 3–12 | po | 3, 6, 9 | — |
| Quetiapine | Seroquel | 300–600 | po | 25, 100, 200, 300 | 125 |
| Quetiapine extended-release | Seroquel XR | 400–800 | po | 200, 300, 400 | 125 |
| Risperidone | Risperdal | 4–6 | po, L, ODT, D | 0.25, 0.5, 1, 2, 3, 4; 1 mg/mL | 1 |
| Ziprasidone | Geodon | 80–160 | po, im | 20, 40, 60, 80 | 40 |
| **Conventional antipsychotics** | | | | | |
| *Butyrophenones* | | | | | |
| Droperidol | Inapsine | 2.5–10 | im | 2.5 mg/mL | — |
| Haloperidol | Haldol | 5–15 | po, im, D | 0.5, 1, 2, 5, 10, 20 | 2 |
| *Dibenzoxazepines* | | | | | |
| Loxapine | Loxitane | 45–90 | po | 5, 10, 25, 50 | 10 |
| *Dihydroindolones* | | | | | |
| Molindone | Moban | 30–60 | po | 5, 10, 25, 50 | 15 |
| *Phenothiazines* | | | | | |
| Aliphatics | | | | | |
| Chlorpromazine | Thorazine | 300–600 | po, L, im | 10, 25, 50, 100, 200; 100 mg/mL | 100 |
| Piperazines | | | | | |
| Fluphenazine | Prolixin | 5–15 | po, L, im, D | 1, 2.5, 5, 10 | 2 |
| Perphenazine | Trilafon, Etrafon | 32–64 | po, L | 2, 4, 8, 16; 16 mg/mL | 10 |
| Trifluoperazine | Stelazine | 15–30 | po | 1, 2, 5, 10 | 5 |
| Piperidines | | | | | |
| Mesoridazine | Serentil | 150–300 | po | 10, 25, 50, 100 | 50 |
| Thioridazine | Mellaril | 300–600 | po, im | 10, 15, 25, 50, 100 | 100 |
| *Diphenylbutylpiperidine* | | | | | |
| Pimozide | Orap | 2–6 | po | 1, 2 | 2 |
| *Thioxanthenes* | | | | | |
| Thiothixene | Navane | 15–30 | po, L | 1, 2, 5, 10, 20; 5 mg/mL | 4 |

*Note.* po=oral tablets or capsules; L=liquid; ODT=oral disintegrating tablets; im=intramuscular injections; D=decanoate.
*Source.* Equivalent doses from Fuller and Sajatovic 2004, pp. 1440–1441. Adapted from Marangell LB, Martinez JM: *Concise Guide to Psychopharmacology*, 2nd Edition. Washington, DC, American Psychiatric Publishing, 2006, pp. 92–93. Used with permission.

have an equivalent dose of less than 5 mg. Compared with low-potency conventional antipsychotics, the high-potency agents generally have a higher degree of EPS but less sedation, fewer anticholinergic side effects, and less hypotension. Low-potency conventional antipsychotic drugs have an equivalent dose of greater than 40 mg. These drugs have a high level of sedation, anticholinergic side effects, and hypotension but a lower degree of acute EPS. Importantly, tardive dyskinesia rates do not differ between high- and low-potency conventional antipsychotics. Antipsychotic drugs with intermediate potency have a side-effect profile that lies between the profiles of these two groups.

The atypical antipsychotics produce fewer EPS than do conventional antipsychotics, particularly clozapine and quetiapine. Additionally, evidence to date suggests that the atypical agents are associated with lower rates of tardive dyskinesia than are the conventional agents. With the exception of risperidone, the atypical antipsychotics also produce substantially less hyperprolactinemia than do the conventional agents. However, several safety and tolerability issues are associated with atypical antipsychotic medications, including the potential for weight gain and metabolic abnormalities. Weight gain is an important side effect associated to varying degrees with all atypical agents, with less weight gain propensity associated with ziprasidone and aripiprazole.

### Optimal Dosages

High-dosage strategies are no longer recommended because controlled studies found that modest dosages of conventional antipsychotic drugs are as effective as higher dosages and are better tolerated. Several reviews of controlled trials of conventional antipsychotics concluded that the optimal dosage for most patients is between 300 and 600 mg/day of chlorpromazine equivalents, with some patients responding to lower doses and with little benefit found at doses greater than 700 mg/day (Appleton and Davis 1980; Baldessarini et al. 1988; J.M. Davis 1985). General guidelines for the acute use of antipsychotics are shown in Table 30–9.

## Risks, Side Effects, and Their Management

### Extrapyramidal Side Effects

EPS include acute dystonic reactions, parkinsonian syndrome, akathisia, tardive dyskinesia, and neuroleptic malignant syndrome (NMS). Although high-potency conventional antipsychotics are more likely than low-potency conventional antipsychotics to cause EPS, all first-gener-

---

**TABLE 30–9.    Guidelines for the acute use of antipsychotic drugs**

Prior to treatment, obtain a medical and psychiatric history. Baseline laboratory studies are also indicated as part of the initial evaluation. An evaluation for the presence of any abnormal movements is also advisable. An electrocardiogram should be considered for patients with a history of cardiac problems.

After discussion with the patient and family about the risks and benefits of treatment, select the appropriate antipsychotic agent on the basis of the patient's physical status, the side-effect profile of the drug, and the patient's previous responses to medication, if known.

Educate the patient and family about the risks of developing metabolic syndrome, diabetes, obesity, dyslipidemia, neuroleptic malignant syndrome, and tardive dyskinesia. Document this discussion in the patient's chart.

Initiate treatment with antipsychotic medication at low to moderate doses, depending on the patient's history and clinical presentation. Titrate as tolerated to the target dose.

If possible, administer the antipsychotic medication at bedtime to increase adherence and minimize daytime side effects.

If the patient has been compliant with treatment and side effects are minimal but no or minimal response to treatment occurs, increase the dose gradually (e.g., every 2–4 weeks). Full response may be delayed for 6 months or longer.

If the patient still has no response, is taking an adequate dose, and is compliant with treatment, consider another antipsychotic medication.

*Source.*  Lehman et al. 2004. Adapted from Marangell LB, Martinez JM: *Concise Guide to Psychopharmacology*, 2nd Edition. Washington, DC, American Psychiatric Publishing, 2006, p. 96. Used with permission.

---

ation antipsychotic drugs are equally likely to cause tardive dyskinesia. The atypical antipsychotics cause substantially fewer EPS, although careful titration of risperidone is necessary to avoid neurological side effects. Although the use of anticholinergic agents or amantadine may prevent or ameliorate EPS, the use of atypical agents is increasingly recommended to avoid these side effects without introducing additional medications. Long-term use of anticholinergic medications should be minimized because these agents can produce significant side effects, includ-

**TABLE 30–10.** Drugs used to treat extrapyramidal side effects

| Generic drug name | Trade name | Drug type (mechanism) | Usual adult dosage | Indications for extrapyramidal side effects |
|---|---|---|---|---|
| Amantadine | Symmetrel | Dopaminergic agent | 100 mg po bid | Parkinsonian syndrome |
| Benztropine | Cogentin | Anticholinergic agent | 1–2 mg po bid | Dystonia, parkinsonian syndrome |
| | | | 2 mg iv[a] | Acute dystonia |
| Diphenhydramine | Benadryl | Anticholinergic agent | 25–50 mg po tid | Dystonia, parkinsonian syndrome |
| | | | 25 mg im or iv[a] | Acute dystonia |
| Propranolol | Inderal | β-Blocker | 20 mg po tid 1 mg iv | Akathisia |
| Trihexyphenidyl | Artane | Anticholinergic agent | 5–10 mg po bid | Dystonia, parkinsonian syndrome |

*Note.* po=oral administration of tablets or capsules; bid=twice daily; iv=intravenous; tid=three times a day; im=intramuscular.
[a]Follow with oral medication.
*Source.* Adapted from Marangell LB, Martinez JM: *Concise Guide to Psychopharmacology*, 2nd Edition. Washington, DC, American Psychiatric Publishing, 2006, p. 98. Used with permission.

ing impairments of memory and attention. Clozapine appears to be the only agent that does not cause tardive dyskinesia, and data suggest that a reduced risk with the atypical agents is possible (Correll et al. 2004; Jeste et al. 1999; Margolese et al. 2005; Tarsy and Baldessarini 2006; Tollefson et al. 1997).

Acute dystonic reactions are among the most disturbing and acutely disabling adverse reactions that can occur with the administration of antipsychotic drugs. These reactions occur within hours or days of initiation of treatment with a high-potency conventional antipsychotic medication. The uncontrollable tightening of muscles typically involves spasms of the neck, back (opisthotonos), tongue, or muscles that control lateral eye movement (oculogyric crisis). Laryngeal involvement may compromise the airway and result in ventilatory difficulties (stridor). Intravenous or intramuscular administration of anticholinergic medication is a rapid and effective treatment for acute dystonia. The drugs and dosages used to treat dystonic reactions are listed in Table 30–10. Because antipsychotic drugs have long half-lives and durations of action, additional oral anticholinergic drugs should be prescribed for several days after an acute dystonic reaction, or longer if treatment with the antipsychotic drug is continued unchanged. Amantadine, 100 mg twice a day, should be considered for treatment of EPS in elderly patients who are highly sensitive to

anticholinergic activity, particularly if a switch to an atypical agent is not appropriate.

Acute dystonic reactions may be treated prophylactically with anticholinergic medications, such as benztropine 1–2 mg twice a day. Parkinsonian syndrome has many of the features of classic idiopathic Parkinson's disease, including a diminished range of facial expression, cogwheel rigidity, slowed movements, drooling, small handwriting (micrographia), and pill-rolling tremor. This side effect may appear weeks after the initiation of the antipsychotic medication. The most common treatments for idiopathic Parkinson's disease restore the dopamine–acetylcholine balance by increasing dopamine availability. The treatment of antipsychotic medication–related parkinsonism most often involves decreasing the level of acetylcholine (although amantadine, a dopaminergic drug, often effectively attenuates parkinsonian side effects without exacerbating the underlying psychotic illness). Drugs used in the treatment of the parkinsonian side effects of antipsychotic agents are listed in Table 30–10.

The rabbit syndrome, consisting of fine, rapid movements of the lips that resemble the chewing movements of a rabbit, is often considered a subset of parkinsonian side effects. This side effect occurs after more prolonged treatment and may be confused with buccolingual tardive dyskinesia. It has been found in approximately 4% of patients receiving antipsychotics without concomitant anticholinergics (Yassa and Lal 1986). Like parkinsonian side effects, the rabbit syndrome is treated effectively with anticholinergic drugs.

Akinesia is a behavioral state of diminished spontaneity characterized by decreased gestures, unspontaneous speech, apathy, and difficulty with initiating usual activities. Akinesia may appear after several weeks of therapy and is often an element of the parkinsonism syndrome. This drug-induced syndrome may be mistaken for depression or for negative symptoms of schizophrenia.

Akathisia is an extrapyramidal disorder consisting of a subjective feeling of restlessness in the lower extremities, often manifested as an inability to sit still. It is a common reaction that most often occurs shortly after initiation of treatment with a conventional antipsychotic medication or aripiprazole. After a single oral dose of 5 mg of haloperidol, 40% of patients in one study experienced akathisia; this rate increased to 75% after patients received a 10-mg nighttime dose for 1 week (van Putten et al. 1984).

Akathisia is among the most treatment resistant of the acute EPS. Benzodiazepines are helpful in some cases. The current treatment of choice for akathisia is either a switch to an atypical agent (with the exception of aripiprazole) or the addition of a β-adrenergic–blocking drug, particularly propranolol. Several well-controlled studies have documented that propranolol, in dosages up to 120 mg/day, is an effective treatment for akathisia (Adler et al. 1985, 1989; Lipinski et al. 1984). In general, the lipophilic β-blockers are more effective in treating akathisia than the hydrophilic ones.

### Tardive Disorders

Tardive dyskinesia is a disorder characterized by involuntary choreoathetoid movements of the face, trunk, or extremities. The syndrome is usually associated with prolonged exposure to dopamine receptor–blocking agents—most frequently, antipsychotic drugs. However, the antidepressant amoxapine and the antiemetic agents metoclopramide and prochlorperazine can also cause tardive dyskinesia. The American Psychiatric Association Task Force on Tardive Dyskinesia estimated a cumulative incidence of 5% per year of exposure among young adults and a prevalence of 30% after 1 year of treatment with conventional antipsychotics among elderly patients (American Psychiatric Association 1992). Clozapine seems to carry little or no risk of inducing tardive dyskinesia. The incidence of tardive dyskinesia associated with other atypical antipsychotics is higher than that associated with clozapine and lower than that associated with conventional antipsy-

chotics (Correll et al. 2004; Jeste et al. 1999; Tollefson et al. 1997). Elderly patients taking antipsychotics are at increased risk for tardive dyskinesia.

Clinicians can use the Abnormal Involuntary Movement Scale (AIMS) to examine a patient for the presence or emergence of tardive dyskinesia (Guy 1976). An evaluation for abnormal movements should be conducted before treatment begins and every 6 or 12 months thereafter. In typical cases, the patient often is unaware of mild involuntary movements. Severe dyskinetic movements are less common and can be disfiguring or even disabling as a result of affecting the muscles involved in the production of speech or swallowing. Although the most common form of tardive disorder is the dyskinetic variety (nonrhythmic, quick choreiform movements), other types have been identified. These include tardive akathisia, tardive dystonia, and tardive tics.

The most significant and consistently documented risk factor for the development of tardive dyskinesia is increasing age of the patient (Branchey and Branchey 1984; Jeste and Wyatt 1982; Kane and Smith 1982). The duration of exposure to a conventional antipsychotic is also an important factor because the cumulative incidence has been shown to remain constant at about 5% for the first 8 years in nonelderly patients. Women have been found to be at greater risk for severe tardive dyskinesia, although the evidence suggests that this finding is limited to geriatric populations (Kennedy et al. 1971; Seide and Muller 1967). Other risk factors may include EPS early in the course of treatment, a history of drug holidays (a greater number of drug-free periods is associated with an increased risk), the presence of brain damage, diabetes mellitus, and a diagnosis of a mood disorder.

Because antipsychotic medications are the most effective treatment for most patients with schizophrenia, the situation often arises in which a patient develops tardive dyskinesia but still requires an antipsychotic medication to function. If discontinuation of the antipsychotic drug is clinically possible, tardive dyskinesia may gradually diminish; however, involuntary movements often worsen initially with tapering of the antipsychotic dose, a phenomenon referred to as withdrawal-emergent dyskinesia (Glazer et al. 1984). Withdrawal-emergent dyskinesia also may occur when a conventional antipsychotic is replaced with an atypical antipsychotic.

No definitive treatment for tardive dyskinesias has been identified to date. α-Tocopherol (vitamin E) was shown to be of some benefit in several small studies (Adler et al. 1993; Akhtar et al. 1993; Dabiri et al. 1994; Egan et al. 1992; Elkashef et al. 1990; Lohr and Caligiuri 1996;

Lohr et al. 1987), but no benefit was discerned with vitamin E in a Department of Veterans Affairs trial (Adler et al. 1998). Still, vitamin E is a relatively benign antioxidant that may protect neurons from the damaging effects of free radicals, which have been implicated in the etiology of tardive dyskinesia. Despite inconsistent evidence for efficacy, prophylaxis with vitamin E has been recommended. The typical dose of vitamin E is 1,600 IU/day.

Clozapine may be useful for certain patients with tardive dyskinesia who need an antipsychotic medication. In a clinical study by Lieberman et al. (1991), 30 patients with severe tardive dyskinesia were given clozapine at a mean dosage of 486 mg/day for 36 months. On follow-up at 100 weeks, 16 of the 30 patients showed a greater than 50% reduction in their tardive dyskinesia symptoms on the Simpson Dyskinesia Scale, and 10 patients had complete remission. According to the investigators, symptoms did not reemerge over the follow-up period, suggesting that clozapine has a therapeutic effect on tardive dyskinesia that is distinct from the effect of neuroleptics, which only mask the pathology. The study by Lieberman and colleagues seems to confirm the benefits of clozapine on tardive dyskinesia reported in an earlier study by Gerbino et al. (1980).

## Neuroleptic Malignant Syndrome

In rare instances, patients taking antipsychotic medications develop a potentially life-threatening disorder known as NMS. Although it occurs most frequently with the use of high-potency conventional antipsychotic drugs, this condition may appear during treatment with any antipsychotic agent, including atypical antipsychotics. Patients with NMS typically have marked muscle rigidity, although this feature may be absent in patients taking atypical antipsychotics. Other features include fever, autonomic instability, increased white blood cell (WBC) counts (>15,000/mm$^3$), increased creatine kinase levels (>300 U/mL), and delirium. The increased creatine kinase concentrations are the result of muscle breakdown, which can lead to myoglobinuria and acute renal failure.

In a large prospective study, Rosebush and Stewart (1989) found that NMS was associated most often with the initiation or increase of antipsychotic medication, and in every case it occurred within 1 month of admission to a psychiatric unit. Episodes that occurred in patients taking stable dosages of antipsychotic medications were almost always associated with antecedent dehydration. Lithium use increases the risk appreciably, as does the presence of a mood disorder. Higher dosages, rapid escalation of dosage, and intramuscular injections of antipsy-

chotics are all associated with the development of NMS (Keck et al. 1989).

Treatment of NMS includes discontinuation of the antipsychotic medication, a thorough medical evaluation, administration of intravenous fluids and antipyretic agents, and the use of cooling blankets. Rosebush et al. (1989) reviewed 20 cases of patients who developed NMS while taking conventional agents and found that delaying reinitiation of an antipsychotic by at least 2 weeks after resolution of symptoms was associated with a markedly decreased risk of relapse. Dantrolene and bromocriptine have been reported to improve symptoms of NMS, but their efficacy over supportive care has not been proven and is controversial (Rosebush et al. 1991). Bromocriptine is a centrally active dopamine agonist that has been used successfully in some cases of NMS (Guze and Baxter 1985). Bromocriptine is administered at an initial dosage of 1.25–2.5 mg twice daily, and the dosage may be increased to 10 mg three times a day. Rigidity may respond rapidly, but the temperature elevation, blood pressure instability, and creatine kinase level may not normalize for several days. Dantrolene sodium, a drug that is also used to treat malignant hyperthermia, is a muscle relaxant that may reduce the thermogenesis of NMS caused by the tonic contraction of skeletal muscles. The manufacturer's recommendation for administration of dantrolene for acute malignant hyperthermia is 1 mg/kg by rapid intravenous push. Administration of the drug should be continued until the symptoms are reversed or until a maximum dose of 10 mg/kg has been given. The oral dosage of dantrolene after a malignant hyperthermic crisis is 4–8 mg/kg/day in four divided doses. This regimen should be continued until all symptoms resolve. The potential for hepatotoxicity is significant with dantrolene therapy; thus, the drug should not be administered to patients with liver dysfunction.

## Anticholinergic Side Effects

Anticholinergic side effects are categorized as peripheral effects or central effects. The most common peripheral side effects are dry mouth, decreased sweating, decreased bronchial secretions, blurred vision, difficulty with urination, constipation, and tachycardia. Bethanechol chloride, a cholinergic drug that does not cross the blood-brain barrier, may effectively treat these side effects at a dosage of 25–50 mg three times a day. Central side effects of anticholinergic drugs include impairment in concentration, attention, and memory. In cases of toxicity, anticholinergic delirium—which includes hot and dry skin, dry mucous membranes, dilated pupils, absent bowel sounds, tachycardia, and confusion—may occur.

## Adrenergic Side Effects

Antipsychotics block $\alpha_1$-adrenergic receptors, which can result in orthostatic hypotension and dizziness. Orthostatic hypotension is commonly associated with low-potency conventional agents. Among the atypical agents, clozapine, quetiapine, risperidone, and ziprasidone require initial dose titration, particularly in the elderly, to avoid orthostatic hypotension.

## Endocrine Effects

Numerous studies have suggested a relation between the use of atypical antipsychotic medications and the development of hyperglycemia, dyslipidemia, and metabolic syndrome (American Diabetes Association et al. 2004; Citrome et al. 2005). The metabolic syndrome comprises several metabolic risk factors that may be associated with an increased cardiovascular risk. One definition of the metabolic syndrome specifies the presence of three or more of the following five clinical or laboratory features: 1) elevated plasma triglyceride levels ($\geq150$ mg/dL); 2) decreased plasma high-density lipoprotein levels ($<50$ mg/dL in women or $<40$ mg/dL in men); 3) elevated fasting glucose levels ($\geq110$ mg/dL); 4) waist circumference greater than 35 inches in women or greater than 40 inches in men; and 5) elevated blood pressure ($\geq130/85$ mm Hg) (Citrome et al. 2005; Expert Panel on Detection, Evaluation, and Treatment of High Blood Cholesterol in Adults 2001).

Hyperglycemia can develop independent of or secondary to weight gain and, in some cases, resolves after discontinuation of the medication. Patients taking clozapine and olanzapine have a higher risk of developing diabetes compared with patients taking other conventional and atypical antipsychotics (see American Diabetes Association et al. 2004). Data indicate that alterations in serum lipids are concordant with changes in body weight. Clozapine and olanzapine are associated with the greatest increases in total cholesterol, low-density lipoprotein, and triglycerides, as well as decreases in high-density lipoprotein. Aripiprazole and ziprasidone do not appear to be associated with dyslipidemia. However, monitoring should be considered for all patients taking an antipsychotic medication.

The National Institute of Mental Health–funded Clinical Antipsychotic Trials of Intervention Effectiveness (CATIE) randomly assigned patients with schizophrenia to treatment with perphenazine, olanzapine, risperidone, quetiapine, or ziprasidone for up to 18 months (Lieberman et al. 2005). With respect to metabolic outcomes, olanza-pine-treated patients had a higher discontinuation rate as a result of weight gain or metabolic effects, whereas ziprasidone was the only medication associated with improvements in metabolic parameters (Lieberman et al. 2005).

At present, it appears appropriate to monitor all patients taking atypical antipsychotics for metabolic changes. Published guidelines recommend monitoring patients taking atypical antipsychotics for several metabolic risk factors, including personal and family history of metabolic risks (baseline and annually), waist circumference (baseline and annually), body mass index (baseline, week 4, week 8, week 12, and quarterly), blood pressure and fasting glucose levels (baseline, week 12, and annually), and lipid panel (baseline, week 12, and every 5 years) (American Diabetes Association et al. 2004).

All conventional antipsychotic medications and risperidone may cause hyperprolactinemia. Clinical signs and symptoms of hyperprolactinemia may include gynecomastia, galactorrhea, amenorrhea, and decreased libido. Although such side effects were frequently associated with hyperprolactinemia resulting from conventional antipsychotics, a review of clinical experience with risperidone found relatively low rates of side effects despite markedly elevated prolactin levels (Kleinberg et al. 1997). Hyperprolactinemia secondarily can lower estrogen levels, resulting in amenorrhea and theoretically placing patients at risk for osteoporosis and pathological fractures (Klibanski et al. 1981).

## Weight Gain

Both conventional and atypical antipsychotic medications can be associated with weight gain. Antipsychotics associated with weight gain include risperidone, quetiapine, chlorpromazine, thioridazine, olanzapine, and clozapine (Allison et al. 1999; American Diabetes Association et al. 2004); however, all patients taking an antipsychotic medication should be monitored for weight gain throughout treatment.

Allison et al. (1999) analyzed results from all published controlled trials of antipsychotic agents and estimated the mean weight change after 10 weeks of treatment for each agent. The effect of conventional antipsychotics ranged from a mean loss of 0.4 kg with molindone to a mean gain of 3.2 kg with thioridazine. Haloperidol produced a mean 1.1-kg weight gain. Among atypical agents, only ziprasidone produced no change in weight; the other atypical agents were associated with the following estimates of weight gain at 10 weeks: risperidone 2.1 kg, olanzapine 4.15 kg, and clozapine 4.45 kg.

## Sexual Effects

A combination of anticholinergic effects, α-adrenergic receptor blockade, and hormonal effects may lead to several types of sexual difficulty. In men, inability to achieve or maintain erections, decreased ability to achieve orgasm, and changes in the pleasurable quality of orgasm have been reported with conventional agents (Ghadirian et al. 1982). Thioridazine may cause painful retrograde ejaculation, in which semen is ejected into the bladder. Priapism, which necessitates immediate urological consultation, has been reported, especially with thioridazine and chlorpromazine, although atypical agents also have been linked to priapism. Women may experience changes in the quality of orgasm, as well as decreased ability to achieve orgasm, with use of antipsychotics. Because sexual side effects are troubling to patients and often interfere with adherence to treatment, regular assessment by the clinician of sexual side effects is important.

## Ocular Effects

Antipsychotics may cause pigmentary changes in the lens and retina, especially if the drugs are administered for long periods. Pigment deposition in the lens of the eye does not affect vision; however, pigmentary retinopathy, which can lead to irreversible blindness, has been associated specifically with the use of thioridazine. Although pigmentary retinopathy has been reported most often in patients taking more than 800 mg/day of thioridazine (the maximum recommended dose), this condition also has occurred at usual clinical doses (Ball and Caroff 1986; Hamilton 1985).

## Dermatological Effects

Patients taking antipsychotics, especially the aliphatic phenothiazines (e.g., chlorpromazine), may become more sensitive to sunlight, which can lead to severe sunburn.

## Cardiac Effects

In materials submitted to the Psychopharmacological Drugs Advisory Committee of the FDA, Pfizer, Inc., reported results from a trial designed to examine the electrocardiographic effects of atypical agents and thioridazine at maximum therapeutic serum concentrations and at the potentially higher concentrations that might occur in clinical practice if these agents were co-prescribed with metabolic inhibitors. After correcting the QT interval for heart rate, thioridazine produced the greatest mean delay in QTc (35.6 msec), followed by ziprasidone (20.6 msec), quetiapine (9.1 msec), olanzapine (6.8 msec), and halo-

peridol (4.7 msec). Quetiapine produced the greatest increase in heart rate (11 beats/minute). Metabolic inhibitors only produced further increases in QTc when added to quetiapine (19.7 msec) and haloperidol (8.9 msec). Although the mean 39% increase in serum ziprasidone concentrations produced by ketoconazole coadministration did not result in an increase in the mean QTc duration, ziprasidone serum concentrations weakly correlated with QTc duration. In 8 cases of overdose reported by the manufacturer and 1 published case (Burton et al. 2000), ziprasidone did not produce significant cardiac toxicity. Only 2 of 3,095 subjects (0.06%) in premarketing trials developed QTc intervals longer than 500 ms; however, participants in these trials were screened to exclude cardiac disease. In 2 reports of overdose with quetiapine, prolongation of the QT interval was observed (Gajwani et al. 2000; Hustey 1999), whereas most reported cases of overdose with risperidone and olanzapine have described relatively benign ECG findings. In the CATIE, ziprasidone was not associated with a greater rate of occurrences of prolonged QTc intervals compared with the other antipsychotics studied, and no instances of torsades de pointes were reported (Lieberman et al. 2005).

In several studies, sudden death attributed to thioridazine or chlorpromazine therapy in young, healthy patients has been reported (Aherwadkar et al. 1974; Giles and Modlin 1968). Thioridazine slows atrial and ventricular conduction and prolongs refractory periods. Thus, thioridazine can be quite dangerous if taken in overdose or in combination with quinidine-like drugs. Chlorpromazine also prolongs QT intervals and atrioventricular conduction, even at relatively low doses (150 mg/day). Pimozide also may produce significant changes in cardiac conduction as a result of its calcium channel–blocking properties. It is recommended that serial ECGs be performed when treatment with pimozide is started, and the drug should be discontinued if the QT interval exceeds 520 msec (in adults) or 470 msec (in children). This strategy should be considered for patients taking thioridazine or ziprasidone, but it is not mandatory in healthy patients. Extremely high doses of intravenous haloperidol have been administered safely in patients with cardiac disease, although rare cases of torsades de pointes have been reported at these doses (Metzger and Friedman 1993).

## Hepatic Effects

Increased levels on liver function tests have been associated with antipsychotic treatment. If abnormalities suggest obstructive liver disease, with increases in bilirubin and alkaline phosphatase, the drug must be immediately discontinued. This reaction appears to be more common with low-potency conventional antipsychotics. Transient elevations in hepatic enzymes have been observed with olanzapine and quetiapine, but these laboratory findings have not been linked to liver injury.

### Hematological Effects

Transient leukopenia and, in rare cases, agranulocytosis have been associated with neuroleptic treatment. Although *agranulocytosis* is strictly defined as a complete absence of all granulocytes in the blood, it also may refer to severe neutropenia, with a neutrophil count of less than 500/mL. This idiosyncratic reaction usually occurs within the first 3–4 weeks after the initiation of treatment with an antipsychotic drug. However, this risk continues for 2–3 months during therapy. A higher risk of agranulocytosis is associated with low-potency conventional antipsychotic drugs and, most significantly, clozapine.

Signs and symptoms of this reaction include high fever, stomatitis, severe pharyngitis, lymphadenopathy, and malaise. Patients should be educated about the signs and symptoms of agranulocytosis and instructed to contact their physician immediately should these symptoms develop.

### Lowered Seizure Threshold

Most conventional antipsychotics are associated with a dose-dependent risk of a lowered seizure threshold, although the incidence of seizures with most of these drugs is quite small. Of all the conventional antipsychotics, molindone and fluphenazine have been shown most consistently to have the lowest potential for this side effect (Itil and Soldatos 1980; Oliver et al. 1982). The atypical antipsychotic clozapine is associated with a dose-dependent risk of seizure and has been estimated to produce seizures in as many as 10% of the patients receiving the drug for 3.8 years.

### Suppressed Temperature Regulation

Antipsychotic drugs directly affect the hypothalamus and suppress temperature regulation. In combination with the α-adrenergic receptor antagonism and cholinergic receptor antagonism of antipsychotics, this effect becomes particularly serious in hot, humid weather. Severe hyperthermia, rhabdomyolysis, renal failure, and death may result. This potentially life-threatening condition requires immediate medical intervention and supportive treatment. A cool environment and adequate amounts of fluids are mandatory for patients taking antipsychotic agents.

### Risks in Elderly Patients With Dementia

Treatment with atypical antipsychotics recently has been associated with an almost twofold increased mortality rate when used in elderly patients with dementia. It is important to note that these medications are often used in clinical practice, but they are not approved by the FDA for the treatment of dementia-related psychosis (Herrmann and Lanctot 2005). The risk associated with atypical antipsychotics is not statistically different from the risk associated with treatment with conventional antipsychotics (Gill et al. 2005).

## Use in Pregnancy

Like most other drugs, antipsychotic agents should be avoided, if possible, during pregnancy and during lactation periods for breast-feeding mothers. The use of low-potency phenothiazine antipsychotics during the first trimester of pregnancy may increase the baseline risk of congenital anomalies by 0.4%, or 4 cases per 1,000 pregnancies (Altshuler et al. 1996). Infants born to mothers who were first exposed to antipsychotic drugs during the sixth to tenth week of gestation may have an increase in birth defects (Edlund and Craig 1984).

Less is known about the risks for teratogenicity, perinatal complications, and neurobehavioral problems associated with atypical antipsychotic medications. Data from a prospective comparative study indicated that treatment with olanzapine, risperidone, quetiapine, and clozapine was not associated with a significantly higher risk of major malformations; however, treatment with these agents was associated with a lower birthrate ($P=0.05$) and higher rate of therapeutic abortions ($P=0.003$) (McKenna et al. 2005). Data related to the use of aripiprazole and ziprasidone are still limited (see review by Gentile 2004). One case of agenesis of the corpus callosum was reported with risperidone use (Physicians' Desk Reference 2001). A possible case of a meningocele and ankyloblepharon associated with olanzapine was reported (Arora and Praharaj 2006).

In addition, antipsychotic agents should be prescribed with great caution in the peripartum period. Extrapyramidal symptoms and neonatal jaundice have been reported in infants following in utero exposure to conventional antipsychotic drugs. Also, neonates may be exposed to small amounts of antipsychotics in breast milk (Stewart et al. 1980). It is therefore necessary to reassess the potential risks and benefits of antipsychotic treatment as the pregnancy comes to term. As a general guideline, antipsychotic drugs should be used in pregnant patients only if absolutely necessary, at the minimal dose required, and for the briefest possible time. Documentation of informed consent from both the mother and the father is necessary. Use of electroconvulsive therapy (ECT) to treat acute psychosis in pregnant mothers should be considered.

## Drug Interactions

Antipsychotic drugs have profound effects on multiple CNS receptors, and these effects are compounded when other medications are added. For example, the α-adrenergic receptor blockade of antipsychotics may affect the efficacy of the antihypertensive drug guanethidine. The sedative and anticholinergic effects of antipsychotic drugs are increased with the addition of other sedating or anticholinergic drugs. As mentioned previously, patients taking drugs with potentially serious adverse effects should be monitored through plasma level determinations when other medications are used concurrently.

Pharmacokinetic interactions with antipsychotic drugs are common and have been reviewed elsewhere (Goff and Baldessarini 1995). Most antipsychotics are metabolized by the hepatic CYP2D6 isoenzyme. Exceptions include ziprasidone and quetiapine, which are metabolized mainly by the CYP3A4 enzyme. The activity of the CYP2D6 enzyme varies greatly (on the basis of genetic polymorphisms) among individuals and can be inhibited by certain drugs, such as SSRIs. For example, the addition of fluoxetine increased serum haloperidol concentrations by 20% and serum fluphenazine concentrations by 65% in one study (Goff et al. 1995). Two categories of potential drug–drug interactions are of particular concern. The first includes interactions that can increase serum concentrations of antipsychotics to dangerous levels. For example, clozapine is metabolized by the CYP2D6, CYP3A4, and CYP1A2 isoenzymes. When the drug is taken with CYP3A4 and CYP1A2 inhibitors, such as erythromycin and fluvoxamine, serum clozapine concentrations can rise to toxic levels (Cohen et al. 1996; Wetzel et al. 1998). The other category of potentially serious interactions includes those that induce metabolism of antipsychotic agents, thereby lowering serum concentrations below a therapeutic threshold. Large reductions in serum clozapine and haloperidol concentrations have been reported with the addition of carbamazepine, phenobarbital, and phenytoin (Arana et al. 1986; Byerly and DeVane 1996). Notably, cigarette smoking can affect antipsychotic metabolism; serum concentrations of clozapine in particular are reduced with smoking and increased after smoking cessation (Byerly and DeVane 1996; Haring et al. 1989).

## Atypical Antipsychotics

The atypical antipsychotics are referred to as *atypical* (compared with conventional antipsychotics) for several reasons, including their receptor binding profiles, improved side-effect profile, and spectrum of efficacy in patients with schizophrenia. In general, the atypical antipsychotic drugs provide superior efficacy for the treatment of negative symptoms, produce fewer acute motor side effects, and may reduce the risk of tardive dyskinesia compared with conventional antipsychotic drugs. These drugs also may improve cognitive function in patients with schizophrenia (Green et al. 1997; Hagger et al. 1993; Purdon et al. 2000; Rossi et al. 1997). In this subsection, we review the atypical antipsychotic medications currently available in the United States: clozapine, olanzapine, risperidone, quetiapine, ziprasidone, aripiprazole, and paliperidone.

### Clozapine

Clozapine was the first medication shown to be efficacious in otherwise nonresponsive patients. In addition, clozapine was the first agent to attenuate significantly the negative symptoms of schizophrenia, such as marked social withdrawal and apathy, thereby helping many patients return to meaningful and productive lives. Also, clozapine rarely produces EPS, and to date it is the only antipsychotic drug that is not associated with treatment-emergent tardive dyskinesia. This important clinical property is concordant with the observation that chronic administration of clozapine results in selective inhibition of dopamine neurons in the mesolimbic pathways, with little functional effect on striatal dopamine tracts. Finally, clozapine has minimal effects on the tuberoinfundibular system, and therefore it does not cause hyperprolactinemia.

Clozapine is the prototype for the atypical antipsychotic medication class. However, because it is associated with a risk for agranulocytosis, clozapine use is restricted to patients who have not adequately responded to or tolerated treatment with two other antipsychotics (Lewis et al. 2006). Several studies have confirmed its efficacy in patients with a history of nonresponse to previous antipsychotic treatment (Kane et al. 1988; Lewis et al. 2006; McEvoy et al. 2006). McEvoy et al. (2006) randomly assigned patients with schizophrenia who had prospectively not responded to an atypical antipsychotic medication in the CATIE to open treatment with clozapine or blinded treatment with olanzapine, risperidone, or quetiapine. They reported that switching to clozapine was more effective in atypical antipsychotic nonresponders than switching to a different atypical agent.

Because clozapine appears to be devoid of parkinsonian side effects, it is also useful in low dosages (25 mg/day) for patients with Parkinson's disease and psychosis induced by dopamine agonists. Other indications require higher dosages, as discussed later, and an extended period of titration to achieve therapeutic dosages and clinical response.

**Mechanism of action.** Clozapine shows high in vitro receptor affinities for the $D_4$, 5-$HT_2$, $\alpha_1$-adrenergic, muscarinic, and $H_1$ receptors and a relatively weak affinity for $D_1$, $D_2$, and $D_3$ receptors. The high 5-$HT_2$-to-$D_2$ ratio is hypothesized to be responsible for many of clozapine's advantages over typical antipsychotic drugs, either directly or indirectly (Meltzer 1991). Other investigators have suggested that clozapine's superior efficacy may be related to the drug's ability to increase norepinephrine outflow (Breier et al. 1994) or may be a result of indirect effects on glutamatergic systems (Goff and Coyle 2001).

**Clinical use.** Because of prominent sedation and orthostatic hypotension, clozapine therapy is initiated at a dosage of 12.5 mg/day, with a rapid increase to 12.5 mg twice a day. The dose is then increased as tolerated, generally in 25- or 50-mg increments every day or every other day. Clozapine is usually added to the previous antipsychotic agent in a cross-titration in which the dose of the previous drug is tapered once a clozapine dosage of approximately 100 mg/day has been achieved. This strategy should be used with caution if the existing medication is a low-potency conventional antipsychotic because of the possibility of additive $\alpha$-adrenergic and anticholinergic side effects. The typical target dose is 300–500 mg/day in divided doses. Although routine blood level monitoring is not recommended, a serum level greater than 350 ng/mL is associated with a higher response rate (Perry et al. 1991). Serum levels should be ascertained in nonresponders. The duration of treatment required to assess response is longer than for most medications—that is, typically 3–6 months (Meltzer 1994). If patients are nonresponsive after 6 months of continuous clozapine treatment, the dosage may be gradually increased to a maximum of 900 mg/day.

**Risks, side effects, and their management.**

*Agranulocytosis.* Agranulocytosis was previously estimated to occur in 0.8% of the patients receiving clozapine during the first year of treatment, with a peak incidence at 3 months. However, a system of hematological monitoring has reduced agranulocytosis-related fatalities to extremely low levels (Honigfeld et al. 1998). The dispensing of cloza-

---

**TABLE 30–11. Hematological monitoring guidelines for patients taking clozapine**

Initial white blood cell (WBC) count must be greater than 3,500/$mm^3$, and absolute neutrophil count (ANC) must be greater than 2,000/$mm^3$.

Weekly WBC count and ANC are required for the first 6 months of treatment and for 4 weeks after discontinuation of clozapine. After 6 months, monitoring is required every 2 weeks; and after 12 months, monitoring is required every 4 weeks.

If WBC count is 2,000–3,000/$mm^3$ or ANC is 1,000–1,500/$mm^3$, interrupt therapy and monitor for signs of infection. Perform WBC and differential counts daily. If no symptoms of infection are seen, if WBC count returns to greater than 3,000/$mm^3$, and if ANC is greater than 1,500/$mm^3$, resume clozapine therapy with twice-weekly WBC and differential counts until total WBC count returns to more than 3,500/$mm^3$ and ANC is greater than 2,000/$mm^3$.

If WBC count is less than 2,000/$mm^3$ or ANC is less than 1,000/$mm^3$, discontinue clozapine and do not rechallenge. Perform WBC and differential counts daily until WBC count is greater than 3,000/$mm^3$ and ANC is greater than 1,500/$mm^3$. Then monitor twice weekly until WBC count returns to more than 3,500/$mm^3$ and ANC is greater than 2,000/$mm^3$. Then monitor weekly for 4 weeks. Treat any infection with antibiotics. Consider bone marrow aspiration to ascertain granulopoietic status. If granulopoiesis is deficient, consider protective isolation.

*Source.* Adapted from Marangell LB, Martinez JM: *Concise Guide to Psychopharmacology*, 2nd Edition. Washington, DC, American Psychiatric Publishing, 2006, p. 112. Used with permission.

---

pine in the United States is linked to weekly WBC counts during the first 6 months and biweekly counts thereafter. Strict guidelines based on WBC and absolute neutrophil counts have been set (Table 30–11). Since the implementation of the Clozaril National Registry in the United States, the rate of agranulocytosis has been estimated to be 0.38% on the basis of data collected from February 1990 to December 1994 (Honigfeld 1996; Honigfeld et al. 1998).

If agranulocytosis develops, prompt consultation with a hematologist is indicated. Reverse isolation and prophylactic antibiotics may be used to prevent infection. Granulocyte colony–stimulating factors may be used to shorten the duration and reduce the morbidity of agranulocytosis (Barnas et al. 1992; Gerson et al. 1992; Nielsen 1993).

Although lithium often causes leukocytosis, it does not appear to treat or prevent clozapine-induced agranulocytosis. Once a patient has developed agranulocytosis while taking clozapine, he or she should not be rechallenged with this medication.

Clozapine is contraindicated in patients who have myeloproliferative disorders or who are immunocompromised as a result of diseases such as active tuberculosis or HIV infection because of their increased risk for agranulocytosis. Concomitant administration of medications that are associated with bone marrow suppression, such as carbamazepine, is also contraindicated.

*Extrapyramidal side effects.* EPS are uncommon with any dose of clozapine, although some patients experience akathisia or hand tremors. NMS has been reported in patients medicated with clozapine (Anderson and Powers 1991; DasGupta and Young 1991; Miller et al. 1991).

*Sedation.* Sedation is the most common side effect of clozapine, and it is particularly prominent early in treatment. Sedation generally attenuates when the dose is reduced, when tolerance to this side effect develops, or when a disproportionate amount is given at bedtime.

*Cardiovascular effects.* Hypotension and tachycardia occur in most patients taking clozapine. Additionally, cases of potentially fatal myocarditis and dilated cardiomyopathy have been reported (Kilian et al. 1999). Myocarditis typically occurs within 3 weeks of starting clozapine, but cardiomyopathy may not be apparent for several years.

*Weight gain.* Body weight increases by 10% or more in many patients. One naturalistic study found that weight gain did not plateau with clozapine therapy until year 4, and the weight gain was not dose related (Henderson et al. 2000).

*Endocrine effects.* As noted earlier, numerous studies suggested a relation between the use of atypical antipsychotic medications and the development of hyperglycemia, dyslipidemia, and metabolic syndrome (American Diabetes Association et al. 2004; review by Citrome et al. 2005).

*Hypersalivation.* Hypersalivation occurs in one-third of the patients taking clozapine. However, because clozapine has potent anticholinergic properties, addition of an anticholinergic agent is not recommended for control of hypersalivation.

*Fever.* Clozapine is associated with benign, transient temperature increases, generally within the first 3 weeks of treatment. Patients taking clozapine who develop fevers should be evaluated for infections, agranulocytosis, and NMS.

*Seizures.* Clozapine is associated with a dose-dependent risk of seizures. The vast majority of clozapine-induced seizures are tonic-clonic, but myoclonic seizures also occur. Doses less than 300 mg/day are associated with a 1%–3% risk of seizures. Doses of 300–600 mg/day carry a 2.7% risk, and doses greater than 600 mg/day are associated with a 4.4% risk (Devinsky et al. 1991). Because of this risk, clozapine doses greater than 600 mg/day are not recommended unless the patient's symptoms have not responded at lower doses.

*Anticholinergic side effects.* Anticholinergic effects, such as dry mouth, blurred vision, constipation, and urinary retention, are common early side effects.

**Drug interactions.** Clozapine should not be combined with any drugs that have the potential to suppress bone marrow function, such as carbamazepine. There have been isolated reports of respiratory arrest in patients taking both clozapine and a high-potency benzodiazepine.

Clozapine is metabolized by hepatic CYP1A2 and, to a lesser degree, CYP3A3/4; therefore, the drug is subject to changes in serum concentration when combined with medications that inhibit or induce these enzymes. Serum clozapine levels increase with coadministration of fluvoxamine or erythromycin and decrease with coadministration of phenobarbital or phenytoin and with cigarette smoking (Byerly and DeVane 1996). These pharmacokinetic interactions are particularly important because of the dose-dependent risk of seizures.

## Olanzapine

Olanzapine represents a modification of the clozapine molecule. Like risperidone, olanzapine is a monoaminergic antagonist with high-affinity binding at the $5HT_2$ and $D_1$, $D_2$, $D_3$, and $D_4$ receptors. Compared with clozapine, olanzapine has greater $D_2$ and weaker $D_4$ and $\alpha$-adrenergic affinity. Despite its structural similarity to clozapine, olanzapine is not associated with higher-than-expected rates of agranulocytosis. Although in vitro binding studies have indicated a high affinity for $M_1$ receptors, anticholinergic side effects are not as prominent as these data would predict.

In the CATIE, which randomly assigned 1,493 patients with chronic schizophrenia to treatment for up to 18 months with olanzapine (range=7.5–30 mg/day; mean modal dose=20.1 mg/day), quetiapine (range=200–800 mg/day; mean modal dose=543.4 mg/day), risperidone (range=1.5–6.0 mg/day; mean modal dose=3.9 mg/day), ziprasidone (range=40–160 mg/day; mean modal dose=112.8 mg/day), or perphenazine (range=8–32 mg/day; mean modal dose=20.8 mg/day), olanzapine showed better effectiveness (lower rates of discontinuation, shorter duration of successful treatment, and lower rates of hospitalizations) compared with other agents (Lieberman et al. 2005).

Acute dystonia is uncommon. Akathisia may occur, but it is significantly less common than with the conventional antipsychotic drugs. In prospective double-blind studies, treatment-emergent tardive dyskinesia was reported to occur in 1% of the olanzapine group compared with 4.6% of the haloperidol group (Tollefson et al. 1997). Olanzapine is associated with modest dose-dependent elevations in serum prolactin levels, but most often these elevations are transient and within the normal reference range (Tollefson et al. 1997).

**Clinical use.** The recommended starting dosage of olanzapine is 10 mg at bedtime for patients with schizophrenia and 10–15 mg at bedtime for acutely manic patients. The clinically effective dosage range is 7.5–20 mg/day (5–20 mg/day in mania). Olanzapine can be administered in a single daily dose at bedtime. It is important to note that meaningful improvement may not be evident for the first several weeks after initiation of treatment. Usual dosages for maintenance treatment in patients with bipolar disorder range from 5 to 20 mg/day. Although no systematic data are available regarding switching from other antipsychotic drugs to olanzapine, early clinical experience favors a gradual cross-titration. Commonly, olanzapine is added to the existing antipsychotic medication, whose dose is tapered after 1–2 weeks.

Olanzapine is available in a short-acting intramuscular injectable form, providing clinicians with another option for treating acute agitation associated with psychosis or mania. Peak plasma concentrations are achieved within 15–45 minutes.

**Risks, side effects, and their management.**

*Somnolence.* Somnolence is a common, dose-dependent side effect of olanzapine. Patients often become tolerant to this side effect over time.

*Anticholinergic side effects.* Anticholinergic side effects are clinically less significant than would be predicted on the basis of in vitro muscarinic receptor–binding affinity. However, dry mouth has been reported in association with olanzapine treatment (Beasley et al. 1996).

*Seizures.* Treatment-emergent seizures are rare in the absence of concomitant medical disorders. Olanzapine should be used with caution in patients with a history of seizures and in patients with conditions that may lower the seizure threshold, such as dementia.

*Hepatic effects.* Transaminase levels were increased in approximately 2% of the patients taking olanzapine in premarketing evaluation. In many cases, these levels normalized without medication discontinuation. Olanzapine should be used with caution in patients with hepatic disease or with additional risk factors for hepatic toxicity. In this group of patients, serum transaminase levels must be monitored if olanzapine is prescribed.

*Weight gain.* Treatment-emergent weight gain is common with olanzapine therapy and averages about 4.15 kg after 10 weeks of treatment (Allison et al. 1999). By 39 weeks, weight gain tends to plateau (Kinon et al. 2001), and approximately 20% of patients may not gain weight. Patients with higher body mass indices ($>27.6$ kg/m$^2$) tend to gain less weight than do those with lower body mass indices. Weight gain is independent of dose (Kinon et al. 2001). In the CATIE, significantly more olanzapine-treated patients gained 7% or more of their baseline body weight compared with those receiving other agents (Lieberman et al. 2005).

**Drug interactions.** Olanzapine is metabolized by several pathways and is unlikely to be affected by concurrent administration of other medications. Additionally, olanzapine does not appear to inhibit any cytochrome P450 enzymes. However, additive pharmacodynamic effects are expected if olanzapine is combined with medications that also have anticholinergic, antihistaminic, or $\alpha_1$-adrenergic side effects.

### Risperidone

Risperidone is an atypical antipsychotic medication that combines $D_2$ receptor antagonism with potent 5-HT$_2$ receptor antagonism. Risperidone has a higher affinity for $D_2$ receptors than does clozapine. Risperidone also antagonizes $D_1$ and $D_4$ receptors, $\alpha_1$- and $\alpha_2$-adrenergic receptors, and $H_1$ receptors. Risperidone was more effective than haloperidol 20 mg/day against both the positive and the negative symptoms of chronic schizophrenia (Chouinard et al. 1993; Marder and Meibach 1994). The optimal dosage of risperidone in the North American trials was 6 mg/day, but subsequent clinical experience has indicated that most patients do well on lower dosages of 3–6 mg/day, and the elderly may require dosages as low as 0.5 mg/day. Clinicians should titrate the dose of risperidone to avoid EPS. Unlike the other atypical agents, risperidone elevates prolactin levels.

**Clinical use.** Risperidone is most effective at total daily doses of 4–6 mg. For initial treatment, we recommend using divided doses, starting at 1 mg twice a day and quickly increasing to 2 mg twice a day. For elderly persons, the initial dose should be much lower (0.25–0.5 mg/day). After the first week of treatment, the entire dose can be given at bedtime. This approach usually helps the patient sleep and reduces daytime side effects. However, we do not suggest this practice for elderly persons, because of an increased risk of falling.

Risperidone is the only atypical antipsychotic currently available in a long-acting injectable form (Risperdal Consta). Results from a 12-week multicenter double-blind study indicated that long-acting risperidone is more effective than placebo for improving the positive and negative symptoms associated with schizophrenia (Kane et al. 2003).

**Risks, side effects, and their management.** Insomnia, hypotension, agitation, headache, and rhinitis are the most common side effects of risperidone. These tend to lessen with time. Overall, the drug tends to be well tolerated. Risperidone does not have significant anticholinergic side effects. Hyperprolactinemia is common.

*Extrapyramidal side effects.* In comparison with relatively high dosages of haloperidol (20 mg/day), risperidone is associated with a lower prevalence of acute extrapyramidal effects and akathisia. EPS occur in a dose-dependent manner, with more frequent occurrence when the dosage is greater than 6 mg/day. Thus, clinicians are advised to titrate the dose of risperidone in a manner that maximizes its clinical benefits and minimizes EPS.

*Cardiovascular effects.* Brief hypotension may occur, as may be expected with $\alpha$-adrenergic receptor blockade. Tachycardia is also common.

*Tardive disorders.* Risperidone at low doses produces few parkinsonian side effects. The incidence of risperidone-induced tardive dyskinesia is not known, but it is assumed to be between that of clozapine and the conventional antipsychotics. In one 9-month study of elderly patients, risperidone produced very low rates of tardive dyskinesia compared with haloperidol (Jeste et al. 1999).

*Weight gain.* Weight gain associated with risperidone treatment is quite variable and is generally less than weight gain associated with olanzapine and clozapine (Allison et al. 1999). The mean weight gain after 10 weeks of exposure to risperidone is approximately 2.1 kg. All patients taking atypical antipsychotics should be monitored for weight gain, particularly during the early course of treatment.

**Drug interactions.** Risperidone is metabolized primarily by CYP2D6 (Byerly and DeVane 1996). Medications that inhibit this enzyme, such as many of the SSRIs, cause increases in plasma risperidone levels. However, there does not appear to be an increase in side effects resulting from such an interaction, possibly because the primary metabolite of risperidone, 9-hydroxyrisperidone, is fully active and is excreted unchanged by the kidneys (Shelton and Stahl 2004). Inhibition of the CYP2D6 enzyme may merely alter the balance between parent drug and metabolite without significantly altering total $D_2$ occupancy. Pharmacodynamic interactions may occur when risperidone is combined with medications that share a similar physiological effect, such as orthostatic hypotension.

### Quetiapine

Quetiapine is a dibenzothiazepine derivative with weak affinity for $5\text{-HT}_{1A}$, $5\text{-HT}_2$, $D_1$, $D_2$, $H_1$, $\alpha_1$, and $\alpha_2$ receptors. Quetiapine has very "loose" binding to $D_2$ receptors. For example, $D_2$ receptor occupancy may decline from approximately 57% when measured 3 hours after an oral quetiapine dose of 400 mg to 20% after 9 hours. In a fixed-dose comparison of quetiapine to haloperidol (12 mg/day) and placebo, quetiapine was superior to placebo at doses of 150–750 mg on most measures but superior to placebo for the treatment of negative symptoms only at the 300-mg dose (Arvanitis and Miller 1997). A comparison of high-dose quetiapine (approximately 500 mg/day) and low-dose quetiapine (approximately 250 mg/day) found significantly greater efficacy with the higher dose (Small et al. 1997). Quetiapine's relatively high $5\text{-HT}_2$–to–$D_2$ ratio is consistent with the hypothesized advantageous properties of the atypical antipsychotics. Antagonism of $H_1$ receptors is associated with sedative side effects, and $\alpha_1$ antagonism is associated with orthostatic hypotension.

**Clinical use.**    Quetiapine therapy is initiated at a dose of 25 mg twice a day for patients with schizophrenia, with increases to 50 mg twice a day on day 2, 100 mg twice a day on day 3, and 100 mg in the morning and 200 mg in the evening on day 4. The optimal dosage for most patients appears to range between 400 and 600 mg/day, although the drug is safe and efficacious for some patients within a dose range of 150–750 mg. Slower titration and lower daily doses may be warranted in patients with hepatic disease and in elderly patients. Because of its relatively short half-life of 6–8 hours, quetiapine is usually administered twice daily.

A new formulation of quetiapine, quetiapine XR (extended-release tablets), is administered once daily, usually in the evening. The recommended initial dosage is 300 mg/day, and the effective dosage range is 400–800 mg/day. The dose can be increased by up to 300 mg/day, and increases can occur at 1-day intervals.

For patients who have acute mania, treatment should be initiated with twice-daily doses totaling 100 mg on day 1, 200 mg on day 2, 300 mg on day 3, and 400 mg on day 4. Additional adjustments up to 800 mg/day by day 6 can be made. Doses should not be increased by more than 200 mg/day on days 5 and 6. Most patients respond to dosages between 400 and 800 mg/day.

**Risks, side effects, and their management.** Quetiapine was no different from placebo in dosages to 750 mg/day regarding EPS and changes in serum prolactin levels (Arvanitis and Miller 1997).

*Somnolence.*    Somnolence and psychomotor slowing are dose dependent, and patients often become tolerant to these side effects over time.

*Cardiovascular effects.*    Given $\alpha_1$-adrenergic receptor antagonism, quetiapine may induce orthostatic hypotension and concomitant symptoms of dizziness, tachycardia, and syncope. Quetiapine should be used with caution in patients with cardiovascular disease, cerebrovascular disease, or other illnesses predisposing to hypotension.

*Hepatic effects.*    In premarketing trials, increased transaminase levels were noted in 6% of the patients taking quetiapine. These changes usually occur in the first weeks of treatment. Routine laboratory monitoring currently is not recommended, but quetiapine should be used with caution in patients with hepatic disease or with additional risk factors for hepatic toxicity.

*Weight gain.*    In premarketing placebo-controlled studies, a weight gain of at least 7% of body weight was observed in 23% of the quetiapine-treated patients with schizophrenia, compared with 6% of the control subjects given placebo. Thus, patients should be educated about the potential risk for weight gain, and weight should be monitored periodically throughout treatment.

**Drug interactions.**    Quetiapine is metabolized by hepatic CYP3A3/4. Concurrent administration of cytochrome P450–inducing drugs, such as carbamazepine, decreases blood levels of quetiapine. In such circumstances, increased doses of quetiapine are appropriate. Quetiapine does not appreciably affect the pharmacokinetics of other medications. Pharmacodynamic effects are expected if quetiapine is combined with medications that also have antihistaminic or $\alpha$-adrenergic side effects. Because of its potential for inducing hypotension, quetiapine also may enhance the effects of certain antihypertensive agents.

## Ziprasidone

Ziprasidone is the only atypical antipsychotic available in capsule form. This medication combines a high affinity for 5-$HT_2$ receptors with an intermediate affinity for $D_2$, resulting in a very high 5-$HT_2$-to-$D_2$ affinity ratio.

**Clinical use.**    For patients with schizophrenia, ziprasidone is usually started at a dosage of 20–40 mg twice a day. In medically healthy nonelderly patients, the dose can be rapidly titrated over 2–4 days to a typical therapeutic dosage of 60–80 mg twice a day. For patients with acute mania, treatment should be initiated at 40 mg twice a day. This dose should be increased to 60 or 80 mg twice a day on day 2 and subsequently adjusted on the basis of individual tolerance and symptoms to between 40 and 80 mg twice a day. Ziprasidone has a half-life of 5–10 hours and is usually administered twice daily with meals. Food increases absorption by approximately 100%. Ziprasidone at a dosage of 80 mg twice a day was comparable to haloperidol 15 mg/day in overall efficacy, and substantially fewer patients receiving ziprasidone required antiparkinsonian medication compared with those receiving haloperidol (10% vs. 53%) (Goff et al. 1998). Ziprasidone also has shown efficacy for negative symptoms in placebo-controlled trials (Daniel et al. 1999; Keck et al. 1998).

Because safety data regarding ziprasidone are largely derived from studies that excluded subjects with cardiac disease, clinicians should screen patients (preferably with a baseline ECG and measurement of serum electrolyte levels) for cardiac risk factors before initiating ziprasidone therapy. Patients with QTc prolongation at baseline must be monitored very closely; a cardiology consultation is recommended.

Ziprasidone is also available for intramuscular administration. The recommended dose for intramuscular injection (for the treatment of acute agitation associated with schizophrenia) is 10–20 mg, with a maximum dosage of 40 mg/day. The 10-mg doses can be administered every 2 hours, whereas the 20-mg doses can be administered every 4 hours. Peak plasma concentrations are achieved by 60 minutes.

**Risks, side effects, and their management.** In general, ziprasidone is well tolerated. The most common side effects are headache, dyspepsia, nausea, constipation, abdominal pain, somnolence, and EPS. Ratings of parkinsonism and akathisia with ziprasidone, 120 mg/day, did not differ from those with placebo. Although dizziness has been reported, rates of orthostatic hypotension have not differed from rates associated with placebo in controlled clinical trials. Ziprasidone produces transient hyperprolactinemia, which returns to predrug baseline levels after 12 hours; prolactin levels are significantly lower with ziprasidone than with haloperidol (Goff et al. 1998).

*Cardiovascular effects.* Ziprasidone delays the QTc interval at maximum therapeutic blood levels by approximately 20 ms, on average, which is a larger effect than with other atypical agents but less than with thioridazine. As noted earlier in this section, ziprasidone was not associated with greater effects on QTc intervals in the CATIE compared with other agents (Lieberman et al. 2005). Although monitoring of ECGs is not routinely required, clinicians should consider the relative risk of cardiac conduction delay compared with the benefits of ziprasidone (which include tolerability and minimal weight gain) when selecting a medication.

*Weight gain.* Ziprasidone is associated with less weight gain than are other atypical antipsychotic agents.

**Drug interactions.** Drugs that inhibit CYP3A4 reduce metabolism of ziprasidone: concurrent treatment with ketoconazole increased blood levels of ziprasidone by approximately 40%. Carbamazepine (and possibly other enzyme inducers) may decrease ziprasidone levels by approximately 35%. Effects of ziprasidone on metabolism of other drugs have not been reported.

Ziprasidone is contraindicated for use in patients taking other medications that can prolong the QT interval, including quinidine, class Ia and II antiarrhythmics, sotalol, dofetilide, dolasetron mesylate, probucol, tacrolimus, certain antibiotics (sparfloxacin, gatifloxacin, moxifloxacin), halofantrine, mefloquine, pentamidine, arsenic trioxide, certain antipsychotics (chlorpromazine, thioridazine, mesoridazine, pimozide), droperidol, and levomethadyl acetate (Geodon 2005).

### Aripiprazole

Aripiprazole has a high affinity for $D_2$ and $D_3$ receptors, as well as $5\text{-HT}_{1A}$ and $5\text{-HT}_{2A}$ receptors. Aripiprazole has partial agonist activity at the $D_2$ and $5\text{-HT}_{1A}$ receptors and antagonist activity at the $5\text{-HT}_{2A}$ receptor.

**Clinical use.** The recommended starting and target dosage for aripiprazole in patients with schizophrenia is 10 or 15 mg/day. The recommended starting dose for treatment of an acute manic or mixed episode is 30 mg; the recommended dosage for maintenance treatment in stable patients is 15 mg/day. The elimination half-life is 75 hours, and steady-state concentrations are reached within 2 weeks. Therefore, dosage adjustments are recommended every 2 weeks, to allow time for clinical assessments of the medication's effects to be observed at steady-state concentrations.

**Risks, side effects, and their management.** The most common side effects associated with aripiprazole include headache, nausea, dyspepsia, agitation, anxiety, insomnia, somnolence, and akathisia. Like all other antipsychotic medications, aripiprazole is associated with a risk for NMS and tardive dyskinesias.

**Drug interactions.** Aripiprazole is hepatically metabolized, mainly by two cytochrome P450 enzymes: CYP2D6 and CYP3A4. Therefore, dosage adjustments are necessary when this medication is given with other medications that either inhibit or induce these enzymes.

## Long-Acting Injectable Antipsychotics

For patients with chronic psychotic symptoms who are not compliant with antipsychotic medication, a long-acting depot preparation should be considered after stabilization is achieved with oral medication. Fluphenazine, haloperidol, and risperidone are the only long-acting injectable antipsychotic medications currently available in the United States.

Conversion to a decanoate preparation is complicated by the highly variable individual pharmacokinetics of the oral and long-term depot agents. Most patients respond to a fluphenazine decanoate dose of 10–30 mg given every 2 weeks. A loading dose strategy has been established for haloperidol decanoate, in which patients receive an initial dose that is 20 times the oral maintenance dose (Ereshefsky et al. 1993). The maximum volume per injection of haloperidol decanoate should not exceed 3 mL, and the maximum dose per injection should not exceed 100 mg. If 20 times the oral dose is greater than 100 mg, the dose is given in divided injections spaced 3–7 days apart. Subsequent doses are decreased monthly, to about 10 times the oral dose by the third or fourth month. Ten times the oral dose, administered every 4 weeks, is a typical maintenance dose for haloperidol decanoate. For elderly or debilitated patients, the initial dose is 10–15 times the previous oral daily dose. Many clinicians prefer to continue giving oral medication at approximately half the previous maintenance dose during the first few months of depot antipsychotic administration rather than administer a loading dose of depot medication. Steady-state serum concentrations are achieved after approximately 10 weeks (five injection intervals) with fluphenazine decanoate and after approximately 20 weeks with haloperidol decanoate. Side effects may take months to subside, and withdrawal dyskinesia may not appear for months after discontinuation of the decanoate formulation.

The recommended starting dose for the risperidone long-acting injection is 25 mg. Although an initial release of medication occurs, the amount released is small, and the main release of the drug begins 3 weeks after the injection. This release is maintained from 4 to 6 weeks and subsides by 7 weeks. Because not much drug is released for the first 3 weeks after the injection, oral antipsychotic supplementation is recommended. Injections are given every 2 weeks, and steady-state plasma concentrations are achieved after four injections. Dosing adjustments should not be made more often than once a month; the maximum dose is 50 mg every 2 weeks. Doses of 25, 37.5, and 50 mg are available, and different dosage strengths should not be combined. Dose titration depends on clinical symptoms. If the patient has not taken risperidone before, a trial of oral risperidone is recommended to determine whether the patient has a hypersensitivity reaction to the medication.

# Mood Stabilizers

The term *mood stabilizer* is used to refer to a group of medications that are effective in the treatment of bipolar disorder. These treatments serve as the foundation for the psychopharmacological treatment of bipolar illnesses. Currently, lithium, valproate, carbamazepine, lamotrigine, and most of the atypical antipsychotic medications are approved by the FDA for the treatment of one or more phases of bipolar disorder.

In order to prescribe mood stabilizers skillfully, the clinician must have a strong knowledge of the pharmacology of each medication and appreciate the differences in efficacy as well as side effects. Compared with most other classes of psychotropic medications, the group referred to as mood stabilizers are much more diverse with respect to their pharmacokinetic and pharmacodynamic properties, side-effect profiles, and potential for drug interactions.

## Lithium

### Mechanism of Action

Lithium is a cation that inhibits several steps in phosphoinositide metabolism, as well as many second and third messengers, including G proteins and protein kinases (Bitran et al. 1995; Lenox et al. 1992; Manji et al. 1993, 1995, 1999). Recent evidence suggests that lithium ultimately stimulates neurite growth, regeneration, and neurogenesis, which is likely related to its therapeutic effect (Coyle and Duman 2003; Kim et al. 2004).

### Indications and Efficacy

Lithium has been proven effective for acute and prophylactic treatment of both manic and depressive episodes in patients with bipolar disorder (American Psychiatric Association 2002), although patients with rapid-cycling bipolar disorder have been reported to respond less well to lithium treatment (Dunner and Fieve 1974). Lithium is also effective in prevention of future depressive episodes in patients with recurrent unipolar depressive disorder (American Psychiatric Association 2002) and as an adjunct to antidepressant therapy in depressed patients whose illness is partially refractory to treatment with antidepressants alone (discussed earlier in this chapter in the "Antidepressant Medications" section). Furthermore, lithium may be useful in maintaining remission of depressive disorders after ECT (Sackeim et al. 2001), as well as in the management of some cases of aggression and behavioral dyscontrol.

## Clinical Use

Lithium carbonate is completely absorbed by the gastrointestinal tract and reaches peak plasma levels in 1–2 hours. The elimination half-life is approximately 24 hours. Steady-state lithium levels are achieved in approximately 5 days. Therapeutic plasma levels for the treatment of bipolar disorder range from 0.5 to 1.2 mEq/L. Although lower plasma levels are associated with less troubling side effects, many clinicians target lithium levels of 0.8 mEq/L or more when treating acute manic episodes. Therefore, treatment of acute mania with lithium should not be considered a failure until the treatment has been tried throughout the therapeutic plasma level range (provided that the treatment is tolerated). Additionally, more severely acutely ill patients may require combination treatment.

Serum concentrations required for prophylaxis are not as well determined. One controlled trial of patients randomly assigned to a low lithium level (0.4–0.6 mEq/L) compared with a standard-dose lithium group (0.8–1.0 mEq/L) found fewer recurrences in the standard-dose group (Gelenberg et al. 1989); however, a reanalysis of these data indicated that an abrupt decrease in serum lithium level may be a more powerful predictor of recurrence of bipolar disorder than is the absolute assignment to a low or a standard dose of lithium (Perlis et al. 2002).

Lithium dosing is based on achieving therapeutic blood levels, targeting clinical response, and minimizing side effects if possible. Lithium can be administered either as a single daily dose or in divided doses. Divided daily dosing with lithium carbonate results in several peak lithium levels a day, whereas a single daily dose is associated with a single, but higher, peak level. Some clinicians prefer evening dosing because some side effects are associated with peak blood levels. Lithium levels should be determined 12 hours after the last lithium dose. After therapeutic lithium levels have been established, levels should be measured every month for the first 3 months and every 3 months thereafter. In patients who have remained stable and who are aware of early signs of both relapse and lithium toxicity, lithium levels may be measured less frequently. In addition, blood urea nitrogen and creatinine levels should be measured before lithium therapy has commenced and every 3–6 months during therapy, with more frequent testing if there are specific complaints or signs of renal dysfunction. As with any treatment, patients should be informed of the potential benefits and risks of lithium treatment and also should be educated about other treatment alternatives.

## Contraindications and Pretreatment Medical Evaluation

Lithium should not be administered to patients with unstable renal function. Because lithium may affect functioning of the cardiac sinus node, patients with sinus node dysfunction (e.g., sick sinus syndrome) should not receive lithium. Although lithium also has acute and chronic effects on the thyroid, patients with hypothyroidism may receive lithium if the thyroid disease is adequately treated and monitored. Laboratory tests that should be performed before initiation of lithium treatment are listed in Table 30–12.

Lithium treatment during pregnancy has been associated with teratogenic effects. The risk of Ebstein's anomaly in infants exposed to lithium in utero is 0.1%–0.7%, compared with 0.01% in the general population.

## Risks, Side Effects, and Their Management

**Renal effects.** In the absence of toxicity, most of the effects of lithium on the kidneys are largely reversible after discontinuation of the drug (although permanent morphological changes in renal structure may occur in some patients). However, lithium inhibits vasopressin and may result in an impairment in renal concentrating ability, called *nephrogenic diabetes insipidus* (NDI). This condition results in polyuria for up to 60% of patients taking lithium. NDI may result in serious complications, including dehydration, lithium toxicity, and electrolyte imbalance.

Preventive and management strategies for NDI include increasing the patient's fluid intake and decreasing the amount of lithium given to the lowest effective dosage. Once-daily dosing also results in lower urinary output than the multiple-dosing schedule (Hetmar et al. 1991; Plenge et al. 1982). For some patients, potassium supplementation, 10–20 mEq/day, may be effective. The nonthiazide diuretic amiloride also may treat lithium-induced NDI. For lithium-induced NDI, amiloride is prescribed in a dosage of 5 mg twice a day and increased to 10 mg twice a day if necessary. Even though amiloride does not appear to increase plasma lithium levels, it is prudent to continue to monitor serum lithium levels with greater frequency (at least every 2 months) when amiloride is combined with lithium.

Interstitial nephritis has been reported to be a consequence of long-term lithium therapy. Hetmar et al. (1987) performed renal biopsies on 46 bipolar patients with a mean of 8 years of lithium therapy and found that the proportion of sclerotic glomeruli, atrophic tubules, and interstitial fibrosis was significantly greater in patients who had

**TABLE 30–12.    Key characteristics of mood stabilizers[a]**

| | Lithium | Valproate | Carbamazepine | Lamotrigine |
|---|---|---|---|---|
| Available preparations | Lithium carbonate (Eskalith, Lithonate, Lithotabs; 150-, 300-, 600-mg tablets; capsules) Lithium citrate liquid (8 mEq/5 mL) Extended-release lithium (Eskalith CR, 450 mg; Lithobid, 300 mg) | Divalproex sodium (Depakote, 125-, 250-, 500-mg tablets; 125-mg sprinkle capsules) Valproate sodium injection (Depacon) Valproic acid (Depakene, 250-mg capsules; 250 mg/5 mL syrup) Extended-release divalproex sodium (Depakote ER, 250, 500 mg) | Carbamazepine (Tegretol; 100-mg chewable tablets; 200-mg tablets) Extended-release carbamazepine capsules (Equetro, 100, 200, 300 mg; Carbatrol, 200, 300 mg) Carbamazepine suspension (100 mg/5 mL) Extended-release carbamazepine tablets (Tegretol XR, 100, 200, 400 mg) | Lamotrigine (Lamictal, 25-, 100-, 150-, 200-mg tablets; Lamictal CD [chewable dispersible], 2-, 5-, 25-mg tablets) |
| Half-life (hours) | 24 | 96 | Initially, 25–65; decreases to 12–17 because of autoinduction | 25–33[b] |
| Starting dosage | 300 mg twice daily | 250 mg three times a day or 20 mg/kg[c] | Tablets/capsules: 200 mg twice daily[d]; suspension: 100 mg four times a day | 25 mg/day[b] |
| Blood level | 0.8–1.2 mEq/L | 45–125 µg/mL | Not helpful; monitor for signs or symptoms of toxicity | Not monitored; target dose of lamotrigine is 200 mg/day |
| Metabolism | Renal | Hepatic | Hepatic | Hepatic |
| Contraindications[e] | Unstable renal function | Hepatic dysfunction | Hepatic dysfunction, bone marrow suppression | Previous hypersensitivity to lamotrigine |

**TABLE 30–12.** Key characteristics of mood stabilizers[a] *(continued)*

| | Lithium | Valproate | Carbamazepine | Lamotrigine |
|---|---|---|---|---|
| Key side effects, risks, and features | Nephrogenic diabetes insipidus<br>Reversible hypothyroidism<br>Tremor<br>Benign leukocytosis<br>Weight gain<br>Narrow therapeutic index<br>Potentially fatal toxicity<br>Risk of Ebstein's anomaly with first-trimester exposure | Titration or loading dose strategies<br>Rare hepatotoxicity<br>Rare pancreatitis<br>Polycystic ovary syndrome<br>Weight gain<br>Tremor<br>Alopecia<br>Rare blood cell dyscrasias<br>Risk of neural tube defects with first-trimester exposure | Cytochrome P450 inducer (oral contraceptive failure)<br>Autoinduction<br>Rare blood cell dyscrasias: aplastic anemia, agranulocytosis<br>Hepatotoxicity<br>Rash risk, including Stevens-Johnson syndrome<br>Risk for SIADH<br>Teratogenicity risk: neural tube defects, craniofacial defects | Rash risk in 5%–10%<br>Rarely, life-threatening rash (including Stevens-Johnson syndrome)<br>Risk minimized by low starting dose and slow titration<br>Metabolism inhibited by valproate<br>Metabolism induced by carbamazepine |
| Pretreatment laboratory evaluation | Chem 20,[f] CBC, TSH level determination, ECG (if patient is 40 years of age or older or has cardiac disease), pregnancy test | AST and ALT level determination, pregnancy test | AST, ALT, CBC, sodium level; pregnancy test | None; might consider a pregnancy test |

*Note.* SIADH=syndrome of inappropriate antidiuretic hormone secretion; CBC=complete blood count; TSH=thyroid-stimulating hormone; ECG=electrocardiogram; AST=aspartate transaminase; ALT=alanine transaminase.

[a]The atypical antipsychotics are not included in this table. Please refer to the antipsychotics section of this chapter for information about their characteristics.

[b]The effective half-life of lamotrigine approximately doubles with valproate and decreases by approximately half with carbamazepine, primidone, phenytoin, phenobarbital, and rifampin; therefore, initial doses may vary depending on concomitant medications. The reader should refer to current product labeling for specific information regarding drug–drug interactions, their effects on lamotrigine, and lamotrigine dosing guidelines.

[c]Increase dose by 10%–20% when converting from valproate, divalproex, or valproic acid to the extended-release formulation of divalproex sodium.

[d]100 mg twice daily if given in combination with a neuroleptic or lithium.

[e]Lithium, valproate, and carbamazepine should be avoided in pregnancy, if possible; see text for discussion. Recent reports also have noted cases of oral clefts with lamotrigine use; see text for discussion.

[f]Especially blood urea nitrogen, creatinine, sodium, and calcium levels.

*Source.* Adapted from Marangell LB, Martinez JM: *Concise Guide to Psychopharmacology,* 2nd Edition. Washington, DC, American Psychiatric Publishing, 2006, pp. 138–141. Used with permission.

received a multiple daily dosing schedule, compared with patients with a history of once-daily dosing and with a control group with no history of lithium exposure. To minimize the risk of renal complications, we recommend frequent patient education about the risks of renal toxicity. Nephrology consultation is warranted if routine laboratory monitoring detects a pattern of rising creatinine levels.

**Thyroid dysfunction.**    Reversible hypothyroidism may occur in as many as 20% of the patients receiving lithium. Therefore, thyroid function should be evaluated every 6–12 months during lithium treatment or if symptoms develop that might be attributable to thyroid dysfunction, including depression or rapid cycling. If laboratory studies indicate the development of hypothyroidism, the patient should be referred to an endocrinologist for further evaluation and management.

**Parathyroid dysfunction.**    The effects of lithium on calcium metabolism may be related to lithium-induced hyperparathyroidism (Ananth and Dubin 1983; Mallette and Eichhorn 1986). Potential neuropsychiatric sequelae include affective changes, anxiety, aggressiveness, sleep disturbance, apathy, psychosis, delirium, dementia, and seizures. When signs or symptoms that might be related to hyperparathyroidism develop, serum calcium ion levels should be checked, and if they are abnormal, parathyroid hormone levels should be measured and an endocrinologist consulted.

**Neurotoxicity.**    Several types of neurological adverse events may occur with lithium treatment. A fine resting tremor is a common side effect of lithium. β-Blockers, such as propranolol (<80 mg/day in divided doses), may effectively treat this tremor (Zubenko et al. 1984). Additionally, subjective memory impairment commonly occurs (Goodwin and Jamison 1990).

**Cardiac effects.**    Benign flattening of the T wave on the ECG occurs in 20%–30% of patients taking lithium (Bucht et al. 1984). In addition, lithium may suppress the function of the sinus node and result in sinoatrial block. Thus, an ECG should be obtained before initiating lithium treatment in patients older than 40 years or in those with a history or symptoms of cardiac disease.

**Weight gain.**    Weight gain is a frequent side effect of lithium treatment.

**Dermatological effects.**    Dermatological reactions to lithium include acne, follicular eruptions, and psoriasis. Hair loss and thinning also have been reported. Except for cases of exacerbation of psoriasis, these reactions are usually benign. Lithium-induced acne responds to topical treatment with retinoic acid, such as tretinoin (Retin-A).

**Gastrointestinal symptoms.**    Gastrointestinal side effects, particularly nausea and diarrhea, are common and occur early during treatment. In general, the slow-release formulations of lithium are more often associated with nausea, whereas the immediate-release preparations are more commonly associated with diarrhea.

**Hematological effects.**    The most frequent hematological change associated with lithium therapy is leukocytosis (approximately 15,000 WBC/mm$^3$). This change is generally benign and typically reversible on lithium discontinuation.

### Overdose and Toxicity

There is a narrow margin between therapeutic and toxic plasma lithium levels. Thus, the physician should educate the patient about the risks for lithium toxicity, the signs and symptoms of lithium toxicity, and the importance of preventing lithium toxicity by ensuring adequate salt and water intake, taking the lithium as prescribed, and following through with recommended laboratory monitoring. The signs and symptoms of lithium toxicity, as well as the recommended management of lithium toxicity, are outlined in Table 30–13.

### Drug Interactions

Because lithium treatment is associated with a narrow therapeutic range, it is crucial that clinicians have good knowledge about the potential drug–drug interactions that may be associated with the concomitant administration of lithium and other drugs. Because lithium is excreted by the kidneys, any medication that alters renal function can affect lithium levels. Thiazide diuretics and nonsteroidal anti-inflammatory agents may increase lithium levels by decreasing renal clearance of lithium. Other medications that may increase lithium levels include angiotensin-converting enzyme inhibitors and cyclooxygenase-2 inhibitors (e.g., celecoxib, rofecoxib). Drugs that may decrease lithium levels include theophylline and aminophylline. Lithium may potentiate the effects of succinylcholine-like muscle relaxants.

## Valproate

Divalproex sodium is approved by the FDA for the treatment of acute mania.

TABLE 30–13. Signs, symptoms, and management of lithium toxicity

## TABLE 30–13. Signs, symptoms, and management of lithium toxicity

Signs and symptoms of lithium toxicity

**Mild to moderate intoxication (lithium level= 1.5–2.0 mEq/L)**

*Gastrointestinal symptoms*

Vomiting

Abdominal pain

Dryness of mouth

*Neurological symptoms*

Ataxia

Dizziness

Slurred speech

Nystagmus

Lethargy or excitement

Muscle weakness

**Moderate to severe intoxication (lithium level= 2.1–2.5 mEq/L)**

*Gastrointestinal symptoms*

Anorexia

Persistent nausea and vomiting

*Neurological symptoms*

Blurred vision

Muscle fasciculations

Clonic limb movements

Hyperactive deep tendon reflexes

Choreoathetoid movements

Convulsions

Delirium

Syncope

Electroencephalographic changes

Stupor

Coma

Circulatory failure (decreased blood pressure, cardiac arrhythmias, conduction abnormalities)

**Severe intoxication (lithium level > 2.5 mEq/L)**

Generalized convulsions

Oliguria and renal failure

Death

## TABLE 30–13. Signs, symptoms, and management of lithium toxicity *(continued)*

Management of lithium toxicity

1. The patient should immediately contact his or her personal physician or go to a hospital emergency department.

2. Lithium should be discontinued, and the patient should ingest fluids if possible.

3. A physical examination (including checking of vital signs) and a neurological examination (including a complete formal mental status examination) should be performed.

4. As soon as possible, lithium and serum electrolyte levels should be measured, renal function tests performed, and an electrocardiogram obtained.

5. In cases of significant acute ingestion, residual gastric contents should be removed by induction of emesis, gastric lavage, and absorption with activated charcoal.[a]

6. Vigorous hydration and maintenance of electrolyte balance are essential.

7. In a patient with a serum lithium level greater than 4.0 mEq/L or with serious manifestations of lithium toxicity, hemodialysis should be initiated.[a]

8. Repeat dialysis may be required every 6–10 hours, until the lithium level is within nontoxic range and the patient has no signs or symptoms of lithium toxicity.

[a]Information from Goldfrank et al. 1986.
*Source.* Adapted from Marangell LB, Martinez JM: *Concise Guide to Psychopharmacology*, 2nd Edition. Washington, DC, American Psychiatric Publishing, 2006, pp. 146–147. Used with permission.

## *Mechanism of Action*

Although many mechanisms of action have been proposed, the basis for the mood-stabilizing effects of valproate is most likely concordant with lithium's mechanism of action—specifically, attenuation of the activity of protein kinase C and other steps in the signal transduction pathway, leading to neuronal adaptation and changes in gene expression (Chen et al. 1994; Manji et al. 1996), including neurotrophic effects (Coyle and Duman 2003).

## *Clinical Use*

Before starting treatment with valproate, patients should be told that they might experience nausea, sedation, and a fine hand tremor. Several valproate preparations are available in the United States, including valproic acid, sodium valproate, divalproex sodium, and an XL preparation of divalproex sodium. Divalproex sodium is a dimer of sodium valproate and valproic acid with an enteric coating, and it is much better tolerated than other oral valproate preparations. The half-life of valproate is 9–16 hours.

Most clinicians use two general dosing strategies when treating acute mania: 1) a gradual dose titration or 2) a more rapid "loading dose" strategy. Most commonly, treatment with valproate is initiated with a gradual titration strategy in which it is started at a dosage of 250 mg three times a day, with subsequent increases of 250 mg every 3 days. Most patients require a daily dosage of 1,250–2,000 mg. Although valproate has a relatively short half-life, moderate doses may be given once a day at bedtime to reduce daytime sedation in patients with bipolar disorder.

When an acutely manic patient requires rapid stabilization, valproate treatment can be initiated at a dose of 20 mg per kilogram of body weight (Keck et al. 1993). Plasma levels of 45–100 µg/mL are recommended for the treatment of acute mania (Bowden et al. 1996); however, dosing should be based on the balance between clinical response and side effects rather than on absolute blood level alone. The XL preparation of divalproex sodium has 80%–90% of the bioavailability of the initial divalproex sodium, so doses may need to be slightly higher when this preparation is used.

### Contraindications

Valproate is relatively contraindicated in patients with hepatitis or liver disease. Valproate has been linked to spina bifida and other neural tube defects in the offspring of patients exposed to this medication in the first trimester of pregnancy (Lammer et al. 1987; Robert and Guibaud 1982).

### Risks, Side Effects, and Their Management

**Hepatotoxicity.**  Although it is estimated that 1 in 118,000 patients dies from non-dose-related hepatic failure, no cases have occurred in patients older than 10 years who were receiving valproate monotherapy. Nonetheless, baseline liver function tests are indicated. If baseline test results are normal, monitoring for clinical signs of hepatotoxicity is more important than routine monitoring of liver enzyme levels, which has little predictive value and may be less effective than clinical monitoring (Pellock and Willmore 1991).

Transient mild increases in liver enzyme levels, up to three times the upper limit of normal, do not necessitate discontinuation of valproate. Although γ-glutamyltransferase levels are often checked by clinicians, these levels are often increased, without clinical significance, in patients receiving valproate and carbamazepine (Dean and Penry 1992). Likewise, plasma ammonia levels are often increased transiently during valproate treatment, but this finding does not necessitate interruption of treatment (Jaeken et al. 1980).

**Hematological effects.**  Valproate has been associated with changes in platelet counts, but clinically significant thrombocytopenia has rarely been documented (Dean and Penry 1992). Coagulation defects also have been reported. Overall, the risk of inducing a coagulation disturbance in an otherwise healthy adult is extremely low. However, in patients in whom anticoagulation is strictly contraindicated and in patients who are already receiving anticoagulation therapy, monitoring of the coagulation profile is required at baseline, after 1 month of therapy, and then at least every 3 months.

**Gastrointestinal symptoms.**  Multiple gastrointestinal side effects may be associated with valproate, including indigestion, nausea, and heartburn. Use of the divalproex sodium preparation and administration of the medication with food may alleviate these effects. Pancreatitis is a rare occurrence in patients receiving relatively high doses of valproate (Murphy et al. 1981). If vomiting and severe abdominal pain develop during valproate therapy, serum amylase levels should be determined immediately.

**Weight gain.**  Weight gain is a common side effect of valproate treatment that does not appear to be dose dependent. Isojarvi et al. (1996) reported significant weight gain with associated hyperinsulinemia in approximately 50% of a cohort of women taking valproate.

**Neurological effects.**  A benign essential tremor is a common side effect of valproate therapy. Drowsiness is another common side effect, but tolerance often develops once a steady-state level of the drug is reached.

**Alopecia.**  Both transient and persistent hair loss have been associated with valproate use. Patients with valproate-induced alopecia may benefit from zinc supplementation, at a dose of 22.5 mg/day (Hurd et al. 1984).

**Polycystic ovary syndrome.**  Polycystic ovary syndrome is characterized by menstrual irregularity, hyperandrogenism, and the exclusion of other etiologies. Isojarvi et al. (1993) reported an association between polycystic ovary syndrome and valproate in women receiving long-term valproate treatment for epilepsy, especially those who were younger than 20 years.

### Overdose

Valproate overdose results in increasing sedation, confusion, and ultimately coma. The patient also may manifest hyperreflexia or hyporeflexia, seizures, respiratory suppression, and supraventricular tachycardia. Treatment should include gastric lavage, electrocardiographic monitoring, treatment of emergent seizures, and respiratory support.

### Drug Interactions

Valproate can inhibit hepatic enzymes, resulting in increased levels of other medications. Valproate is also highly bound to plasma proteins and may displace other highly bound drugs from protein-binding sites. Drugs that may increase valproate levels include cimetidine, macrolide antibiotics (e.g., erythromycin), and felbamate. Valproate may increase concentrations of phenobarbital, ethosuximide, and the active 10,11-epoxide metabolite of carbamazepine, increasing the risk of toxicity. Valproate also may raise lamotrigine levels, increasing the risk of rash (current lamotrigine product labeling provides specific lamotrigine dosing guidelines for patients who are taking valproate). Valproate metabolism may be induced by other anticonvulsants, including carbamazepine, phenytoin, primidone, and phenobarbital, resulting in an increased total clearance of valproate and perhaps decreased efficacy.

## Carbamazepine

Carbamazepine is effective in both acute and prophylactic treatment of mania (Gerner and Stanton 1992; Keck et al. 1992; Weisler et al. 2004, 2005). An XL formulation of carbamazepine, marketed in the United States under the brand name Equetro, is approved by the FDA for the treatment of acute mania. XL preparations of carbamazepine are preferred because the simplified dosage schedules may facilitate patient adherence. Other XL carbamazepine preparations include Tegretol XR and Carbatrol, although neither has been specifically indicated for the treatment of bipolar disorder.

### Clinical Use

Carbamazepine should be initiated at a dosage of 200 mg twice a day, with increments of 200 mg/day every 3–5 days.

Cited plasma levels of 8–12 µg/mL are based on clinical use in patients with seizure disorders and do not correlate with clinical response in patients with psychiatric disorders. We recommend a dose titration strategy that emphasizes achieving a clinical response and minimizes side effects. During the titration phase, patients may be particularly prone to side effects such as sedation, dizziness, and ataxia; if these occur, titration should be more gradual (the dosage might be 100 mg twice a day, for example). Because carbamazepine induces its own metabolism (autoinduction), dosage adjustments may be required for weeks or months after initiation of treatment to maintain therapeutic plasma levels.

### Contraindications

Because of the potential for hematological and hepatic toxicity, carbamazepine should not be administered to patients with liver disease or thrombocytopenia or to those at risk for agranulocytosis. For this reason, carbamazepine is strictly contraindicated in patients receiving clozapine. Because of reports of teratogenicity, including increased risks of spina bifida (Rosa 1991), microcephaly (Bertollini et al. 1987), and craniofacial defects (Jones et al. 1989), carbamazepine is relatively contraindicated in pregnant women. Additionally, because carbamazepine has a tricyclic structure, there are concerns about concomitant use of carbamazepine and MAOIs. Pretreatment evaluation should include a complete blood count and determination of ALT and aspartate transaminase (AST) levels. Because of the risk for teratogenicity, a pregnancy test also should be obtained in women of childbearing potential.

### Risks, Side Effects, and Their Management

**Hematological effects.** The most serious toxic hematological side effects of carbamazepine are agranulocytosis and aplastic anemia, both of which can be fatal. Whereas carbamazepine-induced agranulocytosis or aplastic anemia is extremely rare (Pellock 1987), other hematological effects, such as leukopenia (total WBC count<3,000 cells/mm$^3$), thrombocytopenia, and mild anemia, may occur more frequently. Although it is important to assess hematological function and risk factors before initiating treatment, there appears to be no benefit to ongoing monitoring in the absence of clinical indicators. When carbamazepine-induced agranulocytosis occurs, the onset is rapid. Therefore, it is more important to educate the patient to early signs and symptoms of agranulocytosis and thrombocytopenia and to tell the patient to inform the psychiatrist immediately if these signs and symptoms develop.

If significant leukopenia develops, such as an absolute neutrophil count of less than 1,000, carbamazepine therapy should be discontinued, and a hematologist should be consulted.

**Hepatotoxicity.** Carbamazepine therapy is occasionally associated with hepatic toxicity (Gram and Bentsen 1983), usually a hypersensitivity hepatitis that appears after a latency period of several weeks and involves increases in ALT, AST, and lactate dehydrogenase levels. Cholestasis is also possible, with increases in bilirubin and alkaline phosphatase concentrations. Mild transient increases in transaminase levels generally do not necessitate discontinuation of carbamazepine. If ALT or AST levels increase more than three times the upper limit of normal, carbamazepine should be discontinued.

**Dermatological effects.** Rash is a common side effect of carbamazepine, occurring in 3%–17% of patients (Warnock and Knesevich 1988) and typically occurring within 2–20 weeks after treatment initiation. Carbamazepine is generally discontinued if a rash develops because of the risk of progression to an exfoliative dermatitis or Stevens-Johnson syndrome, a severe bullous form of erythema multiforme (Patterson 1985).

**Endocrine disorders.** Carbamazepine may cause reductions in circulating thyroid hormones (Bentsen et al. 1983; Yeo et al. 1978). SIADH, with resultant hyponatremia, may be induced by carbamazepine treatment. Alcoholic patients may be at greater risk for hyponatremia.

**Gastrointestinal symptoms.** Nausea and occasional vomiting are common side effects of carbamazepine.

**Neurological effects.** Patients taking carbamazepine may develop dizziness, drowsiness, or ataxia, particularly during the early phases of treatment.

### Overdose

Carbamazepine overdose may initially present with neuromuscular disturbances, such as nystagmus, myoclonus, and hyperreflexia, which may then progress to seizures and coma. Cardiac conduction changes, nausea, vomiting, and urinary retention also may occur.

Treatment of carbamazepine overdose should include induction of vomiting, gastric lavage, and supportive care.

### Drug Interactions

Carbamazepine induces hepatic cytochrome P450 enzymes, which may reduce levels of other medications. Importantly, carbamazepine therapy can lead to oral contraceptive failure (Coulam and Annegers 1979). Use of medications or substances that inhibit CYP3A3/4 may result in significant increases in plasma carbamazepine levels (Brodie and MacPhee 1986; Cozza et al. 2003; Ketter et al. 1995).

## Lamotrigine

Lamotrigine is an anticonvulsant medication that decreases sustained high-frequency repetitive firing of the voltage-dependent sodium channel, which may then decrease glutamate release (Leach et al. 1991; Macdonald and Kelly 1995).

### Clinical Use

Lamotrigine treatment is usually initiated at 25 mg once a day. Because the risk of a serious rash increases with rapid titration, it is essential to follow the recommended titration schedule. After 2 weeks, the dosage is increased to 50 mg/day for another 2 weeks. At week 5, the dosage can be increased to 100 mg/day and at week 6 to 200 mg/day. In patients who are taking valproate or other medications that decrease the clearance of lamotrigine, the dosing schedule and target dose are halved. Conversely, the titration schedule and dose are increased in those taking carbamazepine. In the absence of carbamazepine or other enzyme inducers, doses higher than 200 mg are typically not recommended in the treatment of bipolar disorder.

### Risks, Side Effects, and Their Management

**Rash.** Lamotrigine has been associated with both benign and severe rashes. A maculopapular rash develops in 5%–10% of patients taking lamotrigine, usually in the first 8 weeks of treatment. Calabrese et al. (2002) analyzed data from 12 multicenter trials of lamotrigine in patients with mood disorders and reported an 8.3% rate of benign rashes with lamotrigine therapy. Lamotrigine also has been associated with serious rashes requiring hospitalization and discontinuation of treatment. The incidence of these rashes, which have included Stevens-Johnson syndrome, is approximately 0.3% in adults receiving adjunctive treatment for epilepsy, 0.13% in adults receiving adjunctive therapy in mood disorders clinical trials, and 0.08% in adults receiving lamotrigine as initial mono-

**TABLE 30–14.** Atypical antipsychotic dosing in the treatment of acute mania

| Generic drug | Trade name | Dosing in acute mania (mg/day)[a] | | |
| | | Starting dose | Dose titration | Target dose |
| --- | --- | --- | --- | --- |
| Olanzapine | Zyprexa | 10–15 | 5 mg/day increments | 5–20 |
| Risperidone | Risperdal | 2–3 | 1 mg/day increments | 1–6 |
| Aripiprazole | Abilify | 15–30 | 15 mg increments | 30 |
| Quetiapine | Seroquel | 100 | 50–100 mg/day increments | 600 |
| Ziprasidone | Geodon | 80 (divided twice daily) | 40–80 mg/day increments | 120–160 |

[a]Lower doses and slower dose titrations are indicated for the elderly. The reader is referred to current product labeling for specific information regarding approved indications for use and dosing in special populations.
*Source.* Adapted from Marangell LB, Martinez JM: *Concise Guide to Psychopharmacology*, 2nd Edition. Washington, DC, American Psychiatric Publishing, 2006, p. 161. Used with permission.

therapy in mood disorders clinical trials (Lamictal 2005). Before initiating lamotrigine therapy, the patient must be advised of the potential risk of developing a serious rash and the necessity to call the clinician immediately if a rash emerges. To minimize the risk of a rash, the clinician must prescribe lamotrigine in accordance with the current product labeling's recommended starting dose and titration schedule (noting that the titration schedules vary depending on the presence or absence of concomitant medications, particularly valproate).

**Teratogenicity.** Data published from the North American Antiepileptic Drug Registry reported 3 cases of cleft palate and 2 cases of cleft lip in infants from a total of 564 infants exposed in the first trimester to lamotrigine monotherapy (8.9 per 1,000) (Holmes et al. 2006).

### Drug Interactions

Several important potential drug–drug interactions may occur with lamotrigine. Of particular importance to patients with bipolar disorders, valproate will increase lamotrigine levels, and carbamazepine will decrease lamotrigine levels. Many other anticonvulsants interact with lamotrigine as well. Oral contraceptives can result in decreases in lamotrigine concentrations, but lamotrigine does not affect the availability of oral contraceptives.

## Oxcarbazepine

Oxcarbazepine is a keto derivative of carbamazepine but offers several advantages over carbamazepine. Specifically, oxcarbazepine does not require blood cell count,

hepatic, or serum drug level monitoring; causes less cytochrome P450 enzyme induction than does carbamazepine (but may decrease effectiveness of oral contraceptives containing ethinyl estradiol and levonorgestrel); and does not induce its own metabolism. These properties, combined with its similarity to carbamazepine, led many clinicians to use this medication for the treatment of bipolar disorder. However, it is important to note that oxcarbazepine has not been approved by the FDA for the acute or long-term treatment of bipolar disorder. To date, small controlled trials have suggested efficacy in the treatment of acute mania compared with lithium and haloperidol (Emrich 1990).

Oxcarbazepine has been associated with hyponatremia (Pendlebury et al. 1989; Trileptal 2006); thus, serum sodium levels should be monitored in patients at risk. Additionally, Stevens-Johnson syndrome and toxic epidermal necrolysis may occur at rates 3- to 10-fold higher than background incidence rates (Trileptal 2006).

## Other Anticonvulsants

There is considerable interest in the potential usefulness of newer anticonvulsants for the treatment of bipolar disorder. However, positive data from well-designed controlled monotherapy trials to date are lacking for these agents.

## Atypical Antipsychotics

All of the atypical antipsychotic medications (olanzapine, risperidone, quetiapine, ziprasidone, and aripiprazole), except clozapine, are approved by the FDA for the treatment of acute mania. Across randomized controlled trials, atypical antipsychotics have shown efficacy in treating the core symptoms of mania. General dosing guidelines for acute mania are shown in Table 30–14. It is common clinical practice to use lower starting dosages for patients who are less ill, particularly those patients receiving treatment in outpatient settings, but this practice has not been studied in randomized controlled trials. At present, only two of the atypical antipsychotics—olanzapine and aripiprazole—have been approved by the FDA as maintenance-phase treatments for bipolar disorder, although studies are under way with the other agents. The use of these agents for the depressed phase of bipolar disorder is an area of active clinical investigation. Clozapine has not received FDA approval for use in bipolar disorder, but it is a valuable option for patients whose symptoms are otherwise resistant to treatment (Suppes et al. 1999).

## Olanzapine–Fluoxetine Combination

The olanzapine–fluoxetine combination is currently the only medication approved by the FDA specifically for treatment of depression in patients with bipolar disorder. This indication was based on data from a double-blind, randomized study in which the combination was superior to both olanzapine monotherapy and placebo (Tohen et al. 2003). Treatment-emergent mania or hypomania did not occur more frequently in the olanzapine–fluoxetine combination group than in the placebo group during the acute trial.

### Clinical Use

The olanzapine–fluoxetine combination is available in four dosing preparations (6 mg/25 mg, 12 mg/25 mg, 6 mg/50 mg, 12 mg/50 mg) that allow clinicians to tailor treatment individually to provide greater or lesser amounts of each medication component. The typical starting dose for most patients is 6 mg/25 mg. Common side effects include somnolence, weight gain, increased appetite, asthenia, peripheral edema, and tremor. As one might expect, warnings and precautions that apply to either olanzapine or fluoxetine also apply to this combination treatment.

## Key Points: Psychopharmacology

- Accurate diagnosis is the key to a well-informed treatment decision; whenever possible, treat the primary diagnosis and not the symptoms.

- Several factors are important when selecting an appropriate medication, including identifying medication-responsive target symptoms, ruling out nonpsychiatric causes of a patient's symptomatology, noting the presence of other medical problems that will influence drug selection, evaluating concomitant medications that may cause drug–drug interactions, and evaluating personal and family histories of medication response.

- Whenever possible, the clinician should involve the patient in medication decisions and educate the patient and significant others about the illness and potential benefits, risks, and side effects of any medication being prescribed.

- Patients must be educated about the typical time to response for the medication being prescribed and the need for strict adherence to the treatment regimen to ensure an optimal chance for treatment success.

- In addition to pharmacotherapy, other interventions such as disease-specific psychotherapies should be considered.

- In an evaluation of a patient with a history of treatment failures, a detailed treatment history should include a review of the dose, duration, tolerability, adherence, and reason for discontinuation for each prior treatment; many prior medication failures may be a result of inadequate dosing, inadequate treatment duration, noncompliance, or poor tolerability.

- Ongoing psychiatric and medical monitoring during treatment should be individualized to each patient according to several factors, including the severity of the illness, the current clinical status of the patient (e.g., acutely ill, partially remitted), and the specific medication(s) being prescribed.

- The clinician should evaluate response to each prescribed treatment by monitoring symptomatic and functional improvement and strive for complete symptomatic and functional recovery.

- Clinicians should be mindful of the response to each medication and consider discontinuing any treatment that has provided no benefit despite an adequate dose and duration of treatment.

# References

Abernethy DR, Greenblatt DJ, Ochs HR, et al: Benzodiazepine drug-drug interactions commonly occurring in clinical practice. Curr Med Res Opin 8 (suppl 4):80–93, 1984

Adler LA, Angrist B, Peselow E, et al: Efficacy of propranolol in neuroleptic-induced akathisia. J Clin Psychopharmacol 5:164–166, 1985

Adler LA, Angrist B, Reiter S, et al: Neuroleptic-induced akathisia: a review. Psychopharmacology (Berl) 97:1–11, 1989

Adler LA, Peselow E, Rotrosen J, et al: Vitamin E in the treatment of tardive dyskinesia. Am J Psychiatry 150:1405–1407, 1993

Adler LA, Edson R, Lavori P, et al: Long-term treatment effects of vitamin E for tardive dyskinesia. Biol Psychiatry 43:868–872, 1998

Aherwadkar SJ, Efendigil MC, Coulshed N: Chlorpromazine therapy and associated acute disturbances of cardiac rhythm. Br Heart J 36:1251–1252, 1974

Akhtar S, Jajor TR, Kumar S: Vitamin E in the treatment of tardive dyskinesia. J Postgrad Med 39:124–126, 1993

Allison DB, Mentore JL, Heo M, et al: Antipsychotic-induced weight gain: a comprehensive research synthesis. Am J Psychiatry 156:1686–1696, 1999

Altshuler LL, Cohen L, Szuba MP, et al: Pharmacological management of psychiatric illness during pregnancy: dilemmas and guidelines. Am J Psychiatry 153:592–606, 1996

American Diabetes Association, American Psychiatric Association, American Association of Clinical Endocrinologists, North American Association for the Study of Obesity: Consensus development conference on antipsychotic drugs and obesity and diabetes. Diabetes Care 27:596–601, 2004

American Psychiatric Association: Benzodiazepine Dependence, Toxicity, and Abuse: A Task Force Report of the American Psychiatric Association. Washington, DC, American Psychiatric Association, 1990

American Psychiatric Association: Tardive Dyskinesia: A Task Force Report of the American Psychiatric Association. Washington, DC, American Psychiatric Association, 1992

American Psychiatric Association: Practice Guideline for the Treatment of Patients With Major Depresive Disorder, 2nd Edition. Washington, DC, American Psychiatric Association, 2000

American Psychiatric Association: Practice guideline for the treatment of patients with bipolar disorder (revision). Am J Psychiatry 159 (4 suppl):1–50, 2002

Amsterdam JD: A double-blind, placebo-controlled trial of the safety and efficacy of selegiline transdermal system without dietary restrictions in patients with major depressive disorder. J Clin Psychiatry 64:208–214, 2003

Amsterdam J, Berwish NJ: High dose tranylcypromine therapy for refractory depression. Pharmacopsychiatry 22:21–25, 1989

Ananth J, Dubin SE: Lithium and symptomatic hyperparathyroidism. J R Soc Med 96:1026–1029, 1983

Anderson ES, Powers PS: Neuroleptic malignant syndrome associated with clozapine use. J Clin Psychiatry 52:102–104, 1991

Angst F, Stassen HH, Clayton PJ, et al: Mortality of patients with mood disorders: follow-up over 34–38 years. J Affect Disord 68:167–181, 2002

Appleton WS, Davis JM: Practical Clinical Psychopharmacology, 2nd Edition. Baltimore, MD, Williams & Wilkins, 1980

Arana GW, Goff DC, Friedman H, et al: Does carbamazepine-induced reduction of plasma haloperidol levels worsen psychotic symptoms? Am J Psychiatry 143:650–651, 1986

Aronson MD, Hafez H: A case of trazodone-induced ventricular tachycardia. J Clin Psychiatry 47:388–389, 1986

Arora M, Praharaj SK: Meningocele and ankyloblepharon following in utero exposure to olanzapine. Eur Psychiatry 21:345–346, 2006

Arvanitis LA, Miller BG: Multiple fixed doses of "Seroquel" (quetiapine) in patients with acute exacerbation of schizophrenia: a comparison with haloperidol and placebo. The Seroquel Trial 13 Study Group. Biol Psychiatry 42:233–246, 1997

Baldessarini RJ, Cohen BM, Teicher MH: Significance of neuroleptic dose and plasma level in the pharmacological treatment of psychoses. Arch Gen Psychiatry 45:79–91, 1988

Ball WA, Caroff SN: Retinopathy, tardive dyskinesia, and low-dose thioridazine (letter). Am J Psychiatry 143:256–257, 1986

Barnas C, Zwierzina H, Hummer M, et al: Granulocyte-macrophage colony-stimulating factor (GM-CSF) treatment of clozapine-induced agranulocytosis: a case report. J Clin Psychiatry 53:245–247, 1992

Beasley CM Jr, Tollefson G, Tran P, et al: Olanzapine versus placebo and haloperidol: acute phase results of the North American double-blind olanzapine trial. Neuropsychopharmacology 14:111–123, 1996

Bentsen KD, Gram L, Veje A: Serum thyroid hormones and blood folic acid during monotherapy with carbamazepine or valproate: a controlled study. Acta Neurol Scand 67:235–241, 1983

Bertollini R, Källen B, Mastroiacovo P, et al: Anticonvulsant drugs in monotherapy: effect on the fetus. Eur J Epidemiol 3:164–171, 1987

Bitran JA, Manji HK, Potter WZ, et al: Downregulation of PKC alpha by lithium in vitro. Psychopharmacol Bull 31:449–452, 1995

Bodkin J, Amsterdam JD: Transdermal selegiline in major depression: a double-blind, placebo-controlled, parallel-group study in outpatients. Am J Psychiatry 159:1869–1875, 2002

Bowden CL, Janicak PG, Orsulak P, et al: Relation of serum valproate concentration to response in mania. Am J Psychiatry 153:765–770, 1996

Branchey M, Branchey L: Patterns of psychotropic drug use and tardive dyskinesia. J Clin Psychopharmacol 4:41–45, 1984

Breier A, Buchanan RW, Waltrip RW II, et al: The effect of clozapine on plasma norepinephrine: relationship to clinical efficacy. Neuropsychopharmacology 10:1–7, 1994

Bremner JD: A double-blind comparison of Org 3770, amitriptyline, and placebo in major depression. J Clin Psychiatry 56:519–525, 1995

Brodie MJ, MacPhee GJ: Carbamazepine neurotoxicity precipitated by diltiazem. Br Med J (Clin Res Ed) 292:1170–1171, 1986

Bucht G, Smigan L, Wahlin A, et al: ECG changes during lithium therapy: a prospective study. Acta Med Scand 216:101–104, 1984

Burton S, Heslop K, Harrison K, et al: Ziprasidone overdose (letter). Am J Psychiatry 157:835, 2000

Byerly MJ, DeVane CL: Pharmacokinetics of clozapine and risperidone: a review of recent literature. J Clin Psychopharmacol 16:177–187, 1996

Calabrese JR, Sullivan JR, Bowden CL, et al: Rash in multicenter trials of lamotrigine in mood disorders: clinical relevance and management. J Clin Psychiatry 63:1012–1019, 2002

Callahan AM, Marangell LB, Ketter TA: Evaluating the clinical significance of drug interactions: a systematic approach. Harv Rev Psychiatry 4:153–158, 1996

Chambers CD, Hernandez-Diaz S, Van Marter LJ, et al: Selective serotonin-reuptake inhibitors and risk of persistent pulmonary hypertension of the newborn. N Engl J Med 354:579–587, 2006

Chen G, Manji HK, Hawver DB, et al: Chronic sodium valproate selectively decreases protein kinase C alpha and epsilon in vitro. J Neurochem 63:2361–2364, 1994

Chouinard G, Jones BD, Remington G, et al: A Canadian multicenter, placebo-controlled study of fixed doses of risperidone and haloperidol in the treatment of chronic schizophrenic patients. J Clin Psychopharmacol 13:25–40, 1993

Citrome L, Blonde L, Damatarca C: Metabolic issues in patients with severe mental illness. South Med J 98:714–720, 2005

Cohen LG, Chesley S, Eugenio L, et al: Erythromycin-induced clozapine toxic reaction. Arch Intern Med 156:675–677, 1996

Cohn JB, Wilcox CS: Low-sedation potential of buspirone compared with alprazolam and lorazepam in the treatment of anxious patients: a double-blind study. J Clin Psychiatry 47:409–412, 1986

Correll CU, Leucht S, Kane JM: Lower risk for tardive dyskinesia associated with second generation antipsychotics: a systematic review of 1-year studies. Am J Psychiatry 161:414–425, 2004

Coulam CB, Annegers JF: Do anticonvulsants reduce the efficacy of oral contraceptives? Epilepsia 20:519–525, 1979

Coupland NJ, Bell CJ, Potokar JP: Serotonin reuptake inhibitor withdrawal. J Clin Psychopharmacol 16:356–362, 1996

Coyle JT, Duman RS: Finding the intracellular signaling pathways affected by mood disorder treatments. Neuron 38:157–160, 2003

Cozza KL, Armstrong SC, Oesterheld JR: Concise Guide to Drug Interaction Principles for Medical Practice: Cytochrome P450s, UGTs, P-Glycoproteins, 2nd Edition. Washington, DC, American Psychiatric Publishing, 2003

Cymbalta (package insert). Indianapolis, IN, Eli Lilly & Co, 2006

Dabiri LM, Pasta D, Darby JK, et al: Effectiveness of vitamin E for the treatment of long-term tardive dyskinesia. Am J Psychiatry 151:925–926, 1994

Daniel DG, Zimbroff DL, Potkin SG, et al: Ziprasidone 80 mg/day and 160 mg/day in the acute exacerbation of schizophrenia and schizoaffective disorder: a 6-week placebo-controlled trial. Neuropsychopharmacology 20:491–505, 1999

DasGupta K, Young A: Clozapine-induced neuroleptic malignant syndrome. J Clin Psychiatry 52:105–107, 1991

Davis JM: Maintenance therapy and the natural course of schizophrenia. J Clin Psychiatry 46:18–21, 1985

Davis KL, Kahn RS, Ko G, et al: Dopamine in schizophrenia: a review and reconceptualization. Am J Psychiatry 148:1474–1486, 1991

Dean JC, Penry JK: Valproate, in The Medical Treatment of Epilepsy. Edited by Resor SR Jr, Kutt H. New York, Marcel Dekker, 1992, pp 265–278

De Boer T: The pharmacological profile of mirtazapine. J Clin Psychiatry 57 (suppl 4):19–25, 1996

Devinsky O, Honigfeld G, Patin J: Clozapine-related seizures. Neurology 41:369–371, 1991

Di Rocco A, Brannan T, Prikhojan A, et al: Sertraline induced parkinsonism: a case report and an in-vivo study of the effect of sertraline on dopamine metabolism. J Neural Transm 105:247–251, 1998

Dixon J, Power SJ, Grundy EM, et al: Sedation for local anaesthesia: comparison of intravenous midazolam and diazepam. Anaesthesia 39:372–378, 1984

Dolovich LR, Addis A, Vaillancourt JM, et al: Benzodiazepine use in pregnancy and major malformations or oral cleft: meta-analysis of cohort and case-control studies. BMJ 317:839–843, 1998

Drug Facts and Comparisons, 56th Edition. St. Louis, MO, Facts & Comparisons, A Wolters Kluwer Company, 2002, pp 915–921, 1012–1014

Dunner DL, Fieve RR: Clinical factors in lithium carbonate prophylaxis failure. Arch Gen Psychiatry 30:229–233, 1974

Edlund MJ, Craig TJ: Antipsychotic drug use and birth defects: an epidemiologic reassessment. Compr Psychiatry 25:32–37, 1984

Egan MF, Hyde TM, Albers GW, et al: Treatment of tardive dyskinesia with vitamin E. Am J Psychiatry 149:773–777, 1992

Elkashef AM, Ruskin PE, Bacher N, et al: Vitamin E in the treatment of tardive dyskinesia. Am J Psychiatry 147:505–506, 1990

Emrich HM: Studies with oxcarbazepine (Trileptal) in acute mania. Int Clin Psychopharmacol 5:83–88, 1990

EMSAM (product information). Princeton, NJ, Bristol-Myers Squibb Co, 2006

Ereshefsky L, Toney G, Saklad SR, et al: A loading-dose strategy for converting from oral to depot haloperidol. Hosp Community Psychiatry 44:1155–1161, 1993

Expert Panel on Detection, Evaluation, and Treatment of High Blood Cholesterol in Adults: Executive Summary of the Third Report of the National Cholesterol Education Program (NCEP) Expert Panel on Detection, Evaluation, and Treatment of High Blood Cholesterol in Adults (Adult Treatment Panel III). JAMA 285:2486–2497, 2001

Faucette SR, Hawke RL, Lecluyse EL, et al: Validation of bupropion hydroxylation as a selective marker for human cytochrome P450 2B6 catalytic activity. Drug Metab Dispos 28:1222–1230, 2000

Fava M, Rankin MA, Alpert JE, et al: An open trial of oral sildenafil in antidepressant-induced sexual dysfunction. Psychother Psychosom 67:328–331, 1998

Feinberg SS, Holzer B: The monoamine oxidase inhibitor (MAOI) diet and kosher pizza (letter). J Clin Psychopharmacol 17:227–228, 1997

Feinberg SS, Holzer B: Clarifying the safety of the MAOI diet and pizza (letter). J Clin Psychiatry 61:145, 2000

Fuller MA, Sajatovic M: Lexi-Comp's Drug Information Handbook for Psychiatry, 4th Edition. Hudson, OH, Lexi-Comp, 2004

Gajwani P, Pozuelo L, Tesar GE: QT interval prolongation with quetiapine (Seroquel) overdose. Psychosomatics 41:63–65, 2000

Gardner DM, Shulman KI, Walker SE, et al: The making of a user friendly MAOI diet. J Clin Psychiatry 57:99–104, 1996

Gelenberg AJ, Kane JM, Keller MB, et al: Comparison of standard and low serum levels of lithium for maintenance treatment of bipolar disorder. N Engl J Med 321:1489–1493, 1989

Gentile S: Clinical utilization of atypical antipsychotics in pregnancy and lactation. Ann Pharmacother 38:1265–1271, 2004

Geodon (product information). New York, Pfizer, 2005

Gerbino L, Shopsin B, Collora M: Clozapine in the treatment of tardive dyskinesia: an interim report, in Tardive Dyskinesia: Research & Treatment. Edited by Fann WE, Smith RC, Davis JM, et al. New York, SP Medical & Scientific Books, 1980, pp 475–489

Gerner RH, Stanton A: Algorithm for patient management of acute manic states: lithium, valproate, or carbamazepine? J Clin Psychopharmacol 12(suppl):57S–63S, 1992

Gerson SL, Gullion G, Yeh HS, et al: Granulocyte colony-stimulating factor for clozapine-induced agranulocytosis (letter). Lancet 340:1097, 1992

Ghadirian AM, Chouinard G, Annable L: Sexual dysfunction and plasma prolactin levels in neuroleptic-treated schizophrenic outpatients. J Nerv Ment Dis 170:463–467, 1982

Giles TD, Modlin RK: Death associated with ventricular arrhythmia and thioridazine hydrochloride. JAMA 205:108–110, 1968

Gill SS, Rochon PA, Herrmann N, et al: Atypical antipsychotic drugs and risk of ischaemic stroke: population based retrospective cohort study. BMJ 330:445, 2005

Glazer WM, Moore DC, Schooler NR, et al: Tardive dyskinesia: a discontinuation study. Arch Gen Psychiatry 41:623–627, 1984

Glick ID, Marder SR: Long term maintenance therapy with quetiapine versus haloperidol decanoate in patients with schizophrenia or schizoaffective disorder. J Clin Psychiatry 66:638–641, 2005

Goff DC, Baldessarini R: Antipsychotics, in Drug Interactions in Psychiatry, 2nd Edition. Edited by Ciraulo D, Shader R, Greenblatt D, et al. Baltimore, MD, Williams & Wilkins, 1995, pp 129–174

Goff DC, Coyle JT: The emerging role of glutamate in the pathophysiology and treatment of schizophrenia. Am J Psychiatry 158:1366–1377, 2001

Goff DC, Evins AE: Negative symptoms in schizophrenia: neurobiological models and treatment response. Harv Rev Psychiatry 6:59–77, 1998

Goff DC, Midha KK, Sarid-Segal O, et al: A placebo-controlled trial of fluoxetine added to neuroleptic in patients with schizophrenia. Psychopharmacology (Berl) 117:417–423, 1995

Goff D, Posever T, Herz L, et al: An exploratory haloperidol-controlled dose-finding study of ziprasidone in hospitalized patients with schizophrenia or schizoaffective disorder. J Clin Psychopharmacol 18:296–304, 1998

Goldberg HL, Finnerty RJ: The comparative efficacy of buspirone and diazepam in the treatment of anxiety. Am J Psychiatry 136:1184–1187, 1979

Goodwin FK, Jamison R: Manic-Depressive Illness. New York, Oxford University Press, 1990

Gram L, Bentsen KD: Hepatic toxicity of antiepileptic drugs: a review. Acta Neurol Scand Suppl 97:81–90, 1983

Green MF, Marshall BD Jr, Wirshing WC, et al: Does risperidone improve verbal working memory in treatment-resistant schizophrenia? Am J Psychiatry 154:799–804, 1997

Greenblatt DJ, von Moltke LL, Harmatz JS, et al: Drug interactions with newer antidepressants: role of human cytochromes P450. J Clin Psychiatry 59 (suppl 15):19–27, 1998

Greenblatt DJ, von Moltke LL, Harmatz JS, et al: Human cytochromes and some newer antidepressants: kinetics, metabolism, and drug interactions. J Clin Psychopharmacol 19:23S–35S, 1999

Guy W: Abnormal Involuntary Movement Scale (AIMS), in ECDEU Assessment Manual for Psychopharmacology, Revised. Washington, DC, U.S. Department of Health, Welfare, and Education, 1976, pp 534–537

Guze BH, Baxter LR: Current concepts: neuroleptic malignant syndrome. N Engl J Med 313:163–166, 1985

Hagger C, Buckley P, Kenny JT, et al: Improvement in cognitive functions and psychiatric symptoms in treatment-refractory schizophrenic patients receiving clozapine. Biol Psychiatry 34:702–712, 1993

Hamilton JD: Thioridazine retinopathy within the upper dosage limit. Psychosomatics 26:823–824, 1985

Haring C, Barnas C, Saria A, et al: Dose-related plasma levels of clozapine. J Clin Psychopharmacol 9:71–72, 1989

Harvey KV, Balon R: Augmentation with buspirone: a review. Ann Clin Psychiatry 7:143–147, 1995

Henderson DC, Cagliero E, Gray C, et al: Clozapine, diabetes mellitus, weight gain, and lipid abnormalities: a 5-year naturalistic study. Am J Psychiatry 157:975–981, 2000

Herrmann N, Lanctot KL: Do atypical antipsychotics cause stroke? CNS Drugs 19:91–103, 2005

Hetmar O, Bren C, Clemmesen L, et al: Lithium: long-term effects on the kidney, II: structural changes. J Psychiatr Res 21:279–288, 1987

Hetmar O, Poulsen UJ, Ladefoged J, et al: Lithium: long-term effects on the kidney: a prospective follow-up study ten years after kidney biopsy. Br J Psychiatry 158:53–58, 1991

Hodgman MJ, Martin TG, Krenzelok EP: Serotonin syndrome due to venlafaxine and maintenance tranylcypromine therapy. Hum Exp Toxicol 16:14–17, 1997

Holmes LB, Wyszynski DF, Baldwin EJ, et al: Increased risk for non-syndromic cleft palate among infants exposed to lamotrigine during pregnancy (abstract). Birth Defects Res A Clin Mol Teratol 76:318, 2006

Honigfeld G: Clozapine National Registry System: forty years of risk management. J Clin Psychiatry Monogr 14:29–32, 1996

Honigfeld G, Arellano F, Sethi J, et al: Reducing clozapine-related morbidity and mortality: 5 years of experience with the Clozaril National Registry. J Clin Psychiatry 59 (suppl 3): 3–7, 1998

Hurd RW, Van Rinsvelt HA, Wilder BJ, et al: Selenium, zinc, and copper changes with valproic acid: possible relation to drug side effects. Neurology 34:1393–1395, 1984

Hustey FM: Acute quetiapine poisoning. J Emerg Med 17:995–997, 1999

Isojarvi JIT, Laatikainen TJ, Pakarinen AJ, et al: Polycystic ovaries and hyperandrogenism in women taking valproate for epilepsy. N Engl J Med 39:579–584, 1993

Isojarvi JI, Laatikainen TJ, Knip M, et al: Obesity and endocrine disorders in women taking valproate for epilepsy. Ann Neurol 39:579–584, 1996

Itil TM, Soldatos C: Epileptogenic side effects of psychotropic drugs: practical recommendations. JAMA 244:1460–1463, 1980

Jaeken J, Casaer P, Corbeel L: Valproate, hyperammonaemia, and hyperglycinaemia (letter). Lancet 2(8188):260, 1980

Jankowsky D, Curtis G, Zisook S, et al: Trazodone-aggravated ventricular arrhythmias. J Clin Psychopharmacol 3:372–376, 1983

Jenkins SC, Tinsley JA, Van Loon JA: A Pocket Reference for Psychiatrists, 3rd Edition. Washington, DC, American Psychiatric Publishing, 2001, pp 133–134

Jeste DV, Wyatt RJ: Understanding and Treating Tardive Dyskinesia. New York, Guilford, 1982

Jeste DV, Lacro JP, Bailey A, et al: Lower incidence of tardive dyskinesia with risperidone compared to haloperidol in older patients. J Am Geriatr Soc 47:716–719, 1999

Jones KL, Lacro RV, Johnson KA, et al: Pattern of malformations in the children of women treated with carbamazepine during pregnancy. N Engl J Med 320:1661–1666, 1989

Källén B, Otterblad Olausson P: Antidepressant drugs during pregnancy and infant congenital heart defect. Reprod Toxicol 21:221–222, 2006

Kane JM: Treatment-resistant schizophrenic patients. J Clin Psychiatry 57:35–40, 1996

Kane JM, Smith JM: Tardive dyskinesia: prevalence and risk factors, 1959 to 1979. Arch Gen Psychiatry 39:473–481, 1982

Kane JM, Honigfeld G, Singer J, et al: Clozapine for the treatment-resistant schizophrenic: a double-blind comparison vs chlorpromazine/benztropine. Arch Gen Psychiatry 45:789–796, 1988

Kane JM, Eerdekens M, Lindenmayer JP, et al: Long-acting injectable risperidone: efficacy and safety of the first long-acting atypical antipsychotic. Am J Psychiatry 160:1125–1132, 2003

Kapur S, Seeman P: Does fast dissociation from the dopamine D2 receptor explain the action of atypical antipsychotics? A new hypothesis. Am J Psychiatry 158:360–369, 2001

Karoum F, Chuang LW, Eisler T, et al: Metabolism of (−)deprenyl to amphetamine and methamphetamine may be responsible for deprenyl's therapeutic benefit: a biochemical assessment. Neurology 32:503–509, 1982

Keck PE Jr, Pope HG Jr, Cohen BM, et al: Risk factor for neuroleptic malignant syndrome. Arch Gen Psychiatry 46:914–918, 1989

Keck PE Jr, McElroy SL, Nemeroff CB: Anticonvulsants in the treatment of bipolar disorder. J Neuropsychiatry Clin Neurosci 4:395–405, 1992

Keck PE Jr, McElroy SL, Tugrul KC, et al: Valproate oral loading in the treatment of acute mania. J Clin Psychiatry 54:305–308, 1993

Keck P Jr, Buffenstein A, Ferguson J, et al: Ziprasidone 40 and 120 mg/day in the acute exacerbation of schizophrenia and schizoaffective disorder: a 4-week placebo-controlled trial. Psychopharmacology (Berl) 140:173–184, 1998

Kennedy PF, Hershon HI, McGuire RJ: Extrapyramidal disorders after prolonged phenothiazine therapy. Br J Psychiatry 118:509–518, 1971

Ketter TA, Flockhart DA, Post RM, et al: The emerging role of cytochrome P450 3A in psychopharmacology. J Clin Psychopharmacol 15:387–398, 1995

Kilian JG, Kerr K, Lawrence C, et al: Myocarditis and cardiomyopathy associated with clozapine. Lancet 354:1841–1845, 1999

Kim JS, Chang MY, Yu IT, et al: Lithium selectivity increases neuronal differentiation of hippocampal neural progenitor cells both in vitro and in vivo. J Neurochem 89:324–336, 2004

Kinon BJ, Basson BR, Gilmore JA, et al: Long-term olanzapine treatment: weight change and weight-related health factors in schizophrenia. J Clin Psychiatry 62:92–100, 2001

Kleinberg D, Brecher M, Davis J: Prolactin levels and adverse events in patients treated with risperidone. Paper presented at the 150th annual meeting of the American Psychiatric Association, San Diego, CA, May 17–22, 1997

Klibanski A, Neer R, Beitins I: Decreased bone density in hyperprolactinemic women. N Engl J Med 303:1511–1514, 1981

Kolecki P: Venlafaxine induced serotonin syndrome occurring after abstinence from phenelzine for more than two weeks (letter). J Toxicol Clin Toxicol 35:211–212, 1997

Labbate LA, Pollack MH: Treatment of fluoxetine-induced sexual dysfunction with bupropion: a case report. Ann Clin Psychiatry 6:13–15, 1994

Laird LK: Issues in the monopharmacotherapy and polypharmacotherapy of obsessive-compulsive disorder. Psychopharmacol Bull 32:569–578, 1996

Lamictal (product information). Research Triangle Park, NC, GlaxoSmithKline, 2005

Lammer EJ, Sever LE, Oakley GP Jr: Teratogen update: valproic acid. Teratology 35:465–473, 1987

Leach MJ, Baxter MG, Critchley MA: Neurochemical and behavioral aspects of lamotrigine. Epilepsia 32 (suppl 2):S4–S8, 1991

Lehman AF, Lieberman JA, Dixon LB, et al: Practice guideline for the treatment of patients with schizophrenia, 2nd edition. Am J Psychiatry 161 (suppl 2):1–56, 2004

Lenox RH, Watson DG, Patel J, et al: Chronic lithium administration alters a prominent PKC substrate in rat hippocampus. Brain Res 570:333–340, 1992

Lewis SW, Barnes TR, Davies L, et al: Randomized controlled trial of effect of prescription of clozapine versus other second-generation antipsychotic drugs in resistant schizophrenia. Schizophr Bull 32:715–723, 2006

Lieberman JA, Saltz BL, Johns CA, et al: The effects of clozapine on tardive dyskinesia. Br J Psychiatry 158:503–510, 1991

Lieberman JA, Stroup TS, McEvoy JP, et al: Effectiveness of antipsychotic drugs in patients with chronic schizophrenia. N Engl J Med 353:1209–1223, 2005

Linazasoro G: Worsening of Parkinson's disease by citalopram. Parkinsonism Relat Disord 6:111–113, 2000

Lipinski JF, Zubenko GS, Cohen BM, et al: Propranolol in the treatment of neuroleptic induced akathisia. Am J Psychiatry 141:412–415, 1984

Lohr JB, Caligiuri MP: A double-blind placebo-controlled study of vitamin E treatment of tardive dyskinesia. J Clin Psychiatry 57:167–173, 1996

Lohr JB, Cadet JL, Lohr MA, et al: Alpha-tocopherol in tardive dyskinesia. Lancet 1:913–914, 1987

Lucki I, Rickels K, Geller AM: Chronic use of benzodiazepines and psychomotor and cognitive test performance. Psychopharmacology (Berl) 88:426–433, 1986

Lunesta (product information). Marlborough, MA, Sepracor, 2005

Macdonald RL, Kelly KM: Antiepileptic drug mechanisms of action. Epilepsia 36:S2–S12, 1995

Mallette LE, Eichhorn E: Effects of lithium carbonate on human calcium metabolism. Arch Intern Med 146:770–776, 1986

Manji HK, Bebchuk JM, Moore GJ, et al: Modulation of CNS signal transduction pathways and gene expression by mood-stabilizing agents: therapeutic implications. J Clin Psychiatry 60 (suppl 2):27–39, 1993

Manji HK, Chen G, Shimon H, et al: Guanine nucleotide-binding proteins in bipolar affective disorder: effects of long-term lithium treatment. Arch Gen Psychiatry 52:135–144, 1995

Manji HK, Chen G, Hsiao JK, et al: Regulation of signal transduction pathways by mood-stabilizing agents: implications for the delayed onset of therapeutic efficacy. J Clin Psychiatry 57 (suppl 13):34–46, 1996

Manji HK, Chen G, Hsiao JK, et al: Regulation of signal transduction pathways by mood-stabilizing agents: implications for the delayed onset of therapeutic efficacy. J Clin Psychiatry 57:34–46, 1999

Marder SR, Meibach RC: Risperidone in the treatment of schizophrenia. Am J Psychiatry 151:825–835, 1994

Margolese HC, Chouinard G, Kolivakis TT, et al: Tardive dyskinesia in the era of typical and atypical antipsychotics, part 2: incidence and management strategies in patients with schizophrenia. Can J Psychiatry 50:703–714, 2005

McEvoy JP, Lieberman JA, Stroup TS, et al: Effectiveness of clozapine versus olanzapine, quetiapine, and risperidone in patients with chronic schizophrenia who did not respond to prior atypical antipsychotic treatment. Am J Psychiatry 163:600–610, 2006

McKenna K, Koren G, Tetelbaum M, et al: Pregnancy outcome of women using atypical antipsychotic drugs: a prospective comparative study. J Clin Psychiatry 66:444–449, 2005

Meltzer HY: The mechanism of action of novel antipsychotic drugs. Schizophr Bull 17:265–287, 1991

Meltzer HY: An overview of the mechanism of action of clozapine. J Clin Psychiatry 55 (suppl B):47–52, 1994

Metzger E, Friedman R: Prolongation of the corrected QT and torsades de pointes cardiac arrhythmia associated with intravenous haloperidol in the medically ill. J Clin Psychopharmacol 13:128–132, 1993

Michalets EL: Update: clinically significant cytochrome P450 drug interactions. Pharmacotherapy 18:84–112, 1998

Miller DD, Sharafuddin MJ, Kathol RG: A case of clozapine-induced neuroleptic malignant syndrome. J Clin Psychiatry 52:99–101, 1991

Munjack DJ, Bruns J, Baltazar PL, et al: A pilot study of buspirone in the treatment of social phobia. J Anxiety Disord 5:87–98, 1991

Murphy MJ, Lyon IW, Taylor JW, et al: Valproic acid associated pancreatitis in an adult (letter). Lancet 1(8210):41–42, 1981

Nielsen H: Recombinant human granulocyte colony-stimulating factor (rhG-CSF; filgrastim) treatment of clozapine-induced agranulocytosis. J Intern Med 234:529–531, 1993

NIMH/NIH Consensus Development Conference Statement: Mood disorders: pharmacological prevention of recurrences. Consensus Development Panel. Am J Psychiatry 142:469–476, 1985

Nishino S, Mishima K, Mignot E, et al: Sedative-hypnotics, in The American Psychiatric Publishing Textbook of Psychopharmacology, 3rd Edition. Edited by Schatzberg AF, Nemeroff CB. Washington, DC, American Psychiatric Publishing, 2004, pp 651–670

Oldham JM: Guideline Watch: Practice Guidelines for the Treatment of Patients With Borderline Personality Disorder. Arlington, VA, American Psychiatric Association, 2005

Oliver AP, Luchins DJ, Wyatt RJ: Neuroleptic-induced seizures: an in vitro technique for assessing relative risk. Arch Gen Psychiatry 39:206–209, 1982

Patterson JF: Stevens-Johnson syndrome associated with carbamazepine therapy (letter). J Clin Psychopharmacol 5:185, 1985

Pearlstein TB, Halbreich U, Batzar ED, et al: Psychosocial functioning in women with premenstrual dysphoric disorder before and after treatment with sertraline or placebo. J Clin Psychiatry 61:101–109, 2000

Pellock JM: Carbamazepine side effects in children and adults. Epilepsia 28:S64–S70, 1987

Pellock JM, Willmore LJ: A rational guide to routine blood monitoring in patients receiving antiepileptic drugs. Neurology 41:961–964, 1991

Pendlebury SC, Moses DK, Eadie MJ: Hyponatremia during oxcarbazepine therapy. Hum Toxicol 8:337–344, 1989

Perlis RH, Sachs GS, Lafer B, et al: Effect of abrupt change from standard to low serum levels of lithium: a reanalysis of double-blind lithium maintenance data. Am J Psychiatry 159:1155–1159, 2002

Perry PJ, Miller DD, Arndt SV, et al: Clozapine and norclozapine plasma concentrations and clinical response of treatment-refractory schizophrenic patients. Am J Psychiatry 148:231–235, 1991

Physicians' Desk Reference, 51st Edition. Montvale, NJ, Medical Economics, 2001

Pies RW: Handbook of Essential Psychopharmacology. Washington, DC, American Psychiatric Press, 1998

Plenge P, Mellerup ET, Bolwig C, et al: Lithium treatment: does the kidney prefer one daily dose instead of two? Acta Psychiatr Scand 66:121–128, 1982

Preskorn SH, Burke M: Somatic therapy for major depressive disorder: selection of an antidepressant. J Clin Psychiatry 53 (suppl):5–18, 1992

Purdon SE, Jones BDW, Stip E, et al: Neuropsychological change in early phase schizophrenia during 12 months of treatment with olanzapine, risperidone, or haloperidol. Arch Gen Psychiatry 57:249–258, 2000

Quitkin FM, Rifkin A, Klein DF: Monoamine oxidase inhibitors: a review of antidepressant effectiveness. Arch Gen Psychiatry 36:749–760, 1979

Rakel RE: Long-term buspirone therapy for chronic anxiety: a multicenter international study to determine safety. South Med J 83:194–198, 1990

Reitan JA, Porter W, Braunstein M: Comparison of psychomotor skills and amnesia after induction of anesthesia with midazolam or thiopental. Anesth Analg 65:933–937, 1986

Robert E, Guibaud P: Maternal valproic acid and congenital neural tube defects (letter). Lancet 2(8304):937, 1982

Rohatagi S, Barrett JS, DeWitt KE, et al: Integrated pharmacokinetic and metabolic modeling of selegiline and metabolites after transdermal administration. Biopharm Drug Dispos 18:567–584, 1997

Rosa FW: Spina bifida in infants of women treated with carbamazepine during pregnancy. N Engl J Med 324:674–677, 1991

Rosebush PI, Stewart TD: A prospective analysis of 24 episodes of neuroleptic malignant syndrome. Am J Psychiatry 146:717–725, 1989

Rosebush PI, Stewart TD, Gelenberg AJ: Twenty neuroleptic rechallenges after neuroleptic malignant syndrome in 15 patients. J Clin Psychiatry 50:295–298, 1989

Rosebush PI, Stewart T, Mazurek MF: The treatment of neuroleptic malignant syndrome: are dantrolene and bromocriptine useful adjuncts to supportive care? Br J Psychiatry 159:709–712, 1991

Rosenbaum JF, Fava M, Hoog SL, et al: Selective serotonin reuptake inhibitor discontinuation syndrome: a randomized clinical trial. Biol Psychiatry 44:77–87, 1998

Rosenberg L, Mitchell AA, Parsells JL, et al: Lack of relation of oral clefts to diazepam use during pregnancy. N Engl J Med 309:1282–1285, 1983

Rossi A, Mancini F, Stratta P, et al: Risperidone, negative symptoms, and cognitive deficit in schizophrenia: an open study. Acta Psychiatr Scand 95:40–43, 1997

Rothschild AJ: Disinhibition, amnestic reactions, and other adverse reactions secondary to triazolam: a review of the literature. J Clin Psychiatry 53(suppl):69–79, 1992

Sackeim HA, Haskett RF, Mulsant BH, et al: Continuation pharmacotherapy in the prevention of relapse following electroconvulsive therapy: a randomized controlled trial. JAMA 285:1299–1307, 2001

Scher M, Krieger JN, Juergens S: Trazodone and priapism. Am J Psychiatry 140:1362–1363, 1983

Schneier FR, Saoud JB, Campeas RC, et al: Buspirone in social phobia. J Clin Psychopharmacol 13:251–256, 1992

Seide H, Muller HR: Choreiform movements as side effects of phenothiazine medication in elderly patients. J Am Geriatr Soc 15:517–522, 1967

Shader RI, Greenblatt DJ: Approaches to the treatment of anxiety states, in Manual of Psychiatric Therapeutics, 3rd Edition. Edited by Shader RI. Philadelphia, PA, Lippincott Williams & Wilkins, 2003, pp 199–200

Sheehan DV, Raj AB, Sheehan KH, et al: Is buspirone effective for panic disorder? J Clin Psychopharmacol 10:3–11, 1990

Shelton RC, Stahl SM: Risperidone and paroxetine given singly and in combination for bipolar depression. J Clin Psychiatry 65:1715–1719, 2004

Shulman KI, Walker SE: Refining the MAOI diet: tyramine content of pizzas and soy products. J Clin Psychiatry 60:191–193, 1999

Shulman KI, Walker SE: Reply: clarifying the safety of the MAOI diet and pizza (letter). J Clin Psychiatry 61:145–146, 2000

Shulman KI, Tailor SA, Walker SE, et al: Tap (draft) beer and monoamine oxidase inhibitor dietary restrictions. Can J Psychiatry 42:310–312, 1997

Small J, Hirsch S, Arvanitis L, et al: Quetiapine in patients with schizophrenia. Arch Gen Psychiatry 54:549–557, 1997

Smith WT, Glaudin V, Panagides J, et al: Mirtazapine vs. amitriptyline vs. placebo in the treatment of major depressive disorder. Psychopharmacol Bull 26:191–196, 1990

Sramek JJ, Tansman M, Suri A, et al: Efficacy of buspirone in generalized anxiety disorder with coexisting mild depressive symptoms. J Clin Psychiatry 57:287–291, 1996

Stewart RB, Karas B, Springer PK: Haloperidol excretion in human milk. Am J Psychiatry 137:849–850, 1980

Suppes T, Webb A, Paul B, et al: Clinical outcome in a randomized 1-year trial of clozapine versus treatment as usual for patients with treatment-resistant illness and a history of mania. Am J Psychiatry 156:1164–1169, 1999

Tallman JF, Paul SM, Skolnick P, et al: Receptors for the age of anxiety: pharmacology of the benzodiazepines. Science 207:274–281, 1980

Tarsy D, Baldessarini RJ: Epidemiology of tardive dyskinesia: is risk declining with modern antipsychotics? Mov Disord 21:589–598, 2006

Tohen M, Vieta E, Calabrese J, et al: Efficacy of olanzapine-fluoxetine combination in the treatment of bipolar I depression. Arch Gen Psychiatry 60:1079–1088, 2003

Tollefson GD, Beasley CM Jr, Tamura RN: Blind, controlled long-term study of the comparative incidence of treatment-emergent tardive dyskinesia with olanzapine or haloperidol. Am J Psychiatry 154:1248–1254, 1997

Trileptal (product information). East Hanover, NJ, Novartis Pharmaceuticals Corp, 2006

Trivedi MH, Fava M, Wisniewski SR, et al: Medication augmentation after the failure of SSRIs for depression. N Engl J Med 354:1243–1252, 2006

van Putten T, May PRA, Marder SR: Akathisia with haloperidol and thiothixene. Arch Gen Psychiatry 31:67–72, 1984

Vitullo RN, Wharton JM, Allen NB, et al: Trazodone-related exercise-induced nonsustained ventricular tachycardia. Chest 98:247–248, 1990

Walker SE, Shulman KI, Tailor SAN, et al: Tyramine content of previously restricted foods in monoamine oxidase inhibitor diets. J Clin Psychopharmacol 16:383–388, 1996

Walker SE, Shulman KE, Tailor SAN: Reply: tyramine content in Chinese food. J Clin Psychopharmacol 17:227–228, 1997

Warnock JK, Knesevich J: Adverse cutaneous reactions to antidepressants. Am J Psychiatry 145:425–430, 1988

Wecker L, James S, Copeland N, et al: Transdermal selegiline: targeted effects on monoamine oxidases in the brain. Biol Psychiatry 54:1099–1104, 2003

Weisler RH, Kalali AH, Ketter TA, et al: A multicenter, randomized, double-blind, placebo-controlled trial of extended-release carbamazepine capsules as monotherapy for bipolar disorder patients with manic or mixed episodes. J Clin Psychiatry 65:478–484, 2004

Weisler RH, Keck PE Jr, Swann AC, et al: Extended-release carbamazepine capsules as monotherapy for acute mania in bipolar disorder: a multicenter, randomized, double-blind, placebo-controlled trial. J Clin Psychiatry 66:323–330, 2005

Wetzel H, Anghelescu I, Szegedi A, et al: Pharmacokinetic interactions of clozapine with selective serotonin reuptake inhibitors: differential effects of fluvoxamine and paroxetine in a prospective study. J Clin Psychopharmacol 18:2–9, 1998

Wikander I, Sundblad C, Andersch B, et al: Citalopram in premenstrual dysphoria: is intermittent treatment during luteal phases more effective than continuous medication throughout the menstrual cycle? J Clin Psychopharmacol 18:390–398, 1998

Wing YK, Chen CN: Tyramine content in Chinese food (letter). J Clin Psychopharmacol 17:227, 1997

Yassa R, Lal S: Prevalence of the rabbit syndrome. Am J Psychiatry 143:656–657, 1986

Yeo PP, Bates D, Howe JG, et al: Anticonvulsants and thyroid function. Br Med J 1:1581–1583, 1978

Yonkers KA, Halbreich U, Freeman E, et al: Symptomatic improvement of premenstrual dysphoric disorder with sertraline treatment: a randomized controlled trial. Sertraline Premenstrual Dysphoric Collaborative Study Group. JAMA 278:983–988, 1997

Zubenko GS, Cohen BM, Lipinski JF: Comparison of metoprolol and propranolol in the treatment of lithium tremor. Psychiatry Res 11:163–164, 1984

Zyban (package insert). Research Triangle Park, NC, GlaxoSmithKline, 2005

# 31

# Nonpharmacological Somatic Treatments

MARK S. GEORGE, M.D.

ZIAD H. NAHAS, M.D., M.S.C.R.

JEFFREY J. BORCKARDT, Ph.D.

BERRY ANDERSON, B.S.N., R.N.

MILTON J. FOUST JR., M.D.

Psychiatry is developing a third realm of treatment modalities, complementing the well-established realms of psychopharmacology (medications) and psychotherapy. As a class, these methods involve focal electrical brain stimulation of some sort and vary widely in their invasiveness and methods of delivery. Table 31–1 lists the current methods.

## Electroconvulsive Therapy

ECT is the grandfather of this new family of treatments and involves the deliberate induction of a generalized tonic-clonic seizure by electrical means. Contemporary ECT devices typically deliver bidirectional (alternating current), brief-pulse, square-wave stimulation through a pair of electrodes, which are applied externally on the patient's scalp. Because of the risk of bodily harm from the convulsion, ECT is performed under general anesthesia, with the body paralyzed. As with other convulsive therapies that historically preceded ECT, the goal is to produce a seizure. The presence of seizure activity appears to be essential; stimuli that are below the seizure threshold appear to be clinically ineffective. And although the production of a seizure appears to be necessary, a seizure alone is

The authors' work with brain stimulation treatments has been supported over the past 5 years in part by research grants from NARSAD, the Stanley Foundation, the Borderline Personality Disorders Research Foundation (BPDRF), and the Dana Foundation; by National Institute of Neurological Disorders and Stroke (NINDS) grant RO1 AG40956 (George); by National Institutes of Health (NIH) grants RO1 AG409565R01MH069887-02 (George), 1 RO1 MH069887-01 (George), and 1K08MH070915-01A1 (Nahas); and by the Defense Advanced Research Projects Agency (DARPA). The Brain Stimulation Laboratory at the Medical University of South Carolina, Charleston, has also received grant funding from GlaxoSmithKline, Jazz, Cyberonics, Neuronetics, and NeuroPace. Dr. George holds several transcranial magnetic stimulation (TMS)–related patents. These are not in the area of TMS therapeutics, but rather are for new TMS machine designs as well as for combining TMS with magnetic resonance imaging (MRI). Dr. George serves or has served as a paid consultant to several device and pharmaceutical companies.

**TABLE 31–1. Overview of somatic nonpharmacological treatments**

| Acronym (full name) | Convulsive? | Stimulation site | Psychiatric disorders | Clinical use status |
|---|---|---|---|---|
| ECT (electroconvulsive therapy) | Yes | Cortical | Depression, mania, catatonia | Grandfathered FDA approval |
| rTMS (repetitive transcranial magnetic stimulation) | | Cortical | Depression | Pivotal trial in depression complete; FDA review under way; some psychiatrists already use rTMS off-label |
| VNS (vagus nerve stimulation) | | Cervical cranial nerve | Depression | FDA approved for treatment-resistant depression |
| MST (magnetic seizure therapy) | Yes | Cortical | Depression | Experimental for all conditions |
| DBS (deep brain stimulation) | | Subcortical | Depression | FDA approved for Parkinson's disease; pivotal trials in depression under way |
| tDCS (transcranial direct current stimulation) | | Cortical | Substance abuse, depression | Experimental for all conditions |
| TENS (transcutaneous electrical nerve stimulation) | | Peripheral nerve | Pain | FDA approved for pain conditions |
| EPI-fMRI (echoplanar imaging–functional magnetic resonance imaging) | | Unknown; possibly subcortical | Depression | Experimental for all conditions |
| FEAT (focal electrical alternating current therapy); also known as tACS (transcranial alternating current stimulation) | | Cortical | Depression | Experimental for all conditions |
| FEAST (focal electrical alternating current seizure therapy) | Yes | Cortical | Depression | Experimental for all conditions |

*Note.*   FDA=U.S. Food and Drug Administration.

not sufficient. Some forms of seizure induction are in fact clinically ineffective (Sackeim et al. 1993). A variety of psychiatric and neurological conditions respond favorably to ECT, particularly if they are severe or accompanied by psychotic symptoms, although the majority of patients treated with ECT have mood disorders, such as unipolar or bipolar depression. Other conditions, such as mania, schizoaffective disorder, catatonia, neuroleptic malignant syndrome, Parkinson's disease, and intractable seizures, may respond to ECT as well. Patients with schizophrenia who also have a prominent disturbance of mood are likely to respond best to ECT. For a typical series or course of ECT, treatments are usually given two to three times per week for six to eight treatments. This may then be followed by maintenance treatment in the form of medication, additional ECT given at less frequent intervals, or both. New data have suggested that shorter pulse widths are less toxic than the fatter pulse widths used in traditional ECT (Sackeim et al. 2000). (Applying electricity after the neuron has depolarized is not necessary and is perhaps cognitively harmful.) Also, ECT as practiced in the general community has lower response rates (20%–50%) than historical response rates (60%–80%) in the literature published in academic medical settings (Prudic et al. 2004). ECT is unfortunately associated with acute and sometimes chronic memory loss (Lisanby et al. 2000; Sackeim 2000). Because of these limitations, it is underused.

# Transcranial Magnetic Stimulation

TMS is perhaps the most interesting of all the new techniques because the skull does not need to be opened in order to focally stimulate with TMS, no seizure is needed, and, to date, there appear to be only limited side effects (M.S. George 2002; M.S. George et al. 2000, 2002). TMS involves creating a powerful electrical current near the scalp. The electricity flowing in an electromagnetic coil on the scalp creates an extremely potent (near 1.5 Tesla) but brief (microseconds) magnetic field. The TMS magnetic field performs the neat trick of entering the surface of the brain without interference. Although skin and bone act as resistors to impede electrical currents, magnetic fields pass unimpeded through the skull and soft tissue. In the brain, the magnetic pulse encounters nerve cells with resting potentials and induces electrical current to flow. Thus, electrical energy is converted to magnetic fields, which are then converted back into electrical currents in the brain (Bohning 2000). TMS is thus sometimes called "electrodeless electrical stimulation."

## Therapeutic Uses of TMS

### *Depression*

Although there is controversy, and more work is needed, certain brain regions have consistently been implicated in the pathogenesis of depression and mood regulation (M.S. George 1994; M.S. George et al. 1994a, 1994b, 1995a, 1996, 1997, 1998; Ketter et al. 1996; Kimbrell et al. 2002). These include the medial and dorsolateral prefrontal cortex, the cingulate gyrus, and other regions commonly referred to as limbic (amygdala, hippocampus, parahippocampus, septum, hypothalamus, limbic thalamus, insula) and paralimbic (anterior temporal pole, orbitofrontal cortex). A widely held theory over the last decade has been that depression results from a dysregulation of these prefrontal cortical and limbic regions (M.S. George et al. 1994b, 1995b, 1996; Mayberg et al. 1999).

The very first uses of TMS as an antidepressant were not influenced by this regional neuroanatomical literature, and stimulation was applied over the vertex (Beer 1902; Grisaru et al. 1994; Kolbinger et al. 1995). However, working within the prefrontal cortical limbic dysregulation framework outlined above, and given that theories of ECT action emphasize the role of prefrontal cortex effects (Nobler et al. 1994), in 1995 George performed the first open trial of prefrontal TMS as an antidepressant (M.S. George et al. 1995c), followed immediately by a crossover double-blind study (M.S. George et al. 1997). My reasoning was that chronic, frequent subconvulsive stimulation of the prefrontal cortex over several weeks might initiate a therapeutic cascade of events both in the prefrontal cortex and in connected limbic regions, thereby causing the dysregulated circuits to rebalance and normalize, thus alleviating depression symptoms (M.S. George and Wassermann 1994).

The imaging evidence previously discussed now shows that this hunch was largely correct—prefrontal TMS sends direct information to important mood-regulating regions like the cingulate gyrus, orbitofrontal cortex, insula, and hippocampus. Thus, beginning with these prefrontal studies, modern TMS was specifically designed as a focal nonconvulsive, circuit-based approach to therapy.

Since the initial studies, there has been continued high interest in TMS as an antidepressant treatment. There are now more than 29 published randomized clinical trials evaluating TMS as an antidepressant. Because initially there was no large TMS company promoting TMS as a treatment, until recently all of these studies were government or foundation sponsored, and all were conducted at a single site. As in any new field, not all TMS antidepressant treatment studies have been positive (Loo et al. 1999). Five independent meta-analyses of the published or public TMS antidepressant literature, each differing in the articles included and the statistics used (Burt et al. 2002; Holtzheimer et al. 2001; Kozel and George 2002; Martin et al. 2002; McNamara et al. 2001), largely concluded that daily prefrontal TMS delivered over several weeks has antidepressant effects greater than sham treatment. Several small-sample studies have compared TMS with ECT without finding differences in efficacy. TMS was clearly more easily tolerated than ECT, with no cognitive side effects and no need for repeated general anesthesia.

Saxby Pridmore, a TMS pioneer in this area, in 2000 compared the antidepressant effects of standard ECT (three times per week) and one ECT per week followed by TMS on the other 4 weekdays (Pridmore 2000). At 3 weeks, both regimens had produced similar antidepressant effects. Relapse rates in the 6 months following ECT or rTMS were similar (Dannon et al. 2002).

## Vagus Nerve Stimulation

TMS is noninvasive, focal, largely limited to different cortical sites, and intermittent. VNS is in some sense the opposite of TMS, as it is invasive and requires surgical implantation of a device in the chest wall and a wire in the neck. The brain region stimulated always follows the same initial route—the vagus nerve in the neck. It is also a permanent implant that cannot be removed without surgery. Finally, although TMS has not been approved by the U.S. Food and Drug Administration (FDA) to treat any disorder, VNS has been approved for almost 10 years as a treatment for epilepsy (Ben-Menachem et al. 1994; R. George et al. 1994; Salinsky et al. 1996; Uthman et al. 1993; Vagus Nerve Stimulation Study Group 1995) and was FDA approved in 2005 for chronic use in patients with treatment-resistant depression.

## VNS Methods

The broad term *vagus nerve stimulation* refers to any technique used to stimulate the vagus nerve, including animal studies in which the vagus was accessed through the abdomen and diaphragm. However, for virtually all human studies, *VNS* refers to stimulation of the left cervical vagus nerve using a commercial device.

VNS resembles the implantation of a cardiac pacemaker. In both VNS and cardiac pacemakers, a subcutaneous generator sends an electrical signal to an organ through an implanted electrode. With VNS, the electrical stimulation is delivered through the generator, an implantable, multiprogrammable, bipolar pulse generator (about the size of a pocket watch) that is implanted in the left chest wall to deliver electrical signals to the left vagus nerve through a bipolar lead. The electrode is wrapped around the vagus nerve in the neck and is connected to the generator subcutaneously.

VNS implantation surgery is typically an outpatient procedure and is most commonly, but not exclusively, performed by neurosurgeons. The VNS generator can be controlled by a personal computer or personal digital assistant (PDA) connected to an infrared wand. As a safety feature, the VNS generator is designed to shut off in the presence of a constant magnetic field. Each patient is thus given a magnet that, when held over the pulse generator, turns off stimulation. When the magnet is removed, normal programmed stimulation resumes. This allows patients to control and temporarily eliminate stimulation-related side effects during important behaviors such as public speaking (voice tremor) or heavy exercising (mild shortness of breath).

## Therapeutic Uses of VNS

### Depression

Psychiatric research has a long history of demonstrating that anticonvulsant medications (e.g., carbamazepine) or devices (e.g., ECT) have mood-stabilizing or antidepressant effects. In early 1998, several lines of evidence suggested that VNS might have antidepressant effects. Anecdotal reports of mood improvement in VNS-implanted epilepsy patients, knowledge of vagus function and neuroanatomy, brain imaging studies, work in animals, and cerebrospinal fluid studies all supported an initial pilot clinical trial in treatment-resistant depression (M.S. George et al. 2000).

In June 1998, the first patient ever treated with VNS for the indication of depression was implanted at the Medical University of South Carolina (MUSC) in Charleston, launching an open study of VNS for the treatment of chronic or recurrent treatment-resistant depression. This study involved four sites (MUSC–Charleston; New York State Psychiatric Institute; University of Texas Southwestern Medical Center in Dallas; and Baylor College of Medicine in Houston, Texas) and initially involved 30 subjects (Rush et al. 2000), with a later extension of 30 more subjects to clarify the effect size and identify response predictors (Sackeim et al. 2001b). The study design involved selecting patients with treatment-resistant, chronic, or recurrent major depressive episode (unipolar or non-rapid-cycling bipolar) and then adding VNS to a stable regimen of antidepressant medications or no antidepressant medications. No stimulation was given for the first 2 weeks following implantation, creating a single-blind placebo phase and allowing for surgical recovery. All patients met eligibility criteria by failing to respond to at least two adequate-treatment trials in the current episode.

Ten weeks of VNS therapy were provided with medications held constant. Of 59 completers (1 patient improved during the surgical recovery period), the response rates were 30.5% for the primary Hamilton Rating Scale for Depression (HRSD28) measure, 34.0% for the Montgomery-Åsberg Depression Rating Scale, and 37.3% for the Clinical Global Impression—Improvement score (CGI-I of 1 or 2). VNS was well tolerated in this group, with side effects similar to those encountered by epilepsy patients. The most common side effect was voice alteration or hoarseness, 60.0% (36/60), which was generally mild and related to the intensity of the output current. There were no adverse cognitive effects (Sackeim et al. 2001a). The only response predictor was prior antidepressant treatment resistance. VNS as used in this open study was more effective in depressed patients who were less treatment resistant.

These encouraging initial results served as the basis for a recently completed U.S. multisite double-blind trial of VNS for chronic or recurrent treatment-resistant depression. In this trial, active VNS failed to show a statistically significant difference in acute response from the sham group (Rush et al. 2005). The sham response rate was 10%, and the active response rate was 15%.

## Key Points: Nonpharmacological Somatic Treatments

- The brain is fundamentally an electrochemical organ, where electrical impulses serve as the basis for information flow and then cause neurotransmitter release.

- Electrical stimulation of the brain can theoretically cause focal neuropsychopharmacological changes without the side effects of systemic medications.

- Brain stimulation therapies as a class share several common concepts and principles and can be understood by identifying which procedures produce seizures on purpose (ECT, MST, focal electrical alternating current seizure therapy [FEAST]) and which do not (TMS, VNS, DBS).

- ECT is our most effective treatment for acute major depression.

- TMS is an exciting research tool.

- Repeated daily prefrontal TMS has acute antidepressant effects similar to those of medications or ECT, with few side effects.

- VNS is FDA approved for the treatment of epilepsy and treatment-resistant depression.

- VNS is best reserved for patients with a long history of depression (chronic) who cannot be given most other treatment options.

- More research on the fundamental neurobiological effects of brain electrical stimulation will help these new techniques continue to improve and evolve.

## References

Beer B: Uber das Auftreten einer objectiven Lichtempfindung in magnetischen Felde. Klinische Wochenzeitschrift 15:108–109, 1902

Ben-Menachem E, Manon-Espaillat R, Ristanovic R, et al: Vagus nerve stimulation for treatment of partial seizures, I: a controlled study of effect on seizures. Epilepsia 35:616–626, 1994

Bohning DE: Introduction and overview of TMS physics, in Transcranial Magnetic Stimulation in Neuropsychiatry. Edited by George MS, Belmaker RH. Washington, DC, American Psychiatric Press, 2000, pp 13–44

Burt T, Lisanby SH, Sackeim HA: Neuropsychiatric applications of transcranial magnetic stimulation. Int J Neuropsychopharmacol 5:73–103, 2002

Dannon PN, Dolberg OT, Schreiber S, et al: Three- and six-month outcome following courses of either ECT or rTMS in a population of severely depressed individuals—preliminary report. Biol Psychiatry 51:687–690, 2002

George MS: An introduction to the emerging neuroanatomy of depression. Psychiatr Ann 24:635–636, 1994

George MS: Advances in brain stimulation. Guest editorial. J ECT 18:169, 2002

George MS, Wassermann EM: Rapid-rate transcranial magnetic stimulation (rTMS) and ECT. Convuls Ther 10:251–253, 1994

George MS, Ketter TA, Parekh PI, et al: Regional brain activity when selecting a response despite interference: an H215O PET study of the Stroop and an emotional Stroop. Hum Brain Mapp 1:194–209, 1994a

George MS, Ketter TA, Post RM: Prefrontal cortex dysfunction in clinical depression. Depression 2:59–72, 1994b

George MS, Ketter TA, Parekh PI, et al: Brain activity during transient sadness and happiness in healthy women. Am J Psychiatry 152:341–351, 1995a

George MS, Post RM, Ketter TA, et al: Neural mechanisms of mood disorders, in Current Review of Mood Disorders. Edited by Rush AJ. Philadelphia, PA, Current Medicine, 1995b, pp 20–25

George MS, Wassermann EM, Williams WA, et al: Daily repetitive transcranial magnetic stimulation (rTMS) improves mood in depression. Neuroreport 6:1853–1856, 1995c

George MS, Ketter TA, Post RM: What functional imaging studies have revealed about the brain basis of mood and emotion, in Advances in Biological Psychiatry. Edited by Panksepp J. Greenwich, CT, JAI Press, 1996, pp 63–113

George MS, Wassermann EM, Kimbrell TA, et al: Mood improvements following daily left prefrontal repetitive transcranial magnetic stimulation in patients with depression: a placebo-controlled crossover trial. Am J Psychiatry 154:1752–1756, 1997

George MS, Huggins T, McDermut W, et al: Abnormal facial emotion recognition in depression: serial testing in an ultra-rapid-cycling patient. Behavior Modification 22:192–204, 1998

George MS, Sackeim HA, Rush AJ, et al: Vagus nerve stimulation: a new tool for brain research and therapy. Biol Psychiatry 47:287–295, 2000

George MS, Nahas Z, Kozel FA, et al: Mechanisms and state of the art of transcranial magnetic stimulation. J ECT 18:170–181, 2002

George R, Salinsky M, Kuzniecky R, et al: Vagus nerve stimulation for treatment of partial seizures, 3: long-term follow-up on first 67 patients exiting a controlled study. First International Vagus Nerve Stimulation Study Group. Epilepsia 35:637–643, 1994

Grisaru N, Yarovslavsky U, Abarbanel J, et al: Transcranial magnetic stimulation in depression and schizophrenia. European Neuropsychopharmacology 4:287–288, 1994

Holtzheimer PE, Russo J, Avery DH: A meta-analysis of repetitive transcranial magnetic stimulation in the treatment of depression. Psychopharmacol Bull 35:149–169, 2001

Ketter TA, Andreason PJ, George MS, et al: Anterior paralimbic mediation of procaine-induced emotional and psychosensory experiences. Arch Gen Psychiatry 53:59–69, 1996

Kimbrell TA, Ketter TA, George MS, et al: Regional cerebral glucose utilization in patients with a range of severities of unipolar depression. Biol Psychiatry 51:237–252, 2002

Kolbinger HM, Hoflich G, Hufnagel A, et al: Transcranial magnetic stimulation (TMS) in the treatment of major depression—a pilot study. Human Psychopharmacology: Clinical and Experimental 10:305–310, 1995

Kozel FA, George MS: Meta-analysis of left prefrontal repetitive transcranial magnetic stimulation (rTMS) to treat depression. J Psychiatr Pract 8:270–275, 2002

Lisanby SH, Maddox JH, Prudic J, et al: The effects of electroconvulsive therapy on memory of autobiographical and public events. Arch Gen Psychiatry 57:581–590, 2000

Loo C, Mitchell P, Sachdev P, et al: A double-blind controlled investigation of transcranial magnetic stimulation for the treatment of resistant major depression. Am J Psychiatry 156:946–948, 1999

Martin JLR, Barbanoj MJ, Schlaepfer TE, et al: Transcranial magnetic stimulation for treating depression. Cochrane Database Syst Rev (2):CD003493, 2002

Mayberg HS, Liotti M, Brannan SK, et al: Reciprocal limbic-cortical function and negative mood: converging PET findings in depression and normal sadness. Am J Psychiatry 156:675–682, 1999

McNamara B, Ray JL, Arthurs OJ, et al: Transcranial magnetic stimulation for depression and other psychiatric disorders. Psychol Med 31:1141–1146, 2001

Nobler MS, Sackeim HA, Prohovnik I, et al: Regional cerebral blood flow in mood disorders, III: treatment and clinical response. Arch Gen Psychiatry 51:884–897, 1994

Pridmore S: Substitution of rapid transcranial magnetic stimulation treatments for electroconvulsive therapy treatments in a course of electroconvulsive therapy. Depress Anxiety 12:118–123, 2000

Pridmore S, Oberoi G: Transcranial magnetic stimulation applications and potential use in chronic pain: studies in waiting. J Neurol Sci 182:1–4, 2000

Prudic J, Olfson M, Marcus SC, et al: Effectiveness of electroconvulsive therapy in community settings. Biol Psychiatry 55:301–312, 2004

Rush AJ, George MS, Sackeim HA, et al: Vagus nerve stimulation (VNS) for treatment-resistant depressions: a multicenter study. Biol Psychiatry 47:276–286, 2000

Rush AJ, Marangell LB, Sackeim HA, et al: Vagus nerve stimulation for treatment-resistant depression: a randomized, controlled acute phase trial. Biol Psychiatry 58:347–354, 2005

Sackeim HA: Memory and ECT: from polarization to reconciliation. J ECT 16:87–96, 2000

Sackeim HA, Prudic J, Devanand DP, et al: Effects of stimulus intensity and electrode placement on the efficacy and cognitive effects of electroconvulsive therapy. N Engl J Med 328:839–846, 1993

Sackeim HA, Prudic J, Devanand DP, et al: A prospective, randomized, double-blind comparison of bilateral and right unilateral electroconvulsive therapy at different stimulus intensities. Arch Gen Psychiatry 57:425–434, 2000

Sackeim HA, Keilp JG, Rush AJ, et al: The effects of vagus nerve stimulation on cognitive performance in patients with treatment-resistant depression. Neuropsychiatry Neuropsychol Behav Neurol 14:53–62, 2001a

Sackeim HA, Rush AJ, George MS, et al: Vagus nerve stimulation (VNS) for treatment-resistant depression: efficacy, side effects, and predictors of outcome. Neuropsychopharmacology 25:713–728, 2001b

Salinsky MC, Uthman BM, Ristanovic RK, et al: Vagus nerve stimulation for the treatment of medically intractable seizures: results of a 1-year open-extension trial. The Vagus Nerve Stimulation Study Group. Arch Neurol 53:1176–1180, 1996

Uthman BM, Wilder BJ, Penry JK, et al: Treatment of epilepsy by stimulation of the vagus nerve. Neurology 43:1338–1345, 1993

Vagus Nerve Stimulation Study Group: A randomized controlled trial of chronic vagus nerve stimulation for treatment of medically intractable seizures. Neurology 45:224–230, 1995

# 32

# Psychodynamic Psychotherapy

ROBERT J. URSANO, M.D.

STEPHEN M. SONNENBERG, M.D.

SUSAN G. LAZAR, M.D.

## The Focus of Psychodynamic Psychotherapy

Psychodynamic (psychoanalytically oriented) psychotherapy focuses primarily on the effects of past experience on molding patterns of behavior and expectations through particular cognitions (defenses) and interpersonal styles of interaction and perception (transference) that have become repetitive and that interfere with health (Table 32–1).

An individual's past exists in the present through memory and biology. Expectations—the anticipated present and future—are formed by one's past experiences and biology. Likewise, the way in which language is used metaphorically by a patient may reflect a particular organization (cluster of feelings, thoughts, and behaviors) formed in the past and affecting present perception and behavior. By exploring the past and present meaning of events and their context, the psychodynamic psychotherapist aims to alter the organizers of behavior, restructuring how information and experience are organized.

Psychodynamic psychotherapy (also called *psychoanalytic psychotherapy, exploratory psychotherapy,* or *insight-oriented psychotherapy*) is a method of treatment for psychiatric disorders that uses words exchanged between two people to effect changes in behavior. Psychodynamic psychotherapy shares with the other psychotherapies a general defi-

| TABLE 32–1. Psychodynamic psychotherapy |
| --- |
| **Focus** |
| Effects of past experience on present behaviors (cognitions, affects, fantasies, and actions) |
| **Goal** |
| Understanding the defense mechanisms and the transference responses of the patient, particularly as they appear in the doctor–patient relationship |
| **Techniques** |
| Therapeutic alliance |
| Free association |
| Defense and transference interpretation |
| Frequent meetings |
| **Duration of treatment** |
| Months to years |

nition: a two-person interaction, primarily verbal, in which one person is designated the help giver and the other the help receiver. The goal is to elucidate the patient's characteristic problems of living; the hope is to achieve behavioral change. Psychodynamic psychotherapy uses specific techniques and a particular understanding of mental functioning to guide and direct the treatment and the therapist's interventions.

Although the strategic goals of a psychodynamic treatment are to alter symptoms and change behavior to alleviate pain and suffering and decrease morbidity and mortality, the moment-to-moment objective is very different. In psychodynamic psychotherapy it is the therapist's understanding of what is causing the disease process, and of how a particular intervention will affect the recovery in the long run, that directs the tactical moment-to-moment process of treatment.

Psychodynamic psychotherapy is based on the principles of mental functioning and the psychotherapeutic techniques originally developed by Sigmund Freud. Freud began his work by using hypnosis; he later turned to free association as the method by which to understand the unrecognized (unconscious) conflicts that arose from development and continued into adult life. Such conflicts are patterns of behavior—that is, patterns of feelings, thoughts, and behaviors laid down in the brain during childhood. These patterns are the result of the individual's developmental history and biological givens.

Typically, these unconscious conflicts are between libidinal or aggressive desires (wishes) and the fear of loss, the fear of retaliation, the limits imposed by the real world, or the opposition of conflicting desires. *Libidinal wishes* are best thought of as longings for sexual and emotional gratification. *Aggressive wishes*, on the other hand, are destructive wishes that either are primary or are the result of perceived frustration or deprivation (Ursano et al. 1990). The beginning therapist frequently confuses the old terminology of libidinal wishes with the idea of specifically genital feelings. *Sexual gratification* in psychodynamic work refers to the broad concept of bodily pleasure—the states of excitement and pleasure experienced since infancy. The patient talking about happiness, excitement, pleasure, anticipation, love, or longing is describing libidinal wishes. The desire to destroy or the experience of pleasure in anger, hate, and pain is usually the expression of aggressive wishes.

Neurotic conflict (i.e., conflicted feelings/ambivalence derived from past [usually childhood] experiences and usually out of awareness) can result in anxiety, depression, and somatic symptoms; work, social, or sexual inhibitions; or maladaptive interpersonal relations. These unconscious neurotic conflicts are evident as patterns of behavior: feelings, thoughts, fantasies, and actions. These patterns, learned in childhood, may at one time have been appropriate to the patient's childhood view of the world and may have been adaptive or even necessary for survival. Even though these behaviors are not evident to the patient initially, through the psychotherapeutic work

they become clear, and their many ramifications for the patient's life become evident.

Psychodynamic psychotherapy is more focused than psychoanalysis, per se, and somewhat more oriented to the here and now. However, both these techniques share the goal of understanding the nature of the patient's conflicts—maladaptive patterns of behavior derived from childhood (also called the *infantile neurosis*)—and their effects in adult life.

## The Setting of Psychodynamic Psychotherapy

Psychodynamic psychotherapy may be brief, intermittent, or long-term. Intermittent psychotherapy is often the norm. This is the result of episodes of brief or time-limited psychodynamic psychotherapy being given to a patient over a longer period of time. Intermittent psychotherapy may also be necessary due to resources of time, money, or the patient's unwillingness to undertake longer-term treatment. Intermittent psychotherapy can also be planned after the initial evaluation as a joint plan of the therapist and patient to unfold over time, often with medication as a part of the treatment. This type of psychotherapy requires study, because it has become quite common and yet is not often considered as offering both unique opportunities and limitations.

Psychodynamic psychotherapy may take months or years. Typically, a longer-term treatment is open ended; no termination date is set in the beginning of treatment. The length of treatment depends on the number of conflict areas to be addressed and the course of the treatment. Psychotherapy sessions are usually held one, two, or three times a week, although in brief treatments once a week is the norm. The frequent meetings permit a more detailed exploration of the patient's inner life and a fuller development of the transference. The frequent meetings also support the patient during the treatment process.

## The Technique of Psychodynamic Psychotherapy

Behavioral change occurs in psychodynamic psychotherapy primarily through two processes of treatment: understanding the cognitive and affective patterns derived from childhood (defense mechanisms) and understanding the conflicted relationship(s) one had with one's childhood significant figures as they are reexperienced in the doctor–patient relationship (transference). The recovery and understanding of these feelings and perceptions are the focus of treatment. The treatment setting is designed to facilitate the emergence of these patterns in a way that allows them to be analyzed rather than being confused with the reality of the doctor–patient relationship or being dismissed as trivial.

Primary to the success of psychoanalytically oriented psychotherapy is the need for the patient to feel engaged in the work and to trust the relationship with the therapist. This therapeutic alliance is built on the reality-based elements of the treatment, such as the mutual working together toward a common goal and the consistency and reliability of the therapist (Bruch 1974). Only in contrast to a good therapeutic alliance can the patient view the transference feelings and experience the distortion that the transference reveals.

The clinician empathically hears what the patient says in order to understand what an experience means to the patient (Fromm-Reichman 1950). What the patient is able to bring into focus is what is dealt with in the treatment (Coleman 1968). The depth of interpretation and exploration is always at the point of urgency for the patient, not ahead of or behind the patient's thoughts and feelings. Beginning therapists often think that as soon as they see something, it is time to tell the patient. The timing of when to tell the patient is the essence of the skill of the therapist; careful thought and planning are needed to determine the appropriate time. Although the actual event of interpreting—explaining a piece of behavior in the context of the present and past and in relation to transference elements—is spontaneous, it is "spontaneous" after much preparation. When to tell the patient a new piece of information is determined by when the patient can hear and understand what the therapist has to say.

The patient's free association—that is, speaking without censoring or inhibiting his or her thoughts—is encouraged. This encouragement can be as simple as telling a patient that she is free to talk about whatever she wishes. The therapist's main task is to listen to the undercurrents of the patient's associations. Frequently this involves wondering about the connection between one vignette and the next or listening for how the patient is experiencing a particular person she describes or a particular interaction with the therapist. Often, listening to the ambiguity in a patient's associations may open the door to the unconscious conflict and the person from the past to which it relates.

The transference may be experienced by the therapist as a pressure to act in a certain way toward the patient. More often than not, for the beginning therapist it is identified, as in learning to ski, by noticing the direction in which one is about to fall! The transference is a specific example of the tendency of the brain to see the past in the present, to make use of old patterns of perception and response, and to exclude new information. When the transference is alive, it is very real to the patient, and contradictory information is disregarded. For the new therapist it is often difficult to see the irrational elements in the patient's feelings and perceptions about the therapist. Often the transference is built on a seed of accurate perception about the therapist. It is the elaboration of this seed that makes the unconscious evident. The therapist may experience the accuracy of the patient's perceptions and fail to listen to the elements of the past that may be appearing.

Exploring the transference is just a special case of the ongoing work of examining the patterns of relationships that the patient experiences. This is all part of the attempt to understand the inner world of the patient—the world of how the patient sees and experiences people and events, the world of psychic reality. Transference is not unique to the psychotherapeutic setting. It occurs throughout life and in medical treatments of all kinds. In fact, asking someone to come into a hospital (an unfamiliar setting) and take off his clothes, have no one know who he is, and be required to eat when told and go where told is a very powerful way to induce transferences! What is unique is the attempt to understand the transference and to examine it when it occurs rather than to try to undo it (Gabbard 2000; Luborsky and Crits-Christoph 1998).

The therapist may also experience feelings toward the patient that come from the therapist's past. This is called the *countertransference*. The countertransference is increased during times of stressful events and unresolved conflicts in the life of the therapist. The countertransference can be a friend, guiding one to see subtle aspects of the doctor–patient relationship that may have gone unnoticed. It can also be a block to a successful treatment, causing the therapist to misperceive and mishear the patient.

## Evaluation

### Assessment, Diagnosis, and Prescription of Brief, Intermittent, or Long-Term Psychodynamic Psychotherapy

As part of the evaluation for psychodynamic psychotherapy, the clinician must assess the presence or absence of

**TABLE 32–2.    Psychodynamic listening**

### I. Wishes/desires

What is the patient wishing for?

What in the patient's developmental history caused this wish to be prominent?

Are the wishes developmentally appropriate?

### II. Defenses

What in the patient's developmental history disrupted his or her wishes and desires?

How does the patient keep wishes out of awareness?

### III. Self-esteem

Does the patient like him- or herself?

Does he or she feel valued, admired, recognized by others?

How does the patient respond to events in life that decrease self-esteem or the feeling of being valued?

### IV. Interpersonal relations—present and in memory/fantasy

Who are the important people in the patient's past and present?

How are they recalled and spoken of at the different phases of the patient's life and development?

Who from the past does the patient behave and feel and think like (even if the patient is not aware of it)?

Whom does the patient miss and long for?

Who was lost from the patient's life at an early age (by death, moving, illness, conflict, or absence/neglect)?

**TABLE 32–3.    Psychodynamic perspectives**

| Theory | Focus |
| --- | --- |
| Drive theory | Wishes and feelings |
| Ego function | Defense mechanisms, cognitive style, and areas of health in the personality |
| Self psychology | Regulation of self-esteem |
| Object relations | Internalized memories of interpersonal relationships |
| Intersubjectivity and relational theory | Subjective experience and interpersonal relations |
| Attachment theory | Infant–caregiver attachment |

organic causes for the patient's psychiatric disturbance, the need for medication, the risk of untoward outcomes (suicide, homicide, divorce, work disruption), and the possibility that the patient's condition will worsen.

The psychiatric assessment for psychodynamic psychotherapy includes the use of two important techniques: psychodynamic listening (Chessick 2000) and the psychodynamic assessment or evaluation. Both are important to distinguish as techniques because they are applicable to many types of treatment and intervention, not just to psychodynamic psychotherapy. The use of psychodynamic listening and evaluation can be critical in medication management, consultation-liaison evaluation, and inpatient treatment, to name a few.

Psychodynamic listening (Mohl 2003; Sonnenberg 1995) puts the psychiatrist in an attitude of curious inquiry, listening to the meanings, metaphors, developmental sequencing, and interpersonal nuances of the patient's story

and of the doctor–patient interaction (Edelson 1993) (Table 32–2).

Particular attention is paid to stories, present and past, about 1) feelings and wishes; 2) the management of various feelings through the life cycle (e.g., defense mechanisms and cognitive style) and areas of healthy interaction with the world; 3) self-esteem regulation; and 4) interpersonal relationships. These four areas reflect the four psychodynamic perspectives on psychopathology: drives, ego function, self psychology, and object relationships (Pine 1988; Table 32–3).

The psychodynamic assessment or evaluation uses the data obtained from questioning and from psychodynamic listening (MacKinnon et al. 2006; Sullivan 1954; Table 32–4). The evaluation aims to integrate the patient's chief complaint; history of present illness; past history; family history; developmental history, including any traumatic events or deviations from usual developmental patterns; mental status examination; style of doctor–patient interaction; and transference and the psychiatrist's countertransference feelings. The outcome of this evaluation is a psychodynamic understanding of the patient's past and present experiences from the patient's subjective viewpoint. This psychodynamic formulation provides an integrated understanding through the patient's life cycle from the four psychodynamic perspectives on the past and present experiences of the patient, and it makes predictions of potential doctor–patient interactions and the patient's patterns of defense mechanisms and interpersonal interactions.

In this way, the evaluation phase provides information for the assessment of the type and degree of psychiatric illness and impairment, the selection of treatment modal-

**TABLE 32–4. Guidelines for psychodynamic assessment**

Listen to and explore:

> The precipitants of the symptoms, of the illness, and of seeking help
>
> The history of significant events from childhood to the present

Identify the significant people in the patient's history from childhood to present

Ask for the patient's earliest memory

Explore any recurrent or recent dreams and the context of when they were dreamed

Observe how the patient relates to the therapist

Discuss the patient's previous treatments and therapists

Give a trial interpretation

Invite collaboration in "understanding"

**TABLE 32–5. The evaluation**

**Goal**

Educate the patient about the evaluation process

Establish an atmosphere of safety and inquiry

Assess for the appropriate treatment

**Tasks**

Assess for life-threatening behaviors

Assess for organic causes of the patient's illness

Determine the diagnosis

Identify areas of conflict across the life cycle

**Duration**

Meet for one to four sessions

**Techniques**

Use questioning and listening

Listen for the patient's fears about starting treatment

Attend to the precipitants of the illness and of seeking treatment

---

ity, and the conduct of psychotherapy itself. After a well-conducted evaluation, the patient feels respected and safe, believes that his or her best interests are the primary concern of the clinician, and feels that any topic can be talked about (Levinson et al. 1967).

The therapist's asking about medical signs and symptoms and suicidal and homicidal thoughts and actions frequently relieves the patient of the feeling that he or she is the only one worried about these areas. Often the patient is wondering whether the doctor will ask about these issues. Whether the therapist inquires about these particular areas may be used by the patient as a way to assess whether the therapist is serious about listening and being concerned about the patient or whether these are topics that the clinician feels are irrelevant or too dangerous to talk about. "VIP" and physician patients in particular are alert to whether the therapist is thorough in the evaluation. The patient who feels that all areas—medical as well as behavioral—and all risks and concerns have been forthrightly and empathically explored will feel the beginning of a working relationship centered on trust and mutual respect. The beginning of the psychotherapy in the evaluation phase is critical to the psychotherapeutic work to follow that can include many distortions of the doctor-patient relationship. Commonly, long after a therapy has started—and frequently in its termination phase—a patient may reveal, for example, the one question the therapist asked, or the particular way in which the therapist greeted him or her at the door, that led to the feeling that working together would be possible.

## Beginning the Evaluation

The evaluation begins when the therapist meets the patient (Lazare and Eisenthal 1989a, 1989b). In the outpatient setting, it is best for the therapist to introduce him- or herself and explain to the patient what the therapist knows about the patient's problems. One should not assume that a patient knows that a session is an evaluation. Rather, the therapist should set the context of the meeting, explaining that he or she, the therapist, would like to spend some time getting to know the nature of the patient's difficulties and inviting the patient to tell more (see Table 32–5).

The number of evaluation sessions usually ranges from one to four, but more sessions may be needed. The length of the evaluation is determined by the amount of time required to collect the information for the diagnostic and psychodynamic assessment and to address the practical issues of beginning treatment (Table 32–6).

The clinician uses two methods for data collection during the evaluation: asking questions and listening unobtrusively (Silberman and Certa 2003). Both styles must be used to collect the needed information. A patient complaining of depression should not leave the first evaluation session without the clinician's knowing the severity of the depression and the risk of suicide. This usually requires at least some direct questioning. Life-threatening issues must be dealt with early in order to gather the

---

**TABLE 32–6. Helpful hints for the evaluation**

When the clinician is only doing the evaluation and the patient will be referred to another therapist for treatment, it is most helpful to the evaluation and to its successful termination that the patient know this plan at the beginning.

Infrequently, it may be advantageous and important to have the initial evaluation done by a clinician who will not be the treating therapist. In the case where the patient needs a very firm, direct, confrontational approach to enter a much-needed treatment, the evaluating clinician who is not expecting to treat the patient may feel freer to be blunt, in a tactful manner, with the patient.

Patients must be given the time and space in which to paint a picture of their world without the therapist choosing the colors! Being either too intrusive or too silent can lead to missed information and can needlessly confuse the patient.

All therapists also experience certain therapist–patient differences that they cannot bridge, and in such cases they refer the patient to another clinician.

Early termination may be due to defenses against seeking help, a transference reaction, a decision that this is not the right treatment, or, at times, a relief of symptoms as a result of the evaluation.

---

**TABLE 32–7. First session**

By the end of the first session, the clinician should know the answers to these questions:

What further organic workup is needed?

Is psychosis in the differential diagnosis?

Are there any life-threatening issues, either now or possibly in the future?

How many (if any) more sessions will be taken for the evaluation?

---

needed diagnostic information. However, other historical information can be collected as part of the patient's story (Horowitz et al. 1995; Perry et al. 1987).

Frequently, the skill of the therapist lies in how the history and diagnostic information are collected. The more skilled the therapist, the more able he or she is to understand—to reach—and therefore to work with a wider range of patients. The skilled therapist can establish a rapport across a wide array of socioeconomic classes and sexual, racial, religious, cultural, and emotional differences.

In the first session the therapist should listen for the patient's fears of starting psychotherapy. These fears should be explored early, as they appear and are articulated by the patient. The patient will feel safer and be more interested in continuing the evaluation and the treatment when these fears have been heard, respected, and explored by the therapist. In addition, airing these fears will leave the therapist in a better position to interpret any precipitous stopping of the treatment. It is not unusual for a patient to drop out during the evaluation phase before beginning

treatment. That is one reason to view this phase as the candidacy stage. (In clinic settings, about 50% of patients stop before the fifth session [Malan et al. 1973; see Table 32–7].)

## Indications and Selection Criteria

Psychodynamic psychotherapy has its best outcomes with what have been called *neurotic-level disorders*. These individuals have conflicts that are primarily oedipal in nature (e.g., competition, guilt, independence, adult sexuality and intimacy, parental loss and identification) and that are experienced as internal by the patient. DSM-IV-TR disorders that frequently involve a primarily neurotic conflict include obsessive-compulsive disorder, anxiety disorders (Bond and Perry 2004), conversion disorder, psychological factors affecting physical disease, dysthymic disorder, mild to moderate mood disorders (Bond 2006), adjustment disorders, and mild to moderate personality disorders (Gabbard et al. 2002; Leichsenring 2005; Leichsenring and Leibing 2003). Patients who are psychologically minded, who are able to observe feelings without acting on them, and who can obtain symptom relief through understanding may benefit from psychodynamic psychotherapy. The patient who has a supportive environment—family, friends, work—usually does better because he or she is able to use the therapy in a more intensive manner. Such a patient does not need the therapist to be a primary reality support in order to weather the stresses of life or the treatment.

Although psychological mindedness is important, intelligence per se is not a selection criterion; in fact, it can reflect a highly organized obsessional character structure that may be very difficult to treat. Socioeconomic class is also not a good predictor of success in treatment. Rather, the ability to work with patients from diverse socioeconomic classes is usually a part of the therapist's task and skill: to span a range of life experiences and accurately empathize with the patient's world. The patient–therapist match is therefore very important, especially to the opening phase of treatment and the establishment of the therapeutic alliance.

In general, patients who like their therapists, who have had a shorter duration of symptoms, and who are seeking understanding of their problems as well as symptom relief have the best outcomes. The use of a trial interpretation during the evaluation phase can provide much useful information on how the patient makes use of understanding to modify symptoms and to what extent the patient experiences understanding provided through interpretation as supportive and helpful (Malan 1980).

## Treatment

Teaching the patient about the goals and process of psychodynamic psychotherapy is very important to the successful beginning of the psychotherapy. One way to conceptualize this phase of treatment is that an atmosphere of safety must be established. In the opening phase of the treatment, the patient learns that psychodynamic psychotherapy will work because in the relationship with the therapist, the patient will reexperience the past in the present through the transference relationship. By examining feelings in the therapy setting, the patient develops an understanding of how the personal past is continually reexperienced in life. The patient will then begin to understand that psychological pain can result from symbolically reliving the past in the here and now, causing the reawakening of the conflicted feelings and anxieties of childhood. The patient also learns by experience that through recognizing these unconscious processes, the painful feelings diminish and new behaviors are possible.

The patient is educated directly both through teaching and explanation and through example. At times, the clinician should explain very directly and supportively to the patient the process of the treatment. When this has been done, it is best not to continue to repeat the explanations but instead to change into a mode of understanding rather than teaching, listening to the patient's possible emotional blocks to understanding. The skilled clinician is always making decisions early in treatment about whether this is a time to educate or a time to listen to more material from the patient, delaying any further instructive comments. Generally, the new therapist struggles with how much to educate and how much to listen in the opening sessions. Later in treatment, after explanations have been

given clearly, the therapist can assume that cognitive education is not the difficulty the patient is having. However, the therapist cannot assume this in the opening phase, particularly with the naïve patient. Understanding the goals and processes of treatment is important to the patient's feeling safe and comfortable enough to explore and tolerate the anxiety that arises in the treatment setting (Sonnenberg et al. 1996, 2003).

## Abstinence, Neutrality, and Free Association

After the patient has begun to understand the process of treatment, the therapist will, over time, become somewhat less verbally active in order to hear more about how the patient organizes his or her psychological world. Technically this is called being abstinent. Again the therapist may need to explain this to the patient if he or she asks about the therapist's silence. The therapist might say, "I am listening to you very closely. I want to be able to best understand how you see the world and not interfere with what you are telling me." The therapist also encourages the patient to speak as freely as possible and to suspend judgment about the accuracy or logic of what is said. This may be explained to the patient in the following manner: "You are free to say whatever you would like. In fact, it is most helpful if you say whatever comes to mind. I know that is difficult to do." The therapist helps the patient say whatever comes to mind—to speak without editing thoughts—even though the patient may say things that he or she fears would be untrue or hurtful to the therapist or to loved ones.

This method of communication is known as *free association*. It is characteristic of the mode of thinking and talking used by the patient in classical psychoanalysis, although free association in classical psychoanalysis is much freer because of the other elements of the psychoanalytic treatment. However, the psychodynamic psychotherapy patient will come fairly close to that same mode of expression (S. Freud 1917/1963).

Inevitably, free association is only relative, and the unconscious conflicts the patient experiences are the major forces that block the free expression of thoughts, feelings, and fantasies. The therapist, in collaboration with the patient, listens for clues to what may be outside the patient's awareness and may appear as a block to the free expression of thoughts. These ways of thinking that block uncomfortable feelings and conflicts from being experienced are called *defense mechanisms*. The therapist carefully observes, and at the right time shares with the patient, the patterns the patient shows in his or her thoughts and feelings and the blocks to these thoughts and feelings. The therapist observes the changes in the patient's thoughts and feelings and any movement away from the treatment. The therapist experiences the patient's defense mechanisms as a resistance to the work. Through the process of understanding how the resistances—the patient's defense mechanisms—operate, the transference emerges later in treatment.

The clinician and patient work together to recognize the patterns of the patient's thoughts and feelings. This collaborative work allows the patient to experience this task as one he or she can eventually assume, rather than as something magical. This task—the analysis of defenses—forms the basis on which the patient can eventually choose alternative behaviors. At times the enthusiasm of the new therapist can lead to wanting to tell the patient a pattern without working together with the patient to identify it. This can lead to the therapist's being seen as very powerful by the patient and often will create problems later in treatment.

The patient at times experiences feelings of frustration because of the clinician's relative silence. However, the patient should, overall, experience the therapist as standing with him or her, as an ally with whom the patient can master the forces that keep so much outside consciousness (Schafer 1983). Helping the patient understand this during the opening phase of treatment is essential.

In therapy, what the patient says is met with an effort to understand, not with judgment or criticism. The therapist maintains neutrality. The job of the psychodynamic psychotherapist does not involve managing the patient's life (one reason why patient selection is so important) or judging its worth or the value of the way in which it is conducted (Poland 1984).

The therapist's abstinent, neutral demeanor in the therapeutic setting is, in part, a technique, a special form of behavior designed to offer the patient the opportunity to experience his or her own feelings, thoughts, and fantasies. Partly as a result of this unique aspect of the psychotherapeutic setting and partly because of the normal course of life, the patient is able to think in a less well-organized, less structured fashion, giving access to more unconscious feelings and thoughts and thereby acting on the psychotherapeutic stage. Over time, the therapy becomes a laboratory in which the patient can examine in detail the feelings, thoughts, and fantasies he or she experiences toward another person (the therapist) within the safety of the therapeutic alliance (Bender 2005).

Although this goal requires the therapist to be relatively passive and silent, this technical stance is not meant to be harsh or depriving. The collaboration develops in part through the clinician's appropriate concern and through explanations of the special kind of team effort and working together that are a part of the therapy. The therapist and the patient work together to understand the patient's experience, which in turn leads to the amelioration of the patient's psychic pain. The therapist and the patient are more accurately described as trying to develop a working (Greenson 1965) or therapeutic alliance (Curtis 1979; Zetzel 1956).

The psychiatrist doing this form of therapy works from the perspective of the concerned physician, with gentleness and an awareness of the patient's pain (Schafer 1983; Stone 1981). Over and over again, through working together, the physician conveys the awareness that the patient is experiencing psychological pain not only in life outside the therapy but, because of reexperiencing the past, in life inside the therapy as well. The psychiatrist conveys respect for the patient's efforts to understand him- or herself and to keep going in therapy in spite of the pain.

# Transference, Defense Mechanisms, and Resistance

## Transference

Transference is at the core of how psychodynamic psychotherapy works, but it is never easily understood by the patient. Freud developed the idea that all human relationships are transference relationships. By this he meant that all human beings experience others by superimposing their perceptions of figures from the past on new individuals. Today, although within psychoanalysis there exists a range of views on the nature of transference, it is generally felt that memories of the past are activated in all relationships. To some extent, each individual unconsciously plays out in current relationships certain aspects of important past relationships (Table 32–8).

Because the psychodynamic psychotherapist is abstinent and does not share details of his or her personal life with the patient, the therapist creates a kind of blank screen on which the patient may paint a transference picture of his or her own design. Early in the therapy this becomes apparent. By pointing it out, the therapist and the patient create a common focus of attention. In this way the patient's understanding of how therapy works is also deepened.

**TABLE 32–8. Transference**

Transference...

Is part of all relationships

Is a primary focus of psychodynamic psychotherapy

Brings the past alive to the patient in the doctor–patient relationship

Aids in remembering the past

Provides examples of patterns of interpersonal behaviors, fantasies, feelings, and thoughts that influence the patient's present relationships

Can be felt by the therapist as "role pressure"—a pressure to respond in a particular way to the patient

People form transferences in all relationships. This is because we use the past as a pattern for understanding the present and because there seems to be in all people a psychological need to repeat the past in an effort to master that which was difficult or emotionally painful. Therefore, not just in psychoanalysis and psychodynamic psychotherapy but everywhere, people construct their relationships in the present by reproducing emotionally important aspects of their past relationships (S. Freud 1912/1958; McLaughlin 1981).

Thus, another way of conceptualizing transference is to think of the human mind as made up, in part, of sets of memories of important individuals from a person's past. These organized sets of memories are called *object representations*. Whenever a person meets someone new, he or she begins to form a new object representation. Obviously, this process proceeds to a significant extent only when the new person is of some importance to the observer; but whenever the process takes place, the observer, in an effort to understand a new acquaintance, scans his or her memories for standards against which to measure and compare the new individual. Soon, new and old object representations are psychologically connected in response to the observer's need for familiarity and to other psychological needs (explained later). The newcomer is on the receiving end of ideas, thoughts, and feelings that were originally directed toward the old friend, relative, loved one, or enemy.

What we see when we observe individuals and talk with them about their present life or current relationships is the surface of their psychological life. Beneath that surface are the memories of their important past relationships, which—like the muscles, nerves, and bones beneath the skin—constitute vital parts of the organic whole of their interpersonal world, present as well as past (Goldstein and Goldberg 2003; Sandler et al. 1973). The individual, however, perceives his or her current relationship as the whole. The connections of the current relationship to an old relationship and the way in which the present is serving as a vehicle for working out old relationships remain outside conscious awareness. Therefore, the therapist may experience the transference in the therapy as pressure to behave in a certain way toward the patient that is reminiscent of a previous relationship the patient had in childhood.

In psychodynamic psychotherapy, the therapist, through his or her neutrality, abstinence, and encouraging of free association, creates an environment in which conscious transference responses are relatively more intense than in typical relationships (although they are less intense than in a classical psychoanalysis). The development and understanding of the transference is one of the therapist's most important tools. It is the vehicle for bringing alive—in the consulting room—the patient's difficulties and for examining these in depth in an existentially meaningful environment. In fact, it is this process that, more than anything else, distinguishes psychodynamic psychotherapy from other forms of treatment.

From another perspective, the transference is the way the patient remembers what he or she has forgotten—what is unconscious and the source of psychological pain. In popular caricatures of psychiatric treatment, the patient remembers dramatic childhood events in a melodramatic fashion. In reality, this remembering occurs as a result of detailed effort to dissect the frequently small memories of long-forgotten, sometimes repetitively experienced parts of the past as they present in the transference relationship. Through the transference the patient develops an understanding of what was experienced in the past and how that experience lives on in the here and now. To help the patient understand transference and begin to develop the ability to work with it, the psychiatrist must direct the patient's attention to this dimension of his or her thoughts. Thus, the therapist may ask the patient to describe what he or she is thinking or feeling about the therapist when it appears that may be in the patient's near awareness (Halpert 1994; Ogden 1995).

## Defense Mechanisms and Resistance

The psychotherapist attempts to clarify the patient's feelings and the meaning of what the patient is trying to say. At other times, the therapist may supportively confront the patient with attitudes the patient has disavowed but clearly demonstrates. In both cases the therapist is hoping to point out the kinds of thoughts and feelings that the patient obscures and the ways they are obscured, defended against, and kept unconscious. Throughout this process the patient's defensive ways of thinking are elucidated.

In the opening phase the therapist will have the opportunity to identify patterns of defense and resistance and must orient the patient to how awareness of these patterns can be used to advance the patient's knowledge of him- or herself (Loewald 1960).

*Resistance* is a general term referring to all the forces in the patient that oppose the painful work of therapy. There are many different categories of resistance, including general fear of any change, an overly harsh conscience that punishes a patient with the continuation of suffering, and the insistence on the gratification of childish impulses that forms part of an emotional illness. All people, including patients in therapy, employ mechanisms of defense to keep painful feelings and memories outside conscious awareness. These defense mechanisms are specific, discrete maneuvers or ways of thinking that the mind employs to avoid painful emotional material (Nemiah 1961; Shapiro 1965).

Whenever a patient is manifesting resistance, in whatever form, it is because the patient is protecting him- or herself from experiencing, including remembering or reliving, the old dangers and fears associated with the childhood conflicts and developmental difficulties of his or her life. Character (the set of expectable responses from a person in a given setting) is in great part a result of the defense mechanisms each person characteristically uses. Defenses are our cognitive mechanisms of structuring mental and emotional experience to keep psychic pain at a minimum and bring our interpersonal and intrapsychic functioning and relationships into some congruence with external reality.

The patient's defense mechanisms are an important source of resistance in psychotherapy. In 1936, Anna Freud, in *The Ego and the Mechanisms of Defense* (A. Freud 1966), outlined the functioning of many of these defense maneuvers. Since that time, the list has grown and been elaborated upon (Table 32–9).

Several common and important mechanisms of defense are defined in Table 32–10. There are also more primitive mechanisms of defense—splitting, projection, projective identification, omnipotence, devaluing, and primitive idealization—that are seen in severe personality disorders such as borderline personality disorder and psychotic disorders (Kernberg 1975).

**TABLE 32–9.   Defense mechanisms**

| Common defense mechanisms | Primitive defense mechanisms |
| --- | --- |
| Repression | Splitting |
| Denial | Projection |
| Reaction formation | Projective identification |
| Displacement | Omnipotence |
| Identification | Devaluing |
| Identification with the aggressor | Primitive idealization |
| Intellectualization | |
| Isolation of affect | |
| Sublimation | |

## Use of Dreams

The therapist also attends to the dream life of the patient (Brenner 1976; S. Freud 1900/1953). Not all patients in psychotherapy work extensively with dreams, but many do, and for those who can, the work is an important tool. Every patient should be given the opportunity to work with dreams. It is in the opening phase that this road to understanding is introduced and learned. Frequently, dreams reported early in treatment are particularly revealing of the core conflicts of the patient. They can also serve to educate the patient about unconscious processes (Sharpe 1961). Dreams can be presented to the patient as thoughts and concerns the patient is having while asleep, although the rules for how these thoughts and concerns are created are different (i.e., primary process thinking) than during waking life (i.e., secondary process thinking) (Reiser 1994).

## Countertransference

*Countertransference* is the emotional reaction of the therapist to the patient. Historically, countertransference was limited in meaning to the therapist's transference onto the patient. This was felt to be a response to the patient's transference. Like all transferences, the therapist's countertransference was the result of unconscious conflicts; however, these unresolved conflicts were those of the therapist rather than those of the patient. This countertransference was thought to obscure the therapist's judgment in conducting the therapy (Gabbard 1995; Gabbard and Wilkinson 2001).

**TABLE 32–10. Definitions of common mechanisms of defense**

| | |
|---|---|
| Repression | Among the first mechanisms of defense described by Sigmund Freud, this refers to the active pushing out of awareness of painful memories, feelings, and impulses. |
| Denial | Similar to repression, denial averts a patient's attention from painful ideas or feelings without making them completely unavailable to consciousness. A patient using denial simply ignores painful realities and acts as though they do not exist. |
| Reaction formation | Reaction formation consists of exaggerating one emotional trend to help repress the opposite emotion. The obsessional patient may manifest punctuality, parsimony, and cleanliness to defend against wishes to be tardy, extravagant, and messy. |
| Displacement | Displacement is changing the object of one's feelings to a safer one. The worker who is enraged by his boss and comes home, abuses his dog, and shouts at his family is a familiar example. |
| Identification with the aggressor | This is the tendency to imitate what the patient perceives as the aggressive and intimidating manner of someone toward him or her. Children who have been abused may become abusers themselves in adulthood, using identification with the aggressor as a defense. |
| Intellectualization | Intellectualization is the excessively factual, detailed, and cognitive way of talking about and experiencing emotionally charged topics without the feelings and associated affects. |
| Isolation of affect | Related to intellectualization, this is the repression of the feelings connected with a particular thought. Both intellectualization and isolation of affect are typical of obsessional patients in particular. |
| Sublimation | A mature mechanism of defense, sublimation is the hoped-for, healthy, nonconflicted evolution of primitive childhood impulses into a mature level of expression. |

Countertransferences are many and varied. Often they are the result of events occurring in the therapist's life that may make him or her more sensitive to certain themes in the patient's associations. The developmental period of the therapist's life—involving issues of intimacy, achievement, or old age, for example—may also affect how the therapist hears the patient. Intense transferences of all kinds—erotic, aggressive, devaluing, idealizing, and others—are ripe for serving as the stimulus to awaken in the therapist elements of his or her own past (Mitchell and Aron 1999).

When all one's patients seem to be talking about feeling overworked, or angry, or sad, the therapist can reflect on these feelings and wonder whether this theme is being selected by him or her rather than being the central issue for all of his or her patients. Finally, a common countertransference issue in training occurs at the end of training when both the therapist and the patient are dealing with termination. For the patient it is the end of treatment; for the therapist it is both the end of a treatment and the end of a stage of life, usually accompanied by a move and loss of colleagues and friends as well as a sense of new achievement.

The clinician may first note a patient's core conflictual issue through observing subtle emotional reactions stirred in him- or herself (Kernberg 1976; Searles 1979). The clinician can then explore these feelings, through self-analysis, as possible reverberations from the unconscious but also as emerging concerns of the patient that may be hidden in the patient's language, behavior, or fantasies.

The psychodynamic psychotherapist observes his or her own emotional reactions and values and processes them as possible windows on the patient's experience. Frequently, the more intense and even embarrassing the therapist's responses, the more likely they are to reflect a crucial, hidden, conflicted state residing within the patient. There are generally two types of countertransference reactions: concordant and complementary (Racker 1968; Table 32–11).

## Termination

Often, psychodynamic psychotherapy is conducted in an open-ended fashion regardless of whether it is to be short or longer term. At the beginning of the treatment, the therapist explained to the patient that the treatment would

---

**TABLE 32–11.    Countertransference**

**Concordant countertransference**

The therapist experiences and empathizes with the patient's emotional position (e.g., therapist thinks: "Boy, my patient is right! His boss sounds like a terrible person!").

**Complementary countertransference**

The therapist experiences and empathizes with the feelings of an important person from the patient's life (e.g., therapist thinks: "My patient is infuriating—I certainly see why his boss gets so angry at him!").

---

take as long as required to discover and resolve the patient's unconscious core conflicts and for the patient to understand the workings of his or her mind.

There comes a time, however, when the patient and the psychiatrist agree that it is time to end the treatment. At this juncture the troublesome areas of the patient's personality seem to be separate from the core of the patient's sense of self (Alexander 1941). What was once central to the patient's presenting difficulties is now experienced as alien. The patient has learned to use intellect and perception in an affectively rich manner in the service of self-awareness (Dewald 1982).

The therapist must remember and the patient must come to realize that treatment goals are related to, but different from, the patient's life goals (Ticho 1972). Treatment goals are always dependent to some extent on life's demands and possibilities—what is possible at a given time of life and in a given context. Termination does not mean a patient has realized all of his or her hopes and wishes. Rather, the patient entering the end phase of treatment after a successful treatment has experienced substantial relief of psychological suffering, and this relief is evident to both the patient and the therapist. In addition, the internal conflicts of the patient, as well as the presenting symptoms, have been resolved, and reasonably permanent changes in behavior have occurred.

The patient shows a detailed understanding of the working of his or her mind and is beginning to use self-inquiry as a method of problem solving. Often there have been gains in most of these areas, although not necessarily all. The gains are observed by the therapist and shared with the patient as part of the patient's increasing awareness of new areas of strength and conflict resolution (Table 32–12).

---

**TABLE 32–12.    Criteria for termination**

The patient. . .

Experiences relief of symptoms.

Experiences symptoms as alien.

Understands his or her characteristic defenses.

Is able to understand and recognize his or her characteristic transference responses.

Engages in ongoing self-inquiry as a method of resolving internal conflicts.

---

The termination phase has its own tasks to consolidate the treatment and facilitate leave taking while maintaining the therapeutic relationship (Table 32–13).

---

**TABLE 32–13.    Tasks of the termination phase**

**Review the treatment**

The patient reviews the treatment, reconsidering his or her history and conflicts and placing in perspective what has been learned. Frequently the patient experiences a feeling of pride, strength, and gratitude to the therapist in this process while refreshing the "table of contents" of the patient's knowledge about him- or herself.

**Experience the loss of the psychotherapy and the therapist**

In termination, the patient experiences what is an essential and poignant aspect of the human condition: the experience of separation—the loss of a relationship with a person who has been very helpful and who often is perceived as kind and understanding. This loss may reawaken the conflicts of previous losses.

**Reexperience and remaster the transference**

Very often, in the context of termination, there is a recrudescence of the patient's symptoms and a return of old transference patterns and styles of interacting with the therapist.

**Increase skills in self-inquiry as a method of problem solving**

The patient now begins to take over the functions of the therapist. The patient increasingly exercises a greater degree of self-inquiry to resolve now well-known and well-understood internal conflicts.

---

## Key Points: Psychodynamic Psychotherapy

- Transference occurs in all interpersonal relationships.

- *Defense mechanisms* are cognitive mechanisms to decrease anxiety and other distressing feelings.

- Early childhood development structures brain development and leaves patterns of feelings, thoughts, behaviors, and interpersonal relating.

- Psychotherapy is an effective form of treatment, as effective as many other medical interventions.

- The working, reality-based relationship with the patient is called the *therapeutic alliance.*

- Psychodynamic psychotherapy may be brief, intermittent, or longer term.

- The principles of psychodynamic psychotherapy are used in many doctor–patient interactions other than psychodynamic psychotherapy.

## References

Alexander F: The voice of the intellect is soft. Psychoanal Rev 28:12–29, 1941

Bender DS: The therapeutic alliance in the treatment of personality disorders. J Psychiatr Pract 11:73–87, 2005

Bond M: Psychodynamic psychotherapy in the treatment of mood disorders. Curr Opin Psychiatry 19:40–43, 2006

Bond M, Perry C: Long-term changes in defense styles with psychodynamic psychotherapy for depressive, anxiety and personality disorders. Am J Psychiatry 161:1665–1671, 2004

Brenner C: Psychoanalytic Technique and Psychic Conflicts. New York, International Universities Press, 1976

Bruch H: Learning Psychotherapy: Rationale and Ground Rules. Cambridge, MA, Harvard University Press, 1974

Chessick RD: Psychoanalysis: clinical and theoretical. Am J Psychiatry 157:846–848, 2000

Coleman JV: Aims and conduct of psychotherapy. Arch Gen Psychiatry 18:1–6, 1968

Curtis HC: The concept of therapeutic alliance: implications for the "widening scope." J Am Psychoanal Assoc 27 (suppl):159–192, 1979

Dewald PA: The clinical importance of the termination phase. Psychoanal Inq 2:441–461, 1982

Edelson M: Telling and enacting stories in psychoanalysis and psychodynamic psychotherapy. Psychoanal Study Child 48:293–325, 1993

Freud A: The Ego and the Mechanisms of Defense, Revised Edition. New York, International Universities Press, 1966

Freud S: The interpretation of dreams (1900), in The Standard Edition of the Complete Psychological Works of Sigmund Freud, Vols 4 and 5. Translated and edited by Strachey J. London, England, Hogarth, 1953

Freud S: The dynamics of transference (1912), in The Standard Edition of the Complete Psychological Works of Sigmund Freud, Vol 12. Translated and edited by Strachey J. London, England, Hogarth, 1958, pp 97–108

Freud S: Resistance and repression (1917), in The Standard Edition of the Complete Psychological Works of Sigmund Freud, Vol 16. Translated and edited by Strachey J. London, England, Hogarth, 1963, pp 286–302

Fromm-Reichmann F: Principles of Intensive Psychotherapy. Chicago, IL, University of Chicago Press, 1950

Gabbard GO: Countertransference: the emerging common ground. Int J Psychoanal 76:475–485, 1995

Gabbard GO: Psychodynamic Psychiatry in Clinical Practice, 3rd Edition. Washington, DC, American Psychiatric Press, 2000

Gabbard GO, Wilkinson SM: Management of Countertransference With Borderline Patients. Washington, DC, American Psychiatric Publishing, 2001

Gabbard GO, Gunderson JG, Fonagy P: The place of psychoanalytic treatments within psychiatry. Arch Gen Psychiatry 59:505–510, 2002

Goldstein WN, Goldberg ST: The Transference in Psychotherapy. Northvale, NJ, Jason Aronson, 2003

Greenson RR: The working alliance and the transference neurosis. Psychoanal Q 34:155–181, 1965

Halpert E: Asclepius: magic in transference to physicians. Psychoanal Q 63:733–755, 1994

Horowitz MJ, Eells T, Singer J, et al: Role-relationship models for case formulation. Arch Gen Psychiatry 52:625–633, 1995

Kernberg OF: Borderline Conditions and Pathological Narcissism. New York, Jason Aronson, 1975

Kernberg OF: Transference and countertransference in the treatment of borderline patients, in Object-Relations Theory and Clinical Psychoanalysis. New York, Jason Aronson, 1976, pp 161–184

Lazare A, Eisenthal S: Clinician/patient relations, I: attending to the patient's perspective, in Outpatient Psychiatry. Edited by Lazare A. Baltimore, MD, Williams & Wilkins, 1989a, pp 125–136

Lazare A, Eisenthal S, Frank A: Clinician/patient relations, II: conflict and negotiation, in Outpatient Psychiatry. Edited by Lazare A. Baltimore, MD, Williams & Wilkins, 1989b, pp 137–157

Leichsenring F: Are psychodynamic and psychoanalytic therapies effective? A review of empirical data. Int J Psychoanal 86:841–868, 2005

Leichsenring F, Leibing E: The effectiveness of psychodynamic therapy and cognitive behavior therapy in the treatment of personality disorders: a meta analysis. Am J Psychiatry 160:1223–1232, 2003

Levinson D, Merrifield J, Berg K: Becoming a patient. Arch Gen Psychiatry 17:385–406, 1967

Loewald HW: On the therapeutic action of psycho-analysis. Int J Psychoanal 41:16–33, 1960

Luborsky L, Crits-Christoph P: Understanding Transference: The CCRT Method, 2nd Edition. Washington, DC, American Psychological Association Press, 1998

MacKinnon RA, Michels R, Buckley PJ (eds): The Psychiatric Interview in Clinical Practice, 2nd Edition. Washington, DC, American Psychiatric Publishing, 2006

Malan DH: Toward the Validation of Dynamic Psychotherapy. New York, Plenum, 1980

Malan DH, Heath ES, Baral HA, et al: Psychodynamic changes in untreated neurotic patients, II: apparently genuine improvement. Arch Gen Psychiatry 32:110–126, 1973

McLaughlin JT: Transference, psychic reality, and countertransference. Psychoanal Q 50:639–664, 1981

Mitchell S, Aron L (eds): Relational Psychoanalysis: The Emergence of a Tradition. Hillsdale, NJ, Analytic Press, 1999

Mohl PC: Listening to the patient, in Psychiatry, 2nd Edition. Edited by Tasman A, Kaye J, Lieberman J. New York, Wiley, 2003, pp 3–18

Nemiah JC: Foundations of Psychopathology. New York, Oxford University Press, 1961

Ogden TH: Analysing forms of aliveness and deadness of the transference-countertransference. Int J Psychoanal 76:695–709, 1995

Perry S, Cooper AM, Michels R: The psychodynamic formulation: its purpose, structure and clinical application. Am J Psychiatry 144:543–550, 1987

Pine F: The four psychologies of psychoanalysis and their place in clinical work. J Am Psychoanal Assoc 36:571–596, 1988

Poland WS: On the analyst's neutrality. J Am Psychoanal Assoc 32:283–299, 1984

Racker H: Transference and Countertransference. New York, International Universities Press, 1968

Reiser MF: Memory in Mind and Brain: What Dream Imagery Reveals. New Haven, CT, Yale University Press, 1994

Sandler J, Dare C, Holder A: The Patient and the Analyst: The Basis of the Psychoanalytic Process. New York, International Universities Press, 1973

Schafer R: The atmosphere of safety: Freud's "Papers on Technique" (1911–1915), in The Analytic Attitude. New York, Basic Books, 1983, pp 14–33

Searles HF: Countertransference and Related Subjects. New York, International Universities Press, 1979

Shapiro D: Neurotic Styles. New York, Basic Books, 1965

Sharpe EF: Dream Analysis. London, England, Hogarth Press, 1961

Silberman EK, Certa K: The psychiatric interview: settings and techniques, in Psychiatry, 2nd Edition. Edited by Tasman A, Kaye J, Lieberman J. New York, Wiley, 2003, pp 30–51

Sonnenberg SM: Analytic listening and the analyst's self-analysis. Int J Psychoanal 76:335–342, 1995

Sonnenberg SM, Sutton L, Ursano RJ: Physician–patient relationship, in Psychiatry. Edited by Tasman A, Kaye J, Lieberman J. Philadelphia, PA, WB Saunders, 1996, pp 41–49

Sonnenberg SM, Ursano AM, Ursano RJ: Physician–patient relationship, in Psychiatry, 2nd Edition. Edited by Tasman A, Kay J, Lieberman JA. New York, Wiley, 2003, pp 52–63

Stone L: Notes on the noninterpretive elements in the psychoanalytic situation and process. J Am Psychoanal Assoc 29:89–118, 1981

Sullivan HS: The Psychiatric Interview. New York, WW Norton, 1954

Ticho E: Termination of psychoanalysis: treatment goals, life goals. Psychoanal Q 41:315–333, 1972

Ursano RJ, Silberman EK, Diaz A Jr: The psychotherapies: basic theoretical principles, techniques and indications, in Clinical Psychiatry for Medical Students. Edited by Stoudemire A. Philadelphia, PA, JB Lippincott, 1990, pp 855–890

Zetzel ER: Current concepts of transference. Int J Psychoanal 37:369–376, 1956

# 33

# Cognitive Therapy

JESSE H. WRIGHT, M.D., Ph.D.

MICHAEL E. THASE, M.D.

AARON T. BECK, M.D.

## Basic Concepts

### The Cognitive Model

The cognitive therapy (CT) perspective can be summarized in a working model (Figure 33–1) that expands on the well-known stimulus–response paradigm (Wright 1988; Wright et al. 2006). Cognitive mediation is given the central role in this model. However, an interactive relationship between environmental influences, cognition, emotion, and behavior is also recognized. It should be emphasized that this working model does not presume that cognitive pathology is the cause of specific syndromes or that other factors such as genetic predisposition, biochemical alterations, or interpersonal conflicts are not involved in the etiology of psychiatric illnesses. Instead, the model is used simply as a guide for the actions of the cognitive therapist in clinical practice. It is assumed that most forms of psychopathology have complex etiologies involving cognitive, biological, social, and interpersonal influences, and that there are multiple, potentially useful, approaches to treatment. In addition, it is assumed that cognitive changes are accomplished through biological processes and that psychopharmacological treatments can alter cognitions (Wright and Thase 1992). This posi-

tion is consistent with outcome research on CT and pharmacotherapy (Blackburn et al. 1981) and with other studies that have documented neurobiological changes associated with conditioning in animals (Kandel and Schwarz 1982; Mohl 1987) or psychotherapy in humans (Baxter et al. 1992; Goldapple et al. 2004).

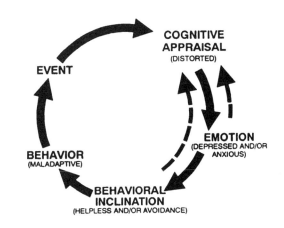

**FIGURE 33–1.** **A working model for cognitive therapy.**

*Source.* Adapted from Wright 1988.

Drs. Wright and Beck receive a portion of profits from sales of the "Good Days Ahead" software for computer-assisted cognitive therapy discussed in this chapter.

TABLE 33–1.    Adaptive and maladaptive schemas

| Adaptive | Maladaptive |
|---|---|
| No matter what happens, I can manage somehow. | I must be perfect to be accepted. |
| If I work at something, I can master it. | If I choose to do something, I must succeed. |
| I'm a survivor. | I'm a fake. |
| Others can trust me. | Without a woman [man], I'm nothing. |
| I'm lovable. | I'm stupid. |
| People respect me. | No matter what I do, I won't succeed. |
| I can figure things out. | Others can't be trusted. |
| If I prepare in advance, I usually do better. | I can never be comfortable around others. |
| I like to be challenged. | If I make one mistake, I'll lose everything. |
| There's not much that can scare me. | The world is too frightening for me. |

## Levels of Dysfunctional Cognitions

Beck and colleagues (Beck 1976; Beck et al. 1979; Dobson and Shaw 1986) have suggested that there are two major levels of dysfunctional information processing: 1) automatic thoughts and 2) basic beliefs incorporated in schemas. Automatic thoughts are the cognitions that occur rapidly while a person is in a situation (or recalling an event). These automatic thoughts usually are not subjected to rational analysis and often are based on erroneous logic. Although the individual may be only subliminally aware of these cognitions, automatic thoughts are accessible through questioning techniques used in CT (Beck et al. 1979; Wright and Beck 1983). The different types of faulty logic in automatic thinking have been termed *cognitive errors* (Beck et al. 1979). Typical cognitive errors include selective abstraction (sometimes termed "mental filter"), arbitrary inference, absolutistic thinking ("all or none" thinking), magnification and minimization, personalization, and catastrophic thinking.

Schemas are deeper cognitive structures that contain the basic rules for screening, filtering, and coding information from the environment (Beck et al. 1979; D.A. Clark et al. 1999; Wright and Beck 1983). These organizing constructs are developed through early childhood experiences and subsequent formative influences. Schemas can play a highly adaptive role in allowing rapid assimilation of data and appropriate decision making. However, in psychiatric disorders there are clusters of maladaptive schemas that perpetuate dysphoric mood and ineffective or self-defeating behavior (Beck 1976; Beck and Freeman 1990). Examples of adaptive and maladaptive schemas are presented in Table 33–1.

One of the basic tenets of CT is that maladaptive schemas often lie dormant until they are triggered by stressful life events (Beck et al. 1979; D.A. Clark et al. 1999). The newly emerged schema then influences the more superficial level of cognitive processing so that automatic thoughts are consistent with the rules of the schema. This theory applies primarily to episodic disorders such as depression. In chronic conditions (e.g., personality disturbances and eating disorders), schemas that pertain to the self may be present consistently and may be more resistant to change than in depression or anxiety disorders (Beck and Freeman 1990).

## Cognitive Pathology in Depression and Anxiety Disorders

The role of cognitive functioning in depression and anxiety disorders has been studied extensively. Information processing also has been examined in eating disorders, characterological problems, and other psychiatric conditions. In general, the results of this investigative effort have confirmed Beck's hypotheses (Beck 1963, 1964, 1976; Beck et al. 1979; D.A. Clark et al. 1999; Wright and Beck 1983). A full review of this research is not attempted here. However, a synthesis of results of significant studies on depression and anxiety is provided (see Table 33–2). These findings have played an important role in both confirming and shaping the treatment procedures used in CT. Cognitive pathology in eating disturbances, personality disorders, and psychoses is described in the section on CT applications.

Reviews of the voluminous research on cognitive processes in depression have found strong evidence for a negative cognitive bias in this disorder (D.A. Clark et al.

TABLE 33–2. Pathological information processing in depression and anxiety disorders

| Predominant in depression | Predominant in anxiety disorders | Common to both depression and anxiety disorders |
| --- | --- | --- |
| Hopelessness | Fears of harm or danger | Demoralization |
| Low self-esteem | High sensitivity to information about potential threat | Self-absorption |
| Negative view of environment | | Heightened automatic information processing |
| Automatic thoughts with negative themes | Automatic thoughts associated with danger, risk, uncontrollability, incapacity | Maladaptive schemas |
| Misattributions | | Reduced cognitive capacity for problem solving |
| Overestimates of negative feedback | Overestimates of risk in situations | |
| Enhanced recall of negative memories | Enhanced recall of memories for threatening situations | |
| Impaired performance on cognitive tasks requiring effort, abstract thinking | | |

1999). Substantial evidence has been collected to support the concept of the negative cognitive triad (D.A. Clark et al. 1999). A particularly well-designed study in this area of research was performed by Blackburn et al. (1986), who used the Cognitive Bias Questionnaire to test distortions in the three areas of the negative cognitive triad (self, world, and future). Depressed individuals scored more than twice as high on this scale as nondepressed control subjects. A large group of investigations has established that one of the elements of the negative cognitive triad, hopelessness, is highly associated with suicide risk (Beck et al. 1975, 1985b; Fawcett et al. 1987).

## Therapeutic Principles

### General Procedures

CT is usually a short-term treatment, lasting from 5 to 20 sessions. In some instances, very brief treatment courses are used for patients with mild or circumscribed problems, or longer series of CT sessions are used for those with chronic or especially severe conditions. However, the typical patient with major depression or an anxiety disorder can be treated successfully within the short-term format. After completion of the initial course of treatment, intermittent booster sessions may be useful in some cases, particularly for individuals with a history of recurrent illness or incomplete remission (Jarrett et al. 2001). Booster sessions can help maintain gains, solidify what has been learned in CT, and decrease the chances of relapse (Thase 1992).

The bulk of the therapeutic effort in CT is devoted to working on specific problems or issues in the patient's present life. The problem-oriented approach is emphasized for several reasons. First, directing the patient's attention to current problems stimulates the development of action plans that can help reverse helplessness, hopelessness, avoidance, or other dysfunctional symptoms. Second, data on cognitive responses to recent life events are more readily accessible and verifiable than for events that happened years in the past. Third, practical work on present problems helps to prevent the development of excessive dependency or regression in the therapeutic relationship. Finally, current problems usually provide ample opportunity to understand and explore the impact of past experiences.

### The Therapeutic Relationship

The therapeutic relationship in CT is characterized by a high degree of collaboration between patient and therapist and an empirical tone to the work of therapy. The therapist and patient function much like an investigative team. They develop hypotheses about the validity of automatic thoughts and schemas or alternately about the effectiveness of patterns of behavior. A series of exercises or experiments is then designed to test the validity of the hypotheses and, subsequently, to modify cognitions or behavior. Beck et al. (1979) have termed this form of therapeutic relationship *collaborative empiricism*. Methods of building a collaborative and empirical relationship are listed in Table 33–3.

---

**TABLE 33–3.    Methods of enhancing collaborative empiricism**

---

Work together as an investigative team.

Adjust therapist activity level to match the severity of illness and phase of treatment.

Encourage self-monitoring and self-help.

Obtain accurate assessment of validity of cognitions and efficacy of behavior.

Develop coping strategies for real losses and actual deficits.

Promote essential "nonspecific" therapist variables (e.g., kindness, empathy, equanimity, positive general attitude).

Provide and request feedback on regular basis.

Recognize and manage transference.

Customize therapy interventions.

Use gentle humor.

---

The therapist usually is more active in CT than in most other psychotherapies. The degree of therapist activity varies with the stage of treatment and the severity of the illness. Generally, a more directive and structured approach is emphasized early in treatment, when symptoms are severe. For example, a markedly depressed patient who is beginning treatment may benefit from considerable direction and structure because of symptoms such as helplessness, hopelessness, low energy, and impaired concentration. As the patient improves and understands more about the methods of CT, the therapist can become somewhat less active. By the end of treatment, the patient should be able to use self-monitoring and self-help techniques with little reinforcement from the therapist.

Collaborative empiricism is fostered throughout the therapy, even when directive work is required. Although the therapist may suggest specific strategies or give homework assignments designed to combat severe depression or anxiety, the patient's input is always solicited and the self-help component of CT is emphasized from the outset of treatment. Also, it is made clear that CT is not an attempt to convert all negative thoughts to positive ones. In fact, bad things do occur to people, and some individuals have behaviors that are ineffective or self-defeating. It is emphasized that in CT one seeks to obtain an accurate assessment of 1) the validity of cognitions, and 2) the adaptive versus maladaptive nature of behavior. If cognitive distortions have occurred, then the patient and therapist will work together to develop a more rational perspective. On the other hand, if actual negative experiences

or characteristics are identified, they will attempt to find ways to cope or to change.

Another characteristic that can influence the therapeutic relationship is the therapist's general attitude. Clinicians with a reasonably positive outlook on life and a belief that individual efforts can lead to significant change are likely to form more adaptive therapeutic relationships than those who may be overly discouraged or pessimistic. If the latter features are present, the therapist may require personal therapy to be able to forge the collaborative and empirical relationships that are necessary for effective CT.

Additional procedures that cognitive therapists use to encourage collaborative empiricism are 1) providing feedback throughout sessions, 2) recognizing and managing transference, 3) customizing therapy interventions, and 4) using gentle humor. The therapist gives feedback to keep the therapeutic relationship anchored in the "here and now" and to reinforce the working aspect of the therapy process. Comments are made frequently throughout the session to summarize major points, to give direction, and to keep the session on target. Also, questions are asked at several intervals in each session to determine how well the patient has understood a concept or has grasped the essence of a therapeutic intervention.

Because CT is highly psychoeducational, the therapist functions to some degree as a teacher. Thus, discreet positive feedback is given to help stimulate and reward the patient's efforts to learn. On a cautionary note, however, the cognitive therapist needs to avoid overzealous coaching or providing inaccurate or overdone positive feedback. Such actions will usually undermine the development of a good collaborative relationship. Some of these structuring procedures for cognitive therapy are summarized in Table 33–4.

---

**TABLE 33–4.    Structuring procedures for cognitive therapy**

---

Set agenda for therapy sessions.

Give constructive feedback to direct the course of therapy.

Employ common cognitive therapy techniques on a regular basis.

Assign homework to link sessions together.

---

A collaborative therapeutic relationship with frequent opportunities for two-way feedback generally discourages the formation of a transference neurosis. CT methodology and the short-term nature of treatment promote pragmatic working relationships as opposed to recapitulations of dysfunctional early relationships. Nevertheless, significant transference reactions can occur. These are more likely with patients who have personality disorders or other chronic illnesses that require longer-term treatment. The formation of negative or problematic transference reactions is rare in conventional short-term CT of persons with uncomplicated depression or anxiety disorders. When transference reactions occur, the cognitive therapist applies CT procedures to understand the phenomenon and to intervene. Typically, automatic thoughts and schemas that pertain to the therapeutic relationship are identified, explored, and modified if possible.

Another feature of CT that increases the collaborative nature of the therapeutic relationship is the customization of therapy interventions to meet the level of the patient's cognitive and social functioning. A profoundly depressed or anxious individual of low average intelligence may require a primarily behavioral approach, with limited efforts at understanding concepts such as automatic thoughts and schemas, especially in the beginning of treatment. Conversely, a less symptomatic patient with higher intelligence and ability to grasp abstract concepts may be able to profit from schema assessment early in therapy. If treatment procedures are pitched at a proper level, the patient is more likely to understand the material of therapy and to form a collaborative relationship with the therapist who is directing the treatment.

## Assessment and Case Conceptualization

Assessment for CT begins with completion of a standard history and mental status examination. Although special attention is paid to cognitive and behavioral elements, a full biopsychosocial evaluation is completed and used in formulating the treatment plan. The Academy of Cognitive Therapy, a certifying organization for cognitive therapists, has outlined a method for assessment and case conceptualization, which involves consideration of developmental influences, family history, social and interpersonal issues, genetic and biological contributions, and strengths and assets, in addition to key automatic thoughts, schemas, and behavioral patterns. The book *Learning Cognitive-Behavior Therapy: An Illustrated Guide* (Wright et al. 2006) provides detailed methods, worksheets, and examples of use of the Academy of Cognitive Therapy formulation methods. Worksheets from this book can be downloaded from the American Psychiatric Publishing Inc. Web site (www.appi.org). Also, the Academy of Cognitive Therapy Web site (www.academyofct.org)

supplies illustrations of how to complete case conceptualizations.

The key elements of the case conceptualization are 1) an outline of the most salient aspects of the history and mental status examination; 2) detailing of at least three examples from the patient's life of the relationship between events, automatic thoughts, emotions, and behaviors (specific illustrations of the cognitive model as it pertains to this patient); 3) identification of important schemas; 4) listing of strengths; 5) a working hypothesis that weaves together all of the information in numbers 1–4 with the cognitive and behavioral theories that most closely fit the patient's diagnosis and symptoms (e.g., models for anxiety disorders, depression, eating disorders, personality disorders, and other conditions; and 6) a treatment plan (including choices for specific CT methods) that is based on the working hypothesis (see Table 33–5). The conceptualization is continually developed throughout therapy and may be augmented or revised as new information is collected and treatment methods are tested.

**TABLE 33–5. Key elements of cognitive therapy case conceptualization**

History and mental status examination

Examples of cognitive-behavioral model from patient's life

Identification of major schemas

List of strengths

Working hypothesis

Treatment plan

## Structuring Therapy

Agenda setting helps to counteract hopelessness and helplessness by reducing seemingly overwhelming problems down into workable segments. The agenda-setting process also encourages patients to take a problem-oriented approach to their difficulties. Simply articulating a problem in a specific manner often can initiate the process of change. In addition, the agenda keeps the patient focused on salient issues and encourages efficient use of the therapy time.

Feedback procedures described earlier are also used in structuring CT sessions. For example, the therapist may observe that the patient is drifting from the established agenda or is spending time discussing a topic of questionable relevance. In situations such as these, constructive

**TABLE 33–6.** Psychoeducational materials and programs for cognitive therapy

| Title | Authors | Description |
|---|---|---|
| "Coping With Anxiety" | A.T. Beck et al. 1985a | Appendix to book |
| "Coping With Depression" | A.T. Beck et al. 1995 | Brief pamphlet |
| *Feeling Good* | Burns 1980, 1999 | Book with self-help program |
| *Getting Your Life Back: The Complete Guide to Recovery From Depression* | Wright and Basco 2002 | Book with self-help program; integrates cognitive therapy and biological approaches |
| *Good Days Ahead: The Multimedia Program for Cognitive Therapy* | Wright et al. 2004 | Computer-assisted therapy and self-help program |
| *Mastery of Your Anxiety and Panic* | Barlow and Craske 1999 | Self-help for anxiety |
| *Mind Over Mood* | Greenberger and Padesky 1995 | Self-help workbook |
| *Never Good Enough* | Basco 1999 | Book on perfectionism |
| *Stop Obsessing! How to Overcome Your Obsessions and Compulsions* | Foa and Wilson 2001 | Self-help for OCD |

feedback is given to direct the patient back to a more profitable area of inquiry. Heavy-handed, negatively oriented feedback is avoided. Instead, the therapist tends to give encouraging remarks that point the patient to issues that provide significant opportunities for change.

Commonly used CT techniques add an additional structural element to the therapy. Examples include activity scheduling, thought recording, and graded task assignments. These interventions, and others of similar nature, provide a clear and understandable method for reducing symptoms. Repeated use of procedures such as recording, labeling, and modifying automatic thoughts helps to link sessions together, especially if they are introduced in therapy and then assigned as homework.

## Psychoeducation

Psychoeducational procedures are a routine component of CT. One of the major goals of the treatment approach is to teach patients a new way of thinking and behaving that can be applied in resolving current symptoms and in managing problems that will be encountered in the future. The psychoeducational effort usually begins with the process of socializing the patient to therapy. In the opening phase of treatment, the therapist explains the basic concepts of CT and introduces the patient to the format of CT sessions. The therapist also devotes time early in treatment to discussing the therapeutic relationship in CT and the expectations for both patient and therapist. Psychoeducational work during a course of CT often involves brief explanations or illustrations coupled with homework assignments. These activities are woven into treatment sessions in a manner that emphasizes a collaborative, active learning approach. Some cognitive therapists have described the use of "mini-lectures," but a heavily didactic approach is generally avoided.

Psychoeducation can be facilitated with reading assignments and computer programs that reinforce learning, deepen the patient's understanding of CT principles, and promote the use of self-help methods. Table 33–6 contains a list of useful psychoeducational tools, including a pamphlet, books, and a computer program, that teach the CT model and encourage self-help. Most cognitive therapists liberally use psychoeducational tools as a basic part of the therapy process.

# Cognitive Techniques

## Identifying Automatic Thoughts

Much of the work of CT is devoted to recognizing and then modifying negatively distorted or illogical automatic thoughts (Table 33–7). The most powerful way of introducing the patient to the effects of automatic thoughts is to find an in vivo example of how automatic thoughts can influence emotional responses. Mood shifts during the therapy session are almost always good places to pause to identify automatic thoughts. The therapist observes that a strong emotion such as sadness, anxiety, or anger has appeared and then asks the patient to describe the thoughts that "went through your head" just prior to the mood shift.

**TABLE 33–7.** **Methods for identifying and modifying automatic thoughts**

Socratic questioning (guided discovery)

Use of mood shifts to demonstrate automatic thoughts in vivo

Imagery exercises

Role-play

Thought recording

Generating alternatives

Examining the evidence

Decatastrophizing

Reattribution

Cognitive rehearsal

Beck has described emotion as the "royal road to cognition" (Beck 1989). The patient usually is most accessible during periods of affective arousal, and cognitions such as automatic thoughts and schemas generally are more potent when they are associated with strong emotional responses. Hence, the cognitive therapist capitalizes on spontaneously occurring affective states during the interview and also pursues lines of questioning that are likely to produce an intense affect. One of the misconceptions about CT is that it is an overly intellectualized form of therapy. In fact, CT, as formulated by Beck et al. (1979), involves efforts to increase affect and to use emotional responses as a core ingredient of therapy.

One of the most frequently used procedures in CT is Socratic questioning. There is no set format or protocol for this technique. Instead, the therapist must rely on his or her experience and ingenuity to formulate questions that will help patients move from having a "closed mind" to a state of inquisitiveness and curiosity. Socratic questioning stimulates recognition of dysfunctional cognitions and development of a sense of dissonance about the validity of strongly held assumptions.

Imagery and role-play are used as alternate methods of uncovering cognitions when direct questions are unsuccessful in generating suspected automatic thinking (Beck et al. 1979). These techniques also are selected when only a limited amount of automatic thoughts can be brought out through Socratic questioning, and the therapist expects that more important automatic thoughts are present. Some patients may be able to use imagery procedures with few prompts or directions. In this case, the clinician only may need to ask the patient to imagine himself or herself back in a particularly troubling or emotion-provoking sit-

uation and then to describe the thoughts that occurred. However, most patients, particularly in the early phases of therapy, can benefit from "setting the scene" for the use of imagery. The patient is asked to describe the details of the setting. When and where did it take place? What happened immediately before the incident? How did the characters in the scene appear? What were the main physical features of the setting? Questions such as these help bring the scene alive in the patient's mind and facilitate recall of cognitive responses to the situation.

Role-play is a related technique for evoking automatic thoughts. When this procedure is used, the therapist first asks a series of questions to try to understand a vignette involving an interpersonal relationship or other social interchange that is likely to stimulate dysfunctional automatic thinking. Then, with the permission of the patient, the therapist briefly steps into the role of the individual in the scene and facilitates the playing out of a typical response set. Role-play is used less frequently than Socratic questioning or imagery and is best suited to therapeutic situations in which there is an excellent collaborative relationship and the patient is unlikely to respond to the role-play exercise with a negative or distorted transference reaction.

Thought recording is one of the most frequently used CT procedures for identifying automatic thoughts (J. Beck 1995; Wright et al. 2006). Patients can be asked to log their thoughts in a number of different ways. The simplest method is the two-column technique—a procedure that often is used when the patient is just beginning to learn how to recognize automatic thoughts. The two-column technique is illustrated in Table 33–8. In this case, the patient was asked to write down automatic thoughts that occurred in stressful or upsetting situations. Alternately, the patient could try to identify emotional reactions in one column and automatic thoughts in the other. A three-column exercise could include a description of the situation, a list of automatic thoughts, and a notation of the emotional response. Thought recording helps the patient to recognize the effects of underlying automatic thoughts and to understand how the basic cognitive model (i.e., relationship between situations, thoughts, feelings, and behaviors) applies to his or her own experiences. This procedure also initiates the process of modifying dysfunctional cognitions.

Thought recording is usually explained and illustrated in a therapy session and then additional exercises are assigned for homework. Depending on the case conceptualization, the therapist may suggest that the patient pay special attention to certain situations or issues (e.g., panic-

| TABLE 33–8. | Two-column thought recording |
| --- | --- |
| **Situation** | **Automatic thoughts** |
| Call from boss to submit a report | I can't do this. I don't know what to do. It won't be acceptable. |
| My wife asks me to help more around the house | Nothing I do is ever enough. She thinks I don't try. |
| Car won't start | I was stupid to buy this car. Nothing works right anymore. This is the last straw. |

inducing environmental cues, recurrent interpersonal problems, or dysfunctional behavioral responses). Also, specific assignments may be made to set up an in vivo experience that is likely to generate automatic thoughts. Examples might include discussing a troubling situation with a family member or attempting to engage in an anxiety-provoking situation or behavior that is usually avoided. Automatic thoughts that are recorded during these homework assignments are brought to the next session for review and discussion.

## Modifying Automatic Thoughts

There usually is no sharp division in CT between the phases of eliciting and modifying automatic thoughts. In fact, the processes involved in identifying automatic thoughts often are enough to initiate substantive change. As the patient begins to recognize the nature of his or her dysfunctional thinking, there typically is an increased degree of skepticism regarding the validity of automatic thoughts. Although patients can start to revise their cognitive distortions without specific additional therapeutic interventions, modification of automatic thoughts can be accelerated if the therapist applies Socratic questioning and other basic CT procedures to the change process.

Techniques used for revising automatic thoughts include 1) generating alternatives, 2) examining the evidence, 3) decatastrophizing, 4) reattribution, 5) thought recording, and 6) cognitive rehearsal (Beck et al. 1979; J. Beck 1995; Wright et al. 2006).

*Examining the evidence* is a major component of the collaborative empirical experience in CT. Specific automatic thoughts or clusters of related automatic thoughts are set forth as hypotheses, and the patient and therapist then search for evidence both for and against the hypothesis. In the case of Ms. D, the thought "If I don't go to school, I'd just be the same—stuck in a rut, not going anywhere"

was selected for an examining the evidence exercise. The therapist believed that returning to school was probably an adaptive action for the patient to take. However, it also was thought that seeing further education as the only route to change would excessively load this activity with a "make or break" mentality and would promote a disregard for other modifications that might increase self-esteem and self-efficacy.

*Decatastrophizing* involves efforts to reconceptualize feared outcomes in a manner that encourages coping and problem solving. This technique can be effective even if there is a reasonably high likelihood that a negative prediction will actually occur. For example, a man might correctly judge his marriage to be so troubled that his wife may ask for a divorce. In this instance, the therapist would help the patient to recognize distorted cognitions about his ability to manage a possible breakup of the marriage. The patient might think, "I couldn't make it without her" or "I'd lose everything." The decatastrophizing procedure would involve examining negative automatic thoughts for their validity; looking for previously unrecognized attributes, interests, or coping mechanisms; reviewing the ways that the patient had managed losses in the past; and stimulating the patient to think beyond the immediate situation. The use of *reattribution techniques* is based on findings of studies on the attributional process in depression explained earlier in this chapter. Depressed individuals have been found to have negatively biased attributions in three dimensions: global versus specific, internal versus external, and fixed versus variable (Abramson et al. 1978). Several different types of reattribution procedures are employed, including psychoeducation about the attributional process, Socratic questioning to stimulate reattribution, written exercises to recognize and reinforce alternate attributions, and homework assignments to test the accuracy of attributions.

Five-column Thought Change Records (TCRs; Beck et al. 1979) or other similar thought-recording devices are standard tools used in modification of automatic thoughts. The five-column TCR is used to encourage both identification and change of dysfunctional cognitions. A fourth (rational thoughts) and fifth (outcome) column are added to the three-column thought record (events, automatic thoughts, and emotions) typically used to identify automatic thoughts. The patient is instructed to use this form to capture and change automatic thoughts. Either a stressful event or a memory of an event or situation is noted in the first column. Automatic thoughts are recorded in the second column and are rated for degree of belief (how much the patient believes them to be true at the moment they occur) on a 0–100 scale. The third column is used to observe the emotional response to the automatic thoughts. The intensity of emotion is rated on a 1–100 scale. The fourth column, rational thoughts, is the most critical part of the TCR. The patient is asked to stand back from the automatic thoughts, assess their validity, and then write out a more rational or realistic set of cognitions. There are a wide variety of procedures that can be used to facilitate the development of rational thoughts for the TCR.

Previously described techniques such as generating alternatives, examining the evidence, and using reattribution also are used by the patient in a self-help format when the TCR is assigned for homework. In addition, the therapist often is able to help the patient refine or add to the list of rational thoughts when the TCR is reviewed at a subsequent therapy session. Repeated attention to generating rational thoughts on the TCR is usually quite helpful in breaking maladaptive patterns of automatic and negatively distorted thinking.

The fifth column of the TCR, outcome, is used to record any changes that have occurred as a result of revising and modifying automatic thoughts. In the case of Mr. E, there was a significant decrease in dysphoric affect. Although the use of the TCR will usually lead to the development of a more adaptive set of cognitions and a reduction in painful affect, on some occasions the initial automatic thoughts will prove to be accurate. In such situations, the therapist helps the patient take a problem-solving approach, including the development of an action plan, to manage the stressful or upsetting event.

*Cognitive rehearsal* is used to help uncover potential negative automatic thoughts in advance and to coach the patient in ways of developing more adaptive cognitions. First, the patient is asked to use imagery or role-play to identify possible distorted cognitions that could occur in a stressful situation. Second, the patient and therapist work together to modify the dysfunctional cognitions. Third, imagery or role-play is used again, this time to practice the more adaptive pattern of thinking. Finally, for a homework assignment, the patient is asked to try out the newly acquired cognitive patterns in vivo.

## Identifying and Modifying Schemas

The process of identifying and modifying schemas is somewhat more difficult than changing negative automatic thoughts because these core beliefs are more deeply embedded, may be largely out of the patient's awareness, and usually have been reinforced through years of life ex-

perience. However, many of the same techniques described for automatic thoughts are employed successfully in therapeutic work at the schema level (Beck et al. 1979; Wright et al. 2006). Procedures such as Socratic questioning, imagery, role-play, and thought recording are used to uncover maladaptive schemas (Table 33–9).

---

**TABLE 33–9.** Methods for identifying and modifying schemas

Socratic questioning

Imagery and role-play

Thought recording

Identifying repetitive patterns of automatic thoughts

Psychoeducation

Listing schemas in therapy notebook

Examining the evidence

Listing advantages and disadvantages

Generating alternatives

Cognitive rehearsal

---

As the patient gains experience in recognizing automatic thoughts, repetitive patterns begin to emerge that may suggest the presence of underlying schemas. Therapists have several options at this point. A psychoeducational approach can be used to explain the concept of schemas (may be alternately termed *core beliefs* or *basic assumptions*) and their linkage to more superficial automatic thoughts. Patients may then start to recognize schemas on their own. However, when the patient first starts to learn about basic assumptions, the therapist may need to suggest that certain schemas might be operative and then engage the patient in collaborative exercises that test these hypotheses.

Modification of schemas may require repeated attention, both in and out of therapy sessions (Table 33–10). One commonly used procedure is to ask the patient to keep a list in a therapy notebook of all the schemas that have been identified to date. The schema list can be reviewed before each session. This technique promotes a high level of awareness of schemas and usually encourages the patient to place issues pertaining to schemas on the agenda for therapy.

CT interventions that are particularly helpful in modifying schemas include examining the evidence, listing advantages and disadvantages, generating alternatives, and using cognitive rehearsal. After a schema has been identified, the therapist may ask the patient to do a pro/con

**TABLE 33–10.    Schema modification through examining the evidence**

**Schema: "I must be perfect to be accepted."**

| Evidence for | Evidence against |
|---|---|
| The better I do, the more people seem to like me. | Others who aren't "perfect" seem to be loved and accepted. Why should I be different? |
| Women who have a perfect figure are most attractive to men. | You don't have to have a perfect figure. Hardly anybody has one—just the models on television. |
| My parents have the highest standards; they are always pushing me to do better. | My parents want me to do well. But they'll probably accept me as long as I try to do my best, even if I don't meet all of their expectations. This statement is absolute and sets me up for failure, because no one can be perfect all the time. |

analysis (examining the evidence) using a double-column procedure. This technique usually induces the patient to doubt the validity of the schema and to start to think of alternate explanations (see Table 33–11).

**TABLE 33–11.    Schema modification through listing advantages and disadvantages**

**Schema: "I must be perfect to be accepted."**

| Advantages | Disadvantages |
|---|---|
| I've tried very hard to be the best. | I never really feel accepted because I've never reached perfection. |
| I've received top marks in school. | I'm always down on myself. I've developed bulimia. I'm obsessed with my body size. |
| I'm in lots of activities, and I've won dancing competitions. | I have trouble accepting my successes. I drive myself too hard and can't enjoy ordinary things. |

The list of alternative schemas will usually include several different options, ranging from rather minor adjustments to extensive revisions in the schema. The therapist uses Socratic questioning and other CT techniques such as imagery and role-play to help the patient recognize potential alternative schemas. A "brainstorming" attitude is encouraged. Instead of trying to be sure that a revised schema is entirely accurate at first glance, the therapist usually suggests that they try to generate a variety of modified schemas without initially considering their validity or practicality. This stimulates creativity and gives the patient further encouragement to step aside from long-standing rigid schemas (see Table 33–12).

After alternatives are generated and discussed, the therapy turns toward examining the potential consequences of changing basic attitudes. Cognitive rehearsal can be used in the therapy session to test a schema modification. This may be followed by a homework assignment to try out the revised schema in vivo. Therapist and patient work together to choose the most reasonable modifications for underlying schemas and to reinforce learning these new constructs through multiple practice sessions in therapy sessions and in real-life experiences.

**TABLE 33–12.    Schema modification through generating alternatives**

Schema: "I must be perfect to be accepted."

Possible alternatives

People who are successful are more likely to be accepted.

If I try to do my best (even if it's not perfect), others are likely to accept me.

I would like to be perfect, but that's an impossible goal. I'll choose certain areas to try to excel (school, work, and career) and not demand perfection everywhere.

You don't need to be perfect to be accepted.

I'm worthy of love and acceptance without trying to be perfect.

## Behavioral Procedures

Behavioral interventions are used in CT to 1) change dysfunctional patterns of behavior (e.g., helplessness, isolation, phobic avoidance, inertia, bingeing and purging); 2) reduce troubling symptoms (e.g., tension, somatic and psychic anxiety, intrusive thoughts); and 3) assist in identifying and modifying maladaptive cognitions. Table 33–13

**TABLE 33–13.  Behavioral procedures used in cognitive therapy**

Questioning to identify behavioral patterns

Activity scheduling with mastery and pleasure recording

Self-monitoring

Graded task assignments

Behavioral rehearsal

Exposure and response prevention

Coping cards

Distraction

Relaxation exercises

Respiratory control

Assertiveness training

Modeling

Social skills training

presents a listing of behavioral techniques. As discussed earlier in this chapter, the cognitive model for therapy suggests that there is an interactive relationship between cognition and behavior. Thus, behavioral initiatives should influence cognition, and cognitive interventions should have an impact on behavior.

The Socratic questions used in cognitively oriented procedures have a direct parallel when the emphasis is on behavioral change. The therapist asks a series of questions that help differentiate actual behavioral deficits from negatively distorted accounts of behavior. Depressed and anxious patients usually overreport their symptomatic distress or the difficulties they have in managing situations. Often, well-framed questions can reveal cognitive distortions and also stimulate change as the patient considers the negative impact of dysfunctional behavior. Four specific behavioral techniques—activity scheduling, graded task assignments, exposure, and coping cards—are explained below. A more detailed description of behavioral methods is available in Wright et al. (2006) or Meichenbaum (1977).

Activity scheduling is a structured method of learning about the patient's behavioral patterns, encouraging self-monitoring, increasing positive mood, and designing strategies for change (Beck et al. 1979; Wright et al. 2006). A daily or weekly activity log is employed in which the patient is asked to record what he or she does during each hour of the day and then to rate each activity for mastery and pleasure on a 0–10 scale. When the activity record is first introduced, the patient usually is asked to make a

record of baseline activities without attempting to make any changes. The data are then reviewed in the next therapy session.

Another behavioral procedure, the graded task assignment, can be used when the patient is facing a situation that seems excessively difficult or overwhelming. A challenging behavioral goal is broken down into small steps that can be taken one at a time. The graded task assignment is somewhat similar to the systematic desensitization protocols that are used in traditional behavior therapy (Wolpe 1969). However, a cognitive component is added to the methodology. There is an added emphasis placed on improving self-esteem and self-efficacy, countering hopelessness and helplessness, and using the graded task assignment to disprove maladaptive thoughts and schemas. With depressed individuals, the graded task assignment typically is used as a problem-solving technique. This stepwise approach, coupled with cognitive techniques such as Socratic questioning and thought recording, can reactivate the patient and focus his or her energy in a productive manner.

Exposure techniques are a central part of cognitive-behavioral approaches to anxiety disorders. For example, a phobia can be conceptualized as an unrealistic fear of an object or a situation coupled with a conditioned pattern of avoidance.

Treatment can proceed along two complementary lines: cognitive restructuring to modify dysfunctional thoughts and exposure therapy to break the pattern of avoidance. Typically, a hierarchy of feared stimuli is developed with the patient. The hierarchy should contain a number of different stimuli that cause varying degrees of distress. Usually the items are ranked by degree of distress. One commonly used system involves rating each item on a scale from 0 to 100, with 100 representing the maximum distress possible. After the hierarchy is established, the therapist and patient work collaboratively to set goals for gradual exposure, starting with the items that are ranked lower on the distress scale. Breathing training, relaxation exercises, and other behavioral methods may be used to enhance the patient's ability to carry out the exposure protocol.

Exposure can be done with imagery in treatment sessions or in vivo. Also, innovative virtual-reality methods have been developed for exposure therapy (Rothbaum et al. 1995). Virtual-reality exposure techniques have been shown to be effective in empirical trials, but they are expensive and are not yet widely available. Clinician-administered exposure therapy is frequently used as part of the cognitive-behavioral approach to simple phobias, panic disorder with agoraphobia, social phobia, and obsessive-compulsive disorder (OCD).

Coping cards are another commonly used method to achieve behavioral change. The therapist helps the patient to identify specific actions that are likely to help her or him cope with an anticipated problem or put CT skills into action. These ideas are then written down on a small card, which the patient carries with her or him as a reminder and as a tool to help in solving problems. Coping cards often contain both cognitive and behavioral interventions.

## Selecting Patients for Cognitive Therapy

CT procedures have been described for a large number of diagnostic categories (Beck 1993). Although there are no contraindications to using this treatment approach, CT is usually not attempted with patients who have marked brain disease. CT can be considered a primary treatment for 1) disorders in which it has been proven to be effective in controlled research (e.g., unipolar depression [nonpsychotic], anxiety disorders, eating disorders, and psychophysiological disorders), and 2) other conditions for which a clearly detailed treatment method has been developed (e.g., personality disorders, substance abuse) and there is some evidence for CT's effectiveness. CT should be considered an adjunctive therapy for disorders such as major depression with psychotic features, bipolar illness, and schizophrenia, in which there is clear evidence for the effectiveness of biological treatments and the effects of CT alone compared with pharmacotherapy have not been studied.

Clinical experience has suggested that patients who do not have severe character pathology (especially borderline or antisocial features), have previously formed trusting relationships with significant others, have a belief in the importance of self-reliance, and have a curious or inquisitive nature are especially suitable for CT (Wright et al. 2006). Above-average intelligence is not associated with better outcome, and CT procedures can be simplified for those with subnormal intellectual skills or impaired learning and memory functioning. Of course, most patients do not have a full combination of the ideal features noted above. A flexible approach can be employed in which CT procedures are customized to match the special characteristics of the patient's social background, intellectual level, personality structure, and clinical disorder (Wright et al. 2006).

# Cognitive Therapy Applications

## Depression

In the opening phase of treatment of depression, the cognitive therapist focuses on establishing a collaborative relationship and introduces the patient to the cognitive model. Agendas, feedback, and psychoeducational procedures are used to structure sessions. The emphasis is placed on two major forms of cognitive dysfunction: negatively distorted thinking and deficits in learning and memory functioning. Early in therapy, a special effort may be placed on relieving hopelessness because of the close link between this element of the negative cognitive triad and suicide risk. Also, reduction in hopelessness can be an important step in reactivating and reenergizing the depressed patient.

Problems with learning and memory functioning are countered with the aforementioned structuring procedures and with learning reinforcement techniques such as written therapy notes, diagrams, and homework assignments. The clinician carefully matches the therapeutic work to the patient's level of cognitive functioning so that learning is encouraged and the patient is not overwhelmed with the material of therapy. Behavioral techniques, such as activity scheduling and graded task assignments, often are a major component of the opening phase of CT of depression.

The middle portion of treatment is usually devoted to eliciting and modifying negatively distorted automatic thoughts. Behavioral techniques continue to be used in most cases. By this point in the therapy, patients should understand the cognitive model and be able to employ thought monitoring techniques to reverse all three elements of the negative cognitive triad (self, world, and future). Typically, the patient is taught to identify cognitive errors (e.g., selective abstraction, arbitrary inference, absolutistic thinking) and to use procedures such as generating alternatives and examining the evidence to alter negatively distorted thinking.

Work on eliciting and testing automatic thoughts continues during the latter portion of treatment. However, if there have been gains in functioning and the patient has grasped the basic principles of CT, therapy can turn primarily to identifying and altering maladaptive schemas. The concept of schemas usually has been introduced earlier in therapy, but the principal efforts at changing these underlying structures are reserved for the late phase of treatment when the patient is more likely to grasp and retain complex therapeutic initiatives. Before therapy concludes, the therapist helps the patient review what has been learned during the course of treatment and also suggests thinking ahead to possible circumstances that could trigger a return of depression. The potential for relapse is recognized, and problem-solving strategies are developed that can be employed in future stressful situations.

## Anxiety Disorders

Although the techniques used in CT for anxiety disorders are similar to those employed in the treatment of depression, treatment efforts are directed toward altering four major types of dysfunctional anxiety-producing cognitions: 1) overestimates of the likelihood of a feared event, 2) exaggerated estimates of the severity of a feared event, 3) underestimation of personal coping abilities, and 4) unrealistically low estimates of the help that others can offer. Most authors have recommended that a mixture of cognitive and behavioral measures be used in patients who have anxiety disorders (Barlow and Cerney 1988; Beck et al. 1985a).

In panic disorder, the emphasis is placed on helping the patient to recognize and change grossly exaggerated estimates of the significance of physiological responses or fears of imminent psychological disaster (Beck et al. 1985a, 1992; D.M. Clark 1986). For example, an individual with panic disorder may begin to perspire or breathe more rapidly, after which cognitions such as "I can't catch my breath….I'll pass out….I'll have a stroke" increase the intensity of the autonomic nervous system activity. The vicious cycle interaction between catastrophic cognitions and physiological arousal can be broken in two complementary ways: 1) altering the dysfunctional cognitions and 2) interrupting the cascading autonomic hyperactivity. Commonly used cognitive interventions include Socratic questioning, imagery, thought recording, generating alternatives, and examining the evidence. Behavioral measures such as relaxation training and respiratory control are used to dampen the physiological arousal associated with panic (D.M. Clark et al. 1985). Also, when panic attacks are stimulated by specific situations (e.g., driving, public speaking, crowds), graded exposure may be particularly useful in helping patients to both master a feared task and overcome their panic symptoms.

CT of phobic disorders centers on modifying unrealistic estimates of risk or danger in situations and engaging the patient in a series of graded exposure assignments. Generally, cognitive and behavioral procedures are used simultaneously. For example, a graded task assignment for an individual with agoraphobia might include a stepwise increase in experiences in a social setting accompa-

nied by use of a TCR to record and revise maladaptive automatic thinking. Patients with generalized anxiety disorder (GAD) usually have diffuse cognitive distortions about many circumstances in their lives (e.g., physical health, finances, loss of control, family issues) coupled with persistent autonomic overarousal (Beck et al. 1985a). The CT approach to GAD is closely related to methods used for panic disorder and phobias. However, special attention is paid to defining the stimuli that are associated with increased anxiety. Breaking down the generalized state of anxiety into workable segments can help the patient gain mastery over what initially appears to be an uncontrollable situation.

Behavioral techniques such as exposure and response prevention are used together with cognitive restructuring for patients with OCD (Salkovskis 1985). Cognitive interventions include challenging the validity of obsessional thoughts, attempting to replace dysfunctional cognitions with positive self-statements, and modifying negative automatic thoughts. Salkovskis and Warwick (1985) have noted that cognitive procedures may be needed in some cases to help the patient engage in exposure and response prevention. A combined approach of cognitive techniques to modify maladaptive thought patterns and behavioral interventions to counter patterns of avoidance is also used in CT for posttraumatic stress disorder (Harvey et al. 2003).

## Eating Disorders

CT is a well-established first-line treatment for bulimia nervosa and binge-eating disorder. CT for both conditions was given a grade A rating by the United Kingdom's National Institute for Clinical Excellence (NICE), indicating that there is strong support for efficacy from empirical trials (Wilson and Shafran 2005). Although methods have been described and tested for anorexia nervosa, NICE made no specific recommendations for this more severe form of eating disorder (Wilson and Shafran 2005). Considerably less research has been conducted on CT for anorexia nervosa than for other eating disorders. However, cognitive and behavioral interventions can be included in comprehensive treatment programs for this difficult-to-treat condition.

Individuals with eating disorders may have many of the same cognitive distortions that are seen in depression. However, they have an additional cluster of cognitive biases about body image, eating behavior, and weight (D.A. Clark et al. 1989). Patients with eating disorders usually place inordinate value on body shape as a measure of self-worth and as a condition for acceptance (e.g., "I must be thin to be accepted"; "If I'm overweight, nobody will want me"; "Fat people are weak"). They also may believe that any variance from their excessive standards means a total loss of control.

CT interventions are used to subject these maladaptive cognitions to empirical testing. Commonly used procedures include eliciting and testing automatic thoughts, examining the evidence, using reattribution, and giving in vivo homework assignments. In addition, behavioral techniques are used to stimulate more adaptive eating behavior and to uncover significant cognitions related to eating. As in treatment of other disorders, the relative emphasis on cognitive procedures compared with behavioral measures is dictated by the severity of the illness and the phase of treatment. An individual with anorexia nervosa who is malnourished and has an electrolyte imbalance may require hospitalization during the initial part of treatment for a contingency management program. Patients with this level of illness may have a significant impairment in learning and memory functioning and therefore have limited capacity to understand thought recording or other cognitive interventions. In contrast, a patient with uncomplicated bulimia nervosa may be able to benefit from relatively demanding cognitively oriented procedures early in treatment.

One of the critical factors in treating patients with eating disorders is the development of an effective working relationship. Compared with individuals with depression or anxiety disorders, those with eating disturbances often are reluctant to fully engage in therapy. Frequently, they have long-standing patterns of hiding their behavior from others and have developed elaborate methods of maintaining their dysfunctional approach to meals, body weight, and exercise. Thus, the patient with an eating disorder poses a special problem for the cognitive therapist. A thorough psychoeducational effort and considerable patience are usually required for the formation of a collaborative empirical relationship. Also, if the therapist focuses in the beginning on problem areas that the patient clearly wants to change (e.g., low self-esteem, hopelessness, loss of interest), struggles over control of eating disorders can be avoided until there have been successful experiences in working together in therapy.

## Personality Disorders

Beck and Freeman (1990) articulated a CT approach to personality disorders that is based on a cognitive conceptualization of characterological disturbances. They sug-

gest that the different personality types have idiosyncratic cognitions in four main areas: basic beliefs, view of self, view of others, and strategies for social interaction. For example, an individual with a narcissistic personality might believe, "I'm special....I'm better than the rest.... Ordinary rules don't apply to me." This cognitive set leads to behavioral strategies such as manipulation, breaking rules, and exploiting others (Beck and Freeman 1990). In contrast, a person with a dependent personality disorder might have core beliefs such as, "I need others to survive. ... I can't manage on my own....I can't be happy if I'm alone." The interpersonal strategies associated with these beliefs would include efforts to cling to or entrap others (Beck and Freeman 1990).

CT methods typically employed in treatment of affective disorders may not be successful with characterological problems (Beck and Freeman 1990). Recommendations that have been made for modifying CT for treatment of personality disorders are summarized in Table 33–14 (Beck and Freeman 1990; Linehan 1993). The problem-oriented, structured, and collaborative empirical characteristics of CT are retained in therapeutic work with patients who have personality disturbances, but there is an added emphasis on the therapeutic relationship. Treatment of personality disorders with CT may take considerably longer than therapy of more circumscribed problems such as depression or anxiety. Patients with personality disturbances have deeply ingrained schemas that are unlikely to change within the short-term format used for other disorders (Brown et al. 2004). When the course of therapy lengthens, there is a greater chance for development of transference and countertransference reactions. In CT, transference is viewed as a manifestation of underlying schemas. Therefore, transferential phenomena are recognized as opportunities for examining and modifying core beliefs.

An individualized case conceptualization is used. This formulation includes hypotheses on the role of maladaptive schemas in symptom production. Consideration also is given to the influences of parent–child conflicts, traumatic experiences, and the current social network on cognitive and behavioral pathology. Patients with personality disorders often have significant real-life problems, including severely disturbed interpersonal relationships and pronounced social skills deficits.

Although an ultimate goal of treatment is to modulate ineffective or maladaptive schemas, initial efforts (using procedures such as behavioral techniques or thought recording) may be directed at more readily accessible targets such as increasing self-efficacy or decreasing dyspho-

**TABLE 33–14. Modifications of cognitive therapy for personality disorders**

Pay special attention to the therapeutic relationship.

Attend to one's own (the therapist's) cognitive responses and emotional reactions.

Develop an individualized case conceptualization (including an assessment of the impact of developmental experiences, significant traumas, and environmental stresses).

Place an initial focus on increasing self-efficacy.

Use behavioral techniques, such as rehearsal and social skills training, to reverse actual deficits in interpersonal functioning.

Set firm, reasonable limits.

Set realistic goals.

Anticipate adherence problems.

Review and repeat treatment interventions.

ric mood. Self-monitoring, self-help exercises, and the structuring procedures used in CT help prevent excessive dependency. However, patients with character disorders (especially those with borderline, narcissistic, or dependent personalities) are prone to have excessive expectations, to be overly demanding, or to exhibit manipulative behavior. Thus, the cognitive therapist needs to set firm but reasonable limits and to help the patient articulate realistic treatment goals (Beck and Freeman 1990).

Adherence to treatment recommendations can be another problem in CT of personality disorders. The therapist can use procedures such as Socratic questioning or schema identification to uncover the reasons for nonadherence and help the patient follow through with homework assignments or other therapeutic work. Reviewing and repeating treatment interventions is another important component of CT for personality disorders. Considerable patience and persistence are required from the therapist as efforts are made to help the patient reverse chronic, deeply imbedded psychopathology.

Dialectical behavior therapy (DBT) is a specialized form of cognitive-behavioral therapy (CBT) developed by Marsha Linehan (1993) for treatment of borderline personality disorder. DBT employs cognitive and behavioral methods in addition to acceptance strategies derived from Zen teaching and practice. Therapy with DBT is long term and involves repeated behavioral analysis, behavioral skills instruction, contingency management, cognitive restructuring, exposure interventions to reduce avoidance

and dysfunctional emotions, and mindfulness training. DBT has been used successfully in borderline patients with suicidal behavior and substance abuse (Linehan et al. 1991, 1993, 1994, 2006).

## Psychosis

Psychotic illnesses are one of the indications for adjunctive CT. In CT of patients who have psychotic symptoms, the therapist conveys that maladaptive cognitions and reactions to life stress may interact with biological factors in the expression of the illness. Therefore, attempts to develop more adaptive cognitions or to learn how to cope better with environmental pressures can assist with efforts toward managing the disorder. During the early part of therapy with a psychotic patient, there is a strong emphasis on building a therapeutic alliance (Kingdon and Turkington 2005). The therapist tries to normalize and destigmatize the condition (Kingdon and Turkington 2005), and the rationale for antipsychotic medication in combination with CT is explained. Attempts may be made to stimulate hope by modifying intensely negative cognitions about the illness or its treatment (e.g., "I'm to blame….Nothing will help….Drugs don't work"). Usually, work on challenging hallucinations or delusions directly is delayed until a solid therapeutic relationship has been established. However, efforts are made to reverse delusional self-destructive cognitions as early as possible in the treatment process.

Reality testing is performed in a gentle, nonconfrontational manner (Kingdon and Turkington 2005). Usually delusions with lowest level of conviction are targeted first. The therapist uses guided discovery as a major intervention, but also may help the patient to record and change distorted automatic thoughts or perform examining the evidence exercises. Behavioral techniques such as activity scheduling, graded task assignments, and social skills training also are used with psychotic patients. These procedures can be used to provide needed structure or to teach adaptive behaviors. Negative symptoms are typically approached slowly in a manner that gives consideration to the difficulty of changing this manifestation of psychotic disorders (Kingdon and Turkington 2005). Other components of the CT approach to psychotic disorders may include 1) use of CT techniques that enhance medication adherence (see, e.g., Lecompte 1995), 2) identification of potential triggers for symptom exacerbation, 3) development of cognitive and behavioral strategies to manage stressful life events, and 4) implementation of family and/or group therapy applications of cognitive therapy (Wykes et al. 2005).

## Bipolar Disorder

CT methods for bipolar disorder focus primarily on attempts to help persons understand and cope with a disease that is thought to have strong genetic and biological influences. For example, Basco and Rush (2005) recommend extensive psychoeducation, in addition to techniques such as mood graphing and symptom summary worksheets. The latter interventions are used to assist patients in recognizing early signs of a mood swing and then devising methods to reduce the risk of cycling into a full depression or mania. To illustrate, a person who notes that decreased sleep typically heralds the onset of a manic episode might be coached on cognitive-behavioral strategies for improving sleep patterns, or a patient who recognizes that pressured activity and distractibility often progress to more severe symptoms of mania may practice cognitive-behavioral methods for slowing down and staying focused on productive task completion. Medication adherence is another important goal of CT for bipolar disorder (Basco and Rush 2005; Cochran 1986). Dysfunctional cognitions about medication can be modified with CT, and behavioral interventions, such as reminder systems and behavioral plans to overcome obstacles to adherence, can be used.

Treatment of depressive episodes in bipolar disorder utilizes many of the same interventions described for CT of major depression. Typically, CT is not used as a mainstay of treatment for severe mania when persons are markedly agitated or grossly psychotic. Instead, the CT effort is greater when symptoms are less extreme and the patient can concentrate on the work of therapy. The overall goals of CT for bipolar disorder are to lower symptoms of both depression and mania, improve psychosocial functioning, gain stress management skills, and reduce the risk for relapse.

## Key Points: Cognitive Therapy

- Studies of information processing in mental disorders have found characteristic patterns of cognitions that are linked with dysphoric emotions and maladaptive behavior.

- Treatment with cognitive therapy involves modification of dysfunctional cognitions and associated behaviors.

- Cognitive therapy is an active treatment characterized by a highly collaborative therapeutic relationship.

- Structure, psychoeducation, and homework are important components of treatment.

- Cognitive therapists help patients identify and change automatic thoughts and core beliefs (schemas).

- Behavioral methods are used to reverse helplessness, anhedonia, avoidance, and other core symptoms of mental disorders.

- Cognitive therapy has been extensively researched. There is strong empirical support for the efficacy of this treatment approach.

- Cognitive therapy methods have been developed for many conditions including mood and anxiety disorders, schizophrenia, eating disorders, substance abuse, and personality disorders.

## References

Abramson LY, Seligman MEP, Teasdale J: Learned helplessness in humans: critique and reformulation. J Abnorm Psychol 87:49–74, 1978

Barlow DH, Cerney JA: Psychological Treatment of Panic. New York, Guilford, 1988

Barlow DH, Craske MG: Mastery of Your Anxiety and Panic (MAP3). Boston, MA, Graywind Publications, 1999

Basco MR: Never Good Enough. New York, Free Press, 1999

Basco MR, Rush AJ: Cognitive-Behavioral Therapy for Bipolar Disorder. New York, Guilford, 2005

Baxter LR Jr, Schwartz JM, Bergman KS, et al: Caudate glucose metabolic rate changes with both drug and behavior therapy for obsessive-compulsive disorder. Arch Gen Psychiatry 49:681–689, 1992

Beck AT: Thinking and depression. Arch Gen Psychiatry 9:324–333, 1963

Beck AT: Thinking and depression, II: theory and therapy. Arch Gen Psychiatry 10:561–571, 1964

Beck AT: Cognitive Therapy and the Emotional Disorders. New York, International Universities Press, 1976

Beck AT: Cognitive therapy and research: a 25-year retrospective. Presented at the World Congress of Cognitive Therapy. Oxford, England, 1989

Beck AT: Cognitive therapy: past, present, and future. J Consult Clin Psychol 61:194–198, 1993

Beck AT, Freeman A: Cognitive Therapy of Personality Disorders. New York, Guilford, 1990

Beck AT, Kovacs M, Weissman A: Hopelessness and suicidal behavior—an overview. JAMA 234:1146–1149, 1975

Beck AT, Rush AJ, Shaw BF, et al: Cognitive Therapy of Depression. New York, Guilford, 1979

Beck AT, Emery GD, Greenberg RL: Anxiety Disorders and Phobias: A Cognitive Perspective. New York, Basic Books, 1985a

Beck AT, Steer RA, Kovacs M, et al: Hopelessness and eventual suicide: a 10-year prospective study of patients hospitalized with suicidal ideation. Am J Psychiatry 142:559–562, 1985b

Beck AT, Sokol L, Clark DA, et al: A cross-over study of focused cognitive therapy for panic disorder. Am J Psychiatry 149:778–783, 1992

Beck AT, Greenberg RL, Beck J: Coping with depression (a booklet). Bala Cynwyd, PA, The Beck Institute, 1995

Beck J: Cognitive Therapy: Basics and Beyond. New York, Guilford, 1995

Blackburn IM, Bishop S, Glen AIM, et al: The efficacy of cognitive therapy in depression: a treatment trial using cognitive therapy and pharmacotherapy, each alone and in combination. Br J Psychiatry 139:181–189, 1981

Blackburn IM, Jones S, Lewin RJP: Cognitive style in depression. Br J Clin Psychol 25:241–251, 1986

Brown GK, Newman CF, Charlesworth SE, et al: An open clinical trial of cognitive therapy for borderline personality disorder. J Personal Disord 18:257–271, 2004

Burns DD: Feeling Good. New York, William Morrow, 1980

Burns DD: Feeling Good: The New Mood Therapy. New York, HarperCollins, 1999

Clark DA, Feldman J, Channon S: Dysfunctional thinking in anorexia and bulimia nervosa. Cognit Ther Res 13:377–387, 1989

Clark DA, Beck AT, Alford BA: Scientific Foundations of Cognitive Theory and Therapy of Depression. New York, Wiley, 1999

Clark DM: A cognitive approach to panic. Behav Res Ther 24:461–470, 1986

Clark DM, Salkovskis PM, Chalkley AJ: Respiratory control as a treatment for panic attacks. J Behav Ther Exp Psychiatry 16:23–30, 1985

Cochran SD: Compliance with lithium regimens in the outpatient treatment of bipolar affective disorders. J Compliance Health Care 1:151–169, 1986

Dobson KS, Shaw BF: Cognitive assessment with major depressive disorders. Cognit Ther Res 10:13–29, 1986

Fawcett J, Scheftner W, Clark D, et al: Clinical predictors of suicide in patients with major affective disorders: a controlled prospective study. Am J Psychiatry 144:35–40, 1987

Foa E, Wilson R: Stop Obsessing! How to Overcome Your Obsessions and Compulsions, Revised Edition. New York, Bantam Books, 2001

Goldapple K, Segal Z, Garson C, et al: Modulation of cortical-limbic pathways in major depression: treatment-specific effects of cognitive behavior therapy. Arch Gen Psychiatry 61:34–41, 2004

Greenberger D, Padesky CA: Mind Over Mood. New York, Guilford, 1995

Harvey AG, Bryant RA, Tarrier N: Cognitive behaviour therapy for posttraumatic stress disorder. Clin Psychol Rev 23:501–522, 2003

Jarrett RB, Kraft D, Doyle J, et al: Preventing recurrent depression using cognitive therapy with and without a continuation phase: a randomized clinical trial. Arch Gen Psychiatry 58:381–388, 2001

Kandel ER, Schwartz JH: Molecular biology of learning: modulation of transmitter release. Science 218:433–443, 1982

Kingdon D, Turkington D: Cognitive Therapy for Schizophrenia. New York, Guilford, 2005

Lecompte D: Drug compliance and cognitive-behavioral therapy in schizophrenia. Acta Psychiatr Belg 95:91–100, 1995

Linehan MM: Cognitive-Behavioral Treatment of Borderline Personality Disorder. New York, Guilford, 1993

Linehan MM, Armstrong HE, Suarez A, et al: Cognitive-behavioral treatment of chronically parasuicidal borderline patients. Arch Gen Psychiatry 48:1060–1064, 1991

Linehan MM, Heard HL, Armstrong HE: Naturalistic follow-up of a behavioral treatment for chronically parasuicidal borderline patients. Arch Gen Psychiatry 50:971–974, 1993

Linehan MM, Tutek DA, Heard HL, et al: Interpersonal outcome of cognitive behavioral treatment for chronically suicidal borderline patients. Am J Psychiatry 151:1771–1776, 1994

Linehan MM, Comtois KA, Murray AM, et al: Two-year randomized controlled trial and follow-up of dialectical behavior therapy vs therapy by experts for suicidal behaviors and borderline personality disorder. Arch Gen Psychiatry 63:757–766, 2006

Meichenbaum DB: Cognitive-Behavior Modification: An Integrative Approach. New York, Plenum, 1977

Mohl PC: Should psychotherapy be considered a biological treatment? Psychosomatics 28:320–326, 1987

Rothbaum BO, Hodges LF, Kooper R, et al: Effectiveness of computer-generated (virtual reality) graded exposure in the treatment of acrophobia. Am J Psychiatry 152:626–628, 1995

Salkovskis PM: Obsessional-compulsive problems: a cognitive-behavioral analysis. Behav Res Ther 25:571–583, 1985

Salkovskis PM, Warwick HM: Cognitive therapy of obsessive-compulsive disorder: treating treatment failures. Behavioural Psychotherapy 13:243–255, 1985

Thase ME: Transition and aftercare, in Cognitive Therapy with Inpatients: Developing a Cognitive Milieu. Edited by Wright JH, Thase ME, Beck AT, et al. New York, Guilford, 1992, pp 414–435

Wilson GT, Shafran R: Eating disorders guidelines from NICE. Lancet 365:79–81, 2005

Wolpe J: The Practice of Behavior Therapy. New York, Pergamon, 1969

Wright JH: Cognitive therapy of depression, in The American Psychiatric Press Review of Psychiatry, Vol 7. Edited by Frances AJ, Hales RE. Washington, DC, American Psychiatric Press, 1988, pp 554–590

Wright JH, Basco MR: Getting Your Life Back: The Complete Guide to Recovery From Depression (Paperback Edition). New York, Touchstone, 2002

Wright JH, Beck AT: Cognitive therapy of depression: theory and practice. Hosp Community Psychiatry 34:1119–1127, 1983

Wright JH, Thase ME: Cognitive and biological therapies: a synthesis. Psychiatr Ann 22:451–458, 1992

Wright JH, Wright AS, Beck AT: Good Days Ahead: The Multimedia Program for Cognitive Therapy. Louisville, KY, MindStreet, 2004

Wright JH, Basco MR, Thase ME: Learning Cognitive-Behavior Therapy: An Illustrated Guide (Core Competencies in Psychotherapy Series, Glen O. Gabbard, series ed). Arlington, VA, American Psychiatric Publishing, 2006

Wykes T, Hayward P, Thomas N, et al: What are the effects of group cognitive behaviour therapy for voices: a randomised control trial. Schizophr Res 77:201–210, 2005

## 34

# Pain Disorders

RAPHAEL J. LEO, M.D.

## Pain Disorder

The diagnostic criteria for pain disorder are summarized in Table 34–1.

## Comorbid Psychiatric Conditions

### Depression

Depression prevalence rates among patients with chronic pain are substantially higher than those in the general population, with estimates varying from 30% to 54% (Banks and Kerns 1996). Depression, therefore, constitutes a common psychiatric comorbidity.

### Anxiety

Research findings suggest a relationship between anxiety states and arthritic conditions (McWilliams et al. 2003), migraine (Swartz et al. 2000), back pain (McWilliams et al. 2004), and fibromyalgia (H. Cohen et al. 2002). The presence of comorbid anxiety may lead to hyperarousal and increased vigilance for pain and somatic concerns. Anxiety may influence the emotional valence associated with somatic sensations and increase proclivity to misinterpret somatic experiences (Derakshan and Eysenck 1997; van der Kolk et al. 1996).

### Sleep Disorders

Sleep disturbances are common among patients with a variety of pain disorders (Moldofsky 2001). The etiology

is likely to be multifactorial, including disruptions due to pain itself, comorbid psychiatric disturbances, effects of pain medications, lack of aerobic exercise, and behavioral conditioning due to protracted reclining and daytime napping (M.J.M.Cohen et al. 2000). As a consequence, patients may report difficulty falling asleep, frequent awakenings and disrupted sleep, decreased total sleep time, and daytime fatigue. Measures to address these difficulties require that patients be educated about development of appropriate sleep hygiene techniques. Dosing of pain medications may need to be adjusted to reduce sleep-interfering effects. Nonbenzodiazepine sedatives, such as zolpidem, may be indicated to facilitate sleep. In conjunction, antidepressants and anticonvulsants required for certain pain states can be useful in augmenting sleep potential due to their sedating effects. Stimulants may be required to reduce excess daytime sedation associated with opiate analgesic use.

## Substance Abuse and Dependence

Rates of substance abuse or dependence among patients with chronic pain have been reportedly higher than those in the general population (Brown et al. 1996). For most, the substance use disorder preceded the onset of the pain disorder (Brown et al. 1996). In fact, a preexisting substance use disorder may predispose the individual to accidents and injuries, some of which may evolve into chronic pain syndromes (Polatin et al. 1993).

Although chronic pain patients may be vulnerable to developing new substance use disorders in the course of treatment (Brown et al. 1996; Dersh et al. 2002; Dunbar and Katz 1996), some contend that this is an extraordinar-

---

**TABLE 34–1.    DSM-IV-TR diagnostic criteria for pain disorder**

---

A.  Pain in one or more anatomical sites is the predominant focus of the clinical presentation and is of sufficient severity to warrant clinical attention.

B.  The pain causes clinically significant distress or impairment in social, occupational, or other important areas of functioning.

C.  Psychological factors are judged to have an important role in the onset, severity, exacerbation, or maintenance of the pain.

D.  The symptom or deficit is not intentionally produced or feigned (as in factitious disorder or malingering).

E.  The pain is not better accounted for by a mood, anxiety, or psychotic disorder and does not meet criteria for dyspareunia.

*Code* as follows:

**307.80   Pain disorder associated with psychological factors:**   psychological factors are judged to have the major role in the onset, severity, exacerbation, or maintenance of the pain. (If a general medical condition is present, it does not have a major role in the onset, severity, exacerbation, or maintenance of the pain.) This type of pain disorder is not diagnosed if criteria are also met for somatization disorder.

*Specify* if:

**Acute:**   duration of less than 6 months

**Chronic:**   duration of 6 months or longer

**307.89   Pain disorder associated with both psychological factors and a general medical condition:**   both psychological factors and a general medical condition are judged to have important roles in the onset, severity, exacerbation, or maintenance of the pain. The associated general medical condition or anatomical site of the pain (see below) is coded on Axis III.

*Specify* if:

**Acute:**   duration of less than 6 months

**Chronic:**   duration of 6 months or longer

**Note:**   The following is not considered to be a mental disorder and is included here to facilitate differential diagnosis.

**Pain disorder associated with a general medical condition:** a general medical condition has a major role in the onset, severity, exacerbation, or maintenance of the pain. (If psychological factors are present, they are not judged to have a major role in the onset, severity, exacerbation, or maintenance of the pain.) The diagnostic code for the pain is selected based on the associated general medical condition if one has been established (see Appendix G) or on the anatomical location of the pain if the underlying general medical condition is not yet clearly established—for example, low back (724.2), sciatic (724.3), pelvic (625.9), headache (784.0), facial (784.0), chest (786.50), joint (719.40), bone (733.90), abdominal (789.0), breast (611.71), renal (788.0), ear (388.70), eye (379.91), throat (784.1), tooth (525.9), and urinary (788.0).

---

ily rare event (Zenz et al. 1992). Risk factors include a prior history of substance abuse, prior physical or sexual abuse, major depression, anxiety disorders, and personality disorders (Dersh et al. 2002; Fishbain et al. 1998). Although opiates have been a predominant focus, several other agents used in pain treatment are likewise prone to abuse and dependence, including the muscle relaxant carisoprodol (Soma), ketamine, ergot alkaloids, and barbiturates employed in migraine treatment, and benzodiazepines.

## Treatment Approaches

### Psychotherapy

The experience of the pain goes beyond mere sensory phenomena. It can shape the manner in which patients make sense about events in their lives. In addition, it can alter how patients perceive themselves and the world. Thus, problematic beliefs about the self (e.g., inadequacy, helplessness, and undesirability), the world (e.g., dangerousness), and the future (e.g., hopelessness) can emerge, producing significant distress. An individual harboring such beliefs may experience a loss of self-esteem and self-efficacy, loss of connections with others, and marked disappointment and disillusionment in addition to physical discomfort. Such beliefs may lead to unhealthy behaviors such as substance abuse, nonadherence with treatment, withdrawal from support systems, and incapacitating emotional states (e.g., marked dysphoria, anger, anxiety) warranting psychotherapeutic intervention. In fact, low self-efficacy is a predictor of perceived disability resulting from persisting pain (Arnstein 2000).

The patient's cognitive style and propensity toward distorted appraisal of life events can impair functioning (Jensen et al. 1991b). Catastrophizing has been associated with increased pain and perceived disability, poor adjustment to pain, and marked emotional distress (Hasenbring et al. 2001; M.J. Sullivan et al. 2001). Other examples of problematic cognitive styles interfering with the adjustment to pain are listed in Table 34–2.

The distress related to pain, unpleasant emotional states, and negative cognitions may be difficult for patients to tolerate. The strategies employed by the individual to self-soothe, reduce distress, and modulate unpleasant physical and emotional states can be quite diverse. Patients who employ passive coping by hoping for relief, praying, avoiding activity, and so on may be at a distinct disadvantage compared with those individuals who employ more proactive coping strategies such as distracting oneself with other activities or engaging in self-statements that can produce relief (Jensen et al. 1991b; Rosenstiel and Keefe 1983). Perceived self-efficacy may be a major determinant of the patient's ability to utilize proactive coping strategies (Jensen et al. 1991a). Evidence of ineffective coping (e.g., a tendency to embellish or magnify somatic complaints; self-medicating inappropriately or abusing substances so as to assuage distress) warrants intervention, because such behaviors can undermine treatment endeavors. Emotion-focused coping strategies can be quite effective and easily taught to patients to facilitate stress management. Those with a limited repertoire of coping abilities may experience despair and even suicidal ideation. Suicide rates are quite high among patients with chronic pain (Chochinov et al. 1998; Fishbain 1999), necessitating the recognition of lethality and appropriate intervention.

It is pertinent to consider significant persons in the patient's life and how those relationships have been influenced by the pain. Changes in role responsibilities in the home as a result of pain may cause marked distress, ac-

---

**TABLE 34–2. Problematic cognitive patterns in pain**

**Catastrophizing:** The tendency to view and expect the worst (e.g., "I am doomed to have pain and misery forever!")

**Helplessness:** The belief that nothing that one does matters, that there is no benefit despite one's best efforts (e.g., "My doctor says that I should exercise to improve my osteoarthritis. I know it won't help!")

**Help-rejecting:** Rejecting efforts of well-meaning others as a means of expressing anger, securing ongoing "support" or attention, and even manipulating others (e.g., "I had problems with the last four medicines you gave me.")

**Labeling:** Ascribing a behavior of an individual to a characteristic or nature of the individual (e.g., the patient who is disappointed with the ineffectiveness of a medication may need to discount the qualifications of the clinician: "The medication the doctor gave me didn't help. What a quack!")

**Magnification:** The exaggeration of the significance of a negative event (e.g., "My pain got worse at work yesterday. I had to leave an hour early. I might as well come to grips with the fact that I am totally disabled!")

**Overgeneralization:** Expanding one adverse event or setback to many or all aspects of his or her life (e.g., "If this medication doesn't help me, nothing will!")

**Personalization:** The interpretation that an event or situation is indicative of something about oneself (e.g., "Because of the pain, I am a worthless failure!")

**Selective abstraction:** The propensity to attend selectively to negative aspects of one's life while ignoring satisfying and rewarding aspects (e.g., "Everything that happens in my life is bad!")

*Source.* Reprinted from Leo RJ: *Clinical Manual of Pain Management in Psychiatry.* Washington, DC, American Psychiatric Publishing, 2003, p. 43. Used with permission.

---

companied by resentment and anger. There may be little emotional reserve to invest in other relationships and loss of intimacy and sexual satisfaction. How pain is communicated, what responses are generated from others, and how the patient perceives those responses may suggest areas warranting intervention. For example, for some patients there may be much to be gained interpersonally by focusing on their complaints, such as avoiding conflicts or communicating displeasure with others (Fishbain 1994; Ford 1986). An inability to negotiate interpersonal diffi-

**TABLE 34–3.    Psychotherapeutic modalities employed in pain management**

| Modality | Techniques | Uses |
|---|---|---|
| Behavioral | Activity scheduling; pacing and graded activity; desensitization | Increase exercise/activity levels; overcome fear–avoidance |
| Cognitive-behavioral | Collaborative process identifying cognitive appraisals; cognitive restructuring; assess utility of coping strategies; coping skills training | Reduce depression and anxiety associated with pain; develop effective coping strategies; reduce problematic cognitive styles |
| Interpersonal | Role-playing, analysis of communication patterns | Address role transitions due to pain; relationship difficulties/conflicts |
| **Adjunctive techniques** | | |
| Biofeedback | Physiological parameters are measured and fed back to patient to facilitate mastery over them | Muscle relaxation; control of physiological parameters contributing to pain (e.g., headache) |
| Guided imagery | Talking patient through pleasant scenarios to produce vivid distracting and relaxing images | Relaxation; distraction from pain |
| Hypnosis | Focused attention and dissociation directed at altering pain experiences | Relaxation; pain severity reduction; distraction |
| Progressive muscle relaxation | Sequential muscle tightening and subsequent relaxation | Muscle relaxation; distraction from pain |

culties, such as through a tendency toward a lack of assertiveness (Lackner and Gurtman 2005) or an inability of the patient's support system to adapt appropriately to the patient's needs, may foster isolation and impair the patient's abilities to cope effectively.

## Psychotherapy Modalities

Cognitive-behavioral therapy (CBT) has dominated the literature in terms of its applicability to pain treatment. However, it should be recognized that other therapeutic approaches have promise in pain management as well (Table 34–3). For example, the individual experiencing marked difficulties in role transitions or relationship difficulties with spouse or other family members as a result of illness may benefit from interpersonal psychotherapy (M.M. Weissman et al. 2000) or marital and family therapies. Operant conditioning techniques may be employed to modify disruptive, pain-associated behaviors that have become incorporated into the patient's customary repertoire through prior environmental contingencies. Excess reclining, avoidance of activity, and immobility may be modifiable with graded exposure, pacing of activities, and judicious implementation of social/environmental reinforcements (Sanders 2003).

CBT involves a collaborative process between the therapist and patient. Initial sessions involve elicitation of the patient's perception of the pain; appraisals of current life situations; beliefs about life, relationships, and the future; and current coping measures. The focus shifts in subsequent sessions to empirically assess the accuracy and overall usefulness of the patient's beliefs and coping strategies, replacing those that are maladaptive with alternative approaches. In so doing, it is expected that there will be resultant improvements in the patient's mood, ability to interpret day-to-day events, and adaptation.

Adjunctive therapeutic techniques such as relaxation training, biofeedback, and hypnosis can be useful in the armamentarium of acute and chronic pain states (Orne 1976; Turk et al. 1979; Turner and Chapman 1982a, 1982b). In general, such measures facilitate relaxation, can reduce physiological parameters linked with the genesis and perpetuation of pain, and, in the case of hypnosis, can lead to dissociative states resulting in modifications of the experience of pain. However, these measures can be limited in their utility among highly distressed and distracted patients (Leo 2007). Interventions to mitigate co-occurring depression or anxiety may be required initially, so as to render patients amenable to participating in and practicing these interventions for reduction of pain severity.

**TABLE 34–4.  Adjuvant medications for pain management**

| Class of medication | Indication | Limitations |
|---|---|---|
| Antidepressants | Neuropathic pain, tension and migraine headaches, fibromyalgia, functional gastrointestinal disorders, comorbid depression/anxiety | Analgesia is best with agents possessing NE/5-HT reuptake influences<br>Side effects: TCAs are perhaps least tolerable; drug interactions |
| Anticonvulsants | Neuropathic pain, migraine headache, central pain, phantom limb pain | Side effects: sedation, motor and gastrointestinal adverse effects, rash, drug interactions |
| Benzodiazepines | Muscle relaxation, anxiety associated with acute pain and procedures/interventions, insomnia | Abuse/dependence potential; sedation |
| Lithium | Cluster headache prophylaxis | Not effective for episodic cluster headache; risk of toxicity if dehydration occurs or with certain drug combinations |
| Stimulants | Opiate analgesia augmentation, opiate-induced fatigue and sedation | Abuse/dependence potential; overstimulation, anorexia, insomnia |
| NMDA antagonists | Opiate analgesia augmentation, neuropathic pain | Side effects: hallucinations with ketamine |
| Muscle relaxants | Acute muscle pain, muscle spasticity, fibromyalgia | Abuse/dependence potential with some agents; delirium from abrupt baclofen withdrawal; questionable utility in long-term use |

*Note.*   5-HT = 5-hydroxytryptamine (serotonin); NE = norepinephrine; NMDA = *N*-methyl-D-aspartate; TCAs = tricyclic antidepressants.

## Pharmacological Approaches

The classes of medications frequently used for pain management are shown at Table 34–4.

### *Nonsteroidal Anti-Inflammatory Drugs and Acetaminophen*

Effective for mild to moderate acute and chronic pain, nonsteroidal anti-inflammatory drugs (NSAIDs; including aspirin) act by interfering with prostaglandin synthesis and pain-inducing inflammatory processes. The exact mechanism of acetaminophen analgesic activity is unclear, but it is thought to be a weak inhibitor of prostaglandin synthesis (Lucas et al. 2005). However, these agents are limited by a ceiling effect—that is, a dosage limit beyond which the analgesic effect is no longer appreciated. Adverse effects associated with NSAIDs include gastric irritation and ulceration, renal dysfunction, and bleeding due to decreased platelet aggregation. The cyclooxygenase-2 inhibitors have a lower incidence of gastrointestinal side effects; however, the risks associated with stroke and cardiovascular complications have resulted in the withdrawal of the commercial availability of two of these agents, rofe-

coxib and valdecoxib. At the time of this writing, only celecoxib (Celebrex) is still available for use. For acetaminophen, there are concerns over hepatotoxicity in dosages beyond 4,000 mg daily (see Table 34–5)

### *Tramadol*

Tramadol (Ultram) is useful in the treatment of mild to moderate acute and chronic pain (see Table 34–5). It is unique in that it possesses dual pharmacological effects: weak opiate agonist effects along with reuptake inhibition of norepinephrine and serotonin. A variant that combines the anti-inflammatory effects of acetaminophen with tramadol (i.e., Ultracet) is available that is effective in moderate to severe pain (Schnitzer 2003). Risks associated with tramadol use include seizures (especially in those with epilepsy), head trauma, alcohol withdrawal (Gardner et al. 2000), and serotonin syndrome, especially when co-administered with serotonergic antidepressants or monoamine oxidase inhibitors (Lange-Asschenfeldt et al. 2002). Reports have emerged indicating that tramadol is an agent on which patients can become quite dependent, particularly patients with preexisting drug or alcohol dependence (Leo et al. 2000).

**TABLE 34–5.   Pharmacological approaches for mild to moderate pain**

| Class of medication | Mechanism | Indication | Limitations |
|---|---|---|---|
| NSAIDs | Prostaglandin synthesis inhibitor | Bone pain, inflammatory pain | Ceiling effect; gastrointestinal and renal effects; increased bleeding |
| Acetaminophen | Prostaglandin synthesis inhibitor | Headache, inflammatory pain | Ceiling effect; hepatotoxic effects |
| Celecoxib | Cyclooxygenase-2 inhibitor | Rheumatoid arthritis and osteoarthritis | High doses may be associated with gastrointestinal effects; patients with cardiovascular risk factors may require aspirin supplementation |
| Tramadol | Weak opiate agonist; NE and 5-HT reuptake inhibitor | Acute and chronic pain, cancer pain | Seizure risk; potential for serotonin syndrome; abuse potential |

*Note.*   5-HT=5-hydroxytryptamine (serotonin); NE=norepinephrine; NSAIDs=nonsteroidal anti-inflammatory drugs.

## Opioids

Opioids are recommended for the management of moderate to severe acute pain and cancer pain (World Health Organization 1990). Increasingly, opioids are employed for management of moderate to severe nonmalignant pain (Clark 2002; Zenz et al. 1992). As a class, these agents stimulate mu, kappa, and delta opiate receptors, resulting in inhibition of pain transmission in the peripheral and central nervous systems.

Generally, opioids are effective when administered on a scheduled basis rather than "as needed" (Portenoy 1996). However, the need for supplemental opioids should be anticipated to address breakthrough pain emerging between scheduled doses (Portenoy and Hagen 1990). Ideally, opioids should be administered in the least invasive route possible. Transmucosal or transdermal applications may be alternatives for patients who are incapable of swallowing orally administered agents. Adverse effects associated with opioid analgesia need to be addressed in order to facilitate patient comfort (McQuay 1997); common interventions are summarized in Table 34–6.

Fear of addiction is often offered as an explanation of why clinicians are inclined to suboptimally manage pain. Such concerns are moot in the context of pain treatment for patients with terminal conditions. Addiction to opiate analgesics is unlikely in the treatment of acute pain and cancer pain, particularly in those patients without a personal or familial history of substance abuse/dependence or those without premorbid psychopathology (Passik and Weinreb 2000). However, addiction concerns are particularly heightened when long-term treatment of chronic,

**TABLE 34–6.   Management strategies for opioid adverse effects**

| Adverse effect | Strategy |
|---|---|
| Delirium | Antipsychotics (e.g., haloperidol) |
| Dysphoria | Stimulants, antidepressants |
| Gastrointestinal | |
|   Constipation | Stool softeners (e.g., bisacodyl) |
|   Nausea | Antiemetics (e.g., metoclopramide) |
| Hypogonadism | Testosterone |
| Pruritis | Antihistamines (e.g., diphenhydramine) |
| Respiratory depression | Naloxone (acutely); lowered opioid doses; use of alternative agonists–antagonists |
| Sedation | Stimulants (e.g., methylphenidate) |

nonmalignant pain is encountered. Psychiatrists may be enlisted in the care of the patient who is perceived to be medication seeking or to address issues pertaining to opioid abuse and dependence.

The presence of substance dependence is suggested by a desire for acquisition of opioids for something other than pain relief (e.g., its psychological effects). The patient who is addicted to analgesics experiences a loss of control over the use of the agent; compulsively consuming or misusing medication that impedes the patient's adaptive function and role responsibilities undermines interpersonal relationships and interferes with rehabilitation. Aberrant drug use behaviors suggestive of abuse or dependence include multiple calls to clinicians requesting additional medications for "lost" or "stolen" prescriptions; multiple unsanctioned dosage escalations without clinical consultation; acquisition of additional opiates "off the street," from friends and family, or from multiple treating sources unknown to the patient's primary treatment provider; concurrent abuse of illicit substances; and adulteration of use of prescribed medications, such as injecting crushed medications intended solely for oral use (Miotto et al. 1996).

Patients with recent or current opiate addictions can pose particular challenges in the context of pain management (Prater et al. 2002). Due to their tolerance for narcotics, these patients' opioid requirements can be quite high, beyond customary dosages. Use of opiate agonists-antagonists should be avoided in the context of recent opiate abuse, because these can precipitate withdrawal, enhancing distress and discomfort. Use of long-acting preparations such as transdermal fentanyl (Duragesic) or controlled-release oral morphine sulfate (MS Contin), among others, and analgesics with less potential of inducing euphoria (e.g., methadone) may be preferable. Despite morphine's long half-life, its analgesic effects appear to be short-lived; thus, morphine should be administered in multiple divided daily doses on a scheduled basis so as to mitigate pain. Detoxification from opiates should be addressed once pain management is no longer indicated. It may be prudent to implement a treatment contract (Dunbar and Katz 1996) stipulating the patient's and clinician's responsibilities regarding ongoing care.

## Antidepressants

Antidepressants can be useful to address pain associated with neuropathy (e.g., postherpetic, diabetic, and post-stroke pain), headache (e.g., tension, migraine), oral-facial pain, fibromyalgia, and functional gastrointestinal disorders (Ansari 2000; Collins et al. 2000; J.L. Jackson et al. 2000; Magni 1991; Onghena and Van Houdenhove 1992; Rowbotham et al. 2005). The pain-mitigating effects of antidepressants remain a subject of intensive investigation and are thought to involve a number of supraspinal, spinal, and peripheral processes. In addition, when concurrently administered, some antidepressants may augment opiate analgesia (Schreiber et al. 2002).

Much of the data on analgesic efficacy of antidepressants has largely focused on tricyclic antidepressants (TCAs). For example, in a review of randomized controlled trials in which TCAs and anticonvulsants were employed to treat pain associated with diabetic and postherpetic neuropa-

thies, it was found that one-third of patients achieved at least 50% pain relief with either antidepressants or anticonvulsants (Collins et al. 2000; McQuay 2002). However, the side effects of the TCAs (e.g., anticholinergic and α-adrenergic influences) limit their utility in pain treatment. When compared with anticonvulsants, adverse effects were slightly more common with TCAs (Collins et al. 2000; McQuay 2002).

The serotonin and norepinephrine reuptake inhibitors (SNRIs) venlafaxine and duloxetine have demonstrated utility as analgesic agents and bypass several of the untoward effects commonly associated with the TCAs. Both agents have been demonstrated to have pain-mitigating effects in randomized, controlled trials of patients with neuropathy (Goldstein et al. 2005; Rowbotham et al. 2004; Sindrup et al. 2003) and fibromyalgia (Arnold et al. 2004; Zijlstra et al. 2002), with and without comorbid depression. Duloxetine has received U.S. Food and Drug Administration (FDA) approval for treatment of diabetic neuropathy. Simultaneous norepinephrine and serotonin influences are achieved at low dosages with duloxetine; dosages as low as 20 mg/day may be sufficient (Goldstein et al. 2005). The serotonin effects predominate at low dosages for venlafaxine. To achieve pain-mitigating effects, antidepressant-level dosing may be required (Zijlstra et al. 2002). Adverse effects of SNRIs can include nausea, dry mouth, nervousness, constipation, and somnolence.

Generally, SSRIs are not as consistently analgesic as the TCAs or SNRIs (Lynch 2001; Sindrup and Jensen 1999). Use of SSRIs is associated with, and may potentially exacerbate, restless legs syndrome (Ohayon and Roth 2002).

Treatment should be initiated early in the course of illness for optimal results. For example, when amitriptyline is initiated within 3 months of developing the rash of herpes zoster infection, patients are less likely to develop the complications of postherpetic neuralgia (Bowsher 1997). Restriction of and delays in the efficacy of TCAs in producing analgesia would be expected if administered after significant peripheral and central pathophysiological mechanisms have set in. It is best to initiate treatment at low dosages; gradual dosage increases are possible approximately every 3–7 days.

## Anticonvulsants

Anticonvulsant drugs historically have demonstrated efficacy in neuropathic pain, including trigeminal neuralgia and phantom limb pain (McQuay et al. 1995), as well as migraine (Pappagallo 2003; Snow et al. 2002). Carbamazepine is FDA approved for the treatment of trigeminal neu-

**TABLE 34–7.** Anticonvulsant mechanisms of action

| Drug | Decrease in sodium channel activity | Increase in CNS GABA activity | Modulation of $Ca^{2+}$ channels | Reduction of excitatory amino acid activity |
|---|---|---|---|---|
| Carbamazepine | + | | | |
| Phenytoin | + | | | |
| Valproate | + | + | + | |
| Gabapentin | + | + | + (?) | |
| Lamotrigine | + | | + | |
| Oxcarbazepine | + | | | |
| Topiramate | + | + | | + |
| Pregabalin | | + | + | |
| Levetiracetam | | | + | |
| Tiagabine | | + | | |
| Zonisamide | + | | + | |

*Note.* $Ca^{2+}$=calcium; CNS=central nervous system; GABA=γ-aminobutyric acid.
*Source.* Adapted from Leo 2006 and Massie 2000.

ralgia; gabapentin for treatment of postherpetic neuralgia; pregabalin for postherpetic neuralgia, diabetic neuropathy, and fibromyalgia; and divalproex sodium for migraine prophylaxis. Emerging evidence suggests potential analgesic roles of newer anticonvulsant drugs, such as lamotrigine (Lamictal), oxcarbazepine (Trileptal), tiagabine (Gabitril), and topiramate (Topamax) (Galer 1995; Khoromi et al. 2005; Novak et al. 2001; Pappagallo 2003), that offer greater tolerability than some of the older anticonvulsant drugs.

Analgesia produced by anticonvulsant drugs can be quite varied (Table 34–7). Analgesia produced by carbamazepine, lamotrigine, and oxcarbazepine is presumed to be related to inhibition of voltage-gated sodium channels, which slows peripheral nerve conduction of primary afferent fibers and dampens the painful sensory information relayed to the central nervous system (Pappagallo 2003). In addition, some anticonvulsant drugs such as pregabalin and gabapentin may have a role in influencing central proneuropathic pain mechanisms mediated through calcium antagonism and γ-aminobutyric acid (GABA)-ergic mechanisms responsible for inhibiting pain processes within the central nervous system (Guay 2003; Vinik 2005).

Because of the differences in presumed mechanisms of action between anticonvulsant drugs and antidepressants, it is plausible that anticonvulsant drugs would be viable alternatives for patients who have persisting pain despite optimal antidepressant use or those for whom antidepressant use proved intolerable. Alternatively, simultaneous administration of antidepressants and anticonvulsant drugs may be employed, capitalizing on complementary mechanisms of action. When co-administered, lower dosages of either or both agents may be sufficiently analgesic, perhaps making it possible to avoid dosages that produce adverse effects.

Selection of anticonvulsant drugs for pain would require careful consideration of the risks and benefits for any given patient. Anticonvulsant drugs have mood-stabilizing effects and may be ideal for patients with bipolar disorder (Chandramouli 2002). On the other hand, certain medical comorbidities may limit use of selected anticonvulsant drugs. In the event of renal dysfunction, dosages of carbamazepine, oxcarbazepine, gabapentin, pregabalin, and topiramate would need to be reduced, and if the condition is severe enough, use of these agents may be precluded. For patients with hepatic disease, dosages of carbamazepine, oxcarbazepine, and lamotrigine should be reduced.

## Other Psychopharmacological Agents

**Benzodiazepines.** Short-term use of benzodiazepines has been employed to mitigate pain arising from muscle spasm (e.g., fibromyalgia), phantom limb pain, restless legs syndrome, tension headache, trigeminal neuralgia, and neuropathic pain (Bartusch et al. 1996; Bouckoms and Litman 1985; Dellemijn and Fields 1994). However, protracted benzodiazepine use may be counterproductive. In a study of chronic pain patients referred to a tertiary pain center, regression analysis revealed that long-term benzodiazepine use predicted low activity levels, high utilization of ambulatory medical services, and high disability levels (Ciccone et al. 2000). In addition, benzodiazepines acting through GABA receptor systems influence serotonin neurotransmitter release, attenuating opioid analgesia (Nemmani and Mogil 2003). Other concerns related to long-term benzodiazepine use in chronic pain include dependence and the potential for secondary depression (King and Strain 1990). Use of benzodiazepines has to be undertaken cautiously, because these agents can contribute to excess sedation, gait instability, and memory impairments. Buspirone (BuSpar) may be useful to treat comorbid anxiety accompanying pain. However, direct pain-mitigating efficacy for buspirone has not been substantiated (Kishore-Kumar et al. 1989).

**Stimulants.** For purposes of pain management, the use of stimulants has been twofold. Although the mechanism of action remains unclear, stimulants (e.g., dextroamphetamine, methylphenidate) have been employed to augment opioid analgesia (Forrest et al. 1977). Additionally, they are employed to reduce the sedation, dysphoria, and cognitive inefficiency that can accompany opiate use. However, use of stimulants may be limited by intervening adverse effects, including overstimulation (e.g., anxiety, insomnia), appetite suppression, confusion, and even paranoia. Taken in overdose, arrhythmias, seizures, hallucinations (e.g., formication), delirium, and death can occur. Because of concerns of abuse liability, caution is advised in patients with current or preexisting substance use disorders, especially prior stimulant abuse (e.g., cocaine).

**Lithium.** Lithium has been employed in the prophylaxis of chronic cluster headache; the effective dosage is approximately 600–900 mg/day (Ekbom and Hardebo 2002). However, a double-blind, placebo-controlled trial found that lithium was not effective for prophylaxis of episodic cluster headache (Steiner et al. 1997).

### Muscle Relaxants

Generally, antispasmodics are employed for acute pain arising from muscle strain or injury, such as low back pain. Included in this category are true muscle relaxants (dantrolene), $GABA_B$ agonists (baclofen [Lioresal]), $GABA_A$ agonists (diazepam), $\alpha_2$ agonists (tizanidine [Zanaflex]), and centrally acting agents that are thought to suppress polysynaptic reflexes, such as carisoprodol (Soma), cyclobenzaprine (Flexeril), methocarbamol (Robaxin), and orphenadrine (Norflex), among others. Baclofen may be indicated for more chronic pain arising from muscle spasticity, such as after stroke or severe spinal cord injury. The utility of these agents over long-term use is unclear; some have been effectively employed in patients with fibromyalgia (Tofferi et al. 2004). There may be abuse potential associated with carisoprodol and methocarbamol; abrupt discontinuation of these muscle relaxants may precipitate withdrawal, including abdominal cramps, insomnia, nausea, headache, and anxiety.

## Key Points: Pain Disorders

- Pain is a complex perception involving sensory as well as psychological components.

- The diagnostic taxonomy of pain disorder in DSM-IV-TR recognizes that psychological factors can contribute to the experience of pain; however, critics contend that the criteria are insufficiently operationalized to distinguish pain disorder from other psychiatric conditions and that the nosology still retains vestiges of mind–body dualism.

- Common psychiatric comorbidities that accompany chronic pain include depression, anxiety, substance abuse, and sleep disorders. Treatment of comorbidities is required as part of comprehensive pain management.

- A complex array of adjuvant agents with different mechanisms of action can be employed for chronic pain treatment, including antidepressants and anticonvulsants, among other agents.

- Antidepressants have direct pain-mitigating effects apart from influences on mood. Those agents with simultaneous norepinephrine and serotonin effects appear to be most efficacious.

- Psychotherapeutic measures can be useful in the comprehensive management of pain to address comorbid psychiatric conditions and subsyndromal psychological states interfering with rehabilitation as well as to reduce the adversity produced by the pain itself.

- Multidisciplinary treatment approaches can be useful in reducing perceived pain, enhancing rehabilitative measures, reducing disability, and addressing the psychological comorbidities accompanying chronic and enduring pain.

# References

Ansari A: The efficacy of newer antidepressants in the treatment of chronic pain: a review of current literature. Harv Rev Psychiatry 7:257–277, 2000

Arnold LM, Lu Y, Crofford LJ, et al: A double-blind, multicenter trial comparing duloxetine with placebo in the treatment of fibromyalgia patients with or without major depressive disorder. Arthritis Rheum 50:2974–2984, 2004

Arnstein P: The mediation of disability by self efficacy in different samples of chronic pain patients. Disabil Rehabil 22:794–801, 2000

Banks SM, Kerns RD: Explaining high rates of depression in chronic pain: a diathesis-stress framework. Psychol Bull 119:95–110, 1996

Bartusch SL, Sanders BJ, D'Alessio JG, et al: Clonazepam for the treatment of lancinating phantom limb pain. Clin J Pain 12:59–62, 1996

Blier P, Abbott FV: Putative mechanisms of action of antidepressant drugs in affective and anxiety disorders and pain. J Psychiatry Neurosci 26:37–43, 2001

Bouckoms AJ, Litman RE: Clonazepam in the treatment of neuralgic pain syndrome. Psychosomatics 26:933–936, 1985

Bowsher D: The effects of preemptive treatment of postherpetic neuralgia with amitriptyline: a randomized, double-blind, placebo-controlled trial. J Pain Symptom Manage 13:327–331, 1997

Brown RL, Patterson JJ, Rounds LA, et al: Substance abuse among patients with chronic back pain. J Fam Pract 43:152–160, 1996

Capuron L, Gumnick JF, Musselman DL, et al: Neurobehavioral effects of interferon-alpha in cancer patients: phenomenology and paroxetine responsiveness of symptom dimensions. Neuropsychopharmacology 26:643–652, 2002

Chandramouli J: Newer anticonvulsant drugs in neuropathic pain and bipolar disorder. J Pain Palliat Care Pharmacother 16:19–37, 2002

Chochinov HM, Wilson KG, Enns M, et al: Depression, hopelessness, and suicidal ideation in the terminally ill. Psychosomatics 39:366–370, 1998

Ciccone DS, Just N, Bandilla EB, et al: Psychological correlates of opioid use in patients with chronic nonmalignant pain: a preliminary test of the downhill spiral hypothesis. J Pain Symptom Manage 20:180–192, 2000

Clark JD: Chronic pain prevalence and analgesic prescribing in a general medical population. J Pain Symptom Manage 23:131–137, 2002

Cohen H, Neumann L, Haiman Y, et al: Prevalence of post-traumatic stress disorder in fibromyalgia patients: overlapping syndromes or post-traumatic fibromyalgia syndrome? Semin Arthritis Rheum 32:38–50, 2002

Cohen MJM, Menefee LA, Doghramji K, et al: Sleep in chronic pain: problems and treatments. Int Rev Psychiatry 12:115–126, 2000

Collins SL, Moore RA, McQuay HJ, et al: Antidepressants and anticonvulsants for diabetic neuropathy and postherpetic neuralgia: a quantitative systematic review. J Pain Symptom Manage 20:449–458, 2000

Dellemijn PL, Fields HL: Do benzodiazepines have a role in chronic pain management? Pain 57:137–152, 1994

Derakshan N, Eysenck MW: Interpretive biases for one's own behavior and physiology in high-trait-anxious individuals and repressors. J Pers Soc Psychol 73:816–825, 1997

Dersh J, Polatin PB, Gatchel RJ: Chronic pain and psychopathology: research findings and theoretical considerations. Psychosom Med 64:773–786, 2002

Doyle CA, Hunt SP: Substance P receptor (neurokinin-1)-expressing neurons in lamina I of the spinal cord encode for the intensity of noxious stimulation: a c-fos study in rat. Neuroscience 89:17–28, 1999

Dunbar SA, Katz NP: Chronic opioid therapy for nonmalignant pain in patients with a history of substance abuse: report of 20 cases. J Pain Symptom Manage 11:163–171, 1996

Ekbom K, Hardebo JE: Cluster headache: aetiology, diagnosis and management. Drugs 62:61–69, 2002

Fishbain DA: Secondary gain concept: definition, problems and its abuse in medical practice. J Pain 3:264–273, 1994

Fishbain DA: The association of chronic pain and suicide. Semin Clin Neuropsychiatry 4:221–227, 1999

Fishbain DA, Cutler R, Rosomoff H: Comorbid psychiatric disorders in chronic pain patients with psychoactive substance use disorders. Pain Clinic 11:79–87, 1998

Ford CU: Somatizing disorders. Psychosomatics 27:327–337, 1986

Forrest WH, Brown BW, Brown CR, et al: Dextroamphetamine with morphine for the treatment of postoperative pain. N Engl J Med 296:712–715, 1977

Galer BS: Neuropathic pain of peripheral origin: advances in pharmacological treatment. Neurology 45 (suppl):17–25, 1995

Gardner JS, Blough D, Drinkard CR, et al: Tramadol and seizures: a surveillance study in a managed care population. Pharmacotherapy 20:1423–1431, 2000

Goldstein DJ, Lu Y, Detke MJ, et al: Duloxetine vs. placebo in patients with painful diabetic neuropathy. Pain 116:109–118, 2005

Guay DR: Oxcarbazepine, topiramate, zonisamide, and levetiracetam: potential use in neuropathic pain. Am J Geriatr Pharmacother 1:18–37, 2003

Hasenbring M, Hallner D, Klasen B: Psychological mechanisms in the transition from acute to chronic pain: over- or underrated? Schmerz 15:442–447, 2001

Jackson JL, O'Malley PG, Tomkins G, et al: Treatment of functional gastrointestinal disorders with antidepressant medications: a meta-analysis. Am J Med 108:65–72, 2000

Jensen MP, Turner JA, Romano JM: Self-efficacy and outcome expectancies: relationship to chronic pain coping strategies and adjustment. Pain 44:263–269, 1991a

Jensen MP, Turner JA, Romano JM, et al: Coping with chronic pain: a critical review of the literature. Pain 47:249–283, 1991b

Khoromi S, Patsalides A, Parada S, et al: Topiramate in chronic lumbar radicular pain. J Pain 6:829–836, 2005

King SA, Strain JJ: Benzodiazepine use by chronic pain patients. Clin J Pain 6:143–147, 1990

Kishore-Kumar R, Schafer SC, Lawlor BA, et al: Single doses of the serotonin agonists buspirone and *m*-chlorophenylpiperazine do not relieve neuropathic pain. Pain 37:223–227, 1989

Lackner JM, Gurtman MB: Patterns of interpersonal problems in irritable bowel syndrome patients: a circumplex analysis. J Psychosom Res 58:523–532, 2005

Lange-Asschenfeldt C, Weigmann H, Hiemke C, et al: Serotonin syndrome as a result of fluoxetine in a patient with tramadol abuse: plasma level-correlated symptomatology. J Clin Psychopharmacol 22:440–441, 2002

Leo RJ: Treatment considerations in neuropathic pain. Curr Treat Options Neurol 8:389–400, 2006

Leo RJ: Clinical Manual of Pain Management in Psychiatry. Washington, DC, American Psychiatric Publishing, 2007

Leo RJ, Narendran R, DeGuiseppe B: Methadone detoxification of tramadol dependence. J Subst Abuse Treat 19:297–299, 2000

Lucas R, Warner TD, Vojnovic I, et al: Cellular mechanisms of acetaminophen: role of cyclo-oxygenase. FASEB J 19:635–637, 2005

Lynch ME: Antidepressants as analgesics: a review of randomized controlled trials. J Psychiatry Neurosci 26:30–36, 2001

Magni G: The use of antidepressants in the treatment of chronic pain: a review of the current evidence. Drugs 42:730–748, 1991

Mantyh PW: Neurobiology of substance P and the NK1 receptor. J Clin Psychiatry 63 (suppl):6–10, 2002

Massie MJ (ed): Pain: What Psychiatrists Need to Know (Review of Psychiatry Series, Vol 19, No 2; Oldham JM, Riba MB, series eds). Washington, DC, American Psychiatric Press, 2000

McQuay HJ: Opioid use in chronic pain. Acta Anaesthesiol Scand 41:175–183, 1997

McQuay HJ: Neuropathic pain: evidence matters. Eur J Pain 6 (suppl):11–18, 2002

McQuay H, Carroll D, Jadad AR, et al: Anticonvulsant drugs for management of pain: a systematic review. BMJ 311:1047–1052, 1995

McWilliams LA, Cox BJ, Enns MW: Mood and anxiety disorders associated with chronic pain: an examination in a nationally representative sample. Pain 106:127–133, 2003

McWilliams LA, Goodwin RD, Cox BJ: Depression and anxiety associated with three pain conditions: results from a nationally representative sample. Pain 111:77–83, 2004

Miotto K, Compton P, Ling W, et al: Diagnosing addictive disease in chronic pain patients. Psychosomatics 37:223–235, 1996

Moldofsky H: Sleep and pain. Sleep Med Rev 5:387–398, 2001

Nemmani KVS, Mogil JS: Serotonin-GABA interactions in the modulation of mu- and kappa-opioid analgesia. Neuropharmacology 44:304–310, 2003

Novak V, Kanard R, Kissel JT, et al: Treatment of painful sensory neuropathy with tiagabine: a pilot study. Clin Auton Res 11:357–361, 2001

Ohayon MM, Roth T: Prevalence of restless legs syndrome and periodic movement disorder in the general population. J Psychosom Res 53:547–554, 2002

Onghena P, Van Houdenhove B: Antidepressant-induced analgesia in chronic non-malignant pain: a meta-analysis of 39 placebo-controlled studies. Pain 49:205–219, 1992

Orne MT: Mechanisms of hypnotic pain control, in Advances in Pain Research and Therapy, Vol 1. Edited by Bonica JJ, Ale-Fessard D. New York, Raven, 1976, pp 717–726

Pappagallo M: Newer antiepileptic drugs: possible uses in the treatment of neuropathic pain and migraine. Clin Ther 25:2506–2538, 2003

Passik SD, Weinreb HJ: Managing chronic nonmalignant pain: overcoming obstacles to the use of opioids. Adv Ther 17:70–83, 2000

Polatin PB, Kinney RK, Gatchel RJ, et al: Psychiatric illness and chronic low-back pain. The mind and the spine: which goes first? Spine 18:66–71, 1993

Portenoy RK: Opioid therapy for chronic nonmalignant pain: a review of the critical issues. J Pain Symptom Manage 11:203–217, 1996

Portenoy RK, Hagen NA: Breakthrough pain: definition, prevalence and characteristics. Pain 41:273–281, 1990

Prater CD, Zylstra RG, Miller KE: Successful pain management for the recovering addicted patient. Prim Care Companion J Clin Psychiatry 4:125–131, 2002

Rosenstiel AK, Keefe FJ: The use of coping strategies in chronic low back pain patients: relationship to patient characteristics and current adjustment. Pain 17:33–44, 1983

Rowbotham MC, Goli V, Kunz NR, et al: Venlafaxine extended release in the treatment of painful diabetic neuropathy: a double-blind, placebo-controlled study. Pain 110:697–706, 2004

Rowbotham MC, Reisner LA, Davies PS, et al: Treatment response in antidepressant-naive postherpetic neuralgia patients: double-blind, randomized trial. J Pain 6:741–746, 2005

Sanders SH: Operant therapy with pain patients: evidence for its effectiveness, in Seminars in Pain Medicine I. Edited by Lebovits AH. Philadelphia, PA, WB Saunders, 2003, pp 90–98

Santarelli L, Gobbi G, Blier P, et al: Behavioral and physiologic effects of genetic or pharmacological inactivation of the substance P receptor (NK1). J Clin Psychiatry 63 (suppl):11–17, 2002

Schnitzer T: The new analgesic combination tramadol/acetaminophen. Eur J Anaesthesiol 20 (suppl):13–18, 2003

Schreiber S, Bleich A, Pick CG: Venlafaxine and mirtazapine: different mechanisms of antidepressant action, common opioid-mediated anti nociceptive effects: a possible opioid involvement in severe depression? J Mol Neurosci 18:143–149, 2002

Sindrup SH, Jensen TS: Efficacy of pharmacological treatments of neuropathic pain: an update and effect related to mechanism of drug action. Pain 83:389–400, 1999

Sindrup SH, Bach FW, Madsen C, et al: Venlafaxine versus imipramine in painful polyneuropathy: a randomized, controlled trial. Neurology 60:1284–1289, 2003

Snow V, Weiss K, Wall EM, et al: Pharmacological management of acute attacks of migraine and prevention of migraine headache. Ann Intern Med 137:840–849, 2002

Steiner TJ, Hering R, Couturier EG, et al: Double-blind placebo-controlled trial of lithium in episodic cluster headache. Cephalalgia 17:673–675, 1997

Sullivan MJ, Thorn B, Haythornthwaite JA, et al: Theoretical perspectives on the relation between catastrophizing and pain. Clin J Pain 17:52–64, 2001

Swartz KL, Pratt LA, Armenian HK, et al: Mental disorders and the incidence of migraine headaches in a community sample: results from the Baltimore Epidemiologic Catchment Area follow-up study. Arch Gen Psychiatry 57:945–950, 2000

Tofferi JK, Jackson JL, O'Malley PG: Treatment of fibromyalgia with cyclobenzaprine: a meta-analysis. Arthritis Rheum 51:9–13, 2004

Turk DC, Meichenbaum DH, Berman WH: Application of biofeedback for the regulation of pain: a critical review. Psychol Bull 86:1322–1338, 1979

Turner JA, Chapman CR: Psychological interventions for chronic pain: a critical review, I: relaxation training and biofeedback. Pain 12:1–21, 1982a

Turner JA, Chapman CR: Psychological interventions for chronic pain: a critical review, II: operant conditioning, hypnosis, and cognitive-behavioral therapy. Pain 12:23–46, 1982b

van der Kolk BA, Pelcovitz D, Roth S, et al: Dissociation, somatization, and affect dysregulation: the complexity of adaptation to trauma. Am J Psychiatry 153:83–93, 1996

Vinik A: Use of antiepileptic drugs in the treatment of chronic painful diabetic neuropathy. J Clin Endocrinol Metab 90:4936–4945, 2005

Weissman MM, Markowitz JC, Klerman GL: Comprehensive Guide to Interpersonal Psychotherapy. New York, Basic Books, 2000

World Health Organization: Cancer pain relief and palliative care: report of a WHO expert committee. World Health Organ Tech Rep Ser 804:1–75, 1990

Zenz M, Strumpf M, Tryba M: Long-term oral opioid therapy in patients with chronic nonmalignant pain. J Pain Symptom Manage 7:69–77, 1992

Zijlstra TR, Barendregt PJ, van de Laar MAF: Venlafaxine in fibromyalgia: results of a randomized, placebo-controlled, double-blind trial (abstract). Arthritis Rheum 46 (suppl): 105, 2002

Zubieta JK, Ketter TA, Bueller JA, et al: Regulation of human affective responses by anterior cingulate and limbic mu-opioid neurotransmission. Arch Gen Psychiatry 60:1145–1153, 2003

# 35

# Suicide

ROBERT I. SIMON, M.D.

## Suicide Statistics

The suicide rate in the United States for the year 2004 was 11.1 per 100,000. The suicide rate for males was 17.7 per 100,000 and for females 4.6 per 100,000 (American Association of Suicidology 2006). Suicide ranks eleventh as a cause of death. It is the eighth leading cause of death in the United States for all men (National Center for Injury Prevention and Control 2006). Women attempt suicide about three times as often as men (Table 35–1). In 2004, there were 3.7 male suicides for each female suicide and 3 female attempts for each male attempt (American Association of Suicidology 2006). Suicide completions occur on an average of one person every 16.6 minutes. For young persons, on average, one person commits suicide every 2 hours and 11 minutes.

**TABLE 35–1.** Suicide statistics, United States (2004)

| Suicide rates | |
| --- | --- |
| Males | 17.7 per 100,000 |
| Females | 4.6 per 100,000 |
| Total | 11.1 per 100,000 |
| **Gender ratios** | |
| Suicide completions | 3.71 male suicides for each female suicide |
| Suicide attempts | 3 female attempts for each male attempt |

*Source.* American Association of Suicidology 2006.

The most common methods of suicide in 2004 were firearms (51.6%), suffocation/hanging (22.6%), and poisoning (17.9%; American Association of Suicidology 2006). Firearms accounted for 16,750 suicides in 2004. Guns in the home substantially increase the risk of suicide in psychiatric patients, as does the recent purchase of a firearm, especially a handgun purchase for women (Brent 2001; Wintemute et al. 1999).

The suicide rate for individuals with bipolar disorders is estimated at 193 per 100,000 (absolute risk), or 18 times higher (relative risk) compared with the suicide rate for the general population (Baldessarini 2003). Reframing these data, of every 100,000 patients with bipolar disorder, 99,807 will *not* commit suicide. Statistical data are static factors that can be useful in supplementing assessment of suicide risk.

## Suicide Risk Assessment

The suicide risk assessment method in Table 35–2 is only one way of *conceptualizing* risk assessment. It is *not* intended to be used as a suicide risk assessment form or protocol. Obviously, suicidal patients may present only with a few risk factors or risk factors not identified on a form or protocol. No form or protocol can encompass all possible risk factors. Using stand-alone risk assessment forms may lead to robotic assessments, failing to capture the highly individual risk and protective factors presented by every patient at risk for suicide. Invariably, crucial risk factors are omitted.

**TABLE 35–2.    Systematic suicide risk assessment: conceptual model**

| Assessment factors[a] | Risk | Protective |
|---|---|---|
| **Individual** | | |
| Unique clinical features | | |
| **Clinical** | | |
| Current attempt (lethality) | | |
| Panic attacks[b] | | |
| Psychic anxiety[b] | | |
| Loss of pleasure and interest[b] | | |
| Alcohol abuse[b] | | |
| Depressive turmoil (mixed states)[b] | | |
| Diminished concentration[b] | | |
| Global insomnia[b] | | |
| Suicide plan | | |
| Suicidal ideation (command hallucinations)[c] | | |
| Suicide intent[c] | | |
| Hopelessness[c] | | |
| Prior attempts (lethality)[c] | | |
| Therapeutic alliance | | |
| Psychiatric diagnoses  (Axis I and Axis II) | | |
| Symptom severity | | |
| Comorbidity | | |
| Recent discharge from psychiatric hospital | | |
| Drug abuse | | |
| Impulsivity | | |
| Agitation | | |
| Physical illness | | |
| Family history of mental illness (suicide) | | |
| Mental competency | | |
| **Interpersonal relations** | | |
| Work or school | | |
| Family | | |
| Spouse or partner | | |
| Children | | |
| **Situational** | | |
| Living circumstances | | |
| Employment or school status | | |
| Financial status | | |
| Availability of guns | | |
| Managed care setting | | |
| **Statistical** | | |
| Age | | |
| Gender | | |
| Marital status | | |
| Race | | |
| **Overall risk ratings**[d] | | |

[a]Rate risk and protective factors present as low (L), moderate (M), high (H), nonfactor (0), or range (e.g., L–M, M–H).
[b]Risk factors statistically significant within 1 year of assessment.
[c]Associated with suicide 2–10 years following assessment.
[d]Judge overall suicide risk as low, moderate, high, or a range of risk.

## Suicide Risk and Protective Factors

### Risk Factors

Suicide is the result of multifaceted determinants, including diagnostic (psychiatric and medical), psychodynamic, genetic, familial, occupational, environmental, social, cultural, and contextual factors. A single risk factor does not have the statistical power upon which to base a suicide risk assessment. General risk assessment factors have been identified through retrospective community-based psychological autopsies and studies of completed suicides (Fawcett et al. 1993). To be useful, general risk factors must be adapted to the clinical presentation of the individual patient. Evidence-based research finds that high-risk factors associated with attempted suicide in adults include depression, prior suicide attempts, hopelessness, suicidal ideation, alcohol abuse, cocaine abuse, and recent loss of an important relationship (Murphy et al. 1992).

Short-term suicide risk factors derived from a 10-year prospective study of patients with affective disorders were statistically significant within 1 year of assessment (Fawcett et al. 1990). The short-term risk factors were panic attacks, psychic anxiety, loss of pleasure and interest, moderate alcohol abuse, depressive turmoil, diminished concentration, and global insomnia. Short-term risk factors were predominantly severe, anxiety driven, and treatable by a variety of drugs (Fawcett 2001). Acute suicide risk factors are usually treatable or modifiable. For example, treating anxiety or severe insomnia in a depressed patient can rapidly lower suicide risk. Modifying just a few acute risk factors can significantly reduce a patient's risk for suicide (Table 35–3).

**TABLE 35–3.** Examples of modifiable and treatable suicide risk factors

| | |
|---|---|
| Depression | Impulsivity |
| Anxiety | Agitation |
| Panic attacks | Physical illness |
| Psychosis | Difficult situations (e.g., family, work) |
| Sleep disorders | Lethal means (e.g., guns, drugs) |
| Substance abuse | |
| Command hallucinations | |

*Source.* Reprinted from Simon RI: *Assessing and Managing Suicide Risk: Guidelines for Clinically Based Risk Management.* Washington, DC, American Psychiatric Publishing, 2004, p. 26.

**TABLE 35–4.** Suicide risk associated with various mental and physical disorders

| Disorder | Standardized mortality ratio[a] |
|---|---|
| Eating disorders | 23.14 |
| Major depression | 20.35 |
| Sedative abuse | 20.34 |
| Mixed drug abuse | 19.23 |
| Bipolar disorder | 15.05 |
| Opioid abuse | 14.00 |
| Dysthymia | 12.12 |
| Obsessive-compulsive disorder | 11.54 |
| Panic disorder | 10.00 |
| Schizophrenia | 8.45 |
| Personality disorders | 7.08 |
| AIDS | 6.58 |
| Alcohol abuse | 5.86 |
| Epilepsy | 5.11 |
| Child and adolescent psychiatric | 4.73 |
| Cannabis abuse | 3.85 |
| Spinal cord injury | 3.82 |
| Neuroses | 3.72 |
| Brain injury | 3.50 |
| Huntington's chorea | 2.90 |
| Multiple sclerosis | 2.36 |
| Malignant neoplasms | 1.80 |
| Mental retardation | 0.88 |

[a]Standardized mortality ratio is calculated by dividing observed mortality by expected mortality.
*Source.* Adapted from Harris and Barraclough 1997.

Long-term suicide risk factors in patients with major affective disorders were associated with suicides completed 2–10 years after assessment (Fawcett et al. 1990). Long-term risk factors include suicidal ideation, suicidal intent, severe hopelessness, and prior suicide attempts.

Suicide risk associated with various mental disorders and physical diseases is shown in Table 35–4.

Patients with Axis I psychiatric disorders such as schizophrenia, anxiety disorders, major affective disorders, and substance abuse disorders (especially alcohol) often present with acute (state) suicide risk factors. Sareen et al. (2005) demonstrated that a preexisting anxiety disorder is an independent risk factor for the onset of suicidal ideation and attempts. Patients with Axis II disorders often display chronic (trait) suicide risk factors. Exacerbation of a personality disorder or comorbidity with an Axis I disorder (including substance abuse) can transform a chronic suicide risk factor into an acute factor. Suicide risk increases with the total number of risk factors, providing a quasi-quantitative dimension to suicide risk assessment (Murphy et al. 1992).

Patients with personality disorders have a sevenfold increased risk of suicide compared with the general population (Harris and Barraclough 1997). Cluster B personality disorders, especially borderline and antisocial personality disorders, place patients at increased risk for suicide (Duberstein and Conwell 1997). In borderline patients, impulsivity was associated with a high number of suicide attempts, after controlling for substance abuse and a lifetime diagnosis of depressive disorder (Brodsky et al. 1997).

The lifetime suicide rate for schizophrenia is between 9% and 13%. The lifetime rate for suicide attempts is between 20% and 40%. The estimated number of suicides annually in the United States among schizophrenic patients is 3,600, or 12% of total suicides. Suicide is the leading cause of death among persons with schizophrenia who are younger than 35 years (Meltzer 2001). Suicide tends to occur in the early stages of a schizophrenic illness and during acute exacerbations (Meltzer 2001). Suicide remains a risk throughout the individual's life cycle. Palmer et al. (2005), in a reexamination of the psychiatric literature, estimated that 4.9% of schizophrenic patients will complete suicide, usually near the onset of illness.

Prior suicide attempts by any method had the highest standardized mortality ratio (38.36). Suicide risk was highest in the 2 years after the first attempt (Harris and Barraclough 1997). Between 7% and 12% of patients who make suicide attempts complete suicide within 10 years. Thus, a suicide attempt is a significant risk factor for suicide. Most suicides, however, occur in patients with no prior history of attempts (Malone et al. 1995).

Suicidal ideation is an important risk factor. Suicidal *ideation* should be differentiated from suicide intent. *Suicidal ideation* can be passive, fleeting, intermittent, active, and intense, with or without the intent to die. *Suicide intent* is the subjective expectation and desire to die by a self-destructive act. *Lethality* refers to the danger to life posed by a suicide method or act.

In the National Comorbidity Survey, the transition from suicide ideation to suicide plan was 34% and from plan to attempt was 72% (Kessler et al. 1999). The transition from suicide ideation to an unplanned attempt was 26%. Approximately 90% of unplanned and 60% of planned first attempts occurred within 1 year of the onset of suicide ideation. Mann et al. (1999) found that the severity of suicidal ideation is an indicator of risk for attempting suicide. Beck et al. (1990) discovered that when patients were asked about suicidal ideation at its worst point, patients with higher scores were 14 times more likely to complete suicide than patients with lower scores.

The offspring of patients with mood disorders who attempt suicide are at a markedly increased risk for suicide (Brent et al. 2002). Genetic and familial transmission of suicide risk is independent of the transmission of psychiatric illnesses (Brent et al. 1996). Trémeau et al. (2005) found that a family history of suicide was associated with an increased risk for suicide attempt, with lethality of method, with repeated attempts, and with the number of attempts. For suicide to occur, a trigger (stress)—usually a psychiatric disorder and a preexisting vulnerability to suicidal behaviors (diathesis)—must be present.

## Protective Factors

The self-report Reasons for Living Inventory measures beliefs that may act as preventive factors against suicide (Linehan et al. 1983). The preventive factors include survival and coping skills, responsibility to family, child-related concerns, fear of suicide, fear of social disapproval, and moral/religious values. Other protective factors may include availability and community access to effective clinical care for mental, physical, and substance abuse disorders; adherence with recommended treatments; family and community support; life-affirming cultural values that discourage suicide; skills in problem solving and nonviolent conflict resolution; children at home; and pregnancy (Goldsmith et al. 2001). Dervic et al. (2004) found that religious affiliation was associated with less suicide behavior in depressed patients. Severely depressed patients, however, may feel angry and abandoned by God or that "God will understand," increasing their risk of suicide.

The presence of a therapeutic alliance can be an important protective factor against suicide (R.I. Simon 1998). The therapeutic alliance is influenced by a number of factors, especially the nature and severity of the patient's mental disorder. It can change from session to session. It cannot be assumed, therefore, that a therapeutic alliance will remain a protective factor between sessions. Clinicians are shocked and bewildered when a patient with whom they believed they had a sustaining therapeutic alliance attempts or completes suicide between sessions. The absence of a therapeutic alliance with a patient at risk for suicide is a significant risk factor (R.I. Simon 2004).

Patients display distinctive suicide risk and protective factors. Suicide patterns can be identified by obtaining a detailed history of the patient's past suicide crises or attempts. Understanding a patient's psychodynamic responses to past and current life stressors is also important. Identifying a patient's recurrent prodromal symptomatology provides the clinician with insight in treating and managing the patient's current clinical condition.

A suicide attempt, especially if recent, may be a rehearsal for completed suicide. Although a patient may repeat the method of prior attempts, there is no assurance that a subsequent attempt will use the same methods. Isometsa and Lonnqvist (1998) found that 82% of suicide attempters used at least two different methods in subsequent suicide attempts and completions. Sixty-two percent of males and 38% of females died in their first attempt. The risk of suicide is highest during the first year after a suicide attempt.

## Populations at Suicide Risk

### Children and Adolescents

Practice parameters are available for the assessment and treatment of children and adolescents with suicidal behavior (American Academy of Child and Adolescent Psychiatry 2001). Risk factors for adolescents' suicide include prior attempts, affective disorder, substance abuse, living alone, male gender, age 16 years or older, and a history of physical and/or sexual abuse. Adverse childhood experiences such as emotional, physical, and sexual abuse are associated with an increased risk of attempted suicide throughout the life span (Dube et al. 2001). More suicidal women than suicidal men experienced childhood abuse (Kaplan et al. 1995).

### The Elderly

In adults older than 65 years, risk factors for late-life suicide include depression, physical illnesses, functional impairment, personality traits of neuroticism, social isolation, and loss of important relationships (Conwell and Duberstein 2001). The suicide rate for men 85 years and older rises substantially. Forty-one percent of older adults had seen their primary care physician within 28 days of committing suicide (Isometsa et al. 1995).

### Sexual Minorities

Recent studies have consistently found that gay, lesbian, and bisexual youths have a greater risk of suicide attempts than matched heterosexual comparison groups (American Psychiatric Association 2003). In HIV-positive men, suicide rates are only moderately elevated and comparable with other medically ill populations since the advent of antiretroviral treatments (American Psychiatric Association 2000; Marzuk et al. 1997).

Suicide risk may be increased in individuals who experience high stress concerning the experiences of homophobia, harassment, and disclosure of sexual orientation to family and friends and other difficulties associated with gender nonconformity (American Psychiatric Association 2003).

### Jail and Prison Inmates

The suicide rate in jails (rural and city jails and police lockups) is high in comparison with that among prison inmates. In 1986 the suicide rate for jail inmates was 107 per 100,000, or approximately nine times greater than in the general population. In 1999, the suicide rate for prison inmates was 14 per 100,000, compared with 55 per 100,000 among jail inmates. The profile of a jail suicide victim is a young, white, single, first-time nonviolent offender who is intoxicated, has a substance abuse history, is in isolated jail housing, hangs him- or herself with bed clothing, and dies within 24 hours of arrest (Metzner and Hayes 2006).

## Treatment

### Psychotherapies

Evidence-based research has identified psychotherapeutic treatments that reduce the risk of suicide attempts or completions in psychiatric patients. In a randomized controlled trial, cognitive therapy was found effective in preventing suicide attempts for adults who had recently attempted suicide (Brown et al. 2005).

Linehan et al. (2006) demonstrated, in a 2-year randomized controlled trial, that dialectical behavior therapy (DBT) was uniquely effective in reducing suicide attempts. In comparison with therapy by experts for suicidal behaviors and borderline personality disorder, DBT was associated with better outcomes during a 2-year treatment and follow-up period.

Treatment of borderline personality disorder using a randomized, controlled trial of psychodynamically based partial hospitalization demonstrated dramatic reductions in suicide behavior (Bateman and Fonagy 2000, 2004). Ninety-five percent of the sample of 39 borderline patients attempted suicide in the 6 months before the beginning of the study. Only 5.3% made attempts in the 6 months after treatment.

## Somatic Therapies

The risk of suicide attempts in bipolar patients taking lithium is more than eight times lower than among patients not taking the medication. Even with lithium, however, the completed suicide rate among bipolar patients is still 10 times higher than the suicide rate in the general population (Baldessarini 2003). The potential for lethal overdose should guide the quantity of lithium prescribed for a patient at risk for suicide. In some responders, antidepressant medication can have a significant therapeutic benefit within several weeks. Most responders require 8–12 weeks for maximum benefit following the initiation of antidepressant treatment (Gelenberg and Chesen 2000).

Clozapine reduces the suicide attempt and completion rates in schizophrenia and schizoaffective disorder (Meltzer 2001; Meltzer et al. 2003). The U.S. Food and Drug Administration (FDA) has approved clozapine for the treatment of recurrent suicidal behaviors in patients with schizophrenia or schizoaffective disorder.

Suicidal ideation, intent, and plan in selected patients with mood and psychotic disorders are indications for electroconvulsive therapy (ECT), especially when alternative treatments are not appropriate or have not been effective (American Psychiatric Association 2001). ECT should be the treatment of choice when rapid results are needed for the patient at high risk for suicide for whom a delay would be life-threatening. A rapid clinical response with reduction or resolution of suicidal behaviors often occurs with ECT, presumably by treating the underlying psychiatric disorder (Prudic and Sackheim 1999).

Baldessarini et al. (2001) asserted that the extensive use of antidepressant and antimanic treatments has not reduced the long-term rates of suicide or premature mortality from other causes of illness. For example, the suicide rate in the United States between 1901 (11.8 per 100,000) and 2000 (10.6 per 100,000) dropped by only 1.2 per 100,000 despite the availability of antidepressants and other treatments since the 1950s (Silverman 2003). Because 90%–95% of individuals who completed suicide were mentally ill before their deaths, psychiatric interventions have not substantially reduced the suicide rate over 99 years (Barraclough et al. 1974).

In contrast, Isacsson (2000) examined the overall suicide rates in Sweden from 1978 to 1996, determining that suicide rates decreased with increased antidepressant use.

In a 22-year prospective study of patients hospitalized with mood disorders, long-term medication (antidepressants, lithium, and neuroleptics alone or in combination) significantly lowered the suicide rates, despite the fact that more severely ill patients were treated (Angst et al. 2002). G.E. Simon et al. (2006) reviewed the computerized health plan records of 65,103 patients with 82,285 episodes of antidepressant treatment between January 1, 1992, and June 30, 2003. They found that risk of suicide was not "significantly" higher in the months following initiation of antidepressant medications than in later months. The patients' risk of suicide was highest in the month prior to starting medication, declining steadily after they started antidepressant treatment.

In 2004, the FDA began requiring black-box warnings of increased suicide risk for children and adolescents with major depressive disorders and other psychiatric disorders during the first few months of treatment with selective serotonin reuptake inhibitors (SSRIs). In 2005, the FDA issued similar warnings for adults treated with antidepressants.

The FDA has told manufacturers of antidepressants to issue stronger warnings on their labels regarding the monitoring of both pediatric and adult patients for the emergence of suicidal ideation and the worsening of depression. Precursors to worsening depression and suicidal ideation include symptoms of activation syndrome such as anxiety, agitation, panic attacks, insomnia, irritability, hostility, impulsivity, akathisia, hypomania, and mania. Psychiatrists should document the rationale, including risk–benefit assessments, for prescribing an antidepressant drug to a child or adolescent. At a minimum, FDA monitoring requirements should be followed. Hopelessness and suicide may be averted by informing all patients and the parents of children and adolescents that activation symptoms can be a drug reaction, a worsening of the psychiatric disorder, or some combination of both. Close follow-up by the clinician is indicated according to the clinical needs of the patient.

A study by Gibbons et al. (2007) demonstrated an association between decreased SSRI prescriptions for children and adolescents and increased suicide cases in this population in the United States and Finland. SSRIs continue to be considered the first-line treatment for depression with associated suicidal behaviors. While psychiatrists wait for further studies to definitively settle the question, the risks and benefits of SSRIs should be thoroughly explained (with documentation) to patients and their families, according to the current state of scientific knowledge.

# Safety Management

Patients who are determined to commit suicide will find a way (Fawcett et al. 2003). Fawcett et al. (2003), in a review of 76 inpatient suicides, found that 42 of these patients were on 15-minute checks. Nine percent of patients were on one-to-one observation or with a staff member at the time of suicide. Deception and lack of patient cooperation complicate safety assessments.

Gun safety management may be necessary. The psychiatrist usually asks a responsible family member to remove and secure guns and ammunition outside the home. Guns may also be kept by the suicidal patient in his or her car or office or at another location. The psychiatrist must receive a timely call-back from the responsible person confirming that the guns and ammunition have been removed and separately secured according to plan. A call-back is essential.

## Outpatients

In outpatient settings, patient safety is usually managed by clinical intervention such as increasing the frequency of visits, strengthening the therapeutic alliance, providing or adjusting medications, and involving family or other concerned persons in the treatment, if the patient permits. Voluntary or, if necessary, involuntary hospitalization remains an option for suicidal patients at high suicide risk who can no longer be safely treated as outpatients. In the managed care era, most suicidal patients at moderate suicide risk and even some patients at high risk are treated in outpatient settings.

The clinician, after systematic suicide risk assessment, may determine that the suicidal patient requires hospitalization. The risks and benefits of continuing outpatient treatment are weighed against the risks and benefits of hospitalization, and these are shared with the patient. If the patient agrees, arrangements for immediate hospitalization are made. The patient must go *directly* to the hospital, accompanied by a responsible person. The patient should not stop to do errands, get clothing, or make last-minute arrangements.

## Involuntary Hospitalization

If the patient rejects the clinician's recommendation for hospitalization, the matter is immediately addressed as a treatment issue. Because the need for hospitalization is acute, a prolonged inquiry into the patient's reasons for rejecting the recommendation for hospitalization is not feasible. Furthermore, the therapeutic alliance may be strained.

Documenting suicide risk assessment and the rationale for involuntary hospitalization represents good clinical care and provides sound risk management. When involuntary hospitalization is sought on reasonable clinical grounds, it must be left to the courts to resolve uncertainty about commitment.

## Inpatients

With patients at risk for suicide, standard safety precautions must be observed where indicated, such as removal of shoelaces, belts, sharps, glass products, and even pillowcases that can be used for suffocation and other potentially lethal instruments. A thorough search for contraband is standard procedure on admission. Psychiatric units are usually fitted, at a minimum, with non-weight-bearing fixtures and shower curtain rods, very short cords for electrical beds (properly insulated), cordless telephones or telephones with safety cords, jump-proof windows, barricade-proof doors, and closed-circuit video cameras.

The most common and available method of committing suicide by inpatients is strangulation, usually accomplished by a belt, articles of clothing, shoelaces, or a bed sheet hooked up to the patient's bed, door, or bathroom fixtures. Safe installation of plumbing pipes for toilets and use of solid ceilings are necessary to diminish the risk of hanging. The most dangerous place on the psychiatric unit is the patient's room, especially the bathroom. Seclusion rooms should have windows or audiovisual surveillance capability (Lieberman et al. 2004).

## Suicide Prevention Contracts

The suicide prevention contract has achieved wide acceptance, although no studies demonstrate that it is effective in preventing suicide (Stanford et al. 1994). It is frequently used by mental health professionals in outpatient and inpatient settings and in hospital emergency departments. In managed care settings, a criterion for admission to an inpatient unit may be based on a patient's refusal to sign a suicide prevention contract. If the patient is willing to sign a no-harm contract, third-party payers may not authorize admission. Suicide prevention contracts are frequently used in nursing assessments (Egan 1997).

Suicide prevention measures work best when a therapeutic alliance exists between the psychiatrist and patient. The therapeutic alliance is a dynamic, changeable interaction between the clinician and the patient that is influenced by the course of the patient's illness as well as situational and other factors. The status of the therapeutic alliance should be assessed regularly and documented. The presence or absence of a therapeutic alliance can be a key preventive or suicide risk factor.

Mental capacity should be assessed as necessary and documented. The existence and terms of agreement (including time limit) of the suicide prevention contract or plan also require documentation. If suicide prevention contracts are used, mental health personnel should be trained in their appropriate use (Chiles and Strosahl 2005).

## Key Points: Suicide

- Systematic suicide risk assessment informs treatment and management for patients at risk for suicide. It is secondarily a risk management technique.

- Treatable and modifiable acute suicide risk factors should be identified early and treated aggressively.

- Systematic suicide assessment identifies and weights the clinical importance of both risk and preventive factors.

- Suicide risk assessment is a process, not an event. Psychiatric inpatients should have suicide risk assessments conducted at admission and discharge and at other important clinical junctures during treatment.

- Suicide prevention contracts must not take the place of conducting systematic suicide risk assessments.

- Contemporaneous documentation of suicide risk assessments is good clinical care and standard practice.

- Systematic suicide risk assessment performed at the time of discharge informs the patient's postdischarge plan.

- During the treatment of patients at significant risk for suicide, it may be necessary to contact family members or others to facilitate hospitalization, to mobilize support, and to acquire information of clinical importance to the clinician. Whenever possible, this should be done with the patient's permission.

- Suicide risk assessment is the responsibility of the psychiatrist. It should not be delegated to others.

- The treatment and management of the patient at risk for suicide require the clinician's full commitment of time and effort, despite denial of services and cost containment policies of third-party payers.

## References

American Academy of Child and Adolescent Psychiatry: Practice parameter for the assessment and treatment of children and adolescents with suicidal behavior. J Am Acad Child Adolesc Psychiatry 40 (7 suppl):24S–51S, 2001

American Association of Suicidology: Suicide Statistics Archive 1996–2002. Available at: http://www.suicideinfo. ca/csp/90/aspx. Accessed February 5, 2006.

American Psychiatric Association: Practice Guideline for the Treatment of Patients with HIV/AIDS. Washington, DC, American Psychiatric Association, 2000

American Psychiatric Association: The Practice of Electroconvulsive Therapy: Recommendations for Treatment, Training, and Privileging. A Task Force Report of the American Psychiatric Association, 2nd Edition. Edited by Weiner RD. Washington, DC, American Psychiatric Association, 2001

American Psychiatric Association: Practice guidelines for the assessment and treatment of patients with suicidal behaviors. Am J Psychiatry 160 (suppl):1–60, 2003

Angst F, Stassen HH, Clayton PJ, et al: Mortality of patients with mood disorders: follow-up over 34–38 years. J Affect Disord 68:167–181, 2002

Baldessarini RJ: Lithium effects on depression and suicide. J Clin Psychiatry (visuals), January 2003

Baldessarini RJ, Tondo L, Henner J: Treating the suicidal patient with bipolar disorder: reducing suicide risk with lithium. Ann NY Acad Sci 932:24–38, 2001

Barraclough B, Bunch J, Nelson B, et al: A hundred cases of suicide: clinical aspects. Br J Psychiatry 125:355–373, 1974

Bateman AW, Fonagy P: Psychotherapy for Borderline Personality Disorder: Mentalization-Based Treatment. Oxford, England, Oxford University Press, 2000

Bateman AW, Fonagy P: Mentalization-based treatment of BPD. J Personal Disord 18:36–51, 2004

Beck AT, Brown G, Berchick RJ, et al: Relationship between hopelessness and ultimate suicide: a replication with psychiatric outpatients. Am J Psychiatry 147:190–195, 1990

Brent DA: Assessment and treatment of the youthful suicidal patient. Ann NY Acad Sci 932:106–131, 2001

Brent DA, Bridge J, Johnson BA, et al: Suicidal behavior runs in families. Arch Gen Psychiatry 53:1145–1152, 1996

Brent DA, Oquendo M, Birmaher B, et al: Familial pathways to early onset suicide attempt. Arch Gen Psychiatry 59:801–807, 2002

Brodsky BS, Malone KM, Ellis SP, et al: Characteristics of borderline personality disorder associated with suicidal behavior. Am J Psychiatry 154:1715–1719, 1997

Brown GK, Ten Have T, Henriques GR, et al: Cognitive therapy for prevention of suicide attempts. JAMA 294:536–570, 2005

Chiles JA, Strosahl KD: Clinical Manual for Assessment and Treatment of Suicidal Patients. Washington, DC, American Psychiatric Publishing, 2005

Conwell Y, Duberstein PR: Suicide in elders. Ann NY Acad Sci 932:132–150, 2001

Dervic K, Oquendo MA, Grunebaum MF, et al: Religious affiliation and suicide attempt. Am J Psychiatry 161:2303–2308, 2004

Dube SR, Anda RF, Felitti VJ, et al: Childhood abuse, household dysfunction and the risk of attempted suicide throughout the lifespan: findings from the Adverse Childhood Experiences Study. JAMA 286:3089–3096, 2001

Duberstein P, Conwell Y: Personality disorders and completed suicide: a methodological and conceptual review. Clinical Psychology: Science and Practice 4:359–376, 1997

Egan MP: Contracting for safety: a concept analysis. Crisis 18:23, 1997

Fawcett J: Treating impulsivity and anxiety in the suicidal patient. Ann NY Acad Sci 932:94–105, 2001

Fawcett J, Scheftner WA, Fogg L, et al: Time-related predictors of suicide in major affective disorder. Am J Psychiatry 147:1189–1194, 1990

Fawcett J, Clark DC, Busch KA: Assessing and treating the patient at suicide risk. Psychiatr Ann 23:244–255, 1993

Fawcett J, Busch KA, Jacobs DG: Clinical correlates of inpatient suicide. J Clin Psychiatry 64:14–19, 2003

Gelenberg AJ, Chesen CL: How fast are antidepressants? J Clin Psychiatry 61:712–721, 2000

Gibbons RD, Brown CH, Hur K, et al: Early evidence on the effects of regulators' suicidality warnings on SSRI prescriptions and suicide in children and adolescents. Am J Psychiatry 164:1356–1363, 2007

Goldsmith SK, Pellman TC, Kleinman AM, et al (eds): Reducing Suicide: A National Imperative. Washington, DC, National Academies Press, 2001

Harris CE, Barraclough B: Suicide as an outcome for mental disorders. Br J Psychiatry 170:205–228, 1997

Isacsson G: Suicide prevention: a medical breakthrough? Acta Psychiatr Scand 102:113–117, 2000

Isometsa ET, Lonnqvist JK: Suicide attempts preceding completed suicide. Br J Psychiatry 173:531–535, 1998

Isometsa ET, Heikkinen ME, Martunen MJ, et al: The last appointment before suicide: is suicide intent communicated? Am J Psychiatry 152:919–922, 1995

Kaplan M, Asnis GM, Lipschitz DS, et al: Suicidal behavior and abuse in psychiatric outpatients. Compr Psychiatry 36:229–235, 1995

Kessler RC, Borges G, Walters EE: Prevalence of and risk factors for lifetime suicide attempts in the National Comorbidity Survey. Arch Gen Psychiatry 55:617–626, 1999

Lieberman DZ, Resnik HLP, Holder-Perkins V: Environmental risk factors in hospital suicide. Suicide Life Threat Behav 34:448–453, 2004

Linehan MM, Goodstein JL, Nielsen SL, et al: Reasons for staying alive when you are thinking of killing yourself: the Reasons for Living Inventory. J Consult Clin Psychol 51:276–286, 1983

Linehan MM, Comtois KA, Murray AM, et al: Two-year randomized controlled trial and follow-up of dialectical behavior therapy vs therapy by experts for suicidal behaviors and borderline personality disorder. Arch Gen Psychiatry 63:757–766, 2006

Malone KM, Haas GL, Sweeney JA, et al: Major depression and the risk of attempted suicide. J Affect Disord 34:173–185, 1995

Mann JJ, Waternaux C, Haas GL, et al: Toward a clinical model of suicidal behavior in psychiatric patients. Am J Psychiatry 156:181–189, 1999

Marzuk PM, Tardiff K, Leon AC, et al: HIV seroprevalence among suicide victims in New York City, 1991–1993. Am J Psychiatry 154:1720–1725, 1997

Meltzer HY: Treatment of suicidality in schizophrenia. Ann NY Acad Sci 932:44–58, 2001

Meltzer HY, Alphs L, Green AI, et al: Clozapine treatment for suicidality in schizophrenia. Arch Gen Psychiatry 60:82–91, 2003

Metzner JL, Hayes LM: Suicide prevention in jails and prisons, in The American Psychiatric Publishing Textbook of Suicide Assessment and Management. Edited by Simon RI, Hales RE. Washington, DC, American Psychiatric Publishing, 2006, pp 139–156

Murphy GE, Wetzel RD, Robins E, et al: Multiple risk factors predict suicide in alcoholism. Arch Gen Psychiatry 49:459–462, 1992

National Center for Injury Prevention and Control: Suicide fact sheet. Available at: http://www.cdc.gov/ncipc/factsheets/suifacts.htm. Accessed February 5, 2006.

Palmer BA, Pankratz S, Bostwick JM: The lifetime risk of suicide in schizophrenia. Arch Gen Psychiatry 62:247–253, 2005

Prudic J, Sackheim H: Electroconvulsive therapy and suicide risk. J Clin Psychiatry 60 (suppl):104–110, 1999

Sareen J, Cox BJ, Afifi TO, et al: Anxiety disorders and risk for suicidal ideation and suicide attempts: a population-based longitudinal study of adults. Arch Gen Psychiatry 62:1249–1257, 2005

Silverman MM: Understanding suicide in the 21st century. Preventing Suicide: The National Journal 2(2), March/April 2003

Simon GE, Savarino J, Opersklaski B, et al: Suicide risk during antidepressant treatment. Am J Psychiatry 163:41–47, 2006

Simon RI: The suicidal patient, in The Mental Health Practitioner and the Law: A Comprehensive Handbook. Edited by Lifson LE, Simon RI. Cambridge, MA, Harvard University Press, 1998, pp 329–343

Simon RI: Assessing and Managing Suicide Risk: Guidelines for Clinically Based Risk Management. Washington, DC, American Psychiatric Publishing, 2004

Stanford EJ, Goetz RR, Bloom JD: The no harm contract in the emergency assessment of suicidal risk. J Clin Psychiatry 55:344–348, 1994

Trémeau F, Staner L, Duval F, et al: Suicide attempts and family history of suicide in three psychiatric populations. Suicide Life Threat Behav 35:702–713, 2005

Wintemute GJ, Parham CA, Beaumont JJ, et al: Mortality among recent purchasers of handguns. N Engl J Med 341:1583–1589, 1999

# 36

# Assessment of Dangerousness

CHARLES L. SCOTT, M.D.

CAMERON D. QUANBECK, M.D.

PHILLIP J. RESNICK, M.D.

When conducting a violence risk assessment, the clinician should consider dividing the concept of dangerousness into the five components outlined in Table 36–1.

---

**TABLE 36–1.** Components of dangerousness

---

Magnitude of harm

Likelihood harm will take place

Imminence of harm

Frequency of aggressive behavior

Situational factors associated with violence

---

In humans, two primary subtypes of aggression have been described: 1) reactive aggression characterized by an emotionally laden, uncontrolled outburst of aggressive behavior that is impulsive in nature, and 2) planned or predatory aggression that is controlled, purposeful, and premeditated, with little associated emotion (Weinshenker and Siegel 2002). In reactive (impulsive) aggression, the violence is often externally provoked, with subsequent feelings of remorse and confusion. In contrast, premeditated aggressive acts are not usually considered to have a large emotional component but are more "cold blooded" in nature. The aggression is goal oriented and requires a degree of forethought or planning (Stanford et al. 2003). Predatory violence is more dangerous because there is

usually an absence of observable antecedent behaviors that foreshadow the aggression (Meloy 1987). The predator usually has no remorse and is comfortable using violence to retaliate against others, to gain a sense of control, or to obtain a desired goal.

## Risk Factors Associated With Violence

### Demographic Factors and Violence Risk

The clinical assessment of dangerousness requires a review of several risk factors that have been associated with an increased likelihood of future violence. Table 36–2 highlights demographic risk factors associated with violence.

Males in the general population perpetrate violent acts approximately 10 times more often than females (Tardiff and Sweillam 1980). However, among people with mental disorders, men and women do not significantly differ in their base rates of violent behavior.

The MacArthur Violence Risk Assessment Study monitored male and female psychiatric inpatients (ages 18–40 years) released into the community for acts of violence toward others (MacArthur Foundation 2001). During the 1-year follow-up, men were "somewhat more

| TABLE 36–2. | Demographic factors associated with violence |
| --- | --- |

Younger age (Swanson et al. 1990)

Male gender (in non–mentally ill individuals)

Lower socioeconomic status (Borum et al. 1996)

Concentrated poverty in neighborhood (E. Silver et al. 1999)

Lower intelligence and mild mental retardation (Borum et al. 1996; Quinsey and Maguire 1986)

Less education (Borum et al. 1996; Link et al. 1992)

likely" than women to be violent, but the difference was not large. Women were more likely than men to target their aggression toward family members in the home environment. Violent acts by men were more likely to result in an arrest or a need for medical treatment (MacArthur Foundation 2001). Research examining the relationship of gender and violence committed by psychiatric inpatients also concluded that both men and women have similar rates of aggression in this setting. In their study of 155 male and 67 female psychiatric inpatients, Krakowski and Czobor (2004) found that a similar percentage of women and men had an incident of physical assault in the hospital. However, women had a higher frequency of physical assaults during the first 10 days of the study period, and men were more likely to perpetrate assaults that resulted in an injury.

## Past Violence History

The evaluator should determine the answers to the questions described in Table 36–3 when conducting an assessment of past violence.

Criminal and court records are particularly useful in evaluating the person's past history of violence and illegal behavior. For example, the age at first arrest for a serious offense is highly correlated with persistence of criminal offending (Borum et al.1996). Each prior episode of violence increases the risk of a future violent act (Borum et al. 1996).

For those individuals who have served in the military, the clinician should review any history of fights, absences without leave (AWOL), and disciplinary measures (Article XV in the Uniform Code of Military Justice), as well as the type of discharge. An evaluation of the work history should review frequency of job changes and reasons for each termination. Frequent terminations increase the risk for violence. Persons who are laid off from work are six

| TABLE 36–3. | Evaluation of past history of violence |
| --- | --- |

What is the most aggressive act you have ever committed?

What are triggers for your anger and violence?

Have your targets of aggression been people, property, or both?

Who are the victims of your aggression?

What weapons have you used when violent?

Were you under the influence of alcohol or another substance when you were aggressive?

Were you experiencing any type of mental health symptom when violent?

If you were on psychiatric medications, were you taking them when you became violent?

What have been the legal consequences of your violence in the past?

What have been the social consequences of your violence in the past?

How do you feel about the violent acts you have committed?

What factors have helped you control your aggression?

times more likely to be violent than their employed peers (Catalano et al. 1993).

The main difference between assault and homicide is the lethality of the weapon used. Loaded guns have the highest lethality of any weapon. An assault with a gun is five times more likely to result in a fatality than an attack with a knife (Zimring 1991). According to the U.S. Department of Justice, an estimated 40% of U.S households contain a gun and 20% of all gun-owning households keep the gun loaded and unlocked (Cook and Ludwig 1997). Subjects should be asked whether they own or have ever owned a weapon. The recent movement of a weapon, such as transferring a gun from a closet to a nightstand, is particularly ominous in a paranoid person.

### Substance Use and Violence Risk

Drugs and alcohol are strongly associated with violent behavior (MacArthur Foundation 2001). The majority of persons involved in violent crimes are under the influence of alcohol at the time of their aggression (Murdoch et al. 1990). At least half of all violent events, including murders, were preceded by alcohol consumption by the perpetrator of a crime, the victim, or both (see Roth 1994). Stimulants such as cocaine, crack, amphetamines, and phencyclidine (PCP) are of special concern. These drugs typically result in feelings of disinhibition, grandiosity, and paranoia. Among psychiatric patients, a coexisting diagnosis of substance abuse is strongly predictive of violence (MacArthur Foundation 2001). In a study comparing discharged psychiatric patients and nonpatients in the community, substance abuse tripled the rate of violence in nonpatients and increased the rates of violence in discharged patients by up to five times (Steadman et al. 1998).

## Psychosis and Violence Risk

The presence of psychosis is of particular concern when evaluating a person's risk of future violence. In paranoid psychotic patients, violence is often well planned and in line with their false beliefs. The violence is usually directed at a specific person who is perceived as a persecutor. Relatives or friends are often the targets of the paranoid individual. In addition, paranoid persons in the community are more likely to be dangerous because they have greater access to weapons (Krakowski et al. 1986) (see Table 36–4).

---

**TABLE 36–4.** **Factors associated with delusionally driven violence**

Associated negative emotional states (Appelbaum et al. 1999):

- Unhappiness
- Fear
- Anxiety
- Anger

Prior history of acting on delusional beliefs (Monahan et al. 2001)

---

In general, the presence of hallucinations is not related to dangerous acts, but certain types of hallucinations may increase the risk of violence (Zisook et al. 1995). Patients with schizophrenia are more likely to be violent if their hallucinations generate negative emotions (anger, anxiety, sadness) and if the patients have not developed successful strategies to cope with their voices (Cheung et al. 1997a).

Although the majority of individuals with schizophrenia do not behave violently (Walsh et al. 2002), there is emerging evidence that a diagnosis of schizophrenia is associated with an increase in criminal offending. In a retrospective review of 2,861 Australian patients with schizophrenia followed over a 25-year period, Wallace et al. (2004) found that patients with schizophrenia accumulated a greater total number of criminal convictions and were significantly more likely to have been convicted of a crim-

inal offense (including violent offenses) relative to matched comparison subjects. In data from the CATIE (Clinical Antipsychotic Trials of Intervention Effectiveness) project, researchers clinically assessed and interviewed 1,410 schizophrenia patients about violent behavior. Definitions of violence were those used in the MacArthur Community Violence Interview. The 6-month prevalence of any violence was 19.1%, with 3.6% of individuals reporting serious violence. Positive symptoms, including persecutory ideation, increased the risk of both minor and serious violence. By contrast, negative symptoms, such as social withdrawal, actually lowered the risk of serious violence (Swanson et al. 2006).

## Mood Disorders and Violence Risk

Depression may result in violent behavior, particularly in depressed individuals who strike out against others in despair. After committing a violent act, the depressed person may attempt suicide. Depression is the most common diagnosis in murder–suicides (Marzuk et al. 1992). One pattern of murder–suicide involves depressed or psychotic parents (particularly mothers of very young children) who kill their children prior to attempting to take their own lives (Resnick 1969). Murder–suicide in couples is associated with feelings of jealousy and possessiveness (Rosenbaum 1990). In murder–suicides, the homicide is often an extension of the suicidal act. The individual can no longer endure life without what is perceived to be a vital element (i.e., spouse, family, or a job). The perpetrator cannot bear the thought of other persons carrying on without him, so he forces others to join him in death.

Patients with mania show a high percentage of assaultive or threatening behavior, but serious violence itself is rare (Krakowski et al. 1986). Additionally, patients with mania show considerably less criminality of all kinds than patients with schizophrenia. Patients with mania most commonly exhibit violent behavior when they are restrained or have limits set on their behavior (Tardiff and Sweillam 1980). However, active manic symptoms appear to play a substantial role in criminal behavior. In a study of 66 inmates with bipolar disorder, 74% were manic and 59% were psychotic at the time of their arrest (Quanbeck et al. 2004).

## Cognitive Impairment and Violence Risk

After a brain injury, formerly normal individuals may become verbally and physically aggressive (National Institutes of Health 1998). Characteristic features of aggression resulting from a brain injury are outlined in Table 36–5.

**TABLE 36–5.    Characteristics of aggression associated with brain injuries**

Reactive behavior triggered by trivial stimuli

Lack of planning or reflection

Nonpurposeful action with no clear aims or goals

Explosive outbursts without a gradual buildup

Episodic pattern with long periods of relative calm

Feelings of concern and remorse following episode

### *Personality Factors and Violence Risk*

While borderline personality disorder (Tardiff and Sweillam 1980) and sadistic personality traits (Meloy 1992) are associated with increased violence, the personality disorder most commonly associated with violence is antisocial personality disorder (MacArthur Foundation 2001). The violence by individuals with antisocial personality disorder is often motivated by revenge or occurs during a period of heavy drinking. Violence among these persons is frequently cold and calculated and lacks emotionality (Williamson et al. 1987). Low IQ and antisocial personality disorder are a particularly ominous combination for increasing the risk of future violence (Heilbrun 1990). It is important to assess for the presence of antisocial personality disorders in individuals with a major mental illness. Compared with schizophrenic patients without antisocial personality disorder, offenders with both schizophrenia and antisocial personality disorder are less likely to have violence that is prompted by psychotic symptoms. Their violence is more likely to be associated with alcohol use, involve an altercation with the victim prior to violence, and be perpetrated against a victim who is not a family member (Joyal et al. 2004).

Adults may have personality traits that increase their risk for violent behavior but may still not meet the criteria for a personality disorder. Personality traits associated with violence include impulsivity (Borum et al. 1996), low frustration tolerance, inability to tolerate criticism, repetitive antisocial behavior, reckless driving, a sense of entitlement, and superficiality. The violence associated with these personality traits usually has a paroxysmal, episodic quality. When interviewed, these people often have poor insight into their behavior and frequently blame others for their difficulties (Reid and Balis 1987).

The term *psychopath* was described by Cleckey (1976) as an individual who is superficially charming, lacks empathy, lacks close relationships, is impulsive, and is concerned primarily with self-gratification. Hare and col-

leagues developed the Psychopathy Checklist—Revised (PCL-R; Hare 1991) as a validated measure of psychopathy in adults. The concept of psychopathy is important, because the presence of psychopathy is a strong predictor of criminal behavior generally and violence among adults (Salekin et al. 1996).

## Assessment of Current Dangerousness

All threats should be taken seriously and details fully elucidated. Table 36–6 outlines important elements to consider when evaluating a particular threat.

**TABLE 36–6.    Components of threat evaluation**

Obtain detailed information regarding how threat is to be carried out.

Evaluate what other steps (if any) the person has taken to solve the situation prior to initiating threat.

Review whether prior threats have been acted on.

Determine what steps have been taken to enact current threat.

Inquire as to the person's expected personal consequences if threat is enacted.

Review any grudge lists, which may include unidentified potential victims.

Investigate person's violent fantasies.

Assess suicide risk, particularly history of violent suicide attempts.

A sample violence risk management chart is shown in Table 36–7.

## Psychiatric Inpatients and Risk of Violence

### Common Characteristics of Assaultive Inpatients

Past research has consistently shown that a small percentage of patients are responsible for the majority of assaults in institutional settings (Cheung et al. 1997b; Convit et al. 1990). In addition, these patients inflict serious injuries at a rate 10 times higher than that of patients who assault less

**TABLE 36–7.  Sample violence risk management chart**

| Risk factor | Intervention | Status |
|---|---|---|
| Paranoia | Antipsychotic medication | Treated for 7 days; symptoms decreased but are still present. |
| Gun at home | Removal of gun | Brother removed all guns from home, and gun is now under lock and key. |
| Cocaine abuse | Substance use treatment Random urine drug screens | Refusing substance groups. Positive urine for cocaine. |
| Marital conflict | Marital therapy | Two marital sessions completed; jealousy of wife persists. |
| Antipsychotic medication nonadherence history | Antipsychotic intramuscular depot injection | Client agreed to depot medication. |

frequently. Identifying characteristics of this high-risk group provides clinicians an opportunity to focus efforts on reducing overall levels of institutional aggression. In contrast to gender ratios of violence in the general population, mentally ill male psychiatric patients are not more violent than their female counterparts. Factors in the literature that have been associated with psychiatric inpatient aggression are summarized in Table 36–8.

**TABLE 36–8.  Common characteristics of assaultive psychiatric inpatients**

Younger age (Flannery 2002; Rabinowitz and Mark 1999)

Prior history of aggression (Klassen and O'Connor 1988; Soliman and Reza 2001)

Previous violent suicide attempt (Flannery 2002)

Victim of childhood physical abuse and/or other deviant upbringing (Hoptman et al. 1999)

Schizophrenia (Tardiff and Sweillam 1982)

Personality disorder (Tardiff and Sweillam 1982)

Impulse-control disorder (Tardiff and Sweillam 1982)

Mental retardation (Tardiff and Sweillam 1982)

Neurological impairment (Tardiff and Sweillam 1982)

Abnormal electroencephalogram (Convit et al. 1988)

## Categories and Motivations for Violent Inpatient Aggression

In a recent study of inpatient assaults, researchers reviewed more than 1,000 aggressive acts committed by chronically assaultive inpatients at a large California state psychiatric hospital (Quanbeck et al. 2007). The three cat-

egories of violent behavior (impulsive, predatory/planned, and psychotic) were also observed in this study. More than 40% of all assaults were impulsive in nature. Specific triggers, such as a staff member directing the patient to go to his or her room or refusing the patient something he or she wanted, were common precipitants to the impulsive act. Organized or planned assaults were the second most common reason inpatients were aggressive and accounted for over 25% of all assaults. These aggressive acts were frequently motivated by the patient's desire to seek revenge or retaliate against another patient or staff member. Psychotic assaults were the least common type (15%) of all assaults. Psychotic aggression was usually committed by patients acting under the paranoid belief that the victim intended to harm them (e.g., by poisoning), was stealing from them, or was talking about/laughing at them (Quanbeck et al. 2007). Characteristics that distinguish impulsive, organized, and psychotic assaults are detailed in Table 36–9.

## Pharmacological Management of Chronic Aggression

In contrast, the primary objective of the pharmacological treatment of chronic aggression is the prevention of future assaultive acts without adversely affecting other areas of functioning. As of September 2007, no medication had been approved by the U.S. Food and Drug Administration (FDA) for the treatment of chronic aggression. Therefore, physicians who prescribe medications to help manage chronic assaultive behavior should consider utilizing the systematic approach outlined in Table 36–10.

**TABLE 36–9.**    Characteristics of impulsive, organized, and psychotic assaults

| Assault type | Impulsive | Organized | Psychotic |
|---|---|---|---|
| Triggering event | Stressor immediately precedes assault | Delay between triggering event and assault | Psychotic misperception of reality, resulting in sudden and unexpected assault |
| Behaviors preceding assault | Agitated, pacing, clenched jaw, yelling, verbally threatening | Calm, minimal signs of emotional escalation, controlled behavior, "surprise attack" on victim | Isolated, pacing, mumbling, disorganized speech, hallucinating, fearful, anxious |
| Motivation for assault | Impulsive reaction with no long-term motive or secondary gain | Clear motive or self-serving goal (e.g., extortion of goods, retaliation, dominance of others) | Psychotic motivation stemming from fear, paranoia, or misperceived need to act in self-defense |
| Insight regarding assaultive behavior | Remorseful and may recognize reaction was in excess of stressor | Limited insight or superficial expression of remorse and minimization of harm to others | Limited insight due to psychotic symptoms |

**TABLE 36–10.**   Systematic approach to the pharmacological treatment of chronic aggression

Choose medication with empirical evidence of antiaggressive effects.

Document informed consent regarding potential risks and benefits.

Utilize an objective measure to record aggressive acts and monitor treatment outcome.

Change medications one at a time when possible.

Use adequate dosage for appropriate time period.

Have modest expectations for treatment improvement.

Medicatons that are frequently used to treat aggression and which are not approved by the FDA for this purpose are shown in Table 36–11.

## Selective Serotonin Reuptake Inhibitors

Selective serotonin reuptake inhibitors (SSRIs) have shown some benefit in reducing impulsivity and aggression in a variety of patient populations. In a study of 51 "normal" individuals (defined as not meeting criteria for an Axis I disorder), 25 "normals" treated with paroxetine over a 4-week period were less hostile, less irritable, and more socially cooperative compared with 26 "normals" treated with placebo (Knutson et al. 1998). Paroxetine has also been shown to decrease the number of aggressive and impulsive responses in a sample of adult males with antiso-

cial personality characteristics playing a computer game (Cherek et al. 2002). Other SSRIs have been shown to decrease measures of aggression in persistently assaultive inpatients with schizophrenia (Vartiainen et al. 1995), a sample of personality disorder patients (Coccaro and Kavoussi 1997), and patients with dementia and brain injury (Kim et al. 2001). The antiaggressive properties of the SSRIs may be mediated by their ability to stabilize mood, reduce negative affects (Knutson et al. 1998), and improve impulse control (Hollander and Rosen 2000).

## Anticonvulsants

Anticonvulsant medications have demonstrated efficacy in decreasing aggressive behavior in individuals with a wide variety of psychiatric symptoms and diagnoses. In a study of prisoners exhibiting impulsive aggression, phenytoin reduced the frequency and intensity of violence among the impulsive group but had no effect on violence committed by prisoners whose aggression was premeditated. Carbamazepine has shown some efficacy in reducing the severity of "rage attacks" in a sample of patients with a variety of diagnoses including antisocial and borderline personality disorders, substance use disorders, attention-deficit disorder, intermittent explosive disorder (Mattes 1984), and aggressive behavior subsequent to traumatic brain injury (Azouvi et al. 1999). Oxcarbazepine had a significant benefit in the treatment of outpatients with clinically significant impulsive aggression (Mattes 2005).

**TABLE 36–11.** Off-label pharmacotherapy interventions for aggression

| Medication class | Target symptoms |
| --- | --- |
| Selective serotonin reuptake inhibitors | Irritability, impulsivity, negative affect–triggered aggression |
| Anticonvulsants | Paroxysmal rage attacks, impulse-control disorders, aggression triggered by poor information processing or head injury |
| Lithium | Aggression triggered by negative affect or head injury, impulsivity, violence associated with mental retardation |
| Antipsychotics | Hostility associated with psychosis, potential use in aggression associated with borderline personality disorder |
| β-Adrenergic blockers | Aggression associated with schizophrenia, akathisia, or head injury |

Impulsive-aggressive behaviors account for a substantial portion of the morbidity and mortality associated with borderline personality disorder (Goodman and New 2000). Several well-designed placebo-controlled studies indicate that anticonvulsants may play a role in treating assaultive behavior by decreasing irritability, anger, and aggression (Frankenburg and Zanarini 2002; Hollander et al. 2001; Nickel et al. 2004, 2005; Tritt et al. 2005). Anticonvulsants are sometimes used as an adjunctive treatment for patients with schizophrenia. Valproic acid is the only mood stabilizer considered to be a first-line augmenting agent for patients with schizophrenia who are persistently aggressive (Volavka 2002).

## Lithium

In a classic study examining the efficacy of lithium in decreasing violence, inmates convicted of a violent offense and engaging in impulsively aggressive acts while in prison were randomly assigned to placebo or Eskalith CR (a slow-release form of lithium) (Sheard et al. 1976). The lithium-treated inmates had a significant decrease in the number of major violent infractions. Lithium has also demonstrated efficacy in open and controlled trials in reducing aggressive behavior in those with mental retardation and brain injury (Volavka 2002). In the above studies,

lithium levels were maintained in a range lower than typically used to treat mania (0.5–1.0 mEq/L). Because this relatively low lithium level is not commonly associated with sedation and impaired cognition, the decrease in aggressive behaviors may be due to specific antiaggressive properties of lithium rather than decreased violence due to sedation.

## Antipsychotics

Clozapine has demonstrated efficacy superior to that of atypical antipsychotics (risperidone and olanzapine) and haloperidol in reducing hostility (Citrome et al. 2001) and reducing the number and severity of aggressive incidents (Volavka et al. 2004) in treatment-resistant patients diagnosed with chronic schizophrenia or schizoaffective disorder. In these studies, the antiaggressive effect of clozapine was independent from measures of sedation and positive psychotic symptoms. Risperidone (Aleman and Kahn 2001) and quetiapine (Volavka 2002) are superior to typical antipsychotics (haloperidol) in reducing hostility in patients with schizophrenia. In one study, atypical antipsychotics (clozapine, risperidone, olanzapine) significantly reduced the risk of violent behavior in persons with schizophrenia in community-based treatment, whereas treatment with conventional neuroleptics did not have the same beneficial effect (Swanson et al. 2004). This positive effect was primarily attributable to fewer adverse side effects and increased medication adherence. The propensity of typical neuroleptics (particularly at high doses) to cause akathisia has been linked to irritability and increased violence (Volavka 2002) and therefore may have the effect of increasing rather than decreasing assaultive behaviors.

Atypical antipsychotics may also have a role in the treatment of aggression in borderline personality disorder. Risperidone significantly reduced self-rated aggression in an open trial of patients with borderline personality disorder and a history of aggression (Rocca et al. 2002). A randomized controlled trial of female patients with borderline personality disorder treated with olanzapine over a 6-month period found a significant improvement on many core symptoms including aggression and hostility (Zanarini and Frankenburg 2001). In both of these studies, the mean dose was lower than would be used in the treatment of schizophrenia (e.g., risperidone 3 mg, olanzapine 5 mg). In a chart review study, the effects of clozapine were examined in a diagnostically heterogeneous group of persistently violent patients (including patients whose primary diagnosis was a personality disorder). Clozapine treatment resulted in marked decreases in violent episodes and the use of seclusion and restraint.

## Beta-Adrenergic Blockers

There is evidence that the adjunctive use of propranolol (J.M. Silver et al. 1999) and nadolol (Ratey et al. 1992) decreases aggressive behavior in schizophrenia. This finding suggests that β-adrenergic blockers may mediate antiaggressive effects by treating the motor symptoms of akathisia (Lipinski et al. 1988). Propranolol has demonstrated efficacy in reducing organically driven aggression (e.g., head injury) but at variable and often high dosages (from 30 to 1,600 mg/day). In addition, the effect may require an extended trial lasting up to 2 months (Greendyke and Kanter 1986; Greendyke et al. 1986; Yudofsky et al. 1981). Subsequently, it is unclear if nonspecific sedation mediates the antiaggressive effects of β-blockers. Further, the use of propranolol requires careful monitoring of blood pressure and heart rate during titration and is contraindicated in certain medical conditions (e.g., asthma, heart failure, bradycardia).

Pindolol, a β-adrenergic blocker with partial agonist effect, has fewer cardiovascular side effects. Studies indicate that pindolol reduced assaultiveness and hostility in patients with dementia without causing lethargy (Greendyke and Kanter 1986) and significantly reduced the number and severity of aggressive incidents in patients with schizophrenia who had been repetitively assaultive (Caspi et al. 2001).

## Benzodiazepines

Chlordiazepoxide and diazepam appeared to exert a general calming effect on state hospital inpatients with a variety of psychiatric diagnoses. A subsequent small randomized controlled trial investigating the use of clonazepam as an augmenting agent in schizophrenia found no benefit. Surprisingly, several patients became aggressive who had no history of aggression in the past (Karson et al. 1982). A number of case reports have appeared in the literature where patients treated with benzodiazepines developed paradoxical "rage reactions" (French 1989; Gutierrez et al. 2000; Mathew et al. 2000). In a randomized clinical trial examining the effects of benzodiazepines on aggressive behavior, researchers compared the willingness of men treated with benzodiazepines or placebo to shock an imaginary opponent in a reaction-time test (Weisman et al. 1998). Surprisingly, subjects treated with benzodiazepines delivered more severe shocks than did subjects on placebo, particularly diazepam-treated subjects. The effect of benzodiazepines on aggression is complex and difficult to predict. Because there is no substantial evidence that the long-term use of benzodiazepines reduces the risk of violence, their use should probably be reserved for the management of acute aggression and agitation.

# Psychotherapeutic Approaches to Treating Chronic Aggression

## Behavioral Interventions

In chronic institutionalized psychiatric patients, social learning programs have been effective in decreasing aggression, the need for seclusion and restraint, and time to discharge (Goodness and Renfro 2002). These programs are based on social learning theory, which holds that social behaviors are learned and acquired over time through two mechanisms: 1) experiencing success or failure as the result of one's own actions, and 2) observing the positive and negative consequences of others' behaviors (Bandura 1977).

The goal of behavioral intervention is to restructure the consequences of a patient's actions so that the link between aggressive behavior and its reinforcers is weakened while the link between alternate prosocial behaviors is reinforced. The token economy is one type of behavioral management approach used to foster the development of prosocial behavior. In this system, a patient's socially appropriate behavior is positively reinforced by earning tokens or points that can be exchanged for rewards (e.g., privileges, games, TV time, snacks). A token can be earned by attending groups, taking medications, and refraining from or reducing aggressive behavior for a specified period of time. Maladaptive aggressive behavior results in a loss of tokens or privileges, or "time-outs" in which a patient is temporarily placed into a calmer environment. This type of program requires a careful assessment of behaviors targeted for change, clearly defined objectives for the patient, and consistent positive reinforcement by staff.

Social skills training is often used in conjunction with a behavioral program to accelerate progress by teaching patients new behaviors to replace dysfunctional interactions. Patients learn assertiveness and self-control skills in individual or group settings. Important elements of social skills training are summarized in Table 36–12.

**TABLE 36–12.  Essential components of social skills training**

Focused education on the specific behavior desired

Modeling of how to perform expected behavior

Rehearsal and role-playing of expected behavior

Positive reinforcement of desired behaviors and corrective actions for inappropriate behaviors

Practicing of skills in real-life situations

## Cognitive-Behavioral Approaches

Treatments of aggression involving cognitive-behavioral techniques have been predominantly based on anger management techniques (Alpert and Spillmann 1997). Novaco's cognitive-behavioral model of anger proposes that anger and aggression are mediated by an individual's perception of threat from others. The treatment assists the person in formulating strategies to managing conflict in a nonaggressive manner (Novaco 1997). This technique has shown efficacy in violent forensic patients (Holbrook 1997; Serin and Kuriychuk 1994) and in those with mild borderline intellectual functioning (Lindsay et al. 2003). A potentially beneficial cognitive-behavioral approach to aggression in those with borderline personality disorder has recently been identified. Male forensic patients with borderline personality disorder who participated in a dialectical behavior therapy program modified to target violence and anger had significant reductions in the seriousness of violence-related incidents and in self-report measures of hostility and anger (Evershed et al. 2003).

Key components of successful anger management treatment are described in Table 36–13.

**TABLE 36–13.  Key components of anger management skills training**

Imagining angry scenarios, then using relaxation techniques

Identifying and challenging cognitive distortions

Identifying personal warning signs of anger

Recognizing potentially provocative situations

Implementing nonaggressive responses to provocative situations

Building a repertoire of behavioral skills for managing conflict

# Key Points: Assessment of Dangerousness

- The best predictor of future violent behavior is a past history of violent behavior.
- Mental disorders, particularly paranoia and suspiciousness, increase the risk of violence.
- Substance use represents a major risk factor for future violent behavior.
- Actuarial risk assessment instruments can assist the evaluator in more accurately predicting future violence.
- Inpatient violence includes impulsive, planned, and psychotic assaults.
- Treatment interventions should match type of assaultive behavior.

# References

Aleman A, Kahn RS: Effects of the atypical antipsychotic risperidone on hostility and aggression in schizophrenia: a meta-analysis of controlled trials. Eur Neuropsychopharmacol 11:289–293, 2001

Alpert JE, Spillmann MK: Psychotherapeutic approaches to aggressive and violent patients. Psychiatr Clin North Am 20:453–472, 1997

Appelbaum PS, Robbins PC, Roth LH: Dimensional approach to delusions: comparison across types and diagnosis. Am J Psychiatry 156:1938–1943, 1999

Azouvi P, Jokic C, Attal N, et al: Carbamazepine in agitation and aggressive behavior following severe closed-head injury: results of an open trial. Brain Inj 13:797–804, 1999

Bandura A: Social Learning Theory. Englewood Cliffs, NJ, Prentice Hall, 1977

Borum R, Swartz M, Swanson J: Assessing and managing violence risk in clinical practice. Journal of Practical Psychiatry and Behavioral Health 4:204–215, 1996

Caspi N, Modai I, Barak P, et al: Pindolol augmentation in aggressive schizophrenic patients: a double-blind crossover study. Int Clin Psychopharmacol 16:111–115, 2001

Catalano R, Dooley D, Navaco RW, et al: Using ECA survey data to examine the effect of job layoffs on violent behavior. Hosp Community Psychiatry 44:874–879, 1993

Cherek DR, Lane SD, Pietras CJ, et al: Effects of chronic paroxetine administration on measures of aggressive and impulsive responses of adult males with a history of conduct
disorder. Psychopharmacology (Berl) 159:266–274, 2002

Cheung P, Schweitzer I, Crowley K, et al: Violence in schizophrenia: role of hallucinations and delusions. Schizophr
Res 26:181–190, 1997a

Cheung P, Schweitzer I, Tuckwell V, et al: A prospective study
of assaults on staff by psychiatric inpatients. Med Sci Law
37:46–52, 1997b

Citrome L, Volavka J, Czobor P, et al: Effects of clozapine, olanzapine, risperidone, and haloperidol on hostility in patients
with schizophrenia. Psychiatr Serv 52:1510–1514, 2001

Cleckley HM: The Mask of Sanity. St. Louis, MO, Mosby, 1976

Coccaro EF, Kavoussi RJ: Fluoxetine and impulsive aggressive
behavior in personality-disordered subjects. Arch Gen Psychiatry 54:1081–1088, 1997

Convit A, Jaeger J, Lin SP, et al: Predicting assaultiveness in psychiatric inpatients: a pilot study. Hosp Community Psychiatry 39:429–434, 1988

Convit A, Isay D, Otis D, et al: Characteristics of repeatedly assaultive psychiatric inpatients. Hosp Community Psychiatry 41:1112–1115, 1990

Cook PJ, Ludwig J: Guns in America: National Survey on Private Ownership and Use of Firearms. May 1997. Available
at: www.ncjrs.org/txtfiles/165476.txt. Accessed June 2005.

Evershed S, Tennant A, Boomer D, et al: Practice-based outcomes of dialectical behavior therapy (DBT) targeting anger and violence, with male forensic patients: a pragmatic
and non-contemporaneous comparison. Crim Behav Ment
Health 13:198–213, 2003

Flannery RB Jr: Repetitively assaultive psychiatric patients: review of published findings, 1978–2001. Psychiatr Q 73:229–
237, 2002

Frankenburg FR, Zanarini MC: Divalproex sodium treatment
of women with borderline personality disorder and bipolar
II disorder: a double-blind placebo-controlled pilot study.
J Clin Psychiatry 63:442–446, 2002

French AP: Dangerously aggressive behavior as a side effect of
alprazolam. Am J Psychiatry 146:276, 1989

Goodman M, New A: Impulsive aggression in borderline personality disorder. Curr Psychiatry Rep 2:56–61, 2000

Goodness KR, Renfro NS: Changing a culture: a brief program analysis of a social learning program on a maximum-
security forensic unit. Behav Sci Law 20:495–506, 2002

Greendyke RM, Kanter DR: Therapeutic effects of pindolol on
behavioral disturbances associated with organic brain disease:
a double-blind study. J Clin Psychiatry 47:423–426, 1986

Greendyke RM, Kanter DR, Schuster DB, et al: Propranolol
treatment of assaultive patients with organic brain disease:
a double-blind crossover, placebo-controlled study. J Nerv
Ment Dis 174:290–294, 1986

Gutierrez MA, Roper JM, Hahn P: Paradoxical reactions to
benzodiazepines. Am J Nurs 101:34–39, 2000

Hare RD: The Hare Psychopathy Checklist—Revised. Toron-
to, ON, Canada, Multi-Health Systems, 1991

Heilbrun AB Jr: The measurement of criminal dangerousness as
a personality construct: further validation of a research index. J Pers Assess 54:141–148, 1990

Holbrook MI: Anger management training in prison inmates.
Psychol Rep 81:623–626, 1997

Hollander E, Rosen J: Impulsivity. J Psychopharmacol 14:S39–
S44, 2000

Hollander E, Allen A, Lopez RP, et al: A preliminary double-
blind, placebo-controlled trial of divalproex sodium in borderline personality disorder. J Clin Psychiatry 62:199–203,
2001

Hoptman MJ, Yates KF, Patalinjug MB, et al: Clinical prediction of assaultive behavior among male psychiatric patients
at a maximum-security forensic facility. Psychiatr Serv
50:1461–1466, 1999

Joyal CC, Putkonen A, Paavola P, et al: Characteristics and circumstances of homicidal acts committed by offenders with
schizophrenia. Psychol Med 34:433–442, 2004

Karson CN, Weinberger DR, Bigelow L, et al: Clonazepam
treatment of chronic schizophrenia: negative results in a
double-blind, placebo-controlled trial. Am J Psychiatry
139:1627–1628, 1982

Kim KY, Moles JK, Hawley JM: Selective serotonin reuptake inhibitors for aggressive behavior in patients with dementia
after head injury. Pharmacotherapy 21:498–501, 2001

Klassen D, O'Connor WA: A prospective study of predictors of
violence in adult male mental health admission. Law Hum
Behav 12:143–158, 1988

Knutson B, Wolkowitz OM, Cole SW, et al: Selective alteration
of personality and social behavior by serotonergic intervention. Am J Psychiatry 155:373–379, 1998

Krakowski M, Czobor P: Gender differences in violent behaviors: relationship to clinical symptoms and psychosocial
factors. Am J Psychiatry 161:459–465, 2004

Krakowski M, Volavka J, Brizer D: Psychopathology and violence: a review of literature. Compr Psychiatry 27:131–148,
1986

Lindsay WR, Allan R, MacLeod F, et al: Long-term treatment
and management of violent tendencies of men with intellectual disabilities convicted of assault. Ment Retard 41:47–
56, 2003

Link BG, Andrews H, Cullen FT: The violent and illegal behavior of mental patients reconsidered. Am Sociol Rev 57:275–
292, 1992

Lipinski JF Jr, Keck PE Jr, McElroy SL: Beta-adrenergic antagonists in psychosis: is improvement due to treatment of
neuroleptic-induced akathisia? J Clin Psychopharmacol
8:409–416, 1988

MacArthur Foundation: The MacArthur Violence Risk Assessment Study Executive Summary. 2001. Available at: http://
macarthur.virginia.edu/risk.html. Accessed August 11,
2002.

Marzuk PM, Tardiff K, Hirsch CS: The epidemiology of murder-suicide. JAMA 267:3179–3183, 1992

Mathew VM, Dursun SM, Reveley MA: Increased aggressive, violent, and impulsive behavior in patients during chronic-prolonged benzodiazepine use. Can J Psychiatry 45:89–90, 2000

Mattes JA: Carbamazepine for uncontrolled rage outbursts. Lancet 2(8415):1164–1165, 1984

Mattes JA: Oxcarbazepine in patients with impulsive aggression: a double-blind, placebo-controlled trial. J Clin Psychopharmacol 25:575–579, 2005

Meloy JR: The prediction of violence in outpatient psychotherapy. Am J Psychother 41:38–45, 1987

Meloy JR: Violent Attachments. Northvale, NJ, Jason Aronson, 1992

Monahan J, Steadman HJ, Silver E, et al: Rethinking Risk Assessment: The MacArthur Study of Mental Disorder and Violence. New York, Oxford University Press, 2001

Murdoch D, Pihl RO, Ross D: Alcohol and crimes of violence: present issues. Int J Addict 25:1065–1081, 1990

National Institutes of Health: Rehabilitation of Persons with Traumatic Brain Injury, National Institutes of Health Consensus Development Conference Statement. October 26–28, 1998. Available at: http://consensus.nih.gov/1998/1998TraumaticBrainInjury109html.htm. Accessed May 31, 2006.

Nickel MK, Nickel C, Mitterlehner FO, et al: Topiramate treatment of aggression in female borderline personality disorder patients: a double-blind, placebo-controlled study. J Clin Psychiatry 65:1515–1519, 2004

Nickel MK, Nickel C, Kaplan P, et al: Treatment of aggression with topiramate in male borderline patients: a double-blind, placebo-controlled study. Biol Psychiatry 57:495–499, 2005

Novaco R: Remediating anger and aggression with violent offenders. Legal and Criminological Psychology 2:77–88, 1997

Quanbeck CD, Stone DC, Scott CL, et al: Clinical and legal correlates of inmates with bipolar disorder at time of criminal arrest. J Clin Psychiatry 65:198–203, 2004

Quanbeck CD, McDermott BE, Lam J, et al: Categorization of aggressive acts committed by chronically assaultive state hospital patients. Psychiatr Serv 58:521–528, 2007

Quinsey VL, Maguire A: Maximum security psychiatric patients: actuarial and clinical prediction of dangerousness. J Interpers Violence 1:143–171, 1986

Rabinowitz J, Mark M: Risk factors for violence among long-stay psychiatric patients: national study. Acta Psychiatr Scand 99:341–347, 1999

Ratey JJ, Sorgi P, O'Driscoll GA, et al: Nadolol to treat aggression and psychiatric symptomatology in chronic psychiatric inpatients: a double-blind, placebo-controlled study. J Clin Psychiatry 53:41–46, 1992

Reid WH, Balis GU: Evaluation of the violent patient, in Psychiatry Update: The American Psychiatric Association Annual Review, Vol 6. Edited by Hales RE, Frances AJ. Washington, DC, American Psychiatric Press, 1987, pp 491–509

Resnick PJ: Child murder by parents: a psychiatric review of filicide. Am J Psychiatry 126:325–334, 1969

Rocca P, Marchiaro L, Cocuzza E, et al: Treatment of borderline personality disorder with risperidone. J Clin Psychiatry 63:241–244, 2002

Rosenbaum M: The role of depression in couples involved in murder–suicide and homicide. Am J Psychiatry 147:1036–1039, 1990

Roth JA: Psychoactive substances and violence (publication NCJ 145534). U.S. Department of Justice, National Institute of Justice, 1994. Available at: http://www.ncjrs.gov/txtfiles/psycho.txt. Accessed June 1, 2006.

Salekin RT, Rogers R, Sewell KW: A review of meta-analysis of the Psychopathy Checklist and Psychopathy Checklist—Revised: predictive validity of dangerousness. Clinical Psychology: Science and Practice 3:203–213, 1996

Serin RC, Kuriychuk M: Social and cognitive processing deficits in violent offenders: implications for treatment. Int J Law Psychiatry 17:431–441, 1994

Sheard MH, Marini JL, Bridges CI, et al: The effect of lithium on impulsive aggressive behavior in man. Am J Psychiatry 133:1409–1413, 1976

Silver E, Mulvey EP, Monahan J: Assessing violence risk among discharged psychiatric patients: toward an ecological approach. Law Hum Behav 2:237–255, 1999

Silver JM, Yudofsky SC, Slater JA, et al: Propranolol treatment of chronically hospitalized aggressive patients. J Neuropsychiatry Clin Neurosci 11:328–335, 1999

Soliman AE, Reza H: Risk factors and correlates of violence among acutely ill adult psychiatric inpatients. Psychiatr Serv 52:75–80, 2001

Stanford MS, Houston R, Villemarette-Pittman N, et al: Premeditated aggression: clinical assessment and cognitive psychophysiology. Pers Individ Diff 34:773–781, 2003

Steadman HJ, Mulvey EP, Monahan J, et al: Violence by people discharged from acute psychiatric inpatient facilities and by others in the same neighborhoods. Arch Gen Psychiatry 55:393–401, 1998

Swanson JW, Holzer CE 3rd, Ganju VK, et al: Violence and psychiatric disorder in the community: evidence from the Epidemiologic Catchment Area surveys. Hosp Community Psychiatry 41:761–770, 1990

Swanson JW, Swartz MS, Elbogen EB: Effectiveness of atypical antipsychotic medications in reducing violent behavior among persons with schizophrenia in community-based treatment. Schizophr Bull 30:3–20, 2004

Swanson JW, Swartz MS, Van Dorn RA, et al: A national study of violent behavior in persons with schizophrenia. Arch Gen Psychiatry 63:490–499, 2006

Tardiff K, Sweillam A: Assault, suicide, and mental illness. Arch Gen Psychiatry 37:164–169, 1980

Tardiff K, Sweillam A: Assaultive behavior among chronic inpatients. Am J Psychiatry 139:212–215, 1982

Tritt K, Nickel C, Lahmann C, et al: Lamotrigine treatment of aggression in female borderline patients: a randomized, double-blind, placebo-controlled study. J Psychopharmacol 19:287–291, 2005

Vartiainen H, Tiihonen J, Putkonen A, et al: Citalopram, a selective serotonin reuptake inhibitor, in the treatment of aggression in schizophrenia. Acta Psychiatr Scand 91:348–351, 1995

Volavka J: Neurobiology of Violence. Washington, DC, American Psychiatric Publishing, 2002

Volavka J, Czobor P, Nolan K, et al: Overt aggression and psychotic symptoms in patients with schizophrenia treated with clozapine, olanzapine, risperidone, or haloperidol. J Clin Psychopharmacol 24:225–228, 2004

Wallace C, Mullen PE, Burgess P: Criminal offending in schizophrenia over a 25-year period marked by deinstitutionalization and increasing prevalence of comorbid substance use disorders. Am J Psychiatry 161:716–727, 2004

Walsh E, Buchanan A, Fahy T: Violence and schizophrenia: examining the evidence. Br J Psychiatry 180:490–495, 2002

Weinshenker N, Siegel A: Bimodal classification of aggression: affective defense and predatory attack. Aggression and Violent Behavior 7:237–250, 2002

Weisman AM, Berman ME, Taylor SP: Effects of clorazepate, diazepam, and oxazepam on a laboratory measurement of aggression in men. Int Clin Psychopharmacol 13:183–188, 1998

Williamson S, Hare R, Wong S: Violence: criminal psychopaths and their victims. Canadian Journal of Behavioral Sciences 19:454–462, 1987

Yudofsky S, Williams D, Gorman J: Propranolol in the treatment of rage and violent behavior in patients with chronic brain syndromes. Am J Psychiatry 138:218–220, 1981

Zanarini MC, Frankenburg FR: Olanzapine treatment of female borderline personality disorder patients: a double-blind, placebo-controlled pilot study. J Clin Psychiatry 62:849–854, 2001

Zimring FE: Firearms, violence, and public policy. Sci Am 265:48–54, 1991

Zisook S, Byrd D, Kuck J, et al: Command hallucinations in outpatients with schizophrenia. J Clin Psychiatry 56:462–465, 1995

# 37

# Ethical Aspects of Psychiatry

JINGER G. HOOP, M.D.

LAURA B. DUNN, M.D.

## Professionalism

Professionalism is an important concept that is applied to physicians. Some definitions are summarized in Table 37–1.

#### TABLE 37–1.    Definitions of professionalism

Being a professional is an ethical matter, entailing devotion to a way of life, in the service of others and of some higher good (Kass 1983).

A profession is a socially sanctioned activity whose primary object is the well-being of others above the professional's personal gain (Racy 1990).

A profession has three features: training that is intellectual and involves knowledge, as distinguished from skill; work that is pursued primarily for others and not for oneself; and success that is measured by more than the amount of financial return (Brandeis 1993).

Professionalism is not a matter of *trying* but of *being* (LaCombe 1993).

A profession is a set of values, attitudes, and behaviors that results in serving the interests of patients and society before one's own (Reynolds 1994).

Professionalism means aspiring to altruism, accountability, excellence, duty, service, honor, integrity, and respect for others (Stobo and Blank 1994).

*Source.*    Adapted from Roberts and Dyer 2004, pp. 15–16.

## Essential Ethical Skills of Psychiatrists

The clinical skills and personal abilities of well-trained psychiatrists translate readily into a natural facility with ethical problem solving that goes beyond a simple adherence to written guidelines, laws, and codes. These skills are summarized in Table 37–2.

#### TABLE 37–2.    Essential ethics skills in clinical practice

Ability to identify the ethical features of a patient's care

Ability to see how the clinician's own life experience, attitudes, and knowledge may influence the care of the patient

Ability to identify one's areas of clinical expertise (i.e., scope of clinical competence) and to work within these boundaries

Ability to anticipate ethically risky or problematic situations

Ability to gather information and to seek consultation and additional expertise in order to clarify and, ideally, to resolve ethical conflicts

Ability to build ethical safeguards into the patient care situation

*Source.*    Reprinted from Roberts LW, Dyer AR: "Clinical Decision-Making and Ethics Skills," in *Concise Guide to Ethics in Mental Health Care.* Washington, DC, American Psychiatric Publishing, 2004, p. 20. Copyright 2004, American Psychiatric Publishing. Used with permission.

**TABLE 37–3.　Ethical tensions in common clinical situations**

| Clinical situation | Relevant ethical principles | Conflicts and tensions |
| --- | --- | --- |
| A patient refuses a medically indicated treatment | Autonomy and beneficence | The patient's right to make his or her own decisions is in tension with the physician's duty to do good by providing medically indicated treatment |
| A patient tells his psychiatrist that he plans to harm another person | Confidentiality and beneficence | The physician's duty to guard his patient's privacy must be balanced against the obligation to protect the threatened third party |
| A close friend asks a psychiatrist to write a prescription for a sleep medicine | Nonmaleficence | The desire to oblige a friend may conflict with the psychiatrist's duty to avoid harm by prescribing without conducting a medical evaluation and establishing a treatment relationship |
| The parent of an adolescent patient asks the psychiatrist for information about the patient's sexual activity and drug or alcohol use | Confidentiality and beneficence | The psychiatrist's duty to guard his patient's privacy may be in tension with the psychiatrist's desire to do good by educating the parent about the child's high-risk behaviors |
| A patient asks a psychiatrist to document a less-stigmatizing diagnosis when filling out insurance forms | Veracity and nonmaleficence | The psychiatrist's obligation to document the truth may be in tension with the desire to avoid the harm that may occur if the insurance company learns of the diagnosis |
| A rural psychiatrist's patient needs a treatment the psychiatrist is not competent to provide; no other practitioner is available | Nonmaleficence | The psychiatrist's duty to avoid harming the patient by practicing outside his scope of competencies is in conflict with the obligation to avoid harming the patient by leaving him without any treatment provider |
| A medical student performs a lumbar puncture for the first time on a patient | Nonmaleficence and beneficence | The medical student's obligation to avoid harming the patient by performing a procedure without sufficient expertise must be balanced against the student's need to "learn by doing" in order to help future patients |
| A psychiatrist treating a physician believes the patient is too impaired to practice medicine safely; the patient/physician refuses to close his practice because he has no other source of income | Confidentiality, nonmaleficence, and beneficence | The psychiatrist's duty to guard his patient's privacy and to avoid harming him is in tension with the obligation to protect the impaired physician's patients by reporting the impairment to the proper authorities |
| A pharmaceutical company offers a psychiatrist a large fee for referring patients to a research trial | Fidelity | Financial self-interest threatens the psychiatrist's duty to remain faithful to the goals of treatment and to the role as a healer |
| A psychiatrist transfers care of a "difficult" patient to another provider | Fidelity, nonmaleficence, and beneficence | The psychiatrist's obligations to remain faithful to the goals of treatment and to avoid the harm of patient abandonment must be balanced against the duty to do good by transferring care to a more competent or appropriate provider when clinically necessary |

**TABLE 37–4.    Key ethical challenges in special clinical circumstances**

| Clinical circumstance | Key ethical challenges |
|---|---|
| Academic psychiatry | Conflicts between clinical and supervisory roles of faculty and between clinical and student roles of trainees |
| | Financial conflicts of interest related to managed care contracts and relationships with industry |
| | Duty to provide competent care despite trainee status of resident physicians and medical students |
| Addiction psychiatry | Confidentiality, due to adverse legal and social consequences of addictive behaviors |
| | Justice, because of the lack of equitable treatment for persons with addictive disorders compared with other conditions |
| Child and adolescent psychiatry | Confidentiality and truth telling for patient and guardians |
| | Informed consent for treatment, which may require the consent of guardians |
| Forensic psychiatry | Conflicts between roles as forensic expert and physician |
| Geriatric psychiatry | Informed consent for treatment when decisional capacity may be impaired |
| | End-of-life issues, including assisted suicide and treatment withdrawal |
| Military psychiatry | Conflicts between roles as physician and member of the military |
| Psychotherapy and psychoanalysis | Confidentiality, due to the intensely private nature of patient disclosures |
| | Maintenance of therapeutic boundaries |
| Public psychiatry | Duty to provide competent care despite limited resources |
| | Justice, in terms of the need to distribute social resources fairly |
| Rural psychiatry | Confidentiality in a setting where "everyone knows everyone" |
| | Conflicts among multiple roles of physician and patients within community |
| | Duty to provide competent care in the absence of specialists |
| | Nonabandonment of patients in a setting in which there may be a lack of qualified clinicians to provide backup coverage |
| Treatment of "difficult" patients | Duty to provide competent care to patients with clinically challenging psychopathology |
| | Nonabandonment despite countertransference feelings or physician burnout |

*Source.*   Adapted from Roberts and Dyer 2004.

Various ethical conflicts and techniques that psychiatrists will encounter in different clinical situations are summarized in Table 37–3.

Many psychiatric subspecialties and selected psychiatric clinical settings (academic, military, and public psychiatry) present unique, ethical challenges to psychiatrists. These key ethical challenges are summarized in Table 37–4.

## Terms Used in Ethics

Psychiatrists will encounter a number of key terms that are applied to ethical issues that they will encounter. These terms are summarized in Table 37–5.

## Practical Ethical Problem Solving

Many clinicians use an eclectic approach to ethical problem solving that intuitively makes use of both principle-based ethics and casuistry through a combination of inductive and deductive reasoning. Such an approach does not typically yield one "right" answer but, rather, an array of possible and ethically justifiable approaches that may be acceptable in the current situation. In the clinical setting, a widely used approach to ethical problem solving is the "four-topics method" described by Jonsen et al. (1998). This method entails gathering and evaluating information about 1) clinical indications, 2) patient preferences, 3) patient quality of life, and 4) contextual or external influences on the ethical decision-making process (Figure 37–1).

---

**TABLE 37–5.    Glossary of ethics terms**

---

**Altruism**    The virtue of acting for the good of another rather than for oneself, at times entailing self-sacrifice.

**Autonomy**    Literally, "self-rule." In medical ethics, autonomy is the ability to make deliberated or reasoned decisions for oneself and to act on the basis of such decisions.

**Beneficence**    An action done to benefit others. The principle of beneficence in medicine signifies an obligation to benefit patients and to seek their good.

**Coercion**    The use of some form of pressure to persuade or compel an individual to agree to a belief or action.

**Compassion**    Literally, "suffering with" another person, with kindness and an active regard for his or her welfare. Compassion is more closely related to empathy than to sympathy, as sympathy connotes the more distanced experience of "feeling sorry for" the individual.

**Confidentiality**    The obligation of physicians not to disclose information obtained from patients or observed about them without their permission. In clinical care, it entails taking precautions to protect the personal information of patients. Confidentiality is a privilege linked to the legal right of privacy and may at times be overridden by exceptions stipulated in law.

**Conflict of interest**    In medicine, a situation in which a physician has competing roles, relationships, or interests that could potentially interfere with the ability to care for patients. Such situations may naturally occur in clinical care and research, and they are not inherently unethical but must be recognized and managed appropriately to safeguard the well-being of vulnerable individuals (e.g., patients, research participants) and to prevent exploitative practices.

**Empathy**    The act of entering into someone else's frame of reference in terms of thoughts, feelings, and experiences, to gain an authentic understanding of the other person's experiences imaginatively as one's own.

**Euthanasia**    A form of physician-assisted death in which the physician deliberately and with compassionate intent acts to end the life of a person with an incurable and progressive disease that will cause imminent death.

**Fidelity**    The virtue of promise keeping, truthfulness, and honor. In clinical care, it refers to the faithfulness with which a clinician commits to the duty of helping patients and acting in a manner that is in keeping with the ideals of the profession.

**Fiduciary**    An entity in a position of trust with a duty to act on behalf of another, for the other's good. Physicians are fiduciaries with respect to their patients.

**Honesty**    A virtue in which one conveys the truth fully, without misrepresentation through deceit, bias, or omission.

**Human dignity**    The belief that every person, intrinsically, is valued and worthy of respect. In medical ethics, every patient is believed to have innate and inalienable worth as a human being that requires he or she be treated with respect and compassion and full interpersonal regard as expressed in attitudes, behaviors, and nondiscriminatory practices.

**Informed consent**    In the clinical setting, a legal and ethical obligation for clinicians to inform patients about their illness and alternatives for care and to assist them in making reasoned, authentic decisions about treatment. In the research setting, a similar obligation for a researcher to inform participants about the research protocol and help them make reasoned, authentic decisions about research participation.

**Integrity**    A virtue literally defined as wholeness or coherence. It connotes professional soundness and reliability of intention and action.

**Justice**    The ethical principle of fairness. Distributive justice refers to the fair and equitable distribution of resources and burden throughout society.

**Medical decision making**    The intentional process associated with making a choice in clinical care. It pertains to a patient's capacity to make decisions related to his or her health or health care and to the clinician's process of deliberation, consultation, and data gathering that results in the development of a diagnosis and of therapeutic alternatives for a patient.

**Medical negligence**    The legal concept of a breach of duty of medical care. It rests on the existence of a duty of care, failure to fulfill that duty, and the existence of harm.

**TABLE 37–5.   Glossary of ethics terms *(continued)***

**Nonmaleficence**   The duty to avoid doing harm.

**Personhood**   Having full moral status as a human being.

**Quality of life**   The expression of a value judgment regarding the experience of life as a whole or some aspect of it by an individual.

**Respect**   The virtue of fully regarding and according intrinsic value to someone or something. In clinical care, it is reflected in treating another individual with genuine consideration and attentiveness to that person's life history, values, and goals.

**Self-understanding**   The awareness of one's own values and motivations. Self-understanding based on insight and careful self-scrutiny is a key ethical skill of special importance to mental health care ethics.

**Therapeutic boundaries**   The set of concepts, rules, and duties that structures the clinician–patient relationship to ensure psychological safety, to optimize therapeutic benefit, and to prevent potentially exploitative practices.

**Trustworthiness**   A virtue that pertains to a disposition that inspires confident belief in and reliance upon the physician's character and ability to act beneficently and honestly.

**Voluntary**   The attribute in which a belief or act derives from one's own free will and is not coerced or unduly influenced by others.

**Vulnerability**   The capacity to be wounded or hurt physically, emotionally, spiritually, or socially and being without the means to defend or advocate for oneself fully.

*Source.*   Adapted from Roberts and Dyer 2004, p. 319.

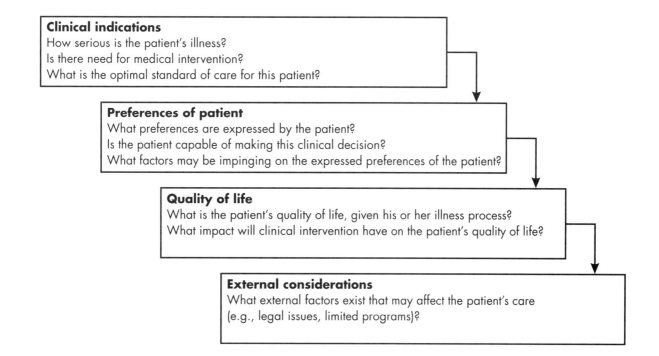

**FIGURE 37–1.   A model for ethical decision making.**

*Source.*   Reprinted from Roberts LW, Dyer AR: *Concise Guide to Ethics in Mental Health Care.* Washington, DC, American Psychiatric Publishing, 2004, p. 307. Used with permission.

**TABLE 37–6.    Selections from The Principles of Medical Ethics With Annotations Especially Applicable to Psychiatry**

**Section 1:**    "A physician shall be dedicated to providing competent medical service with compassion and respect for human dignity."

**Section 1.2:**    "A psychiatrist should not be a party to any type of policy that excludes, segregates, or demeans the dignity of any patient because of ethnic origin, race, sex, creed, age, socioeconomic status, or sexual orientation."

**Section 1.4:**    "A psychiatrist should not be a participant in a legally authorized execution."

**Section 2:**    "A physician shall uphold the standards of professionalism, be honest in all professional interactions and strive to report physicians deficient in character or competence, or engaging in fraud or deception to appropriate entities."

**Section 2.1:**    "Sexual activity with a current or former patient is unethical."

**Section 2.3:**    "A psychiatrist who regularly practices outside his/her area of professional competence should be considered unethical."

**Section 2.4:**    "Special consideration should be given to those psychiatrists who, because of mental illness, jeopardize the welfare of their patients and their own reputations and practices. It is ethical, even encouraged, for another psychiatrist to intercede in such situations."

**Section 4.2:**    "A psychiatrist may release confidential information only with the authorization of the patient or under proper legal compulsion."

**Section 4.14:**    "Sexual involvement between a faculty member or supervisor and a trainee or student, in those situations in which an abuse of power can occur, often takes advantages of inequalities in the working relationship and may be unethical because (a) any treatment of a patient being supervised may be deleteriously affected; (b) it may damage the trust relationship between teacher and student; and (c) teachers are important professional role models for their trainees and affect their trainees' future professional behavior."

**Section 7.3:**    "On occasion, psychiatrists are asked for an opinion about an individual who is in the light of public attention, or who has disclosed information about himself/herself through public media. In such circumstances, a psychiatrist may share with the public his/her expertise about psychiatric issues in general. However, it is unethical for a psychiatrist to offer a professional opinion unless he/she has conducted an examination and been granted proper authorization for such a statement."

*Source.*    Reprinted from American Psychiatric Association: *The Principles of Medical Ethics With Annotations Especially Applicable to Psychiatry*, 2006 Edition. Washington, DC, American Psychiatric Association, 2006 (available at: http://www.psych.org/psych_pract/ethics/ppaethics. cfm). Used with permission.

## Codes of Ethical Conduct

### Ethical Codes for Clinicians

Table 37–6 shows key situations from *Principles of Medical Ethics With Annotations Especially Applicable to Psychiatry*.

## Research Ethics

When physicians are involved in research involving human subjects, three research codes are applied: the Nuremberg Code, Declaration of Helsinki, and Belmont Report. These codes are summarized in Table 37–7.

## Key Ethical Issues in Clinical Psychiatry

Ethical decision making can be extremely challenging in the field of psychiatry because of the complexities of the doctor–patient relationship in this medical specialty, the need for careful attention to ethical safeguards when working with people with disorders and treatments that affect mental processes, and the legally authorized power of psychiatrists to use involuntary treatment and hospitalization.

*Boundary violations* are actions by the psychiatrist that are outside normal professional limits and that have the potential to harm patients.

**TABLE 37–7.** Major codes of research ethics

| Code | Major principles articulated |
| --- | --- |
| **Nuremberg Code** (Katz 1972) | Voluntary participation, legal capacity for informed consent, elements of informed consent |
| | Results must be useful to society and unobtainable by other means |
| | Human research must be justified based on animal research and other knowledge informing the basis of the planned study |
| | Must avoid unnecessary physical and mental suffering |
| | Must not occur if there is reason to believe that death or disabling injury will occur |
| | Degree of risk should be justified by the importance of the research question |
| | Even remote possibilities of injury should be protected against |
| | Qualified people must conduct the experiment |
| | Voluntary withdrawal by participant at any time |
| | Termination of study by researcher if continuation is likely to result in injury, disability, or death |
| **Declaration of Helsinki** (World Medical Association 1964) | Physician duty to protect life, health, privacy, and dignity of the human subject |
| | Scientific basis and validity of methods of medical research |
| | Respect for environment and animals |
| | Independent protocol review and monitoring |
| | Qualified and supervised persons must conduct the research |
| | Assessment of risks and burdens must precede the research; risks must be managed; termination of study if positive and conclusive evidence of benefit |
| | Favorable risk–benefit ratio |
| | Voluntary informed consent |
| | Protection of privacy, confidentiality |
| | Elements of informed consent |
| | Safeguards for informed consent process |
| | Provision for informed consent from legally authorized representative in the case of minors or individuals who are legally incompetent because of physical or mental incapacity |
| | Other provisions for proxy consent: requirement of scientific necessity of enrolling the decisionally incapable population, assent from incompetent individual |
| | Ethical obligations of authors and publishers: accuracy, publication of negative findings, sources of funding and possible conflict of interests declared |
| | Provisions for combining of research with clinical care |
| | New method should be tested against best currently available methods; access at end of study to best methods identified by study (placebo-controlled trial acceptable in specific circumstances: "Where for compelling and scientifically sound methodological reasons its use is necessary to determine the efficacy or safety of a prophylactic, diagnostic or therapeutic method"; or for minor condition with no additional risk of serious harm to those receiving placebo) |
| | Inform patients which aspects of clinical care are research |
| | Ability, based on physician judgment, to use unproven or new methods in some situations; ideally should be focus of research |
| **Belmont Report** (National Commission for Protection of Human Subjects of Biomedical and Behavioral Research 1979) | Respect for persons: Treat individuals as autonomous agents; protect those with diminished autonomy |
| | Beneficence: Do no harm; maximize possible benefits/minimize possible harms |
| | Justice: Addresses principles of fairness in recruitment and in distribution of fruits of knowledge gained |

Sexual contact with *former* patients is also understood as inherently exploitative, as there has been growing recognition that transference feelings do not disappear when treatment ends (American Psychiatric Association 2001a). In addition, sexual or romantic involvement with key third parties to a treatment, such as the parent or spouse of a patient, threatens the therapeutic relationship and presents a conflict of interest that should be avoided (American Psychiatric Association 2001b).

The term *boundary crossing* has been used to describe a subtle nonsexual transgression that is helpful to the patient because it advances the treatment (Gutheil and Gabbard 1993, 1998). As an example of a boundary crossing, Gabbard describes a guarded, paranoid patient who offers her psychiatrist a cookie. By accepting this token gift graciously, the psychiatrist helps the patient feel more relaxed in the treatment setting and more willing to discuss her symptoms. See Table 37–8 for a list of warning signs for boundary violations.

## Patient Nonabandonment

According to accepted ethical standards in medicine, except in emergencies, physicians are "free to choose whom to serve" (American Psychiatric Association 2001a). Once an ongoing doctor–patient relationship has been established, however, the physician may not ethically abandon the patient. As a practical matter, this means that psychiatrists must arrange for clinical coverage when on vacation and must give adequate notice to patients when closing their practices (American Psychiatric Association 2001b).

---

**TABLE 37–8.    Warning signs of problems maintaining therapeutic boundaries**

Doing any of the following for your family members or social acquaintances: prescribing medication, making diagnoses, offering psychodynamic explanations for their behavior

Accepting gifts or bequests from patients

Engaging in a personal relationship with patients after treatment is terminated

Making exceptions for a patient, such as providing special scheduling or reducing fees, because you find the patient attractive, appealing, or impressive

Touching patients (other than shaking hands or performing appropriate medical procedures)

Using information learned from patients, such as business tips or political information, for your own financial or career gain

Asking patients to do personal favors for you (e.g., bring lunch, mail a letter)

Arranging business deals with patients

Accepting for treatment persons with whom you have had social involvement

Disclosing sensational aspects of a patient's life to others (even when protecting the patient's identity)

Accepting a medium of exchange other than money for professional services (e.g., work on your office or home, trading of professional services)

Making exceptions in the conduct of treatment because you feel sorry for a patient or because you believe that the patient is in such distress or so disturbed that there is no other choice

Recommending treatment procedures or referrals that you do not believe to be necessarily in the patient's best interests but that may instead be to your own direct or indirect financial benefit

Making exceptions for a patient because you are afraid that the patient will otherwise become extremely angry or self-destructive

Failing to deal with the following patient behavior(s): Paying the fee late, missing appointments on short notice and refusing to pay for the time (as agreed), seeking to extend the length of sessions

Telling patients personal things about yourself

Trying to influence patients to support political causes or positions in which you have a personal interest

Seeking social contact with patients outside of clinically scheduled visits

Joining in an activity with a patient that may serve to deceive a third party (e.g., misleading an insurance company)

---

*Source.*    Adapted from Epstein and Simon 1990.

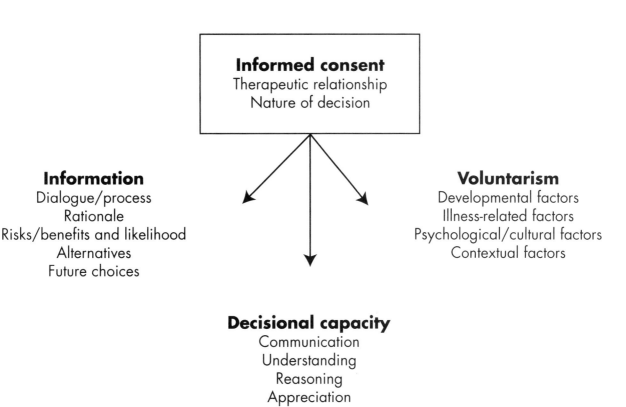

FIGURE 37–2.  **Elements of informed consent.**

*Source.*  Reprinted from Roberts LW, Dyer AR: *Concise Guide to Ethics in Mental Health Care.* Washington, DC, American Psychiatric Publishing, 2004, p. 52. Used with permission.

## Informed Consent

Informed consent is the process by which individuals make free, knowledgeable decisions about whether to accept a proposed psychiatric treatment or whether to participate in a medical research study. Informed consent is thus a cornerstone of ethical practice in both treatment and research settings. While informed consent is a legal requirement in both contexts, its philosophical roots as a medicolegal doctrine are deeply embedded in our societal and cultural respect for individual persons, in affirming individuals' freedom of self-determination. An adequate process of informed consent thus reflects and promotes the ethical principle of autonomy.

### Standards for Consent

Informed consent has been conceptualized as consisting of three distinct yet related features: information, decisional capacity, and voluntarism (Figure 37–2) (Faden et al. 1986). Each of these is discussed in turn below.

Although there is no clear index for deciding how stringent the standard for consent should be, a general rule of thumb is to use a "sliding scale" approach, titrating the expectation for consent to the potential risk of the decision (see Figure 37–3).

**Information.** *Information provision,* or information sharing, the first element, refers to a dialogue in which the patient or potential research participant is given all relevant information about treatment options, proposed tests, or the research protocol.

**Decisional capacity.** Decisional capacity can be described as a "sociocultural construct" (Dunn et al. 2007) consisting of intrapersonal elements, aspects related to the quality of the consent process (deriving from the information-sharing component described above as well as from the professionalism of the physician), and the complexity of the information and the decision at hand.

Decisional capacity has been defined by experts as consisting of four standards (Appelbaum and Grisso 1995). The first ability, communication of a preference, is the least stringent standard, requiring that a person be able to express or state a decision. This standard was originally

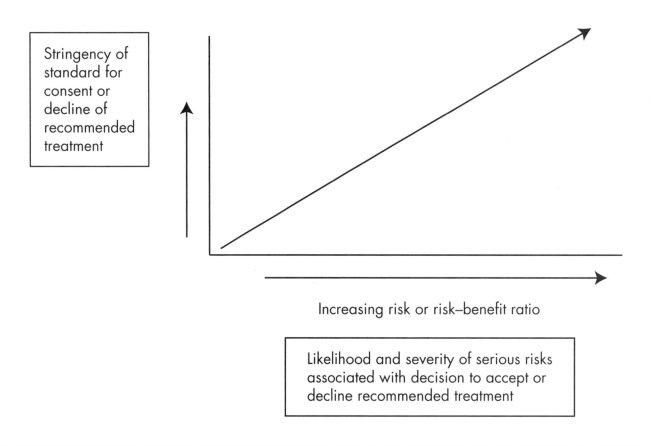

FIGURE 37–3.    **The "sliding scale" of consent standards.**
*Source.*    Reprinted from Roberts LW, Dyer AR: *Concise Guide to Ethics in Mental Health Care.* Washington, DC, American Psychiatric Publishing, 2004, p. 61. Used with permission.

conceived as a basic physical ability to communicate—a capability that is sometimes lost when a patient is experiencing catatonia or in patients who are comatose, poststroke, or post–spinal injury. Some have come to view this standard differently and as relating to the ability to communicate a stable choice, and there are certainly circumstances where even this standard is not met—for example, a patient with delirium whose attention waxes and wanes, affecting her ability to focus on a discussion of her treatment options; or a patient who is ambivalent or erratic by virtue of his illness process.

The second standard, understanding or comprehension of the information necessary for the specific decision at hand, is primarily a cognitive ability and has been shown to be correlated with cognitive functioning in people with a variety of psychiatric illnesses (Carpenter et al. 2000; Kovnick et al. 2003; Moser et al. 2002; Palmer et al. 2005). Cognitive disorders such as dementia clearly affect the ability to understand relevant information (Kim et al.

2001). It is important to note additionally that sociocultural factors, such as literacy, numeracy, and educational background, clearly influence the ability to understand health decision information. It is thus critical that psychiatrists strive to communicate health information in ways that can be more readily understood by patients (Roberts and Dyer 2004).

The third ability or standard is "appreciation." This generally is considered to refer to the patient's awareness of the implications and significance of the information provided or the choice being made for his or her own life circumstances. Appreciation is a concept tightly linked with the psychiatric notion of insight, a patient's knowledge that his or her symptoms are abnormal or the product of illness. Insight is often eroded in diverse mental illnesses, personality disorders, and disabling conditions. Lack of insight may create a situation in which an individual has an understanding of factual information but cannot apply it to his or her own situation, in which case appreciation would be lacking. An example is the patient who can demonstrate an understanding that an untreated infection could lead to death but who believes that this information does not apply to him—for example, because he has supernatural powers that will protect him.

The fourth standard is the ability to reason—to weigh information, comparing options and considering their consequences. An assessment of reasoning abilities should include evaluating whether the patient understands the consequences of alternative treatment choices and also of no treatment. A patient does not need to be able to calculate probabilities but should be able to weigh options. The patient also need not come to the "rational" choice as a result of the reasoning process. A patient who refuses treatment but whose understanding, appreciation, reasoning, and indication of a choice are adequate has the right to refuse treatment. Involuntary treatment is predicated, in part, on the absence of intact decision-making capacity, and thus careful assessment of these component abilities is key in evaluating the appropriateness of seeking involuntary treatment for a given patient.

**Voluntarism.** The third key part of informed consent is voluntarism. Being able to make an authentic, free decision—a decision that is most concordant with an individual's own values, history, and circumstances—is a fundamental aspect of autonomy. The four domains of potential influences for voluntarism are shown in Figure 37–4.

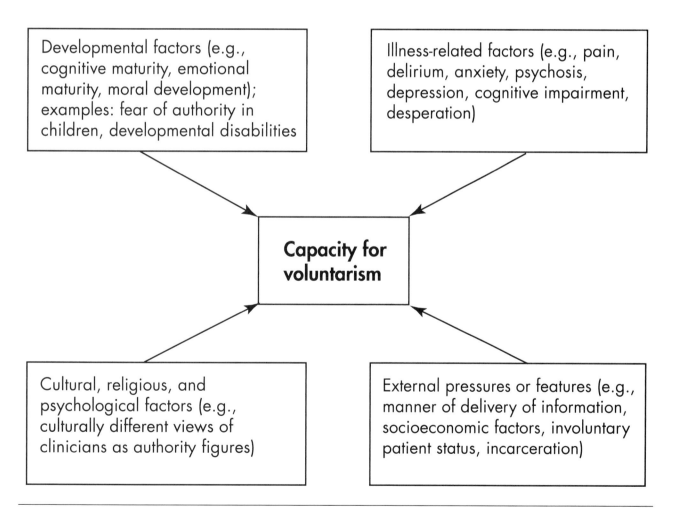

FIGURE 37–4. **Conceptual model of voluntarism: four domains of potential influences.**

*Source.* Adapted from Roberts LW: "Informed Consent and the Capacity for Voluntarism." *American Journal of Psychiatry* 159:705–712, 2002. Used with permission.

### Alternative Decision Making and Advance Directives

In cases where an individual is deemed, via a clinical assessment or legal decision, to lack the ability to make a particular decision or set of decisions related to his or her care, a surrogate, proxy, or alternative decision maker is asked to step in and make choices for that person.

Advance directives are documents that describe an individual's wishes regarding future care in the event that the person loses decisional capacity. Advance directives are typically used to help in end-of-life decision making. The existence of an advance directive does not necessarily increase the accuracy of an alternative decision maker's choices, as one study showed (Ditto et al. 2001).

## Ethical Use of Power

The relationship between physician and patient is inherently one of inequity. Relative to the population at large, the psychiatrist holds a position of power because of his or her education and socioeconomic standing, by the role as healer and keeper of confidences, and by the special powers granted by the state—the ability to involuntarily hospitalize patients and to stand as a gatekeeper to health care services such as prescribed medication.

### Involuntary Treatment

Far more subtle but nonetheless important ethical issues surround the use of power in high-risk situations by well-meaning and thoughtful clinicians. An example of such a high-risk situation is psychiatrists' legally authorized use of involuntary treatment which is sometimes necessary in the care of patients whose mental illness makes them a danger to themselves or others. Involuntary treatment is a clear example of conflicting ethical principles: the obligation to respect patient autonomy and the obligation of beneficence.

In recognition of the needs of many seriously psychiatrically ill individuals for outpatient treatment, and spurred by the tragic death of a young woman in New York City, a new mandatory outpatient treatment program was signed into law in New York State in 1999 (New York State Office of Mental Health 2005). Known as "Kendra's Law," this legislation provided mechanisms for identifying and providing care to individuals with a treatment history of nonadherence, who were unlikely to voluntarily engage in treatment and whose current behavior indicated that without assisted outpatient treatment, they were at risk of clinical deterioration that was likely to re-

sult in harm to themselves or others. Table 37–9 summarizes key strategies for providing ethical care in involuntary treatment.

---

**TABLE 37–9.    Working therapeutically in the setting of involuntary treatment**

Understand treatment refusal as a possible expression of distress

Ascertain the reasons for refusal

Allow the patient to discuss his or her preferences and fears

Explain the reason for the intervention in simple language

Offer options for the disposition of treatment

Appropriately enlist the assistance of family and friends

Request support from nursing and support staff

Assess decisional capacity and if necessary have recourse to the courts

Attend to side effects—both long-term and short-term, serious and bothersome

Employ emergency treatment options where available

Work to preserve the therapeutic alliance

Utilize treatment guardians where appropriate

---

*Source.*    Adapted from Roberts LW, Dyer AR: "Ethical Use of Power in High-Risk Situations," in *Concise Guide to Ethics in Mental Health Care.* Washington, DC, American Psychiatric Publishing, 2004, p. 93. Used with permission.

## Confidentiality

From the standpoint of U.S. law, doctor–patient confidentiality is a legal privilege granted to patients. The privilege requires physicians to keep patient information private, unless the doctor is legally compelled to make a disclosure or the patient waives the privilege. Although this may sound straightforward, in practice there are many gray areas in which a physician's legal and ethical duties may conflict. In remote rural settings, where clinicians and their patients are also neighbors, lifelong friends, and even relatives by blood or by marriage, confidentiality poses extraordinary challenges (Roberts et al. 1999). With the Health Insurance Portability and Accountability Act (HIPAA) of 1996, specific protections for personal health information, including a higher level of protection for psychotherapy notes, were also enacted (see U.S. Department of Health and Human Services 1996).

There are other instances when a nonconsenting patient may have the privilege of confidentiality suspended, based on the physician's overriding duties to others. These situations typically involve breaching patient confidentiality in order to protect third parties in cases of child or elder abuse or threatened violence. The notion that psychiatrists have a "duty to protect" members of the public from the violent intentions of their patients was demonstrated by the legal case *Tarasoff v. Regents of the University of California, 1974 and 1976.* From an ethical standpoint, the *Tarasoff* ruling gives more weight to the importance of beneficence (preventing harm to a third party) than to fidelity and confidentiality (protecting the confidences of one's own patient). A useful list of do's and don'ts for safeguarding patient confidentiality related to specific issues has been compiled by Roberts et al. (2002).

## Management of Dual Roles and Conflicts of Interest

### *Financial Conflicts of Interest Pertaining to Patient Care*

Among the most obviously unacceptable conflicts of interest are those in which physicians have a clear-cut financial arrangement that could adversely influence how they treat patients.

### *Relations With Industry*

The possibility of conflicts of interest arising from accepting gifts or other forms of support from industry is the subject of much controversy in all of medicine. A meta-analysis of 29 studies on physician–pharmaceutical company interactions demonstrated that physicians' attitudes toward a medication and/or their prescribing practices are influenced by having personal contact with pharmaceutical sales representatives, attending sales presentations, attending continuing medical education (CME) conferences sponsored by pharmaceutical companies, and using industry funding for travel and housing expenses to attend professional meetings (Wazana 2000).

### *Dual Agency*

Another type of conflict of interest arises for psychiatrists who have additional professional duties that may not be fully congruent with the role of physician. Such conflicts are sometimes referred to as "dual agency" situations.

## Social Stigmatization of Mental Illness

AMA and APA ethics codes state that a physician "shall recognize a responsibility to participating in activities contributing to an improved community" (American Psychiatric Association 2001a). Many psychiatrists feel ethically compelled to speak out against social injustice that harms psychiatric patients, such as mental health insurance nonparity, stigmatization and discrimination, and public policies that neglect the needs of the mentally ill.

## Ethical Interactions With Colleagues and Trainees

As members of a profession, psychiatrists are expected to behave ethically toward their colleagues individually and collectively. The AMA *Principles of Medical Ethics* explicitly states that physicians should "deal honestly" with colleagues, "respect the rights" of colleagues, and "strive to expose those physicians deficient in character or competence, or who engage in fraud or deception" (American Psychiatric Association 2006) (see Table 37–6). While the first two statements in the ethics code encourage collegial behavior, the third suggests the importance of self-governance in the medical professions and the need to report colleague misconduct and impairment.

### *Ethical Issues of Concern to Medical Faculty and Trainees*

The ethical obligations of psychiatric faculty toward trainees involve many of the same requirements as relations with colleagues, plus the added obligations of a "fiduciary-like" relationship with trainees (Mohamed et al. 2005).

## Ethical Concerns in Psychiatric Research

In general, concerns have centered on issues of scientific design (e.g., the use of medication washout periods, the use of placebo controls), research safeguards (institutional review practices, study monitoring, and debriefing), and informed consent (Dunn and Roberts 2005). In addition, the nature of psychiatric illnesses—which may cause some individuals to have impaired decision-making abilities, to have decreased insight into the need for and potential benefits of treatment, and to be subject to involuntarily imposed treatments—raises ethical concerns about the recruitment and enrollment of those with serious psychiatric disorders into clinical research protocols.

# Key Points: Ethical Aspects of Psychiatry

- Ethical decision making is a skill that can be taught and learned.

- Key moral principles that provide a foundation for contemporary discussions of medical ethics are autonomy, respect for persons, beneficence, nonmaleficence, justice, veracity, fidelity, and privacy.

- Psychiatrists have an ethical duty to provide competent care, treat patients with respect and dignity, and uphold ethical and professional obligations of confidentiality and truth telling.

- Sexual contact with patients and former patients is unethical.

- Physicians have an ethical duty to report the improper behavior of colleagues.

- Informed consent represents not only a legal and ethical requirement but also an opportunity to enhance physician–patient communication, assess patient preferences and values, and optimize treatment planning through a process of shared decision making.

- Individuals with psychiatric diagnoses are heterogeneous in terms of their decision-making abilities for treatment and research and should not be presumed to lack decisional capacity.

- Information about decisions should be provided in a manner that is appropriate to the individual patient.

- A "sliding scale" approach should be used for assessing decision-making capacity: a higher level of capacity may be needed for higher-risk or risk–benefit ratio decisions.

- The ethical use of involuntary treatment and hospitalization balances the duties of trying to do good, avoiding harm, and respecting autonomy.

# References

American Psychiatric Association: Ethics Primer of the American Psychiatric Association. Washington, DC, American Psychiatric Association, 2001a

American Psychiatric Association: Opinions of the Ethics Committee on The Principles of Medical Ethics. Washington, DC, American Psychiatric Association, 2001b

American Psychiatric Association: The Principles of Medical Ethics With Annotations Applicable to Psychiatry. Washington, DC, American Psychiatric Association, 2006

Appelbaum PS, Grisso T: The MacArthur Competence Study I, II, III. Law Hum Behav 19:105–174, 1995

Brandeis LD: Business: A Profession. Boston, MA, Hole, Cushman & Flint, 1993

Carpenter WT, Gold JM, Lahti AC, et al: Decisional capacity for informed consent in schizophrenia research. Arch Gen Psychiatry 57:533–538, 2000

Ditto PH, Danks JH, Smucker WD, et al: Advance directives as acts of communication: a randomized controlled trial. Arch Intern Med 161:421–430, 2001

Dunn LB, Roberts LW: Emerging findings in ethics of schizophrenia research. Curr Opin Psychiatry 18:111–119, 2005

Dunn LB, Palmer BW, Karlawish JHT: Frontal dysfunction and capacity to consent to treatment or research: conceptual considerations and empirical evidence, in The Human Frontal Lobes: Functions and Disorders, 2nd Edition. Edited by Miller B, Cummings JL. New York, Guilford, 2007, pp 335–344

Faden RR, Beauchamp TL, King N: A History and Theory of Informed Consent. New York, Oxford University Press, 1986

Gutheil TH, Gabbard GO: The concept of boundaries in clinical practice: theoretical and risk-management dimensions. Am J Psychiatry 150:188–196, 1993

Gutheil TH, Gabbard GO: Misuses and misunderstandings of boundary theory in clinical and regulatory settings. Am J Psychiatry 155:409–414, 1998

Jonsen AR, Siegler M, Winslade WJ: Clinical Ethics, 4th Edition. New York, McGraw-Hill, 1998

Kass LR: Professing ethically: on the place of ethics in defining medicine. JAMA 249:1305–1310, 1983

Katz J: Experimentation With Human Beings. New York, Russell Sage Foundation, 1972

Kim SY, Caine ED, Currier GW, et al: Assessing the competence of persons with Alzheimer's disease in providing informed consent for participation in research. Am J Psychiatry 158:712–717, 2001

Kovnick JA, Appelbaum PS, Hoge SK, et al: Competence to consent to research among long-stay inpatients with chronic schizophrenia. Psychiatr Serv 54:1247–1252, 2003

LaCombe MA: On professionalism. Am J Med 94:329, 1993

Mohamed M, Punwani M, Clay M, et al: Protecting the residency training environment: a resident's perspective on the ethical boundaries in the faculty-resident relationship. Acad Psychiatry 29:368–373, 2005

Moser DJ, Schultz SK, Arndt S, et al: Capacity to provide informed consent for participation in schizophrenia and HIV research. Am J Psychiatry 159:1201–1207, 2002

National Commission for the Protection of Human Subjects of Biomedical and Behavioral Research: The Belmont Report: ethical principles and guidelines for the protection of human subjects of research, 1979. Available at: http://www.hhs.gov/ohrp/humansubjects/guidance/belmont.htm. Accessed June 12, 2006.

New York State Office of Mental Health: Kendra's Law: final report on the status of assisted outpatient treatment. New York, Office of Mental Health, 2005

Palmer BW, Dunn LB, Appelbaum PS, et al: Assessment of capacity to consent to research among older persons with schizophrenia, Alzheimer disease, or diabetes mellitus: comparison of a 3-item questionnaire with a comprehensive standardized capacity instrument. Arch Gen Psychiatry 62:726–733, 2005

Racy J: Professionalism: sane and insane. J Clin Psychiatry 51:138–140, 1990

Reynolds PP: Reaffirming professionalism through the education community. Ann Intern Med 120:609–614, 1994

Roberts LW, Dyer AR (eds): Concise Guide to Ethics in Mental Health Care. Washington, DC, American Psychiatric Publishing, 2004

Roberts LW, Battaglia J, Smithpeter M, et al: An office on Main Street. Health care dilemmas in small communities. Hastings Cent Rep 29:28–37, 1999

Stobo JD, Blank LL: American Board of Internal Medicine's Project Professionalism: staying ahead of the wave. Am J Med 97:1–3, 1994

U.S. Department of Health and Human Services: Health Insurance Portability and Accountability Act of 1996. Available at: http://aspe.hhs.gov/admnsimp/pl104191.htm. Accessed November 21, 2006.

Wazana A: Physicians and the pharmaceutical industry: is a gift ever just a gift? JAMA 283:373–380, 2000

World Medical Association: Declaration of Helsinki: ethical principles for medical research involving human subjects. Ferney-Voltaire, France, World Medical Association, 1964. Available at: http://www.wma.net/e/policy/b3.htm. Accessed June 12, 2006.

# 38

# Traumatic Brain Injury

JONATHAN M. SILVER, M.D.

ROBERT E. HALES, M.D., M.B.A.

STUART C. YUDOFSKY, M.D.

Those at the highest risk for brain injury are men ages 15–24 years. Alcohol use is common in brain injury; a positive blood alcohol concentration was demonstrated in 56% of one sample of victims (J.F. Kraus et al. 1989). Motor vehicle accidents account for approximately one-half of traumatic injuries; other common causes are falls (21%), assaults and violence (20%), and accidents associated with sports and recreation (3%) (although up to 90% of injuries in this category may be unreported) (NIH Consensus Development Panel 1999). Studies examining psychosocial functioning and adjustment at 1 month, 2 years, or 7 years after severe traumatic brain injury (TBI) have shown that patients have extreme difficulty in numerous critical areas of functioning, including work, school, familial, interpersonal, and avocational activities (Crawford 1983; McLean et al. 1984; Oddy et al. 1985; Weddell et al. 1980).

## Neuropsychiatric Assessment of Traumatic Brain Injury

### History-Taking

Confusion, intellectual changes, affective lability, or psychosis may occur directly after the trauma or as long as many years afterward. Individuals who present for emergency treatment for blunt trauma may not be adequately screened for TBI (Chambers et al. 1996).

## Documentation and Rating of Symptoms

Symptom rating scales, electrophysiological imaging, and neuropsychiatric assessments should be used to define symptoms and signs that result from TBI (Table 38–1).

The severity of injury may be determined by several parameters, including duration of unconsciousness, initial score on the Glasgow Coma Scale (GCS) (Teasdale and Jennett 1974), and degree of posttraumatic amnesia. The GCS (Table 38–2) is a 15-point scale that documents eye opening, verbal responsiveness, and motor response to stimuli and may be used to measure the depth of coma, both initially and longitudinally.

In severe TBI, posttraumatic amnesia or loss of consciousness (LOC) may persist for at least 1 week or longer or, in extreme cases, may last weeks to months. GCS scores for severe TBI are less than 10. Mild head injury is usually defined as LOC for less than 15–20 minutes, GCS score of 13–15, brief or no hospitalization, and no prominent residual neurobehavioral deficits. LOC is not required for the diagnosis of traumatic brain injury; however, there must be some evidence of alteration in consciousness, including feeling dazed or experiencing a period of posttraumatic amnesia (Committee on Head Injury Nomenclature 1966; Mild Traumatic Brain Injury Committee 1993; Quality Standards Subcommittee 1997).

A specific grading scale has been developed for concussions that occur during sports: Grade 1—confusion with-

| TABLE 38–1. | Assessment of traumatic brain injury |
| --- | --- |

**Behavioral assessment**

Structured interviews (e.g., Structured Clinical Interview for DSM-IV Diagnoses [SCID], Mini-International Neuropsychiatric Inventory [MINI])

Neurobehavioral Rating Scale (NBRS)

Positive and Negative Syndrome Scale (PANSS)

Glasgow Coma Scale (GCS)

Galveston Orientation and Amnesia Test (GOAT)

Rancho Los Amigos Cognitive Scale

Rating scales for depression (Hamilton)

Rating scales for aggression (Overt Aggression Scale/Agitated Behavior Scale)

Neuropsychiatric Inventory/Neuropsychiatric Inventory Questionnaire

Brain Injury Screening Questionnaire

Rivermead Post Concussion Symptoms Questionnaire

**Brain imaging**

Computed tomography (CT)

Magnetic resonance imaging (MRI) with fluid-attenuated inversion recovery (FLAIR)

Functional magnetic resonance imaging (fMRI)

Single-photon emission computed tomography (SPECT)

Regional cerebral blood flow (rCBF)

Positron emission tomography (PET)

Proton magnetic resonance spectroscopy (MRS)

Diffusion tensor imaging (DTI)

**Electrophysiological assessment**

Electroencephalogram (EEG), including special leads

Computerized EEG

Brain electrical activity mapping (BEAM)

**Neuropsychological assessment**

Attention and concentration

Premorbid intelligence

Memory

Executive functioning

Verbal capacity

Problem-solving skills

| TABLE 38–2. | Glasgow Coma Scale |
| --- | --- |

**Eye opening**

| | |
| --- | --- |
| None | Not attributable to ocular swelling |
| To pain | Pain stimulus is applied to chest or limbs |
| To speech | Nonspecific response to speech or shout, does not imply the patient obeys command to open eyes |
| Spontaneous | Eyes are open, but this does not imply intact awareness |

**Motor response**

| | |
| --- | --- |
| No response | Flaccid |
| Extension | "Decerebrate." Adduction, internal rotation of shoulder, and pronation of the forearm |
| Abnormal flexion | "Decorticate." Abnormal flexion, adduction of the shoulder |
| Withdrawal | Normal flexor response; withdraws from pain stimulus with adduction of the shoulder |
| Localizes pain | Pain stimulus applied to supraocular region or fingertip causes limb to move so as to attempt to remove it |
| Obeys commands | Follows simple commands |

**Verbal response**

| | |
| --- | --- |
| No response | (Self-explanatory) |
| Incomprehensible | Moaning and groaning, but no recognizable words |
| Inappropriate | Intelligible speech (e.g., shouting or swearing), but no sustained or coherent conversation |
| Confused | Patient responds to questions in a conversational manner, but the responses indicate varying degrees of disorientation and confusion |
| Oriented | Normal orientation to time, place, and person |

Source.  Adapted from Teasdale and Jennett 1974.

out amnesia and no LOC; Grade 2—confusion with amnesia and no LOC; and Grade 3—LOC (Kelly 1995).

## Laboratory Evaluation

### Imaging Techniques

Computed tomography (CT) is used for the acute assessment of the patient with head trauma to document hemorrhage, edema, midline shifts, herniation, fractures, and contusions. Thus, for a significant number of patients with severe brain injury, initial CT evaluations may not detect lesions that are observable on CT scans performed 1 and 3 months after the injury (Cope et al. 1988).

Magnetic resonance imaging (MRI) has been shown to detect clinically meaningful lesions in patients with severe brain injury when CT scans have not demonstrated anatomical bases for the degree of coma (Levin et al. 1987a; Wilberger et al. 1987). MRI is especially sensitive in detecting lesions in the frontal and temporal lobes that are not visualized by CT, and these loci are frequently related to the neuropsychiatric consequences of the injury (Levin et al. 1987a). MRI has been found to be more sensitive for the detection of contusions, shearing injury, and subdural and epidural hematomas (Orrison et al. 1994), and it has been able to document evidence of diffuse axonal injury in patients who have a normal CT scan after experiencing mild TBI (Mittl et al. 1994). MR imaging in the chronic stage is better correlated with neuropsychiatric symptoms (Bigler 2005).

### Electrophysiological Techniques

Electroencephalography can detect the presence of seizures or abnormal areas of functioning. To enhance the sensitivity of this technique, the electroencephalogram (EEG) should be performed after sleep deprivation, with photic stimulation and hyperventilation and with anterotemporal and/or nasopharyngeal leads (Goodin et al. 1990). Computed interpretation of the EEG and brain electrical activity mapping (BEAM) may be useful in detecting areas of dysfunction not shown in the routine EEG (Watson et al. 1995).

### Neuropsychological Testing

Neuropsychological assessment of the patient with TBI is essential to document cognitive and intellectual deficits and strengths. Tests are administered to assess the patient's attention, concentration, memory, verbal capacity, and executive functioning. This latter capacity is the most difficult to assess and includes problem-solving skills, abstract

**TABLE 38–3.** Major factors affecting neuropsychological test findings

Original endowment
Environment
Motivation (effort)
Physical health
Psychological distress
Psychiatric disorders
Medications
Qualifications and experience of neuropsychologist
Errors in scoring
Errors in interpretation

*Source.* Reprinted from Simon RI: "Ethical and Legal Issues," in *Textbook of Traumatic Brain Injury.* Edited by Silver JM, McAllister TW, Yudofsky SC. Washington, DC, American Psychiatric Publishing, 2005, pp. 583–605. Used with permission.

thinking, planning, and reasoning abilities. A valid interpretation of these tests includes assessment of the patient's preinjury intelligence and other higher levels of functioning. Because multiple factors affect the results of testing (Table 38–3), tests must be performed and interpreted by a clinician with skill and experience.

## Clinical Features

The neuropsychiatric sequelae of TBI include problems with attention and arousal, concentration, and executive functioning; intellectual changes; memory impairment; personality changes; affective disorders; anxiety disorders; psychosis; posttraumatic epilepsy; sleep disorders; aggression; and irritability. Physical problems such as headache, chronic pain, vision impairment, and dizziness complicate recovery. Factors influencing outcome after TBI are summarized in Table 38–4.

Morbidity and mortality rates after brain injury increase with age. Elderly persons who experience TBI have longer periods of agitation and greater cognitive impairment and are more likely to develop mass lesions and permanent disability than are younger victims (Kim 2005). Individuals who have a previous brain injury do not recover as well from subsequent injuries (Carlsson et al. 1987).

Social conditions and support networks that existed before the injury affect the symptoms and course of recovery. In general, individuals with greater preinjury intelligence recover better after injury (G. Brown et al. 1981). Factors such as level of education, level of income, and

---

**TABLE 38–4. Factors influencing outcome after brain injury**

Severity of injury

Type of injury

Anosmia

Intellectual functioning

Psychiatric diagnosis

Sociopathy

Premorbid behavioral problems (children)

Social support

Substance use

Neurological disorder

Age

Apolipoprotein E status

---

socioeconomic status are positive factors in the ability to return to work after minor head injury (Rimel et al. 1981).

## Personality Changes

Thomsen (1984) found that 80% of 40 patients with severe TBI had personality changes that persisted for 2–5 years, and 65% had changes lasting 10–15 years after the injury. These changes included childishness (60% and 25%, respectively), emotional lability (40% and 35%, respectively), and restlessness (25% and 38%, respectively). Approximately two-thirds of patients had less social contact, and one-half had loss of spontaneity and poverty of interests after 10–15 years.

Because of the vulnerability of the prefrontal and frontal regions of the cortex to contusions, injury to these regions is common and gives rise to changes in personality known as the frontal lobe syndrome. For the prototypic patient with frontal lobe syndrome, the cognitive functions are preserved while personality changes abound. Psychiatric disturbances associated with frontal lobe injury commonly include impaired social judgment, labile affect, uncharacteristic lewdness, inability to appreciate the effects of one's behavior or remarks on others, a loss of social graces (such as eating manners), a diminution of attention to personal appearance and hygiene, and boisterousness. Impaired judgment may take the form of diminished concern for the future, increased risk taking, unrestrained drinking of alcohol, and indiscriminate selection of food. Patients may appear shallow, indifferent, or apathetic, with a global lack of concern for the consequences of their behavior.

Certain behavioral syndromes have been related to damage to specific areas of the frontal lobe (Auerbach 1986). The orbitofrontal syndrome is associated with behavioral excesses, such as impulsivity, disinhibition, hyperactivity, distractibility, and mood lability. Injury to the dorsolateral frontal cortex may result in slowness, apathy, and perseveration. This may be considered similar to the negative (deficit) symptoms associated with schizophrenia, wherein the patient may exhibit blunted affect, emotional withdrawal, social withdrawal, passivity, and lack of spontaneity (S. R. Kay et al. 1987). As with TBI, deficit symptoms in patients with schizophrenia are thought to result from disordered functioning of the dorsolateral frontal cortex (Berman et al. 1988). Outbursts of rage and violent behavior occur after damage to the inferior orbital surface of the frontal lobe and anterior temporal lobes.

Patients also develop changes in sexual behavior after brain injury, most commonly decreased sex drive, erectile function, and frequency of intercourse (Zasler 1994). Kleine-Levin syndrome—characterized by periodic hypersomnolence, hyperphagia, and behavioral disturbances that include hypersexuality—has also been reported to occur subsequent to brain injury (Will et al. 1988).

In DSM-IV-TR (American Psychiatric Association 2000), these personality changes would be diagnosed as personality change due to traumatic brain injury. Specific subtypes are provided as the most significant clinical problems (Table 38–5).

## Intellectual Changes

Changes can occur in the ability to attend, concentrate, remember, abstract, calculate, reason, plan, and process information (McCullagh and Feinstein 2005). Problems with arousal can take the form of inattentiveness, distractibility, and difficulty switching and dividing attention (Ponsford and Kinsella 1992). Mental sluggishness, poor concentration, and memory problems are common complaints of both patients and relatives (Brooks et al. 1986; McKinlay et al. 1981; Thomsen 1984). High-level cognitive functions, termed *executive functions*, are frequently impaired, although such impairments are difficult to detect and diagnose with cursory cognitive testing (Table 38–6) (McCullagh and Feinstein 2005). Studies suggest that among the long-term sequelae of brain trauma is Alzheimer's disease (Amaducci et al. 1986; Graves et al. 1990).

**TABLE 38–5. DSM-IV-TR diagnostic criteria for personality change due to traumatic brain injury**

A. A persistent personality disturbance that represents a change from the individual's previous characteristic personality pattern. (In children, the disturbance involves a marked deviation from normal development or a significant change in the child's usual behavior patterns lasting at least 1 year).

B. There is evidence from the history, physical examination, or laboratory findings that the disturbance is the direct physiological consequence of a general medical condition.

C. The disturbance is not better accounted for by another mental disorder (including other Mental Disorders Due to a General Medical Condition).

D. The disturbance does not occur exclusively during the course of a delirium.

E. The disturbance causes clinically significant distress or impairment in social, occupational, or other important areas of functioning.

*Specify* type:

**Labile Type:** if the predominant feature is affective lability

**Disinhibited Type:** if the predominant feature is poor impulse control as evidenced by sexual indiscretions, etc.

**Aggressive Type:** if the predominant feature is aggressive behavior

**Apathetic Type:** if the predominant feature is marked apathy and indifference

**Paranoid Type:** if the predominant feature is suspiciousness or paranoid ideation

**Other Type:** if the presentation is not characterized by any of the above subtypes

**Combined Type:** if more than one feature predominates in the clinical picture

**Unspecified Type**

Children who survive head trauma often return to school with behavioral and learning problems (Mahoney et al. 1983). Children with behavioral disorders are much more likely to have a history of prior head injury (Michaud et al. 1993). In addition, children who sustained injury at or before age 2 years had significantly lower IQ scores (Michaud et al. 1993).

**TABLE 38–6. Aspects of executive functions potentially impaired after traumatic brain injury**

Goal establishment, planning, and anticipation of consequences

Initiation, sequencing, and inhibition of behavioral responses

Generation of multiple response alternatives (in contrast to perseverative or stereotyped responses)

Conceptual/inferential reasoning, problem solving

Mental flexibility/ease of mental and behavioral switching

Transcending the immediately salient aspects of a situation (in contrast to "stimulus-bound behavior" or "environmental dependency")

Executive attentional processes

Executive memory processes

Self-monitoring and self-regulation, including emotional responses

Social adaptive functioning: sensitivity to others, using social feedback, engaging in contextually appropriate social behavior

*Source.* Reprinted from McCullagh S, Feinstein A: "Cognitive Changes," in *Textbook of Traumatic Brain Injury.* Edited by Silver JM, McAllister TW, Yudofsky SC. Washington, DC, American Psychiatric Publishing, 2005, pp. 321–335. Used with permission.

## Psychiatric Disorders

Histories of prior psychiatric disorders in individuals with TBI have varied between 17% and 44%, and pre-TBI substance use figures have ranged from 22% to 30% (Jorge et al. 1994; van Reekum et al. 1996). Fann et al. (1995) found that 50% of individuals who had sustained TBI reported a history of psychiatric problems prior to the injury. The Research and Training Center for the Community Integration of Individuals with TBI at Mt. Sinai Medical Center in New York found that in a group of 100 individuals with TBI, 51% had pre-TBI psychiatric disorders, most commonly major depression or substance use disorders, which occurred at rates more than twice those reported in community samples (Hibbard et al. 1998). Fann et al. (2002) analyzed the HMO database of 450,000 members for the occurrence of a TBI and evidence of a psychiatric condition. They found that the relative risk for TBI was 1.3- to 4-fold higher in individuals with a preceding psychiatric diagnosis (24.2% vs. 14.3%).

## Affective Changes

Depression occurs frequently after TBI. There are several diagnostic issues that must be considered in the evaluation of the patient who appears depressed after TBI. Sadness is a common reaction after TBI, as patients describe "mourning" the loss of their "former selves," often a reflection of deficits in intellectual functioning and motoric abilities. Careful psychiatric evaluation is required to distinguish grief reactions, sadness, and demoralization from major depression.

### *Prevalence of Depression After TBI*

The prevalence of depression after brain injury has been assessed through self-report questionnaires, rating scales, and assessments by relatives. For mild TBI, estimates of depressive complaints range from 6% to 39%. For depression after severe TBI, in which patients often have concomitant cognitive impairments, reported rates of depression vary from 10% to 77%.

### *Mania After TBI*

Manic episodes and bipolar disorder have also been reported to occur after TBI (Burstein 1993), although the occurrence is less frequent than that of depression after brain injury (Bakchine et al. 1989; Bamrah and Johnson 1991; Bracken 1987; Clark and Davison 1987; Nizamie et al. 1988). Predisposing factors for the development of mania after brain injury include damage to the basal region of the right temporal lobe (Starkstein et al. 1990) and right orbitofrontal cortex (Starkstein et al. 1988) in patients who have family histories of bipolar disorder.

## Delirium

When a psychiatrist is consulted during the period when a patient with a brain injury is emerging from coma, the usual clinical picture is one of delirium with restlessness, agitation, confusion, disorientation, delusions, and/or hallucinations. Although delirium in patients with TBI is most often the result of the effects of the injury on brain tissue chemistry, the psychiatrist should be aware that there may be other causes for the delirium (such as side effects of medication, withdrawal, or intoxication from drugs ingested before the traumatic event) and environmental factors (such as sensory monotony). Table 38–7 lists common factors that can result in posttraumatic delirium.

**TABLE 38–7.  Causes of delirium in patients with traumatic brain injury**

Mechanical effects (acceleration or deceleration, contusion, and others)

Cerebral edema

Hemorrhage

Infection

Subdural hematoma

Seizure

Hypoxia (cardiopulmonary or local ischemia)

Increased intracranial pressure

Alcohol intoxication or withdrawal, Wernicke's encephalopathy

Reduced hemoperfusion related to multiple trauma

Fat embolism

Change in pH

Electrolyte imbalance

Medications (barbiturates, steroids, opioids, and anticholinergics)

*Source.* Reprinted from Trzepacz PT, Kennedy RE: "Delirium and Posttraumatic Amnesia," in *Textbook of Traumatic Brain Injury*. Edited by Silver JM, McAllister TW, Yudofsky SC. Washington, DC, American Psychiatric Publishing, 2005, pp. 175–200. Used with permission.

## Psychotic Disorders

There is evidence of an interaction between genetic predisposition to schizophrenia and TBI. Malaspina et al. (2001) analyzed data from their study of the effect of TBI on the development of schizophrenia in families with bipolar disorder or schizophrenia. They found that members of the schizophrenia pedigrees, even those without a schizophrenia diagnosis, had greater exposure to TBI compared with members of the bipolar disorder pedigrees. Within the schizophrenia pedigrees, TBI was associated with a greater risk of schizophrenia, consistent with synergistic effects between genetic vulnerability for schizophrenia and TBI.

## Posttraumatic Epilepsy

Posttraumatic epilepsy, with repeated seizures and the requirement for anticonvulsant medication, occurs in approximately 12%, 2%, and 1% of patients with severe, moderate, and mild head injuries, respectively, within

5 years of the injury (Annegers et al. 1980). Risk factors for posttraumatic epilepsy include skull fractures and wounds that penetrate the brain, a history of chronic alcohol use, intracranial hemorrhage, and increased severity of injury (Yablon 1993). Posttraumatic epilepsy is associated with psychosis, especially when seizures arise from the temporal lobes. Brief episodic psychoses may occur with epilepsy; about 7% of patients with epilepsy have persistent psychoses (McKenna et al. 1985). These psychoses exhibit a number of atypical features, including confusion and rapid fluctuations in mood.

## Anxiety Disorders

Several anxiety disorders may develop after TBI (Warden and Labatte 2005). Because of the potential life-threatening nature of many of the causes of TBI, including motor vehicle accidents and assaults, one would expect that these patients are at increased risk of developing posttraumatic stress disorder (PTSD). There is a 9.2% risk of developing PTSD after exposure to trauma, highest for assaultive violence (Breslau et al. 1998).

## Sleep Disorders

It is common for individuals with TBI to complain of disrupted sleep patterns, ranging from hypersomnia to difficulty maintaining sleep (Rao et al. 2005). Fichtenberg and colleagues (2000) assessed 91 individuals with TBI who were admitted to an outpatient neurorehabilitation clinic. The presence of depression (as indicated by score on the Beck Depression Inventory) and mild severity of the TBI were correlated with the occurrence of insomnia.

## Mild Traumatic Brain Injury and Postconcussion Syndrome

Patients with mild TBI may present with somatic, perceptual, cognitive, and emotional symptoms that have been characterized as the *postconcussion syndrome* (Table 38–8). By definition, mild TBI is associated with a brief duration of LOC (less than 20 minutes) or no LOC, and posttraumatic amnesia of less than 24 hours; the patient usually does not require hospitalization after the injury.

Individuals with mild TBI have an increased incidence of somatic complaints, including headache, dizziness, fatigue, sleep disturbance, and sensitivity to noise and light (S.J. Brown et al. 1994; Dikmen et al. 1986; Levin et al. 1987b; Rimel et al. 1981).

**TABLE 38–8.** **Postconcussion syndrome**

**Somatic symptoms**
Headache
Dizziness
Fatigue
Insomnia
**Cognitive symptoms**
Memory difficulties
Impaired concentration
**Perceptual symptoms**
Tinnitus
Sensitivity to noise
Sensitivity to light
**Emotional symptoms**
Depression
Anxiety
Irritability

*Source.* Adapted from Lishman 1988.

Therefore, there may be two groups of mild TBI patients: those who recover by 3 months and those who have persistent symptoms. It is not known whether the persistent symptoms are part of a cohesive syndrome or simply represent a collection of loosely related symptoms resulting from the vagaries of an individual injury (Alves et al. 1986). However, it is increasingly recognized that "mild" TBI and concussions that occur in sports injuries result in clinically significant neuropsychological impairment (Freeman et al. 2005).

In an extensive review of the literature, Alexander (1995) highlighted several important aspects regarding patients who develop prolonged postconcussion syndrome: 1) they are more likely to have been under stress at the time of the accident, 2) they develop depression and/or anxiety soon after the accident, 3) they have extensive social disruption after the accident, and 4) they have problems with physical symptoms such as headache and dizziness.

The treatment of patients with mild TBI involves initiating several key interventions (T. Kay 1993). In the early phase of treatment, the major goal is prevention of the postconcussion syndrome. This involves providing information and education about understanding and predicting symptoms and their resolution and actively managing a gradual process of return to functioning. Education about the postconcussion syndrome and its natural history improves prognosis (Wade et al. 1998).

## Aggression

Individuals who have traumatic brain injury may experience irritability, agitation, and aggressive behavior (Silver et al. 2005). These episodes range in severity from irritability to outbursts that result in damage to property or assaults on others. In severe cases, affected individuals cannot remain in the community or with their families and often are referred to long-term psychiatric or neurobehavioral facilities. Increased isolation and separation from others often occur.

In the acute recovery period, 35%–96% of patients are reported to have exhibited agitated behavior (Silver et al. 2005). After the acute recovery phase, irritability or bad temper is common.

Carlsson et al. (1987) examined the relationship between the number of traumatic brain injuries associated with LOC and various symptoms, and they demonstrated that irritability increases with subsequent injuries. Of the men who did not have head injuries with LOC, 21% reported irritability, whereas 31% of men with one injury with LOC and 33% of men with two or more injuries with LOC admitted to this symptom ($P<0.0001$).

Explosive and violent behaviors have long been associated with focal brain lesions as well as with diffuse damage to the central nervous system (Anderson and Silver 1999). The current diagnostic category in DSM-IV-TR is personality change due to a general medical condition (American Psychiatric Association 2000). Patients with aggressive behavior would be specified as aggressive type, whereas those with mood lability are specified as labile type. Characteristic behavioral features occur in many individuals who exhibit aggressive behavior after brain injury (Yudofsky et al. 1990). Typically, violence seen in these patients is *reactive* (i.e., triggered by modest or trivial stimuli). It is *nonreflective*, in that it does not involve premeditation of planning, and *nonpurposeful*, in the sense that the aggression serves no obvious long-term aims or goals. The violence is *periodic*, with brief outbursts of rage and aggression interspersed between long periods of relatively calm behavior. The aggression is *ego-dystonic*, such that the individual is often upset or embarrassed after the episode. Finally, it is generally *explosive*, occurring suddenly with no apparent buildup.

## Psychopharmacological Treatment

There are several general guidelines that should be followed in the pharmacological treatment of patients with the psychiatric syndromes that occur after TBI: 1) start low, go slow, 2) conduct a therapeutic trial of all medications, 3) maintain continuous reassessment of clinical condition, 4) monitor drug-drug interactions, 5) augment partial response, and 6) discontinue or lower the dose of the most recently prescribed medication if there is a worsening of the treated symptom soon after the medication had been initiated (or increased).

## Affective Illness

### Depression

**Guidelines for using antidepressants for patients with TBI.** The choice of an antidepressant depends predominantly on the desired side-effect profile. Usually, antidepressants with the fewest sedative, hypotensive, and anticholinergic side effects are preferred. Thus, the selective serotonin reuptake inhibitors (SSRIs) are usually the first-line medications prescribed.

ECT remains a highly effective and underused modality for the treatment of depression overall, and ECT can be used effectively after acute or severe TBI (Kant et al. 1999; Ruedrich et al. 1983). If the patient has preexisting memory impairment, nondominant unilateral ECT should be used.

**Side effects.** The most common and disabling antidepressant side effects in patients with TBI are the anticholinergic effects, especially with the older heterocyclic antidepressants. These medications may impair attention, concentration, and memory, especially in patients with brain lesions. SSRIs, venlafaxine, and bupropion all have minimal or no anticholinergic action.

In some individuals, SSRIs may result in word-finding problems or apathy. This may be due to the effects of SSRIs in decreasing dopaminergic functioning, and it may be reversible with the addition of a dopaminergic or stimulant medication.

The available evidence suggests that, overall, antidepressants may be associated with a greater frequency of seizures in patients with brain injury. The antidepressants maprotiline and bupropion may be associated with a higher incidence of seizures (Davidson 1989; Pinder et al. 1977).

### Mania

Manic episodes that occur after TBI have been successfully treated with lithium carbonate, carbamazepine (Stewart and Nemsath 1988), valproic acid (Pope et al.

1988), clonidine (Bakchine et al. 1989), and ECT (Clark and Davison 1987). Lamotrigine and gabapentin are other options. Because of the increased incidence of side effects when lithium is used in patients with brain lesions, we limit the use of lithium in patients with TBI to those with mania or with recurrent depressive illness that preceded their brain damage.

### Lability of Mood and Affect

The classic disorder of affective dysregulation is pathological laughing and/or crying (PLC), also sometimes referred to as "emotional incontinence" or "pseudobulbar affect." Patients with this condition experience episodes of involuntary crying and/or laughing that may occur many times per day, are often provoked by trivial (i.e., not sentimental) stimuli, are quite stereotyped in their presentation, are uncontrollable, do not evoke a concordant subjective affective experience, and do not produce a persistent change in the prevailing mood (Poeck 1985).

## Cognitive Function and Arousal

Stimulants, such as dextroamphetamine and methylphenidate, and dopamine agonists, such as amantadine and bromocriptine, may be beneficial in treating the patient with apathy and impaired concentration to increase arousal and to diminish fatigue. These medications all act on the catecholaminergic system but in different ways. Dextroamphetamine blocks the reuptake of norepinephrine and, in higher doses, also blocks the reuptake of dopamine. Methylphenidate has a similar mechanism of action. Amantadine acts both presynaptically and postsynaptically at the dopamine receptor and may also increase cholinergic and GABAergic activity (Cowell and Cohen 1995). In addition, amantadine is an $N$-methyl-D-aspartate (NMDA) glutamate receptor antagonist (Weller and Kornhuber 1992). Bromocriptine is a dopamine type 1 receptor antagonist and a dopamine type 2 receptor agonist. It appears to be a dopamine agonist at midrange doses (Berg et al. 1987).

### Dextroamphetamine and Methylphenidate

Several reports have indicated that impairments in verbal memory and learning, attention, and behavior are alleviated with either dextroamphetamine or methylphenidate (Bleiberg et al. 1993; Evans et al. 1987; Kaelin et al. 1996; Lipper and Tuchman 1976; Weinberg et al. 1987; Weinstein and Wells 1981).

When used, methylphenidate should be initiated at 5 mg twice daily and dextroamphetamine at 2.5 mg twice daily. Maximum dosage of each medication is usually 60 mg/day, administered twice daily or three times daily. However, we have seen some patients who have required higher dosages of methylphenidate to obtain a reasonable serum level of 15 mg/mL.

### Amantadine

Amantadine may be beneficial in the treatment of anergia, abulia, mutism, and anhedonia subsequent to brain injury (Chandler et al. 1988; Cowell and Cohen 1995; Gualtieri et al. 1989; Nickels et al. 1994). M.F. Kraus and Maki (1997) administered amantadine 400 mg/day to six patients with TBI. Improvement was found in motivation, attention, and alertness, as well as executive function and dyscontrol. Dosages should initially be 50 mg twice daily and should be increased every week by 100 mg/day to a maximum dosage of 400 mg/day.

### Side Effects of Medications for Impaired Concentration and Arousal

Adverse reactions to medications for impaired concentration and arousal are most often related to increases in dopamine activity. Dexedrine and methylphenidate may lead to paranoia, dysphoria, agitation, and irritability. Depression often occurs on discontinuation, so stimulants should be discontinued using a slow regimen. Interestingly, there may be a role for stimulants to increase neuronal recovery subsequent to brain injury (Crisostomo et al. 1988). Side effects of bromocriptine include sedation, nausea, psychosis, headaches, and delirium. Amantadine may cause confusion, hallucinations, edema, and hypotension; these reactions occur more often in elderly patients.

## Problems With Processing Multiple Stimuli

Although individuals with TBI may have difficulty with maintaining attention on single tasks, they can also have difficulty in processing multiple stimuli. This difficulty has been called an abnormality in auditory gating, and it is consistent with an abnormal response in processing auditory stimuli that are given 50 milliseconds apart (P50 response) (Arciniegas et al. 2000). Preliminary evidence suggests that this response normalizes after treatment with donepezil 5 mg, which also results in symptomatic improvement (Arciniegas et al. 2001).

## Fatigue

Stimulants (methylphenidate and dextroamphetamine) and amantadine can diminish the profound daytime fatigue experienced by patients with TBI. Dosages utilized would be similar to those used for treatment of diminished arousal and concentration. Modafinil, a medication recently approved for the treatment of excessive daytime somnolence in patients with narcolepsy, also may have a role in treatment of post-TBI fatigue.

## Cognition

### *Cholinesterase Inhibitors*

TBI may produce cognitive impairments via disruption of cholinergic function (Arciniegas et al. 1999), and the relative sensitivity of TBI patients to medications with anticholinergic agents has prompted speculation that cognitively impaired TBI patients may have a relatively reduced reserve of cholinergic function. With the advent of relatively centrally selective acetylcholinesterase inhibitors such as donepezil, the issue of cholinergic augmentation strategies in the treatment of cognitive impairment following TBI is currently being revisited, and preliminary reports suggest that donepezil may improve memory and global functioning (Kaye et al. 2003; Morey et al. 2003; Taverni et al. 1998; Whelan et al. 2000; Zhang et al. 2004).

## Psychosis

The psychotic ideation resulting from TBI is generally responsive to treatment with antipsychotic medications. However, side effects such as hypotension, sedation, and confusion are common. Also, brain-injured patients are particularly subject to dystonia, akathisia, and other parkinsonian side effects—even at relatively low doses of antipsychotic medications (Wolf et al. 1989). Antipsychotic medications have also been reported to impede neuronal recovery after brain injury (Feeney et al. 1982). Therefore, we advise that antipsychotics should be used sparingly during the acute phases of recovery after the injury. Of the newer "atypical" antipsychotic medications, quetiapine has the fewest extrapyramidal effects. Risperidone, olanzapine, aripiprazole, and ziprasidone may all have a role in the treatment of post-TBI psychosis, although published literature is limited. In general, we recommend a low-dose neuroleptic strategy for all patients with neuropsychiatric disorders. Clozapine is a novel and effective antipsychotic medication that does not produce extrapyramidal side effects.

Among all the first-generation antipsychotic drugs, molindone and fluphenazine have consistently demonstrated the lowest potential for lowering the seizure threshold (Oliver et al. 1982). Clozapine treatment is associated with a significant dose-related incidence of seizures (ranging from 1% to 2% of patients who receive doses below 300 mg/day and 5% of patients who receive 600–900 mg/day); thus, in patients with TBI it must be used with extreme caution and for most carefully considered indications (Lieberman et al. 1989).

## Sleep

Sleep patterns of patients with brain damage are often disordered, with impaired rapid eye movement (REM) recovery and multiple nocturnal awakenings (Prigatano et al. 1982). Hypersomnia that occurs after severe missile head injury most often resolves within the first year after injury, whereas insomnia that occurs in patients with long periods of coma and diffuse injury has a more chronic course (Askenasy et al. 1989). Barbiturates and long-acting benzodiazepines should be prescribed for sedation with great caution, if at all. These drugs interfere with REM and Stage IV sleep patterns and may contribute to persistent insomnia (Buysse and Reynolds 1990). Clinicians should warn patients of the dangers of using over-the-counter preparations for sleeping and for colds because of the prominent anticholinergic side effects of these agents.

Trazodone, a sedating antidepressant medication that is devoid of anticholinergic side effects, may be used for nighttime sedation. A dose of 50 mg should be administered initially; if this is ineffective, doses up to 150 mg may be prescribed. Nonpharmacological approaches should be considered. These include minimizing daytime naps, adhering to regular sleep times, and engaging in regular physical activity during the day.

## Aggression and Agitation

Although there is no medication approved by the U.S. Food and Drug Administration (FDA) that is specifically for the treatment of aggression, medications are widely used (and commonly misused) in the management of patients with acute or chronic aggression. (e.g., as with anticonvulsants), to reduce "hyperactive" limbic monoaminergic neurotransmission (e.g., noradrenergic blockade with propranolol, dopaminergic blockade with haloperidol), to augment orbitofrontal and/or dorsolateral prefrontal cortical activity with monoaminergic agonists (e.g., amantadine, methylphenidate, and perhaps buspirone), or to increase serotonergic input (SSRIs). Unfortunately, there is a paucity of rigorous double-blind, placebo-controlled studies (i.e., "Level I" studies) or even prospective cohort studies (i.e., "Level II" studies) to guide clinicians in the use of pharmacological interventions.

### Chronic Aggression

If a patient continues to exhibit periods of agitation or aggression beyond several weeks, the use of specific anti-aggressive medications should be initiated to prevent these episodes from occurring. Because no medication has been approved by the FDA for treatment of aggression, the clinician must use medications that may be anti-aggressive but that have been approved for other uses (e.g., seizure disorders, depression, hypertension) (Silver and Yudofsky 1994; Yudofsky et al. 1998).

**Antipsychotic medications.** If, after thorough clinical evaluation, it is determined that the aggressive episodes result from psychosis, such as paranoid delusions or command hallucinations, then antipsychotic medications will be the treatment of choice. Risperidone has been used to treat agitation in elderly patients with dementia with good results (Goldberg and Goldberg 1995). Olanzapine appears to be more sedating, and quetiapine may have fewer extrapyramidal symptoms than does risperidone. Clozapine may have greater antiaggressive effects than other antipsychotic medications (Michals et al. 1993; Ratey et al. 1993). However, the increased risk of seizures must be carefully assessed.

**Antianxiety medications.** Serotonin appears to be a key neurotransmitter in the modulation of aggressive behavior. In preliminary reports, buspirone, a serotonin type 1A agonist, has been reported to be effective in the management of aggression and agitation for patients with head injury, dementia, and developmental disabilities and autism (Silver and Yudofsky 1994; Yudofsky et al. 1998). In rare instances, some patients become more aggressive when treated with buspirone. Therefore, buspirone should be initiated at low dosages (i.e., 5 mg twice daily) and increased by 5 mg every 3–5 days. Dosages of 45–60 mg/day may be required before there is improvement in aggressive behavior, although we have noted dramatic improvement within 1 week.

Clonazepam may be effective in the long-term management of aggression, although controlled, double-blind studies have not yet been conducted.

**Anticonvulsive medications.** Several open studies have indicated that carbamazepine may be effective in decreasing aggressive behavior associated with TBI dementia (Chatham-Showalter 1996), developmental disabilities, and schizophrenia and in patients with a variety of other organic brain disorders (Silver and Yudofsky 1994; Yudofsky et al. 1998).

Valproic acid may also be helpful to some patients with organically induced aggression (Geracioti 1994; Giakas et al. 1990; Horne and Lindley 1995; Mattes 1992; Wroblewski et al. 1997). For patients with aggression and epilepsy whose seizures are being treated with anticonvulsant drugs such as phenytoin and phenobarbital, switching to carbamazepine or to valproic acid may treat both conditions.

Gabapentin may be beneficial for the treatment of agitation in patients with dementia (Herrmann et al. 2000; Roane et al. 2000). Dosages have ranged from 200–2400 mg/day.

**Antimanic medications.** Patients with brain injury have increased sensitivity to the neurotoxic effects of lithium (Hornstein and Seliger 1989; Moskowitz and Altshuler 1991). Because of lithium's potential for neurotoxicity and its relative lack of efficacy in many patients with aggression secondary to brain injury, we limit the use of lithium in patients whose aggression is related to manic effects or recurrent irritability related to cyclic mood disorders.

**Antidepressants.** The antidepressants that have been reported to control aggressive behavior are those that act preferentially (amitriptyline) or specifically (trazodone and fluoxetine) on serotonin. Fluoxetine has been reported to be effective in the treatment of aggressive behavior in a patient who sustained brain injury as well as in patients with personality disorders and depression, and adolescents with mental retardation and self-injurious behavior (Silver and Yudofsky 1994; Yudofsky et al. 1998). We have used SSRIs with considerable success in aggressive patients with brain lesions. The dosages used are similar to those for the treatment of mood lability and depression.

We have evaluated and treated many patients with emotional lability that is characterized by frequent episodes of tearfulness and irritability and the full symptomatic picture of neuroaggressive syndrome (Silver and Yudofsky 1994). These patients—who would be diagnosed under DSM-IV with personality change, labile type, due to traumatic brain injury—have responded well to antidepressants.

**Antihypertensive medications: beta-blockers.**
Since the first report of the use of β-adrenergic receptor blockers in the treatment of acute aggression in 1977, more than 25 articles have appeared in the neurologic and psychiatric literature reporting experience in using β-blockers with more than 200 patients with aggression (Yudofsky et al. 1987). Most of these patients had been unsuccessfully treated with antipsychotics, minor tranquilizers, lithium, and/or anticonvulsants before being treated with β-blockers. The β-blockers that have been investigated in controlled prospective studies include propranolol (a lipid-soluble, nonselective receptor antagonist), nadolol (a water-soluble, nonselective receptor antagonist), and pindolol (a lipid-soluble, nonselective β receptor antagonist with partial sympathomimetic activity).

A growing body of preliminary evidence suggests that β-adrenergic receptor blockers are effective agents for the treatment of aggressive and violent behaviors, particularly those related to organic brain syndrome. The effectiveness of propranolol in reducing agitation has been demonstrated during the initial hospitalization after TBI (Brooke et al. 1992). When a patient requires the use of a once-a-day medication because of compliance difficulties, long-acting propranolol (i.e., Inderal LA) or nadolol (Corgard) can be used. When patients develop bradycardia that prevents prescribing therapeutic dosages of propranolol, pindolol (Visken) can be substituted, using one-tenth the dosage of propranolol. The intrinsic sympathomimetic activity of pindolol stimulates the β receptor and restricts the development of bradycardia.

## Behavioral and Cognitive Treatments

Behavioral treatments are important in the care of patients who have sustained TBI. These programs require careful design and execution by a staff well versed in behavioral techniques. Behavioral methods can be used in response to aggressive outbursts and other maladaptive social behaviors (Corrigan and Bach 2005). One study (Eames and Wood 1985) found that behavior modification was 75% effective in dealing with disturbed behavior after severe brain injury.

After brain injury, patients may need specific cognitive strategies to assist with impairments in memory and concentration (Cicerone et al. 2005; Gordon and Hibbard 2005). As opposed to earlier beliefs that cognitive therapy should "exercise" the brain to develop skills that have been damaged, current therapies involve teaching the patient new strategies to compensate for lost or impaired functions. Salazar et al. (2000) for the Defense and Veterans Head Injury Program Study Group compared an intensive 8-week in-hospital cognitive rehabilitation program to a limited home program. Both groups improved, but there was no significant difference between the two treatments.

## Key Points: Traumatic Brain Injury

- Traumatic brain injury (TBI) is associated with impairment in several domains of neuropsychiatric function, including personality changes and intellectual deficits.
- The initial psychiatric presentation of the TBI patient emerging from coma is usually delirium, which is attributed to many factors.
- Patients with mild TBI may present with somatic and neuropsychiatric symptoms referred to as the *postconcussion syndrome.*
- Psychopharmacological treatment of TBI patients often includes modifications of typical psychopharmacological strategies.
- TBI patients may experience chronic aggression and/or agitation.

## References

Alexander MP: Mild traumatic brain injury: pathophysiology, natural history, and clinical management. Neurology 45:1253–1260, 1995

Alves WM, Coloban ART, O'Leary TJ, et al: Understanding posttraumatic symptoms after minor head injury. J Head Trauma Rehabil 1:1–12, 1986

Amaducci LA, Fratiglioni L, Rocca WA, et al: Risk factors for clinically diagnosed Alzheimer's disease: a case control study of an Italian population. Neurology 36:922–931, 1986

American Psychiatric Association: Diagnostic and Statistical Manual of Mental Disorders, 4th Edition, Text Revision. Washington, DC, American Psychiatric Association, 2000

Anderson KE, Silver JM: Neurological and mental diseases and violence, in Medical Management of the Violent Patient. Edited by Tardiff K. New York, Marcel Dekker, 1999, pp 87–124

Annegers JF, Grabow JD, Groover RV, et al: Seizures after head trauma: a population study. Neurology 30:683–689, 1980

Arciniegas D, Adler L, Topkoff J, et al: Attention and memory dysfunction after traumatic brain injury: cholinergic mechanisms, sensory gating, and a hypothesis for further investigation. Brain Inj 13:1–13, 1999

Arciniegas DB, Topkoff J, Silver JM: Neuropsychiatric aspects of traumatic brain injury. Curr Treat Options Neurol 2:169–186, 2000

Arciniegas DB, Topkoff JL, Anderson CA, et al: Normalization of P50 physiology by donepezil hydrochloride in traumatic brain injury patients (abstract). J Neuropsychiatry Clin Neurosci 13:140, 2001

Askenasy JJM, Winkler I, Grushkiewicz J, et al: The natural history of sleep disturbances in severe missile head injury. J Neurol Rehabil 3:93–96, 1989

Auerbach SH: Neuroanatomical correlates of attention and memory disorders in traumatic brain injury: an application of neurobehavioral subtypes. J Head Trauma Rehabil 1:1–12, 1986

Bakchine S, Lacomblez L, Benoit N, et al: Manic-like state after bilateral orbitofrontal and right temporoparietal injury: efficacy of clonidine. Neurology 39:777–781, 1989

Bamrah JS, Johnson J: Bipolar affective disorder following head injury. Br J Psychiatry 158:117–119, 1991

Berg MJ, Ebert B, Willis DK, et al: Parkinsonism—drug treatment: part I. Drug Intell Clin Pharm 21:10–21, 1987

Berman KF, Illowsky BP, Weinberger DR: Physiological dysfunction of dorsolateral prefrontal cortex in schizophrenia, IV: further evidence for regional and behavioral specificity. Arch Gen Psychiatry 45:616–622, 1988

Bigler ED: Structural imaging, in Textbook of Traumatic Brain Injury. Edited by Silver JM, McAllister TW, Yudofsky SC. Washington, DC, American Psychiatric Publishing, 2005, pp 79–106

Bleiberg J, Garmoe W, Cederquist J, et al: Effects of Dexedrine on performance consistency following brain injury: a double-blind placebo crossover case study. Neuropsychiatry Neuropsychol Behav Neurol 6:245–248, 1993

Bracken P: Mania following head injury. Br J Psychiatry 150:690–692, 1987

Breslau N, Kessler RC, Chilcoat HD, et al: Trauma and post-traumatic stress disorder in the community: the 1996 Detroit Area Survey of Trauma. Arch Gen Psychiatry 55:626–632, 1998

Brooke MM, Patterson DR, Questad KA, et al: The treatment of agitation during initial hospitalization after traumatic brain injury. Arch Phys Med Rehabil 73:917–921, 1992

Brooks N, Campsie L, Symington C, et al: The five year outcome of severe blunt head injury: a relative's view. J Neurol Neurosurg Psychiatry 49:764–770, 1986

Brown G, Chadwick O, Shaffer D, et al: A prospective study of children with head injuries, III: psychiatric sequelae. Psychol Med 11:63–78, 1981

Brown SJ, Fann JR, Grant I: Postconcussional disorder: time to acknowledge a common source of neurobehavioral morbidity. J Neuropsychiatry Clin Neurosci 6:15–22, 1994

Burstein A: Bipolar and pure mania disorders precipitated by head trauma. Psychosomatics 34:194–195, 1993

Buysse DJ, Reynolds CF III: Insomnia, in Handbook of Sleep Disorders. Edited by Thorpy MJ. New York, Marcel Dekker, 1990, pp 373–434

Carlsson GS, Svardsudd K, Welin L: Long-term effects of head injuries sustained during life in three male populations. J Neurosurg 67:197–205, 1987

Chambers J, Cohen SS, Hemminger L, et al: Mild traumatic brain injuries in low-risk trauma patients. J Trauma 41:976–979, 1996

Chandler MC, Barnhill JL, Gualtieri CT: Amantadine for the agitated head-injury patient. Brain Inj 2:309–311, 1988

Chatham-Showalter PE: Carbamazepine for combativeness in acute traumatic brain injury. J Neuropsychiatry Clin Neurosci 8:96–99, 1996

Cicerone KD, Dahlberg C, Malec JF, et al: Evidence-based cognitive rehabilitation: updated review of the literature from 1998 through 2002. Arch Phys Med Rehabil 86:1681–1692, 2005

Clark AF, Davison K: Mania following head injury: a report of two cases and a review of the literature. Br J Psychiatry 150:841–844, 1987

Committee on Head Injury Nomenclature: Report of the Ad Hoc Committee to study head injury nomenclature: proceedings of the Congress of Neurological Surgeons in 1964. Clin Neurosurg 12:386–394, 1966

Cope DN, Date ES, Mar EY: Serial computerized tomographic evaluations in traumatic head injury. Arch Phys Med Rehabil 69:483–486, 1988

Corrigan PW, Bach PA: Behavioral treatment, in Textbook of Traumatic Brain Injury. Edited by Silver JM, McAllister TW, Yudofsky SC. Washington, DC, American Psychiatric Publishing, 2005, pp 661–678

Cowell LC, Cohen RF: Amantadine: a potential adjuvant therapy following traumatic brain injury. J Head Trauma Rehabil 10:91–94, 1995

Crawford C: Social problems after severe head injury. NZ Med J 96:972–974, 1983

Crisostomo EA, Duncan PW, Propst M, et al: Evidence that amphetamine with physical therapy promotes recovery of motor function in stroke patients. Ann Neurol 23:94–97, 1988

Dikmen S, Machamer JE: Neurobehavioral outcomes and their determinants. J Head Trauma Rehabil 10:74–86, 1995

Dikmen S, McLean A, Temkin N: Neuropsychological and psychosocial consequences of minor head injury. J Neurol Neurosurg Psychiatry 49:1227–1232, 1986

Eames P, Wood R: Rehabilitation after severe brain injury: a follow-up study of a behavior modification approach. J Neurol Neurosurg Psychiatry 48:613–619, 1985

Evans RW, Gualtieri CT, Patterson D: Treatment of chronic closed head injury with psychostimulant drugs: a controlled case study and an appropriate evaluation procedure. J Nerv Ment Dis 175:106–110, 1987

Fann JR, Katon WJ, Uomoto JM, et al: Psychiatric disorders and functional disability in outpatients with traumatic brain injuries. Am J Psychiatry 152:1493–1499, 1995

Fann JR, Leonetti A, Jaffe K, et al: Psychiatric illness and subsequent traumatic brain injury: a case control study. J Neurol Neurosurg Psychiatry 72:615–620, 2002

Feeney DM, Gonzalez A, Law WA: Amphetamine, haloperidol, and experience interact to affect rate of recovery after motor cortex injury. Science 217:855–857, 1982

Fichtenberg NL, Millis SR, Mann NR, et al: Factors associated with insomnia among post-acute traumatic brain injury survivors. Brain Inj 14:659–667, 2000

Freeman JR, Barth JT, Broshek DK, et al: Sports injuries, in Textbook of Traumatic Brain Injury. Edited by Silver JM, McAllister TW, Yudofsky SC. Washington, DC, American Psychiatric Publishing, 2005, pp 453–476

Geracioti TD: Valproic acid treatment of episodic explosiveness related to brain injury. J Clin Psychiatry 55:416–417, 1994

Giakas WJ, Seibyl JP, Mazure CM: Valproate in the treatment of temper outbursts (letter). J Clin Psychiatry 51:525, 1990

Goldberg RJ, Goldberg JS: Low-dose risperidone for dementia related disturbed behavior in nursing home. Paper presented at the annual meeting of the American Psychiatric Association, Miami, FL, May 20–25, 1995

Goodin DS, Aminoff MJ, Laxer KD: Detection of epileptiform activity by different noninvasive EEG methods in complex partial epilepsy. Ann Neurol 27:330–334, 1990

Gordon WA, Hibbard MR: Cognitive rehabilitation, in Textbook of Traumatic Brain Injury. Edited by Silver JM, McAllister TW, Yudofsky SC. Washington, DC, American Psychiatric Publishing, 2005, pp 655–660

Graves AB, White E, Koepsell TD, et al: The association between head trauma and Alzheimer's disease. Am J Epidemiol 131:491–501, 1990

Gualtieri T, Chandler M, Coons TB, et al: Amantadine: a new clinical profile for traumatic brain injury. Clin Neuropharmacol 12:258–270, 1989

Herrmann N, Lanctot K, Myszak M: Effectiveness of gabapentin for the treatment of behavioral disorders in dementia. J Clin Psychopharmacol 20:90–93, 2000

Hibbard MR, Uysal S, Kepler K, et al: Axis I psychopathology in individuals with traumatic brain injury. J Head Trauma Rehabil 13:24–39, 1998

Horne M, Lindley SE: Divalproex sodium in the treatment of aggressive behavior and dysphoria in patients with organic brain syndromes. J Clin Psychiatry 56:430–431, 1995

Hornstein A, Seliger G: Cognitive side effects of lithium in closed head injury (letter). J Neuropsychiatry Clin Neurosci 1:446–447, 1989

Jorge RE, Robinson RG, Starkstein SE, et al: Influence of major depression on 1-year outcome in patients with traumatic brain injury. J Neurosurg 81:726–733, 1994

Kaelin DL, Cifu DX, Matthies B: Methylphenidate effect on attention deficit in the acutely brain-injured adult. Arch Phys Med Rehabil 77:6–9, 1996

Kant R, Coffey CE, Bogyi AM: Safety and efficacy of ECT in patients with head injury: a case series. J Neuropsychiatry Clin Neurosci 11:32–37, 1999

Kay SR, Fiszbein A, Opler LA: The Positive and Negative Syndrome Scale (PANSS) for schizophrenia. Schizophr Bull 13:261–276, 1987

Kay T: Neuropsychological treatment of mild traumatic brain injury. J Head Trauma Rehabil 8:74–85, 1993

Kaye NS, Townsend JB 3rd, Ivins R: An open-label trial of donepezil (Aricept) in the treatment of persons with mild traumatic brain injury. J Neuropsychiatry Clin Neurosci 15:383–384, 2003

Kelly JP: Concussion, in Current Therapy in Sports Medicine, 3rd Edition. Edited by Torg JS, Shephard RJ. Philadelphia, PA, CV Mosby, 1995, pp 21–24

Kim E: Elderly, in Textbook of Traumatic Brain Injury. Edited by Silver JM, McAllister TW, Yudofsky SC. Washington, DC, American Psychiatric Publishing, 2005, pp 495–508

Kraus MF, Maki PM: Effect of amantadine hydrochloride on symptoms of frontal lobe dysfunction in brain injury: case studies and review. J Neuropsychiatry Clin Neurosci 9:222–230, 1997

Kraus JF, Morgenstern H, Fife D, et al: Blood alcohol tests, prevalence of involvement, and outcomes following brain injury. Am J Public Health 79:294–299, 1989

Levin HS, Amparo E, Eisenberg HM, et al: Magnetic resonance imaging and computerized tomography in relation to the neurobehavioral sequelae of mild and moderate head injuries. J Neurosurg 66:706–713, 1987a

Levin HS, Mattis S, Ruff RM, et al: Neurobehavioral outcome following minor head injury: a three-center study. J Neurosurg 66:234–243, 1987b

Lieberman JA, Kane JM, Johns CA: Clozapine: guidelines for clinical management. J Clin Psychiatry 50:329–338, 1989

Lipper S, Tuchman MM: Treatment of chronic post-traumatic organic brain syndrome with dextroamphetamine: first reported case. J Nerv Ment Dis 162:366–371, 1976

Lishman WA: Physiogenesis and psychogenesis in the "post-concussional syndrome." Br J Psychiatry 153:460–469, 1988

Mahoney WJ, D'Souza BJ, Haller JA, et al: Long-term outcome of children with severe head trauma and prolonged coma. Pediatrics 71:754–762, 1983

Malaspina D, Goetz RR, Friedman JH, et al: Traumatic brain injury and schizophrenia in members of schizophrenia and bipolar disorder pedigrees. Am J Psychiatry 36:1278–1285, 2001

Mattes JA: Valproic acid for nonaffective aggression in the mentally retarded. J Nerv Ment Dis 180:601–602, 1992

McCullagh S, Feinstein A: Cognitive changes, in Textbook of Traumatic Brain Injury. Edited by Silver JM, McAllister TW, Yudofsky SC. Washington, DC, American Psychiatric Publishing, 2005, pp 321–335

McKenna PJ, Kane JM, Parrish K: Psychotic syndromes in epilepsy. Am J Psychiatry 142:895–904, 1985

McKinlay WW, Brooks DN, Bond MR, et al: The short-term outcome of severe blunt head injury as reported by the relatives of the injured person. J Neurol Neurosurg Psychiatry 44:527–533, 1981

McLean A Jr, Dikmen S, Temkin N, et al: Psychosocial functioning at 1 month after head injury. Neurosurgery 14:393–399, 1984

Michals ML, Crismon ML, Roberts S, et al: Clozapine response and adverse effects in nine brain-injured patients. J Clin Psychopharmacol 13:198–203, 1993

Michaud LJ, Rivara FP, Jaffe KM, et al: Traumatic brain injury as a risk factor for behavioral disorders in children. Arch Phys Med Rehabil 74:368–375, 1993

Mild Traumatic Brain Injury Committee of the Head Injury Interdisciplinary Special Interest Group of the American Congress of Rehabilitation Medicine: Definition of mild traumatic brain injury. J Head Trauma Rehabil 8:86–87, 1993

Mittl RL, Grossman RI, Hiehle JF, et al: Prevalence of MR evidence of diffuse axonal injury in patients with mild head injury and normal head CT findings. AJNR Am J Neuroradiol 15:1583–1589, 1994

Morey CE, Cilo M, Berry J, et al: The effect of Aricept in persons with persistent memory disorder following traumatic brain injury: a pilot study. Brain Inj 17:809–816, 2003

Moskowitz AS, Altshuler L: Increased sensitivity to lithium-induced neurotoxicity after stroke: a case report. J Clin Psychopharmacol 11:272–273, 1991

Nickels JL, Schneider WN, Dombovy ML, et al: Clinical use of amantadine in brain injury rehabilitation. Brain Inj 8:709–718, 1994

NIH Consensus Development Panel on Rehabilitation of Persons With Traumatic Brain Injury: Rehabilitation of persons with traumatic brain injury. JAMA 282:974–983, 1999

Nizamie SH, Nizamie A, Borde M, et al: Mania following head injury: case reports and neuropsychological findings. Acta Psychiatr Scand 77:637–639, 1988

Oddy M, Coughlan T, Tyerman A, et al: Social adjustment after closed head injury: a further follow-up seven years after injury. J Neurol Neurosurg Psychiatry 48:564–568, 1985

Oliver AP, Luchins DJ, Wyatt RJ: Neuroleptic-induced seizures: an in vitro technique for assessing relative risk. Arch Gen Psychiatry 39:206–209, 1982

Orrison WW, Gentry LR, Stimac GK, et al: Blinded comparison of cranial CT and MR in closed head injury evaluation. AJNR Am J Neuroradiol 15:351–356, 1994

Pinder RM, Brogden RN, Speight TM, et al: Maprotiline: a review of its pharmacological properties and therapeutic efficacy in mental states. Drugs 13:321–352, 1977

Poeck K: Pathological laughter and crying, in Handbook of Clinical Neurology, Vol. 45: Clinical Neuropsychology, No 1. Edited by Fredericks JAM. Amsterdam, Elsevier, 1985, pp 219–225

Ponsford J, Kinsella G: Attention deficits following closed head injury. J Clin Exp Neuropsychol 14:822–838, 1992

Pope HG Jr, McElroy SL, Satlin A, et al: Head injury, bipolar disorder, and response to valproate. Compr Psychiatry 29:34–38, 1988

Prigatano GP, Stahl ML, Orr WC, et al: Sleep and dreaming disturbances in closed head injury patients. J Neurol Neurosurg Psychiatry 45:78–80, 1982

Quality Standards Subcommittee of the American Academy of Neurology: Practice parameter. Neurobiology (Bp) 48:1–5, 1997

Rao V, Rollings P, Spiro J: Fatigue and sleep problems, in Textbook of Traumatic Brain Injury. Edited by Silver JM, McAllister TW, Yudofsky SC. Washington, DC, American Psychiatric Publishing, 2005, pp 369–384

Ratey JJ, Leveroni C, Kilmer D, et al: The effects of clozapine on severely aggressive psychiatric inpatients in a state hospital. J Clin Psychiatry 54:219–223, 1993

Rimel RW, Giordani B, Barht JT, et al: Disability caused by minor head injury. Neurosurgery 9:221–228, 1981

Roane DM, Feinberg TE, Meckler L, et al: Treatment of dementia-associated agitation with gabapentin. J Neuropsychiatry Clin Neurosci 12:40–43, 2000

Ruedrich I, Chu CC, Moore SI: ECT for major depression in a patient with acute brain trauma. Am J Psychiatry 140:928–929, 1983

Salazar AM, Warden DL, Schwab K, et al: Cognitive rehabilitation for traumatic brain injury: a randomized trial. Defense and Veterans Head Injury Program (DVHIP) Study Group. JAMA 283:3075–3081, 2000

Silver JM, Yudofsky SC: Aggressive disorders, in Neuropsychiatry of Traumatic Brain Injury. Edited by Silver JM, Yudofsky SC, Hales RE. Washington, DC, American Psychiatric Press, 1994, pp 313–356

Silver JM, Yudofsky SC, Anderson KE: Aggressive disorders, in Textbook of Traumatic Brain Injury. Edited by Silver JM, McAllister TW, Yudofsky SC. Washington, DC, American Psychiatric Publishing, 2005, pp 259–278

Starkstein SE, Boston JD, Robinson RG: Mechanisms of mania after brain injury: 12 case reports and review of the literature. J Nerv Ment Dis 176:87–100, 1988

Starkstein SE, Mayberg HS, Berthier ML, et al: Mania after brain injury: neuroradiological and metabolic findings. Ann Neurol 27:652–659, 1990

Stewart JT, Nemsath RH: Bipolar illness following traumatic brain injury: treatment with lithium and carbamazepine. J Clin Psychiatry 49:74–75, 1988

Taverni JP, Seliger G, Lichtman SW: Donepezil mediated memory improvement in traumatic brain injury during post acute rehabilitation. Brain Inj 12:77–80, 1998

Teasdale G, Jennett B: Assessment of coma and impaired consciousness: a practical scale. Lancet 2:81–84, 1974

Thomsen IV: Late outcome of very severe blunt head trauma: a 10–15 year second follow-up. J Neurol Neurosurg Psychiatry 47:260–268, 1984

van Reekum R, Bolago I, Finlayson MA, et al: Psychiatric disorders after traumatic brain injury. Brain Inj 10:319–327, 1996

Wade DT, King NS, Crawford S, et al: Routine follow up after head injury: a second randomised clinical trial. J Neurol Neurosurg Psychiatry 65:177–183, 1998

Warden DL, Labbate LA: Posttraumatic stress disorder and other anxiety disorders, in Textbook of Traumatic Brain Injury. Edited by Silver JM, McAllister TW, Yudofsky SC. Washington, DC, American Psychiatric Publishing, 2005, pp 231–243

Watson MR, Fenton GW, McClelland RJ, et al: The postconcussional state: neurophysiological aspects. Br J Psychiatry 167:514–521, 1995

Weddell R, Oddy M, Jenkins D: Social adjustment after rehabilitation: a two year follow-up of patients with severe head injury. Psychol Med 10:257–263, 1980

Weinberg RM, Auerbach SH, Moore S: Pharmacologic treatment of cognitive deficits: a case study. Brain Inj 1:57–59, 1987

Weinstein GS, Wells CE: Case studies in neuropsychiatry: posttraumatic psychiatric dysfunction—diagnosis and treatment. J Clin Psychiatry 42:120–122, 1981

Weller M, Kornhuber J: A rationale for NMDA receptor antagonist therapy of the neuroleptic malignant syndrome. Med Hypotheses 38:329–333, 1992

Whelan FJ, Walker MS, Schulz SK: Donepezil in the treatment of cognitive dysfunction associated with traumatic brain injury. Ann Clin Psychiatry 12:131–135, 2000

Wilberger JE, Deeb A, Rothfus W: Magnetic resonance imaging in cases of severe head injury. Neurosurgery 20:571–576, 1987

Will RG, Young JPR, Thomas DJ: Klein-Levin syndrome: report of two cases with onset of symptoms precipitated by head trauma. Br J Psychiatry 152:410–412, 1988

Wolf B, Grohmann R, Schmidt LG, et al: Psychiatric admissions due to adverse drug reactions. Compr Psychiatry 30:534–545, 1989

Wroblewski BA, Joseph AB, Kupfer J, et al: Effectiveness of valproic acid on destructive and aggressive behaviours in patients with acquired brain injury. Brain Inj 11:37–47, 1997

Yablon SA: Posttraumatic seizures. Arch Phys Med Rehabil 74:983–1001, 1993

Yudofsky SC, Silver JM, Schneider SE: Pharmacologic treatment of aggression. Psychiatric Annals 17:397–407, 1987

Yudofsky SC, Silver JM, Hales RE: Pharmacologic management of aggression in the elderly. J Clin Psychiatry 51 (suppl 10):22–28, 1990

Yudofsky SC, Silver JM, Hales RE: Treatment of agitation and aggression, in Textbook of Psychopharmacology, 2nd Edition. Edited by Schatzberg AF, Nemeroff CB. Washington, DC, American Psychiatric Press, 1998, pp 881–900

Zasler N: Sexual dysfunction, in Neuropsychiatry of Traumatic Brain Injury. Edited by Silver JM, Yudofsky SC, Hales RE. Washington, DC, American Psychiatric Press, 1994, pp 443–470

Zhang L, Plotkin RC, Wang G, et al: Cholinergic augmentation with donepezil enhances recovery in short-term memory and sustained attention after traumatic brain injury. Arch Phys Med Rehabil 85:1050–1055, 2004

# 39

# Cerebrovascular Disease

## ROBERT G. ROBINSON, M.D.
## SERGIO E. STARKSTEIN, M.D., Ph.D.

## Neuropsychiatric Syndromes Associated With Cerebrovascular Disease

A number of emotional disorders, many of which are discussed in this section, have been associated with cerebrovascular disease (Table 39–1). The neuropsychiatric disorder that has received the greatest amount of investigation, however, is poststroke depression (PSD).

### Poststroke Depression

#### Diagnosis

Poststroke major depression is now categorized in DSM-IV-TR (American Psychiatric Association 2000) as "mood disorder due to stroke with major depressive-like episode." For patients with less severe forms of depression, there are "research criteria" in DSM-IV for minor depression (i.e., subsyndromal major depression; depression or anhedonia with at least one but fewer than four additional symptoms of major depression) or, alternatively, a diagnosis of mood disorder due to stroke with depressive features (i.e., depressed mood but criteria for major depression not met).

#### Prevalence

Over the past 10 years, there have been a large number of studies around the world examining the prevalence of

PSD. The mean frequency of major depression among patients in acute and rehabilitation hospitals was 22% for major depression and 20% for minor depression. Among patients studied in community settings, however, the mean prevalence of major depression was 14% and minor depression was 9%. Thus, PSD is common both among patients who are receiving treatment for stroke and among community samples.

The available data suggest that PSD is not transient but is usually a long-standing disorder with a natural course of approximately 9–10 months for most major cases of depression. Lesion location and severity of associated impairments may influence the longitudinal evolution of PSD.

Two factors have been identified that can influence the natural course of PSD. One factor is treatment of depression with antidepressant medications (discussed below). The second factor is lesion location. Starkstein et al. (1988) compared two groups of depressed patients: one group (n=6) had spontaneously recovered from depression by 6 months after stroke, whereas the other group (n=10) remained depressed at this point. There were, however, two significant between-group differences. One was lesion location: the recovered group had a higher frequency of subcortical and cerebellar–brain stem lesions; the nonrecovered group had a higher frequency of cortical lesions (P<0.01). Impairments in activities of daily living (ADL) were also significantly different between the two groups: the nonrecovered group had significantly

**TABLE 39–1.** Clinical syndromes associated with cerebrovascular disease

| Syndrome | Prevalence | Clinical symptoms | Associated lesion location |
|---|---|---|---|
| Major depression | 20% | Depressed mood, diurnal mood variation, loss of energy, anxiety, restlessness, worry, weight loss, decreased appetite, early morning awakening, delayed sleep onset, social withdrawal, and irritability | Left front lobe and left basal ganglia during the acute period after stroke |
| Minor depression | 19% | Depressed mood, anxiety, restlessness, worry, diurnal mood variation, hopelessness, loss of energy, delayed sleep onset, early morning awakening, social withdrawal, weight loss, and decreased appetite | Left posterior parietal and occipital regions during the acute poststroke period |
| Mania | Unknown, rare | Elevated mood, increased energy, increased appetite, decreased sleep, feeling of well-being, pressured speech, flight of ideas, and grandiose thoughts | Right basotemporal or right orbitofrontal lesions |
| Bipolar mood disorder | Unknown, rare | Symptoms of major depression alternating with mania | Right basal ganglia or right thalamic lesions |
| Anxiety disorder | 27% | Symptoms of major depression plus intense worry and anxious foreboding in addition to depression, associated light-headedness or palpitations and muscle tension or restlessness, and difficulty concentrating or falling asleep | Left cortical lesions, usually dorsolateral frontal lobe |
| Psychotic disorder | Unknown, rare | Hallucinations or delusions | Right temporoparietal-occipital junction |
| Apathy | | | |
|    Without depression | 11% | Loss of drive, motivation, interest, low energy, and unconcern | Posterior internal capsule |
|    With depression | 11% | | |
| Pathological laughing and crying | 20% | Frequent, usually brief, laughing and/or crying; crying not caused by sadness or out of proportion to it; and social withdrawal secondary to emotional outbursts | Frequently, bilateral hemispheric lesions; can occur with almost any lesion location |
| Anosognosia | 24% | Denial of impairment related to motor function, sensory perception, visual perception, or other modality with an apparent lack of concern | Right hemisphere and enlarged ventricles |
| Catastrophic reaction | 19% | Anxiety reaction, tears, aggressive behavior, swearing, displacement, refusal, renouncement, and compensatory boasting | Left anterior-subcortical |
| Aprosodias | | | |
|    Motor | Unknown | Poor expression of emotional prosody and gesturing, good prosodic comprehension and gesturing, and denial of feelings of depression | Right hemisphere: posterior inferior frontal lobe and basal ganglia |
|    Sensory | 32% | Good expression of emotional prosody and gesturing, poor prosodic comprehension and gesturing, and difficulty empathizing with others | Right hemisphere: posterior inferior parietal lobe and posterior superior temporal lobe |

more severe impairments in ADL in hospital than did the recovered group (*P*<0.01).

## Relationship to Lesion Variables and Premorbid Risk Factors

Although a significant proportion of patients with left anterior or right posterior lesions develop PSD, not every patient with a lesion in these locations developed a depressive mood. This observation raises the question of why clinical variability occurs and why some but not all patients with lesions in these locations develop depression. In summary, lesion location is not the only factor that influences the development of PSD. Subcortical atrophy that probably precedes the stroke and a family or personal history of affective disorders also seem to play an important role. The most consistently identified risk factor for depression, however, is severity of functional physical impairment.

## Relationship to Cognitive Impairment

Numerous investigators have reported that elderly patients with functional major depression have intellectual deficits that improve with treatment of depression (Wells 1979). This issue was first examined in patients with PSD by Robinson et al. (1986). Patients with major depression after a left hemisphere infarct were found to have significantly lower (more impaired) scores on the Mini-Mental State Examination (MMSE) (Folstein et al. 1975) than did a comparable group of nondepressed patients. Both the size of patients' lesions and their depression scores correlated independently with severity of cognitive impairment.

## Mechanism of Poststroke Depression

Although the cause of PSD remains unknown, one of the mechanisms that has been hypothesized to play an etiological role is dysfunction of the biogenic amine system. The noradrenergic and serotonergic cell bodies are located in the brain stem and send ascending projections through the median forebrain bundle to the frontal cortex. The ascending axons then arc posteriorly and run longitudinally through the deep layers of the cortex, arborizing and sending terminal projections into the superficial cortical layers (Morrison et al. 1979). Lesions that disrupt these pathways in the frontal cortex or the basal ganglia may affect many downstream fibers. On the basis of these neuroanatomical facts and the clinical findings that the severity of depression correlates with the proximity of the lesion to the frontal pole, Robinson et al. (1984)

suggested that PSD may be the consequence of depletions of norepinephrine and/or serotonin produced by lesions in the frontal lobe or basal ganglia.

## Treatment of Poststroke Depression

On the basis of the available data, if there are no contraindications to nortriptyline such as heart block, cardiac arrhythmia, narrow-angle glaucoma, sedation, or orthostatic hypotension, nortriptyline remains the first-line treatment for PSD. Doses of nortriptyline should be increased slowly and blood levels should be monitored with a goal of achieving serum concentrations between 50 and 150 ng/mL. If there are contraindications to the use of nortriptyline, citalopram (20 mg under age 66 years, 10 mg age 66 years and over) or reboxetine (2 mg bid) would be alternate choices. Electroconvulsive therapy has also been reported to be effective for treating PSD (Murray et al. 1986). It causes few side effects and no neurological deterioration. Psychostimulants have also been reported in open-label trials to be effective for the treatment of PSD. Finally, psychological treatment using cognitive-behavioral therapy (CBT) in 123 stroke patients has been found by Lincoln et al. (2003) to be no more effective than an attention placebo treatment (*n*=39, CBT completers; *n*=43, placebo completers).

## Psychosocial Adjustment

Thompson et al. (1989) examined 40 stroke patients and their caregivers at an average of 9 months after the occurrence of stroke. They found that a lack of meaningfulness in life and overprotection by the caregiver were independent predictors of depression. Kotila et al. (1998) examined depression after stroke as part of the Finnstroke study. This study examined the effect of active rehabilitation programs after discharge together with support and social activities on the frequency of depression among patients and caregivers at 3 months and 1 year after stroke. At both 3 months and 1 year, the frequency of depression was significantly lower among patients receiving active outpatient treatment than among patients without active rehabilitation programs (41% vs. 54% at 3 months and 42% vs. 55% at 1 year). Although there were no significant differences between districts with and without active programs in the rate of depression among caregivers at 3 months, at 12 months there were significantly more severely depressed caregivers in districts without active programs (*P*=0.036). Greater severity of impairment as measured by the Rankin Scale (Rankin 1957) was also associated with increased depression among caregivers at 3 months after stroke.

## Poststroke Mania

Although poststroke mania occurs much less frequently than depression (we have observed only 3 cases among a consecutive series of more than 300 stroke patients), manic syndromes are sometimes associated with stroke. Among 366 patients with bipolar disorder, Cassidy and Carroll (2002) found that late-onset mania (i.e., after age 47 years) was significantly associated with risk factors for vascular disease.

### *Phenomenology of Secondary Mania*

Starkstein et al. (1988) examined a series of 12 consecutive patients who met DSM-III criteria for an organic affective syndrome, manic type. These patients, who developed mania after a stroke, traumatic brain injury, or tumors, were compared with patients with functional (i.e., no known neuropathology) mania (Starkstein et al. 1987). Both groups of patients showed similar frequencies of elation, pressured speech, flight of ideas, grandiose thoughts, insomnia, hallucinations, and paranoid delusions.

### *Lesion Location*

Several studies of patients with brain damage have found that patients who develop secondary mania have a significantly greater frequency of lesions in the right hemisphere than patients with depression or no mood disturbance. The right hemisphere lesions that lead to mania tend to be in specific right hemisphere structures that have connections to the limbic system.

### *Risk Factors*

The relatively rare occurrence of mania after stroke suggests that there are premorbid risk factors that have an impact on the expression of this disorder. Studies thus far have identified two such factors. One is a genetic vulnerability for affective disorder, and the other is a mild degree of subcortical atrophy.

### *Mechanism of Secondary Mania*

Although the mechanism of secondary mania remains unknown, both lesion studies and metabolic studies suggest that the right basotemporal cortex may play an important role.

### *Treatment of Secondary Mania*

Bakchine et al. (1989) carried out a double-blind, placebo-controlled treatment study in a single patient with secondary mania. Clonidine (0.6 mg/day) rapidly reversed the manic symptoms, whereas carbamazepine, at 1,200 mg/day, was associated with no mood changes and levodopa (375 mg/day) was associated with an increase in manic symptoms. In other treatment studies, however, the anticonvulsants valproic acid and carbamazepine as well as antipsychotics and lithium therapy have been reported to be useful in treating secondary mania (Starkstein et al. 1991).

## Poststroke Bipolar Disorder

In an effort to examine the crucial factors in determining which patients have bipolar as opposed to unipolar disorder, Starkstein et al. (1991) examined 19 patients with the diagnosis of secondary mania. The bipolar (manic-depressive) group consisted of patients who, after the occurrence of the brain lesion, met DSM-III-R criteria for organic mood syndrome, mania, followed or preceded by organic mood syndrome, depressed. The unipolar-mania group consisted of patients who met the criteria for mania described previously (i.e., DSM-III-R organic mood syndrome, mania), not followed or preceded by depression.

## Poststroke Anxiety Disorder

Studies of patients with functional depression (i.e., of no known neuropathology) have demonstrated that it is important to distinguish depression associated with significant anxiety symptoms (i.e., agitated depressions) from depression without these symptoms (i.e., retarded depressions) because their cause and course may be different (Stavrakaki and Vargo 1986).

## Poststroke Psychosis

In a study of acute organic psychosis occurring after stroke lesions, Rabins et al. (1991) found a very low prevalence of psychosis among stroke patients (only 5 in more than 300 consecutive admissions). All 5 of these patients, however, had right hemisphere lesions, primarily involving frontoparietal regions. When compared with 5 age-matched patients with cerebrovascular lesions in similar locations but no psychosis, patients with secondary psychosis had significantly greater subcortical atrophy, as manifested by significantly larger areas of both the frontal horn of the lateral ventricle and the body of the lateral ventricle (measured on the side contralateral to the brain lesion). Several investigators have also reported a high frequency of seizures among patients with secondary psychosis (Levine and Finkelstein 1982). These seizures usually started after the occurrence of the brain lesion but before the onset of psychosis.

It has been hypothesized that three factors may be important in the mechanism of organic hallucinations, namely 1) a right hemisphere lesion involving the temporoparietal cortex, 2) seizures, and/or 3) subcortical brain atrophy (Starkstein et al. 1992).

## Apathy

Apathy is the absence or lack of motivation as manifested by decreased motor function, cognitive function, emotional feeling, and interest and has been reported frequently among patients with brain injury. Using the Apathy Scale, Starkstein et al. (1993) examined a consecutive series of 80 patients with single-stroke lesions and no significant impairment in comprehension. Of 80 patients, 9 (11%) showed apathy as their only psychiatric disorder, whereas another 11% had both apathy and depression. The only demographic correlate of apathy was age, as apathetic patients (with or without depression) were significantly older than nonapathetic patients. In addition, apathetic patients showed significantly more severe deficits in ADL, and a significant interaction was noted between depression and apathy on ADL scores, with the greatest impairment found in patients who were both apathetic and depressed.

Patients with apathy (without depression) showed a significantly higher frequency of lesions involving the posterior limb of the internal capsule than did patients without apathy (Starkstein et al. 1993). Lesions in the internal globus pallidus and the posterior limb of the inter-

nal capsule have been reported to produce behavioral changes, such as motor neglect, psychic akinesia, and akinetic mutism (Helgason et al. 1988). The ansa lenticularis is one of the main internal pallidal outputs, and it ends in the pedunculopontine nucleus after going through the posterior limb of the internal capsule (Nauta 1989). Angelelli et al. (2004), in a study of 124 poststroke patients, found apathy in 27%, depression in 61%, and irritability in 33%. Ghika-Schmidt and Bogousslavsky (2000) studied 12 patients with anterior thalamic infarcts. Within a few months' follow-up, the persisting abnormalities included memory dysfunction and apathy. Kobayashi and coworkers, using xenon inhalation, showed that patients with poststroke apathy had decreased blood flow bilaterally in the frontal lobes (Okada et al. 1997) and impaired frontal lobe function (i.e., impaired fluency and prolonged latency of novelty P3 response to auditory stimuli on electroencephalogram) (Yamagata et al. 2004).

## Pathological Emotions

Emotional lability is a common complication of stroke lesions. It is characterized by sudden, easily provoked episodes of crying that, although frequent, generally occur in appropriate situations and are accompanied by a congruent mood change. Pathological laughing and crying is a more severe form of emotional lability and is characterized by episodes of laughing and/or crying that are not appropriate to the context. They may appear spontaneously or may be elicited by nonemotional events and do not correspond to underlying emotional feelings. These disorders have also been termed *emotional incontinence*, *pathologic emotions*, and *involuntary emotional expression disorder*.

## Key Points: Cerebrovascular Disease

- Poststroke depression is a common conseqeuence of stroke.

- The reported prevalences of major depression and minor depression are similar in poststroke mood disorders.

- Poststroke mania and poststroke psychosis are both much less common than poststroke depression.

- Poststroke apathy and pathological emotions may occur in the absence of a full poststroke mood disorder.

## References

American Psychiatric Association: Diagnostic and Statistical Manual of Mental Disorders, 4th Edition, Text Revision. Washington, DC, American Psychiatric Press, 2000

Angelelli P, Paolucci S, Bivona Y, et al: Development of neuropsychiatric symptoms in poststroke patients: a cross-sectional study. Acta Psychiatr Scand 110:55–63, 2004

Bakchine S, Lacomblez L, Benoit N, et al: Manic-like state after orbitofrontal and right temporoparietal injury: efficacy of clonidine. Neurology 39:778–781, 1989

Cassidy F, Carroll BJ: Vascular risk factors in late onset mania. Psychol Med 32:359–362, 2002

Folstein MF, Folstein SE, McHugh PR: Mini-Mental State: a practical method for grading the cognitive state of patients for the clinician. J Psychiatr Res 12:189–198, 1975

Ghika-Schmid F, Bogousslavsky J: The acute behavioral syndrome of anterior thalamic infarction: prospective study of 12 cases. Ann Neurol 48:220–227, 2000

Helgason C, Wilbur A, Weiss A, et al: Acute pseudobulbar mutism due to discrete bilateral capsular infarction in the territory of the anterior choroidal artery. Brain 111 (part 3):507–524, 1988

Kotila M, Numminen H, Waltimo O, et al: Depression after stroke: results of the FINNSTROKE study. Stroke 29:368–372, 1998

Levine DN, Finklestein S: Delayed psychosis after right temporoparietal stroke or trauma: relation to epilepsy. Neurology 32:267–273, 1982

Lincoln NB, Flannaghan T: Cognitive behavioral psychotherapy for depression following stroke: a randomized controlled trial. Stroke 34:111–115, 2003

Morrison JH, Molliver ME, Grzanna R: Noradrenergic innervation of the cerebral cortex: widespread effects of local cortical lesions. Science 205:313–316, 1979

Murray GB, Shea V, Conn DK: Electroconvulsive therapy for poststroke depression. J Clin Psychiatry 47:258–260, 1986

Nauta WJH: Reciprocal links of the corpus striatum with the cerebral cortex and the limbic system: a common substrate for movement and thought? In Neurology and Psychiatry: A Meeting of Minds. Edited by Mueller J. Basel, Switzerland, Karger, 1989, pp 43–63

Okada K, Kobayashi S, Yamagata S, et al: Poststroke apathy and regional cerebral blood flow. Stroke 28:2437–2441, 1997

Rabins PV, Starkstein SE, Robinson RG: Risk factors for developing atypical (schizophreniform) psychosis following stroke. J Neuropsychiatry Clin Neurosci 3:6–9, 1991

Rankin J: Cerebral vascular accidents in patients over the age of 60, III: diagnosis and treatment. Scott Med J 2:254–268, 1957

Robinson RG, Kubos KL, Starr LB, et al: Mood disorders in stroke patients: importance of location of lesion. Brain 107:81–93, 1984

Robinson RG, Bolla-Wilson K, Kaplan E, et al: Depression influences intellectual impairment in stroke patients. Br J Psychiatry 148:541–547, 1986

Starkstein SE, Pearlson GD, Boston J, et al: Mania after brain injury: a controlled study of causative factors. Arch Neurol 44:1069–1073, 1987

Starkstein SE, Robinson RG, Price TR: Comparison of spontaneously recovered versus non-recovered patients with poststroke depression. Stroke 19:1491–1496, 1988

Starkstein SE, Fedoroff JP, Berthier MD, et al: Manic depressive and pure manic states after brain lesions. Biol Psychiatry 29:149–158, 1991

Starkstein SE, Robinson RG, Berthier ML: Post-stroke hallucinatory delusional syndromes. Neuropsychiatry Neuropsychol Behav Neurol 5:114–118, 1992

Starkstein SE, Fedoroff JP, Price TR, et al: Apathy following cerebrovascular lesions. Stroke 24:1625–1630, 1993

Stavrakaki C, Vargo B: The relationship of anxiety and depression: a review of the literature. Br J Psychiatry 149:7–16, 1986

Thompson SC, Sobolew-Shobin A, Graham MA, et al: Psychosocial adjustment following stroke. Soc Sci Med 28:239–247, 1989

Wells CE: Pseudodementia. Am J Psychiatry 136:895–900, 1979

Yamagata S, Yamaguchi S, Kobayashi S: Impaired novelty processing in apathy after subcortical stroke. Stroke 35:1935–1940, 2004

# Section IV

# Exams and Answer Guides

# Exam 1

*Select the single best response for each question.*

1. All of the following psychiatric disorders are common comorbid conditions in Huntington's disease *except*

    A. Schizophreniform disorder.
    B. Intermittent explosive disorder.
    C. Major depression.
    D. Obsessive-compulsive disorder.
    E. Bipolar disorder.

2. Which of the following statements is *true* regarding gender differences in schizophrenia?

    A. The onset of illness tends to be more acute in males than in females.
    B. Men tend to have a higher level of premorbid functioning than women.
    C. Women generally have a more favorable outcome than men.
    D. The age at onset is, on average, 5 years earlier in women than in men.
    E. There are no differences between men and women in onset, tempo of onset, and level of premorbid functioning.

3. Which of the following diagnoses is found at increased prevalence among the first-degree relatives of patients with schizophrenia?

    A. Antisocial personality disorder.
    B. Generalized anxiety disorder.
    C. Borderline personality disorder.
    D. Schizotypal personality disorder.
    E. Attention-deficit/hyperactivity disorder.

4. A 39-year-old woman was prescribed and started taking carbamazepine for trigeminal neuralgia. Several months later, she developed symptoms of recurrent depression. Because she had a history of excellent response to this medication, her psychiatrist restarted the patient on nefazodone. Six weeks later the nefazodone was increased to a dose higher than her previously effective dose because her symptoms had not improved. Two weeks later she reported no improvement of her depression and complained of increased fatigue and "forgetfulness." Which of the following statements is *false* regarding this case?

    A. Both nefazodone and carbamazepine are substrates of the P450 3A4 enzyme.
    B. Carbamazepine is a potent 3A4 inducer.
    C. The patient's blood level of nefazodone is likely to be subtherapeutic.
    D. The patient's blood level of carbamazepine is likely to be decreased.
    E. Venlafaxine may be an appropriate alternative to nefazodone if the patient continues to take carbamazepine.

5. Which of the following is *true* regarding conducting a psychiatric interview with an adolescent?

    A. Avoid interviewing parents alone, because this could disrupt rapport-building with the patient, who may fear that the clinician is colluding with caregivers.
    B. Seeing the adolescent alone first tends to alienate the patient, who may already be anxious about the visit.
    C. Joint interviews with the adolescent and parents are rarely recommended.
    D. The parent interview is an essential part of the initial visit, even with highly functional, communicative adolescents.
    E. To ensure that adequate information is obtained in interviews with adolescents, who tend to be distractible, it is important to focus mostly on the difficulties of the adolescent during the initial interview.

6. In response to amphetamine challenge, individuals with which of the following diagnoses are more likely than control subjects to become psychotic?

A. Antisocial personality disorder.

B. Generalized anxiety disorder.

C. Borderline personality disorder.

D. Avoidant personality disorder.

E. Attention-deficit/hyperactivity disorder.

7. The diagnosis of schizophrenia with childhood onset

   A. Is a common presentation for this disorder.

   B. Is five times more likely in females than in males.

   C. Requires no mood disorder exclusion.

   D. Can be made when signs of disturbance have been present for at least 3 months.

   E. May have a prevalence of less than 1 in 1,000.

8. Classic Munchausen syndrome includes all of the following components *except*

   A. Travel from hospital to hospital.

   B. Simulation of disease.

   C. Unconscious self-induction of disease.

   D. Pseudologia fantastica.

   E. Use of aliases to disguise identity.

9. Which of the following statements is *false* regarding the dopaminergic system?

   A. The cerebral cortex is a major projection site of dopaminergic neurons.

   B. The mediodorsal nucleus of the thalamus and the posterior vermis of the cerebellum contain low densities of dopamine axons.

   C. The majority of dopamine cells are located in the anterior midbrain (mesencephalon).

   D. Subcortical structures receive projections from dopaminergic neurons.

   E. The major projection target of dopamine neurons in the substantia nigra is the striatum.

10. Regarding choice of an antipsychotic for a patient with acute psychosis in schizophrenia, all of the following statements are true *except*

   A. Generally, second-generation (atypical) agents are preferred.

   B. All of the second-generation (atypical) agents are more effective than the first-generation (typical) agents in the treatment of positive and negative symptoms.

   C. It is acceptable to use a first-generation agent if a particular patient has responded to that agent in the past.

   D. The main advantage of second-generation agents is their overall lower risk of causing extrapyramidal symptoms and tardive dyskinesia.

   E. Clozapine may be therapeutically superior to any other antipsychotic medications.

11. DSM-IV-TR suggests that malingering should be strongly suspected if all of the following are present *except*

   A. Medicolegal context of presentation.

   B. Marked discrepancy between the person's claimed stress or disability and the objective findings.

   C. Lack of cooperation during the diagnostic evaluation and in complying with the prescribed treatment regimen.

   D. Diagnosis of antisocial personality disorder associated with the evaluee.

   E. Axis I disorder.

12. A 32-year-old man with schizophrenia has had good control of his psychotic symptoms for the past 2 years while taking quetiapine 600 mg/day. One month ago he was started on phenytoin for a newly diagnosed seizure disorder. The man is admitted to an inpatient psychiatric facility because of worsening paranoia and other psychotic symptoms. His caregiver confirms that the patient has been adhering to his medication regimen. Of the following, which is the best treatment option on this patient's admission?

   A. Increase the dosage of quetiapine to 800 mg/day and add 25–50 mg of quetiapine every 4–6 hours as needed for agitation. Continue the phenytoin at the current dosage.

   B. Increase the dosage of quetiapine to 800 mg/day and add 25–50 mg of quetiapine every 4–6 hours as needed for agitation. Discontinue the phenytoin and start valproic acid.

   C. Continue the current dosage of quetiapine and start ziprasidone 160 mg/day. Continue the phenytoin at the current dosage.

   D. Discontinue quetiapine and start ziprasidone 160 mg/day. Continue the phenytoin at the current dosage.

   E. Continue the current dosage of quetiapine and augment with valproic acid for mood stabilization. Continue phenytoin at the current dosage.

13. Which of the following statements is *false* regarding the data obtained during a psychiatric interview?

    A. The content of the interview can be transmitted verbally and nonverbally.
    B. A patient's language style—his use of active or passive verb forms, technical jargon, colloquialisms, or frequent injunctives—refers to the process data of the interview.
    C. The process of the interview refers to the developing relationship between the interviewer and patient, including the patient's fantasies about the interviewer.
    D. An intervention by the interviewer is considered to be part of the content of the interview.
    E. An interviewer's reactions and attentiveness during the interview may be indicative of important content and process data.

14. Which of the following is a physical sign of phencyclidine (PCP) use intoxication?

    A. Vertical, but not horizontal, nystagmus.
    B. Hypotension.
    C. Hyperacusis.
    D. Bradycardia.
    E. Muscle flaccidity.

15. Aging is associated with increased risk of developing various sleep disorders. Which of the following is *true?*

    A. A parasomnia, obstructive sleep apnea (OSA) is significantly more common than central sleep apnea (CSA).
    B. Insomnia is usually not associated with OSA.
    C. Dyssomnias are often caused by medical conditions or medications.
    D. Clinically significant periodic limb movement disorder (PLMD) is five to six times more common in elderly patients compared with younger adults.
    E. Polysomnography is required for the diagnosis of both PLMD and restless legs syndrome (RLS).

16. The psychiatric interview of older adults can be complicated by

    A. Their not equating present distress with past episodes that are symptomatically similar.
    B. Their becoming angry or irritated when a clinician continues to probe previous periods of overt disability in usual activities.

    C. Their having experienced a major illness or trauma in childhood but viewing this information as being of no relevance to the present episode.
    D. A histrionic personality style.
    E. All of the above.

17. The leading cause of medical morbidity in patients with schizophrenia is

    A. Obesity.
    B. Diabetes.
    C. HIV-associated hepatitis.
    D. Cigarette smoking.
    E. Lack of exercise.

18. Which of the following statements is *true* regarding brain neuroanatomy?

    A. The anterior commissure and massa intermedia structures that connect the right and left hemispheres tend to be the same in women and men.
    B. Language functions are less lateralized in women than in men.
    C. Abnormalities in brain structure and function associated with specific disorders do not differ between men and women.
    D. A larger number of sex differences in brain neuroanatomy have been identified in humans compared with other vertebrates.
    E. The evidence strongly supports the hypothesis that females have a larger corpus callosum than do males.

19. There is substantial comorbidity between which of the following diagnoses?

    A. Generalized social phobia and avoidant personality disorder.
    B. Panic disorder and avoidant personality disorder.
    C. Generalized social phobia and schizotypal personality disorder.
    D. Generalized social phobia and borderline personality disorder.
    E. Generalized anxiety disorder and avoidant personality disorder.

20. The primary receptor site of action of ethanol is

    A. Dopamine transporter (DAT).
    B. Vesicular monoamine transporter (VMAT).

C. Nicotinic acetylcholine (ACh) receptors.

D. Gamma-aminobutyric acid (GABA) and
   $N$-methyl-D-aspartate (NMDA) receptors.

E. Mu receptors.

21. Which of the following characteristics is *true* regarding assault and psychosis?

A. The triggering event usually involves a situational stressor that does not involve hallucinations or delusions.

B. The behavior preceding the assault is typified by agitation, pacing, clenched jaw, yelling, and verbal threats.

C. More than 40% of assaults by chronically assaultive inpatients at a psychiatric facility were psychotic in nature, followed by impulsive then organized assaults.

D. Psychotic assaults are relatively uncommon when compared with impulsive or predatory/planned assaults.

E. Examples of triggers of violent acts by psychotic individuals include a staff member telling a patient to return to his or her room.

22. Which of the following statements is *true* regarding male sexual dysfunction?

A. Men with low or absent gonadal function show little interest in sex and are impotent regardless of exposure to stimuli.

B. Diseases that interfere with neural control over the hypothalamic-pituitary-gonadal (HPG) axis are not believed to affect sexual desire.

C. Common risk factors for erectile dysfunction (ED) directly or indirectly compromise the process of smooth muscle relaxation.

D. Risk factors for premature ejaculation include commonly identifiable conditions such as specific procedures or disorders.

E. Tobacco use is a risk factor for premature ejaculation.

23. Which of the following findings does *not* suggest a psychogenic or "nonorganic" etiology for a neurologic deficit?

A. Tongue deviation away from the hemiparetic side.

B. Complete loss of smell, including of noxious substances.

C. Peripheral facial palsy and ipsilateral hemiparesis.

D. Unilateral hearing loss in the ear ipsilateral to a hemiparesis.

E. Presence of optokinetic nystagmus in a blind patient.

24. Structural magnetic resonance imaging (MRI) studies of subjects with schizotypal personality disorder have shown which of the following?

A. Larger left and right caudate nucleus volumes compared with those in subjects without schizotypal personality disorder.

B. Larger relative size of putamen compared with that in subjects with schizophrenia or control subjects.

C. Higher regional glucose metabolic rate in caudate compared with control subjects.

D. Ventricular enlargement intermediate between that in control subjects and subjects with schizophrenia.

E. Smaller hippocampal volumes compared with those in control subjects.

25. The leading cause of premature death in patients with schizophrenia is

A. Comorbidities associated with obesity.

B. Alcohol and drug use.

C. Comorbidities associated with cigarette smoking.

D. Risky sexual behaviors.

E. Suicide.

26. Recent "right to die" discussions relate to decision making at the end of life. There are important distinctions between incompetent and competent patients in this issue. Regarding right to die and incompetent patients, which of the following is *true?*

A. The *Cruzan v. Director, Missouri Department of Health* (1990) decision allowed the state to remove a feeding tube from an incompetent patient to respect the family's wishes.

B. The *Cruzan* decision found that the state did *not* have the right to maintain an incompetent individual's life against family wishes.

C. When treating severely impaired and/or ill patients, physicians must seek clear and competent instructions regarding foreseeable treatment decisions.

D. Expression of treatment preferences can be valid only with a durable power of attorney agreement.

E. Civil liability may only result from stopping life-sustaining treatment, not from overtreatment.

27. Medication history of the older adult should

A. Involve having the older person bring in all pill bottles.
B. Involve a double check between the written schedule and pill containers.
C. Assess alcohol intake.
D. Assess substance abuse.
E. All of the above.

28. The leading conception of the principles of biomedical ethics includes all of the following *except*

A. Respect for patient autonomy.
B. Beneficence.
C. Honesty.
D. Nonmaleficence.
E. Justice.

29. A test of which of the following specimens is generally least expensive and completed at most clinical laboratories?

A. Blood.
B. Hair.
C. Oral fluid.
D. Sweat.
E. Urine.

30. Which of the following is *false* regarding mood disorders and gender?

A. Depression is the second leading cause of disability for women in the world, followed by ischemic heart disease.
B. The lifetime risk of major depression in the United States has ranged from 10% to 25% for women.
C. In the United States, nearly twice as many women (12%) as men (6.6%) have a depressive disorder each year.
D. In established market economies, schizophrenia and bipolar disorder are among the top 10 causes of disability-adjusted life years for men but not for women.

E. It is projected that by the year 2020, major depression will be the leading cause of disease burden in women.

31. Evaluation of the family of the psychiatrically ill older adult includes all of the following parameters of support *except*

A. Availability of the family member.
B. Tangible services provided by the family.
C. Patient's perception of family support.
D. Tolerance by the family of specific behaviors derived from the psychiatric disorder.
E. Consideration only of those individuals genetically related to the patient.

32. Which of the following second-generation antipsychotics is most effective for treatment-resistant schizophrenia?

A. Clozapine.
B. Risperidone.
C. Olanzapine.
D. Quetiapine.
E. Ziprasidone.

33. Borderline personality disorder is associated with which of the following cognitive and perceptual disturbances?

A. Odd thinking and speech.
B. Ideas of reference.
C. Odd beliefs.
D. Transient, stress-related paranoid ideation.
E. Superstitiousness.

34. Which of the following statements is *true* regarding neurologic exam findings?

A. Patients with slowly developing cerebral hemisphere lesions usually develop spasticity and weakness simultaneously.
B. Patients with strokes or spinal cord injury tend to develop spasticity, weakness, and flaccidity simultaneously.
C. Spasticity is a sign of upper motor neuron disease, the severity of which correlates well with the degree of weakness or hyperreflexia.
D. In hemiplegia, there tends to be excess tone in the extensors of the arms and flexors of the legs.
E. After a large stroke, persistent flaccid hemiplegia rarely occurs with hyperreflexia.

35. Memory loss is often insidious in onset and well established clinically by the time a patient is brought to care. Which of the following statements is *false* regarding the dementia syndromes?

    A. More than half of people with chronic memory loss will, at autopsy, exhibit the changes of Alzheimer's disease only and not other dementias.
    B. The most common dementia syndrome is caused by Alzheimer's disease, followed by vascular dementia.
    C. Approximately 5% of older persons experience memory loss as a result of alcohol-induced amnestic disorder.
    D. Vascular dementia is more common in women than in men.
    E. At autopsy, many individuals with Alzheimer's disease are also found to have changes in the substantia nigra.

36. Adjustment disorder is characterized by

    A. Symptoms that develop within 2 months of the onset of a stressor.
    B. Symptoms that resolve within 12 months of the stressor's ending.
    C. Symptoms that develop within 3 months of the stressor's onset.
    D. Symptoms of distress that are proportional to the stressor.
    E. Symptoms that, if persistent for 7 months, would be considered acute adjustment disorder.

37. Electroconvulsive therapy (ECT) can be a lifesaving treatment in catatonia due to all of the following *except*

    A. Severe unipolar depression.
    B. Neuroleptic malignant syndrome.
    C. Hypercalcemia.
    D. Severe mixed mood disorder episode.
    E. None of the above.

38. Drug dependence has been modeled both as an impulse-control disorder and as a compulsive disorder, two models that feature different drug-related behaviors. Which of the following behaviors is associated with impulse-control disorder as opposed to compulsive disorder?

    A. Tension/arousal.
    B. Anxiety/stress.

C. Repetitive behaviors.
D. Relief of anxiety/relief of stress.
E. Obsessions.

39. Regarding use of antidepressants in treating borderline personality disorder patients, which of the following statements is *true?*

    A. Tricyclic antidepressants (TCAs) and monoamine oxidase inhibitors (MAOIs) pose serious risks of overdose and dangerous adverse effects that are of particular concern in an unstable and an impulsive population.
    B. Selective serotonin reuptake inhibitors (SSRIs) lose efficacy for aggression and irritability after 2 months of treatment.
    C. SSRIs have not been found to decrease suicidality and self-injury in patients with borderline personality disorder.
    D. The MAOI tranylcypromine was found to be inferior to placebo in treating symptoms of borderline personality disorder.
    E. Phenelzine has modest efficacy in borderline personality disorder for depression, psychotic symptoms, and global borderline severity.

40. For severe tardive dyskinesia, which of the following medications may be useful?

    A. Pimozide.
    B. Clozapine.
    C. Haloperidol.
    D. L-Serine.
    E. L-Carnitine.

41. Attention includes an interaction between all of the following processes *except*

    A. Attentional capacity.
    B. Selective consciousness.
    C. Response selection and executive control.
    D. Selective attention.
    E. Sustained attention.

42. The form of malingering most frequently encountered by psychosomatic medicine specialists is

    A. Falsification of laboratory reports.
    B. Production of new illness.
    C. Contamination of laboratory samples.
    D. Embellishment of previous or concurrent illness.
    E. Multiple organ system complaints.

43. Which of the following sensory modalities is impaired consistently in individuals with schizophrenia?

    A. Sight.
    B. Hearing.
    C. Touch.
    D. Taste.
    E. Smell.

44. A 35-year-old man who has been clean from heroin comes to the methadone maintenance clinic to pick up his usual 50-mg-per-day dosage of methadone. Despite taking his usual methadone dose every day, the man reports worsening anxiety, muscle cramps, nausea, diarrhea, and insomnia that started a week ago. Two weeks ago, he was prescribed and started taking a new medication for "really bad pain" on one side of his face, which has resolved completely. What is the name of the new medication?

    A. Phenytoin
    B. Phenobarbital.
    C. Carbamazepine.
    D. Valproic acid.
    E. Gabapentin.

45. The three most useful classes of medications in the treatment of borderline personality disorder are

    A. Benzodiazepines, azapirones, and serotonergic and noradrenergic reuptake inhibitors (SNRIs).
    B. Selective serotonin reuptake inhibitors (SSRIs), mood stabilizers, and atypical antipsychotics.
    C. Mood stabilizers, SSRIs, and benzodiazepines.
    D. Benzodiazepines, SSRIs, and azapirones.
    E. Benzodiazepines, mood stabilizers, and SSRIs.

46. Rapid-eye movement (REM) sleep behavior disorder is a rare condition in which patients "act out their dreams" because of a failure of REM-associated atonia. This condition has been associated with use of all of the following medication classes or agents *except*

    A. Clozapine.
    B. Amitriptyline.
    C. Selegiline.
    D. Venlafaxine.
    E. Fluvoxamine.

47. Reduced volume of anterior, posterior, and (less consistently) total superior temporal gyrus has been correlated with which of the following clinical measures?

    A. Persistence of negative symptoms.
    B. Severity of auditory hallucinations and thought disorder.
    C. Deficits in working memory.
    D. Impaired processing of auditory-evoked potentials.
    E. Magnitude of comorbid mood dysregulation.

48. Regarding the effect of major depression on medically ill patients, which of the following statements is *false?*

    A. Major depression in medically ill patients often makes them incapacitated to make decisions.
    B. Untreated depression has been linked to poor compliance with medical care.
    C. Depression produces more subtle distortions of decision making than does delirium or psychosis.
    D. Refusal of life-saving treatment by a depressed patient cannot be assumed to constitute lack of capacity.
    E. None of the above.

49. Examples of depressive delusions would be *least* likely to involve which of the following statements?

    A. "I've lost my mind."
    B. "My body is disintegrating."
    C. "I ought to be promoted."
    D. "I have an incurable illness."
    E. "I have caused some great harm."

50. Which of the following is *true* regarding the psychotic disorder of late life referred to as *late-life paraphrenia?*

    A. It is the late-life recurrence of an earlier onset of schizophrenia in a patient who had been symptom-free for many years.
    B. According to Kraepelin's original description, most patients were male.
    C. Psychotic symptoms of the late-life episode typically include delusions, but hallucinations are not experienced.
    D. Patients have been reported to have simultaneous sensory deficits.
    E. Antipsychotics have been demonstrated to be effective for late-life delusional disorder.

51. Conventional antipsychotics may be helpful in borderline personality disorder for which of the following problems?

    A. Suicidality.
    B. Ideas of reference.
    C. Social functioning.
    D. All of the above.
    E. None of the above.

52. Which of the following is *true* regarding the treatment of anxiety disorders with buspirone?

    A. Buspirone, a partial agonist at the $5-HT_{1A}$ receptor, interacts with the gamma-aminobutyric acid (GABA) receptor and chloride ion channels and therefore should be used with caution when prescribed with benzodiazepines.
    B. Buspirone interacts with alcohol, and its side effects include sedation and impairment of psychomotor performance. However, it does not pose a risk of abuse.
    C. The efficacy of buspirone is not statistically different from that of benzodiazepines for the treatment of generalized anxiety.
    D. Buspirone has been found to be effective in the treatment of generalized anxiety disorder and panic disorder.
    E. Buspirone is safe to be used in patients with hepatic impairment but not renal impairment.

53. In Project Match, a large randomized trial of alcohol treatment modalities and predictive pretreatment variables, investigators found that the best potential predictor of a treatment outcome was

    A. Social status of the patient.
    B. Patient self-selection of treatment type.
    C. Severity of addiction.
    D. Number of previous treatment attempts.
    E. No specific predictors between specific treatments and indicators were found.

54. Which of the following statements is *false* regarding brain regions and activity?

    A. The dorsolateral prefrontal region is important for cognition, executive function, and focused attention.
    B. The orbital prefrontal region is important for social conduct, insight, judgment, and mood.
    C. The hippocampal complex is key to memory formation and storage functions.
    D. The parietal lobe is important for sensation, speech production/conduction, and deficit recognition.
    E. The thalamus modulates physiological response to emotional stimuli, temperature control, sleep, water metabolism, hormone secretion, satiety, and circadian rhythms.

55. The developmental histories of individuals with schizophrenia reveal higher rates of all of the following *except*

    A. Heavy maternal alcohol use during the first trimester.
    B. Maternal starvation during the first trimester.
    C. Maternal influenza infection during the second trimester.
    D. Rhesus and ABO blood-type incompatibility.
    E. Perinatal anoxic birth injuries.

56. The greatest threat to response to antidepressant treatment is

    A. Drug-drug interactions.
    B. Family history of preferential response.
    C. Suicidal ideation.
    D. Preexisting medical factors.
    E. Nonadherence to medication regimen.

57. Electroconvulsive therapy (ECT) has been shown to be safe and effective in treating all of the following *except*

    A. Comorbid mood disorders in patients with closed head injuries.
    B. Comorbid mood disorders in patients with mental retardation or dementia.
    C. Comorbid mood disorders in patients with intractable seizure disorders.
    D. Obsessive-compulsive disorder (OCD) or a mood disorder during pregnancy.
    E. None of the above.

58. Which of the following agents used in the treatment of opioid dependence is itself a partial agonist of the mu opioid receptor?

    A. Naltrexone.
    B. Buprenorphine.

C. Methadone.

D. Clonidine.

E. Hydromorphone.

59. The personality structure of the elderly shows

A. Remarkable stability over long periods of the life span, with increases on dimensions of neuroticism.

B. Declines on dimensions of neuroticism and increases on dimensions of openness to experience.

C. Increases on dimensions of openness to experience and of extraversion.

D. Remarkable stability over long periods of the life span, with declines on dimensions of neuroticism.

E. Declines in dimensions of neuroticism and of agreeableness.

60. One of the most consistent neuroanatomic findings in schizophrenia has been

A. Enlarged hippocampal volumes.

B. Underdevelopment of the corpus callosum.

C. Enlarged amygdala.

D. Enlarged lateral ventricles.

E. Pituitary hyperplasia.

61. All of the following features are common in families with Munchausen syndrome by proxy *except*

A. A dominant and aggressive husband and a caretaking and supportive wife.

B. Intense family–group loyalty, with little protective concern for the child.

C. A multigenerational pattern of abnormal illness behavior.

D. Enmeshment of parent–child relationships.

E. No gender bias of the child victims.

62. Which of the following statements is *true* regarding prevalence of selective mutism in children?

A. Prevalence estimates in children range from 3% to 5%.

B. Selective mutism symptoms that occur upon starting school are likely to be unremitting.

C. Variability in prevalence estimates may be because of vagueness in the DSM regarding the level of impairment required to meet diagnostic criteria.

D. Scandinavian prevalence studies have reported lower rates of selective mutism than have U.S. studies among school-age children.

E. Variability in prevalence estimates is unlikely to be related to differences in the consistent application of diagnostic criteria in study populations.

63. A lesion in the right frontal operculum will *most likely* lead to

A. Loss of emotional tone of speech (gesturing, prosody, inflection).

B. Nonfluent aphasia.

C. Lack of awareness of deficits.

D. Inability to comprehend speech.

E. Impaired initiation and synchronization of speech.

64. A 53-year-old man with a history of recurrent mild major depressive disorder has avoided psychiatric treatment for "years" because of his earlier experience with a medication. The antidepressant significantly reduced libido and contributed to his gaining 30 lb., so he completely stopped taking it. He does not recall the name of the medication or any other side effects but threatens to stop taking any medications that cause either of these symptoms. Of the following, which pair of antidepressants did the patient *most likely* take in the past?

A. Amitriptyline or nefazodone.

B. Phenelzine or venlafaxine.

C. Mirtazapine or bupropion.

D. Trazodone or paroxetine.

E. Fluoxetine or sertraline

65. Which of the following is *true* regarding personality disorders in older patients?

A. As research into personality disorders has increased, the phenomenon of personality disorders in the elderly has been thoroughly examined.

B. Unlike in younger patients, comorbid personality disorders in elderly patients do not appear to affect outcomes of mood disorders.

C. When an older patient's personality changes significantly because of dementia, the diagnosis is personality change due to a general medical condition.

D. In Alzheimer's disease, the change in personality is usually an exaggeration of premorbid personality traits.

E. Personality disorder not otherwise specified is diagnosed rarely in elderly patients.

66. Which of the following statements best describes the state of current knowledge about genetic markers for bipolar disorder?

A. Chromosome 21 has definitely been implicated.

B. Chromosome 21 and the Y chromosome have definitely been implicated.

C. Although studies implicating chromosome 11 and the X chromosome were published, further studies have not supported these findings.

D. Although studies implicating chromosome 11 and the Y chromosome were published, further studies have not supported these findings.

E. Chromosome 21 and the X chromosome have definitely been implicated.

67. Alzheimer's disease and Parkinson's disease are associated with many neuropsychiatric complications. Among these is disturbed sleep; when sleep disturbance is associated with behavioral agitation, the term *sundowning* is used. Which of the following is *true* regarding sleep disorders commonly seen in patients with Alzheimer's disease and Parkinson's disease?

A. The risk of sudden death usually exceeds the potential benefits of atypical antipsychotic agents in treating sundowning.

B. Sundowning can typically be easily managed at home with light therapy, elimination of daytime napping, and a structured activity program.

C. Sundowning has been linked with disturbed circadian rhythms and a phase delay of body temperature in dementia of Alzheimer's type.

D. Patients with Parkinson's disease have an increased risk of restless leg syndrome but not rapid eye movement (REM) sleep behavior disorder.

E. Although carbidopa/levodopa combinations may cause initial insomnia, they do not increase risk of nightmares.

68. All of the following are theorized to be causes of chronic pain *except*

A. Ongoing activation of pain pathways from the periphery that causes pain to become chronic.

B. Dysfunctional peripheral nerves.

C. Failure of motor reflexes to inhibit pain.

D. Sensitization of the dorsal horn.

E. Sympathetic nervous system input.

69. All of the following are associated with better response rates to lithium in the treatment of acute mania *except*

A. Few lifetime manic episodes.

B. Classic manic or elated symptoms.

C. Rapid-cycling symptoms.

D. Presentation with psychotic symptoms.

E. Presentation with no psychotic symptoms.

70. The primary receptor site of action of cocaine is

A. Dopamine transporter (DAT).

B. Vesicular monoamine transporter (VMAT).

C. Nicotinic acetylcholine (ACh) receptors.

D. Gamma-aminobutyric acid (GABA) receptors.

E. *N*-methyl-D-aspartate (NMDA) receptors.

71. All of the following statements are true regarding possible effects of antidepressants *except*

A. Bupropion causes seizures in about one-third of overdoses.

B. Tricyclic antidepressants (TCAs) may be lethal at doses only three to five times the therapeutic dose.

C. Multidrug overdoses that include fluvoxamine have been known to be lethal in about 50% of cases.

D. Of individuals intentionally overdosing on paroxetine, an overwhelming majority recover without incident.

E. Of the selective serotonin reuptake inhibitors (SSRIs), fluoxetine and sertraline have the highest risk of inducing sudden, violent suicidal ideation.

72. Which of the following statements is *true* regarding schizophrenia?

    A. Approximately 30% of patients achieve remission of psychotic symptoms within 3–4 months.
    B. First-episode patients are generally more resistant to the therapeutic effects and side effects of medication than patients with chronic schizophrenia.
    C. Nearly one-third of patients with schizophrenia have comorbid substance use disorders, excluding nicotine use.
    D. More than one-half of patients with schizophrenia have comorbid nicotine abuse/dependence.
    E. Second-generation antipsychotic agents seem to have similar efficacy for depressive symptoms as first-generation antipsychotics.

73. Which of the following is *true* regarding the obtaining of informed consent for forensic evaluations in minors?

    A. If a forensic evaluation of a minor is court ordered, parental consent is not required.
    B. If a forensic evaluation of a minor is requested by a parent, consent is implied and need not be further explored or documented.
    C. A minor cannot provide consent for an evaluation under any circumstances, and parental consent must be obtained.
    D. When parental consent is obtained, the psychiatrist need not explain to the child the nature of the evaluation and with whom the information will be shared.
    E. Adolescents are not allowed to provide informed consent under any circumstances.

74. Characteristic signs and symptoms are often associated with lesions in specific central nervous system regions. All of the following are correctly paired localizations *except*

    A. Cerebral hemisphere: hemiparesis, hyperactive deep tendon reflexes, spasticity, Babinski sign.
    B. Basal ganglia: parkinsonism, athetosis, chorea, hemiballismus.
    C. Brainstem: cranial nerve palsy with ipsilateral hemiparesis; nystagmus; bulbar palsy.
    D. Cerebellum: ataxic gait, scanning speech, dysdiadochokinesia.

    E. Cerebral hemisphere: hemisensory loss, partial seizures, pseudobulbar palsy.

75. All of the following are true regarding schizophrenia *except*

    A. Men and women have the same overall incidence and lifetime prevalence of schizophrenia.
    B. The onset of symptoms occurs sooner in men than in women.
    C. Schizophrenia in women tends to be relatively mild at first, with increasing severity later on. In men, symptoms tend to taper off with advancing years.
    D. During pregnancy, many women with severe schizophrenia have worsening of psychotic symptoms.
    E. Late-life schizophrenia is more common in women than in men.

76. When a person taking disulfiram drinks alcohol, the subsequent toxic reaction is caused by accumulation of which of the following?

    A. Acetone.
    B. Aldehyde dehydrogenase
    C. Acetaldehyde.
    D. Glutamate.
    E. Dopamine.

77. A 35-year-old Latino woman with no prior psychiatric treatment was diagnosed with a single episode of mild major depressive disorder and was prescribed 10 mg of paroxetine, a selective serotonin reuptake inhibitor (SSRI). The dose of paroxetine was increased to 20 mg after 1 week. Six weeks later, the patient reports that her mood is the "same." She has more difficulty focusing/concentrating at work and worse libido. She constantly berates herself for being a "failure" as a mother despite evidence to the contrary, and has had difficulty falling asleep since increasing the dose of the SSRI, which she takes at bedtime. She has had minimal side effects from the medication. Which of the following strategies would be most recommended at this time?

    A. Increase the dosage of paroxetine to 40 mg/day, and switch to morning dosing.
    B. Discontinue paroxetine and start 20 mg of fluoxetine.
    C. Augment with bupropion.

D. Refer the patient for cognitive-behavioral therapy (CBT).

E. Start weaning the patient off of paroxetine and start an adequate trial of bupropion.

78. The incidence of serious rashes, including Stevens-Johnson syndrome, in pediatric patients taking lamotrigine is approximately

A. 10%.
B. 5%.
C. 1%.
D. 0.1%.
E. 0.01%.

79. Which class of drugs showed an increase in abuse by U.S. adolescents from 1992 to 1997?

A. Alcohol.
B. Marijuana.
C. Cocaine.
D. Hallucinogens.
E. Prescription opiates.

80. Approximately what percentage of persons admitted from the community to a geropsychiatry unit may have a urinary tract infection that may result in a delirium?

A. 10%.
B. 20%.
C. 35%.
D. 45%.
E. 55%.

81. Which of the following antipsychotic agents is recommended in the American Psychiatric Association (APA) practice guideline as a first-line agent to treat delirium?

A. Aripiprazole.
B. Haloperidol.
C. Olanzapine.
D. Risperidone.
E. Quetiapine.

82. A 32-year-old man with multiple sclerosis (MS) comes for an evaluation of his depression. A recent magnetic resonance imaging (MRI) noted a lesion in the cerebellum but nowhere else. When meeting you, he offers his left, not right, hand to shake your hand. You wonder if he has a right-sided dysmetria, which would suggest that

A. A right finger-to-nose test, and possibly a right heel-to-shin test, would likely be abnormal.
B. He has an intention tremor caused by an MS plaque in the left cerebellar hemisphere.
C. A finger-to-nose test would be abnormal, and a left heel-to-shin test may be abnormal.
D. His gait could be characterized as broad based, unsteady, and uncoordinated.
E. On exam, he may also have some paresis, hyperactive deep tendon reflexes (DTRs), or Babinski sign.

83. In treating patients with schizophrenia and co-occurring substance use disorder, which of the following medications shows promise?

A. Haloperidol.
B. Aripiprazole.
C. Risperidone.
D. Clozapine.
E. Quetiapine.

84. In general, which of the following is associated with late-onset depressive disorders?

A. Rates of depressive disorders are higher in older adult populations (15%–20%) than in younger adult populations (5%–12%).
B. Brain imaging that is consistent with significant cerebrovascular disease.
C. Rates of atypical and delusional subtypes that are higher in older adult populations than in younger adult populations.
D. Decreased testosterone levels.
E. Symptom pattern and frequency of specific depressive subtypes similar to those in younger adult populations.

85. Magnetic resonance imaging (MRI) studies in children with schizophrenia have reported all of the following findings except

A. Decreases in total cerebral volume.
B. Cerebral asymmetry.
C. Decreases in ventricular volume.
D. Increases in temporal lobe volume.
E. Decreases in midsagittal thalamic area.

86. According to Kandel's gateway theory of adolescent drug use, drug use often follows a stereotypical escalation among various substances of abuse. Which substance is usually the first abused substance in this cascade?

    A. Illicit drug other than marijuana.
    B. Marijuana.
    C. Hard liquor.
    D. Cigarettes.
    E. Beer or wine.

87. Intermittent explosive disorder may be associated with

    A. Decreased dopamine levels.
    B. Decreased serotonin levels.
    C. Low testosterone levels.
    D. Increased gamma-aminobutyric acid (GABA) levels.
    E. Increased acetylcholine levels.

88. A neurologist refers a 65-year-old woman to you for a 3-month history of "depression" after she had a stroke. On examination, you notice that the woman's left arm is persistently flexed at the elbow, and her left foot is outgoing. She walks slowly as if she is dragging her left foot at times. Extraocular muscles are intact on the left eye, but her right eye is deviated medially throughout the visit. She most likely had an infarct in the

    A. Basal ganglia.
    B. Cerebellum.
    C. Lateral medulla of the brainstem.
    D. Midbrain part of the brainstem.
    E. Right pontine part of the brainstem.

89. Which of the following clinical features is *least often* reported in delirium?

    A. Perceptual changes/hallucinations.
    B. Poor attention/vigilance.
    C. Memory impairment.
    D. Acute onset.
    E. Diffuse cognitive impairment.

90. A 45-year-old woman who is considering moving out of state soon presents to the outpatient clinic for evaluation of depression. She reports depressed mood, hopelessness, increased self-criticism, and indecision about moving. The severity is judged to be mild by the clinician. Before the episode of depression began, she had been ruminating about being "a failure" with regard to home and work issues. Which psychotherapeutic interventions would best help this patient to address her symptoms in general and specifically her feeling that she is "a failure"?

    A. Address information processing distortions arising from dysfunctional schemas, and alter these schemas.
    B. Address conditioned patterns of emotion and behavior triggered by internal and environment cues, and focus on firsthand experiences of mastery.
    C. Address internalized relationship conflicts and patterns by focusing on altering interpersonal patterns in current relationships.
    D. Address specific personality traits by focusing on insight.
    E. Identify key defense mechanisms, and observe and interpret significant transference data.

91. Which of the following neurotransmitter changes is widely accepted to play a role in delirium?

    A. Excess acetylcholine activity.
    B. Reduced glutamate activity.
    C. Excess dopamine activity.
    D. Reduced dopamine activity.
    E. Excess serotonin activity.

92. Factors distinguishing patients with very late-onset schizophrenia from the "true" schizophrenia of younger patients include all of the following *except*

    A. Lower genetic load.
    B. Less evidence of early childhood maladjustment.
    C. Relative lack of formal thought disorder and negative symptoms.
    D. Lesser risk of tardive dyskinesia.
    E. Evidence of a neurodegenerative rather than a neurodevelopmental process.

93. Misdiagnosis of delirium, a common clinical problem, has been found to be more likely among certain patient populations. Misdiagnosis is more likely in patients with all of the following *except*

    A. Hyperactive patient presentation.
    B. Advanced patient age.

C. Sensory impairments.

D. Preexisting dementia.

E. Intensive care unit (ICU) setting.

94. Workplace drug testing conducted under federal guidelines is limited to a small number of drugs. Which of the following drugs is *not* included for testing under these guidelines?

A. Codeine/morphine.

B. Amphetamine/methamphetamine.

C. Synthetic opioids (oxycodone and others).

D. Phencyclidine (PCP).

E. Cocaine.

95. Of the following, the most significant risk factor for Alzheimer's disease is

A. Presence of apolipoprotein-E (APOE) ε4 allele.

B. Poor linguistic and cognitive abilities in early life, and lack of education.

C. Aging.

D. Mutations in the amyloid precursor protein (APP) gene on chromosome 21, the presenilin 1 (PS1) gene on chromosome 4, and the presenilin 2 (PS2) gene on chromosome 1.

E. History of severe traumatic brain injury and/or Down syndrome.

96. Which of the following statements is *false* regarding the noradrenergic system?

A. Norepinephrine (NE)–containing neurons in the central nervous system (CNS) are predominantly located in the brainstem.

B. The locus coeruleus is the largest group of NE-containing neurons in the mammalian brain.

C. Brain regions innervated by the locus coeruleus include the thalamus, cerebellar cortex, and hypothalamus, but not the amygdala.

D. NE-containing cells are present in the lateral ventral tegmental fields.

E. The primary motor cortex contains high densities of both dopaminergic and noradrenergic axons.

97. Diabetes mellitus is a metabolic disorder with substantial neuropsychiatric comorbidity. Which of the following is *true* regarding the neuropsychiatric aspects of diabetes mellitus?

A. Facilitating the identification of automatic thoughts by techniques such as Socratic questioning, use of mood shifts that occur in vivo, thought recording, and guided imagery have been shown to be effective in treating depression in patients with type 2 diabetes.

B. In controlled studies, symptoms of depression occur in 15%–20% of patients with diabetes.

C. The increased prevalence of psychiatric disorders in a community sample of patients with diabetes was attributed to an increase in depressive disorder.

D. The prevalence of depression in diabetes is much higher than in other chronic diseases.

E. When symptoms of depression that may be attributed to the diabetic condition are excluded from a diagnosis of a mood disorder, the prevalence of depression in patients with diabetes is decreased by 50%.

98. A test of which of the following specimens is most subject to cheating?

A. Blood.

B. Hair.

C. Oral fluid.

D. Sweat.

E. Urine.

99. Regarding medical decision making, which of the following statements is *true?*

A. The parents of a disabled adult automatically remain the patient's legal guardians after their child's 18th birthday.

B. Studies have found that most (75%–80%) individuals fill out an advance directive for health care when given the opportunity to do so.

C. When an unmarried, incapacitated patient has an adult child, that adult child automatically is given medical decision making for the patient.

D. The completion of an advance directive for health care allows patients to specify in writing the medical care they wish to receive under various catastrophic medical conditions.

E. Substitute decision makers tend to base their decisions on what the patient would have wanted and not on what they themselves would have wanted had they been in the patient's place.

100. Which of the following is an example of a circumstance in which a drug-using defendant may claim settled insanity as a criminal defense strategy?

    A. Intoxication resulted from trickery.
    B. Long-term drug use has led to a chronic brain injury that is different from acute intoxication or toxic psychosis.
    C. Intoxication occurred under duress.
    D. Intoxication was caused by a previously unknown vulnerability to an atypical reaction to a substance.
    E. Intoxication occurred as a previously unknown side effect of a medication.

101. In bulimia nervosa

    A. Illness onset typically follows a period of dieting.
    B. The majority of patients abuse diuretics.
    C. The average binge episode lasts more than 2 hours.
    D. Comorbid depressive symptoms are seen in a minority of patients.
    E. Impulsivity in other spheres of behavior is infrequent.

102. Which of the following statements is *true* regarding psychiatric interviewing of children?

    A. Children between the ages of 3 and 6 years usually cannot provide correct information when questioned in a way commensurate with their developmental level.
    B. Reports of children between the ages of 3 and 6 years can provide correct information when questioned in a way commensurate with their developmental level.
    C. Young children tend not to be suggestible and tend not to repeat inaccurate information fed to them by hostile parents involved in a bitter custody battle.
    D. For diagnostic purposes, if parents or other caregivers are unavailable to be interviewed, the examination of a child alone usually can suffice for patients who are at least 8 years old.
    E. In most circumstances, it is best to interview children first and then the parents.

103. Which of the following statements is *true* regarding the acetylcholinergic system?

    A. The acetylcholine (ACh)–containing neurons are located mostly in the basal forebrain and the pontomesencephalotegmental region.
    B. Few ACh-containing neurons project to the cerebral cortex.
    C. The two main receptors of ACh are muscarinic and glutaminergic.
    D. ACh is known only to be part of neuronal tissue.
    E. ACh is synthesized by the enzyme acetylcholinesterase.

104. What approximate percentage of patients with Alzheimer's disease present with psychotic symptoms, typically in the middle stages of the disease?

    A. 10%–20%.
    B. 15%–25%.
    C. 25%–30%.
    D. 35%–50%.
    E. 55%–65%.

105. All of the following antidepressants may be appropriate for a patient with bulimia nervosa *except*

    A. Desipramine.
    B. Imipramine.
    C. Phenelzine.
    D. Fluoxetine.
    E. Topiramate

106. A patient is referred to you by an oncologist. One month after receiving the diagnosis, the patient denies the diagnosis and has become noncompliant with the oncologist's treatment recommendations. In your initial psychiatric interview, you uncover no other mood, anxiety, or behavioral symptoms. On the basis of this limited information, what might be a reasonable initial diagnosis for this patient?

    A. Acute stress disorder.
    B. Bereavement.
    C. Adjustment disorder with depressed mood.
    D. Adjustment disorder with mixed disturbance of emotions and conduct.
    E. Adjustment disorder unspecified.

107. Which of the following is considered a dyssomnia?

    A. Circadian rhythm sleep disorder.
    B. Sleepwalking disorder.
    C. Sleep terror disorder.
    D. Nightmare disorder.
    E. Rapid-eye movement (REM) sleep behavior disorder.

108. The most common anxiety disorder in later life is

    A. Posttraumatic stress disorder.
    B. Agoraphobia.
    C. Panic disorder.
    D. Social phobia.
    E. Generalized anxiety disorder, which may be co-morbid with major depression.

109. A test of which of the following specimens can detect drug use for up to 90 days?

    A. Blood.
    B. Hair.
    C. Oral fluid.
    D. Sweat.
    E. Urine.

110. Which of the following statements is *true* regarding the hypothalamic-pituitary-adrenal (HPA) axis and mood?

    A. The data are unclear regarding the relationship between endogenously elevated cortisol and exogenous administration of glucocorticoids with alterations in the regulation of emotion, psychotic symptoms, and clinical depression.
    B. Patients with severe depression tend to have elevated serum cortisol levels, especially in the morning.
    C. Data suggest that gestational stress or prolonged periods of maternal separation early in life increase the magnitude of the neuroendocrine response to stress and the vulnerability for stress-related illness.
    D. Antiglucocorticoid therapy might be useful in the treatment of major depression but not psychotic depression.
    E. Monoamine oxidase inhibitors (MAOIs), tricyclic antidepressants (TCAs), and selective serotonin reuptake inhibitors (SSRIs) tend to "upregulate" the HPA axis.

111. All of the following agents are considered first-line treatments for periodic limb movement disorder and restless legs syndrome *except*

    A. Pramipexole.
    B. Bromocriptine.
    C. Pergolide.
    D. Ropinirole.
    E. Carbidopa/levodopa.

112. Risk factors for development of adjustment disorders include which of the following?

    A. Race, younger age, female gender, chronic medical or psychiatric illness, and poverty.
    B. Older age, male gender, chronic medical or psychiatric illness, and poverty, but not race.
    C. Race, older age, chronic medical or psychiatric illness, and poverty, but not gender.
    D. Race, chronic medical or psychiatric illness, and poverty, but not age or gender.
    E. Chronic medical or psychiatric illness, and poverty, but not race, age, or gender.

113. One common method of classifying malingering includes all of the following categories *except*

    A. Pure malingering.
    B. Partial malingering.
    C. False imputation.
    D. Factitious disorders.
    E. All of the above are considered subcategories of malingering.

114. Evidence of malingered posttraumatic stress disorder (PTSD) may include all of the following *except*

    A. Claims of severe insomnia that does not respond to medication.
    B. Discrepancies in factual data.
    C. Pleasure or enjoyment in reviewing the events associated with the trauma.
    D. Single, repeating dreams that revisit the trauma.
    E. Evidence that the patient is not avoiding reminders of the trauma or not experiencing anxiety when exposed to reminders.

115. This threshold model suggests that the presence of all of the following in the clinical evaluation should trigger the clinicians' suspicion that an individual is malingering *except*

    A. Suspicion of voluntary control over symptoms.
    B. Bizarre or absurd symptoms.
    C. Symptom fluctuation over time.
    D. Complaints grossly in excess of clinical findings.
    E. Substantial noncompliance with treatment.

116. A 34-year-old woman is diagnosed with severe major depressive disorder. Clinical studies indicate that at the time of diagnosis her labwork would include

    A. Decreased cortisol levels in the evening and through the night.
    B. Elevated levels of thyroid-stimulating hormone (TSH); decreased serum levels of $T_3$ and $T_4$.
    C. Normal TSH levels; elevated serum levels of $T_4$; decreased serum levels of $T_3$.
    D. Normal levels of TSH; decreased serum levels of $T_4$; elevated serum levels of $T_3$.
    E. Decreased baseline prolactin level.

117. Mr. Jones reports that he stole a car because he was hearing a voice inside his head telling him that if he did not steal the car, the world would be destroyed. The evaluating psychiatrist would be suspicious of malingering if Mr. Jones reported that this auditory hallucination

    A. Was continuous and incessant.
    B. Was spoken in fluent and grammatical language.
    C. Could be ignored or avoided by turning up the volume on a radio or television.
    D. Was associated with a delusion.
    E. Was associated with a documented history of psychotic episodes of similar content.

118. A thorough psychological evaluation of a child with a physical illness must include an assessment of somatic symptoms. All of the following questionnaires have been developed to assess specifically physically ill children and families *except*

    A. Eating Attitudes Test.
    B. High Sensitivity Cognitive Screen.
    C. Coping Health Inventory for Parents.
    D. McCarthy Scales of Children's Abilities.
    E. Varni-Thompson Pediatric Pain Questionnaire.

119. Which of the following sequences states the correct order of the continuum of decision-making capacity from incapacitated to fully capacitated?

    A. Able to assign a substitute decision maker → unable to make decisions → able to make medical decisions → able to appreciate the differences between clinical care and clinical research → fully capacitated.
    B. Unable to make decisions → able to make medical decisions → able to assign a substitute decision maker → able to appreciate the difference between clinical care and clinical research → fully capacitated.
    C. Unable to make decisions → able to assign a substitute decision maker → able to make medical decisions → able to appreciate the differences between clinical care and clinical research → fully capacitated.
    D. Unable to make decisions → able to appreciate the differences between clinical care and clinical research → able to make medical decisions → able to assign a substitute decision maker → fully capacitated.
    E. Able to assign a substitute decision maker → able to make medical decisions → unable to make decisions → able to appreciate the differences between clinical care and clinical research → fully capacitated.

120. Patients with factitious disorder are characterized by all of the following *except*

    A. Often have a cluster C personality disorder.
    B. May have an Axis I disorder, especially schizophrenia.
    C. Have a need to be the center of attention.
    D. Long to be cared for.
    E. Derive pleasure from deceiving others.

121. Which of the following statements is *true* regarding the diagnosis of adjustment disorder?

    A. The adjustment disorder diagnosis should never be used if the patient's symptoms meet the criteria for another Axis I diagnosis.
    B. Adjustment disorder may be diagnosed if the symptoms are secondary to the direct physiological effects of a general medical condition.
    C. The diagnosis requires the development of symptoms within 6 months of an identifiable stressor's occurrence.

    D. Adjustment disorders are coded by subtype, according to whether symptoms predominantly involve depressed mood, anxiety, disturbance of conduct, or a mixture of these.

    E. The diagnosis does not require that symptoms be time limited or in response to a stressor.

122. Both positron emission tomography (PET) and functional magnetic resonance imaging (fMRI) rely on the empirical relationship between neuronal activity and regional blood flow. Which of the following statements is *false* when comparing PET with fMRI?

    A. PET is quieter but more sensitive to movement artifact than fMRI.

    B. PET is significantly less expensive than fMRI.

    C. PET has superior spatial resolution when compared with fMRI images.

    D. PET has a temporal resolution of minutes compared with fMRI, which has a temporal resolution on the order of seconds.

    E. Both PET and fMRI scans typically take less than an hour.

123. A 27-year-old man reports lifelong intermittent symptoms of worry, muscle tension, irritability, and difficulty falling asleep. Which of the following statements is *true* regarding possible pharmacological interventions?

    A. If a benzodiazepine is prescribed, psychiatric symptoms will be treated more effectively than somatic ones.

    B. If a benzodiazepine is prescribed, somatic symptoms will be more effectively treated than psychiatric ones.

    C. If buspirone is prescribed, alleviation of anxiety symptoms will likely occur within 2 weeks.

    D. If venlafaxine is prescribed, alleviation of anxiety symptoms likely will occur only after the fifth week.

    E. If a tricyclic antidepressant (TCA) is prescribed, only depressive symptoms will remit.

124. Which of the following definitions/statements is *false*?

    A. Physical dependence is a state of adaptation that manifests as a specific withdrawal syndrome.

    B. Withdrawal syndromes are characterized by symptoms similar to those characteristic of use of the substance.

    C. Tolerance is the need for increasing amounts of a substance to obtain the desired effect.

    D. Addiction is characterized by craving and impaired control of drug use despite harm.

    E. Psychological dependence is the feeling of need for a specific substance.

125. All of the following are laboratory findings associated with alcohol abuse *except*

    A. Increased serum gamma-glutamyltransferase (SGGT) level.

    B. Increased serum carbohydrate-deficient transferrin level.

    C. Decreased serum carbohydrate-deficient transferrin level.

    D. Increased uric acid level.

    E. Increased mean corpuscular volume.

126. Buprenorphine is

    A. A schedule IV narcotic.

    B. An opioid agonist at higher doses.

    C. A short-acting opioid receptor partial agonist.

    D. A mu-opioid receptor partial agonist.

    E. An opioid antagonist regardless of dosage.

127. The neural substrates of drug reward and reinforcement include which of the following?

    A. Extrapyramidal system.

    B. Dorsal raphe nuclei.

    C. Tegmental fields.

    D. Mesolimbic projections to the nucleus accumbens.

    E. Amygdala.

128. The evidence base is *least* supportive of which of the following agents for the treatment of child and adolescent attention-deficit/hyperactivity disorder (ADHD)?

    A. Psychostimulants.

    B. Tricyclic antidepressants (TCAs).

    C. Selective serotonin reuptake inhibitors (SSRIs).

    D. Atomoxetine.

    E. Bupropion.

129. In patients with hepatic impairment that has diminished their ability to metabolize medications, which of the following agents would be the best choice for prophylaxis of delirium tremens?

    A. Diazepam.
    B. Clonazepam.
    C. Alprazolam.
    D. Triazolam.
    E. Oxazepam.

130. According to findings from a meta-analysis of 15 studies, patients who are taking second-generation antipsychotics demonstrate

    A. Improved memory.
    B. Less weight gain than with first-generation antipsychotics.
    C. Better verbal fluency.
    D. Better overall clinical outcome.
    E. Similar improvements in neurocognitive symptoms of schizophrenia when compared with those taking first-generation antipsychotics.

131. Which of the following statements is *true* regarding aphasia syndromes?

    A. Broca's aphasia syndrome usually includes normal speech fluency, but Wernicke's aphasia syndrome does not.
    B. Wernicke's aphasia is characterized by relatively normal auditory comprehension, but Broca's aphasia is not.
    C. Anomic aphasia syndrome includes normal fluency, auditory comprehension, repetition, and naming.
    D. Conduction aphasia includes normal auditory comprehension and repetition.
    E. Global aphasia syndrome includes abnormal fluency and auditory comprehension.

132. In comparing lithium with divalproex in the treatment of acute mania, which of the following statements is *false?*

    A. Divalproex works better in patients with depressive symptoms.
    B. Divalproex works better in patients with previous multiple mood episodes.

C. Both lithium and divalproex can help with psychotic symptoms in acute mania.
    D. Both are efficacious for acute mania in comparison with placebo, but lithium is generally superior to divalproex in head-to-head trials.
    E. Both agents have better long-term efficacy in the treatment of acute mania in combination with other medications.

133. Double-blind studies have supported moderate benefit for which of the following medications in preventing relapse to cocaine abuse?

    A. Desipramine.
    B. Bupropion.
    C. Fluoxetine.
    D. Amantadine.
    E. Pergolide.

134. Which of the following statements best describes the usual course of illness in schizophrenia?

    A. After the acute onset, the first 2–5 years are marked by little change in severity.
    B. Negative symptoms usually respond to medication treatment better than positive symptoms.
    C. Positive symptoms usually respond to medication treatment better than negative symptoms.
    D. Positive symptoms usually become increasingly prominent during the course of illness.
    E. All of the above statements are accurate.

135. Which of the following statements is *not* true regarding anxiety disorders?

    A. Generalized anxiety disorder, posttraumatic stress disorder, specific phobias, and agoraphobia have a 2:1 female-to-male lifetime prevalence ratio.
    B. Lifetime prevalence of specific phobias is 10%.
    C. Social phobia is associated with a twofold risk for comorbid alcohol dependence or mood disorders.
    D. Of patients diagnosed with generalized anxiety disorder, 90% have comorbid psychiatric diagnoses.
    E. Obsessive-compulsive disorder has a 1:1 female-to-male lifetime prevalence ratio.

136. The hallucinogen methylenedioxymethamphet-amine (MDMA, Ecstasy) is related to what class of drugs?

    A. Amphetamines.
    B. Opioids.
    C. Dissociative anesthetics.
    D. Cannabinoids.
    E. Benzodiazepine reverse agonists.

137. Efficacy in smoking cessation has been demonstrated by all of the following *except*

    A. Transdermal nicotine.
    B. Bupropion.
    C. Nortriptyline.
    D. Propranolol.
    E. Clonidine.

138. The adjustment disorder diagnosis in DSM-IV-TR (American Psychiatric Association 2000) has been found to have certain advantages and disadvantages for patients and clinicians. Which of the following is the major disadvantage of using the diagnosis?

    A. The concept of temporary emotional symptoms resulting from a stressful life event seems more of a normal human reaction than a pathological diagnostic state.
    B. The more benign course implied by this diagnosis allows clinicians to be more prognostically optimistic.
    C. The diagnosis is less stigmatizing.
    D. Medical insurance carriers do not consider the diagnosis to be a preexisting condition when evaluating a patient's risk.
    E. The concept of the stressor lacks quantifiable and qualifiable guidelines, contributing to the vague and nonspecific nature of the diagnosis.

139. The two best predictors of antidepressant response for the treatment of a depressive disorder are

    A. Choice of antidepressants that have proven to have the most efficacy with major depressive disorder.
    B. Medication side-effect profile and comorbid psychiatric symptoms.
    C. A history of prior response to an agent and sedating versus activating properties.

    D. Family history of response and symptoms such as comorbid insomnia or anxiety.
    E. A history of prior response to an agent and a family history of preferential response.

140. Which of the following statements is *true* regarding memory?

    A. Declarative memory includes semantic and episodic memory.
    B. Declarative memory is unable to be assessed clinically by recall or recognition.
    C. Semantic memories are can usually be associated with specific times or incidents.
    D. Semantic memory are not required for episodic memory.
    E. Procedural memory is a type of declarative memory.

141. In regard to National Institute of Mental Health studies comparing patients with childhood-onset schizophrenia and patients with adult-onset schizophrenia, all of the following findings are correct *except*

    A. Childhood-onset patients show greater delay in language development than do adult-onset patients.
    B. Childhood-onset patients evidence more disruptive behavior disorders than do adult-onset patients.
    C. Childhood-onset patients evidence more learning disorders than do adult-onset patients.
    D. Childhood-onset patients evidence high rates of specific developmental disorders such as autism.
    E. Childhood-onset schizophrenia appears to represent a more malignant form of the disorder.

142. Published open-label treatment studies in children and adolescents with posttraumatic stress disorder (PTSD) have supported the efficacy of all of the following agents *except*

    A. Citalopram.
    B. Clonidine.
    C. Carbamazepine.
    D. Propranolol.
    E. Alprazolam.

143. Orthostatic hypotension is a common side effect of all of the following antidepressants *except*

    A. Trazodone.
    B. Mirtazapine.
    C. Venlafaxine.
    D. Imipramine.
    E. Phenelzine.

144. Which of the following functional or anatomic brain abnormalities have been associated with depression?

    A. Increased hippocampal volumes.
    B. Decreased left lateral prefrontal cortex activity.
    C. Smaller amygdala volumes.
    D. Increased activity of the caudate and putamen.
    E. Neuroimaging evidence of associations between depression and brain abnormalities are equivocal at best.

145. All of the following drugs have shown efficacy in the treatment of acute mania in randomized, placebo-controlled trials *except*

    A. Olanzapine.
    B. Chlorpromazine.
    C. Carbamazepine.
    D. Lamotrigine.
    E. Divalproex.

146. The relationship between mental illness, substance abuse, and violent behavior remains controversial. Which of the following statements is *false?*

    A. Patients with comorbid substance abuse and major mental illness are more frequently violent than persons in the general population.
    B. Patients with comorbid substance abuse and major mental illness are more frequently violent than patients with mental illness alone.
    C. Among all reported violence, over 10% is a result of mental illness in isolation (i.e., no comorbid substance abuse).
    D. When mentally ill patients abuse substances, their risk of violence increase dramatically.
    E. Psychiatric patients who are noncompliant with treatment are at an increased risk of being violent.

147. Which of the following is *true* regarding electroconvulsive therapy (ECT)?

    A. ECT should be considered in the treatment of treatment-resistant mixed mood disorders, delirious mania, catatonic psychosis, and drug-induced psychotic disorder.
    B. ECT should be considered the treatment of last resort in even severely depressed patients.
    C. ECT has been shown to be effective in >80% of cases of treatment-resistant unipolar or bipolar major depression.
    D. In recent years, a large amount of data have emerged comparing the efficacy of ECT to mood stabilizing medications in the treatment of acute and maintenance treatment.
    E. ECT is not effective in the treatment of the motor symptoms of patients with Parkinson's disease.

148. The classic clinical presentation of middle cerebral artery infarction in the dominant hemisphere includes all of the following *except*

    A. Contralateral hemiparesis.
    B. Neglect.
    C. Aphasia.
    D. Sensory loss of a cortical type.
    E. Hemianopsia.

149. Which phase of illness in schizophrenic patients is best described by the following definition: a 1- to 6-month (or longer) period when symptoms of hallucinations, delusions, thought disorder, or disorganized behavior are predominant?

    A. Prodrome.
    B. Acute phase.
    C. Recovery phase.
    D. Residual phase.
    E. Chronicity.

150. What two medications have been approved by the U.S. Food and Drug Administration (FDA) for the treatment of Tourette's syndrome?

    A. Risperidone and haloperidol.
    B. Clonidine and fluphenazine.
    C. Pimozide and clonidine.
    D. Pimozide and haloperidol.
    E. Haloperidol and fluoxetine.

151. Serum vitamin B$_{12}$ and folate levels

    A. Are rarely important in the evaluation of the elderly patient.
    B. May point to etiologies of a range of neuropsychiatric disturbances.
    C. Would not be thought etiologic if recorded as normal.
    D. Are not related to hyperhomocysteinemia.
    E. Are not related to one-carbon metabolism in brain tissue.

152. Systemic complications of anorexia nervosa include

    A. Leukocytosis.
    B. Hyperkalemic alkalosis.
    C. Hyperchloremia.
    D. Decreased serum bicarbonate levels.
    E. Cardiac arrhythmias.

153. The most common anxiety disorder in later life is

    A. Posttraumatic stress disorder.
    B. Agoraphobia.
    C. Panic disorder.
    D. Social phobia.
    E. Generalized anxiety disorder, which may be comorbid with major depression.

154. A 28-year-old man presenting to your outpatient clinic began taking a new antipsychotic medication for undifferentiated schizophrenia 1 week ago. He complains of mild daytime sedation, mild abdominal cramping, nausea, and "weird muscle aches" that make it difficult for him to turn his neck from side to side. On exam, his gaze appears fixated in one position, and he has a facial grimace. You notice that his speech is dysarthric and is occasionally interrupted by what appears to be uncomfortable swallowing as if he's gulping air. He should be treated with

    A. Intramuscular thiamine.
    B. Intravenous diphenhydramine.
    C. Oral benztropine.
    D. IV beta-blockers.
    E. Oral or intravenous lorazepam.

155. A 36-year-old woman who had been fired from her job in March presents to the outpatient medical clinic in August with a 1-month history of depressed

mood and insomnia. She also reports decreased appetite but no other symptoms of depression. She relates her symptoms to the job loss. The most likely diagnosis is

    A. No diagnosis.
    B. Acute adjustment disorder with depressed mood.
    C. Anxiety disorder not otherwise specified.
    D. Acute stress disorder.
    E. Chronic adjustment disorder with depressed mood.

156. Which of the following clinical findings has been demonstrated in patients with bipolar disorder?

    A. Decreased plasma cortisol concentration.
    B. Decreased cortisol in cerebrospinal fluid.
    C. Suppression of plasma glucocorticoid concentration after dexamethasone administration.
    D. Nonsuppression of plasma glucocorticoid concentration after dexamethasone administration.
    E. Increased diurnal variation of plasma cortisol concentrations.

157. Which of the following statements is *false* regarding the noradrenergic system?

    A. The initial steps in the biosynthesis of norepinephrine are similar, but not identical to, those of dopamine.
    B. Norepinephrine-containing neurons in the central nervous system are located predominantly in the medulla and pons.
    C. In the hypothalamus, the paraventricular nucleus contains the highest density of norepinephrine axons.
    D. In the amygdala, the basolateral nuclei contain the highest density of norepinephrine axons.
    E. Norepinephrine elicits responses in the postsynaptic cell via G-protein–mediated second-messenger systems.

158. The genetic contributions to schizophrenia may be best described as

    A. Sex-linked.
    B. Multifactorial.
    C. Mendelian.
    D. Mutations.
    E. Iatrogenic.

159. All of the following tests measure aspects of executive functioning *except*

    A. Tower of London.
    B. Behavioral Assessment of the Dysexecutive Syndrome.
    C. Twenty Questions Test.
    D. Wisconsin Card Sorting Test.
    E. Complex Figure Test.

160. The primary forensic issue in a child custody evaluation in the context of a divorce is

    A. What custodial arrangements will be least disruptive to the child's life.
    B. To what custodial arrangements will the child agree.
    C. What custodial arrangements are in the best interests of the child.
    D. Which parent has been more involved in caretaking of the child.
    E. Which parent is more motivated to do what is best for the child.

161. Which of the following is *true* regarding immune function in patients with depression?

    A. Peripheral blood findings in depressed patients have included decreased lymphocytes, neutrophils, and natural killer (NK) cell activity.
    B. A syndrome of "sickness behavior" mimicking major depression follows administration of interferon-α (IFN-α) and interleukin-2 (IL-2).
    C. Cerebrospinal fluid (CSF) studies of depressed patients have demonstrated increased levels of interleukin-6 (IL-6) and soluble IL-6 receptor.
    D. Decreases in acute phase proteins such as C-reactive protein, serum haptoglobin, the complement protein C4, $\alpha_1$-antitrypsin, and $\alpha_1$-acid glycoprotein.
    E. The high rates of depression in autoimmune and other immune-related diseases demonstrate that depression is associated with a suppression of the immune response.

162. A 77-year-old Caucasian man with no known previous psychiatric history is brought by his caregiver for an evaluation because of his worsening short-term memory and "strange behaviors." The caregiver reports that the patient was recently seen chuckling to himself. When asked why he was laughing, the patient responded, "These little green squirrels are so funny when they square dance with the elephants!" and proceeded to give a detailed description of their activities. To the caregiver's surprise, the patient mentions having been seeing these dancing animals for the past several months. He has a history of hypertension that is well-controlled with medications, with no recent changes in his drug regimen. His vital signs are normal, he appears to be in no apparent physical distress, and his gait is normal. On examination, the patient is intermittently drowsy, easily distracted, and disinhibited at times. Despite multiple introductions, he asks for a third time who you are. Of the following, which is the most likely diagnosis?

    A. Delirium.
    B. Normal pressure hydrocephalus.
    C. Vascular dementia
    D. Lewy Body dementia.
    E. Decompensated schizophrenia.

163. Which of the following characteristics is *not* associated with an increased risk of adolescent substance abuse?

    A. High levels of behavioral activity.
    B. Reduced attention span.
    C. High impulsivity.
    D. Lack of emotional reactivity (i.e., "blunting").
    E. Irritability.

164. Which of the following choices accurately lists, from most common to least common, the four most commonly used substances among patients with schizophrenia?

    A. Nicotine, alcohol, cocaine, cannabis.
    B. Alcohol, nicotine, cocaine, cannabis.
    C. Nicotine, cannabis, alcohol, cocaine.
    D. Alcohol, nicotine, cannabis, cocaine.
    E. Nicotine, alcohol, cannabis, cocaine.

165. About what percentage of serotonin (5-hydroxytryptamine [5-HT]) in the body is found in the cerebrum?

    A. 95%.
    B. 70%.
    C. 35%.
    D. 10%.
    E. 2%.

166. All of the following features are common to all dementias *except*

    A. Memory impairment and aphasia.
    B. Apraxia.
    C. Agnosia.
    D. Disturbed executive functioning.
    E. None of the above.

167. All of the following clinical features are characteristic of cortical dementias *except*

    A. Apraxia.
    B. Agnosia.
    C. Visuospatial deficits.
    D. Prominent motor signs.
    E. Language deficits.

168. Hypothyroidism is an example of a metabolic illness with neuropsychiatric symptoms. Which of the following is *true?*

    A. Anxiety occurs in about one-third of patients with hypothyroidism.
    B. The two most common psychiatric manifestations in hypothyroidism are depression and psychosis.
    C. Replacement of thyroid hormone in the form of $T_3$ (rather than $T_4$) has a specific effect on improving depressed mood but a negligible effect on cognitive performance.
    D. Physical symptoms typically precede psychiatric symptoms in patients with hypothyroidism.
    E. Hypomanic or manic symptoms occur in about one-third of patients with hypothyroidism.

169. Regarding the use of nonsteroidal anti-inflammatory drugs (NSAIDs) in treating or preventing Alzheimer's disease, which of the following statements is *true?*

    A. NSAIDs have been found to increase the risk of developing Alzheimer's disease by 30%–80%.
    B. In prospective clinical trials, NSAIDs have shown no benefit in treating patients with Alzheimer's disease.
    C. No prospective studies have been conducted, only retrospective studies.
    D. NSAID use has proven too risky because of the side effects of these agents.

E. With long-term use of NSAIDs, the risk of Alzheimer's disease is higher.

170. A test of which of the following specimens has the shortest window of detection?

    A. Blood.
    B. Hair.
    C. Oral fluid.
    D. Sweat.
    E. Urine.

171. You are called to provide a psychiatric consultation on patient end-stage pancreatic cancer whose treatment team is considering referral to a hospice program. Of the following, the most relevant ethical principles to consider are

    A. Fidelity and beneficence.
    B. Justice and autonomy.
    C. Nonmaleficence and fidelity.
    D. Confidentiality and nonmalficence.
    E. Autonomy and beneficence.

172. In forensic practice, the clinician needs to be mindful of the possible differences in the definitions of common clinical terms. Which of the following statements is *true?*

    A. The term *narcotic* refers to an addictive drug that is controlled or prohibited by law.
    B. The terms *narcotic* and *opioid* are synonymous clinically and legally.
    C. The terms *addiction* and *substance dependence* are legally interchangeable.
    D. The clinical definition of *chemical dependency* relates to deleterious effects of drug use.
    E. The terms *chemical dependency* and *addiction* are legally, but not necessarily clinically, interchangeable.

173. What percentage of patients treated for apparent major depression in the outpatient setting subsequently receive a diagnosis of bipolar I or II disorder?

    A. 5%–10%.
    B. 15%–30%.
    C. >40%.
    D. <5%.
    E. Unknown.

174. A nonpharmacological treatment indicated for pyromania is

   A. Aversive conditioning.
   B. Cognitive-behavioral psychotherapy.
   C. Interpersonal psychotherapy.
   D. Psychodynamic psychotherapy.
   E. Psychoanalytic psychotherapy.

175. Patients with Alzheimer's disease with and without psychosis differ in all of the following *except*

   A. Patients with Alzheimer's disease with psychosis show greater impairment in executive functioning.
   B. Patients with Alzheimer's disease with psychosis have a greater prevalence of extrapyramidal signs.
   C. Patients with Alzheimer's disease with psychosis have shown increased norepinephrine levels and reduced serotonin levels in subcortical regions.
   D. Patients with Alzheimer's disease with psychosis typically warrant very long term maintenance therapy with antipsychotics.
   E. Patients with Alzheimer's disease with psychosis have more prevalent behavioral disturbances such as agitation than hallucinations and paranoid delusions.

176. A young man is brought to the emergency room by his friends, who report that the patient was at a fraternity party and was "partying" with other partygoers, when he started "acting weird," saying he wanted to kill himself. His roommate recalled that the patient has been increasingly depressed since he was injured in a car accident a week ago, especially in the past few days. The patient binges on alcohol occasionally and has been taking "some pain meds" since his accident but does not use other substances. He quit smoking "cold turkey" 2–3 days ago. He has no known history of a mood disorder. On examination, the young man has slurred speech and an ataxic gait. He has nystagmus bilaterally, and his pupils are constricted. When you gently start examining the leg that was injured, he yells, "What are you doing?! Trying to kill me?!" and wimpers in pain. In addition to alcohol intoxication, which of the following are other conditions in your differential diagnosis?

   A. Opioid withdrawal and/or nicotine withdrawal.
   B. Opioid intoxication and/or phencyclidine (PCP) intoxication.
   C. Nicotine withdrawal and/or opioid intoxication.
   D. Benzodiazepine intoxication, hallucinogen intoxication.
   E. Inhalant intoxication, and/or amphetamine intoxication.

177. Ten seconds after starting an electroconvulsive therapy (ECT) procedure, the ECT is abruptly discontinued becase of the patient inexplicably awakening from anesthesia. No seizure was induced. The procedure was not resumed because the patient then refused to continue the treatment. Which of the following statements is *true?*

   A. Even though a seizure was not induced, it is likely that the patient will derive some benefit from the procedure because he received at least 10 seconds of electrical stimulation.
   B. The patient may not derive any benefit from the procedure because at least 20 seconds of electrical stimulation is required in order for ECT to be of any benefit.
   C. It is unlikely that the patient will derive any therapeutic benefit from the procedure because seizure induction is essential for ECT.
   D. It is difficult to predict whether this patient will derive any benefit from the procedure because 50% of patients do not require seizure-induction in order for ECT to be effective.
   E. All of the above.

178. All of the following statements regarding positive symptoms of schizophrenia are correct *except*

   A. Studies show that a high degree of positive symptoms correlates with a worse long-term prognosis.
   B. Positive symptoms include hallucinations.
   C. Positive symptoms respond to antipsychotic medications.
   D. Positive symptoms are not the first set of symptoms that typically present in schizophrenia.
   E. Positive symptoms are traditionally the focus of medication treatment.

179. In a forensic evaluation, the role of the evaluating psychiatrist is to

    A. Focus on a thorough clinical evaluation to develop a solid diagnostic impression of the patient.
    B. Meet the needs of a third party whose goals are legal or financial.
    C. Ensure that the patient's needs are foremost while conducting the evaluation.
    D. Ensure patient confidentiality, beneficence, and nonmaleficence
    E. None of the above.

180. A 32-year-old woman presents to the emergency room with new onset of myoclonic jerking of her extremities, flushing, fever, nausea, and tremor after she took one dose of sumatriptan that she had recently been prescribed for migraine headaches. Besides sumatriptan, her medication list includes sertraline 100 mg/day, which she has been taking for the past 3 years for a mild depressive disorder. Which of the following medications will likely be of benefit for this patient at this time?

    A. Benztropine.
    B. Propranolol.
    C. Dantrolene.
    D. Phenobarbital.
    E. Lorazepam.

181. A diagnosis of personality disorder in elderly persons is subject to some specific clinical and epidemiological considerations. Which of the following is *true*?

    A. The prevalence of personality disorders in the elderly population is approximately the same as in younger patients, about 10%.
    B. The prevalence of personality disorders among elderly patients with another psychiatric condition is between 25% and 65%.
    C. In the older population, the association between personality and anxiety disorders is the most often reported comorbidity.
    D. Cluster B personality disorders do not improve with age.
    E. The association between comorbid personality disorder and mood disorder is stronger for late-onset than for early-onset depression.

182. Which of the following statements is *true* regarding the differential diagnosis of childhood psychotic disorders?

    A. The diagnostic criteria for schizophreniform disorder require an illness duration of less than 6 months.
    B. Once a diagnosis of schizophreniform disorder is made, a diagnosis of schizophrenia can never be given.
    C. A diagnosis of schizophreniform disorder requires the presence of a decline in function.
    D. Brief psychotic disorder requires a symptom duration of at least 1 month but no more than 6 months.
    E. The diagnosis of psychotic disorder not otherwise specified is very rare in the hospitalized adolescent population.

183. Which of the following statements is *true* regarding patterns of abuse and dependence for different classes of drugs?

    A. The age at highest risk for marijuana and alcohol initiation is between 14 and 17 years.
    B. The age at highest risk for dependence on alcohol is between 24 and 26 years.
    C. The age at highest risk for dependence on marijuana is 3 years older than the corresponding age at risk for alcohol dependence.
    D. The age at highest risk for cocaine initiation is between 15 and 18 years.
    E. The developmental period for alcohol dependence is longer than those for marijuana and cocaine dependence.

184. Outpatient therapy as an initial approach has the *best* chance of success in patients with anorexia nervosa who

    A. Have had the illness for more than 6 months.
    B. Are bingeing.
    C. Are vomiting.
    D. Have medical complications.
    E. Have parents who will participate in family therapy.

185. Which of the following structures is *not* involved in the central processing of pain?

     A. Spinothalamic tracts.
     B. Anterior cingulate gyrus.
     C. Insular cortex.
     D. Prefrontal cortex.
     E. Somatosensory cortex.

186. A number of macroscopic and histological findings in the brain of patients with schizophrenia have been reported. For which of the following findings has the evidence been confirmed by meta-analysis and reported to be strong?

     A. Maldistribution of white matter neurons.
     B. Decreased thalamic volume.
     C. Reduced synaptic and dendritic markers in hippocampus.
     D. Entorhinal cortex dysplasia.
     E. Enlarged lateral and third ventricles.

187. Which of the following statements is *true* regarding epidemiological findings in somatization disorder?

     A. Somatization disorder is diagnosed predominantly in men.
     B. The lifetime risk of somatization disorder is estimated at 10% in women.
     C. Somatization disorder in men shares a common etiology with antisocial personality disorder.
     D. Somatization disorder in women may be related more to anxiety disorder.
     E. Some authors believe that somatization disorder may be more of a personality disorder than an Axis I disorder.

188. Which of the following criteria is found in the diagnosis of substance dependence but *not* substance abuse?

     A. Tolerance and withdrawal.
     B. Recurrent substance-related failure in fulfilling social role obligations.
     C. Recurrent substance use in physically hazardous circumstances.
     D. Recurrent substance-related legal problems.
     E. Continued substance use despite social/interpersonal problems.

189. Which of the following statements is *true* regarding anorexia nervosa?

     A. Obsessive-compulsive behavior rarely develops after the onset of anorexia nervosa.
     B. There is a relatively frequent association with impulsive behavior, such as suicide attempts and self-mutilation, among individuals with the bulimic type of anorexia.
     C. Amenorrhea occurs after noticeable weight loss.
     D. Most adolescent anorexia patients do not have delayed psychosexual development.
     E. Patients with the restrictive type of anorexia are more likely to have a discrete personality disorder diagnosis.

190. Within central processing, the "medial" system is responsible for generating the affective/emotional component of pain, whereas the "lateral" system is responsible for the discriminative sensory components. Which of the following structures is part of the medial system?

     A. Primary somatosensory cortex (SI).
     B. Secondary somatosensory cortex (SII).
     C. Anterior cingulate.
     D. Parietal cortex.
     E. Premotor cortex.

191. A 39-year-old male patient presenting to an outpatient clinic has falsely believed for the past 4–5 years that he is a professional football player. He describes in detail a few of his best plays as a quarterback for the Chicago Bears. He has told similar tales for the past few years and denies other psychotic symptoms. The introverted single man has lived alone in the same apartment for the past 7 years and has counted parts in the inventory department for the same company during that time. His symptoms have been refractory to previous treatments. On the basis of this limited clinical information, the most likely diagnosis is

     A. Paranoid schizophrenia.
     B. Schizophreniform disorder.
     C. Brief psychotic disorder.
     D. Delusional disorder.
     E. Schizoaffective disorder.

192. Several psychological factors have been implicated in conversion disorder, and terminology has evolved to describe these factors. The description "Anxiety is reduced by keeping an internal conflict out of conscious awareness through production of a symptom that is involuntarily produced and not under conscious control" applies to which of the following terms?

    A. Primary gain.
    B. Secondary gain.
    C. Tertiary gain.
    D. La belle indifférence.
    E. Factitious disorder.

193. Regarding family factors and substance abuse among youth, which of the following is *not* considered a characteristic that is related to the incidence of substance abuse?

    A. Parental level of income.
    B. Parental substance dependence.
    C. Parental personality.
    D. Parent–child relationship.
    E. Family cohesion.

194. Which of the following statements is *false* regarding trichotillomania?

    A. Psychiatric comorbidity is quite common among adults with trichotillomania.
    B. The prevalence of clinically significant hair pulling among college students has been estimated to be 1%–3.5%.
    C. Approximately 75% of adult trichotillomania patients report that most of their hair-pulling behavior takes place outside of awareness.
    D. Individuals with trichotillomania often report that hair pulling is painful.
    E. Hair pulling is often preceded by negative internal states involving unpleasant emotions, aversive physiological sensations, or dysregulated arousal.

195. All of the following statements are true regarding the relationship between pain and mood disorders *except*

    A. Patients with pain score higher on measures of depression than do patients without pain.

    B. In cancer patients, depressive symptoms are more highly correlated with pain than with a history of previous clinical depression.
    C. Depression is the most common psychiatric diagnosis among chronic pain patients.
    D. The presence or absence of mood symptoms has a differential effect on the opioid responsiveness of pain.
    E. Emotional aspects of pain, such as depression, are modulated by the insular cortex.

196. Which of the five subtypes of schizophrenia is associated with better premorbid functioning, older age at onset, and higher social and occupational function after illness onset?

    A. Catatonic.
    B. Disorganized.
    C. Paranoid.
    D. Residual.
    E. Undifferentiated.

197. In a patient who presents with a preoccupation with an imagined defect in appearance or markedly excessive concern with a slight physical anomaly, what is the most likely diagnosis?

    A. Hypochondriasis.
    B. Undifferentiated somatoform disorder.
    C. Conversion disorder.
    D. Body dysmorphic disorder.
    E. Somatoform disorder not otherwise specified.

198. Among the following classes of substance use disorders, which one was reported by the National Epidemiologic Survey on Alcohol and Related Conditions to have the highest rate of occurrence, at 2% of the population?

    A. Sedatives.
    B. Tranquilizers.
    C. Opioids.
    D. Amphetamines.
    E. Benzodiazepines.

199. All of the following statements concerning lateral specialization are true *except*

    A. In the vast majority of people, the left hemisphere is specialized for language and for processing verbally coded information.

B. The right hemisphere processes nonverbal information such as visual patterns or auditory signals.

C. The left hemisphere is specialized for the perception of our bodies in space.

D. The right hemisphere is dedicated to the mapping of feeling states.

E. The left hemisphere is involved in the processing of verbal information apprehended through either auditory or visual channels.

200. The MATRICS (measurement and treatment research to improve cognition in schizophrenia) program was developed to identify potential molecular targets to treat cognitive deficits in schizophrenia (Geyer and Tamminga 2004). The molecular targets identified as having the greatest promise to improve cognition include all of the following *except*

A. Dopamine$_1$ (D$_1$) receptor.
B. Dopamine$_2$ (D$_2$) receptor.
C. $\alpha_7$ Nicotinic receptor.
D. Muscarinic receptor.
E. *N*-methyl-D-aspartate (NMDA) receptor.

201. Which of the following is a warning sign for factitious disorder by proxy?

A. The episodes of illness occur only when the child is alone with the parent.
B. The other parent is quite involved with the care of the child.
C. The parent refuses painful or risky diagnostic tests for the child.
D. Signs and symptoms occur even when the child is separated from the parent.
E. There is a negative personal history of factitious disorder in the parent.

202. Various personality characteristics have been associated with substance abuse and dependence. Which of the following personality characteristics is *not* associated with increased risk of substance abuse?

A. Risk taking.
B. Novelty seeking.
C. Impulsivity.
D. Lack of emotional control.
E. Secure interpersonal attachment with dependency.

203. Which of the following descriptors characterizes the Munchausen subtype of factitious disorder?

A. Patients are mostly young women.
B. Patients have been described as passive and immature.
C. Most patients have single-system complaints.
D. Multiple hospitalizations with dramatic and often life-threatening presentations are prominent.
E. Many patients have health-related jobs.

204. Which of the following statements is *false* regarding mood disorders and substance abuse?

A. Both unipolar and bipolar mood disorders are associated with increased risk of substance abuse/dependence.
B. Dysthymic disorder is associated with an increased risk of substance abuse/dependence.
C. Mood disorder patients have a higher rate of abuse of alcohol, tranquilizers, and stimulants.
D. There is a reciprocal relationship between mood disorders and substance abuse; some studies demonstrate that depression precedes substance abuse, whereas other studies demonstrate the opposite.
E. Comorbid depression and substance use disorders are associated with greater functional impairment but not worse treatment outcomes.

205. Patients with delirium typically exhibit abnormalities in all of the following language functions *except*

A. Writing.
B. Word-list generation.
C. Motor speech.
D. Automatic speech.
E. Content of speech.

206. Positron emission tomography (PET) scanning in hallucinating persons with schizophrenia has provided clues to the anatomic structures that may be involved in a "psychosis neural circuit." The proposed psychosis circuit consists of all of the following structures *except*

A. Amygdala.
B. Medial prefrontal cortex.
C. Thalamus.
D. Anterior hippocampus.
E. Anterior cingulate.

# Answer Guide to Exam 1

1.  All of the following psychiatric disorders are common comorbid conditions in Huntington's disease *except*

    A. Schizophreniform disorder.
    B. Intermittent explosive disorder.
    C. Major depression.
    D. Obsessive-compulsive disorder.
    E. Bipolar disorder.

**The correct response is option D.**

Obsessive-compulsive disorder is *infrequently* comorbid with Huntington's disease. Schizophreniform disorder is more common in advanced cases but less common generally than the other disorders listed above. Studies using explicit diagnostic criteria and standardized assessments suggest that *intermittent explosive disorder* and *mood disorders* (especially unipolar depression, but also bipolar disorder) are the most prevalent psychiatric disorders in Huntington's disease.

> Lerner AJ, Riley D: Neuropsychiatric aspects of dementias associated with motor dysfunction, in The American Psychiatric Publishing Textbook of Neuropsychiatry and Behavioral Neurosciences, 5th Edition. Edited by Yudofsky SC, Hales RE. Washington, DC, American Psychiatric Publishing, 2008, p 913

2.  Which of the following statements is *true* regarding gender differences in schizophrenia?

    A. The onset of illness tends to be more acute in males than in females.
    B. Men tend to have a higher level of premorbid functioning than women.
    C. Women generally have a more favorable outcome than men.
    D. The age at onset is, on average, 5 years earlier in women than in men.

    E. There are no differences between men and women in onset, tempo of onset, and level of premorbid functioning.

**The correct response is option C.**

Schizophrenia is a chronic illness, with onset of psychotic symptoms usually occurring around late adolescence and early adulthood. The age at onset is approximately 5 years later in women than in men. The onset of illness also tends to be more acute in women, as compared with the typically more insidious onset in men, and women tend to have had a higher level of premorbid functioning. Although there may be no clear sex differences in cross-sectional symptomatology of the illness, the differences in the age at onset, tempo of onset, and level of premorbid functioning, all of which are prognostic factors, are consistent with the fact that women in general tend to have a more favorable outcome.

> Woo T-UW, Zimmet SV, Wojcik JD, et al: Treatment of schizophrenia, in The American Psychiatric Publishing Textbook of Psychopharmacology, 3rd Edition. Edited by Schatzberg AF, Nemeroff CB. Washington, DC, American Psychiatric Publishing, 2004, pp 888–889

3.  Which of the following diagnoses is found at increased prevalence among the first-degree relatives of patients with schizophrenia?

    A. Antisocial personality disorder.
    B. Generalized anxiety disorder.
    C. Borderline personality disorder.
    D. Schizotypal personality disorder.
    E. Attention-deficit/hyperactivity disorder.

**The correct response is option D.**

Schizotypal personality disorder is more prevalent among first-degree relatives of persons with schizophrenia. This also may be true, although to a lesser extent, of paranoid, schizoid, and avoidant personality disorders but not borderline personality disorder.

Royce L, Coccaro EF: Biology of personality disorders, in The American Psychiatric Publishing Textbook of Psychopharmacology, 3rd Edition. Edited by Schatzberg AF, Nemeroff CB. Washington, DC, American Psychiatric Publishing, 2004, p 837

4.  A 39-year-old woman was prescribed and started taking carbamazepine for trigeminal neuralgia. Several months later, she developed symptoms of recurrent depression. Because she had a history of excellent response to this medication, her psychiatrist restarted the patient on nefazodone. Six weeks later the nefazodone was increased to a dose higher than her previously effective dose because her symptoms had not improved. Two weeks later she reported no improvement of her depression and complained of increased fatigue and "forgetfulness." Which of the following statements is *false* regarding this case?

    A.  Both nefazodone and carbamazepine are substrates of the P450 3A4 enzyme.
    B.  Carbamazepine is a potent 3A4 inducer.
    C.  The patient's blood level of nefazodone is likely to be subtherapeutic.
    D.  The patient's blood level of carbamazepine is likely to be decreased.
    E.  Venlafaxine may be an appropriate alternative to nefazodone if the patient continues to take carbamazepine.

**The correct response is option D.**

Multiple drug-drug interactions occur between nefazodone and carbamazepine, leading to low, subtherapeutic levels of nefazodone and elevated carbamazepine levels. Nefazodone is both a *substrate* and a *competitive inhibitor* of the 3A4 enzyme. Carbamazepine is both a *substrate* and a *potent inhibitor* of the 3A4 enzyme. The presence of carbamazepine, as a 3A4 inducer, led to increased metabolism of nefazodone, the blood level of which may drop 10-fold in the presence of carbamazepine. As a competitive inhibitor of 3A4, nefazodone interfered with the metabolism of carbamazepine, the dose of which increased because of the presence of nefazodone, which caused the fatigue and cognitive problems for the patient. Thus, options A, B, and C are true. Option E is true because venla-

faxine, a 2D6 substrate whose metabolism is not readily inducible by carbamazepine, may be an appropriate alternative to nefazodone.

Sandson NB: Drug-Drug Interaction Primer: A Compendium of Case Vignettes for the Practicing Clinician. Washington, DC, American Psychiatric Publishing, 2007, pp 32–33

5.  Which of the following is *true* regarding conducting a psychiatric interview with an adolescent?

    A.  Avoid interviewing parents alone, because this could disrupt rapport-building with the patient, who may fear that the clinician is colluding with caregivers.
    B.  Seeing the adolescent alone first tends to alienate the patient, who may already be anxious about the visit.
    C.  Joint interviews with the adolescent and parents are rarely recommended.
    D.  The parent interview is an essential part of the initial visit, even with highly functional, communicative adolescents.
    E.  To ensure that adequate information is obtained in interviews with adolescents, who tend to be distractible, it is important to focus mostly on the difficulties of the adolescent during the initial interview.

**The correct response is option D.**

Regardless of an adolescent's competency to provide information, parental interview is an essential part of an adolescent's evaluation. In addition to providing information such as developmental, medical, and family history, parents can provide useful information regarding the purpose of the patient's visit and the interactivity with the family unit. Therefore, option A is incorrect. Option B is incorrect because seeing the adolescent alone may actually allay his or her anxieties regarding the interview. Option C is incorrect because joint interviews may yield very useful information regarding the relationship between the parents and the patient as well as provide reassurance regarding issues such as confidentiality and patient expectations during the joint interview. Option E is incorrect because the opposite is actually recommended, particularly with adolescents, who tend to appreciate when adults, including clinicians, show a genuine interest in them as individuals.

King RA, Schowalter JE: The clinical interview of the adolescent, in The American Psychiatric Publishing Textbook of Child and Adolescent Psychiatry, 3rd Edition. Edited by Wiener JM, Dulcan MK. Washington, DC, American Psychiatric Publishing, 2004, pp 113–114

6.   In response to amphetamine challenge, individuals with which of the following diagnoses are more likely than control subjects to become psychotic?

     A.   Antisocial personality disorder.
     B.   Generalized anxiety disorder.
     C.   Borderline personality disorder.
     D.   Avoidant personality disorder.
     E.   Attention-deficit/hyperactivity disorder.

**The correct response is option C.**

Individuals with borderline personality disorder are more likely than control subjects without borderline personality disorder to develop psychotic symptoms in response to amphetamine challenge (Schulz et al. 1985). Those with comorbid schizotypal personality disorder are more likely than those without it to become psychotic.

Royce L, Coccaro EF: Biology of personality disorders, in The American Psychiatric Publishing Textbook of Psychopharmacology, 3rd Edition. Edited by Schatzberg AF, Nemeroff CB. Washington, DC, American Psychiatric Publishing, 2004, p 838

Schulz SC, Schulz P, Dommisse C, et al: Amphetamine response in borderline patients. Psychiatry Res 15:97–108, 1985

7.   The diagnosis of schizophrenia with childhood onset

     A.   Is a common presentation for this disorder.
     B.   Is five times more likely in females than in males.
     C.   Requires no mood disorder exclusion.
     D.   Can be made when signs of disturbance have been present for at least 3 months.
     E.   May have a prevalence of less than 1 in 1,000.

**The correct response is option E.**

Population studies suggest the prevalence of childhood-onset schizophrenia may be less than 1 in 1,000. Spencer and Campbell (1994) reported a male-to-female ratio of 3.8 to 1 in a sample of 24 children. When diagnosing schizophrenia, the clinician must rule out mood disorders and schizoaffective disorders. The diagnosis can be made when signs of the disturbance have been present for at least 6 months, with at least 1 month of active-phase symptoms.

Spencer EK, Campbell M: Children with schizophrenia: diagnosis, phenomenology, and pharmacotherapy. Schizophr Bull 20:713–725, 1994

Tsai LK, Champine DJ: Schizophrenia and other psychotic disorders, in The American Psychiatric Publishing Textbook of Child and Adolescent Psychiatry, 3rd Edition. Edited by Wiener JM, Dulcan MK. Washington, DC, American Psychiatric Publishing, 2004, p 380

8.   Classic Munchausen syndrome includes all of the following components *except*

     A.   Travel from hospital to hospital.
     B.   Simulation of disease.
     C.   Unconscious self-induction of disease.
     D.   Pseudologia fantastica.
     E.   Use of aliases to disguise identity.

**The correct response is option C.**

Classic Munchausen syndrome consists of 1) the simulation or self-induction of disease, 2) pseudologia fantastica, and 3) travel from hospital to hospital. *Pseudologia fantastica* is a form of pathological lying characterized by a matrix of fact and fiction. Patients with this syndrome frequently present to the emergency room with dramatic symptoms such as hemoptysis, acute chest pain suggestive of a myocardial infarction, or coma from self-induced hypoglycemia. The patient frequently will use aliases to disguise his or her identity. The production of symptoms is not unconscious but involves the intentional production of physical symptoms.

Ford CV: Deception syndromes: factitious disorders and malingering, in The American Psychiatric Publishing Textbook of Psychosomatic Medicine: Official Textbook of the Academy of Psychosomatic Medicine. Edited by Levenson JL. Washington, DC, American Psychiatric Publishing, 2005, pp 298–299

9.   Which of the following statements is *false* regarding the dopaminergic system?

     A.   The cerebral cortex is a major projection site of dopaminergic neurons.
     B.   The mediodorsal nucleus of the thalamus and the posterior vermis of the cerebellum contain low densities of dopamine axons.
     C.   The majority of dopamine cells are located in the anterior midbrain (mesencephalon).

D. Subcortical structures receive projections from dopaminergic neurons.

E. The major projection target of dopamine neurons in the substantia nigra is the striatum.

## The correct response is option B.

Identification of dopamine axons in specific brain regions may be of importance to the pathophysiology and treatment of certain psychiatric disorders. Most of the dopaminergic cells, which synthesize approximately three-fourths of all the dopamine in the brain, are located in the anterior midbrain, or mesencephalon, where the dopamine-dense *substantia nigra* and *ventral tegmental area* are located. Dopamine neurons then project from these regions to several projection sites, including the *striatum*

(caudate, putamen, and nucleus accumbens), *cerebral cortex*, *subcortical structures* (amygdala and hippocampus), and portions of the *thalamus* and *cerebellum*.

The mediodorsal nucleus of the thalamus and the posterior vermis of the cerebellum are areas that are theorized to be dysfunctional in schizophrenia. Previously believed not to receive dopamine innervation, these two regions contain a high density of dopamine axons, so the statement in option B is false and therefore is the correct answer.

Melchitzky DS, Austin MC, Lewis DA: Chemical neuroanatomy of the primate brain, in The American Psychiatric Publishing Textbook of Psychopharmacology, 3rd Edition. Edited by Schatzberg AF, Nemeroff CB. Washington, DC, American Psychiatric Publishing, 2004, pp 70–71, 73

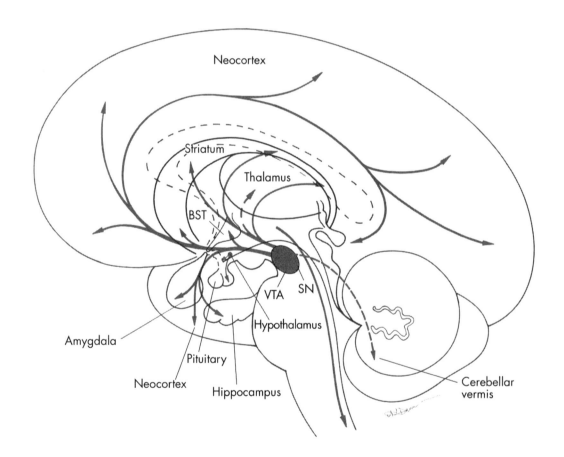

**Dopamine-containing projections from the substantia nigra (SN) and ventral tegmental area (VTA) in the human brain. BST = bed nucleus of the stria terminalis.**

*Source.* Melchitzky DS, Austin MC, Lewis DA: "Chemical Neuroanatomy of the Primate Brain," in *The American Psychiatric Publishing Textbook of Psychopharmacology*, 3rd Edition. Edited by Schatzberg AF, Nemeroff CB. Washington, DC, American Psychiatric Publishing, 2004, p. 71.

10. Regarding choice of an antipsychotic for a patient with acute psychosis in schizophrenia, all of the following statements are true *except*

    A. Generally, second-generation (atypical) agents are preferred.
    B. All of the second-generation (atypical) agents are more effective than the first-generation (typical) agents in the treatment of positive and negative symptoms.
    C. It is acceptable to use a first-generation agent if a particular patient has responded to that agent in the past.
    D. The main advantage of second-generation agents is their overall lower risk of causing extrapyramidal symptoms and tardive dyskinesia.
    E. Clozapine may be therapeutically superior to any other antipsychotic medications.

## The correct response is option B.

The second-generation agents, with the exception of clozapine in patients with treatment-resistant illness, may not be substantially better in the treatment of positive symptoms of schizophrenia compared with first-generation agents. Controversial evidence suggests that some of the newer agents may improve negative symptoms and/or cognitive deficits. Because of the presumed clinical advantages of these agents (including their side-effect profile), they are often preferred for patients who have never been exposed to antipsychotic medication. First-generation drugs may be preferable, however, if a patient has been stable while taking these agents without noticeable neurologic side effects and/or has shown better response to these drugs than to newer ones.

Woo T-UW, Zimmet SV, Wojcik JD, et al: Treatment of schizophrenia, in The American Psychiatric Publishing Textbook of Psychopharmacology, 3rd Edition. Edited by Schatzberg AF, Nemeroff CB. Washington, DC, American Psychiatric Publishing, 2004, p 891

11. DSM-IV-TR suggests that malingering should be strongly suspected if all of the following are present *except*

    A. Medicolegal context of presentation.
    B. Marked discrepancy between the person's claimed stress or disability and the objective findings.
    C. Lack of cooperation during the diagnostic evaluation and in complying with the prescribed treatment regimen.

    D. Diagnosis of antisocial personality disorder associated with the evaluee.
    E. Axis I disorder.

## The correct response is option E.

Malingering should be strongly suspected if any combination of the factors listed in options A, B, C, and D is present. Some investigators believe that the presence of some Axis I disorder increases the risk of malingering, but DSM-IV-TR does not include this as a risk factor.

American Psychiatric Association: Diagnostic and Statistical Manual of Mental Disorders, 4th Edition, Text Revision. Washington, DC, American Psychiatric Association, 2000, p 739

Thompson JW, LeBourgeois HW III, Black FW: Malingering, in The American Psychiatric Publishing Textbook of Forensic Psychiatry. Edited by Simon RI, Gold LH. Washington, DC, American Psychiatric Publishing, 2004, pp 433–444

12. A 32-year-old man with schizophrenia has had good control of his psychotic symptoms for the past 2 years while taking quetiapine 600 mg/day. One month ago he was started on phenytoin for a newly diagnosed seizure disorder. The man is admitted to an inpatient psychiatric facility because of worsening paranoia and other psychotic symptoms. His caregiver confirms that the patient has been adhering to his medication regimen. Of the following, which is the best treatment option on this patient's admission?

    A. Increase the dosage of quetiapine to 800 mg/day and add 25–50 mg of quetiapine every 4–6 hours as needed for agitation. Continue the phenytoin at the current dosage.
    B. Increase the dosage of quetiapine to 800 mg/day and add 25–50 mg of quetiapine every 4–6 hours as needed for agitation. Discontinue the phenytoin and start valproic acid.
    C. Continue the current dosage of quetiapine and start ziprasidone 160 mg/day. Continue the phenytoin at the current dosage.
    D. Discontinue quetiapine and start ziprasidone 160 mg/day. Continue the phenytoin at the current dosage.
    E. Continue the current dosage of quetiapine and augment with valproic acid for mood stabilization. Continue phenytoin at the current dosage.

## The correct response is option D.

This is an example of a P450 3A4 inducer added to a substrate. Quetiapine is primarily a 3A4 substrate, and phenytoin is an inducer of multiple P450 enzymes, including 3A4. The addition of phenytoin led to an increase in the amount of 3A4 available to metabolize the quetiapine, resulting in more rapid metabolism of the quetiapine and, consequently, a sharp decrease in the blood level of quetiapine. The significant decrease in quetiapine in the blood that ensued over the next several weeks led to the emergence of paranoid delusions.

Options A, B, C, and E are incorrect because maintaining or increasing the quetiapine dose would not be of benefit. The strategy in option B to discontinue phenytoin is also not desirable because this medication has led to good seizure control, and valproic acid may not adequately treat the seizure disorder. The plan to continue quetiapine and add ziprasidone is not preferred because the quetiapine is mostly ineffective, and the addition of a relatively high dose of another atypical antipsychotic agent would expose the patient to quetiapine's side effects without being of much benefit.

Sandson NB: Drug-drug Interaction Primer: A Compendium of Case Vignettes for the Practicing Clinician. Washington, DC, American Psychiatric Publishing, 2007, pp 187–188

13. Which of the following statements is *false* regarding the data obtained during a psychiatric interview?

A. The content of the interview can be transmitted verbally and nonverbally.
B. A patient's language style—his use of active or passive verb forms, technical jargon, colloquialisms, or frequent injunctives—refers to the process data of the interview.
C. The process of the interview refers to the developing relationship between the interviewer and patient, including the patient's fantasies about the interviewer.
D. An intervention by the interviewer is considered to be part of the content of the interview.
E. An interviewer's reactions and attentiveness during the interview may be indicative of important content and process data.

**The correct response is option B.**

The patient's language style is considered to be part of the factual information provided by the patient, or content. All the other statements are true. The content of an interview refers both to the factual information provided by the patient and to the specific interventions of the interview. Much of the content is transmitted verbally but also may be communicated nonverbally. Often the verbal content may be unrelated to the real message of the interview. Content involves more than the actual definitions of a patient's words and includes a patient's language style.

MacKinnon RA, Michels R, Buckley PJ: The Psychiatric Interview in Clinical Practice, 2nd Edition. Washington, DC, American Psychiatric Publishing, pp 7–8

14. Which of the following is a physical sign of phencyclidine (PCP) use intoxication?

A. Vertical, but not horizontal, nystagmus.
B. Hypotension.
C. Hyperacusis.
D. Bradycardia.
E. Muscle flaccidity.

**The correct response is option C.**

Option A is incorrect because PCP may cause either vertical or horizontal nystagmus. Nystagmus may also be seen in alcohol or inhalant intoxication. Options B, D, and E are incorrect because PCP intoxication also manifests with hypertension (not hypotension), tachycardia (not bradycardia), muscle rigidity (not flaccidity), and ataxia. Note that at high doses PCP causes dilated pupils (mydriasis), hypersalivation, hyperthermia, involuntary movements, and coma. Pupillary dilation is also found in opioid withdrawal and in cocaine, amphetamine, or hallucinogen intoxication (see table below and on next page).

| Pupillary reaction | Intoxication | Withdrawal |
|---|---|---|
| Mydriasis (dilation) | Amphetamines, hallucinogens, cocaine, high-dose PCP | Opioids |
| Miosis (constriction) | Opioids (severe overdose with opioids may cause dilation if anoxic) | |

Franklin JE Jr, Levenson JL, McCance-Katz EF: Substance-related disorders, in The American Psychiatric Publishing Textbook of Psychosomatic Medicine: The Official Textbook of the Academy of Psychosomatic Medicine. Edited by Levenson JL. Washington, DC, American Psychiatric Publishing, 2005 p 407

| Substance | Intoxication | Withdrawal |
|---|---|---|
| Alcohol | Slurred speech, incoordination, unsteady gait, nystagmus, impaired attention/memory, stupor/coma | Autonomic hyperactivity, increased hand tremor, insomnia, nausea/vomiting, transient visual/tactile/auditory hallucinations, psychomotor agitation, anxiety, grand mal seizures |
| Amphetamine | Tachycardia or bradycardia, pupillary dilation, high or low blood pressure, perspiration or chills, nausea or vomiting, weight loss, psychomotor agitation or retardation, muscular weakness, respiratory depression, chest pain/cardiac arrhythmias, confusion/seizures/dyskinesias/dystonias/coma | Fatigue, vivid and unpleasant dreams, insomnia or hypersomnia, increased appetite, psychomotor retardation or agitation |
| Caffeine | Restlessness, nervousness, excitement, insomnia, flushed face, diuresis, gastrointestinal disturbance, muscle twitching, rambling flow of thought and speech, tachycardia or cardiac arrhythmia, periods of inexhaustibility, psychomotor agitation | None |
| Cannabis | Conjunctival injection, increased appetite, dry mouth, tachycardia | None |
| Cocaine | Tachycardia or bradycardia, pupillary dilation, elevated or lowered blood pressure, perspiration or chills, nausea or vomiting, weight loss, psychomotor agitation or retardation, muscular weakness, respiratory depression, chest pain, cardiac arrhythmias, confusion, seizures, dyskinesias, dystonias or coma | Fatigue, vivid and unpleasant dreams, insomnia or hypersomnia, increased appetite, psychomotor retardation or agitation |
| Hallucinogen | Pupillary dilation, tachycardia, sweating, palpitations, blurring of vision, tremors, incoordination | None |
| Inhalant | Dizziness, nystagmus, incoordination, slurred speech, unsteady gait, lethargy, depressed reflexes, psychomotor retardation, tremor, generalized muscle weakness, blurred vision or diplopia, stupor or coma, euphoria | None |
| Nicotine | | Dysphoric mood, insomnia, irritability/frustration or anger, anxiety, difficulty concentrating, restlessness, bradycardia, increased appetite/weight gain |
| Opioid | Pupillary constriction, drowsiness or coma, slurred speech, impaired attention or memory | Dysphoric mood, nausea or vomiting, muscle aches, lacrimation or rhinorrhea, pupillary dilation/piloerection/sweating, diarrhea, yawning, fever, insomnia |
| Phencyclidine | Vertical or horizontal nystagmus, hypertension or tachycardia, numbness or diminished responsiveness to pain, ataxia, dysarthria, muscle rigidity, seizures or coma, hyperacusis | None |
| Sedative, hypnotic, or anxiolytic | Slurred speech, incoordination, unsteady gait, nystagmus, impaired attention or memory, stupor or coma | Autonomic hyperactivity, increased hand tremor, insomnia, nausea or vomiting, transient visual/tactile/auditory hallucinations or illusions, psychomotor agitation, anxiety, grand mal seizures |

*Source.* American Psychiatric Association: *Diagnostic and Statistical Manual of Mental Disorders*, 4th Edition, Text Revision. Washington, DC, American Psychiatric Association, 2000.

15. Aging is associated with an increased risk of developing various sleep disorders. Which of the following is *true?*

   A. A parasomnia, obstructive sleep apnea (OSA) is significantly more common than central sleep apnea (CSA).
   B. Insomnia is usually not associated with OSA.
   C. Dyssomnias are often caused by medical conditions or medications.
   D. Clinically significant periodic limb movement disorder (PLMD) is five to six times more common in elderly patients compared with younger adults.
   E. Polysomnography is required for the diagnosis of both PLMD and restless legs syndrome (RLS).

**The correct response is option D.**

PLMD occurs in 30%–45% of adults age 60 years or older compared with only 5%–6% of all adults. Option A is incorrect because OSA is a *dyssomnia*, not a *parasomnia*. Option B is incorrect because *insomnia*, defined as difficulty initiating or maintaining sleep or of nonrestorative sleep lasting greater than 1 month, is commonly comorbid with OSA. Option C is incorrect because according to DSM-IV-TR, dyssomnias (and parasomnias) are, by definition, major subcategories of sleep disorders that are *not* caused by secondary factors such as medical illness, medications, or mental illnesses. Option E is incorrect because although necessary to confirm PLMD, polysomnography is not required to diagnose RLS.

American Psychiatric Association: Diagnostic and Statistical Manual of Mental Disorders, 4th Edition, Text Revision. Washington, DC, American Psychiatric Association, 2000, pp 597–661

Benjamin L, Bourgeois JA, Shahrokh NC, et al: Study Guide to Geriatric Psychiatry: A Companion to The American Psychiatric Publishing Textbook of Geriatric Psychiatry, 3rd Edition. Washington, DC, American Psychiatric Publishing, 2006, p 130

16. The psychiatric interview of older adults can be complicated by

   A. Their not equating present distress with past episodes that are symptomatically similar.
   B. Their becoming angry or irritated when a clinician continues to probe previous periods of overt disability in usual activities.
   C. Their having experienced a major illness or trauma in childhood but viewing this information as being of no relevance to the present episode.
   D. A histrionic personality style.
   E. All of the above.

**The correct response is option E.**

Unfortunately, the older adult may not equate present distress with past episodes that are symptomatically similar. Therefore, the perspective of the family is especially valuable in the attempt to link current and past episodes. An older person sometimes becomes angry or irritated when the clinician continues to probe. Not infrequently, the older adult has experienced a major illness or trauma in childhood or as a younger adult, but he or she views this information as being of no relevance to the present episode and therefore dismisses it. Older persons who have chronic and moderately severe anxiety or a histrionic personality style, as well as distressed patients with Alzheimer's disease, tolerate their symptoms poorly.

Blazer DG: The psychiatric interview of older adults, in The American Psychiatric Publishing Textbook of Geriatric Psychiatry, 3rd Edition. Edited by Blazer DG, Steffens DC, Busse EW. Washington, DC, American Psychiatric Publishing, 2004, p 167

17. The leading cause of medical morbidity in patients with schizophrenia is

   A. Obesity.
   B. Diabetes.
   C. HIV-associated hepatitis.
   D. Cigarette smoking.
   E. Lack of exercise.

**The correct response is option D.**

Cigarette smoking, which is consistently reported to be associated with cardiovascular and pulmonary diseases, is the leading cause of morbidity in schizophrenia patients, up to 90% of whom smoke.

Woo T-UW, Zimmet SV, Wojcik JD, et al: Treatment of schizophrenia, in The American Psychiatric Publishing Textbook of Psychopharmacology, 3rd Edition. Edited by Schatzberg AF, Nemeroff CB. Washington, DC, American Psychiatric Publishing, 2004, p 895

18. Which of the following statements is *true* regarding brain neuroanatomy?

    A. The anterior commissure and massa intermedia structures that connect the right and left hemispheres tend to be the same in women and men.
    B. Language functions are less lateralized in women than in men.
    C. Abnormalities in brain structure and function associated with specific disorders do not differ between men and women.
    D. A larger number of sex differences in brain neuroanatomy have been identified in humans compared with other vertebrates.
    E. The evidence strongly supports the hypothesis that females have a larger corpus callosum than do males.

**The correct response is option B.**

Language functions are less lateralized in women than in men. Positron emission tomography and functional magnetic resonance imaging studies have demonstrated that during phonological language processing, brain activation is lateralized to the left inferior frontal gyrus in men but diffusely involves both the left and right inferior frontal gyri in women. During recognition of visual and auditory emotional stimuli, men show unilateral frontal activation, whereas women exhibit bilateral frontal and limbic activation.

Option A is incorrect because these brain structures tend to be larger in women than in men. Option C is incorrect because evidence is emerging that abnormalities in brain structure and function associated with specific disorders are different between men and women. Option D is incorrect because a smaller, not larger, number of sex differences in brain neuroanatomy have been identified in humans compared to other vertebrates. Option E is incorrect because there are conflicting reports regarding females having a larger corpus callosum than males.

Altemus M: Neurobiology and sex/gender, in Age and Gender Considerations in Psychiatric Diagnosis: A Research Agenda for DSM-V. Edited by Narrow WE, First MB, Sirovatka PJ, et al. Washington, DC, American Psychiatric Publishing, 2007, pp 49–50

19. There is substantial comorbidity between which of the following diagnoses?

    A. Generalized social phobia and avoidant personality disorder.
    B. Panic disorder and avoidant personality disorder.
    C. Generalized social phobia and schizotypal personality disorder.
    D. Generalized social phobia and borderline personality disorder.
    E. Generalized anxiety disorder and avoidant personality disorder.

**The correct response is option A.**

There is substantial comorbidity between generalized social phobia and avoidant personality disorder. Substantial comorbidity does not exist between the other pairs of disorders shown in answers B, C, D, and E.

Royce L, Coccaro EF: Biology of personality disorders, in The American Psychiatric Publishing Textbook of Psychopharmacology, 3rd Edition. Edited by Schatzberg AF, Nemeroff CB. Washington, DC, American Psychiatric Publishing, 2004, p 840

20. The primary receptor site of action of ethanol is

    A. Dopamine transporter (DAT).
    B. Vesicular monoamine transporter (VMAT).
    C. Nicotinic acetylcholine (ACh) receptors.
    D. Gamma-aminobutyric acid (GABA) and *N*-methyl-D-aspartate (NMDA) receptors.
    E. Mu receptors.

**The correct response is option D.**

Ethanol's primary molecular targets are GABA and NMDA receptors. Cocaine's three known molecular targets are the DAT, the serotonin transporter (5-HTT), and the norepinephrine transporter (NET), so option A is incorrect. Options B, C, and E are incorrect because VMAT is a primary site of action for amphetamines, ACh for nicotine, and mu (and gamma) opioid receptors for opiates.

Clinton K: Neurobiology of substance abuse disorders, in The American Psychiatric Publishing Textbook of Psychopharmacology, 3rd Edition. Edited by Schatzberg AF, Nemeroff CB. Washington, DC, American Psychiatric Publishing, 2004, p 811; Table 49–1

21. Which of the following characteristics is *true* regarding assault and psychosis?

    A. The triggering event usually involves a situational stressor that does not involve hallucinations or delusions.
    B. The behavior preceding the assault is typified by agitation, pacing, clenched jaw, yelling, and verbal threats.
    C. More than 40% of assaults by chronically assaultive inpatients at a psychiatric facility were psychotic in nature, followed by impulsive then organized assaults.
    D. Psychotic assaults are relatively uncommon when compared with impulsive or predatory/planned assaults.
    E. Examples of triggers of violent acts by psychotic individuals include a staff member telling a patient to return to his or her room.

**The correct response is option D.**

A recent review of more than 1,000 aggressive acts in chronically assaultive patients at a large California state psychiatric hospital suggested that there are three categories of violent behaviors in these settings: impulsive, predatory/planned, and psychotic (Quanbeck et al. 2007). Option A is incorrect because the triggering event of psychotic assaults usually involves psychotic misperception of reality, resulting in sudden and unexpected assault. Option B is incorrect because statement describes behaviors common in impulsive, but not psychotic, assaults. Option C is incorrect because of the three types of assaults, the psychotic type is the least common (15%). More than 40% of assaults by chronically assaultive inpatients are impulsive in nature, followed by predatory/planned assaults (25%). Option E is incorrect because the example describes a typical trigger seen in impulsive, not psychotic, assault.

Quanbeck CD, McDermott BE, Lam J, et al: Categorization of aggressive acts committed by chronically assaultive state hospital patients. Psychiatr Serv 58:521–528, 2007

Scott CL, Quanbeck CD, Resnick PJ: Assessment of dangerousness, in The American Psychiatric Publishing Textbook of Psychiatry, 5th Edition. Edited by Hales RE, Yudofsky SC, Gabbard GO. Washington, DC, American Psychiatric Publishing, 2008, pp 1659–1660; Table 44–6

22. Which of the following statements is *true* regarding male sexual dysfunction?

    A. Men with low or absent gonadal function show little interest in sex and are impotent regardless of exposure to stimuli.
    B. Diseases that interfere with neural control over the hypothalamic-pituitary-gonadal (HPG) axis are not believed to affect sexual desire.
    C. Common risk factors for erectile dysfunction (ED) directly or indirectly compromise the process of smooth muscle relaxation.
    D. Risk factors for premature ejaculation include commonly identifiable conditions such as specific procedures or disorders.
    E. Tobacco use is a risk factor for premature ejaculation.

**The correct response is option C.**

Common risk factors for ED directly or indirectly compromise the process of smooth muscle relaxation (e.g., arteriole dilatation) necessary for penile engorgement. Thus, ED is often associated with cardiovascular disease.

Option A is incorrect because although men with low or absent gonadal function show little interest in sex, they are not necessarily impotent, and they may attain erections when presented with certain kinds of psychosexual stimuli. However, these men are less likely to seek sexual stimulation and fulfillment because of their hormone deficiency. Option B is incorrect because diseases that interfere with neural control over the HPG axis, such as Parkinson's disease and dopamine, and result in high levels of prolactin may interfere with sexual desire. Option D is incorrect because risk factors for premature ejaculation are relatively unclear in contrast with ED, which has common risk factors. Option E is incorrect because tobacco use is a risk factor for ED but not premature ejaculation.

Rowland DL: Sexual health and problems, in Textbook of Men's Mental Health. Edited by Grant JE, Potenza MN. Washington, DC, American Psychiatric Publishing, 2007, pp 179–180

23. Which of the following findings does *not* suggest a psychogenic or "nonorganic" etiology for a neurologic deficit?

    A. Tongue deviation away from the hemiparetic side.
    B. Complete loss of smell, including of noxious substances.
    C. Peripheral facial palsy and ipsilateral hemiparesis.
    D. Unilateral hearing loss in the ear ipsilateral to a hemiparesis.
    E. Presence of optokinetic nystagmus in a blind patient.

## The correct response is option A.

In cerebral hemispheric disease, the tongue deviates *toward* the hemiparetic side, so if the deviation occurs away from the hemiparetic side, suspect a psychogenic neurologic deficit. Options B, C, D, and E are incorrect because these findings are very unusual and/or defy neuroanatomic explanations, suggesting a psychogenic etiology of a neurologic deficit. Patients can develop anosmia (loss of smell), but detection of noxious substances is usually retained because chemicals such as ammonia irritate the nasal mucosa endings of the trigeminal nerve rather than the olfactory nerve. If a single lesion causes peripheral facial weakness and hemiparesis, the lesion is in the brainstem, and the findings should be on opposite sides of the body, so option C suggests a psychogenic origin. Extensive auditory tract synapses in the pons ensure that some tracts reach the upper brainstem and cerebrum despite central nervous system lesions. Hearing loss in one ear is rare. Patients with intact vision cannot suppress optokinetic nystagmus, so the presence of this nystagmus suggests a "functional," not anatomical, blindness.

Kaufman DM: Clinical Neurology for Psychiatrists, 6th Edition. Philadelphia, PA, Saunders Elsevier, 2007, pp 23–24

McGee S: Evidence-Based Physical Diagnosis. Philadelphia, PA, WB Saunders, 2001, pp 825–826

24. Structural magnetic resonance imaging (MRI) studies of subjects with schizotypal personality disorder have shown which of the following?

    A. Larger left and right caudate nucleus volumes compared with those in subjects without schizotypal personality disorder.
    B. Larger relative size of putamen compared with that in subjects with schizophrenia or control subjects.
    C. Higher regional glucose metabolic rate in caudate compared with control subjects.
    D. Ventricular enlargement intermediate between that in control subjects and subjects with schizophrenia.
    E. Smaller hippocampal volumes compared with those in control subjects.

## The correct response is option D.

Structural MRI studies have found evidence of ventricular enlargement in subjects with schizotypal personality disorder compared with control subjects, the extent of which is intermediate between those of schizophrenia patients and control subjects.

Option A is incorrect because those with schizotypal personality disorder tend to have smaller, not larger, caudate nucleus volumes. Option B is incorrect became schizotypal patients have relatively smaller, not larger, putamen sizes compared with individuals with and without schizophrenia. Option C is incorrect because glucose metabolic rate was found decreased in the caudate. Option E is incorrect because no changes in the hippocampal volumes were noted in the patients with schizotypal disorder as compared with controls.

Royce L, Coccaro EF: Biology of personality disorders, in The American Psychiatric Publishing Textbook of Psychopharmacology, 3rd Edition. Edited by Schatzberg AF, Nemeroff CB. Washington, DC, American Psychiatric Publishing, 2004, p 838

25. The leading cause of premature death in patients with schizophrenia is

    A. Comorbidities associated with obesity.
    B. Alcohol and drug use.
    C. Comorbidities associated with cigarette smoking.
    D. Risky sexual behaviors.
    E. Suicide.

## The correct response is option E.

Suicide is the leading cause of premature death in patients with schizophrenia, who have a 10% lifetime risk of suicide.

Woo T-UW, Zimmet SV, Wojcik JD, et al: Treatment of schizophrenia, in The American Psychiatric Publishing Textbook of Psychopharmacology, 3rd Edition. Edited by Schatzberg AF, Nemeroff CB. Washington, DC, American Psychiatric Publishing, 2004, p 900

26. Recent "right to die" discussions relate to decision making at the end of life. There are important distinctions between incompetent and competent patients in this issue. Regarding right to die and incompetent patients, which of the following is *true?*

    A. The *Cruzan v. Director, Missouri Department of Health* (1990) decision allowed the state to remove a feeding tube from an incompetent patient to respect the family's wishes.
    B. The *Cruzan* decision found that the state did *not* have the right to maintain an incompetent individual's life against family wishes.
    C. When treating severely impaired and/or ill patients, physicians must seek clear and competent instructions regarding foreseeable treatment decisions.
    D. Expression of treatment preferences can be valid only with a durable power of attorney agreement.
    E. Civil liability may only result from stopping life-sustaining treatment, not from overtreatment.

**The correct response is option C.**

The U.S. Supreme Court ruled in *Cruzan v. Director, Missouri Department of Health* (1990) that the state of Missouri could refuse to remove a food and water tube surgically implanted in the stomach of Nancy Cruzan without clear and convincing evidence of her wishes. Without clear and convincing evidence of a patient's decision to have life-sustaining measures withheld in a particular circumstance, the state has the right to maintain that individual's life, even to the exclusion of the family's wishes.

The *Cruzan* decision set the precedent that physicians treating severely or terminally impaired patients must seek clear and competent instructions regarding foreseeable treatment decisions. This information is best provided in the form of a living will, durable power-of-attorney agreement, or health care proxy. Although physicians may fear civil or criminal liability for stopping life-sustaining treatment, liability may also arise from overtreating critically or terminally ill patients.

Simon RI, Shuman DW: Psychiatry and the law, in The American Psychiatric Publishing Textbook of Psychiatry, 5th Edition. Edited by Hales RE, Yudofsky SC, Gabbard GO. Washington, DC, American Psychiatric Publishing, 2008, p 1563

27. Medication history of the older adult should

    A. Involve having the person bring in all pill bottles.
    B. Involve a double check between the written schedule and pill containers.
    C. Assess alcohol intake.
    D. Assess substance abuse.
    E. All of the above.

**The correct response is option E.**

The clinician should ask the older person to bring in all pill bottles as well as a list of medications taken and the dosage schedule. A double check between the written schedule and the pill containers will frequently expose some discrepancy. Older persons are less likely than younger persons to abuse alcohol, but a careful history of alcohol intake is essential to the diagnostic workup. Substance abuse beyond alcohol and prescription drugs is rare in older adults, but abuse is not entirely absent.

Blazer DG: The psychiatric interview of older adults, in The American Psychiatric Publishing Textbook of Geriatric Psychiatry, 3rd Edition. Edited by Blazer DG, Steffens DC, Busse EW. Washington, DC, American Psychiatric Publishing, 2004, pp 167–168

28. The leading conception of the principles of biomedical ethics includes all of the following *except*

    A. Respect for patient autonomy.
    B. Beneficence.
    C. Honesty.
    D. Nonmaleficence.
    E. Justice.

**The correct response is option C.**

The four principles that guide biomedical ethics are 1) respect for patient autonomy (option A), which requires that professionals recognize the right of competent adults to make their own decisions about health care; 2) beneficence (option B), to promote the health and well-being of the patient; 3) nonmaleficence (option D), to avoid harming patients or research subjects; and 4) justice (option E), which requires that medical care and research be performed in a fair and equitable way.

Rosenstein DL, Miller FG: Ethical issues, in The American Psychiatric Publishing Textbook of Psychosomatic Medicine: Official Textbook of the Academy of Psychosomatic Medicine. Edited by Levenson JL. Washington, DC, American Psychiatric Publishing, 2005, pp 56–57

29. A test of which of the following specimens is gener-ally least expensive and completed at most clinical laboratories?

    A. Blood.
    B. Hair.
    C. Oral fluid.
    D. Sweat.
    E. Urine.

**The correct response is option E.**

When considered as a part of a total patient assessment, costs of analysis are similar, although hair, oral fluid, sweat, and blood testing are somewhat more expensive than urine testing. Sweat, oral fluid, and hair testing are done only at a limited number of specialized laboratories at present, but urine testing is done at most clinical labora-tories and dozens of federally accredited specialized urine drug-testing laboratories.

DuPont RI, Selavka CM: Testing to identify recent drug use, in The American Psychiatric Publishing Textbook of Substance Abuse Treatment, 4th Edition. Edited by Gal-anter M, Kleber HD. Washington, DC, American Psychi-atric Publishing, 2008, pp 657, 661; Table 46–2

30. Which of the following is *false* regarding mood dis-orders and gender?

    A. Depression is the second leading cause of disability for women in the world, followed by ischemic heart disease.
    B. The lifetime risk of major depression in the United States has ranged from 10% to 25% for women.
    C. In the United States, nearly twice as many women (12%) as men (6.6%) have a depressive disorder each year.
    D. In established market economies, schizophrenia and bipolar disorder are among the top 10 causes of disability-adjusted life years for men but not for women.
    E. It is projected that by the year 2020, major de-pression will be the leading cause of disease bur-den in women.

**The correct response is option D.**

The statements in options A, B, C, and E are all *true*. The statement in option D is incorrect because in established market economies, schizophrenia and bipolar disorder are among the top 10 causes of disability-adjusted life years for *women*. The disability caused by major depres-sion was found to be equivalent to that of blindness or paraplegia. Currently, depression is the second leading cause of disability for women, but by 2020 it is projected that it will be the leading cause of disability for women throughout the world.

Wisner KL, Dolan-Sewell R: Why gender matters, in Age and Gender Considerations in Psychiatric Diagnosis: A Research Agenda for DSM-V. Edited by Narrow WE, First MB, Sirovatka PJ, et al. Washington, DC, American Psychiatric Publishing, 2007, pp 12–13

31. Evaluation of the family of the psychiatrically ill older adult includes all of the following parameters of support *except*

    A. Availability of the family member.
    B. Tangible services provided by the family.
    C. Patient's perception of family support.
    D. Tolerance by the family of specific behaviors derived from the psychiatric disorder.
    E. Consideration only of those individuals geneti-cally related to the patient.

**The correct response is option E.**

For clinical purposes, the family consists of not only indi-viduals genetically related but also those who have devel-oped relationships and are living together as if they were related. At least four parameters of support are important for the clinician to evaluate as the treatment plan evolves: 1) availability of family members to the older person over time, 2) the tangible services provided by the family to the disturbed older person, 3) the perception of family sup-port by the older patient (and subsequently the willing-ness of the patient to cooperate and accept support), and 4) tolerance by the family of specific behaviors that derive from the psychiatric disorder.

Blazer DG: The psychiatric interview of older adults, in The American Psychiatric Publishing Textbook of Geriat-ric Psychiatry, 3rd Edition. Edited by Blazer DG, Steffens DC, Busse EW. Washington, DC, American Psychiatric Publishing, 2004, pp 168–169

32. Which of the following second-generation anti-psychotics is most effective for treatment-resistant schizophrenia?

    A. Clozapine.
    B. Risperidone.

C. Olanzapine.

D. Quetiapine.

E. Ziprasidone.

## The correct response is option A.

Most available data suggest that clozapine is the most effective drug for treatment-resistant schizophrenia.

Woo T-UW, Zimmet SV, Wojcik JD, et al: Treatment of schizophrenia, in The American Psychiatric Publishing Textbook of Psychopharmacology, 3rd Edition. Edited by Schatzberg AF, Nemeroff CB. Washington, DC, American Psychiatric Publishing, 2004, p 892

33. Borderline personality disorder is associated with which of the following cognitive and perceptual disturbances?

    A. Odd thinking and speech.

    B. Ideas of reference.

    C. Odd beliefs.

    D. Transient, stress-related paranoid ideation.

    E. Superstitiousness.

## The correct response is option D.

Borderline personality disorder is associated with transient, stress-related paranoid ideation or severe dissociative symptoms. Schizotypal personality disorder is associated with odd thinking, beliefs, and speech; ideas of reference; and superstitiousness.

Royce L, Coccaro EF: Biology of personality disorders, in The American Psychiatric Publishing Textbook of Psychopharmacology, 3rd Edition. Edited by Schatzberg AF, Nemeroff CB. Washington, DC, American Psychiatric Publishing, 2004, p 837

34. Which of the following statements is *true* regarding neurologic exam findings?

    A. Patients with slowly developing cerebral hemisphere lesions usually develop spasticity and weakness simultaneously.

    B. Patients with strokes or spinal cord injury tend to develop spasticity, weakness, and flaccidity simultaneously.

    C. Spasticity is a sign of upper motor neuron disease, the severity of which correlates well with the degree of weakness or hyperreflexia.

    D. In hemiplegia, there tends to be excess tone in the extensors of the arms and flexors of the legs.

    E. After a large stroke, persistent flaccid hemiplegia rarely occurs with hyperreflexia.

## The correct response is option A.

Patients with slowly developing cerebral hemisphere lesions usually develop spasticity and weakness together. In contrast, patients with strokes or spinal cord injury develop immediate weakness and flaccidity, but spasticity occurs days to weeks later, so option B is incorrect. Option C is incorrect because although it is *true* that spasticity is a sign of upper motor neuron disease, its severity correlates *poorly* with the degree of weakness or hyperreflexia. Option E is incorrect because some patients with large strokes have hyperreflexia but still have persistent flaccid hemiplegia. Option D is incorrect because patients with complete spinal cord lesions have excess tone in the flexors of the arms and extensors of the legs. On examination, the arm and hand are fixed against the chest, flexed, and internally rotated; the foot is pointed; and the leg is extended.

McGee S: Evidence-Based Physical Diagnosis. Philadelphia, PA, WB Saunders, 2001, pp 726–727

35. Memory loss is often insidious in onset and well established clinically by the time a patient is brought to care. Which of the following statements is *false* regarding the dementia syndromes?

    A. More than half of people with chronic memory loss will, at autopsy, exhibit the changes of Alzheimer's disease only and not other dementias.

    B. The most common dementia syndrome is caused by Alzheimer's disease, followed by vascular dementia.

    C. Approximately 5% of older persons experience memory loss as a result of alcohol-induced amnestic disorder.

    D. Vascular dementia is more common in women than in men.

    E. At autopsy, many individuals with Alzheimer's disease are also found to have changes in the substantia nigra.

## The correct response is option D.

In contrast to Alzheimer's disease, vascular dementia is more common in men than in women. In addition to male gender, other risk factors for vascular dementia include hypertension and, possibly, black race.

Option A is incorrect because this statement about Alzheimer's disease is *true*. Alzheimer's disease is the most common disorder contributing to the dementia syndrome and has prevalence estimates of 6%–8% in individuals 65 years and older and more than 30% in those 85 years and older. Alzheimer's disease is characterized by neurofibrillary tangles, deposition of β-amyloid, and brain atrophy.

Option B is incorrect because after Alzheimer's disease, vascular dementia is the second most common syndrome. Vascular dementia is characterized by multiple small infarcts of the brain. Clinically and pathophysiologically, it is difficult to disaggregate the vascular dementias. Vascular dementia frequently is comorbid with Alzheimer's disease. The statements in options C and E are *true*, so these answers are incorrect.

Blazer DG: Treatment of seniors, in The American Psychiatric Publishing Textbook of Psychiatry, 5th Edition. Edited by Hales RE, Yudofsky SC, Gabbard GO. Washington, DC, American Psychiatric Publishing, 2008, p 1452

36. Adjustment disorder is characterized by

A. Symptoms that develop within 2 months of the onset of a stressor.
B. Symptoms that resolve within 12 months of the stressor's ending.
C. Symptoms that develop within 3 months of the stressor's onset.
D. Symptoms of distress that are proportional to the stressor.
E. Symptoms that, if persistent for 7 months, would be considered acute adjustment disorder.

**The correct response is option C.**

According to DSM-IV-TR, adjustment disorder is characterized by the development of emotional or behavioral symptoms in response to an identifiable stressor(s) occurring within 3 months of the onset of the stressor(s). Option B is incorrect because once the stressor has terminated, the symptoms do not persist for more than an additional 6 months. Option D is incorrect because the distress is in excess of what would be expected. Option E is incorrect because the disorder is considered acute if the disturbance lasts less than 6 months and chronic if it lasts more than 6 months.

American Psychiatric Association: Diagnostic and Statistical Manual of Mental Disorders, 4th Edition, Text Revision. Washington, DC, American Psychiatric Association, 2000, p 679

37. Electroconvulsive therapy (ECT) can be a lifesaving treatment in catatonia due to all of the following *except*

A. Severe unipolar depression.
B. Neuroleptic malignant syndrome.
C. Hypercalcemia.
D. Severe mixed mood disorder episode.
E. None of the above.

**The correct response is option E.**

ECT can be a lifesaving treatment for catatonia regardless of the etiology, including medical disorders such as systemic lupus erythematosus, hypercalcemia or other metabolic encephalopathies, status epilepticus, and viral encephalitides.

Garlow SJ, Purselle D, D'Orio B: Psychiatric emergencies, in The American Psychiatric Publishing Textbook of Psychopharmacology, 3rd Edition. Edited by Schatzberg AF, Nemeroff CB. Washington, DC, American Psychiatric Publishing, 2004, p 1075

McDonald WM, Thompson TR, McCall WV, et al: Electroconvulsive therapy, in The American Psychiatric Publishing Textbook of Psychopharmacology, 3rd Edition. Edited by Schatzberg AF, Nemeroff CB. Washington, DC, American Psychiatric Publishing, 2004, p 691

38. Drug dependence has been modeled both as an impulse-control disorder and as a compulsive disorder, two models that feature different drug-related behaviors. Which of the following behaviors is associated with impulse-control disorder as opposed to compulsive disorder?

A. Tension/arousal.
B. Anxiety/stress.
C. Repetitive behaviors.
D. Relief of anxiety/relief of stress.
E. Obsessions.

**The correct response is option A.**

In impulse-control disorders, an increasing tension and arousal occurs before the impulsive act, with pleasure, gratification, or relief during the act. Following the act there may or may not be regret or guilt. In compulsive disorders, there are recurrent and persistent thoughts (obsessions) that cause marked anxiety and stress followed by repetitive behaviors (compulsions) that are aimed at preventing or reducing distress. Positive reinforcement (pleasure/gratification) is more closely associated with impulse-control disorders. Negative reinforcement (relief of anxiety or relief of stress) is more closely associated with compulsive disorders.

Koob GF: Neurobiology of addiction, The American Psychiatric Publishing Textbook of Substance Abuse Treatment, 4th Edition. Edited by Galanter M, Kleber HD. Washington, DC, American Psychiatric Publishing, 2008, p 5; Figure 1–1

39. Regarding use of antidepressants in treating borderline personality disorder patients, which of the following statements is *true?*

   A. Tricyclic antidepressants (TCAs) and monoamine oxidase inhibitors (MAOIs) pose serious risks of overdose and dangerous adverse effects that are of particular concern in an unstable and an impulsive population.
   B. Selective serotonin reuptake inhibitors (SSRIs) lose efficacy for aggression and irritability after 2 months of treatment.
   C. SSRIs have not been found to decrease suicidality and self-injury in patients with borderline personality disorder.
   D. The MAOI tranylcypromine was found to be inferior to placebo in treating symptoms of borderline personality disorder.
   E. Phenelzine has modest efficacy in borderline personality disorder for depression, psychotic symptoms, and global borderline severity.

**The correct response is option A.**

Regardless of efficacy, both TCAs and MAOIs pose serious overdose and dangerous adverse effect risks that are of particular concern in this unstable, impulsive population. Compared with placebo, fluoxetine led to a consistent and significant decrease in aggression and irritability and to global improvement apparent by the second month of treatment, and this effect was independent of changes in depression or anxiety. Option D is incorrect because tranylcypromine was found to be *superior* to placebo in treating symptoms of borderline personality disorder. Option E is incorrect because phenelzine appears to be superior to placebo for anger and hostility but not on measures of depression, atypical depression, psychoticism, impulsivity, or global borderline severity.

Simeon D, Hollander E: Treatment of personality disorders, in The American Psychiatric Publishing Textbook of Psychopharmacology, 3rd Edition. Edited by Schatzberg AF, Nemeroff CB. Washington, DC, American Psychiatric Publishing, 2004, pp 1053, 1055; see also Table 61–1

40. For severe tardive dyskinesia, which of the following medications may be useful?

   A. Pimozide.
   B. Clozapine.
   C. Haloperidol.
   D. L-Serine.
   E. L-Carnitine.

**The correct response is option B.**

Second-generation antipsychotics, especially clozapine, may be helpful in patients who are prone to tardive dyskinesia. Tardive dyskinesia is a syndrome of potentially irreversible involuntary movements that can be induced by antipsychotic medications.

Woo T-UW, Zimmet SV, Wojcik JD, et al: Treatment of schizophrenia, in The American Psychiatric Publishing Textbook of Psychopharmacology, 3rd Edition. Edited by Schatzberg AF, Nemeroff CB. Washington, DC, American Psychiatric Publishing, 2004, p 896

41. Attention includes an interaction between all of the following processes *except*

   A. Attentional capacity.
   B. Selective consciousness.
   C. Response selection and executive control.
   D. Selective attention.
   E. Sustained attention.

**The correct response is option B.**

Attention depends on the interaction between the four components listed in options A, C, D, and E. Humans have a limited capacity for attention (or attentional capacity); we are only able to perform a small number of tasks concurrently. The intensity of attentional focus that can be allocated at one point in time is limited. Attentional capacity governs both the amount of information that can be handled and the intensity of cognitive processing that can be performed on that information. Capacity limits constrain other attentional processes, influencing the efficiency of both sensory and response selection and control. Attentional capacity is not constant over time but fluctuates as function of both extrinsic and intrinsic factors. Extrinsic factors include perceived value of stimuli and prevailing response demands; intrinsic processes include energetic and structural factors such as processing speed, memory capacity, spatial dynamics, and temporal dynamics of the system.

Cohen RA, Salloway S, Sweet LH: Neuropsychiatric aspects of disorders of attention, in The American Psychiatric Publishing Textbook of Neuropsychiatry and Behavioral Neurosciences, 5th Edition. Edited by Yudofsky SC, Hales RE. Washington, DC, American Psychiatric Publishing, 2008, p 406

42. The form of malingering most frequently encountered by psychosomatic medicine specialists is

    A. Falsification of laboratory reports.
    B. Production of new illness.
    C. Contamination of laboratory samples.
    D. Embellishment of previous or concurrent illness.
    E. Multiple organ system complaints.

**The correct response is option D.**

Embellishment of previous or concurrent illness is the most frequently encountered form of malingering by psychosomatic subspecialists.

Ford CV: Deception syndromes: factitious disorders and malingering, in The American Psychiatric Publishing Textbook of Psychosomatic Medicine: Official Textbook of the Academy of Psychosomatic Medicine. Edited by Levenson JL. Washington, DC, American Psychiatric Publishing, 2005, p 305

43. Which of the following sensory modalities is impaired consistently in individuals with schizophrenia?

    A. Sight.
    B. Hearing.
    C. Touch.
    D. Taste.
    E. Smell.

**The correct response is option E.**

Olfactory deficits have been noted in schizophrenia. Olfactory deficits are present at the onset of illness, do not relate to disease severity or treatment, and are possibly progressive. It is unclear whether the deficits are part of the generalized neurocognitive impairment. The neuroanatomic differences noted in patients suggest that olfactory bulb changes and medial temporal lobe abnormalities could mediate the observed behavioral aberrations.

Gur RE, Arnold SE: Neurobiology of schizophrenia, in The American Psychiatric Publishing Textbook of Psychopharmacology, 3rd Edition. Edited by Schatzberg AF, Nemeroff CB. Washington, DC, American Psychiatric Publishing, 2004, p 766

44. A 35-year-old man who has been clean from heroin comes to the methadone maintenance clinic to pick up his usual 50-mg-per-day dosage of methadone. Despite taking his usual methadone dose every day, the man reports worsening anxiety, muscle cramps, nausea, diarrhea, and insomnia that started a week ago. Two weeks ago, he was prescribed and started taking a new medication for "really bad pain" on one side of his face, which has resolved completely. What is the name of the new medication?

    A. Phenytoin
    B. Phenobarbital.
    C. Carbamazepine.
    D. Valproic acid.
    E. Gabapentin.

**The correct response is option C.**

The man was prescribed carbamazepine for trigeminal neuralgia. Carbamazepine is an inducer of several P450 enzymes, specifically 3A4. Because methadone is a substrate for 3A4, there was an increased production of 3A4 after the man started the carbamazepine. Over the ensuing weeks, the blood level of methadone decreased because of the increased availability of 3A4, leading to the development of opioid withdrawal symptoms. After stopping the carbamazepine, the patient's methadone will need to be increased back to his usual dosage over a 2- to 3-week period. Options B and D are incorrect because phenobarbital and valproic acid are 3A4 *inhibitors*, which would have led to increased, not decreased, methadone levels. Phenytoin, a 3A4 inducer, could have theoretically decreased the patient's methadone level. Phenytoin may be used for acute relief of trigeminal neuralgia symptoms, but carbamazepine is typically used for long-term treatment of the condition, so option A is incorrect. Option E is incorrect because gabapentin does not affect blood levels of the 3A4 enzyme and may actually be an appropriate alternative for this patient.

Sandson NB: Drug-Drug Interaction Primer: A Compendium of Case Vignettes for the Practicing Clinician. Washington, DC, American Psychiatric Publishing, 2007, pp 188–189

45. The three most useful classes of medications in the treatment of borderline personality disorder are

    A. Benzodiazepines, azapirones, and serotonergic and noradrenergic reuptake inhibitors (SNRIs).
    B. Selective serotonin reuptake inhibitors (SSRIs), mood stabilizers, and atypical antipsychotics.
    C. Mood stabilizers, SSRIs, and benzodiazepines.
    D. Benzodiazepines, SSRIs, and azapirones.
    E. Benzodiazepines, mood stabilizers, and SSRIs.

**The correct response is option B.**

Three classes of medications have emerged as the most useful in treating borderline personality disorder: SSRIs, mood stabilizers, and atypical antipsychotics. Of these, the fewest controlled data to date are available for the atypical antipsychotics. Thus far, the SSRI fluoxetine and the mood stabilizer valproate have the most data documenting their efficacy.

Simeon D, Hollander E: Treatment of personality disorders, in The American Psychiatric Publishing Textbook of Psychopharmacology, 3rd Edition. Edited by Schatzberg AF, Nemeroff CB. Washington, DC, American Psychiatric Publishing, 2004, p 1059

46. Rapid-eye movement (REM) sleep behavior disorder is a rare condition in which patients "act out their dreams" because of a failure of REM-associated atonia. This condition has been associated with use of all of the following medication classes or agents *except*

    A. Clozapine.
    B. Amitriptyline.
    C. Selegiline.
    D. Venlafaxine.
    E. Fluvoxamine.

**The correct response is option A.**

Serotonin antagonists such as clozapine and risperidone are *not* associated with REM sleep behavior disorder. Options B, C, D, and E are incorrect because tricyclic antidepressnts (e.g., amitriptyline), monoamine oxidase inhibitors (e.g., selegiline), serotonin norepinephrine reuptake inhibitors (venlafaxine), and SSRIs (e.g, fluvoxamine) can induce or exacerbate REM sleep behavior disorder. First-line treatment for REM sleep behavior disorder is a benzodiazepine, mostly commonly clonazepam. Caffeine can also precipitate or exacerbate REM sleep behavior disorder, which can also occur during withdrawal from alcohol, meprobamate, pentazocine, and nitrazepam.

Buysse DJ, Strollo PJ, Black JE, et al: Sleep disorders, in The American Psychiatric Publishing Textbook of Psychiatry, 5th Edition. Edited by Hales RE, Yudofsky SC, Gabbard GO. Washington, DC, 2008, p 956

Hirshkowitz M, Sharafkhaneh A: Neuropsychiatric aspects of sleep and sleep disorders, in The American Psychiatric Publishing Textbook of Neuropsychiatry and Behavioral Neurosciences, 5th Edition, Edited by Yudofsky SC, Hales RE. Washington, DC, 2008, p 700

47. Reduced volume of anterior, posterior, and (less consistently) total superior temporal gyrus has been correlated with which of the following clinical measures?

    A. Persistence of negative symptoms.
    B. Severity of auditory hallucinations and thought disorder.
    C. Deficits in working memory.
    D. Impaired processing of auditory-evoked potentials.
    E. Magnitude of comorbid mood dysregulation.

**The correct response is option B.**

Cortical temporal regions, especially the superior temporal gyrus, have been examined in patients with schizophrenia. Reduced volume has been observed in anterior, posterior, and total superior temporal gyrus and has been related to severity of auditory hallucinations and thought disorder.

Gur RE, Arnold SE: Neurobiology of schizophrenia, in The American Psychiatric Publishing Textbook of Psychopharmacology, 3rd Edition. Edited by Schatzberg AF, Nemeroff CB. Washington, DC, American Psychiatric Publishing, 2004, p 767

48. Regarding the effect of major depression on medically ill patients, which of the following statements is *false*?

    A. Major depression in medically ill patients often makes them incapacitated to make decisions.
    B. Untreated depression has been linked to poor compliance with medical care.

C. Depression produces more subtle distortions of decision making than does delirium or psychosis.

D. Refusal of life-saving treatment by a depressed patient cannot be assumed to constitute lack of capacity.

E. None of the above.

**The correct response is option A.**

Major depression in medically ill patients does not usually make them incapacitated. Untreated depression has been linked to poor medical compliance, increased pain and disability, and greater likelihood of considering euthanasia. Depression produces more subtle distortions of decision making than does delirium or psychosis, but refusal of life-saving treatment cannot be assumed to represent lack of capacity or suicidality.

Rosenstein DL, Miller FG: Ethical issues, in American Psychiatric Publishing Textbook of Psychosomatic Medicine: Official Textbook of the Academy of Psychosomatic Medicine. Edited by Levenson JL. Washington, DC, American Psychiatric Publishing, 2005, pp 56–57, 61

49. Examples of depressive delusions would be *least* likely to involve which of the following statements?

A. "I've lost my mind."

B. "My body is disintegrating."

C. "I ought to be promoted."

D. "I have an incurable illness."

E. "I have caused some great harm."

**The correct response is option C.**

Of 161 patients with endogenous depression studied by Meyers and colleagues (Meyers and Greenberg 1986; Meyers et al. 1985), 72 (45%) were found to be delusional as determined by research diagnostic criteria. These delusions included beliefs such as "I've lost my mind," "My body is disintegrating," "I have an incurable illness," and "I have caused some great harm." Option C is unlikely because depressive delusions are most frequently mood congruent. In this case, a delusion that he was being promoted would be mood incongruent.

Blazer DG: The Psychiatric interview of older adults, in The American Psychiatric Publishing Textbook of Geriatric Psychiatry, 3rd Edition. Edited by Blazer DG, Steffens DC, Busse EW. Washington, DC, American Psychiatric Publishing, 2004, p 170

Meyers BS, Greenberg R: Late-life delusional depression. J Affect Disord 11:133–137, 1986

Meyers BS, Greenberg R, Varda M: Delusional depression in the elderly, in Treatment of Affective Disorders in the Elderly. Edited by Shamoian CA. Washington, DC, American Psychiatric Press, 1985, pp 37–63

50. Which of the following is *true* regarding the psychotic disorder of late life referred to as *late-life paraphrenia?*

A. It is the late-life recurrence of an earlier onset of schizophrenia in a patient who had been symptom-free for many years.

B. According to Kraepelin's original description, most patients were male.

C. Psychotic symptoms of the late-life episode typically include delusions, but hallucinations are not experienced.

D. Patients have been reported to have simultaneous sensory deficits.

E. Antipsychotics have been demonstrated to be effective for late-life delusional disorder.

**The correct response is option D.**

Patients with late-life paraphrenia may have comorbid sensory deficits.

Late-life paraphrenia identifies psychosis that has a late age at onset. According to Kraepelin, most patients were women, usually living alone. Paranoid ideation is sometimes accompanied by hallucinations. Neuroleptics are usually the first-line treatment.

Gwyther LP, Steffens DC: Agitation and suspiciousness, in The American Psychiatric Publishing Textbook of Geriatric Psychiatry, 3rd Edition. Edited by Blazer DG, Steffens DC, Busse EW. Washington, DC, American Psychiatric Publishing, 2004, p 377

51. Conventional antipsychotics may be helpful in borderline personality disorder for which of the following problems?

A. Suicidality.

B. Ideas of reference.

C. Social functioning.

D. All of the above.

E. None of the above.

**The correct response is option D.**

In one large trial (Serban and Siegel 1984) in patients with personality disorder, treatment with thiothixene or haloperidol resulted in improvement on multiple domains, including cognitive disturbance, derealization, ideas of reference, anxiety, depression, and self-esteem and social functioning, suggesting that pharmacotherapy for target symptoms may have a wide-reaching effect. In a placebo-controlled study in patients with personality disorders, mostly borderline, presenting acutely with a suicide attempt and with a history of at least two prior attempts, treatment with a low-dose depot antipsychotic (flupenthixol 20 mg every 4 weeks) was highly effective in reducing suicide attempts at 4–6 months of treatment.

Serban G, Siegel S: Response of borderline and schizotypal patients to small doses of thiothixene and haloperidol. Am J Psychiatry 141:1455–1458, 1984

Simeon D, Hollander E: Treatment of personality disorders , in The American Psychiatric Publishing Textbook of Psychopharmacology, 3rd Edition. Edited by Schatzberg AF, Nemeroff CB. Washington, DC, American Psychiatric Publishing, 2004, p 1052

52.  Which of the following is *true* regarding the treatment of anxiety disorders with buspirone?

A.  Buspirone, a partial agonist at the $5\text{-HT}_{1A}$ receptor, interacts with the gamma-aminobutyric acid (GABA) receptor and chloride ion channels and therefore should be used with caution when prescribed with benzodiazepines.
B.  Buspirone interacts with alcohol, and its side effects include sedation and impairment of psychomotor performance. However, it does not pose a risk of abuse.
C.  The efficacy of buspirone is not statistically different from that of benzodiazepines for the treatment of generalized anxiety.
D.  Buspirone has been found to be effective in the treatment of generalized anxiety disorder and panic disorder.
E.  Buspirone is safe to be used in patients with hepatic impairment but not renal impairment.

**The correct response is option C.**

The efficacy of buspirone is not statistically different from that of benzodiazepines for the treatment of generalized anxiety. However, its onset of therapeutic action is less rapid than that of benzodiazepines, with up to 6 weeks needed for therapeutic effectiveness. Option A is incorrect because although it *is* a partial agonist at the $5\text{-HT}_{1A}$ receptor, buspirone does not interact with the GABA receptor or chloride ion channels. Therefore, buspirone does *not* interact with alcohol, cause sedation, or impair psychomotor performance, so option B is incorrect. However, as stated, buspirone does not pose a risk of abuse. Option D is incorrect because although found to be effective for treating generalized anxiety disorder, it does not appear to effective for the treatment of panic disorder. Buspirone may be helpful as an augmenting agent in the treatment of obsessive-compulsive disorder and depression, and some evidence suggests that it may be effective for the treatment of social phobia. Option E is incorrect because buspirone is metabolized in the liver and excreted by the kidneys, and its use is contraindicated in patients with severe liver or kidney impairments.

Martinez M, Marangell LB, Martinez JM: Psychopharmacology, in The American Psychiatric Publishing Textbook of Psychiatry, 5th Edition. Edited by Hales RE, Yudofsky SC, Gabbard GO. Washington, DC, American Psychiatric Publishing, 2008, pp 1080–1081

Ninan PT, Muntasser S: Buspirone and gepirone, in The American Psychiatric Publishing Textbook of Psychopharmacology, 3rd Edition. Edited by Schatzberg AF, Nemeroff CB. Washington, DC, American Psychiatric Publishing, 2004, p 397

53.  In Project Match, a large randomized trial of alcohol treatment modalities and predictive pretreatment variables, investigators found that the best potential predictor of a treatment outcome was

A.  Social status of the patient.
B.  Patient self-selection of treatment type.
C.  Severity of addiction.
D.  Number of previous treatment attempts.
E.  No specific predictors between specific treatments and indicators were found.

**The correct response is option E.**

Project Match investigators did not find a robust association between specific treatments and specific indicators (Project Match Research Group 1998). Potential predictors, such as severity of addiction, social status, number of previous treatment attempts, coping style, family history, and patient self-selection of treatment type, have not been shown to have consistent associations with treatment outcome.

Franklin JE Jr, Levenson JL, McCance-Katz EF: Substance-related disorders, in The American Psychiatric Publishing Textbook of Psychosomatic Medicine: Official Textbook of the Academy of Psychosomatic Medicine. Edited by Levenson JL. Washington, DC, American Psychiatric Publishing, 2005, p 391

Project Match Research Group: Matching alcoholism treatments to client heterogeneity: treatment main effects and matching effects on drinking during treatment. J Stud Alcohol 59:631–639, 1998

54. Which of the following statements is *false* regarding brain regions and activity?

    A. The dorsolateral prefrontal region is important for cognition, executive function, and focused attention.
    B. The orbital prefrontal region is important for social conduct, insight, judgment, and mood.
    C. The hippocampal complex is key to memory formation and storage functions.
    D. The parietal lobe is important for sensation, speech production/conduction, and deficit recognition.
    E. The thalamus modulates physiological response to emotional stimuli, temperature control, sleep, water metabolism, hormone secretion, satiety, and circadian rhythms.

## The correct response is option E.

These characteristics describe the hypothalamus, not the thalamus. The thalamus has been conceived as the key "relay station" for memory emotion, cognition, behavior, and motor and sensory functions.

Taber KH, Hurley RA: Neuroanatomy for the psychiatrist, in The American Psychiatric Publishing Textbook of Psychiatry, 5th Edition. Edited by Hales RE, Yudofsky SC, Gabbard GO. Washington, DC, American Psychiatric Publishing, 2008, p 188

55. The developmental histories of individuals with schizophrenia reveal higher rates of all of the following *except*

    A. Heavy maternal alcohol use during the first trimester.
    B. Maternal starvation during the first trimester.
    C. Maternal influenza infection during the second trimester.
    D. Rhesus and ABO blood-type incompatibility.
    E. Perinatal anoxic birth injuries.

## The correct response is option A.

Higher frequencies of gestational and perinatal events and obstetrical complications have been noted in prospective studies of people who later manifest schizophrenia. Thus, for example, maternal starvation during the first trimester of pregnancy, maternal influenza infection during the second trimester, rhesus and ABO blood-type incompatibility, and perinatal anoxic birth injuries have been observed to occur at higher rates in the early development of persons who subsequently develop schizophrenia.

Gur RE, Arnold SE: Neurobiology of schizophrenia, in The American Psychiatric Publishing Textbook of Psychopharmacology, 3rd Edition. Edited by Schatzberg AF, Nemeroff CB. Washington, DC, American Psychiatric Publishing, 2004, p 770

56. The greatest threat to response to antidepressant treatment is

    A. Drug-drug interactions.
    B. Family history of preferential response.
    C. Suicidal ideation.
    D. Preexisting medical factors.
    E. Nonadherence to medication regimen.

## The correct response is option E.

The greatest threat to treatment response is nonadherence to an agent, often because of intolerance of common side effects. Dropout rates are an estimated 7%–44% for various tricyclic antidepressants (TCAs) and 7%–23% in selective serotonin reuptake inhibitors (SSRIs). Choosing an agent that will be well tolerated by an individual increases the likelihood of adherence. Options A and D are incorrect because in general, drug-drug interactions and medical factors are less significant to overall treatment response than medication adherence. Option B is incorrect because although family history is a key factor in predicting the efficacy of response for a particular agent, family history is not a threat to antidepressant treatment in general. Studies indicate that the risk of an antidepressant specifically inducing suicide in an otherwise nonsuicidal individual is extremely rare. Option C is incorrect because suicidal ideation itself does not affect antidepressant response to treatment.

Boland RJ, Keller MB: Treatment of depression, in The American Psychiatric Publishing Textbook of Psychopharmacology, 3rd Edition. Edited by Schatzberg AF, Nemeroff CB. Washington, DC, American Psychiatric Publishing, 2004, p 853

Cozza KL, Armstrong SC, Oesterheld JR, et al: Study Guide to Clinical Psychopharmacology: A Companion to The American Psychiatric Publishing Textbook of Psychopharmacology, 3rd Edition, Washington, DC, American Psychiatric Publishing, 2004, pp 270–271

57. Electroconvulsive therapy (ECT) has been shown to be safe and effective in treating all of the following *except*

    A. Comorbid mood disorders in patients with closed head injuries.
    B. Comorbid mood disorders in patients with mental retardation or dementia.
    C. Comorbid mood disorders in patients with intractable seizure disorders.
    D. Obsessive-compulsive disorder (OCD) or a mood disorder during pregnancy.
    E. None of the above.

**The correct response is option E.**

Options A, B, C, and D are incorrect because ECT has been shown to be safe and effective in treating patients with comorbid closed head injuries, mental retardation, dementia, seizure disorders, and during pregnancy. ECT raises the seizure threshold, can interrupt status epilepticus, and can effectively treat intractable seizures. ECT also has been shown to be effective in the treatment of OCD and OCD complicated by schizophrenia.

McDonald WM, Thompson TR, McCall WV, et al: Electroconvulsive therapy, in The American Psychiatric Publishing Textbook of Psychopharmacology, 3rd Edition. Edited by Schatzberg AF, Nemeroff CB. Washington, DC, American Psychiatric Publishing, 2004, pp 690–691

58. Which of the following agents used in the treatment of opioid dependence is itself a partial agonist of the mu opioid receptor?

    A. Naltrexone.
    B. Buprenorphine.
    C. Methadone.
    D. Clonidine.
    E. Hydromorphone.

**The correct response is option B.**

Buprenorphine is a partial agonist of the mu opioid receptor and is a clinically effective analgesic agent, with an estimated potency 25–40 times that of morphine. Buprenorphine in sublingual formulation has been approved by the U.S. Food and Drug Administration (FDA) for treating opioid dependence. Other FDA-approved drugs for this purpose include methadone and L-alpha-acetylmethadol (LAAM), which is a long-acting opioid agonist.

Cornish JW, McNicholas LF, O'Brien CP: Treatment of substance-related disorders, in The American Psychiatric Publishing Textbook of Psychopharmacology, 3rd Edition. Edited by Schatzberg AF, Nemeroff CB. Washington, DC, American Psychiatric Publishing, 2004, p 1018

59. The personality structure of the elderly shows

    A. Remarkable stability over long periods of the life span, with increases on dimensions of neuroticism.
    B. Declines on dimensions of neuroticism and increases on dimensions of openness to experience.
    C. Increases on dimensions of openness to experience and of extraversion.
    D. Remarkable stability over long periods of the life span, with declines on dimensions of neuroticism.
    E. Declines in dimensions of neuroticism and of agreeableness.

**The correct response is option D.**

The American pattern of declines on the dimensions of neuroticism, extraversion, and openness to experience and increases in agreeableness and conscientiousness was consistently replicated in various cultures and nations, suggesting that these cross-sectional age differences were caused by intrinsic maturational processes.

Contrary to popular conceptions that personality changes dramatically throughout adulthood, several longitudinal studies have shown remarkable stability over long periods of the life span.

Siegler IC, Poon LW, Madden DJ, et al: Psychological aspects of normal aging, in The American Psychiatric Publishing Textbook of Geriatric Psychiatry, 3rd Edition. Edited by Blazer DG, Steffens DC, Busse EW. Washington, DC, American Psychiatric Publishing, 2004, pp 127–128

60. One of the most consistent neuroanatomic findings in schizophrenia has been

    A. Enlarged hippocampal volumes.
    B. Underdevelopment of the corpus callosum.
    C. Enlarged amygdala.
    D. Enlarged lateral ventricles.
    E. Pituitary hyperplasia.

**The correct response is option D.**

One of the most consistent neuroanatomic findings in schizophrenia has been an increase in size of the lateral ventricles. The degree of ventricular enlargement correlates with poor premorbid adjustment, and the enlargement has been found at the initial presentation.

Gur RE, Arnold SE: Neurobiology of schizophrenia, in The American Psychiatric Publishing Textbook of Psychopharmacology, 3rd Edition. Edited by Schatzberg AF, Nemeroff CB. Washington, DC, American Psychiatric Publishing, 2004, p 770

61. All of the following features are common in families with Munchausen syndrome by proxy *except*

    A. A dominant and aggressive husband and a caretaking and supportive wife.
    B. Intense family–group loyalty, with little protective concern for the child.
    C. A multigenerational pattern of abnormal illness behavior.
    D. Enmeshment of parent–child relationships.
    E. No gender bias of the child victims.

**The correct response is option A.**

Studies of families with Munchausen syndrome by proxy have revealed that the wife tends to be more dominant and aggressive, whereas the husband is more caretaking and supportive. Commonly observed features include enmeshment of parent–child relationships; multigenerational themes of dominance and submission in parent–child relationships; intense family–group loyalty, with little protective concern for the needs of the developing child; and a multigenerational pattern of abnormal illness behavior on the maternal side of the family. Victims are either male or female and tend to be age 4 years and younger.

Ford CV: Deception syndromes: factitious disorders and malingering, in The American Psychiatric Publishing Textbook of Psychosomatic Medicine: Official Textbook of the Academy of Psychosomatic Medicine. Edited by Levenson JL. Washington, DC, American Psychiatric Publishing, 2005, pp 303–304

62. Which of the following statements is *true* regarding prevalence of selective mutism in children?

    A. Prevalence estimates in children range from 3% to 5%.
    B. Selective mutism symptoms that occur upon starting school are likely to be unremitting.
    C. Variability in prevalence estimates may be because of vagueness in the DSM regarding the level of impairment required to meet diagnostic criteria.
    D. Scandinavian prevalence studies have reported lower rates of selective mutism than have U.S. studies among school-age children.
    E. Variability in prevalence estimates is unlikely to be related to differences in the consistent application of diagnostic criteria in study populations.

**The correct response is option C.**

Variability in prevalence estimates may be a function of the age of the children sampled, differences in the application of the diagnostic criteria, and vagueness of the DSM criteria in terms of the degree of impairment required for the diagnosis.

Black B, Garcia AM, Freeman JB, et al: Specific phobia, panic disorder, social phobia, and selective mutism, in The American Psychiatric Publishing Textbook of Child and Adolescent Psychiatry, 3rd Edition. Edited by Wiener JM, Dulcan MK. Washington, DC, American Psychiatric Publishing, 2004, p 596

63. A lesion in the right frontal operculum will *most likely* lead to

    A. Loss of emotional tone of speech (gesturing, prosody, inflection).
    B. Nonfluent aphasia.
    C. Lack of awareness of deficits.
    D. Inability to comprehend speech.
    E. Impaired initiation and synchronization of speech.

**The correct response is option A.**

Right frontal operculum lesions result in expressive aphasia with loss of emotion in the speech. Option B is incorrect because lesions of the *left* frontal operculum, which contains Broca's area, lead to *nonfluent aphasia*, characterized by difficulty producing fluent speech, defective naming, and impaired repetition. Options C and D are incorrect because patients with lesions in the right frontal operculum are usually aware of the deficits and comprehension of spoken speech is intact. Option E is incorrect because the impaired initiation and synchronization of speech, as well as akinetic mutism, occur with lesions in the superior mesial region.

> Taber KH, Hurley RA: Neuroanatomy for the psychiatrist, in The American Psychiatric Publishing Textbook of Psychiatry, 5th Edition. Edited by Hales RE, Yudofsky SC, Gabbard GO. Washington, DC, American Psychiatric Publishing, 2008, p 161

64.  A 53-year-old man with a history of recurrent mild major depressive disorder has avoided psychiatric treatment for "years" because of his earlier experience with a medication. The antidepressant significantly reduced libido and contributed to his gaining 30 lb., so he completely stopped taking it. He does not recall the name of the medication or any other side effects but threatens to stop taking any medications that cause either of these symptoms. Of the following, which pair of antidepressants did the patient *most likely* take in the past?

A.  Amitriptyline or nefazodone.
B.  Phenelzine or venlafaxine.
C.  Mirtazapine or bupropion.
D.  Trazodone or paroxetine.
E.  Fluoxetine or sertraline

### The correct response is option D.

Trazodone and paroxetine are both associated with significant weight gain and sexual side effects. Of the selective serotonin reuptake inhibitors (SSRIs), paroxetine is the most prone to causing weight gain. Studies show that fluoxetine, sertraline, citalopram, and escitalopram have equivocal effect on weight gain.

Option A is incorrect because amitriptyline causes both weight gain and sexual side effects, but nefazodone has a relatively low risk of sexual side effects. Option B is incorrect because phenelzine causes weight gain, but venlafaxine has a low risk of weight gain. Neither is associated with substantial sexual side effects. Option C is incorrect because mirtazapine is associated with weight gain and sexual side effects, but bupropion has a low risk of both sexual side effects and weight gain. Option E is incorrect because fluoxetine is associated with significant sexual side effects, but sertraline is not associated strongly with either side effect. Based on side-effect profile alone, in order of preference, the patient would most likely adhere to bupropion

(neither side effect), venlafaxine (no weight gain, low risk sexual side effects), and possibly nefazodone (equivocal risk of weight gain, low risk sexual side effects). Thereafter, the SSRIs sertraline, citalopram, and escitalopram may be acceptable options for this patient.

> Boland RJ, Keller M: Treatment of depression, in The American Psychiatric Publishing Textbook of Psychopharmacology, 3rd Edition. Edited by Schatzberg AF, Nemeroff CB. Washington, DC, American Psychiatric Publishing, 2004, pp 858–859; Tables 52–6 and 52–7

===

**BOTTOM LINE**
**Antidepressant Side Effects**

*Most* likely to cause both weight gain *and* sexual side effects: most tricyclic antidepressants (TCAs), paroxetine, trazodone, and mirtazapine.

*Most* likely to cause weight gain: TCAs, especially tertiary TCAs such as clomipramine and doxepin. Weight gain is less common with secondary TCAs such as desipramine, nortriptyline, and protriptyline; phenelzine; paroxetine; trazodone; and mirtazapine.

*Most* likely to cause sexual side effects: TCAs, paroxetine, fluoxetine, trazodone, and mirtazapine.

*Least* likely to cause weight gain: bupropion and venlafaxine.

*Least* likely to cause sexual side effects: bupropion and nefazodone.

===

65.  Which of the following is *true* regarding personality disorders in older patients?

A.  As research into personality disorders has increased, the phenomenon of personality disorders in the elderly has been thoroughly examined.
B.  Unlike in younger patients, comorbid personality disorders in elderly patients do not appear to affect outcomes of mood disorders.
C.  When an older patient's personality changes significantly because of dementia, the diagnosis is personality change due to a general medical condition.
D.  In Alzheimer's disease, the change in personality is usually an exaggeration of premorbid personality traits.
E.  Personality disorder not otherwise specified is diagnosed rarely in elderly patients.

## The correct response is option D.

In Alzheimer's disease, the change in personality is usually an exaggeration of preexisting traits. Although general research in personality disorders has increased, not much has been done with respect to elderly patients. Substantial evidence shows the negative effect of personality disorders on the outcome of depressive disorders. When an older patient's personality changes significantly because of dementia, the diagnosis of personality change due to a general medical condition does not apply. Because older patients commonly show symptoms of more than one personality disorder, the diagnosis of personality disorder not otherwise specified is quite common.

Oxman TE, Ferrell RB: Personality disorders, in The American Psychiatric Publishing Textbook of Geriatric Psychiatry, 3rd Edition. Edited by Blazer DG, Steffens DC, Busse EW. Washington, DC, American Psychiatric Publishing, 2004, pp 369–370

66. Which of the following statements best describes the state of current knowledge about genetic markers for bipolar disorder?

    A. Chromosome 21 has definitely been implicated.
    B. Chromosome 21 and the Y chromosome have definitely been implicated.
    C. Although studies implicating chromosome 11 and the X chromosome were published, further studies have not supported these findings.
    D. Although studies implicating chromosome 11 and the Y chromosome were published, further studies have not supported these findings.
    E. Chromosome 21 and the X chromosome have definitely been implicated.

## The correct response is option C.

Two teams of investigators have reported two different genes associated with bipolar disorder. In a Pennsylvania Amish community, the gene reported to produce bipolar disorder was found to be positioned on chromosome 11 and inherited by autosomal dominant transmission. Unfortunately, subsequent analysis did not confirm this finding in an expanded data set of the same population.

Flores BH, Musselman DL, DeBattista C, et al: Biology of mood disorders, in The American Psychiatric Publishing Textbook of Psychopharmacology, 3rd Edition. Edited by Schatzberg AF, Nemeroff CB. Washington, DC, American Psychiatric Publishing, 2004, p 723

67. Alzheimer's disease and Parkinson's disease are associated with many neuropsychiatric complications. Among these is disturbed sleep; when sleep disturbance is associated with behavioral agitation, the term *sundowning* is used. Which of the following is *true* regarding sleep disorders commonly seen in patients with Alzheimer's disease and Parkinson's disease?

    A. The risk of sudden death usually exceeds the potential benefits of atypical antipsychotic agents in treating sundowning.
    B. Sundowning can typically be easily managed at home with light therapy, elimination of daytime napping, and a structured activity program.
    C. Sundowning has been linked with disturbed circadian rhythms and a phase delay of body temperature in dementia of Alzheimer's type.
    D. Patients with Parkinson's disease have an increased risk of restless leg syndrome but not rapid eye movement (REM) sleep behavior disorder.
    E. Although carbidopa/levodopa combinations may cause initial insomnia, they do not increase risk of nightmares.

## The correct response is option C.

Option A is incorrect because of all medications prescribed for sundowning, antipsychotics have the most evidence of efficacy. Although a black box warning cautions that atypical antipsychotic agents have been associated with an increased risk of sudden death, the risk is relatively small compared with the potential benefits. Light therapy, elimination of daytime napping, and structured activities can decrease the risk of sundowning. However, option B is incorrect because sundowning itself often precipitates nursing home care placement of patients with dementia of Alzheimer's type.

Option D is incorrect because Parkinson's disease is associated with *both* restless legs syndrome and REM sleep behavior disorder. Option E is incorrect because carbidopa/levodopa may cause initial insomnia *and* nightmares.

Krystal AD, Edinger JD, Wohlgemuth WK, et al: Sleep and circadian rhythm disorders, in The American Psychiatric Publishing Textbook of Geriatric Psychiatry, 3rd Edition. Edited by Blazer DG, Steffens DC, Busse EW. Washington, DC, American Psychiatric Publishing, 2004, pp 342–343

68. All of the following are theorized to be causes of chronic pain *except*

    A. Ongoing activation of pain pathways from the periphery that causes pain to become chronic.
    B. Dysfunctional peripheral nerves.
    C. Failure of motor reflexes to inhibit pain.
    D. Sensitization of the dorsal horn.
    E. Sympathetic nervous system input.

**The correct response is option C.**

Motor reflexes may *potentiate* pain, but they are not believed to be involved in the inhibition of pain. Options A, B, D, and E are *true* statements and therefore incorrect. In addition to these factors, cortical and limbic activity is also believed to be involved in chronic pain.

Leo RJ: Clinical Manual of Pain Management in Psychiatry. Washington, DC, American Psychiatric Publishing, 2007, p 23; Table 2–4

69. All of the following are associated with better response rates to lithium in the treatment of acute mania *except*

    A. Few lifetime manic episodes.
    B. Classic manic or elated symptoms.
    C. Rapid-cycling symptoms.
    D. Presentation with psychotic symptoms.
    E. Presentation with no psychotic symptoms.

**The correct response is option C.**

Lithium exerts improvement in psychotic and manic symptoms. Patients with elated or classic manic symptoms and relatively few lifetime mood episodes appear to have a better response rate to lithium than do patients with mixed episodes and rapid cycling.

Keck PE, McElroy SL: Treatment of bipolar disorder, in The American Psychiatric Publishing Textbook of Psychopharmacology, 3rd Edition. Edited by Schatzberg AF, Nemeroff CB. Washington, DC, American Psychiatric Publishing, 2004, p 867

70. The primary receptor site of action of cocaine is

    A. Dopamine transporter (DAT).
    B. Vesicular monoamine transporter (VMAT).
    C. Nicotinic acetylcholine (ACh) receptors.
    D. Gamma-aminobutyric acid (GABA) receptors.
    E. *N*-methyl-D-aspartate (NMDA) receptors.

**The correct response is option A.**

Cocaine's three known molecular targets are the DAT, the serotonin transporter (5-HTT), and the norepinephrine transporter (NET). VMAT is a primary site of action for amphetamines, not cocaine, so option B is incorrect. Options C, D, and E are incorrect because ACh receptors are the primary sites for nicotine, and GABA and NMDA are sites for ethanol, not cocaine.

Clinton K: Neurobiology of substance abuse disorders, in The American Psychiatric Publishing Textbook of Psychopharmacology, 3rd Edition. Edited by Schatzberg AF, Nemeroff CB. Washington, DC, American Psychiatric Publishing, 2004, p 811; see Table 49–1

71. All of the following statements are true regarding possible effects of antidepressants *except*

    A. Bupropion causes seizures in about one-third of overdoses.
    B. Tricyclic antidepressants (TCAs) may be lethal at doses only three to five times the therapeutic dose.
    C. Multidrug overdoses that include fluvoxamine have been known to be lethal in about 50% of cases.
    D. Of individuals intentionally overdosing on paroxetine, an overwhelming majority recover without incident.
    E. Of the selective serotonin reuptake inhibitors (SSRIs), fluoxetine and sertraline have the highest risk of inducing sudden, violent suicidal ideation.

**The correct response is option E.**

In the early 1990s, a great deal of concern was generated by reports of sudden, violent suicidal ideation associated with administration of the SSRIs fluoxetine and sertraline. These reports were followed by a similar report involving sertraline. The result was speculation among some that SSRIs were "suicide pills." Subsequent reports showed that if any prosuicide effect exists, it is extremely rare and not unique to any one antidepressant.

Option A is incorrect because bupropion can cause seizures in about one-third of overdoses. Option B is incorrect because TCAs can be fatal at doses of only three to five times the therapeutic dose. The ratio is lower in children, in whom TCAs can be toxic in doses of 5 mg/kg. Because overdosing on medications is a common method of self-injurious behavior among suicidally depressed individuals, antidepressants with relatively wide safety margins should be chosen for patients at high risk for suicide. Thus, TCAs should be avoided in suicidal patients.

Option C is incorrect because multidrug overdoses that include fluvoxamine have been known to be lethal in about 50% of cases in the past two decades. In the past two decades, death was reported in 253 patients taking fluvoxamine (0.9 of 100,000 patients) in multidrug overdoses. However, only 6 of these patients (1.2% of all reported overdoses) had ingested fluvoxamine alone. Therefore, fluvoxamine itself is unlikely to be especially prosuicidal in comparison with other SSRIs. Option D is incorrect because intentional overdoses with paroxetine are rarely fatal, and the vast majority of patients who overdose on this SSRI recover completely.

Boland RJ, Keller MB: Treatment of depression, in The American Psychiatric Publishing Textbook of Psychopharmacology, 3rd Edition. Edited by Schatzberg AF, Nemeroff CB. Washington, DC, American Psychiatric Publishing, 2004, pp 855–856

72. Which of the following statements is *true* regarding schizophrenia?

    A. Approximately 30% of patients achieve remission of psychotic symptoms within 3–4 months.
    B. First-episode patients are generally more resistant to the therapeutic effects and side effects of medication than patients with chronic schizophrenia.
    C. Nearly one-third of patients with schizophrenia have comorbid substance use disorders, excluding nicotine use.
    D. More than one-half of patients with schizophrenia have comorbid nicotine abuse/dependence.
    E. Second-generation antipsychotic agents seem to have similar efficacy for depressive symptoms as first-generation antipsychotics.

## The correct response is option D.

Option A is incorrect because more than 70%, not 30%, of patients achieve remission of psychotic symptoms within 3–4 months, and 83% achieve stable remission at the end of 1 year. Option B is incorrect because first-episode patients are generally more sensitive to the therapeutic effects and side effects of medication and require lower doses of psychotropics than patients with chronic schizo

phrenia. Option C is incorrect because nearly one-half (not only one-third) of patients with schizophrenia have comorbid substance use disorders, excluding nicotine use. Option E is incorrect because second-generation antipsychotic agents seem to have *better* efficacy for depressive symptoms than do first-generation antipsychotics.

Lehman AF, Lieberman JA, Dixon LB, et al: Practice guideline for the treatment of patients with schizophrenia, second edition, in Practice Guidelines for the Treatment of Psychiatric Disorders: Compendium 2006. Arlington, VA, American Psychiatric Association, 2006, p 577

73. Which of the following is *true* regarding the obtaining of informed consent for forensic evaluations in minors?

    A. If a forensic evaluation of a minor is court ordered, parental consent is not required.
    B. If a forensic evaluation of a minor is requested by a parent, consent is implied and need not be further explored or documented.
    C. A minor cannot provide consent for an evaluation under any circumstances, and parental consent must be obtained.
    D. When parental consent is obtained, the psychiatrist need not explain to the child the nature of the evaluation and with whom the information will be shared.
    E. Adolescents are not allowed to provide informed consent under any circumstances.

## The correct response is option A.

If a forensic evaluation of a minor is court ordered, parental consent is not required. Option B is incorrect because if an evaluation is requested by a parent, then the evaluator should obtain the informed consent of the parent, which should include a signed release to send the report to designated recipients. In limited situations, an adolescent can provide consent for the evaluation. Such situations arise if the adolescent is emancipated, the case is waived to an adult criminal jurisdiction, or the adolescent can consent to treatment. In any event, the evaluator should explain to the child or adolescent in developmentally appropriate terms the nature of the evaluation and the parties with whom information will be shared.

Ash P: Children and adolescents, in The American Psychiatric Publishing Textbook of Forensic Psychiatry. Edited by Simon RI, Gold LH. Washington, DC, American Psychiatric Publishing, 2004, p 455

74. Characteristic signs and symptoms are often associated with lesions in specific central nervous system regions. All of the following are correctly paired localizations *except*

    A. Cerebral hemisphere: hemiparesis, hyperactive deep tendon reflexes, spasticity, Babinski sign.
    B. Basal ganglia: parkinsonism, athetosis, chorea, hemiballismus.
    C. Brainstem: cranial nerve palsy with ipsilateral hemiparesis; nystagmus; bulbar palsy.
    D. Cerebellum: ataxic gait, scanning speech, dysdiadochokinesia.
    E. Cerebral hemisphere: hemisensory loss, partial seizures, pseudobulbar palsy.

**The correct response is option C.**

The brainstem is associated with cranial nerve palsy with contralateral (not ipsilateral) hemiparesis, nystagmus, and bulbar palsy, as well as internuclear ophthalmoplegia. All the other associations are correct.

Kaufman DM: Clinical Neurology for Psychiatrists, 6th Edition. Philadelphia, PA, Saunders Elsevier, 2007, p 5

75. All of the following are true regarding schizophrenia *except*

    A. Men and women have the same overall incidence and lifetime prevalence of schizophrenia.
    B. The onset of symptoms occurs sooner in men than in women.
    C. Schizophrenia in women tends to be relatively mild at first, with increasing severity later on. In men, symptoms tend to taper off with advancing years.
    D. During pregnancy, many women with severe schizophrenia have worsening of psychotic symptoms.
    E. Late-life schizophrenia is more common in women than in men.

**The correct response is option D.**

During pregnancy, when estrogen levels are very high, many women with severe schizophrenia have an improvement in their symptoms, supporting the hypothesis that estrogen has a protective effect against psychotic symptoms. There is also a striking correlation between waning estrogen levels in the fourth decade and the exacerbation of existing illness or the increasingly common presenta-

tion of schizophrenia in postmenopausal women. Studies have thus far not definitively linked decreased estrogen levels to this phenomenon. Schizophrenia in women tends to be relatively mild at first, with increasing severity later on, whereas in men, symptoms tend to taper off with advancing years.

Kulkarni J: Psychotic illness in women at perimenopause and menopause, in Menopause: A Mental Health Practitioner's Guide. Edited by Stewart DE. Washington, DC, American Psychiatric Publishing, 2005, p 88

76. When a person taking disulfiram drinks alcohol, the subsequent toxic reaction is caused by accumulation of which of the following?

    A. Acetone.
    B. Aldehyde dehydrogenase.
    C. Acetaldehyde.
    D. Glutamate.
    E. Dopamine.

**The correct response is option C.**

Disulfiram inhibits a key enzyme, aldehyde dehydrogenase, involved in the breakdown of ethyl alcohol. After drinking, the alcohol–disulfiram reaction produces an excess blood level of acetaldehyde, which is toxic and produces facial flushing, tachycardia, hypotension, nausea and vomiting, and physical discomfort.

Cornish JW, McNicholas LF, O'Brien CP: Treatment of substance-related disorders, in The American Psychiatric Publishing Textbook of Psychopharmacology, 3rd Edition. Edited by Schatzberg AF, Nemeroff CB. Washington, DC, American Psychiatric Publishing, 2004, p 1010

77. A 35-year-old Latino woman with no prior psychiatric treatment was diagnosed with a single episode of mild major depressive disorder and was prescribed 10 mg of paroxetine, a selective serotonin reuptake inhibitor (SSRI). The dose of paroxetine was increased to 20 mg after 1 week. Six weeks later, the patient reports that her mood is the "same." She has more difficulty focusing/concentrating at work and worse libido. She constantly berates herself for being a "failure" as a mother despite evidence to the contrary, and has had difficulty falling asleep since increasing the dose of the SSRI, which she takes at bedtime. She has had minimal side effects from the medication. Which of the following strategies would be most recommended at this time?

Answer Guide to Exam 1745

A. Increase the dosage of paroxetine to 40 mg/day, and switch to morning dosing.
B. Discontinue paroxetine and start 20 mg of fluoxetine.
C. Augment with bupropion.
D. Refer the patient for cognitive-behavioral therapy (CBT).
E. Start weaning the patient off of paroxetine and start an adequate trial of bupropion.

**The correct response is option E.**

Some depressed patients with minimal or no treatment response after an adequate trial of an antidepressant agent may respond to a second agent within the same class. However, the best evidence supports changing to an alternative class agent after an adequate trial. Option A is incorrect because further increasing the dose of paroxetine, which is an SSRI, will be unlikely to lead to further efficacy. If the patient had at least a partial response to the SSRI, however, increasing the dose and switching the dosing time may be of benefit in terms of improving her mood while ameliorating the SSRI's "activating" side effect.

Option B is incorrect because switching from one SSRI to another will probably be less effective than switching to another class of medication. Augmenting an SSRI with bupropion seems to have limited efficacy in treating the sexual side effects caused by antidepressant treatment. Nevertheless, option C is incorrect because her worsening libido is likely to be a symptom of worsening depression, which has thus far not benefited from the SSRI. The patient made statements suggesting a potential focus of CBT ("I'm a failure").

However, option D is incorrect because her worsening depressive symptoms, especially her cognitive symptoms, will preclude her from participating meaningfully in CBT at this time. Once her mood improves, however, referral for CBT should be considered.

Boland RJ, Keller MB: Treatment of depression, in The American Psychiatric Association Textbook of Psychopharmacology, 3rd Edition. Edited by Schatzberg AF, Nemeroff CB. Washington, DC, American Psychiatric Publishing, 2004, p 853

*Nonresponse* in antidepressant treatment is a lack of clinically significant symptom improvement after an adequate trial of an antidepressant agent.

*Adequate* trial in antidepressant treatment is the adequate dose of an antidepressant for an adequate length of time or a minimum of 4–6 weeks. (Some researchers now suggest that an adequate trial requires up to 8–12 weeks.)

78. The incidence of serious rashes, including Stevens-Johnson syndrome, in pediatric patients taking lamotrigine is approximately

A. 10%.
B. 5%.
C. 1%.
D. 0.1%.
E. 0.01%.

**The correct response is option C.**

Common side effects of lamotrigine in children are ataxia, nausea, vomiting, and constipation. Of particular concern is the incidence of serious rash (reported to be 1% in pediatric patients), including Stevens-Johnson syndrome. This high incidence of serious rash may be attributable to the prior use of high doses of lamotrigine with concomitant divalproex.

Wagner KD: Treatment of childhood and adolescent disorders, in The American Psychiatric Publishing Textbook of Psychopharmacology, 3rd Edition. Edited by Schatzberg AF, Nemeroff CB. Washington, DC, American Psychiatric Publishing, 2004, p 1004

79. Which class of drugs showed an increase in abuse by U.S. adolescents from 1992 to 1997?

A. Alcohol.
B. Marijuana.
C. Cocaine.
D. Hallucinogens.
E. Prescription opiates.

**The correct response is option E.**

Substance abuse among adolescents differs from that in adults. Substance use among American youth rose to alarming rates between 1992 and 1997. Since then it has decreased significantly for alcohol, tobacco, and all drug classes but prescription opiates, the use of which continues to increase.

Kaminer Y: Adolescent substance abuse, in The American Psychiatric Publishing Textbook of Substance Abuse Treatment, 4th Edition. Edited by Galanter M, Kleber HD. Washington, DC, American Psychiatric Publishing, 2008, p 525

80. Approximately what percentage of persons admitted from the community to a geropsychiatry unit may have a urinary tract infection that may result in a delirium?

    A. 10%.
    B. 20%.
    C. 35%.
    D. 45%.
    E. 55%.

**The correct response is option B.**

Approximately 20% of people admitted from the community to a geropsychiatry unit may have a urinary tract infection, and in many cases it may result in delirium.

Taylor WD, Doraiswamy PM: Use of the laboratory in the diagnostic workup of older adults, in The American Psychiatric Publishing Textbook of Geriatric Psychiatry, 3rd Edition. Edited by Blazer DG, Steffens DC, Busse EW. Washington, DC, American Psychiatric Publishing, 2004, p 182

81. Which of the following antipsychotic agents is recommended in the American Psychiatric Association (APA) practice guideline as a first-line agent to treat delirium?

    A. Aripiprazole.
    B. Haloperidol.
    C. Olanzapine.
    D. Risperidone.
    E. Quetiapine.

**The correct response is option B.**

Haloperidol has been the most studied treatment for delirium. The APA practice guideline supported haloperidol as a first-line agent for delirium because of its minimal anticholinergic effects, minimal orthostasis, limited sedation, and flexibility in dosing and administration with oral, intramuscular, and intravenous routes.

The recommended dosage of haloperidol is 1–2 mg every 2–4 hours as needed, with further titration until desired effects are seen. Once stabilized, patients are often transitioned to a twice-daily or a daily bedtime oral dose, which is then continued or slowly tapered until the delirium has resolved. Patients with AIDS are sensitive to developing extrapyramidal side effects; thus, low dosages of haloperidol or atypical antipsychotics with lower risk are recommended.

In severe delirium refractory to boluses, continuous haloperidol infusions of 3–25 mg per hour have been used safely, although a ceiling of 5–10 mg per hour is suggested in the practice guideline. Electrocardiographic monitoring is recommended with continuous infusion because of concerns about torsades de pointes, although no specific dosage threshold has been designated. Awareness and management of risk factors for QTc (hypokalemia, hypomagnesemia, bradycardia, congenital long-QT syndrome, preexisting cardiac disease, and drug–drug interactions) is advised. Prolonged QTc intervals beyond 450 msec or 25% above baseline should prompt a cardiology consultation, a dosage reduction, or discontinuation of the antipsychotic agent.

Options A, C, D, and E are incorrect because current APA practice guidelines do not explicly recommend the use of atypical antipsychotics for delirium at this time. However, specialists in psychosomatic medicine have been successfully using these agents in clinical practice for the past decade despite scanty literature support and other pressures. The advantages are the lowered risk of extrapyramidal symptoms or electrocardiographic abnormalities, mood-modulating effects, and possibly enhanced efficacy in select patients.

The use of antipsychotics in elderly patients with dementia has raised some controversy since the U.S. Food and Drug Administration (FDA) released a "black box" warning for these agents because of the increased risk of stroke and mortality in this population. Risk stratification data, however, have found no difference between antipsychotic agents, including haloperidol.

The relative risk of treating or not treating delirium in elderly patients with dementia has not been sufficiently studied to warrant cessation of all antipsychotic use in these individuals.

Bourgeois JA, Seaman JS, Servis ME: Delirium, dementia, and amnestic and other cognitive disorders, in The American Psychiatric Publishing Textbook of Psychiatry, 5th Edition. Edited by Hales RE, Yudofsky SC, Gabbard GO. Washington, DC, American Psychiatric Publishing, 2008, pp 318–320

82.  A 32-year-old man with multiple sclerosis (MS) comes for an evaluation of his depression. A recent magnetic resonance imaging (MRI) noted a lesion in the cerebellum but nowhere else. When meeting you, he offers his left, not right, hand to shake your hand. You wonder if he has a right-sided dysmetria, which would suggest that

A.  A right finger-to-nose test, and possibly a right heel-to-shin test, would likely be abnormal.
B.  He has an intention tremor caused by an MS plaque in the left cerebellar hemisphere.
C.  A finger-to-nose test would be abnormal, and a left heel-to-shin test may be abnormal.
D.  His gait could be characterized as broad based, unsteady, and uncoordinated.
E.  On exam, he may also have some paresis, hyperactive deep tendon reflexes (DTRs), or Babinski sign.

## The correct response is option A.

Dysmetria is a coarse, irregular rhythm of movement that could be detected with the finger-to-nose test. He may have an intention tremor, which is a tremor that reveals itself when a patient moves willfully but is absent during rest and can be tested with the finger-to-nose and heel-to-shin tests. Option B is incorrect because a right-sided intention tremor would suggest a right, not left, cerebellar lesion. Cerebellar lesions lead to ipsilateral, not contralateral, movement and other disorders. Option C is incorrect because both tests would be abnormal on the right side because cerebellar lesions lead to ipsilateral movement disorders. Option D is incorrect because this describes an *ataxic gait*, which is seen in diffuse cerebellar degeneration such as in patients with chronic alcoholism. However, a right-sided cerebellar lesion may cause limb ataxia, which could be revealed in a heel-to-shin test (e.g., right heel wobbles as he slides it along his left shin). Option E is incorrect because a discrete cerebellar lesion would not cause paresis, hyperactive DTRs, or Babinski signs, which are evidence of lesion(s) in the cerebral hemispheres.

Kaufman DM: Clinical Neurology for Psychiatrists, 6th Edition. Philadelphia, PA, Saunders Elsevier, 2007, pp 11, 13

83.  In treating patients with schizophrenia and co-occurring substance use disorder, which of the following medications shows promise?

A.  Haloperidol.
B.  Aripiprazole.
C.  Risperidone.
D.  Clozapine.
E.  Quetiapine.

## The correct response is option D.

In contrast to atypical agents, which appear to decrease substance use among patients with schizophrenia, typical (first-generation) antipsychotics do not appear to decrease substance use in this population. Some data suggest that typical agents may even increase substance use in these patients. Of the second-generation antipsychotics, clozapine is the most promising medication in patients with schizophrenia and co-occurring substance use disorders and has been associated with decreased psychosis, increased abstinence, and decreased substance use, including decreased cocaine and nicotine intake.

Ross S: The mentally ill substance abuser, in The American Psychiatric Publishing Textbook of Substance Abuse Treatment, 4th Edition. Edited by Galanter M, Kleber HD. Washington, DC, American Psychiatric Publishing, 2008 p 547

84.  In general, which of the following is associated with late-onset depressive disorders?

A.  Rates of depressive disorders are higher in older adult populations (15%–20%) than in younger adult populations (5%–12%).
B.  Brain imaging that is consistent with significant cerebrovascular disease.
C.  Rates of atypical and delusional subtypes that are higher in older adult populations than in younger adult populations.
D.  Decreased testosterone levels.
E.  Symptom pattern and frequency of specific depressive subtypes similar to those in younger adult populations.

## The correct response is option B.

*Late-onset depression,* defined as having a first episode after age 60 years, is associated with brain imaging findings consistent with significant vascular disease. Option A is incorrect because the prevalence of major depressive disorder and dysthymia in late life (5%–12%) is similar to that in younger adult populations. Option C is incorrect because melancholic and delusional subtypes are more common in late-life depressive disorders than in depressive disorders in younger adult populations. Option D is incorrect because late-life dysthymia is associated with low testosterone levels in men, not in general. Option E is incorrect because older patients have more somatic symptoms, and both the melancholic and delusional subtypes increase in frequency with age.

Roose SP, Pollock BG, Devanand DP: Treatment during late life, in The American Psychiatric Publishing Textbook of Psychopharmacology, 3rd Edition. Edited by Schatzberg AF, Nemeroff CB. Washington, DC, American Psychiatric Publishing, 2004, p 1086

85. Magnetic resonance imaging (MRI) studies in children with schizophrenia have reported all of the following findings *except*

    A. Decreases in total cerebral volume.
    B. Cerebral asymmetry.
    C. Decreases in ventricular volume.
    D. Increases in temporal lobe volume.
    E. Decreases in midsagittal thalamic area.

**The correct response is option C.**

MRI studies in children with schizophrenia have reported *increases* in ventricular volume and decreases in total cerebral volume. Other findings reported in children with childhood-onset schizophrenia are larger volumes of the superior temporal lobe gyrus and a smaller midsagittal thalamic area.

Tsai LK, Champine DJ: Schizophrenia and other psychotic disorders, in The American Psychiatric Publishing Textbook of Child and Adolescent Psychiatry, 3rd Edition. Edited by Wiener JM, Dulcan MK. Washington, DC, American Psychiatric Publishing, 2004, p 396

86. According to Kandel's gateway theory of adolescent drug use, drug use often follows a stereotypical escalation among various substances of abuse. Which substance is usually the first abused substance in this cascade?

    A. Illicit drug other than marijuana.
    B. Marijuana.
    C. Hard liquor.
    D. Cigarettes.
    E. Beer or wine.

**The correct response is option E.**

Kandel (1982), the initial proponent of the gateway theory, argued that there are at least four distinct developmental stages of drug use: 1) beer or wine consumption, 2) cigarette smoking or hard liquor consumption, 3) marijuana use, and 4) other illicit drug use.

Kaminer Y: Adolescent substance abuse, in The American Psychiatric Publishing Textbook of Substance Abuse Treatment, 4th Edition. Edited by Galanter M, Kleber HD. Washington, DC, American Psychiatric Publishing, 2008, p 526

Kandel DB: Epidemiological and psychosocial perspectives on adolescent drug use. J Am Acad Child Psychiatry 21:328–347, 1982

87. Intermittent explosive disorder may be associated with

    A. Decreased dopamine levels.
    B. Decreased serotonin levels.
    C. Low testosterone levels.
    D. Increased gamma-aminobutyric acid (GABA) levels.
    E. Increased acetylcholine levels.

**The correct response is option B.**

Aggressive and impulsive acts appear to be associated with increased dopamine and testosterone, and with decreased levels of serotonin and GABA, which appear to inhibit predatory aggression.

Wakai ST, Trestman RL: Impulsivity and aggression, in Textbook of Violence Assessment and Management. Edited by Simon RI, Tardiff K. Washington, DC, American Psychiatric Publishing, 2008, p 215

88. A neurologist refers a 65-year-old woman to you for a 3-month history of "depression" after she had a stroke. On examination, you notice that the woman's left arm is persistently flexed at the elbow, and her left foot is outgoing. She walks slowly as if she is dragging her left foot at times. Extraocular muscles are intact on the left eye, but her right eye is deviated medially throughout the visit. She most likely had an infarct in the

    A. Basal ganglia.
    B. Cerebellum.
    C. Lateral medulla of the brainstem.
    D. Midbrain part of the brainstem.
    E. Right pontine part of the brainstem.

## The correct response is option E.

A right pontine infarct damages the abducens nerve (cranial nerve VI), which supplies the ipsilateral eye, and the adjacent corticospinal tract, which supplies the contralateral limbs. Options A and B are incorrect because discrete infarcts in the basal ganglia or cerebellum usually do not cause paresis, which this patient has. Lesions in these regions also do not lead to abnormal hyperactive deep tendon reflexes or Babinski sign. Option C is incorrect because a lateral medullary infarction causes difficulty swallowing and slurred speech. Also, the patient may have absence of pain on the ipsilateral side of the face, as well as an absent corneal reflex. Option D is incorrect because a discrete lesion in the midbrain would cause an ipsilateral cranial nerve III (not cranial nerve VI) palsy with contralateral limb paresis.

Kaufman DM: Clinical Neurology for Psychiatrists, 6th Edition. Philadelphia, PA, Saunders Elsevier, 2007, pp 8, 10

89. Which of the following clinical features is *least often* reported in delirium?

    A. Perceptual changes/hallucinations.
    B. Poor attention/vigilance.
    C. Memory impairment.
    D. Acute onset.
    E. Diffuse cognitive impairment.

## The correct response is option A.

Perceptual changes and hallucinations are least often reported in delirium. For the various clinical features of delirium, the range of reported frequencies is as follows: poor attention/vigilance, 100%; memory impairment, 64%–100%; clouding of consciousness, 45%–100%; disorientation, 43%–100%; acute onset, 93%; disorganized thinking/thought disorder, 59%–95%; diffuse cognitive impairment, 77%; language disorder, 41%–93%; sleep disturbance, 25%–96%; delusions, 18%–68%; mood lability, 43%–63%; psychomotor changes, 38%–55%; and perceptual changes/hallucinations, 17%–55%.

Bourgeois JA, Seaman JS, Servis ME: Delirium, dementia, and amnestic and other cognitive disorders, in The American Psychiatric Publishing Textbook of Psychiatry, 5th Edition. Edited by Hales RE, Yudofsky SC, Gabbard GO. Washington, DC, American Psychiatric Publishing, 2008, p 305; Table 8–2

90. A 45-year-old woman who is considering moving out of state soon presents to the outpatient clinic for evaluation of depression. She reports depressed mood, hopelessness, increased self-criticism, and indecision about moving. The severity is judged to be mild by the clinician. Before the episode of depression began, she had been ruminating about being "a failure" with regard to home and work issues. Which psychotherapeutic interventions would best help this patient to address her symptoms in general and specifically her feeling that she is "a failure"?

    A. Address information processing distortions arising from dysfunctional schemas, and alter these schemas.
    B. Address conditioned patterns of emotion and behavior triggered by internal and environment cues, and focus on firsthand experiences of mastery.
    C. Address internalized relationship conflicts and patterns by focusing on altering interpersonal patterns in current relationships.
    D. Address specific personality traits by focusing on insight.
    E. Identify key defense mechanisms, and observe and interpret significant transference data.

## The correct response is option A.

Option A describes a learning model of treatment that includes a wide range of cognitive-behavioral therapies (CBT) such as cognitive therapy. The premise of cognitive therapy is that early experience leads to the development of global negative assumptions, called *schemas*. The schema in this case is "I'm a failure." Depressive schemas involve distorted assumptions such as "If I'm not perfect, I'm a failure." Option B is incorrect because it describes *exposure therapy*, another learning model that includes the identification of environmental triggers and symptoms, and skills training for symptom management. This patient's main complaints revolved around negative thought patterns (schemas) and not on circumstantially triggered symptoms such as panic symptoms.

Option C is incorrect because it describes *interpersonal therapy*, which would be a better choice if the patient had complained primarily about relational problems. Option D is incorrect because it describes *psychodynamic psychotherapy*, which includes an exhaustive exploration of the past as a primary context for change efforts. Because psychodynamic psychotherapy would ideally span several months or years, this would not be the ideal option for this patient, who may move out of state soon. Option E is incorrect because it also describes components of psychodynamic psychotherapy.

Dewan MJ, Steenbarger BN, Greenberg RP: Brief psychotherapies, in The American Psychiatric Publishing Textbook of Psychiatry, 5th Edition. Edited by Hales RE, Yudofsky SC, Gabbard GO. Washington, DC, American Psychiatric Publishing, 2008, pp 1155–1161

91. Which of the following neurotransmitter changes is widely accepted to play a role in delirium?

    A. Excess acetylcholine activity.
    B. Reduced glutamate activity.
    C. Excess dopamine activity.
    D. Reduced dopamine activity.
    E. Excess serotonin activity.

**The correct response is option C.**

Dopamine has important roles in attention, mood, motor activity, perception, and executive functioning. Dopamine may be particularly valuable in facilitating cortical circuit activity during times of change, stress, or disequilibrium. Excess dopamine activity can lead to delirium, as seen with drugs such as L-dopa or cocaine.

Option A is incorrect because acetylcholine has long been known to be *decreased* in delirium as well as in hypoxia. Arousal, the sleep–wake cycle, attention, learning, and memory are heavily dependent on acetylcholine via its nicotinic and muscarinic receptors. Option B is incorrect because glutamate excess is notably also seen in hypoxia. The glutamate transporter fails in periods of energy deprivation, with a resultant loss of reuptake compounded by massive glutamate efflux. The excess glutamate then induces neuronal injury and necrosis in conjunction with calcium overload, reactive oxygen species, and the mitochondrial permeability transition cascade.

Bourgeois JA, Seaman JS, Servis ME: Delirium, dementia, and amnestic and other cognitive disorders, in The American Psychiatric Publishing Textbook of Psychiatry, 5th Edition. Edited by Hales RE, Yudofsky SC, Gabbard GO. Washington, DC, American Psychiatric Publishing, 2008, pp 307–308

92. Factors distinguishing patients with very late-onset schizophrenia from the "true" schizophrenia of younger patients include all of the following *except*

    A. Lower genetic load.
    B. Less evidence of early childhood maladjustment.
    C. Relative lack of formal thought disorder and negative symptoms.
    D. Lesser risk of tardive dyskinesia.
    E. Evidence of a neurodegenerative rather than a neurodevelopmental process.

**The correct response is option D.**

Factors distinguishing patients with very late-onset schizophrenia from "true" schizophrenia patients include a lower genetic load, less evidence of early childhood maladjustment, a relative lack of thought disorder and negative symptoms (including blunted affect), greater risk of tardive dyskinesia, and evidence of a neurodegenerative rather than a neurodevelopmental process.

Jeste DV, Wetherell JL, Dolder CR: Schizophrenia and paranoid disorders, in The American Psychiatric Publishing Textbook of Geriatric Psychiatry, 3rd Edition. Edited by Blazer DG, Steffens DC, Busse EW. Washington, DC, American Psychiatric Publishing, 2004, p 271

93. Misdiagnosis of delirium, a common clinical problem, has been found to be more likely among certain patient populations. Misdiagnosis is more likely in patients with all of the following *except*

    A. Hyperactive patient presentation.
    B. Advanced patient age.
    C. Sensory impairments.
    D. Preexisting dementia.
    E. Intensive care unit (ICU) setting.

**The correct response is option A.**

A diagnosis of delirium in patients with a *hypoactive* presentation is more likely to be missed. Options B, C, D, and E are incorrect because all of these patient characteristics increase the risk of a missed diagnosis of delirium.

Delirium is commonly misdiagnosed as depression by nonpsychiatrists. Prevalence rates of delirium in the ICU setting are 40%–87%.

Trzepacz PT, Meagher DJ: Neuropsychiatric aspects of delirium, in The American Psychiatric Publishing Textbook of Neuropsychiatry and Behavioral Neurosciences, 5th Edition. Edited by Yudofsky SC, Hales RE. Washington, DC, American Psychiatric Publishing, 2008, p 449

94. Workplace drug testing conducted under federal guidelines is limited to a small number of drugs. Which of the following drugs is *not* included for testing under these guidelines?

    A. Codeine/morphine.
    B. Amphetamine/methamphetamine.
    C. Synthetic opioids (oxycodone and others).
    D. Phencyclidine (PCP).
    E. Cocaine.

### The correct response is option C.

Workplace drug testing conducted under federal guidelines is limited to codeine/morphine, amphetamine/methamphetamine, PCP, marijuana, and cocaine. These federal guidelines apply only to federally mandated drug testing (for federal workers and for Department of Transportation–mandated tests). All other drug testing, including testing in drug treatment programs, is not limited by the currently antiquated federal drug-testing standards.

> DuPont RL, Selavka CM: Testing to identify recent drug use, in The American Psychiatric Publishing Textbook of Substance Abuse Treatment, 4th Edition. Edited by Galanter M, Kleber HD. Washington, DC, American Psychiatric Publishing, 2008, p 659

95. Of the following, the most significant risk factor for Alzheimer's disease is

    A. Presence of apolipoprotein-E (APOE) ε4 allele.
    B. Poor linguistic and cognitive abilities in early life, and lack of education.
    C. Aging.
    D. Mutations in the amyloid precursor protein (APP) gene on chromosome 21, the presenilin 1 (PS1) gene on chromosome 4, and the presenilin 2 (PS2) gene on chromosome 1.
    E. History of severe traumatic brain injury and/or Down syndrome.

### The correct response is option C.

Aging is the biggest risk factor for Alzheimer's disease. Inheritance of the APOE ε4 allele; poor linguistic and cognitive abilities in early life; relatively low educational level; mutations in the APP, PS1, and PS2 genes; and a history of a severe traumatic brain injury or Down syndrome do confer possible risks for Alzheimer's disease, but not to the degree that age does.

> Lah JJ, Levy OA, Levey AI: Biology of Alzheimer's disease, in The American Psychiatric Publishing Textbook of Psychopharmacology, 3rd Edition. Edited by Schatzberg AF, Nemeroff CB. Washington, DC, American Psychiatric Publishing, 2004, pp 797–798

96. Which of the following statements is *false* regarding the noradrenergic system?

    A. Norepinephrine (NE)–containing neurons in the central nervous system (CNS) are predominantly located in the brainstem.
    B. The locus coeruleus is the largest group of NE-containing neurons in the mammalian brain.
    C. Brain regions innervated by the locus coeruleus include the thalamus, cerebellar cortex, and hypothalamus, but not the amygdala.
    D. NE-containing cells are present in the lateral ventral tegmental fields.
    E. The primary motor cortex contains high densities of both dopaminergic and noradrenergic axons.

### The correct response is option C.

Innervated regions include the thalamus, cerebellar cortex, hypothalamus, *and* amygdala. NE-containing neurons in the CNS are predominantly located in the medulla and pons of the brainstem. The locus coeruleus is the principal noradrenergic cell group. NE-containing cells are present in the lateral ventral tegmental fields, which includes the intermediate reticular zone, lateral paragigantocellularis nucleus, and the nucleus ambiguus.

> Melchitzky DS, Austin MC, Lewis DA: Chemical neuroanatomy of the primate brain, in The American Psychiatric Publishing Textbook of Psychopharmacology, 3rd Edition. Edited by Schatzberg AF, Nemeroff CB. Washington, DC, American Psychiatric Publishing, 2004, pp 74–75

97. Diabetes mellitus is a metabolic disorder with substantial neuropsychiatric comorbidity. Which of the following is *true* regarding the neuropsychiatric aspects of diabetes mellitus?

    A. Facilitating the identification of automatic thoughts by techniques such as Socratic questioning, use of mood shifts that occur in vivo, thought recording, and guided imagery have been shown to be effective in treating depression in patients with type 2 diabetes.

B. In controlled studies, symptoms of depression occur in 15%–20% of patients with diabetes.

C. The increased prevalence of psychiatric disorders in a community sample of patients with diabetes was attributed to an increase in depressive disorder.

D. The prevalence of depression in diabetes is much higher than in other chronic diseases.

E. When symptoms of depression that may be attributed to the diabetic condition are excluded from a diagnosis of a mood disorder, the prevalence of depression in patients with diabetes is decreased by 50%.

## The correct response is option A.

Socratic questioning, thought recording, and guided imagery are methods to identify automatic thoughts. This approach is used in cognitive-behavioral therapy, which has shown to be effective in treating major depression in patients with type 2 diabetes. Option B is incorrect because *symptoms* of depression are extremely common in patients with diabetes, occurring in 22%–60%. Although estimates of major depression meeting the full criteria for diagnosis are lower in this population (8.5%–27.3%), the disorder is still relatively common and should be screened for. Option D is incorrect because the prevalence of depression in patients with diabetes is no greater than in patients with other chronic diseases. However, data indicate that the prevalence of psychiatric disorders in patients with diabetes (43.1%) and other chronic medical conditions (50.7%) was higher when compared with the prevalence in healthy individuals (26.2%). Option E is incorrect because investigators have found only a modest decrease when overlapping symptoms are excluded.

Cowles MK, Boswell EB, Anfinson TJ, et al: Neuropsychiatric aspects of endocrine disorders, in The American Psychiatric Publishing Textbook of Neuropsychiatry and Behavioral Neurosciences, 5th Edition. Edited by Yudofsky SC, Hales RE. Washington, DC, American Psychiatric Publishing, 2008, pp 803–807

98. A test of which of the following specimens is most subject to cheating?

A. Blood.
B. Hair.
C. Oral fluid.
D. Sweat.
E. Urine.

## The correct response is option E.

Cheating can be reduced by direct observation of collection, but cheating is an inherent problem with urine tests.

DuPont RL, Selavka CM: Testing to identify recent drug use, in The American Psychiatric Publishing Textbook of Substance Abuse Treatment, 4th Edition. Edited by Galanter M, Kleber HD. Washington, DC, American Psychiatric Publishing, 2008, p 659, Table 46–2

99. Regarding medical decision making, which of the following statements is *true*?

A. The parents of a disabled adult automatically remain the patient's legal guardians after their child's 18th birthday.

B. Studies have found that most (75%–80%) individuals fill out an advance directive for health care when given the opportunity to do so.

C. When an unmarried, incapacitated patient has an adult child, that adult child automatically is given medical decision making for the patient.

D. The completion of an advance directive for health care allows patients to specify in writing the medical care they wish to receive under various catastrophic medical conditions.

E. Substitute decision makers tend to base their decisions on what the patient would have wanted and not on what they themselves would have wanted had they been in the patient's place.

## The correct response is option D.

The completion of a living will or advance directive for health care allows patients to specify their wishes about medical care under catastrophic circumstances.

The parents of a disabled adult do not automatically retain legal guardianship of their child after his or her 18th birthday, nor does an adult child automatically become the decision maker for an unmarried, incapacitated parent. Only 15%–20% of individuals fill out an advance directive for health care when given the opportunity to do so. Substitute decision makers tend to base their decisions on what they would want to have happen to them, rather than what the patient would have wanted.

Rosenstein DL, Miller FG: Ethical issues, in The American Psychiatric Publishing Textbook of Psychosomatic Medicine: Official Textbook of the Academy of Psychosomatic Medicine. Edited by Levenson JL. Washington, DC, American Psychiatric Publishing, 2005, p 60

100. Which of the following is an example of a circumstance in which a drug-using defendant may claim settled insanity as a criminal defense strategy?

    A. Intoxication resulted from trickery.
    B. Long-term drug use has led to a chronic brain injury that is different from acute intoxication or toxic psychosis.
    C. Intoxication occurred under duress.
    D. Intoxication was caused by a previously unknown vulnerability to an atypical reaction to a substance.
    E. Intoxication occurred as a previously unknown side effect of a medication.

**The correct response is option B.**

*Settled insanity* is considered an exculpatory situation in which long-term use has led to a chronic brain injury that led to the commission of a crime. *Involuntary intoxication* is another exculpatory defense and reflects situations in which intoxication occured via trickery, under duress, or as a result of a previously unknown vulnerability to an atypical reaction to a substance or side effect of medication. Some jurisdictions have specific guidelines and limitations for an acceptable involuntary intoxication defense. Over time, case law and statutes have almost completely eliminated voluntary intoxication as a defense against responsibility for any crime.

Mack AH, Barros M: Forensic addiction psychiatry, in The American Psychiatric Publishing Textbook of Substance Abuse Treatment, 4th Edition. Edited by Galanter M, Kleber HD. Washington, DC, American Psychiatric Publishing, 2008, p 693

101. In bulimia nervosa

    A. Illness onset typically follows a period of dieting.
    B. The majority of patients abuse diuretics.
    C. The average binge episode lasts more than 2 hours.
    D. Comorbid depressive symptoms are seen in a minority of patients.
    E. Impulsivity in other spheres of behavior is infrequent.

**The correct response is option A.**

Illness onset typically follows a period of dieting, which may or may not have been successful. Option B is incorrect because most individuals with bulimia nervosa do not abuse diuretics. Option C is incorrect because the average binge episode lasts about 1 hour. Option D is incorrect because comorbid depression is found in most patients with bulimia. Option E is incorrect because impulsive actions such as stealing food, clothing, or jewelry occur in about one-fourth of patients prior to the onset of bulimia.

Halmi KA: Eating disorders, in The American Psychiatric Publishing Textbook of Psychiatry, 5th Edition. Edited by Hales RE, Yudofsky SC, Gabbard GO. Washington, DC, American Psychiatric Publishing, 2008, p 983

102. Which of the following statements is *true* regarding psychiatric interviewing of children?

    A. Children between the ages of 3 and 6 years usually cannot provide correct information when questioned in a way commensurate with their developmental level.
    B. Reports of children between the ages of 3 and 6 years can provide correct information when questioned in a way commensurate with their developmental level.
    C. Young children tend not to be suggestible and tend not to repeat inaccurate information fed to them by hostile parents involved in a bitter custody battle.
    D. For diagnostic purposes, if parents or other caregivers are unavailable to be interviewed, the examination of a child alone usually can suffice for patients who are at least 8 years old.
    E. In most circumstances, it is best to interview children first and then the parents.

**The correct response is option B.**

Option A is incorrect because children between the ages of 3 and 6 years usually can provide correct information when questioned in a way commensurate with their developmental level. Option C is incorrect because although children between the ages of 3 and 6 years can provide correct information, younger children are suggestible, and the validity of a child's report can be influenced by hostile parents. Option D is incorrect because for diagnostic purposes, the examination of the patient alone rarely suffices for children and adolescents, regardless of age. Other informants are necessary to corroborate a child's history—in particular, to provide crucial developmental, medical, and family history. Option E is incorrect because even brief interviews with parents prior to meeting the child may provide useful information to help develop rapport with the patient.

Kestenbaum CJ: The clinical interview of the child, in The American Psychiatric Publishing Textbook of Child and Adolescent Psychiatry, 3rd Edition. Edited by Wiener JM, Dulcan MK. Washington, DC, American Psychiatric Publishing, 2004, pp 103, 106

103. Which of the following statements is *true* regarding the acetylcholinergic system?

    A. The acetylcholine (ACh)–containing neurons are located mostly in the basal forebrain and the pontomesencephalotegmental region.
    B. Few ACh-containing neurons project to the cerebral cortex.
    C. The two main receptors of ACh are muscarinic and glutaminergic.
    D. ACh is known only to be part of neuronal tissue.
    E. ACh is synthesized by the enzyme acetylcholinesterase.

**The correct response is option A.**

The ACh-containing neurons are located mostly in the basal forebrain complex, which is near the inferior surface of the telencephalon between the hypothalamus and orbital cortex, and the pontomesencephalotegmental complex, which consists of the pedunculopontine nucleus and the laterodorsal tegmental nucleus in the ventral part of the periaqueductal gray. Option B is incorrect because the cerebral cortex is a major recipient of cholinergic projections. Option C is incorrect because the two main receptor classes for ACh are muscarinic and nicotinic. Option D is incorrect because ACh is found in many nonneuronal tissues, in which it appears to modulate basic cellular actions. Option E is incorrect because acetylcholinesterase is an enzyme in the synaptic cleft that rapidly inactivates ACh and is the site of action of various drugs. ACh is formed by the synthesis of acetyl coenzyme A and choline via the enzyme choline acetyltransferase.

Melchitzky DS, Austin MC, Lewis DA: Chemical neuroanatomy of the primate brain, in The American Psychiatric Publishing Textbook of Psychopharmacology, 3rd Edition. Edited by Schatzberg AF, Nemeroff CB. Washington, DC, American Psychiatric Publishing, 2004, pp 78–79

104. What approximate percentage of patients with Alzheimer's disease present with psychotic symptoms, typically in the middle stages of the disease?

    A. 10%–20%.
    B. 15%–25%.
    C. 25%–30%.
    D. 35%–50%.
    E. 55%–65%.

**The correct response is option D.**

Approximately 35%–50% of Alzheimer's disease patients manifest psychotic symptoms, typically in the middle stages of the disease. Psychotic symptoms in elderly individuals may arise secondary to Alzheimer's disease or other dementias. Delusions, particularly of a persecutory nature, tend to be more common than hallucinations, the latter being more common in nursing homes and other institutional settings.

Jeste DV, Wetherell JL, Dolder CR: Schizophrenia and paranoid disorders, in The American Psychiatric Publishing Textbook of Geriatric Psychiatry, 3rd Edition. Edited by Blazer DG, Steffens DC, Busse EW. Washington, DC, American Psychiatric Publishing, 2004, pp 272–273

105. All of the following antidepressants may be appropriate for a patient with bulimia nervosa *except*

    A. Desipramine.
    B. Imipramine.
    C. Phenelzine.
    D. Fluoxetine.
    E. Topiramate

**The correct response is option C.**

Patients with bulimia tend to be impulsive and therefore have difficulty adhering to special diets such as a tyramine-restricted diet for monoamine oxidase inhibitors (MAOIs) such as phenelzine. Several deaths have been associated with phenelzine use in bulimia patients. Bupropion should also be avoided because of the increased risk of seizures in patients with electrolyte abnormalities such as in patients with eating disorders. Desipramine, imipramine, fluoxetine, amitriptyline, and nortriptyline have been found to reduce bingeing and purging by about 22% as well as to improve mood in the short term. The long-term efficacy of these medications in treating bulimia nervosa is unknown. Topiramate has also been shown to reduce binge-purge behavior in patients with bulimia nervosa.

Halmi KA: Eating disorders, in The American Psychiatric Publishing Textbook of Psychiatry, 5th Edition. Edited by Hales RE, Yudofsky SC, Gabbard GO. Washington, DC, American Psychiatric Publishing, 2008, p 989

106. A patient is referred to you by an oncologist. One month after receiving the diagnosis, the patient denies the diagnosis and has become noncompliant with the oncologist's treatment recommendations. In your initial psychiatric interview, you uncover no other mood, anxiety, or behavioral symptoms. On the basis of this limited information, what might be a reasonable initial diagnosis for this patient?

    A. Acute stress disorder.
    B. Bereavement.
    C. Adjustment disorder with depressed mood.
    D. Adjustment disorder with mixed disturbance of emotions and conduct.
    E. Adjustment disorder unspecified.

## The correct response is option E.

This patient meets criteria for an adjustment disorder, which is unspecified because of the apparent lack of anxiety or mood symptoms. Thus, option C is incorrect. Option A is incorrect because the diagnosis does not meet criteria for an acute stress disorder, which requires the presence of a life-threatening or horrifying witnessed or personal traumatic event. Option B is incorrect because bereavement requires the death of another individual that has led to symptoms. The patient's nonadherence to the oncologist's recommendations does not violate societal norms or the rights of others and is therefore not considered a "disturbance of conduct," so option D is incorrect.

Strain JJ, Klipstein KG, Newcorn JH: Adjustment disorders, in The American Psychiatric Publishing Textbook of Psychiatry, 5th Edition. Edited by Hales RE, Yudofsky SC, Gabbard GO. Washington, DC, American Psychiatric Publishing, 2008, p 764; see Table 18–4

107. Which of the following is considered a dyssomnia?

    A. Circadian rhythm sleep disorder.
    B. Sleepwalking disorder.
    C. Sleep terror disorder.
    D. Nightmare disorder.
    E. Rapid-eye movement (REM) sleep behavior disorder.

## The correct response is option A.

DSM-IV-TR classifies primary sleep disorders into two subcategories: dyssomnias and parasomnias. In addition to primary sleep disorders, the DSM-IV-TR includes three other major subsections (see inset below).

American Academy of Sleep Medicine: The International Classification of Sleep Disorders, Second Edition: Diagnostic and Coding Manual. Westchester, IL, American Academy of Sleep Medicine, 2005

American Psychiatric Association: Diagnostic and Statistical Manual of Mental Disorders, 4th Edition, Text Revision. Washington, DC, American Psychiatric Association, 2000, p 597

Buysse DJ, Strollo PJ, Black JE, et al: Sleep disorders, in The American Psychiatric Publishing Textbook of Psychiatry, 5th Edition. Edited by Hales RE, Yudofsky SC, Gabbard GO. Washington, DC, American Psychiatric Publishing, 2008, p 930

### DSM-IV-TR–DEFINED SLEEP DISORDERS

#### Primary sleep disorders

*Dyssomnias:* defined as abnormalities in the amount, quality, or timing of sleep. Includes 1) circadian rhythm sleep disorder, 2) breathing-related sleep disorder, 3) narcolepsy, 4) primary insomnia, 5) primary hypersomnia, and 6) dyssomnia not otherwise specified (NOS).

*Parasomnias:* abnormal behavioral or physiological events occurring in association with sleep, specific sleep stages, or sleep-wake transitions. Includes 1) nightmare disorder, 2) sleep terror disorder, 3) sleepwalking disorder, and 4) parasomnia NOS.

#### Sleep disorder related to another mental disorder

#### Sleep disorder due to a general medical condition

#### Substance-induced sleep disorder

A type of parasomnia, REM sleep behavior disorder, is characterized by enactment of dreams that can result in physical injury to the sleep or bed partner. (Note that REM sleep behavior disorder does not have a DSM-IV-TR diagnostic code and could be considered as parasomnia NOS.) Nightmare disorder, also a parasomnia that occurs during REM sleep, is characterized by recurrent distressing dreams that are followed by an awakening and full recall of the dream. For diagnostic and billing purposes, general medical and sleep specialist physicians tend to use the *International Classification of Sleep Disorders, Second Edition,* published by the American Academy of Sleep Medicine, and not DSM-IV-TR.

108. The most common anxiety disorder in later life is

    A. Posttraumatic stress disorder.
    B. Agoraphobia.
    C. Panic disorder.
    D. Social phobia.
    E. Generalized anxiety disorder, which may be co-morbid with major depression.

**The correct response is option E.**

Although anxiety disorders can affect persons at all life stages, many of the anxiety disorders are relatively less frequent in the elderly. Anxiety is a frequent symptom among older persons secondary to physical illness such as hyperthyroidism, comorbid with other psychiatric disorders such as depression, or as the primary symptom of a disorder such as generalized anxiety disorder. Generalized anxiety disorder is a common diagnosis regardless of age, and generalized anxiety is often comorbid with other psychiatric disorders such as major depression.

Posttraumatic stress disorder can occur at any age but is found more frequently in younger persons than older persons. Although phobia disorders can affect persons at all stages of the life cycle, the more severe phobias, such as agoraphobia and social phobia, begin early in life and are more common in children and young adults than in older persons. Panic disorder is relatively frequent and severe among younger persons but much less so among older persons (although data documenting a lower prevalence among older persons are sparse). Obsessive-compulsive traits are common throughout the life cycle, although the severe manifestations of this disorder are less likely to be observed in older persons.

Blazer DG: Treatment of seniors, in The American Psychiatric Publishing Textbook of Psychiatry, 5th Edition. Edited by Hales RE, Yudofsky SC, Gabbard GO. Washington, DC, American Psychiatric Publishing, 2008, p 1458

109. A test of which of the following specimens can detect drug use for up to 90 days?

    A. Blood.
    B. Hair.
    C. Oral fluid.
    D. Sweat.
    E. Urine.

**The correct response is option B.**

A standard 1.5-inch sample of head hair contains drug residuals from the prior 90 days, minus the week immediately before sample collection. A drug user has to refrain from nonmedical drug use for only 3–5 days before submitting a urine sample to pass a urine test for abused drugs.

DuPont RL, Selavka CM: Testing to identify recent drug use, in The American Psychiatric Publishing Textbook of Substance Abuse Treatment, 4th Edition. Edited by Galanter M, Kleber HD. Washington, DC, American Psychiatric Publishing, 2008, pp 657, 661, Table 46–2

110. Which of the following statements is *true* regarding the hypothalamic-pituitary-adrenal (HPA) axis and mood?

    A. The data are unclear regarding the relationship between endogenously elevated cortisol and exogenous administration of glucocorticoids with alterations in the regulation of emotion, psychotic symptoms, and clinical depression.
    B. Patients with severe depression tend to have elevated serum cortisol levels, especially in the morning.
    C. Data suggest that gestational stress or prolonged periods of maternal separation early in life increase the magnitude of the neuroendocrine response to stress and the vulnerability for stress-related illness.
    D. Antiglucocorticoid therapy might be useful in the treatment of major depression but not psychotic depression.
    E. Monoamine oxidase inhibitors (MAOIs), tricyclic antidepressants (TCAs), and selective serotonin reuptake inhibitors (SSRIs) tend to "upregulate" the HPA axis.

**The correct response is option C.**

Data increasingly support the hypothesis that developmental events such as fetal exposure to various maternal hormone states and genetic influences increase the risk of stress-related conditions such as depressive disorders. Option A is incorrect because the data strongly establish the link between, on the one hand, endogenously elevated cortisol levels and exogenous administration of glucocorticoids and, on the other, alterations in the regulation of emotion, psychotic symptoms, and clinical depression. Option B is incorrect because although it is *true* that patients with severe depression tend to have elevated serum cortisol levels, the levels tend to be especially elevated in the evening and during the night when the activity of the axis is usually low, suggesting that the depressed patients are highly stressed. Option D is incorrect because anti-glucocorticoid therapy might be useful in treating major depressive disorders with or without psychotic features. Data are emerging to suggest that normalization of the HPA system might be the final step necessary for stable remission of depression. Option E is incorrect because antidepressant agents, including MAOIs, TCAs, and SSRIs, tend to downregulate the HPA axis.

Gertsik L, Poland RE: Psychoneuroendocrinology, in The American Psychiatric Publishing Textbook of Psychopharmacology, 3rd Edition. Edited by Schatzberg AF, Nemeroff CB. Washington, DC, American Psychiatric Publishing, 2004, pp 118–119

111. All of the following agents are considered first-line treatments for periodic limb movement disorder and restless legs syndrome *except*

    A. Pramipexole.
    B. Bromocriptine.
    C. Pergolide.
    D. Ropinirole.
    E. Carbidopa/levodopa.

**The correct response is option B.**

The first-line treatment for periodic limb movement disorder and restless legs syndrome is dopaminergic agents such as pergolide, carbidopa/levodopa, and the newer-generation dopamine agonists, pramipexole and ropinirole (Hening et al. 1999). Option B is incorrect because there is little evidence that bromocriptine or dantrolene, both dopamine agonists, would be beneficial for either of these disorders. Alternative treatments have included benzodiazepines and anticonvulsant agents.

Hening W, Allen R, Earley C, et al: The treatment of restless legs syndrome and periodic limb movement disorder: an American Academy of Sleep Medicine review. Sleep 22:970–999, 1999

Reite M: Treatment of insomnia, in The American Psychiatric Publishing Textbook of Psychopharmacology, 3rd Edition. Edited by Schatzberg AF, Nemeroff CB. Washington, DC, American Psychiatric Publishing, 2004, p 1158

112. Risk factors for development of adjustment disorders include which of the following?

    A. Race, younger age, female gender, chronic medical or psychiatric illness, and poverty.
    B. Older age, male gender, chronic medical or psychiatric illness, and poverty, but not race.
    C. Race, older age, chronic medical or psychiatric illness, and poverty, but not gender.
    D. Race, chronic medical or psychiatric illness, and poverty, but not age or gender.
    E. Chronic medical or psychiatric illness, and poverty, but not race, age, or gender.

**The correct response is option E.**

No race, age, or gender differences have been found to be risk factors for adjustment disorder.

Powell AD: Grief, bereavement, and adjustment disorders, in Massachusetts General Hospital Comprehensive Clinical Psychiatry. Edited by Stern TA, Rosenbaum JF, Fava M, et al. Philadelphia, PA, Mosby Elsevier, p 522

113. One common method of classifying malingering includes all of the following categories *except*

    A. Pure malingering.
    B. Partial malingering.
    C. False imputation.
    D. Factitious disorders.
    E. All of the above are considered subcategories of malingering.

**The correct response is option D.**

Subcategories of malingering include 1) pure malingering, 2) partial malingering, and 3) false imputation. *Pure malingering* is when a patient feigns a disorder that does not exist at all. Pure malingering tends to occur in criminal forensic contexts. *Partial malingering* is when a patient consciously exaggerates existing symptoms. *False imputation* is when a patient intentionally attributes symptoms to an etiology that has no relationship to the development of symptoms. An example of a false imputation is when an individual seeks compensation by claiming that an unlikely variety of symptoms of a specific injury began after a specific accident. Partial malingering and false imputation may be encountered more often in civil forensic evaluations and clinical settings.

American Psychiatric Association: Diagnostic and Statistical Manual of Mental Disorders, 4th Edition, Text Revision. Washington, DC, American Psychiatric Association, 2000, p 739

Thompson JW, LeBourgeois HW III, Black FW. Malingering, in The American Psychiatric Publishing Textbook of Forensic Psychiatry. Edited by Simon RI, Gold LH. Washington, DC, American Psychiatric Publishing, 2004, pp 428–429

*Malingering* is the intentional production of false or grossly exaggerated physical or psychological symptoms, motivated by external incentives such as avoiding military duty, avoiding work, obtaining financial compensation, evading criminal prosecution, or obtaining drugs. Malingering differs from factitious disorders, such as Munchausen's syndrome, in that the motivation for symptom production in malingering is an external incentive (e.g., financial gain). In factitious disorders, the motivation for intentionally producing or feigning illness is to assume the sick role. (American Psychiatric Association 2000, p. 739)

114. Evidence of malingered posttraumatic stress disorder (PTSD) may include all of the following *except*

 A. Claims of severe insomnia that does not respond to medication.
 B. Discrepancies in factual data.
 C. Pleasure or enjoyment in reviewing the events associated with the trauma.
 D. Single, repeating dreams that revisit the trauma.
 E. Evidence that the patient is not avoiding reminders of the trauma or not experiencing anxiety when exposed to reminders.

**The correct response is option A.**

Clues to the presence of malingered PTSD include the factors in options B, C, D, and E.

Thompson JW, LeBourgeois HW III, Black FW. Malingering, in The American Psychiatric Publishing Textbook of Forensic Psychiatry. Edited by Simon RI, Gold LH. Washington, DC, American Psychiatric Publishing, 2004, pp 434–435

115. This threshold model suggests that the presence of all of the following in the clinical evaluation should trigger the clinicians' suspicion that an individual is malingering *except*

 A. Suspicion of voluntary control over symptoms.
 B. Bizarre or absurd symptoms.
 C. Symptom fluctuation over time.
 D. Complaints grossly in excess of clinical findings.
 E. Substantial noncompliance with treatment.

**The correct response is option C.**

The threshold model is based entirely on clinical presentation, which makes it a suitable initial screening tool for

malingering. Malingering should be suspected when psychological or physical symptoms are accompanied by suspicion of voluntary control over symptoms as demonstrated by bizarre or absurd symptomatology, atypical symptomatic fluctuation consistent with external incentives, or unusual symptomatic response to treatment; atypical presentation in the presence of environmental incentives or noxious environmental conditions; complaints grossly in excess of clinical findings; and substantial noncompliance with treatment. Fluctuation of psychiatric symptoms over time itself is not indicative of malingering. However, malingering should be considered if symptoms fluctuate in such a way as to indicate voluntary control over those symptoms.

Thompson JW, LeBourgeois HW III, Black FW. Malingering, in The American Psychiatric Publishing Textbook of Forensic Psychiatry. Edited by Simon RI, Gold LH. Washington, DC, American Psychiatric Publishing, 2004, pp 439–440

116. A 34-year-old woman is diagnosed with severe major depressive disorder. Clinical studies indicate that at the time of diagnosis her labwork would include

 A. Decreased cortisol levels in the evening and through the night.
 B. Elevated levels of thyroid-stimulating hormone (TSH); decreased serum levels of $T_3$ and $T_4$.
 C. Normal TSH levels; elevated serum levels of $T_4$; decreased serum levels of $T_3$.
 D. Normal levels of TSH; decreased serum levels of $T_4$; elevated serum levels of $T_3$.
 E. Decreased baseline prolactin level.

**The correct response is option C.**

Although chemically euthyroid—normal TSH and serum $T_3$ and $T_4$—most patients with depression have some alteration in thyroid function. These changes include a slight elevation of serum $T_4$ levels, reductions in $T_3$ levels, and a predisposition to autoimmune thyroiditis. The combined elevation of $T_4$ levels and decreased $T_3$ has been referred to as a form of "euthyroid hyperthyroxinemia." Approximately 25% of patients with depression show a blunted TSH response to thyroid-releasing hormone, which is opposite to that observed in subjects with primary hypothyroidism. Depressed and primary hypothyroid patients also tend to show reduced prolactin and cortisol responses to fenfluramine, which is thought to reflect reduced central serotonin activity. Reduced levels of transthyretin, the carrier protein that transports $T_4$ in the brain, have been found in the cerebrospinal fluid of depressed patients. Option A is incorrect because severely depressed individuals tend to have elevated cortisol levels in the evening and through the night. Option E is incorrect because although the prolactin response to stimulatory tests such as fenfluramine is compromised (i.e., decreased prolactin in response to fenfluramine), the baseline prolactin level tends to be normal.

Gertsik L, Poland RE: Psychoneuroendocrinology, in The American Psychiatric Publishing Textbook of Psychopharmacology, 3rd Edition. Edited by Schatzberg AF, Nemeroff CB. Washington, DC, American Psychiatric Publishing, 2004, pp 119–121

117. Mr. Jones reports that he stole a car because he was hearing a voice inside his head telling him that if he did not steal the car, the world would be destroyed. The evaluating psychiatrist would be suspicious of malingering if Mr. Jones reported that this auditory hallucination

A. Was continuous and incessant.
B. Was spoken in fluent and grammatical language.
C. Could be ignored or avoided by turning up the volume on a radio or television.
D. Was associated with a delusion.
E. Was associated with a documented history of psychotic episodes of similar content.

### The correct response is option A.

Malingerers of schizophrenia often attempt to feign positive symptoms of schizophrenia such as hallucinations and delusions, but skilled examiners can detect whether these symptoms are typical or feigned, and therefore atypical. Atypical hallucinations that suggest malingering include auditory hallucinations that are continuous rather than intermittent, vague, or inaudible, spoken in stilted language, and are not associated with a delusion; lack of strategies to diminish auditory hallucinations; and visual hallucinations that are seen in black. In general, imitating negative symptoms and disordered forms of thinking, such as derailment, neologisms, incoherence, and perseveration, is more difficult than mimicking positive symptoms.

Thompson JW, LeBourgeois HW III, Black FW: Malingering, The American Psychiatric Publishing Textbook of Forensic Psychiatry. Edited by Simon RI, Gold LH. Washington, DC, American Psychiatric Publishing, 2004, p 438

118. A thorough psychological evaluation of a child with a physical illness must include an assessment of somatic symptoms. All of the following questionnaires have been developed to assess specifically physically ill children and families *except*

A. Eating Attitudes Test.
B. High Sensitivity Cognitive Screen.
C. Coping Health Inventory for Parents.
D. McCarthy Scales of Children's Abilities.
E. Varni-Thompson Pediatric Pain Questionnaire.

### The correct response is option D.

The McCarthy Scales comprise a verbal scale, perceptual-performance scale, quantitative scale, memory scale, motor scale, and an overall general cognitive scale, which yields a general cognitive index equivalent to an IQ standard score. However, the McCarthy Scales do not focus specifically on children with physical illnesses. Standard assessment instruments may be of limited use with children who are physically ill because disease-related symptoms (e.g., fatigue) complicate efforts to quantify psychological phenomena such as depression and anxiety. The tests mentioned in options A, B, C, and E are assessments that may be useful in the evaluation of children with medical illnesses.

Brown LK, Bruning K, Fritz GK, et al: Somatoform disorders, in The American Psychiatric Publishing Textbook of Child and Adolescent Psychiatry, 3rd Edition. Edited by Wiener JM, Dulcan MK. Washington, DC, American Psychiatric Publishing, 2004, p 757

119. Which of the following sequences states the *correct* order of the continuum of decision-making capacity from incapacitated to fully capacitated?

A. Able to assign a substitute decision maker → unable to make decisions → able to make medical decisions → able to appreciate the differences between clinical care and clinical research → fully capacitated.
B. Unable to make decisions → able to make medical decisions → able to assign a substitute decision maker → able to appreciate the difference between clinical care and clinical research → fully capacitated.
C. Unable to make decisions → able to assign a substitute decision maker → able to make medical decisions → able to appreciate the differences between clinical care and clinical research → fully capacitated.

D. Unable to make decisions → able to appreciate the differences between clinical care and clinical research → able to make medical decisions → able to assign a substitute decision maker → fully capacitated.

E. Able to assign a substitute decision maker → able to make medical decisions → unable to make decisions → able to appreciate the differences between clinical care and clinical research → fully capacitated.

**The correct response is option C.**

The correct order of the continuum of decision-making capacity is as follows: unable to make decisions → able to assign a substitute decision maker → able to make medical decisions → able to appreciate the differences between clinical care and clinical research → fully capacitated.

Rosenstein DL, Miller FG: Ethical issues, in The American Psychiatric Publishing Textbook of Psychosomatic Medicine: Official Textbook of the Academy of Psychosomatic Medicine. Edited by Levenson JL. Washington, DC, American Psychiatric Publishing, 2005, p 58; Figure 4–1

120. Patients with factitious disorder are characterized by all of the following *except*

A. Often have a cluster C personality disorder.
B. May have an Axis I disorder, especially schizophrenia.
C. Have a need to be the center of attention.
D. Long to be cared for.
E. Derive pleasure from deceiving others.

**The correct response is option A.**

The large majority of patients with factitious disorder have an underlying severe personality disorder, usually of the cluster B type, *not* cluster C type, which includes avoidant, dependent, and obsessive-compulsive personality disorders. These patients often feel a need to be the center of attention, long to be cared for by others, and may derive pleasure from deceiving others. Factitious behavior can be seen as a form of acting out, similar to other acting-out behaviors observed in cluster B personality disorders. Axis I comorbidity is not common.

Ford CV: Deception syndromes: factitious disorders and malingering, in The American Psychiatric Publishing Textbook of Psychosomatic Medicine: Official Textbook of the Academy of Psychosomatic Medicine. Edited by Levenson JL. Washington, DC, American Psychiatric Publishing, 2005, p 301

121. Which of the following statements is *true* regarding the diagnosis of adjustment disorder?

A. The adjustment disorder diagnosis should never be used if the patient's symptoms meet the criteria for another Axis I diagnosis.
B. Adjustment disorder may be diagnosed if the symptoms are secondary to the direct physiological effects of a general medical condition.
C. The diagnosis requires the development of symptoms within 6 months of an identifiable stressor's occurrence.
D. Adjustment disorders are coded by subtype, according to whether symptoms predominantly involve depressed mood, anxiety, disturbance of conduct, or a mixture of these.
E. The diagnosis does not require that symptoms be time limited or in response to a stressor.

**The correct response is option D.**

DSM-IV-TR adjustment disorder encompasses six subtypes, classified according to clinical features: with depressed mood, with anxiety, with mixed anxiety and depressed mood, with disturbance of conduct, with mixed disturbance of emotions and conduct, and unspecified.

Option A is incorrect because the adjustment disorder diagnosis *can* be used with another Axis I diagnosis if the symptoms of that diagnosis meet criteria for a major diagnosis (e.g., major depressive disorder), even if a stressor had precipitated that major depressive disorder. Option B is incorrect because the diagnosis of an adjustment disorder is precluded if the symptoms are secondary to the direct physiological effects of a general medical condition and/or its treatment.

Option C is incorrect because the symptom onset is within 3 months of the stressor(s) and can have a duration of <6 months (acute) or >6 months (chronic). Option E is incorrect because adjustment disorder is a stress-related phenomenon in which the stressor has precipitated maladaptation and symptoms (within 3 months of the occurrence of the stressor) that are time limited until the stressor is removed or a new state of adaptation has occurred.

Strain JJ, Klipstein KG, Newcorn JH: Adjustment disorders, in The American Psychiatric Publishing Textbook of Psychiatry, 5th Edition. Edited by Hales RE, Yudofsky SC, Gabbard GO. Washington, DC, American Psychiatric Publishing, 2008, pp 756, 758

122. Both positron emission tomography (PET) and functional magnetic resonance imaging (fMRI) rely on the empirical relationship between neuronal activity and regional blood flow. Which of the following statements is *false* when comparing PET with fMRI?

    A. PET is quieter but more sensitive to movement artifact than fMRI.
    B. PET is significantly less expensive than fMRI.
    C. PET has superior spatial resolution when compared with fMRI images.
    D. PET has a temporal resolution of minutes compared with fMRI, which has a temporal resolution on the order of seconds.
    E. Both PET and fMRI scans typically take less than an hour.

**The correct response is option E.**

PET scans typically take approximately 3 hours, and fMRIs take less than 1 hour. PET has a temporal resolution of minutes compared with fMRI, which has a temporal resolution on the order of seconds.

Because of the relatively lengthy time required for resolution of PET, this prevents the use of sophisticated event-related designs. The number of images collected with PET on a single subject is rarely >12, limiting the statistical treatment in the analysis of the data. Most cognitive neuroscience studies implicitly assume that blood flow increases in areas in which neuronal activity increases.

Pagnoni G, Berns GS: Brain imaging psychopharmacology, in The American Psychiatric Publishing Textbook of Psychopharmacology, 3rd Edition. Edited by Schatzberg AF, Nemeroff CB. Washington, DC, American Psychiatric Publishing, 2004, p 166

123. A 27-year-old man reports lifelong intermittent symptoms of worry, muscle tension, irritability, and difficulty falling asleep. Which of the following statements is *true* regarding possible pharmacological interventions?

    A. If a benzodiazepine is prescribed, psychiatric symptoms will be treated more effectively than somatic ones.
    B. If a benzodiazepine is prescribed, somatic symptoms will be more effectively treated than psychiatric ones.
    C. If buspirone is prescribed, alleviation of anxiety symptoms will likely occur within 2 weeks.
    D. If venlafaxine is prescribed, alleviation of anxiety symptoms likely will occur only after the fifth week.
    E. If a tricyclic antidepressant (TCA) is prescribed, only depressive symptoms will remit.

**The correct response is option B.**

Some evidence suggests that benzodiazepines may be more effective in treating the autonomic arousal and somatic symptoms of generalized anxiety disorder (GAD) but less effective for the psychiatric symptoms of worry and irritability. The use of benzodiazepines over longer periods is controversial, and long-term use can be associated with the development of tolerance, physiological dependence, and withdrawal, especially if abruptly discontinued. Side effects of benzodiazepines include ataxia, sedation, motor dysfunction, and cognitive impairment. An adequate trial of buspirone in GAD would be 3–4 weeks of treatment at a dosage of up to 60 mg/day, in divided doses. In one placebo-controlled trial of venlafaxine (Allgulander et al. 2001), significant improvement in symptoms of psychic anxiety was noted by week 2 of treatment. Potential advantages of the TCAs over the benzodiazepines include their ability to treat symptoms of both anxiety and depression, their absence of potential for abuse and physiological dependence, and their effectiveness in the management of discontinuation of long-term benzodiazepine therapy.

Allgulander C, Hackett D, Salinas E: Venlafaxine extended release (ER) in the treatment of generalised anxiety disorder: twenty-four-week placebo-controlled dose-ranging study. Br J Psychiatry 17:15–22, 2001

Davidson JRT, Connor KM: Treatment of anxiety disorders, in The American Psychiatric Publishing Textbook of Psychopharmacology, 3rd Edition. Edited by Schatzberg AF, Nemeroff CB. Washington, DC, American Psychiatric Publishing, 2004, pp 921, 922, 923

124. Which of the following definitions/statements is *false?*

    A. Physical dependence is a state of adaptation that manifests as a specific withdrawal syndrome.
    B. Withdrawal syndromes are characterized by symptoms similar to those characteristic of use of the substance.

C. Tolerance is the need for increasing amounts of a substance to obtain the desired effect.

D. Addiction is characterized by craving and impaired control of drug use despite harm.

E. Psychological dependence is the feeling of need for a specific substance.

**The correct response is option B.**

Withdrawal encompasses a substance-specific constellation of symptoms that may occur after cessation of or decrease in use of drugs by dependent individuals. Option B is the correct answer because withdrawal syndromes manifest with symptoms *opposite* to those characteristic of use of the substance.

Franklin JE Jr, Levenson JL, McCance-Katz EF: Substance-related disorders, in The American Psychiatric Publishing Textbook of Psychosomatic Medicine: Official Textbook of the Academy of Psychosomatic Medicine. Edited by Levenson JL. Washington, DC, American Psychiatric Publishing, 2005, p 388

125. All of the following are laboratory findings associated with alcohol abuse *except*

A. Increased serum gamma-glutamyltransferase (SGGT) level.

B. Increased serum carbohydrate-deficient transferrin level.

C. Decreased serum carbohydrate-deficient transferrin level.

D. Increased uric acid level.

E. Increased mean corpuscular volume.

**The correct response is option C.**

Levels of serum carbohydrate-deficient transferrin are *increased* in alcohol abuse. Other typical findings are increased SGGT level (particularly sensitive); decreased albumin, vitamin $B_{12}$, and folic acid levels; increased uric acid and amylase levels; evidence of bone marrow suppression; increased mean corpuscular volume; increased aspartate transaminase, alanine transaminase, and lactate dehydrogenase levels; and prolonged prothrombin time (cirrhosis).

Franklin JE Jr, Levenson JL, McCance-Katz EF: Substance-related disorders, in The American Psychiatric Publishing Textbook of Psychosomatic Medicine: Official Textbook of the Academy of Psychosomatic Medicine. Edited by Levenson JL. Washington, DC, American Psychiatric Publishing, 2005, p 397, Table 18–4

126. Buprenorphine is

A. A schedule IV narcotic.

B. An opioid agonist at higher doses.

C. A short-acting opioid receptor partial agonist.

D. A mu-opioid receptor partial agonist.

E. An opioid antagonist regardless of dosage.

**The correct response is option D.**

Buprenorphine is a long-acting mu-opioid receptor partial agonist that was approved by the U.S. Food and Drug Administration in 2003 for treating opioid dependence. Options B and E are incorrect because at lower doses buprenorphine functions as an opioid agonist, but at higher doses it has antagonist properties. Option A is incorrect because it is a schedule III, not schedule IV, narcotic. Option C is incorrect because it is a *long-acting* opioid receptor partial agonist.

Franklin JE Jr, Levenson JL, McCance-Katz EF: Substance-related disorders, in The American Psychiatric Publishing Textbook of Psychosomatic Medicine: Official Textbook of the Academy of Psychosomatic Medicine. Edited by Levenson JL. Washington, DC, American Psychiatric Publishing, 2005, p 403

The Controlled Substances Act (CSA), which was enacted into law by the U.S. Congress in 1970, created five schedules (classifications), with varying qualifications for a drug to be included in each. Classifications are made on the criteria of potential for abuse, accepted medical use in the United States, and potential for dependence.

127. The neural substrates of drug reward and reinforcement include which of the following?

A. Extrapyramidal system.

B. Dorsal raphe nuclei.

C. Tegmental fields.

D. Mesolimbic projections to the nucleus accumbens.

E. Amygdala.

**The correct response is option D.**

Animal models have implicated brain dopamine systems, specifically the mesolimbic projection to the nucleus accumbens (a component of the ventral striatum), as the neural substrate of drug reward and reinforcement.

| Schedule | Criteria | Examples |
|---|---|---|
| I | High potential for abuse; no currently accepted medical use in treatment in the United States; lack of accepted safety for use under medical supervision. Prescriptions may not be written for schedule I substances. | Gamma-hydroxybutyric acid, cannabis, MDMA (3,4 methylenedioxymeth-amphetamine, Ecstasy) |
| II | Has a high potential for abuse; accepted medical use in the United States with severe restrictions; abuse may lead to severe psychological or physical dependence. | Cocaine (topical); methylphenidate, opium, methadone, oxycodone, fentanyl |
| III | Potential for abuse less than substances in schedules I and II; accepted for medical use in the United States; abuse of substance may lead to moderate or low physical dependence or high psychological dependence; may be refilled <5 times within a 6-month period. | Anabolic steroids, intermediate-acting barbiturates, buprenorphine, dihydrocodeine, ketamine, Vicodin, Marinol |
| IV | Low potential for abuse relative to schedule III drugs; accepted for medical use in the United States; abuse may lead to relatively limited physical or psychological dependence compared to schedule III substances; may be refilled <5 times within a 6-month period. | Benzodiazepines, benzodiazepine-like "Z-drugs" (e.g., zolpidem, zopiclone), long-acting barbiturates, "diet drugs" (e.g., phentermine), nonamphetamine stimulants (pemoline, modafinil) |
| V | Low potential for abuse relative to schedule IV substances; currently accepted for medical use in the United States; abuse may lead to relatively limited physical or psychological dependence compared with schedule IV substances. | Cough suppressants with small amounts of codeine, opium or diphenoxylate, pregabalin, centrally acting antidiarrheals (e.g., Lomotil) |

*Source.* Courtwright DT: "The Controlled Substances Act: How a 'Big Tent' Reform Became a Punitive Drug Law." *Drug and Alcohol Dependence* 76:9–15, 2004.

Clinton K: Neurobiology of substance abuse disorders, in The American Psychiatric Publishing Textbook of Psychopharmacology, 3rd Edition. Edited by Schatzberg AF, Nemeroff CB. Washington, DC, American Psychiatric Publishing, 2004, p 810

128. The evidence base is *least* supportive of which of the following agents for the treatment of child and adolescent attention-deficit/hyperactivity disorder (ADHD)?

    A. Psychostimulants.
    B. Tricyclic antidepressants (TCAs).
    C. Selective serotonin reuptake inhibitors (SSRIs).
    D. Atomoxetine.
    E. Bupropion.

**The correct response is option C.**

Results have been mixed regarding the efficacy of SSRIs in the treatment of childhood ADHD. Randomized, controlled studies have found that approximately 70% of school-aged subjects demonstrate significant improvement in ADHD symptoms on psychostimulants.

Of the nonstimulant treatments for ADHD, TCAs have been the most widely studied in children and adolescents, with 15 double-blind, placebo-controlled studies demonstrating their efficacy.

Bupropion's efficacy in improving hyperactivity, impulsivity, conduct problems, and attention in ADHD has been reported in several studies.

Atomoxetine, a selective noradrenergic enhancer being investigated for the treatment of ADHD in children, has been shown to produce statistically significant improvement in hyperactivity and inattention. In open-label trials of atomoxetine, response rates in children with ADHD ranged from 70% to 75%.

Wagner KD: Treatment of childhood and adolescent disorders, in The American Psychiatric Publishing Textbook of Psychopharmacology, 3rd Edition. Edited by Schatzberg AF, Nemeroff CB. Washington, DC, American Psychiatric Publishing, 2004, pp 964–967

129. In patients with hepatic impairment that has dimin-ished their ability to metabolize medications, which of the following agents would be the best choice for prophylaxis of delirium tremens?

    A. Diazepam.
    B. Clonazepam.
    C. Alprazolam.
    D. Triazolam.
    E. Oxazepam.

## The correct response is option E.

Pharmacotherapy with a benzodiazepine is the treatment of choice for the prevention and treatment of the signs and symptoms of alcohol withdrawal. Oxazepam, along with lorazepam and temazepam, does not require hepatic bio-transformation. Oxazepam may be particularly useful in the outpatient setting because it is associated with less abuse.

Cornish JW, McNicholas LF, O'Brien CP: Treatment of substance-related disorders, in The American Psychiatric Publishing Textbook of Psychopharmacology, 3rd Edition. Edited by Schatzberg AF, Nemeroff CB. Washington, DC, American Psychiatric Publishing, 2004, p 1010

---

Benzodiazepines that do not require hepatic biotransformation: remember **"LOT,"** for lorazepam, oxazepam, temazepam.

---

130. According to findings from a meta-analysis of 15 stud-ies, patients who are taking second-generation anti-psychotics demonstrate

    A. Improved memory.
    B. Less weight gain than with first-generation antipsychotics.
    C. Better verbal fluency.
    D. Better overall clinical outcome.
    E. Similar improvements in neurocognitive symp-toms of schizophrenia when compared with those taking first-generation antipsychotics.

## The correct response is option C.

Conventional antipsychotics do not appear to alleviate neurocognitive symptoms of schizophrenia. In contrast, a meta-analysis of 15 studies indicated that second-genera-tion antipsychotics have notable effects on verbal fluency

and executive function, with limited improvement in mem-ory. Second-generation antipsychotics appear to be asso-ciated with more weight gain compared with first-gener-ation antipsychotics. Option D is incorrect because the data, *except* for clozapine, do not show that second-gener-ation agents are superior overall to older drugs.

Woo T-UW, Zimmet SV, Wojcik JD, et al: Treatment of schizophrenia, in The American Psychiatric Publishing Textbook of Psychopharmacology, 3rd Edition. Edited by Schatzberg AF, Nemeroff CB. Washington, DC, American Psychiatric Publishing, 2004, pp 893, 897

131. Which of the following statements is *true* regarding aphasia syndromes?

    A. Broca's aphasia syndrome usually includes nor-mal speech fluency, but Wernicke's aphasia syn-drome does not.
    B. Wernicke's aphasia is characterized by relatively normal auditory comprehension, but Broca's aphasia is not.
    C. Anomic aphasia syndrome includes normal flu-ency, auditory comprehension, repetition, and naming.
    D. Conduction aphasia includes normal auditory comprehension and repetition.
    E. Global aphasia syndrome includes abnormal flu-ency and auditory comprehension.

## The correct response is option E.

Global aphasia includes a severe impairment in all modal-ities of speech, which includes verbal fluency, compre-hension, repetition, naming, reading, and writing. Option A is incorrect because Broca's aphasia is characterized by abnormal fluency, and Wernicke's aphasia is characterized by normal or paraphasic fluency. Option B is incorrect because auditory comprehension is abnormal in Wer-nicke's aphasia and normal in Broca's aphasia. Option C is incorrect because naming is abnormal in anomic aphasia. Option D is incorrect because conduction aphasia is char-acterized by abnormal repetition, naming, and writing, but includes normal fluency, auditory comprehension, and reading comprehension.

Mendez MF, Clark DG: Neuropsychiatric aspects of aphasia and related disorders, in The American Psychiatric Publish-ing Textbook of Neuropsychiatry and Behavioral Neuro-sciences, 5th Edition. Edited by Yudofsky SC, Hales RE. Washington, DC, American Psychiatric Publishing, 2008, pp 522–524

**Principal aphasia syndromes**

| Aphasia syndrome | Fluency | Auditory comprehension | Repetition | Naming | Reading comprehension | Writing |
|---|---|---|---|---|---|---|
| Broca's | Abnormal | Relatively normal | Abnormal | Abnormal | Normal or abnormal | Abnormal |
| Wernicke's | Normal, paraphasic | Abnormal | Abnormal | Abnormal | Abnormal | Abnormal |
| Global | Abnormal | Abnormal | Abnormal | Abnormal | Abnormal | Abnormal |
| Conduction | Normal, paraphasic | Relatively normal | Abnormal | Usually abnormal | Relatively normal | Abnormal |
| Transcortical motor | Abnormal | Relatively normal | Relatively normal | Abnormal | Relatively normal | Abnormal |
| Transcortical sensory | Normal, echolalic | Abnormal | Relatively normal | Abnormal | Abnormal | Abnormal |
| Anomic | Normal | Relatively normal | Normal | Abnormal | Normal or abnormal | Normal or abnormal |

*Source.* Mendez MF, Clark DG: "Neuropsychiatric Aspects of Aphasia and Related Disorders," in *The American Psychiatric Publishing Textbook of Neuropsychiatry and Behavioral Neurosciences*, 5th Edition. Edited by Yudofsky SC, Hales RE. Washington, DC, American Psychiatric Publishing, 2008, pp. 522–524.

132. In comparing lithium with divalproex in the treatment of acute mania, which of the following statements is *false?*

    A. Divalproex works better in patients with depressive symptoms.
    B. Divalproex works better in patients with previous multiple mood episodes.
    C. Both lithium and divalproex can help with psychotic symptoms in acute mania.
    D. Both are efficacious for acute mania in comparison with placebo, but lithium is generally superior to divalproex in head-to-head trials.
    E. Both agents have better long-term efficacy in the treatment of acute mania in combination with other medications.

**The correct response is option D.**

Divalproex and related formulations of valproic acid had superior efficacy compared with placebo and comparable efficacy compared with lithium.

Keck PE, McElroy SL: Treatment of bipolar disorder, in The American Psychiatric Publishing Textbook of Psychopharmacology, 3rd Edition. Edited by Schatzberg AF, Nemeroff CB. Washington, DC, American Psychiatric Publishing, 2004, p 868

133. Double-blind studies have supported moderate benefit for which of the following medications in preventing relapse to cocaine abuse?

    A. Desipramine.
    B. Bupropion.
    C. Fluoxetine.
    D. Amantadine.
    E. Pergolide.

**The correct response is option A.**

Although no medication has been clearly identified as beneficial in the treatment of cocaine abuse, the tricyclic antidepressant desipramine, which has been studied in several double-blind studies, appears to be moderately effective in inducing abstinence. Medications found to be ineffective include fluoxetine, bupropion, amantadine, risperidone, pergolide, and ecopipam; therefore, options B, C, D, and E are incorrect.

Cornish JW, McNicholas LF, O'Brien CP: Treatment of substance-related disorders, in The American Psychiatric Publishing Textbook of Psychopharmacology, 3rd Edition. Edited by Schatzberg AF, Nemeroff CB. Washington, DC, American Psychiatric Publishing, 2004, pp 1013, 1014

134. Which of the following statements best describes the usual course of illness in schizophrenia?

    A. After the acute onset, the first 2–5 years are marked by little change in severity.
    B. Negative symptoms usually respond to medication treatment better than positive symptoms.
    C. Positive symptoms usually respond to medication treatment better than negative symptoms.
    D. Positive symptoms usually become increasingly prominent during the course of illness.
    E. All of the above statements are accurate.

**The correct response is option C.**

Schizophrenia is a chronic illness, with onset of psychotic symptoms usually occurring around late adolescence and early adulthood. After the first episode of psychosis, the course of the illness is often characterized by a gradual and at times continuous deterioration, especially during the first 2–5 years. After an initial period of functional deterioration, symptoms tend to stabilize. An amelioration of positive symptoms (and to a lesser extent of disorganized symptoms) may be seen in older patients. However, findings of amelioration of psychotic symptoms should be interpreted in light of the fact that these are also symptoms most responsive to neuroleptic treatment, making it difficult to distinguish between the natural course of the disorder and the accumulated response to treatment. Positive symptoms usually respond to treatment, whereas negative symptoms are believed to be relatively treatment-resistant and may tend to become increasingly prominent during the course of the illness.

Woo T-UW, Zimmet SV, Wojcik JD, et al: Treatment of schizophrenia, in The American Psychiatric Publishing Textbook of Psychopharmacology, 3rd Edition. Edited by Schatzberg AF, Nemeroff CB. Washington, DC, American Psychiatric Publishing, 2004, pp 888–889

135. Which of the following statements is *not* true regarding anxiety disorders?

    A. Generalized anxiety disorder, posttraumatic stress disorder, specific phobias, and agoraphobia have a 2:1 female-to-male lifetime prevalence ratio.
    B. Lifetime prevalence of specific phobias is 10%.
    C. Social phobia is associated with a twofold risk for comorbid alcohol dependence or mood disorders.

    D. Of patients diagnosed with generalized anxiety disorder, 90% have comorbid psychiatric diagnoses.
    E. Obsessive-compulsive disorder has a 1:1 female-to-male lifetime prevalence ratio.

**The correct response is option C.**

Social phobia, which has a lifetime prevalence in the United States of 13%–16%, is associated with a twofold risk for comorbid alcohol dependence, but a three- to sixfold risk of mood disorders. Option A is incorrect because this statement is true. Options B, D, and E are incorrect because they reflect true statements. Generalized anxiety disorder is associated with the highest psychiatric comorbidity rate (90%), 50%–60% of whom have comorbid major depression or other anxiety disorders. All of the anxiety disorder diagnoses in DSM-IV-TR have a 2:1 female-to-male ratio, except obsessive-compulsive disorder (1:1) and social phobia (1+:1).

Hollander E, Simeon D: Anxiety disorders, in The American Psychiatric Publishing Textbook of Psychiatry, 5th Edition. Edited by Hales RE, Yudofsky SC, Gabbard GO. Washington, DC, American Psychiatric Publishing, 2008, p 506

136. The hallucinogen methylenedioxymethamphetamine (MDMA, Ecstasy) is related to what class of drugs?

    A. Amphetamines.
    B. Opioids.
    C. Dissociative anesthetics.
    D. Cannabinoids.
    E. Benzodiazepine reverse agonists.

**The correct response is option A.**

The hallucinogen MDMA is an amphetamine congener.

Cornish JW, McNicholas LF, O'Brien CP: Treatment of substance-related disorders, in The American Psychiatric Publishing Textbook of Psychopharmacology, 3rd Edition. Edited by Schatzberg AF, Nemeroff CB. Washington, DC, American Psychiatric Publishing, 2004, p 1020

137. Efficacy in smoking cessation has been demonstrated by all of the following *except*

    A. Transdermal nicotine.
    B. Bupropion.
    C. Nortriptyline.

D. Propranolol.

E. Clonidine.

## The correct response is option D.

A placebo-controlled, double-blind trial of propranolol found it to be no better than placebo for smoking cessation. By contrast, the effectiveness of transdermal nicotine in smoking cessation has been well documented. Clonidine, an $\alpha_2$-adrenergic agonist used to treat opiate and alcohol withdrawal symptoms, has also been found to decrease nicotine withdrawal symptoms and tobacco craving. Nortriptyline has been reported to produce significantly higher rates of smoking cessation, independent of depression, compared with placebo; this antidepressant is recommended as a second-line medication for smoking cessation by the Tobacco Use and Dependence Clinical Practice Guideline Panel, Staff, and Consortium Representatives (2000).

Cornish JW, McNicholas LF, O'Brien CP: Treatment of substance-related disorders, in The American Psychiatric Publishing Textbook of Psychopharmacology, 3rd Edition. Edited by Schatzberg AF, Nemeroff CB. Washington, DC, American Psychiatric Publishing, 2004, pp 1021, 1022

Tobacco Use and Dependence Clinical Practice Guideline Panel, Staff, and Consortium Representatives

138. The adjustment disorder diagnosis in DSM-IV-TR (American Psychiatric Association 2000) has been found to have certain advantages and disadvantages for patients and clinicians. Which of the following is the major disadvantage of using the diagnosis?

    A. The concept of temporary emotional symptoms resulting from a stressful life event seems more of a normal human reaction than a pathological diagnostic state.

    B. The more benign course implied by this diagnosis allows clinicians to be more prognostically optimistic.

    C. The diagnosis is less stigmatizing.

    D. Medical insurance carriers do not consider the diagnosis to be a preexisting condition when evaluating a patient's risk.

    E. The concept of the stressor lacks quantifiable and qualifiable guidelines, contributing to the vague and nonspecific nature of the diagnosis.

## The correct response is option E.

The concept of the stressor lacks quantifiable and qualifiable guidelines thus contributing to the vague and nonspecific nature of the adjustment disorder diagnosis. The lack of specificity in the diagnosis of adjustment disorders may be alternatively considered an advantage. It allows clinicians to "tag" early or temporary mental states when the clinical picture may be the earliest sign of an evolving major mental disorder. Therefore, the adjustment disorders occupy an essential place in the psychiatric taxonomic spectrum.

The idea of temporary emotional symptoms resulting directly from a stressful life event seems more of a normal human reaction than a pathological psychiatric state and thus is less stigmatizing. Additionally, the disorder's more benign course (especially in adults) allows a clinician to be more prognostically optimistic. This optimism is shared by medical insurance carriers, who do not consider the diagnosis to be a preexisting condition when evaluating patients' risk.

American Psychiatric Association: Diagnostic and Statistical Manual of Mental Disorders, 4th Edition, Text Revision. Washington, DC, American Psychiatric Association, 2000

Strain JJ, Klipstein KG, Newcorn JH: Adjustment disorders, in The American Psychiatric Publishing Textbook of Psychiatry, 5th Edition. Edited by Hales RE, Yudofsky SC, Gabbard GO. Washington, DC, American Psychiatric Publishing, 2008, p 756

139. The two best predictors of antidepressant response for the treatment of a depressive disorder are

    A. Choice of antidepressants that have proven to have the most efficacy with major depressive disorder.

    B. Medication side-effect profile and comorbid psychiatric symptoms.

    C. A history of prior response to an agent and sedating versus activating properties.

    D. Family history of response and symptoms such as comorbid insomnia or anxiety.

    E. A history of prior response to an agent and a family history of preferential response.

## The correct response is option E.

A history of prior response to an agent and a family history of preferential response are the two best predictors of antidepressant response. Option A is incorrect because, on average, all antidepressants have approximately equal efficacy, although individuals may preferentially respond to a particular class of agents or even to a single agent. Comorbid psychiatric symptoms may influence medication choice but should not supersede the patient's personal and family history. For example, generally a patient with comorbid obsessive-compulsive disorder (OCD) may benefit from a serotonergic agent such as clomipramine, or one of the selective serotonin reuptake inhibitors (SSRIs). Although any of the SSRIs may be effective in general, if a patient with comorbid depressive disorder and OCD has a family history of responsiveness to fluvoxamine, it is prudent to preferentially start with fluvoxamine versus another SSRI.

Options B, C, and D are incorrect because the combination of personal and family history are more strongly predictive than either of these factors alone or in combination with other factors.

Boland RJ, Keller MB: Treatment of depression, in The American Psychiatric Publishing Textbook of Psychopharmacology, 3rd Edition. Edited by Schatzberg AF, Nemeroff CB. Washington, DC, American Psychiatric Publishing, 2004, p 851

Cozza KL, Armstrong SC, Oesterheld JR, et al: Study Guide to Clinical Psychopharmacology: A Companion to The American Psychiatric Publishing Textbook of Psychopharmacology, 3rd Edition. Washington, DC, American Psychiatric Publishing, p 270

140. Which of the following statements is *true* regarding memory?

    A. Declarative memory includes semantic and episodic memory.
    B. Declarative memory is unable to be assessed clinically by recall or recognition.
    C. Semantic memories are can usually be associated with specific times or incidents.
    D. Semantic memory are not required for episodic memory.
    E. Procedural memory is a type of declarative memory.

**The correct response is option A.**

Option B is incorrect because declarative memory is most often assessed clinically with tests of recall or recognition. Option C is incorrect because semantic memory, which is the acquisition of factual information about the world, cannot be fixed as having been acquired at a specific time. For example, many people would recognize George Washington as being the first President of the United States, but few would recall when they learned this fact. Option D

is incorrect because semantic memory is required for episodic memory, which refers to the recording and conscious recollection of personal experiences. Option E is incorrect because procedural memory is a type of *nondeclarative memory*.

Stern Y, Sackeim HA: Neuropsychiatric aspects of memory and amnesia, in The American Psychiatric Publishing Textbook of Neuropsychiatry and Behavioral Neurosciences, 5th Edition. Edited by Yudofsky SC, Hales RE. Washington, DC, American Psychiatric Publishing, 2008, pp 568–569

---

*Declarative memory* describes the conscious recollection of words, scenes, faces, stories, and events. Includes semantic and episode memory.

*Nondeclarative memory* is a collection of memory processes that are not declarative. This type of memory allows individuals to learn information without having to explicitly memorize it. Nondeclarative memory is evidenced by the ability to learn and change behaviors by experience without requiring a conscious access to the experience. Includes procedural (motor, cognitive), priming, and conditioning memories.

(Stern and Sackeim 2008, pp. 568–569)

---

141. In regard to National Institute of Mental Health studies comparing patients with childhood-onset schizophrenia and patients with adult-onset schizophrenia, all of the following findings are correct *except*

    A. Childhood-onset patients show greater delay in language development than do adult-onset patients.
    B. Childhood-onset patients evidence more disruptive behavior disorders than do adult-onset patients.
    C. Childhood-onset patients evidence more learning disorders than do adult-onset patients.
    D. Childhood-onset patients evidence high rates of specific developmental disorders such as autism.
    E. Childhood-onset schizophrenia appears to represent a more malignant form of the disorder.

**The correct response is option D.**

Patients with childhood-onset schizophrenia commonly present with transient early symptoms of autism, especially motor stereotypies. Individuals with childhood-onset

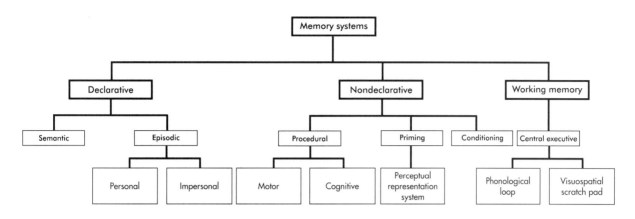

**An outline of the components of memory.**

*Source.* Stern Y, Sackeim HA: "Neuropsychiatric Aspects of Memory and Amnesia," in *The American Psychiatric Publishing Textbook of Neuropsychiatry and Behavioral Neurosciences*, 5th Edition. Edited by Yudofsky SC, Hales RE. Washington, DC, American Psychiatric Publishing, 2008, p. 568.

schizophrenia show greater delays in language development, more premorbid speech and language disorders, disruptive behavior disorders, and learning disorders. However, the statement in option D is false because even though a high percentage of childhood-onset patients show signs and symptoms of developmental delay, these symptoms usually do not meet DSM-IV-TR criteria for autism.

Tsai LK, Champine DJ: Schizophrenia and other psychotic disorders, in The American Psychiatric Publishing Textbook of Child and Adolescent Psychiatry, 3rd Edition. Edited by Wiener JM, Dulcan MK. Washington, DC, American Psychiatric Publishing, 2004, p 382

142. Published open-label treatment studies in children and adolescents with posttraumatic stress disorder (PTSD) have supported the efficacy of all of the following agents *except*

A. Citalopram.
B. Clonidine.
C. Carbamazepine.
D. Propranolol.
E. Alprazolam.

**The correct response is option E.**

Citalopram, clonidine, carbamazepine, and propranolol have all been shown to improve core symptoms and to be well tolerated in children and adolescents with PTSD.

Wagner KD: Treatment of childhood and adolescent disorders, in The American Psychiatric Publishing Textbook of Psychopharmacology, 3rd Edition. Edited by Schatzberg AF, Nemeroff CB. Washington, DC, American Psychiatric Publishing, 2004, pp 960, 961, 962

143. Orthostatic hypotension is a common side effect of all of the following antidepressants *except*

A. Trazodone.
B. Mirtazapine.
C. Venlafaxine.
D. Imipramine.
E. Phenelzine.

**The correct response is option C.**

The most common cardiac side effect of antidepressants is their effect on blood pressure. Venlafaxine causes sustained increases in blood pressure, particularly at dosages >300 mg/day. Although this may diminish over time, the effect can persist. Tricyclic antidepressants such as imipramine and amitriptyline, tetracyclic antidepressants such as trazodone, and mirtazapine all can cause decreases in blood pressure, particularly orthostatic blood pressure. Phenelzine, an MAOI, is associated with orthostatic hypotension, which may lead to discontinuation of treatment.

Boland RJ, Keller MB: Treatment of depression, in The American Psychiatric Publishing Textbook of Psychopharmacology, 3rd Edition. Edited by Schatzberg AF, Nemeroff CB. Washington, DC, American Psychiatric Publishing, 2004, pp 850–854

144. Which of the following functional or anatomic brain abnormalities have been associated with depression?

    A. Increased hippocampal volumes.
    B. Decreased left lateral prefrontal cortex activity.
    C. Smaller amygdala volumes.
    D. Increased activity of the caudate and putamen.
    E. Neuroimaging evidence of associations between depression and brain abnormalities are equivocal at best.

**The correct response is option B.**

Positron emission tomography (PET) and single photon emission computed tomography (SPECT) investigators have repeatedly documented that compared with nondepressed individuals, patients with unipolar depression have a lateralized decrease in left lateral prefrontal cortex activity. Magnetic resonance imaging (MRI) studies have also documented the association between abnormalities in the prefrontal cortex and unipolar depression.

Option A is incorrect because decreased, not increased, hippocampal volumes have been found in individuals with major depression. Option C is incorrect because larger, not smaller, amygdala volumes are associated with depression. Option D is incorrect because depression is associated with decreased, not increased, activity of the caudate and putamen. Option E is incorrect because structural (computed tomography and MRI) and functional (PET and SPECT) imaging studies increasingly are demonstrating the association between mood disorders and various structural and functional brain abnormalities.

Flores BH, Musselman DL, DeBattista C, et al: Biology of mood disorders, in The American Psychiatric Publishing Textbook of Psychopharmacology, 3rd Edition. Edited by Schatzberg AF, Nemeroff CB. Washington, DC, American Psychiatric Publishing, 2004, p 744; Tables 45–10, 45–12, 45–13, and 45–14

145. All of the following drugs have shown efficacy in the treatment of acute mania in randomized, placebo-controlled trials *except*

    A. Olanzapine.
    B. Chlorpromazine.
    C. Carbamazepine.
    D. Lamotrigine.
    E. Divalproex.

**The correct response is option D.**

All except lamotrigine have been shown to be efficacious in treating acute mania (McElroy and Keck 2000). Lamotrigine may help in depression associated with bipolar disorder (American Psychiatric Association 2002).

American Psychiatric Association: Practice guideline for the treatment of patients with bipolar disorder (revision). Am J Psychiatry 159 (suppl):1–50, 2002

Keck PE, McElroy SL: Treatment of bipolar disorder, in The American Psychiatric Publishing Textbook of Psychopharmacology, 3rd Edition. Edited by Schatzberg AF, Nemeroff CB. Washington, DC, American Psychiatric Publishing, 2004, p 867

McElroy SL, Keck PE Jr: Pharmacological agents for the treatment of acute bipolar mania. Biol Psychiatry 48:539–557, 2000

146. The relationship between mental illness, substance abuse, and violent behavior remains controversial. Which of the following statements is *false?*

    A. Patients with comorbid substance abuse and major mental illness are more frequently violent than persons in the general population.
    B. Patients with comorbid substance abuse and major mental illness are more frequently violent than patients with mental illness alone.
    C. Among all reported violence, over 10% is a result of mental illness in isolation (i.e., no comorbid substance abuse).
    D. When mentally ill patients abuse substances, their risk of violence increase dramatically.
    E. Psychiatric patients who are noncompliant with treatment are at an increased risk of being violent.

**The correct response is option C.**

Recent evidence indicates that only 4% of reported violence is the result of mental disorders. Results of the 1998 MacArthur Violence Risk Assessment Study showed that individuals with comorbid substance use and psychiatric disorders are more frequently violent than those in the general population with severe mental illness alone or who have neither of these conditions. Treatment nonadherence increases the risk of violence and substance use increases treatment nonadherence.

Mack AH, Barros M: Forensic addiction psychiatry, in The American Psychiatric Publishing Textbook of Substance Abuse Treatment, 4th Edition. Edited by Galanter M, Kleber HD. Washington, DC, American Psychiatric Publishing, 2008, p 692

147. Which of the following is *true* regarding electro-convulsive therapy (ECT)?

    A. ECT should be considered in the treatment of treatment-resistant mixed mood disorders, delirious mania, catatonic psychosis, and drug-induced psychotic disorder.
    B. ECT should be considered the treatment of last resort in even severely depressed patients.
    C. ECT has been shown to be effective in >80% of cases of treatment-resistant unipolar or bipolar major depression.
    D. In recent years, a large amount of data have emerged comparing the efficacy of ECT to mood stabilizing medications in the treatment of acute and maintenance treatment.
    E. ECT is not effective in the treatment of the motor symptoms of patients with Parkinson's disease.

## The correct response is option C.

ECT has been shown to be effective in >80% of cases of treatment-resistant unipolar and bipolar major depression. Option A is incorrect because although possibly indicated in treatment-resistant mixed mood disorders, delirious mania, and catatonic psychosis, ECT should not be considered for most cases of drug-induced psychotic disorder because it often resolves spontaneously and/or with a relatively brief course of antipsychotic medication management. Option B is incorrect because its high efficacy and rapid clinical response are essential in the treatment of some severely depressed patients in whom it should be considered a first-line treatment. Option D is incorrect because despite the plethora of research comparing various antimanic medications with one another, there is a lack of data comparing the efficacy of these medications to ECT. Option E is incorrect because ECT has been shown to be effective in the treatment of the motor symptoms of patients with Parkinson's disease.

McDonald WM, Thompson TR, McCall WV, et al: Electroconvulsive therapy, in The American Psychiatric Publishing Textbook of Psychopharmacology, 3rd Edition. Edited by Schatzberg AF, Nemeroff CB. Washington, DC, American Psychiatric Publishing, 2004, pp 685–689

148. The classic clinical presentation of middle cerebral artery infarction in the dominant hemisphere includes all of the following *except*

    A. Contralateral hemiparesis.
    B. Neglect.
    C. Aphasia.
    D. Sensory loss of a cortical type.
    E. Hemianopsia.

## The correct response is option B.

Lesions of the middle cerebral artery in the nondominant hemisphere may be accompanied by neglect or perceptual disturbances, therefore the statement in option B is false. Options A, D, and E are incorrect because the classic presentation of middle cerebral artery infarction includes contralateral hemiparesis, and sensory loss of a cortical type. These are often accompanied by hemianopsia if the optic radiation is affected. If the lesion is in the dominant hemisphere, then aphasia may be expected.

Carson AJ, Zeman A, Myles L, et al: Neurology and neurosurgery, in The American Psychiatric Publishing Textbook of Psychosomatic Medicine: Official Textbook of the Academy of Psychosomatic Medicine. Edited by Levenson JL. Washington, DC, American Psychiatric Publishing, 2005, p 702

149. Which phase of illness in schizophrenic patients is best described by the following definition: a 1- to 6-month (or longer) period when symptoms of hallucinations, delusions, thought disorder, or disorganized behavior are predominant?

    A. Prodrome.
    B. Acute phase.
    C. Recovery phase.
    D. Residual phase.
    E. Chronicity.

## The correct response is option B.

During the acute phase, which usually lasts 1–6 months or longer, positive symptoms (i.e., hallucinations, delusions, thought disorder, and disorganized behavior) are predominant. The prodrome phase may be days to weeks or months to years and includes some degree of functional deterioration. The prodrome period does not include frankly psychotic symptoms such as those that occur during the acute phase, but it does include unusual behaviors, bizarre preoccupations, social withdrawal and isolation, poor academic performance, dysphoria, or problems with sleep and appetite. Option C is incorrect because the recovery phase, which occurs after remission of the acute-phase period, lasts several months. The recovery phase often includes impairments such as negative symptoms of flattened affect, apathy, anergia, and social withdrawal. This phase may include a postpsychotic depressive disorder that is characterized by dysphoria and flat affect. Positive symptoms may still be present to some degree during the recovery phase. Option D is incorrect because the residual phase, which follows the recovery phase, is defined as periods of several months or more between acute phases during which there are few positive symptoms but some degree of persisting impairment because of negative symptoms.

Tsai LK, Champine DJ: Schizophrenia and other psychotic disorders, in The American Psychiatric Publishing Textbook of Child and Adolescent Psychiatry, 3rd Edition. Edited by Wiener JM, Dulcan MK. Washington, DC, American Psychiatric Publishing, 2004, p 388

---

Prodrome (days to weeks, or months to years) → acute phase (1–6 months) → recovery phase (several months) → residual phase (several months or more) → chronic (years).

---

150. What two medications have been approved by the U.S. Food and Drug Administration (FDA) for the treatment of Tourette's syndrome?

    A. Risperidone and haloperidol.
    B. Clonidine and fluphenazine.
    C. Pimozide and clonidine.
    D. Pimozide and haloperidol.
    E. Haloperidol and fluoxetine.

**The correct response is option D.**

Although haloperidol and pimozide are FDA-approved medications for the treatment of Tourette's syndrome, the side-effect profile of haloperidol limits its usefulness with children. There is increasing evidence to support the efficacy of atypical antipsychotics for the treatment of children with Tourette's syndrome.

Wagner KD: Treatment of childhood and adolescent disorders, in The American Psychiatric Publishing Textbook of Psychopharmacology, 3rd Edition. Edited by Schatzberg AF, Nemeroff CB. Washington, DC, American Psychiatric Publishing, 2004, p 975

151. Serum vitamin $B_{12}$ and folate levels

    A. Are rarely important in the evaluation of the elderly patient.
    B. May point to etiologies of a range of neuropsychiatric disturbances.
    C. Would not be thought etiologic if recorded as normal.
    D. Are not related to hyperhomocysteinemia.
    E. Are not related to one-carbon metabolism in brain tissue.

**The correct response is option B.**

Vitamin $B_{12}$ and folate deficiencies may result in neuropsychiatric disturbances, including depression, psychosis, and cognitive deficits. Measurement of serum vitamin $B_{12}$ and folate levels is an integral part of the laboratory evaluation because the prevalence of $B_{12}$ deficiency increases with age: the deficiency is present in up to 15% of the elderly population. $B_{12}$ deficiency may have various clinical signs, including macrocytic anemia and neuropathy. Serum homocysteine levels may serve as a functional indicator of $B_{12}$ and folate status because vitamin $B_{12}$ is needed to convert homocysteine to methionine in one-carbon metabolism in brain tissue.

Taylor WD, Doraiswamy PM: Use of the laboratory in the diagnostic workup of older adults, in American Psychiatric Publishing Textbook of Geriatric Psychitry, 3rd Edition. Edited by Blazer DG, Steffens DC, Busse EW. Washington, DC, American Psychiatric Publishing, 2004, pp 181–182

152. Systemic complications of anorexia nervosa include

    A. Leukocytosis.
    B. Hyperkalemic alkalosis.
    C. Hyperchloremia.
    D. Decreased serum bicarbonate levels.
    E. Cardiac arrhythmias.

**The correct response is option E.**

Individuals with anorexia nervosa have an increased risk of cardiac arrhythmias. Options A, B, C, and D are incorrect because leukopenia, hypokalemia, hypochloremia, and elevated serum bicarbonate levels are associated with anorexia nervosa. Patients with electrolyte disturbances experience physical symptoms of weakness and lethargy and, at times, have cardiac arrhythmias.

Halmi KA, Falk JR: Common physiological changes in anorexia nervosa. Int J Eat Disord 1:16–27, 1981

153. The most common anxiety disorder in later life is

    A. Posttraumatic stress disorder.
    B. Agoraphobia.
    C. Panic disorder.
    D. Social phobia.
    E. Generalized anxiety disorder, which may be comorbid with major depression.

**The correct response is option E.**

Although anxiety disorders can affect persons at all life stages, many of the anxiety disorders are relatively less frequent in the elderly. Anxiety is a frequent symptom among older persons because of physical illnesses such as hyperthyroidism, comorbid with other psychiatric disorders such as depression, or as the primary symptom of a disorder such as generalized anxiety disorder. Generalized anxiety disorder is a common diagnosis regardless of age, and generalized anxiety is often comorbid with other psychiatric disorders such as major depression.

Posttraumatic stress disorder can occur at any age but is found more frequently in younger persons than older persons. Although phobia disorders can affect persons at all stages of the life cycle, the more severe phobias, such as agoraphobia and social phobia, begin early in life and are more common in children and young adults than in older persons. Panic disorder is relatively frequent and severe among younger persons but much less so among older persons (although data documenting a lower prevalence among older persons are sparse). Obsessive-compulsive traits are common throughout the life cycle, although the severe manifestations of this disorder are less likely to be observed in older persons.

Blazer DG: Treatment of seniors, in The American Psychiatric Publishing Textbook of Psychiatry, 5th Edition. Edited by Hales RE, Yudofsky SC, Gabbard GO. Washington, DC, American Psychiatric Publishing, 2008, p 1458

154. A 28-year-old man presenting to your outpatient clinic began taking a new antipsychotic medication for undifferentiated schizophrenia 1 week ago. He complains of mild daytime sedation, mild abdominal cramping, nausea, and "weird muscle aches" that make it difficult for him to turn his neck from side to side. On exam, his gaze appears fixated in one position, and he has a facial grimace. You notice that his speech is dysarthric and is occasionally interrupted by what appears to be uncomfortable swallowing as if he's gulping air. He should be treated with

    A. Intramuscular thiamine.
    B. Intravenous diphenhydramine.
    C. Oral benztropine.
    D. IV beta-blockers.
    E. Oral or intravenous lorazepam.

**The correct response is option B.**

Acute dystonic reactions (ADRs) are generally the first type of extrapyramidal side effects (EPSs) to appear and are often the most dramatic. ADRs tend to occur suddenly and usually involve the head and neck, as in this case (e.g., torticollis, facial grimacing, and oculogyric crisis). About 90% of ADRs occur within 4 days of starting an antipsychotic or increasing its dose, and nearly 100% occur by day 10 of starting the medication. Dystonic reactions are characterized by extreme muscle contraction and rigidity in a patient with stable vital signs and a clear sensorium; they occur most frequently as an adverse effect of high-potency, first-generation antipsychotics.

ADRs that include laryngeal spasms, as in this case, should be treated promptly with 50 mg of intravenous diphenhydramine for rapid relief of symptoms. Maintenance treatment of benztropine 1–2 mg twice a day or diphenhydramine 25–50 mg twice a day should be initiated after the acute reaction has resolved. Less severe dystonic reactions can be treated with benztropine 1–2 mg via the oral or intramuscular route. An alternative is diphenhydramine in doses of 25–50 mg via the oral or intramuscular route. Intramuscular thiamine (before glucose) is routinely administered to prevent Wernicke's encephalopathy but not ADRs, therefore option A is incorrect. Option C is incorrect because the oral benztropine would be more appropriate for less severe ADR and/or for maintenance treatment but not in this severe presentation. Option D is incorrect because beta-blockers may be useful in treating akathisia, another type of EPS but is generally not effective for dystonia. Option E is incorrect because intravenous lorazepam will not reverse the ADR.

Garlow SJ, Purselle D, D'Orio B: Psychiatric emergencies, in The American Psychiatric Publishing Textbook of Psychopharmacology, 3rd Edition. Edited by Schatzberg AF, Nemeroff CB. Washington, DC, American Psychiatric Publishing, 2004, p 1069; see Table 62–3

Stanilla JK, Simpson GM: Drugs to treat extrapyramidal side effects, in The American Psychiatric Publishing Textbook of Psychopharmacology, 3rd Edition. Edited by Schatzberg AF, Nemeroff CB. Washington, DC, American Psychiatric Publishing, 2004, p 520

---

*Dystonias* are involuntary sustained or spasmodic muscle contractions that cause abnormal twisting or rhythmical movements and/or postures.

---

155. A 36-year-old woman who had been fired from her job in March presents to the outpatient medical clinic in August with a 1-month history of depressed mood and insomnia. She also reports decreased appetite but no other symptoms of depression. She relates her symptoms to the job loss. The most likely diagnosis is

    A. No diagnosis.
    B. Acute adjustment disorder with depressed mood.
    C. Anxiety disorder not otherwise specified.
    D. Acute stress disorder.
    E. Chronic adjustment disorder with depressed mood.

**The correct response is option B.**

According to DSM-IV-TR, adjustment disorder is characterized by the development of emotional or behavioral symptoms in response to an identifiable stressor occurring within 3 months of the onset of the stressor. This patient is experiencing depressed mood, insomnia, and decreased appetite, all within 3 months of a stressor (loss of job). Apart from insomnia, the patient has no anxiety symptoms.

Option C is incorrect because her fulfilling criteria for adjustment disorder precludes this diagnosis. Option D is incorrect because acute stress disorder requires exposure to a traumatic event in which the person experienced, witnessed, or was confronted with an event that involved actual or threatened death or serious injury, or a threat to the physical integrity of self or others, or a response involving intense fear, helplessness, or horror. For this diagnosis, an individual would also have to experience at least three dissociative symptoms such as derealization or depersonalization. The only criterion that this individual meets for acute stress disorder is the onset and duration of symptoms, which for acute stress disorder is a minimum

of 2 days and a maximum of 4 weeks. Option E is incorrect because symptoms must persist for more than 6 months to be specified as chronic.

American Psychiatric Association: Diagnostic and Statistical Manual of Mental Disorders, 4th Edition, Text Revision. Washington, DC, American Psychiatric Association, 2000, p 679

156. Which of the following clinical findings has been demonstrated in patients with bipolar disorder?

    A. Decreased plasma cortisol concentration.
    B. Decreased cortisol in cerebrospinal fluid.
    C. Suppression of plasma glucocorticoid concentration after dexamethasone administration.
    D. Nonsuppression of plasma glucocorticoid concentration after dexamethasone administration.
    E. Increased diurnal variation of plasma cortisol concentrations.

**The correct response is option D.**

Alterations in the activity of the hypothalamic-pituitary-adrenal axis in bipolar disorder include increased plasma cortisol concentrations, increased cortisol in cerebrospinal fluid, nonsuppression of plasma glucocorticoid concentrations after dexamethasone administration, and blunted diurnal variation of plasma cortisol concentrations.

Flores BH, Musselman DL, DeBattista C, et al: Biology of mood disorders, in The American Psychiatric Publishing Textbook of Psychopharmacology, 3rd Edition. Edited by Schatzberg AF, Nemeroff CB. Washington, DC, American Psychiatric Publishing, 2004, p 725; see Table 45–2

157. Which of the following statements is *false* regarding the noradrenergic system?

    A. The initial steps in the biosynthesis of norepinephrine are similar, but not identical to, those of dopamine.
    B. Norepinephrine-containing neurons in the central nervous system are located predominantly in the medulla and pons.
    C. In the hypothalamus, the paraventricular nucleus contains the highest density of norepinephrine axons.
    D. In the amygdala, the basolateral nuclei contain the highest density of norepinephrine axons.
    E. Norepinephrine elicits responses in the postsynaptic cell via G-protein–mediated second-messenger systems.

## The correct response is option A.

The initial steps in the biosynthesis of norepinephrine are identical to those of dopamine, therefore the statement in option A is false. The precursor for dopamine and all catecholamines (see sidebar) is tyrosine, which is then converted to L-dihydroxyphenylanine (L-dopa), then to dopamine, then to norepinephrine, and then to epinephrine (tyrosine → L-dopa → dopamine → norepinephrine → epinephrine).

All areas of the cerebral cortex receive noradrenergic projections; however, certain areas have higher densities of norepinephrine axons than do other areas. For example, primary somatosensory and visual cortices have a very high density of norepinephrine axons. Within the hypothalamus and amygdala, the paraventricular and basolateral nuclei, respectively, contain the highest density of norepinephrine axons in these structures.

Melchitzky DS, Austin MC, Lewis DA: Chemical neuroanatomy of the primate brain, in The American Psychiatric Publishing Textbook of Psychopharmacology, 3rd Edition. Edited by Schatzberg AF, Nemeroff CB. Washington, DC, American Psychiatric Publishing, 2004, pp 70–71, 73

---

*Catecholamines* are a group of biogenic amines derived from tyrosine that includes the neurotransmitters dopamine, epinephrine, and norepinephrine that exert an important influence on peripheral and central nervous system activity.

---

158. The genetic contributions to schizophrenia may be best described as

    A. Sex-linked.
    B. Multifactorial.
    C. Mendelian.
    D. Mutations.
    E. Iatrogenic.

## The correct response is option B.

Schizophrenia is a heritable brain disorder with evidence of complex neural aberrations affecting frontotemporal brain networks. Current views are that genetic liability and environmental factors combine to produce the symptomatic manifestations. To date, no single gene has been associated with schizophrenia, although positive linkage results have been found for several chromosomal loci. A problem in linkage studies is that "schizophrenia" encompasses a broad range of complex behaviors, with variability even within families.

Gur RE, Arnold SE: Neurobiology of schizophrenia, in The American Psychiatric Publishing Textbook of Psychopharmacology, 3rd Edition. Edited by Schatzberg AF, Nemeroff CB. Washington, DC, American Psychiatric Publishing, 2004, pp 768, 769

159. All of the following tests measure aspects of executive functioning *except*

    A. Tower of London.
    B. Behavioral Assessment of the Dysexecutive Syndrome.
    C. Twenty Questions Test.
    D. Wisconsin Card Sorting Test.
    E. Complex Figure Test.

## The correct response is option E.

Executive functions include the ability to formulate a goal, to plan, to carry out goal-directed plans effectively, and to monitor and self-correct spontaneously and reliably. The Complex Figure Test is a neuropsychological assessment that measures visuospatial processing, not executive functioning.

Howieson DB, Lezak MD: The neuropsychological evaluation, in The American Psychiatric Publishing Textbook of Neuropsychiatry and Behavioral Neurosciences, 5th Edition. Edited by Yudofsky SC, Hales RE. Washington, DC, American Psychiatric Publishing, 2008, p 230

160. The primary forensic issue in a child custody evaluation in the context of a divorce is

    A. What custodial arrangements will be least disruptive to the child's life.
    B. To what custodial arrangements will the child agree.
    C. What custodial arrangements are in the best interests of the child.
    D. Which parent has been more involved in caretaking of the child.
    E. Which parent is more motivated to do what is best for the child.

## The correct response is option C.

The central issue before the court in a custody dispute is a comparison of custody options and a determination of which of these is in the best interest of the child.

Most custody disputes reflect marital disputes that compromise one or both parents' abilities to reason about their children's best interests. However, few divorces stem from disagreements about how to raise children.

Clinicians conducting such evaluations should be aware that current standards for conducting custody evaluations strongly recommend that all parties to a custody case (including both parents and all children) be interviewed before rendering an opinion on child custody matters. The clinician presenting an opinion based on the assessment of only one parent is not likely to have a basis for comparing the custody options or making a well-informed recommendation regarding the child's best interest.

Ash P: Children and adolescents, in The American Psychiatric Publishing Textbook of Forensic Psychiatry. Edited by Simon RI, Gold LH. Washington, DC, American Psychiatric Publishing, 2004, pp 457–458

161. Which of the following is *true* regarding immune function in patients with depression?

 A. Peripheral blood findings in depressed patients have included decreased lymphocytes, neutrophils, and natural killer (NK) cell activity.
 B. A syndrome of "sickness behavior" mimicking major depression follows administration of interferon-$\alpha$ (IFN-$\alpha$) and interleukin-2 (IL-2).
 C. Cerebrospinal fluid (CSF) studies of depressed patients have demonstrated increased levels of interleukin-6 (IL-6) and soluble IL-6 receptor.
 D. Decreases in acute phase proteins such as C-reactive protein, serum haptoglobin, the complement protein C4, $\alpha_1$-antitrypsin, and $\alpha_1$-acid glycoprotein.
 E. The high rates of depression in autoimmune and other immune-related diseases demonstrate that depression is associated with a suppression of the immune response.

**The correct response is option B.**

A syndrome of "sickness behavior" resembling major depression occurs with the administration of cytokine therapies such as IFN-$\alpha$ and IL-2. Prominent features of sickness behavior include depressed mood, anhedonia, sleep and appetite disturbances, malaise, and poor concentration. Option A is incorrect because peripheral blood

findings in depressed patients have included *decreased* lymphocytes and NK cell activity but *increased* neutrophils. Option C is incorrect because depressed patients have *decreased* levels of the cytokine IL-6 in the CSF. Option D is incorrect because depression is associated with immune activation, or increases in acute phase proteins such as C-reactive protein, serum haptoglobin, the complement protein C4, $\alpha_1$-antitrypsin, and $\alpha_1$-acid glycoprotein. Option E is incorrect because immune-related diseases are associated with immune activation (not suppression), which is also seen in depression.

Bourgeois JA, Hales RE, Yudofsky SC: The American Psychiatric Publishing Board Prep and Review Guide for Psychiatry. Washington, DC, American Psychiatric Publishing, 2007, p 35

162. A 77-year-old Caucasian man with no known previous psychiatric history is brought by his caregiver for an evaluation because of his worsening short-term memory and "strange behaviors." The caregiver reports that the patient was recently seen chuckling to himself. When asked why he was laughing, the patient responded, "These little green squirrels are so funny when they square dance with the elephants!" and proceeded to give a detailed description of their activities. To the caregiver's surprise, the patient mentions having been seeing these dancing animals for the past several months. He has a history of hypertension that is well-controlled with medications, with no recent changes in his drug regimen. His vital signs are normal, he appears to be in no apparent physical distress, and his gait is normal. On examination, the patient is intermittently drowsy, easily distracted, and disinhibited at times. Despite multiple introductions, he asks for a third time who you are. Of the following, which is the most likely diagnosis?

 A. Delirium.
 B. Normal pressure hydrocephalus.
 C. Vascular dementia
 D. Lewy Body dementia.
 E. Decompensated schizophrenia.

**The correct response is option D.**

This case is most consistent with Lewy body dementia. Lewy body dementia mimics delirium with its fluctuating symptom severity, confusion, hallucinations (especially visual), and delusions. The lack of risk factors for delirium and the detailed nature of this patient's visual hallucinations that have persisted for several months make delirium an unlikely diagnosis at this time; therefore, option A is incorrect. Nevertheless, because of the patient's age, altered mental status, and unsubstantiated medical history, delirium should still be on the differential diagnosis.

Option B is incorrect because normal pressure hydrocephalus (NPH) usually does not include visual hallucinations. The patient only has one of the three clinical findings (dementia) that is consistent with NPH, and lacks a gait disturbance and (apparently, because it was not mentioned) urinary incontinence. Option C is incorrect because visual hallucinations typically are not seen in vascular dementia. Option E is incorrect because a new diagnosis of schizophrenia is highly unlikely at this older age. In addition, schizophrenia usually does not include impairment of consciousness, attention, and short-term memory (with the exception of the pseudodelirium that can occur as a result of marked perplexity in the acute stage of illness).

Apostolova LG, Cummings JL: Neuropsychiatric aspects of Alzheimer's disease and other dementing illnesses, in The American Psychiatric Publishing Textbook of Neuropsychiatry and Behavioral Neurosciences, 5th Edition. Edited by Yudofsky SC, Hales RE. Washington, DC, American Psychiatric Publishing, pp 925, 953

163. Which of the following characteristics is *not* associated with an increased risk of adolescent substance abuse?

    A. High levels of behavioral activity.
    B. Reduced attention span.
    C. High impulsivity.
    D. Lack of emotional reactivity (i.e., "blunting").
    E. Irritability.

**The correct response is option D.**

Various psychological factors are associated with problematic substance abuse in adolescents. Lack of emotional reactivity is not associated with increased risk of adolescent substance abuse. High levels of behavioral activity have been noted in youth at high risk for substance abuse as well as in those with a substance use disorder. High levels of behavioral activity also correlate with disorder severity. Other temperamental trait deviations found in youth at high risk include reduced attention span, high impulsivity, negative affect states such as irritability, and emotional reactivity.

Kaminer Y: Adolescent substance abuse, in The American Psychiatric Publishing Textbook of Substance Abuse Treatment, 4th Edition. Edited by Galanter M, Kleber HD. Washington, DC, American Psychiatric Publishing, 2008, p 526

164. Which of the following choices accurately lists, from most common to least common, the four most commonly used substances among patients with schizophrenia?

    A. Nicotine, alcohol, cocaine, cannabis.
    B. Alcohol, nicotine, cocaine, cannabis.
    C. Nicotine, cannabis, alcohol, cocaine.
    D. Alcohol, nicotine, cannabis, cocaine.
    E. Nicotine, alcohol, cannabis, cocaine.

**The correct response is option A.**

In the Epidemiological Catchment Area study, 47% of patients with schizophrenia had a lifetime history of a substance use disorder, with 34% having an alcohol use disorder and 28% having a drug use disorder. In mental health treatment settings, the rate of current substance use disorders among persons with schizophrenia ranges from 25% to 75%. According to the recent National Institute of Mental Health Clinical Antipsychotic Trials of Intervention Effectiveness project, 60% of schizophrenia patients were actively using substances of abuse and 37% met criteria for a current substance use disorder. Furthermore, in that study, substance use disorders were strongly associated with male gender and a history of conduct disorder. The most common substances used by persons with schizophrenia are nicotine (75%–90%), alcohol (25%–45%), cocaine (15%–50%), and cannabis (31%).

Ross S: The mentally ill substance abuser, in The American Psychiatric Publishing Textbook of Substance Abuse Treatment, 4th Edition. Edited by Galanter M, Kleber HD. Washington, DC, American Psychiatric Publishing, 2008 p 540

165. About what percentage of serotonin (5-hydroxytryptamine [5-HT]) in the body is found in the cerebrum?

    A. 95%.
    B. 70%.
    C. 35%.
    D. 10%.
    E. 2%.

**The correct response is option E.**

Only 2% of the body's 5-HT is found in the brain. The highest concentration of 5-HT–containing neurons in the mammalian brain is in the raphe nuclei of the brainstem.

Melchitzky DS, Austin MC, Lewis DA: Chemical neuroanatomy of the primate brain, in The American Psychiatric Publishing Textbook of Psychopharmacology, 3rd Edition. Edited by Schatzberg AF, Nemeroff CB. Washington, DC, American Psychiatric Publishing, 2004, p 76

166. All of the following features are common to all dementias *except*

    A.  Memory impairment and aphasia.
    B.  Apraxia.
    C.  Agnosia.
    D.  Disturbed executive functioning.
    E.  None of the above.

**The correct response is option E.**

All of the features listed are common to all dementias.

Bourgeois JA, Seamon JS, Servis ME: Delirium, dementia, and amnestic and other cognitive disorders, in The American Psychiatric Publishing Textbook of Psychiatry, 5th Edition. Edited by Hales RE, Yudofsky SC, Gabbard GO. Washington, DC, American Psychiatric Publishing, 2008, p 323

167. All of the following clinical features are characteristic of cortical dementias *except*

    A.  Apraxia.
    B.  Agnosia.
    C.  Visuospatial deficits.
    D.  Prominent motor signs.
    E.  Language deficits.

**The correct response is option D.**

All dementias have common features such as memory impairment, aphasia, apraxia, agnosia, and disturbed executive functioning. For diagnostic purposes, however dementias have been categorized into subcortical versus cortical dementias. Cortical dementias are characterized by prominent memory impairment (recall and recognition), language deficits, apraxia, agnosia, and visuospatial deficits. Cortical dementias include dementia of the Alzheimer's type, frontotemporal dementia (e.g., Pick's dis-

ease), dementia caused by Creutzfeldt-Jakob disease, and dementia caused by chronic subdural hematoma. Cortical dementias generally lack prominent motor signs, which typically occur in subcortical dementias.

Subcortical dementias include dementias caused by HIV, Parkinson's disease, Huntington's disease, and multiple sclerosis. Subcortical dementias include impairment in recall memory, decreased verbal fluency without anomia, bradyphrenia (slowed thinking), depressed mood, affective lability, apathy, and decreased attention/concentration.

The cortical–subcortical dichotomy is not absolute, however, because aphasia, apraxia, and agnosia (in isolation) have a low sensitivity in distinguishing cortical from subcortical dementia, and several dementia types may express both cortical and subcortical features at some point in the course of illness.

Bourgeois JA, Seamon JS, Servis ME: Delirium, dementia, and amnestic and other cognitive disorders, in The American Psychiatric Publishing Textbook of Psychiatry, 5th Edition. Edited by Hales RE, Yudofsky SC, Gabbard GO. Washington, DC, American Psychiatric Publishing, 2008, pp 322–323

168. Hypothyroidism is an example of a metabolic illness with neuropsychiatric symptoms. Which of the following is *true*?

    A.  Anxiety occurs in about one-third of patients with hypothyroidism.
    B.  The two most common psychiatric manifestations in hypothyroidism are depression and psychosis.
    C.  Replacement of thyroid hormone in the form of $T_3$ (rather than $T_4$) has a specific effect on improving depressed mood but a negligible effect on cognitive performance.
    D.  Physical symptoms typically precede psychiatric symptoms in patients with hypothyroidism.
    E.  Hypomanic or manic symptoms occur in about one-third of patients with hypothyroidism.

**The correct response is option A.**

Anxiety occurs in approximately 30% of patients and tends to be generalized.

Option B is incorrect because the most common psychiatric manifestations of hypothyroidism are depressed mood and delirium, both of which occur in nearly 50% of psychiatrically ill hypothyroid patients. Data indicate that only approximately 5% of patients manifest psychosis.

Note that early case studies of hypothyroid patients reported psychosis in up to 52.9% of patients, leading to the misconception that psychosis is common. Option C is incorrect because replacement of $T_3$ has specific effects on both mood and cognition. $T_4$ replacement may improve mood but does not appear to improve cognition. Option D is incorrect because physical symptoms do not necessarily precede psychiatric symptoms, which are often the first symptoms of thyroid disturbance. Option E is incorrect because hypomania and mania are extremely rare in patients with hypothyroidism.

Bourgeois JA, Hales RE, Yudofsky SC: The American Psychiatric Publishing Board Prep and Review Guide for Psychiatry. Washington, DC, American Psychiatric Publishing, 2007, p 40

169. Regarding the use of nonsteroidal anti-inflammatory drugs (NSAIDs) in treating or preventing Alzheimer's disease, which of the following statements is *true?*

    A. NSAIDs have been found to increase the risk of developing Alzheimer's disease by 30%–80%.
    B. In prospective clinical trials, NSAIDs have shown no benefit in treating patients with Alzheimer's disease.
    C. No prospective studies have been conducted, only retrospective studies.
    D. NSAID use has proven too risky because of the side effects of these agents.
    E. With long-term use of NSAIDs, the risk of Alzheimer's disease is higher.

## The correct response is option B.

Prospective clinical trials of NSAIDs have thus far been negative in treating Alzheimer's disease. However, several epidemiological investigations, including a large prospective population-based study, found that the relative risk of Alzheimer's disease was lower with long-term use of NSAIDs. The magnitude of the reduced risk associated with NSAIDs ranged from 30% to 80%. Nonetheless, it is posited that anti-inflammatory agents may have a protective role in earlier preclinical stages of Alzheimer's disease, and prospective studies examining this possibility are currently under way.

Lah JJ, Levy OA, Levey AI: Biology of Alzheimer's disease, in The American Psychiatric Publishing Textbook of Psychopharmacology, 3rd Edition. Edited by Schatzberg AF, Nemeroff CB. Washington, DC, American Psychiatric Publishing, 2004, pp 798, 803

170. A test of which of the following specimens has the shortest window of detection?

    A. Blood.
    B. Hair.
    C. Oral fluid.
    D. Sweat.
    E. Urine.

## The correct response is option A.

Blood has the shortest window of detection because most drugs are cleared from the blood at measurable levels in 12 hours or less. Urine has a detection window of about 1–3 days because most drugs are cleared within this time after the most recent use of the drug.

DuPont RL, Selavka CM: Testing to identify recent drug use, in The American Psychiatric Publishing Textbook of Substance Abuse Treatment, 4th Edition. Edited by Galanter M, Kleber HD. Washington, DC, American Psychiatric Publishing, 2008, p 661; Table 46–2.

171. You are called to provide a psychiatric consultation on patient end-stage pancreatic cancer whose treatment team is considering referral to a hospice program. Of the following, the most relevant ethical principles to consider are

    A. Fidelity and beneficence.
    B. Justice and autonomy.
    C. Nonmaleficence and fidelity.
    D. Confidentiality and nonmalficence.
    E. Autonomy and beneficence.

## The correct response is option E.

Autonomy and beneficence are important ethical principles to consider in this case. *Autonomy* literally means "self rule." In medical ethics, autonomy is the ability to make deliberated or reasoned decisions for oneself and to act on the basis of such decisions (Roberts et al. 2008). *Beneficence* is an action done to benefit others. The principle of beneficence in medicine signfies an obligation to benefit patients and to seek their good. It is important for the consultant to determine the patient's mental capacity to make a reasoned decision regarding his or her transfer to a hospice program.

Hospice care is designed to maximize a sense of self-efficacy in managing as much as possible one's final transition in a minimally medical environment. The philosophy of hospice emphasizes the importance of a homelike environment for terminal care, effective pain control, the absence of high-technology medical and surgical interventions characteristic of hospitals, and emotional support for dying patients and their families (Maddox and Golda 2004).

Fidelity, justice, nonmaleficence, and confidentiality are ethical principles that are less important to this case at this time; therefore, options A, B, C, and D are incorrect. *Fidelity* is the virtue of promise keeping, truthfulness, and honor. In clinical care, it refers to the faithfulness with which a clinician commits to the duty of helping patients and acting in a manner that is in keeping with the ideals of the profession. *Justice* is the ethical principle of fairness. *Nonmaleficence* is the duty to avoid doing harm. *Confidentiality* is the obligation of physicians not to disclose information obtained from patients or observed about them without their permission.

Maddox GL, Golda EJ: The continuum of care, in The American Psychiatric Publishing Textbook of Geriatric Psychiatry, 3rd Edition. Edited by Blazer DG, Steffens DC, Busse EW. Washington, DC, American Psychiatric Publishing, 2004, p 504

Roberts LW, Hoop JG, Dunn LB: Ethical aspects of psychiatry, in The American Psychiatric Publishing Textbook of Psychiatry, 5th Edition. Edited by Hales RE, Yudofsky SC, Gabbard GO. Washington, DC, American Psychiatric Publishing, 2008, pp 1606–1609

172. In forensic practice, the clinician needs to be mindful of the possible differences in the definitions of common clinical terms. Which of the following statements is *true?*

A. The term *narcotic* refers to an addictive drug that is controlled or prohibited by law.
B. The terms *narcotic* and *opioid* are synonymous clinically and legally.
C. The terms *addiction* and *substance dependence* are legally interchangeable.
D. The clinical definition of *chemical dependency* relates to deleterious effects of drug use.
E. The terms *chemical dependency* and *addiction* are legally, but not necessarily clinically, interhangeable.

**The correct response is option A.**

Clinically, the term *narcotic* is often synonymous with *opioid,* and *addiction* is often synonymous with *chemical dependency.* However, these terms are differentiated le-

gally, with *narcotic* referring to an addictive drug that is controlled or prohibited by law. In contrast, *opioid* does not have any legal implications and simply refers to drugs that act on the opioid receptors. Thus, option B is incorrect. Option C is incorrect because clinically addiction is often interchangeable for substance dependence, with demonstrable alterations in neural activity. Legally, however, addiction refers to the state of taking drugs that are prohibited by law and therefore has legal and social implications. Option D is incorrect because legally chemical dependency relates to deleterious effects of drug use. Option E is incorrect because dependency and addiction are not legally interchangeable but often are used synonymously in clinical arenas.

Mack AH, Barros M: Forensic addiction psychiatry, in The American Psychiatric Publishing Textbook of Substance Abuse Treatment, 4th Edition. Edited by Galanter M, Kleber HD. Washington, DC, American Psychiatric Publishing, 2008, pp 690–691

173. What percentage of patients treated for apparent major depression in the outpatient setting subsequently receive a diagnosis of bipolar I or II disorder?

A. 5%–10%.
B. 15%–30%.
C. >40%.
D. <5%.
E. Unknown.

**The correct response is option B.**

Studies suggest that 15%–30% of the patients treated for apparent major depressive disorder in outpatient settings subsequently receive a diagnosis of bipolar I or bipolar II disorder.

Keck PE, McElroy SL: Treatment of bipolar disorder, in The American Psychiatric Publishing Textbook of Psychopharmacology, 3rd Edition. Edited by Schatzberg AF, Nemeroff CB. Washington, DC, American Psychiatric Publishing, 2004, p 866

174. A nonpharmacological treatment indicated for pyromania is

A. Aversive conditioning.
B. Cognitive-behavioral psychotherapy.
C. Interpersonal psychotherapy.
D. Psychodynamic psychotherapy.
E. Psychoanalytic psychotherapy.

## The correct response is option A.

Treatment modalities that have been implemented for pyromania include behavior therapy with aversive conditioning, positive reinforcement, social skills training, and use of relapse prevention plans. Furthermore, educational programs focusing on the medical, financial, legal, and societal impacts of fire-setting behavior have found to decrease recidivisim in individuals with pyromanic behaviors.

Hollander E, Berlin HA, Stein DJ: Impulse-control disorders not elsewhere classified, in American Psychiatric Publishing Textbook of Psychiatry, 5th Edition. Edited by Hales RE, Yudofsky SC, Gabbard GO. Washington, DC, American Psychiatric Publishing, 2008, p 794

175. Patients with Alzheimer's disease with and without psychosis differ in all of the following *except*

    A. Patients with Alzheimer's disease with psychosis show greater impairment in executive functioning.
    B. Patients with Alzheimer's disease with psychosis have a greater prevalence of extrapyramidal signs.
    C. Patients with Alzheimer's disease with psychosis have shown increased norepinephrine levels and reduced serotonin levels in subcortical regions.
    D. Patients with Alzheimer's disease with psychosis typically warrant very long term maintenance therapy with antipsychotics.
    E. Patients with Alzheimer's disease with psychosis have more prevalent behavioral disturbances such as agitation than hallucinations and paranoid delusions.

## The correct response is option D.

Because psychotic symptoms in patients with dementia tend to remit in the late stages of the disease, very long term maintenance therapy with antipsychotics is typically unnecessary.

Patients with Alzheimer's disease with psychosis and those without psychosis differ in several important ways. Neuropsychologically, patients with Alzheimer's disease with psychosis show greater impairment in executive functioning and a more rapid cognitive decline. Psychosis is associated with a greater prevalence of extrapyramidal signs in Alzheimer's disease. Neuropathologically, dementia patients with psychosis have shown increased neu-

rodegenerative changes in the cortex, increased norepinephrine levels in subcortical regions, and reduced serotonin levels in both cortical and subcortical areas. Hallucinations and paranoid delusions appear to be more persistent than depressive symptoms but less prevalent and persistent than behavioral disturbances, particularly agitation.

Jeste DV, Wetherell JL, Dolder CR: Schizophrenia and paranoid disorders, in The American Psychiatric Publishing Textbook of Geriatric Psychiatry, 3rd Edition. Edited by Blazer DG, Steffens DC, Busse EW. Washington, DC, American Psychiatric Publishing, 2004, p 273

176. A young man is brought to the emergency room by his friends, who report that the patient was at a fraternity party and was "partying" with other partygoers, when he started "acting weird," saying he wanted to kill himself. His roommate recalled that the patient has been increasingly depressed since he was injured in a car accident a week ago, especially in the past few days. The patient binges on alcohol occasionally and has been taking "some pain meds" since his accident but does not use other substances. He quit smoking "cold turkey" 2–3 days ago. He has no known history of a mood disorder. On examination, the young man has slurred speech and an ataxic gait. He has nystagmus bilaterally, and his pupils are constricted. When you gently start examining the leg that was injured, he yells, "What are you doing?! Trying to kill me?!" and wimpers in pain. In addition to alcohol intoxication, which of the following are other conditions in your differential diagnosis?

    A. Opioid withdrawal and/or nicotine withdrawal.
    B. Opioid intoxication and/or phencyclidine (PCP) intoxication.
    C. Nicotine withdrawal and/or opioid intoxication.
    D. Benzodiazepine intoxication, hallucinogen intoxication.
    E. Inhalant intoxication, and/or amphetamine intoxication.

## The correct response is option C.

An important clue to the differential is that the patient's mood has become increasingly dysphoric in the past few days since he quit smoking. The relatively sudden onset of dysphoric mood suggests a substance-induced condition, especially because the patient does not have a history of depression. Of the listed substances, withdrawal from opioids and/or nicotine can cause dysphoric mood, but the finding of pinpoint pupils rules out opioid withdrawal, so option A is incorrect. His history is consistent with the patient being intoxicated with opioids, which is an important piece of evidence suggesting opioid intoxication. Option B is incorrect because his hypersensitivity to pain is incompatible with PCP intoxication, which tends to numb pain.

Option D is incorrect because although benzodiazepine intoxication is possible, the finding of constricted pupils rules out a hallucinogen intoxication, which causes pupil dilation. Option E is incorrect because although an inhalant intoxication is possible (albeit improbable, because inhalants tend to cause euphoria), the patient is unlikely to be intoxicated with amphetamines, which also causes pupil dilation.

American Psychiatric Association: Diagnostic and Statistical Manual of Mental Disorders, 4th Edition, Text Revision. Washington, DC, American Psychiatric Association, 2000, pp 215–216, 227–228, 232, 238, 245–246, 253, 260, 266, 272–273, 281, 287, 289

177. Ten seconds after starting an electroconvulsive therapy (ECT) procedure, the ECT is abruptly discontinued becase of the patient inexplicably awakening from anesthesia. No seizure was induced. The procedure was not resumed because the patient then refused to continue the treatment. Which of the following statements is *true?*

    A. Even though a seizure was not induced, it is likely that the patient will derive some benefit from the procedure because he received at least 10 seconds of electrical stimulation.
    B. The patient may not derive any benefit from the procedure because at least 20 seconds of electrical stimulation is required in order for ECT to be of any benefit.
    C. It is unlikely that the patient will derive any therapeutic benefit from the procedure because seizure induction is essential for ECT.
    D. It is difficult to predict whether this patient will derive any benefit from the procedure because 50% of patients do not require seizure-induction in order for ECT to be effective.
    E. All of the above.

**The correct response is option C.**

Seizure induction is essential for ECT to be clinically effective, therefore all statements except option C are incorrect. In theory, the number of seconds of subseizure threshold electrical stimulation is irrelevant in terms of ECT efficacy; therefore, options A, B, D, and E are incorrect.

George MS, Nahas ZH, Borckardt JJ, et al: Nonpharmacological somatic treatments, in The American Psychiatric Publishing Textbook of Psychiatry, 5th Edition. Edited by Hales RE, Yudofsky SC, Gabbard GO. Washington, DC, American Psychiatric Publishing, 2008, p 1134

178. All of the following statements regarding positive symptoms of schizophrenia are correct *except*

    A. Studies show that a high degree of positive symptoms correlates with a worse long-term prognosis.
    B. Positive symptoms include hallucinations.
    C. Positive symptoms respond to antipsychotic medications.
    D. Positive symptoms are not the first set of symptoms that typically present in schizophrenia.
    E. Positive symptoms are traditionally the focus of medication treatment.

**The correct response is option A.**

Traditionally, the onset of schizophrenia is clinically synonymous with the emergence of positive, or overt psychotic, symptoms. Positive symptoms include hallucinations, delusions, and disorganized thinking, although disorganization also can be conceptualized as an independent symptom dimension. Evidence now indicates that schizophrenia begins long before the onset of psychosis. For example, subtle neurological abnormalities and intellectual and cognitive difficulties have been observed in children who later show symptoms of schizophrenia. As a general rule, positive symptoms tend to respond to treatment with antipsychotic medications and have been the focus of treatment. Although dramatic and often severely disruptive, positive symptoms do not appear to bear any significant association with or predict the long-term functional outcome of the illness.

Woo T-UW, Zimmet SV, Wojcik JD, et al: Treatment of schizophrenia, in The American Psychiatric Publishing Textbook of Psychopharmacology, 3rd Edition. Edited by Schatzberg AF, Nemeroff CB. Washington, DC, American Psychiatric Publishing, 2004, p 886

179. In a forensic evaluation, the role of the evaluating psychiatrist is to

    A. Focus on a thorough clinical evaluation to develop a solid diagnostic impression of the patient.
    B. Meet the needs of a third party whose goals are legal or financial.
    C. Ensure that the patient's needs are foremost while conducting the evaluation.
    D. Ensure patient confidentiality, beneficence, and nonmaleficence
    E. None of the above.

**The correct response is option B.**

Forensic evaluators are retained by third parties whose goals are not clinical but legal or financial. Those third parties may have adverse effects on the evaluee's legal or financial interests, such as prosecution, incarceration, and loss of child custody. Forensic evaluators adopt an objective and skeptical approach to the evaluee's self-report and presentation and seek input from collateral sources of information as well as testing. Options A and C are incorrect because unlike in usual psychiatric evaluations, the focus of a forensic evaluation must not be the evaluation and treatment of the patient. Option D is incorrect because due to the purpose of the forensic evaluation, confidentiality must be breached to provide information to the third parties. In addition, nonmaleficence and beneficence may not be guaranteed because the results of the evaluation may cause financial or legal harm to the patient.

Simon RI, Gold LG: The American Psychiatric Publishing Textbook of Forensic Psychiatry. Washington, DC, American Psychiatric Publishing, pp 139–140

180. A 32-year-old woman presents to the emergency room with new onset of myoclonic jerking of her extremities, flushing, fever, nausea, and tremor after she took one dose of sumatriptan that she had recently been prescribed for migraine headaches. Besides sumatriptan, her medication list includes sertraline 100 mg/day, which she has been taking for the past 3 years for a mild depressive disorder. Which of the following medications will likely be of benefit for this patient at this time?

    A. Benztropine.
    B. Propranolol.
    C. Dantrolene.
    D. Phenobarbital.
    E. Lorazepam.

**The correct response is option E.**

The patient has serotonin syndrome caused by the additive effects of the selective serotonin reuptake inhibitor (SSRI) sertraline and sumatriptan, also a potent inhibitor of serotonin reuptake. Sumatriptan also nonspecifically mobilizes more serotonin to bind with multiple postsynaptic serotonin receptors, including the 5-HT$_{1D}$ receptor, for which sumatriptan is a potent agonist. The combination of increased mobilization of serotonin binding and sumatriptan's specific 5-HT$_{1D}$ agonist effect produced serotonin syndrome, the symptoms of which typically resolve after 24–48 hours of treatment with a benzodiazepine such as lorazepam. Options A, B, C, and D are incorrect because these medications are indicated for other drug-induced conditions, not serotonin syndrome: benztropine or diphenhydramine for acute dystonic reaction or neuroleptic malignant syndrome (NMS), propranolol for akathisia, dantrolene for malignant hyperthermia (e.g., in NMS), and phenobarbital for sedative-hypnotic withdrawal.

Martinez M, Marangell LB, Martinez JM: Psychopharmacology, in The American Psychiatric Publishing Textbook Textbook of Psychiatry, 5th Edition. Edited by Hales RE, Yudofsky SC, Gabbard GO. Washington, DC, American Psychiatric Publishing, 2008, p 1091

Sandson NB: Drug-Drug Interaction Primer: A Compendium of Case Vignettes for the Practicing Clinician. Washington, DC, American Psychiatric Publishing, 2007, p 204

181. A diagnosis of personality disorder in elderly persons is subject to some specific clinical and epidemiological considerations. Which of the following is *true?*

    A. The prevalence of personality disorders in the elderly population is approximately the same as in younger patients, about 10%.
    B. The prevalence of personality disorders among elderly patients with another psychiatric condition is between 25% and 65%.
    C. In the older population, the association between personality and anxiety disorders is the most often reported comorbidity.
    D. Cluster B personality disorders do not improve with age.
    E. The association between comorbid personality disorder and mood disorder is stronger for late-onset than for early-onset depression.

**The correct response is option B.**

The prevalence of personality disorders in older patients with other psychiatric conditions is between 25% and 65%. The prevalence of personality disorders is lower (by about half) in older persons generally compared with younger persons. Cluster B personality disorders improve with age. The association of personality disorders with depressive disorders in the elderly population is probably the single most reported comorbidity and is higher for early-onset than for late-onset depression.

Oxman TE, Ferrell RB: Personality disorders, in The American Psychiatric Publishing Textbook of Geriatric Psychiatry, 3rd Edition. Edited by Blazer DG, Steffens DC, Busse EW. Washington, DC, American Psychiatric Publishing, 2004, pp 370–371

182. Which of the following statements is *true* regarding the differential diagnosis of childhood psychotic disorders?

    A. The diagnostic criteria for schizophreniform disorder require an illness duration of less than 6 months.
    B. Once a diagnosis of schizophreniform disorder is made, a diagnosis of schizophrenia can never be given.
    C. A diagnosis of schizophreniform disorder requires the presence of a decline in function.
    D. Brief psychotic disorder requires a symptom duration of at least 1 month but no more than 6 months.
    E. The diagnosis of psychotic disorder not otherwise specified is very rare in the hospitalized adolescent population.

**The correct response is option A.**

To qualify for a schizophreniform disorder diagnosis, a child must have an illness duration of less than 6 months. With time, a child with schizophreniform disorder may warrant a diagnosis of schizophrenia. Option B is incorrect because schizophreniform disorder may progress to schizophrenia. Option C is incorrect because by definition schizophreniform disorder does not require a decline in function. Option D is incorrect because brief psychotic disorder lasts longer than 1 day but less than 1 month. Option E is incorrect because a diagnosis of psychotic disorder not otherwise specified is common in the hospitalized adolescent population.

Tsai LK, Champine DJ: Schizophrenia and other psychotic disorders, in The American Psychiatric Publishing Textbook of Child and Adolescent Psychiatry, 3rd Edition. Edited by Wiener JM, Dulcan MK. Washington, DC, American Psychiatric Publishing, 2004, p 391

| DSM-IV-TR diagnosis | Duration | Characteristics |
|---|---|---|
| Brief psychotic disorder | >1 day–<1 month | Usually follow severe stress. |
| Schizophreniform disorder | >1 month, <6 months | No decline in functioning. Good prognostic features: 1) onset of prominent psychotic symptoms within 4 weeks of the first noticeable change in usual behavior or functioning; 2) confusion or perplexity at the height of the psychotic episode; 3) good premorbid social and occupational functioning; and 4) absence of blunted or flat affect. |

183. Which of the following statements is *true* regarding patterns of abuse and dependence for different classes of drugs?

    A. The age at highest risk for marijuana and alcohol initiation is between 14 and 17 years.
    B. The age at highest risk for dependence on alcohol is between 24 and 26 years.
    C. The age at highest risk for dependence on marijuana is 3 years older than the corresponding age at risk for alcohol dependence.
    D. The age at highest risk for cocaine initiation is between 15 and 18 years.
    E. The developmental period for alcohol dependence is longer than those for marijuana and cocaine dependence.

**The correct response is option E.**

The developmental period for becoming alcohol dependent seems to be substantially longer than the developmental period for marijuana and cocaine dependence. Using data from the National Comorbidity Survey, Wagner and Anthony (2002) reported that the highest risk for initiating alcohol and marijuana use occurs at around age 18 years, and the highest risk for cocaine initiation occurs at around age 20 years. In addition, a greater percentage of the population is at risk for alcohol initiation than for marijuana and cocaine initiation, and this risk is spread out over a longer age span. The highest risk for meeting dependence criteria, as defined by DSM-III-R, for the entire population was estimated to occur between ages 20 and 21 years for alcohol, between ages 17 and 18 years for marijuana, and between ages 24 and 26 years for cocaine. The approximate period for developing marijuana dependence was completed by age 30 years and for developing cocaine dependence was completed by age 35 years, and the risk of developing alcohol dependence extended through midlife.

Brook JS, Pahl K, Rubenstone E: Epidemiology of addiction, in The American Psychiatric Publishing Textbook of Substance Abuse Treatment, 4th Edition. Edited by Galanter M, Kleber HD. Washington, DC, American Psychiatric Publishing, 2008, p 32

Wagner FA, Anthony JC: From first drug use to drug dependence: developmental periods of risk for dependence upon marijuana, cocaine, and alcohol. Neuropsychopharmacology 26:479–488, 2002

184. Outpatient therapy as an initial approach has the *best* chance of success in patients with anorexia nervosa who

    A. Have had the illness for more than 6 months.
    B. Are bingeing.
    C. Are vomiting.
    D. Have medical complications.
    E. Have parents who will participate in family therapy.

**The correct response is option E.**

Outpatient therapy as an initial approach has the best chance for success in patients with anorexia who 1) have had the illness for less than 6 months, 2) are not bingeing and vomiting, and 3) have parents who are likely to cooperate and effectively participate in family therapy. The more severely ill patient with anorexia may present an extremely difficult medical management challenge and should be hospitalized and undergo daily monitoring of weight, food and calorie intake, and urine output.

Halmi KA: Eating disorders, in The American Psychiatric Publishing Textbook of Psychiatry, 5th Edition. Edited by Hales RE, Yudofsky SC, Gabbard GO. Washington, DC, American Psychiatric Publishing, 2008, p 980

185. Which of the following structures is *not* involved in the central processing of pain?

    A. Spinothalamic tracts.
    B. Anterior cingulate gyrus.
    C. Insular cortex.
    D. Prefrontal cortex.
    E. Somatosensory cortex.

**The correct response is option A.**

Central processing does not involve the spinothalamic tracts. Cortical or central processing involves several key areas: the anterior cingulate gyrus and the insular, prefrontal, inferior parietal, primary and secondary somatosensory, primary motor, and premotor cortices. Disruption of any of these pathways may lead to the perception of pain. The neuromatrix model states that the pain experience itself is created as a matrix of perception, modulated by multiple components with the central nervous system. This matrix includes three key components: ascending modulation within the spinal cord, central processing, or descending inhibition.

Golianu, B, Bhandari R, Shaw RJ, et al: Neuropsychiatric aspects of pain management, in The American Psychiatric Publishing Textbook of Neuropsychiatry and Behavioral Neurosciences, 5th Edition. Edited by Yudofsky SC, Hales RE. Washington, DC, American Psychiatric Publishing, 2008, pp 366–367

186. A number of macroscopic and histological findings in the brain of patients with schizophrenia have been reported. For which of the following findings has the evidence been confirmed by meta-analysis and reported to be strong?

    A. Maldistribution of white matter neurons.
    B. Decreased thalamic volume.
    C. Reduced synaptic and dendritic markers in hippocampus.
    D. Entorhinal cortex dysplasia.
    E. Enlarged lateral and third ventricles.

**The correct response is option E.**

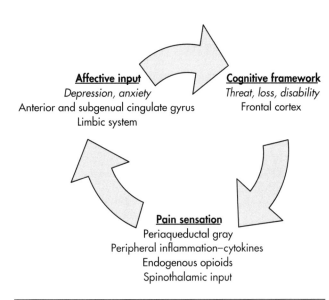

**The circuitous, mutually reinforcing nature of the pain experience: the neuromatrix model includes three key components—ascending modulation with the spinal cord, central processing, and descending inhibition.**
*Source.* Golianu, B, Bhandari R, Shaw RJ, et al.: "Neuropsychiatric Aspects of Pain Management," in *The American Psychiatric Publishing Textbook of Neuropsychiatry and Behavioral Neurosciences,* 5th Edition. Edited by Yudofsky SC, Hales RE. Washington, DC, American Psychiatric Publishing, 2008, p. 366.

Evidence for enlarged lateral and third ventricles in schizophrenia is strong and has been confirmed by meta-analysis. Although evidence for decreased thalamic volume and reduced synaptic and dendritic markers in the hippocampus is good, these findings have not been confirmed by meta-analysis. Only moderate evidence has been reported for maldistribution of white matter neurons, and the evidence for entorhinal cortex dysplasia is weak.

Minzenberg MJ, Yoon JH, Carter CS: Schizophrenia, in The American Psychiatric Publishing Textbook of Psychiatry, 5th Edition. Edited by Hales RE, Yudofsky SC, Gabbard GO. Washington, DC, American Psychiatric Publishing, 2008, p 432, Table 10–6

187. Which of the following statements is *true* regarding epidemiological findings in somatization disorder?

A. Somatization disorder is diagnosed predominantly in men.
B. The lifetime risk of somatization disorder is estimated at 10% in women.
C. Somatization disorder in men shares a common etiology with antisocial personality disorder.

D. Somatization disorder in women may be related more to anxiety disorder.
E. Some authors believe that somatization disorder may be more of a personality disorder than an Axis I disorder.

**The correct response is option E.**

Studies in the 1990s support the hypothesis that somatization disorder is more of a personality disorder than an Axis I disorder. Option A is incorrect because somatization disorder is diagnosed predominantly in women and rarely in men. Option B is incorrect because the lifetime risk for somatization disorder was estimated at about 2% in women. In women, somatization disorder seems to share a common etiology with antisocial personality disorder; in men, this disorder appears to be related to anxiety.

Yutzy SH, Parish BS: Somatoform disorders, in The American Psychiatric Publishing Textbook of Psychiatry, 5th Edition. Edited by Hales RE, Yudofsky SC, Gabbard GO. Washington, DC, American Psychiatric Publishing, 2008, pp 618–620

188. Which of the following criteria is found in the diagnosis of substance dependence but *not* substance abuse?

A. Tolerance and withdrawal.
B. Recurrent substance-related failure in fulfilling social role obligations.
C. Recurrent substance use in physically hazardous circumstances.
D. Recurrent substance-related legal problems.
E. Continued substance use despite social/interpersonal problems.

**The correct response is option A.**

DSM-IV-TR criteria indicate that tolerance and withdrawal are characteristic of substance dependence, not substance abuse. The remaining characteristics listed above pertain to DSM-IV-TR criteria for substance abuse.

Greenfield SF, Hennessy G: Assessment of the patient, in The American Psychiatric Publishing Textbook of Substance Abuse Treatment, 4th Edition. Edited by Galanter M, Kleber HD. Washington, DC, American Psychiatric Publishing, 2008, pp 59–60, 61; Tables 5–1 and 5–2

189. Which of the following statements is *true* regarding anorexia nervosa?

    A. Obsessive-compulsive behavior rarely develops after the onset of anorexia nervosa.
    B. There is a relatively frequent association with impulsive behavior, such as suicide attempts and self-mutilation, among individuals with the bulimic type of anorexia.
    C. Amenorrhea occurs after noticeable weight loss.
    D. Most adolescent anorexia patients do not have delayed psychosexual development.
    E. Patients with the restrictive type of anorexia are more likely to have a discrete personality disorder diagnosis.

**The correct response is option B.**

There is a relatively frequent association with impulsive behavior such as suicide attempts, self-mutilation, stealing, and substance abuse among bulimic individuals with anorexia. Obsessive-compulsive behavior often develops after the onset of anorexia nervosa. Amenorrhea can appear before noticeable weight loss occurred. Many adolescent patients with anorexia have delayed psychosocial sexual development. Bulimic patients with anorexia are more likely to have discrete personality disorder diagnoses.

Halmi KA: Eating disorders, in The American Psychiatric Publishing Textbook of Psychiatry, 5th Edition. Edited by Hales RE, Yudofsky SC, Gabbard GO. Washington, DC, American Psychiatric Publishing, 2008, p 974

190. Within central processing, the "medial" system is responsible for generating the affective/emotional component of pain, whereas the "lateral" system is responsible for the discriminative sensory components. Which of the following structures is part of the medial system?

    A. Primary somatosensory cortex (SI).
    B. Secondary somatosensory cortex (SII).
    C. Anterior cingulate.
    D. Parietal cortex.
    E. Premotor cortex.

**The correct response is option C.**

The anterior cingulate and the insular cortex are thought to be a part of the "medial pain system," responsible for generating the affective/emotional component of pain.

The medial pain system, along with the lateral pain system, is theorized to be involved in the remodeling that takes place over time that makes treatment of pain increasingly difficult.

Options A, B, and D are incorrect because the primary and secondary somatosensory (SI and SII) cortex and the parietal cortex form the "lateral" pain system, which is thought to be involved in the discriminative sensory components of pain. Option E is incorrect because the premotor cortex is part of cortical, or central, processing of pain. Other structures involved in central processing include the anterior cingulate gyrus and insular, prefrontal, inferior parietal, primary motor, and SI and SII cortex.

Golianu, B, Bhandari R, Shaw RJ, et al: Neuropsychiatric aspects of pain management, in The American Psychiatric Publishing Textbook of Neuropsychiatry and Behavioral Neurosciences, 5th Edition. Edited by Yudofsky SC, Hales RE. Washington, DC, American Psychiatric Publishing, 2008, pp 366–367

191. A 39-year-old male patient presenting to an outpatient clinic has falsely believed for the past 4–5 years that he is a professional football player. He describes in detail a few of his best plays as a quarterback for the Chicago Bears. He has told similar tales for the past few years and denies other psychotic symptoms. The introverted single man has lived alone in the same apartment for the past 7 years and has counted parts in the inventory department for the same company during that time. His symptoms have been refractory to previous treatments. On the basis of this limited clinical information, the most likely diagnosis is

    A. Paranoid schizophrenia.
    B. Schizophreniform disorder.
    C. Brief psychotic disorder.
    D. Delusional disorder.
    E. Schizoaffective disorder.

**The correct response is option D.**

In delusional disorder, the psychosis is confined to one or more delusions, usually nonbizarre, as in this case; function remains largely intact; there is minimal decline in function or change in symptoms over time; and symptoms are more refractory to treatment than in schizophrenia.

For paranoid schizophrenia, schizophrenia disorder, brief psychotic disorder, and schizoaffective disorder, the psychosis is exhibited by two or more characteristic symptoms: delusions, hallucinations, disorganized speech, grossly diorganized behavior, and negative symptoms. There is also a significant decline in fuctioning.

Minzenberg MJ, Yoon JH, Carter CS: Schizophrenia, in The American Psychiatric Publishing Textbook of Psychiatry, 5th Edition. Edited by Hales RE, Yudofsky SC, Gabbard GO. Washington, DC, American Psychiatric Publishing, 2008, pp 420–421; Table 10–5

192. Several psychological factors have been implicated in conversion disorder, and terminology has evolved to describe these factors. The description "Anxiety is reduced by keeping an internal conflict out of conscious awareness through production of a symptom that is involuntarily produced and not under conscious control" applies to which of the following terms?

    A. Primary gain.
    B. Secondary gain.
    C. Tertiary gain.
    D. La belle indifférence.
    E. Factitious disorder.

**The correct response is option A.**

In *primary gain*, anxiety is theoretically reduced by keeping an internal conflict or need out of conscious awareness through production of a symptom; the symptom is involuntarily produced and not under conscious control. Several psychological factors have been implicated in the pathogenesis, or at least pathophysiology, of conversion disorder. *Conversion* refers to the hypothesized transformation of a psychological conflict into a somatic complaint. In *secondary gain*, the symptom is voluntarily produced and under conscious control; production is for the purpose of a goal, such as avoiding work or obtaining money (i.e., malingering). In the phenomenon termed *la belle indifférence*, the individual seems indifferent to or disinterested in personal medical issues that should concern him or her.

Yutzy SH, Parish BS: Somatoform disorders, in The American Psychiatric Publishing Textbook of Psychiatry, 5th Edition. Edited by Hales RE, Yudofsky SC, Gabbard GO. Washington, DC, American Psychiatric Publishing, 2008, p 628; Table 13–10

193. Regarding family factors and substance abuse among youth, which of the following is *not* considered a characteristic that is related to the incidence of substance abuse?

    A. Parental level of income.
    B. Parental substance dependence.
    C. Parental personality.
    D. Parent–child relationship.
    E. Family cohesion.

**The correct response is option A.**

Parental level of income is not a factor in the incidence of juvenile substance abuse. Research has identified several aspects of the family environment that are consistently related to substance use, abuse, or dependence, including the factors listed in options B, C, D, and E.

Brook JS, Pahl K, Rubenstone E: Epidemiology of addiction, in The American Psychiatric Publishing Textbook of Substance Abuse Treatment, 4th Edition. Edited by Galanter M, Kleber HD. Washington, DC, American Psychiatric Publishing, 2008, p 35

194. Which of the following statements is *false* regarding trichotillomania?

    A. Psychiatric comorbidity is quite common among adults with trichotillomania.
    B. The prevalence of clinically significant hair pulling among college students has been estimated to be 1%–3.5%.
    C. Approximately 75% of adult trichotillomania patients report that most of their hair-pulling behavior takes place outside of awareness.
    D. Individuals with trichotillomania often report that hair pulling is painful.
    E. Hair pulling is often preceded by negative internal states involving unpleasant emotions, aversive physiological sensations, or dysregulated arousal.

**The correct response is option D.**

Individuals with trichotillomania often report that hair pulling is not painful and pleasurable for some individuals. Psychiatric comorbidity is quite common among adults with trichotillomania. Of the patients with comorbid disorders, there was a lifetime prevalence rate of 65% for mood disorders, 57% for anxiety disorders, 22% for substance abuse disorders, 20% for eating disorders, and 42% for personality disorders. The most frequently cited comorbid personality disorders are histrionic, borderline, and obsessive-compulsive. In studies involving college samples, 10%–13% of students reported hair pulling, with the prevalence of clinically significant pulling ranging between 1% and 3.5%. Approximately 75% of adult trichotillomania patients report that most of their hair-pulling behavior takes place "automatically" or outside of awareness, whereas the remaining 25% describe themselves as primarily focused on hair pulling when they pull. Hair pulling is often preceded by negative internal states such as unpleasant emotions, aversive physiological sensations, or dysregulated arousal.

Hollander E, Berlin HA, Stein DJ: Impulse-control disorders not elsewhere classified, in The American Psychiatric Publishing Textbook of Psychiatry, 5th Edition. Edited by Hales RE, Yudofsky SC, Gabbard GO. Washington, DC, American Psychiatric Publishing, 2008, pp 801, 803, 804

195. All of the following statements are true regarding the relationship between pain and mood disorders *except*

    A. Patients with pain score higher on measures of depression than do patients without pain.
    B. In cancer patients, depressive symptoms are more highly correlated with pain than with a history of previous clinical depression.
    C. Depression is the most common psychiatric diagnosis among chronic pain patients.
    D. The presence or absence of mood symptoms has a differential effect on the opioid responsiveness of pain.
    E. Emotional aspects of pain, such as depression, are modulated by the insular cortex.

**The correct response is option E.**

The emotional aspects of pain are mediated by the anterior cingulate gyrus in conjunction with amygdala and limbic structures, whereas the sensory aspects are controlled by the parietal and insular cortices. Patients with pain score higher on measures of depression, anxiety, and other signs of mood disturbance than those with little or no pain. The presence of significant pain among cancer patients is more strongly associated with major depressive symptoms than is a prior life history of depression. Depression is the most frequently reported psychiatric diagnosis among chronic pain patients. In a study conducted by Wasan et al. in 2004, 48% of patients with a low level of psychiatric symptoms had a good response to opioid analgesia, whereas only 20% of patients with a high level of psychiatric symptoms experienced relief.

Golianu B, Bhandari R, Shaw RJ, et al: Neuropsychiatric aspects of pain management, in The American Psychiatric Publishing Textbook of Neuropsychiatry and Behavioral Neurosciences, 5th Edition. Edited by Yudofsky SC, Hales RE. Washington, DC, American Psychiatric Publishing, 2008, pp 368–369

Wasan A, Davar G, Jamison R, et al: Psychiatric comorbidity diminishes opioid analgesia in patients with discogenic low back pain (abstract no 845). J Pain 5 (suppl 1):S70, 2004

196. Which of the five subtypes of schizophrenia is associated with better premorbid functioning, older age at onset, and higher social and occupational function after illness onset?

    A. Catatonic.
    B. Disorganized.
    C. Paranoid.
    D. Residual.
    E. Undifferentiated.

**The correct response is option C.**

Research suggests that compared with other subtypes, *paranoid schizophrenia* has better premorbid functioning, an older age at onset, higher social and occupational function after illness onset, and fewer cognitive and affective deficits. The diagnosis of *catatonic schizophrenia*, made when catatonia is the most prominent clinical feature, requires the presence of at least two of the following: immobility (cataplexy or stupor); motor hyperactivity without purpose or external influence; extreme negativism or mutism; peculiar voluntary movement or postures, stereotyped movements, or prominent mannerisms or grimacing; and echophenomena (echolalia or echopraxia). *Disorganized schizophrenia* is associated with earlier onset, low levels of social and occupational functioning, and poor long-term prognosis. *Undifferentiated schizophrenia* is the most frequently encountered subtype in clinical practice. *Residual schizophrenia* is thought to represent a relatively attenuated state of schizophrenia in which the positive symptoms are relatively quiescent or less symptomatic.

Minzenberg MJ, Yoon JH, Carter CS: Schizophrenia, in The American Psychiatric Publishing Textbook of Psychiatry, 5th Edition. Edited by Hales RE, Yudofsky SC, Gabbard GO. Washington, DC, American Psychiatric Publishing, 2008, pp 416–418

197. In a patient who presents with a preoccupation with an imagined defect in appearance or markedly excessive concern with a slight physical anomaly, what is the most likely diagnosis?

   A. Hypochondriasis.
   B. Undifferentiated somatoform disorder.
   C. Conversion disorder.
   D. Body dysmorphic disorder.
   E. Somatoform disorder not otherwise specified.

**The correct response is option D.**

Body dysmorphic disorder is a preoccupation (possibly of delusional intensity) with an imagined defect in appearance or markedly excessive concern with a slight physical anomaly. Hypochondriasis is the preoccupation with fears of having a serious disease based on the misinterpretation of bodily symptoms. Undifferentiated somatoform disorder is diagnosed when the patient has one or more physical complaints. Conversion disorder is characterized by symptoms or deficits affecting voluntary motor or sensory function, suggesting a neurological or other general medical condition. Somatoform disorder not otherwise specified includes disorders with specified somatoform symptoms such as pseudocyesis, disorders of less than 6 months duration with fatigue or body weakness, nonpsychotic hypochondrical symptoms, or other physical complaints.

Yutzy SH, Parish BS: Somatoform disorders, in The American Psychiatric Publishing Textbook of Psychiatry, 5th Edition. Edited by Hales RE, Yudofsky SC, Gabbard GO. Washington, DC, American Psychiatric Publishing, 2008, pp 610–611; Table 13–1

198. Among the following classes of substance use disorders, which one was reported by the National Epidemiologic Survey on Alcohol and Related Conditions to have the highest rate of occurrence, at 2% of the population?

   A. Sedatives.
   B. Tranquilizers.
   C. Opioids.
   D. Amphetamines.
   E. Benzodiazepines.

**The correct response is option D.**

According to findings of the 2006 National Epidemiologic Survey on Alcohol and Related Conditions, the lifetime prevalence of sedative, tranquilizer, opioid, and amphetamine use disorders, as assessed by DSM-IV-TR criteria, were 1.1%, 1%, 1.4%, and 2%, respectively. Lifetime prevalence of benzodiazepine use was not reported.

Brook JS, Pahl K, Rubenstone E: Epidemiology of addiction, in The American Psychiatric Publishing Textbook of Substance Abuse Treatment, 4th Edition. Edited by Galanter M, Kleber HD. Washington, DC, American Psychiatric Publishing, 2008, p 30

199. All of the following statements concerning lateral specialization are true *except*

   A. In the vast majority of people, the left hemisphere is specialized for language and for processing verbally coded information.
   B. The right hemisphere processes nonverbal information such as visual patterns or auditory signals.
   C. The left hemisphere is specialized for the perception of our bodies in space.
   D. The right hemisphere is dedicated to the mapping of feeling states.
   E. The left hemisphere is involved in the processing of verbal information apprehended through either auditory or visual channels.

**The correct response is option C.**

The left and right hemispheres of the human brain differ in several fundamental ways. The right hemisphere is specialized for the perception of our bodies in space. In the vast majority of adults, the left side of the brain is specialized for language and for processing verbally coded information. This is true of nearly all (88%) right-handed individuals, the majority (75%) of left-handed persons, and 43% of mixed-handed persons. Thus, verbal information learned through either the auditory or visual channel is processed preferentially by the left hemisphere. The right hemisphere processes nonverbal information such as complex visual patterns or auditory signals that are not coded in verbal form, and it is also dedicated to the mapping of feeling states.

Harel BT, Tranel D: Functional neuroanatomy, in The American Psychiatric Publishing Textbook of Neuropsychiatry and Behavioral Neurosciences, 5th Edition. Edited by Yudofsky SC, Hales RE. Washington, DC, American Psychiatric Publishing, 2008, pp 46–47

200. The MATRICS (measurement and treatment research to improve cognition in schizophrenia) program was developed to identify potential molecular targets to treat cognitive deficits in schizophrenia (Geyer and Tamminga 2004). The molecular targets identified as having the greatest promise to improve cognition include all of the following *except*

    A. Dopamine$_1$ (D$_1$) receptor.
    B. Dopamine$_2$ (D$_2$) receptor.
    C. $\alpha_7$ Nicotinic receptor.
    D. Muscarinic receptor.
    E. *N*-methyl-D-aspartate (NMDA) receptor.

**The correct response is option B.**

The D$_2$ receptor has not been identified as a molecular target to treat cognitive deficits in schizophrenia.

The D$_1$ receptor, the $\alpha_7$ nicotinic receptor, the muscarinic receptor, the 5-hydroxytryptamine$_{1A}$ (5-HT$_{1A}$) and 5-HT$_{2A}$ receptors, the noradrenergic receptors, and the NMDA receptor are believed to have the greatest promise as potential molecular targets in treating cognitive deficits in schizophrenia.

Geyer MA, Tamminga CA: Measurement and treatment research to improve cognition in schizophrenia: neuropharmacological aspects. Psychopharmacology (Berl) 174:1–2, 2004

Tamminga CA, Shad MJ, Ghose S: Neuropsychiatric aspects of schizophrenia, in The American Psychiatric Publishing Textbook of Neuropsychiatry and Behavioral Neurosciences, 5th Edition. Edited by Yudofsky SC, Hales RE. Washington, DC, American Psychiatric Publishing, 2008, p 986

201. Which of the following is a warning sign for factitious disorder by proxy?

    A. The episodes of illness occur only when the child is alone with the parent.
    B. The other parent is quite involved with the care of the child.
    C. The parent refuses painful or risky diagnostic tests for the child.

    D. Signs and symptoms occur even when the child is separated from the parent.
    E. There is a negative personal history of factitious disorder in the parent.

**The correct response is option A.**

In factitious disorder by proxy, episodes occur only when the child is, or has recently been, alone with the parent. The following clusters of warning signs can suggest a diagnosis of factitious disorder by proxy:

- The episodes of illness occur only when the child is, or has recently been, alone with the parent.
- The parent has taken the child to numerous caregivers, resulting in multiple diagnostic evaluations but neither cure nor definitive diagnosis.
- The other parent (usually the father) is notably uninvolved despite the ostensive health crises.
- It has been proven that the parent has provided false information to health care professionals or others.
- The parent continually advocates for painful or risky diagnostic tests for the child.
- The child persistently fails to tolerate or respond to usual medical therapies.
- Signs and symptoms abate or do not occur when the child is separated from the parent.
- Another child in the family has had unexplained illness or childhood death.
- The parent has a personal history of factitious disorder.

McDermott BE, Leamon MH, Feldman MD, et al: Factitious disorder and malingering, in The American Psychiatric Publishing Textbook of Psychiatry, 5th Edition. Edited by Hales RE, Yudofsky SC, Gabbard GO. Washington, DC, American Psychiatric Publishing, 2008, pp 650, 651; Table 14–4

202. Various personality characteristics have been associated with substance abuse and dependence. Which of the following personality characteristics is *not* associated with increased risk of substance abuse?

    A. Risk taking.
    B. Novelty seeking.
    C. Impulsivity.
    D. Lack of emotional control.
    E. Secure interpersonal attachment with dependency.

## The correct response is option E.

Three dimensions of an individual's personality and psychiatric disorders have been found to be related to substance use, abuse, and dependence. The first personality dimension encompasses an orientation toward risk taking and sensation- or novelty-seeking behavior. The second personality dimension consists of a relative lack of emotional control. Individuals who were impulsive and lacked emotional control were more likely to abuse or be dependent on alcohol or drugs. The third personality dimension associated with drug use, abuse, and dependence is interpersonal relatedness. Individuals who have problems establishing or maintaining relationships with others are at elevated risk for drug abuse or dependence.

Brook JS, Pahl K, Rubenstone E: Epidemiology of addiction, in The American Psychiatric Publishing Textbook of Substance Abuse Treatment, 4th Edition. Edited by Galanter M, Kleber HD. Washington, DC, American Psychiatric Publishing, 2008, pp 33–34

203. Which of the following descriptors characterizes the Munchausen subtype of factitious disorder?

    A. Patients are mostly young women.
    B. Patients have been described as passive and immature.
    C. Most patients have single-system complaints.
    D. Multiple hospitalizations with dramatic and often life-threatening presentations are prominent.
    E. Many patients have health-related jobs.

## The correct response is option D.

About 10% of patients with factitious disorder manifest the Munchausen presentation. In this subtype of factitious disorder, multiple hospitalizations with dramatic and often life-threatening presentation, wandering from hospital to hospital (peregrination), and pathological lying (pseudologia fantastica, the telling of dramatic tales that merge truth and falsehood and that the listener initially finds intriguing) are prominent. The vast majority of cases of factitious disorder are of the non-Munchausen type. Patients with this type are mostly young women with conforming lifestyles and more family support and involvement than Munchausen patients. Non-Munchausen patients have been described as passive and immature, and a significant proportion have health-related jobs or training. Most have single-system complaints, are not wanderers, and generate fewer hospitalizations than do

Munchausen patients (although the overall severity and morbidity of their illness may be just as great).

McDermott BE, Leamon MH, Feldman MD, et al: Factitious disorder and malingering, in The American Psychiatric Publishing Textbook of Psychiatry, 5th Edition. Edited by Hales RE, Yudofsky SC, Gabbard GO. Washington, DC, American Psychiatric Publishing, 2008, pp 644–645

204. Which of the following statements is *false* regarding mood disorders and substance abuse?

    A. Both unipolar and bipolar mood disorders are associated with increased risk of substance abuse/dependence.
    B. Dysthymic disorder is associated with an increased risk of substance abuse/dependence.
    C. Mood disorder patients have a higher rate of abuse of alcohol, tranquilizers, and stimulants.
    D. There is a reciprocal relationship between mood disorders and substance abuse; some studies demonstrate that depression precedes substance abuse, whereas other studies demonstrate the opposite.
    E. Comorbid depression and substance use disorders are associated with greater functional impairment but not worse treatment outcomes.

## The correct response is option E.

Comorbid depression and substance use disorders are associated with greater functional impairment and worse treatment outcomes. Major depressive disorder, bipolar disorder, dysthymic disorder, and depressed mood are highly comorbid with substance use disorders. There is evidence of a reciprocal relationship between affective disorders and substance use disorders.

Brook JS, Pahl K, Rubenstone E: Epidemiology of addiction, in The American Psychiatric Publishing Textbook of Substance Abuse Treatment, 4th Edition. Edited by Galanter M, Kleber HD. Washington, DC, American Psychiatric Publishing, 2008, p 34

205. Patients with delirium typically exhibit abnormalities in all of the following language functions *except*

    A. Writing.
    B. Word-list generation.
    C. Motor speech.
    D. Automatic speech.
    E. Content of speech.

## The correct response is option D.

Automatic speech is normal in delirious patients. Options A, B, C, and E are incorrect because they reflect true statements about language functions in patients with delirium.

Mendez MF, Clark DG: Neuropsychiatric aspects of aphasia and related disorders, in The American Psychiatric Publishing Textbook of Neuropsychiatry and Behavioral Neurosciences, 5th Edition. Edited by Yudofsky SC, Hales RE. Washington, DC, American Psychiatric Publishing, 2008, p 525; Table 12–2

206. Positron emission tomography (PET) scanning in hallucinating persons with schizophrenia has provided clues to the anatomic structures that may be involved in a "psychosis neural circuit." The proposed psychosis circuit consists of all of the following structures *except*

A. Amygdala.
B. Medial prefrontal cortex.
C. Thalamus.
D. Anterior hippocampus.
E. Anterior cingulate.

## The correct response is option A.

The amygdala is not involved in the proposed "psychosis neural circuit"; rather, it is implicated in the emotional processing of schizophrenia and is believed to be involved in a "negative affect neural circuit." The proposed psychosis circuit consists of the anterior hippocampus, anterior cingulate, medial prefrontal cortex, thalamus, ventral pallidum, striatum, and substantia nigra/ventral tegmental area. PET scanning in hallucinating persons with schizophrenia has found activations in the medial prefrontal cortex, left superior temporal gyrus, right medial temporal gyrus, left hippocampus/parahippocampal region, thalamus, putamen, and cingulate. These studies provide clues to the anatomic structures that may be involved in a "psychosis neural circuit."

Tamminga CA, Shad MJ, Ghose S: Neuropsychiatric aspects of schizophrenia, in The American Psychiatric Publishing Textbook of Neuropsychiatry and Behavioral Neurosciences, 5th Edition. Edited by Yudofsky SC, Hales RE. Washington, DC, American Psychiatric Publishing, 2008, pp 987, 988; Figure 26–4

# Exam 2

*Select the single best response for each question.*

1. Which of the following is not one of Eugen Bleuler's "four As" of schizophrenia?

    A. Affective flattening.
    B. Alogia.
    C. Ambivalence.
    D. Loosening of associations.
    E. Autism.

2. Which of the following physical signs is *not* characteristic of opioid withdrawal?

    A. Dysphoria.
    B. Muscle aches.
    C. Nausea and vomiting.
    D. Miotic ("pinpoint") pupils.
    E. Piloerection (gooseflesh).

3. Which of the following criteria is *not* necessary in order to diagnose factitious disorder?

    A. Intentional production of physical or psychological signs and symptoms.
    B. Unconscious production of signs or symptoms.
    C. Motivation to assume the sick role.
    D. Absence of external incentives beyond assumption of the sick role.
    E. Factitious symptoms of predominantly physical or psychological origin.

4. Which of the following is a definition of acculturation?

    A. A diversity of cultural backgrounds, in which people from each background share a common national culture.
    B. Identity with a natural and/or shared language of origin, religious practice, dress, diet, holidays, family rituals, and leisure activities.

    C. The accumulative social learning process in which people assimilate the values of the host culture while retaining the values of the original culture.
    D. The comparison of characteristics across culture groups.
    E. Distinct groupings resulting, for example in the context of addiction, from substance use, abuse, or dependence.

5. A 72-year-old woman lost two brothers to cancer, one 12 months ago and the other 10 months ago. Following each loss, the woman experienced a 3- to 4-week period of mildly depressed mood and sleep disturbance, and had visual hallucinations of her brothers walking around in her home. Eight months ago, she voluntarily retired from running a small business that she thoroughly enjoyed for the previous 20 years in order to spend more time with her grandchildren. Two months later, this formerly physically and socially active woman underwent routine urologic surgery that led to multiple medical complications and has prevented her from participating in a bowling league and other activities. She denies depressed mood, but family members have noticed that in the past 6 months she has been more "weepy" than usual, crying at the slightest provocation; watches television all day, rarely leaving the house; and does not seem to be as talkative as before. Of the following, which is the *most* likely current diagnosis?

    A. Bereavement and major depressive disorder.
    B. Chronic adjustment disorder with depressed mood.
    C. Acute adjustment disorder with depressed mood.
    D. Bereavement and adjustment disorder with depressed mood.
    E. Major depressive disorder.

796 THE AMERICAN PSYCHIATRIC PUBLISHING BOARD REVIEW GUIDE FOR PSYCHIATRY

6. Which of the following statements is *true* regarding selective mutism?

   A. Most children with selective mutism do not meet DSM-IV-TR criteria for either social phobia or avoidant disorder.
   B. Social situations are usually difficult to dichotomize into mute versus nonmute situations.
   C. Early trauma has been shown to be a significant risk factor for selective mutism.
   D. Selective mutism is associated with a history of delayed speech and language development and high incidences of enuresis, encopresis, depression, and separation anxiety.
   E. Selective mutism has been associated with oppositional, stubborn, and negative personality traits.

7. A number of tasks place demands on attentional capacity and focus because of the requirement to divide attention or to inhibit interfering stimuli or responses. An example is a test in which the subject is required to name the color of a word while ignoring the actual word. What is the name of this test?

   A. Wisconsin Card Sorting Test.
   B. Trail Making Test.
   C. Controlled Word Association Test.
   D. Continuous Performance Test.
   E. Stroop Test.

8. Which of the following is *least* likely to be associated with psychosis?

   A. Stroke.
   B. Complex partial seizures.
   C. Huntington's disease.
   D. HIV disease.
   E. Late-stage Parkinson's disease.

9. All of the following medications have been shown to have little to no efficacy in the treatment of acute mania *except*

   A. Gabapentin.
   B. Topiramate.
   C. Clonazepam.
   D. Carbamazepine.
   E. Lamotrigine.

10. Which of the following is not considered a risk factor for adolescent suicide?

    A. Prior suicide attempts.
    B. Mood disorder.
    C. Substance abuse.
    D. Female gender.
    E. Age 16 years or older.

11. Delirium is frequently mistaken for a depressive disorder. Which of the following statements is *true* regarding delirium compared to depression?

    A. Hypoactive delirium is frequently mistaken for depression in the acute medical setting.
    B. Delirium tends to have a diurnal course, whereas depression has a fluctuating course.
    C. Level of consciousness is usually impaired in both delirium and depression in acutely ill hospitalized patients.
    D. Acutely ill patients with depressed mood usually have auditory, tactile, gustatory, and olfactory hallucinations, if at all. Patients with delirium usually only have auditory hallucinations.
    E. If present, the delusions seen in acutely ill patients with depressed mood tend to be fleeting and fragmented; delusions in delirium tend to be complex and mood congruent.

12. Which of the following is *true* of essential tremor, also called benign essential tremor and familial tremor?

    A. Essential tremor is defined as a rhythmic oscillation across a joint resulting from voluntary, alternating activation of agonist and antagonist muscles.
    B. The prevalence of essential tremor increases with age and by definition cannot result in severe impairment in activities of daily living.
    C. Early on, a key feature of essential tremor is that the tremor is usually present at rest.
    D. Essential tremor tends to manifest as postural and kinetic tremors of the arms and hands and occasionally of the head and neck.
    E. Essential tremor is similar to the type of tremors that are seen in Parkinson's disease.

13. Twin studies of schizophrenia have contributed a great deal to our understanding of the genetic transmission of this illness. Which of the following statements is *true* regarding twin studies of schizophrenia?

    A. The risk of schizophrenia in monozygotic (MZ) cotwins of affected probands is at least three times that of dizygotic (DZ) cotwins.
    B. About 95% of MZ twin pairs are concordant for schizophrenia despite being genetically identified.
    C. The risk of schizophrenia in MZ cotwins of affected probands is about five times that in the general population.
    D. Monochorionic MZ twins are less likely to be concordant than are dichorionic MZ twins.
    E. Most (up to 75%) nonschizophrenic MZ cotwins of affected probands show a variety of psychiatric disorders.

14. Dementia with Lewy bodies includes all of the following neuropathological correlates *except*

    A. Neurofibrillary tangles.
    B. Neuritic plaques.
    C. More Lewy bodies in the substantia nigra than in idiopathic Parkinson's disease.
    D. Alpha-synuclein expressed in Lewy bodies.
    E. Weight of the brain typically less than the weight of the brain of the patient with Alzheimer's disease.

15. Symptoms of neurological illness may mimic or mask the symptoms of mood disturbance. All of the following symptoms are relatively nonspecific, commonly occurring in neurologic illness but not necessarily a symptom of a primary mood disorder, *except*

    A. Apathy.
    B. Mood disturbance with incongruent affect.
    C. Mood disturbance with congruent affect.
    D. Agitation.
    E. Decreased psychomotor speed.

16. Based on a variety of studies, it appears that patients with psychiatric complaints alone, without other medical problems or symptoms, would benefit from which of the following screening tests?

    A. Serum glucose.
    B. Serum B$_{12}$.

C. Serum calcium.
D. Computed tomography scan.
E. Serum folate.

17. Sanctions by the American Psychiatric Association for misconduct include all of the following *except*

    A. Admonishment.
    B. Reprimand.
    C. Suspension of membership.
    D. Expulsion from membership.
    E. Direction for state medical board to suspend medical license.

18. Which of the following is *not* true regarding federal regulation of nursing homes in the United States?

    A. Regulatory concern in the 1980s focused on the inappropriate use of chemical restraints.
    B. Regulatory concern in the 1980s focused on the inappropriate use of physical restraints.
    C. In the 1980s, there was concern that antidepressants were being prescribed excessively in nursing homes.
    D. The Omnibus Budget Reconciliation Act of 1987, which contained the Nursing Home Reform Act, addressed mental health care issues in nursing homes.
    E. Nursing home applicants must now have a preadmission assessment to establish psychiatric needs and appropriate placement.

19. According to DSM-IV-TR (American Psychiatric Association 2000), sexual aversion disorder is an example of which of the following sexual dysfunctions?

    A. Sexual desire disorder.
    B. Sexual arousal disorder.
    C. Orgasmic disorder.
    D. Sexual pain disorder.
    E. Sexual dysfunction due to a general medical condition.

20. Barriers to effective communication between the older patient and clinician can include

    A. Physician perceiving the older adult patient incorrectly because of personal fears of aging and death.
    B. Patient having perceptual problems.

C. Patient taking longer to respond to inquiries, resisting the physician who attempts to hurry through the interview.

D. Patient perceiving the physician unrealistically.

E. All of the above.

21. Which of the following is *true* regarding serotonin (5-hydroxytryptamine [5-HT]) receptors?

A. To date, three 5-HT receptors have been identified.

B. 5-HT is synthesized from the essential fatty acid (EFA) tyrosine.

C. The $5\text{-HT}_{2A}$ receptor is most abundant in the cerebral cortex.

D. No 5-HT receptors are known to project to the dorsal raphe, median raphe, or subcortical structures.

E. 5-HT is metabolized to 5-hydroxyindoleacetic acid (5-HIAA) via the enzyme catechol-*O*-methyltransferase (COMT).

22. In the evaluation of personality disorders in the elderly patient, the physician can be assisted by several objective and semistructured instruments. Which of the following clinical assessment instruments is a *semistructured interview* rather than an ancillary self-report measure?

A. Millon Clinical Multiaxial Inventory–III.

B. Personality Disorders Examination.

C. Personality Diagnostic Questionnaire.

D. Schedule for Nonadaptive and Adaptive Personality.

E. Wisconsin Personality Disorders Inventory.

23. When the physician evaluates the older patient with suspicious and/or paranoid complaints, which of the following is *not* recommended?

A. Determine whether suspicious behavior is warranted; for example, consider the possibility of neglect or abuse.

B. Challenge the delusion to verify that it is indeed fixed in the patient's mind.

C. Obtain routine laboratory studies, including chemistry and complete blood count.

D. Consider use of neuroimaging (e.g., computed tomography or magnetic resonance imaging of the head).

E. Consider specialty referrals for vision and hearing examination and correction.

24. Sleep disturbances in major depression include all of the following *except*

A. Increased sleep latency.

B. Decrease in slow-wave sleep in the first non–rapid eye movement (NREM)–rapid eye movement (REM) cycle.

C. Increased latency to REM sleep.

D. Occurrence of REM sleep earlier in the night.

E. Increase in REM density.

25. Which of the following is *true* regarding somatization disorder in geriatric patients?

A. Paralleling the relative risk for depressive disorders, the risk for somatization disorder in women is twice that in men.

B. Somatization disorder is common in patients with irritable bowel disease.

C. As patients with somatization disorder age, their reported symptoms tend to change and symptoms are reported in a less consistent pattern.

D. Prominent pain symptoms are the typical "pseudoneurological" presentation.

E. Another term for somatization disorder is *Munchausen syndrome*.

26. Several neurobiological substrates have been identified to explain the acute reinforcing effects of abused drugs. These models include both specific neurotransmitters and anatomical foci. Which drug of abuse is associated with the neurotransmitters glutamate, dopamine, gamma-aminobutyric acid (GABA), and opioid peptides and the anatomic loci of the nucleus accumbens, ventral tegmental area, and amygdala?

A. Alcohol.

B. Nicotine.

C. Cocaine.

D. Amphetamines.

E. Opioids.

27. All of the following symptoms may be present in neuroleptic malignant syndrome (NMS) *except*

A. Autonomic instability that may include labile blood pressure, tachycardia, hyperthermia, and diaphoresis.

B. Altered level of consciousness.

C. Muscular rigidity.

D. Elevated creatine phosphokinase level and white blood cell count.

E. Hyperreflexia and nystagmus.

28. Which of the following is *true* regarding widowhood and widowerhood in the United States?

A. The mean age at spousal loss is 3 years older for women than for men.
B. The mean duration of widowhood for women is twice that of widowerhood for men.
C. The rates of widowhood among persons older than 65 are much higher for Hispanic and Asian Americans than for Caucasian individuals.
D. Among those older than 65, women are twice as likely as men (30% vs. 15%) to have lost a spouse.
E. Following the loss of a spouse, women are at a higher risk for mortality than are men.

29. Panic disorder has been associated with all of the following *except*

A. Hyperreactivity of the locus coeruleus.
B. Dysregulated serotonergic modulation.
C. Decreased GABA–benzodiazepine receptor complex binding.
D. Hypersensitive brainstem carbon dioxide chemoreceptors.
E. Elevated plasma levels of epinephrine.

30. Recent studies suggest that the antidepressant-associated switch rate—the proportion of bipolar disorder patients who switch to manic symptoms in response to antidepressant treatment—is lower than the previously believed 70%. Which of the following best represents the current estimate of this rate?

A. 20%.
B. 30%.
C. 5%–15%.
D. <2%.
E. 50%.

31. Although definitive data on birth defects and selective serotonin reuptake inhibitors (SSRIs) are lacking, a range of transient perinatal symptoms (which may require admission to special care nurseries) have been reported. These perinatal symptoms include all of the following *except*

A. Jitteriness.
B. Poor muscle tone.
C. Weak/absent cry.
D. Hyperglycemia.
E. Low Apgar scores.

32. In their study examining differences in symptom profile between patients with delirium and patients with dementia, which of the following symptoms or disorders were more common in delirium than in dementia?

A. Delusions.
B. Affective lability.
C. Thought process abnormalities.
D. Disorders of short-term memory.
E. Disorders of long-term memory.

33. When handling diagnostic/prognostic communications and while recommending additional services to the family of patients with dementia, which of the following is *true?*

A. Some Asian American families regard use of formal supportive services as a moral failure.
B. Families rarely tolerate the demands of terminal care of an immobile and incontinent patient but usually can manage the disruptive sleep and behavior of moderate dementia.
C. Combined interventions, although appealing, have not been shown to decrease caregiver depression.
D. Health care decisions should not be made until the diagnosis of dementia is clear and there have been several months of follow-up to estimate rapidity of progression.
E. Families should be advised that judgment about financial matters is usually unimpaired in early dementia.

34. Compared with control subjects, depressed patients perform relatively poorly in measures of

A. Incidental learning.
B. Automatic cognitive processing.
C. Declarative memory.
D. Nondeclarative memory.
E. Procedural memory.

35. According to DSM-IV-TR (American Psychiatric Association 2000) diagnostic criteria for somatoform disorders, pseudocyesis falls under which specific diagnostic category?

    A. Undifferentiated somatoform disorder.
    B. Conversion disorder.
    C. Somatoform disorder not otherwise specified (NOS).
    D. Body dysmorphic disorder.
    E. Hypochondriasis.

36. Which of the following statements is *true* regarding sociodemographic variables or migration?

    A. Because Mexican societal attitudes toward women's alcohol consumption are more negative than in other ethnic groups, the rates of alcohol abuse among Mexican women is likely to be less than that of other cultural groups.
    B. The higher proportion of youth within Native American populations should lead to lower substance abuse rates.
    C. Differences in family stability and the occurrence of domestic violence in a given ethnic group are unlikely to influence the prevalence of substance use in that group.
    D. The stronger the ties to Hispanic culture among persons born outside the United States who speak Spanish, the more likely that group is to use drugs, compared with Hispanics born in the United States who speak mostly English.
    E. Hawaiian residents of Chinese and Japanese ancestry have higher levels of alcohol use if born in Asia than if born in Hawaii.

37. When should a screening electrocardiogram (ECG) be ordered for a psychiatric patient?

    A. All psychiatric patients should receive an ECG.
    B. An ECG should be obtained for all psychiatric patients older than 50 years.
    C. An ECG should be obtained for a psychiatric patient prior to receiving a selective serotonin reuptake inhibitor.
    D. An ECG should be obtained for a psychiatric patient prior to initiating treatment with a psychotropic drug such as an atypical antipsychotic,

which is known to increase cardiac conduction times.
    E. Medically healthy psychiatric patients without cardiovascular symptoms would benefit from routine screening.

38. Several key principles apply to the exercise of moral behavior and are especially applicable to medical ethics. The movement toward "parity" legislation to ensure that provision of care for mental illness is analogous to care for systemic illness illustrates the ethical principle of

    A. Nonmaleficence.
    B. Beneficence.
    C. Autonomy.
    D. Respect for persons.
    E. Justice.

39. Which of the following is *true* regarding advance directives?

    A. Patients receiving care funded by Medicare or Medicaid are required to execute advance directives.
    B. Notarization is required for a power of attorney for health care in all 50 states.
    C. "Durable power of attorney" is synonymous with "legal guardianship."
    D. A living will confers a wider scope of decision making than a power of attorney for health care.
    E. Compliance with advance directives by medical institutions remains poor.

40. Which of the following statements is *false* regarding hypoactive sexual desire disorder?

    A. Hypoactive sexual desire disorder is the most common sexual complaint among females.
    B. Hypoactive sexual desire disorder is the most difficult of all the sexual dysfunctions to treat.
    C. There is no consistent evidence to indicate that testosterone increases sexual interest in men.
    D. Bupropion has been found to be beneficial for more than 50% of women with hypoactive sexual desire disorder in women.
    E. Low-dose testosterone therapy has been found to increase sexual interest and desire in women.

41. Which of the following statements is *false* regarding suicide in the United States?

    A. The male suicide rate is approximately four times the female rate.
    B. The rate of suicide attempts among females is three times the rate of attempts among males.
    C. Suicide attempts are far more common than suicide deaths, approximately 25 attempts for each suicide death.
    D. The most common method of suicide death is poisoning.
    E. The suicide death rate in bipolar disorder is nearly 20 times that of the general population.

42. The inhibitory postsynaptic potentials in the brain are mediated primarily by which of the following receptors?

    A. *N*-methyl-D-aspartate (NMDA) receptors.
    B. Non-NMDA receptors.
    C. Alpha-amino-3-hydroxy-5-methylisoxazole-4-propionic acid (AMPA) receptors.
    D. Kainate receptors.
    E. Gamma-aminobutyric acid (GABA) receptors.

43. Vaillant's studies of the hierarchy of psychological defenses have been cited to explain personality function in old age. All of the following defense mechanisms are considered to be mature and thus adaptive *except*

    A. Humor.
    B. Altruism.
    C. Repression.
    D. Sublimation.
    E. Suppression.

44. The clinical evaluation of the suspicious and/or paranoid older patient requires consideration of specific concerns about psychotic disorders in older patients. Which of the following is *true?*

    A. Because of schizophrenia patients' tendency to isolate and have a shorter life expectancy, chronic paranoid schizophrenia is an infrequent cause of suspiciousness in elderly patients.
    B. Elderly schizophrenia patients are best managed with medication alone, rather than comprehensive treatment models.

    C. New-onset delusions in older patients are usually bizarre in nature.
    D. Antipsychotic medication should be used in all cases of sporadic agitation related to delusions.
    E. Agitation may follow family members' challenging of the patient's delusions.

45. Many changes in sleep architecture are seen in aging, and these changes may play a role in late-life insomnia. Which of the following is a typical sleep architecture change affecting the elderly?

    A. Increased total sleep time.
    B. Decreased percentages of Stage 1 and 2 sleep.
    C. Increased percentages of Stage 3 and 4 sleep.
    D. Increased arousal threshold.
    E. Decreased absolute amounts of rapid eye movement (REM) sleep.

46. Undifferentiated somatoform disorder and hypochondriasis may present in the geriatric psychiatric patient. Which of the following statements is *true?*

    A. Undifferentiated somatoform disorder requires the presence of persistent physical complaints for at least 12 months.
    B. Patients with chronic pain rarely also qualify for a diagnosis of undifferentiated somatoform disorder.
    C. The psychological preoccupation in hypochondriasis relates to the symptoms experienced, rather than the possible disease "represented" by the symptoms.
    D. High educational level and high socioeconomic status predispose individuals to hypochondriasis.
    E. Comorbid depressive and anxiety disorders are common in hypochondriasis.

47. Many neurotransmitters are involved in the development of drug dependence, both in the acute reinforcing effects of drugs and in the recruitment of the brain stress system. All of the following neurotransmitters have been identified as being involved in the acute reinforcing effects of drugs *except*

    A. Norepinephrine.
    B. Dopamine.
    C. Opioid peptides.
    D. Serotonin.
    E. Gamma-aminobutyric acid (GABA).

48. A 43-year-old man with a long history of treatment-resistant major depressive disorder was precribed and started taking a new antidepressant about 2 months ago. For the first time he has had some improvement in his symptoms after adequate trials of multiple antidepressant agents. Twenty-four hours after undergoing outpatient arthroscopic knee surgery, he goes to the emergency department, saying he "doesn't feel right" after taking an unknown pain medication by mouth. He has barely eaten anything in the past 48 hours. His blood pressure is 210/120 mmHg, heart rate 140 bpm, and temperature 103°F. On exam, the patient is somnolent and disoriented and noted to have nystagmus, myoclonus, hyperreflexia, and muscle rigidity. All of the following treatments may be beneficial *except*

    A. Benzodiazepines.
    B. Cyproheptadine
    C. Chlorpromazine.
    D. Bromocriptine.
    E. Propranolol.

49. Which of the following statements is *true* regarding bereavement and theories of attachment?

    A. Bowlby's (1961) attachment theory holds that separation anxiety and pining serve to facilitate emotional withdrawal from the lost object.
    B. In accordance with theories of adaptation, grief symptoms typically abate in elderly widows and widowers within 6 months of a spouse's death.
    C. Visual, but not auditory, hallucination-like experiences are a common part of grieving.
    D. The survivor who maintains abstract rather then concrete ties with the lost partner is more likely to manifest healthy adaptation to loss.
    E. Bowlby (1980) found that preoccupation with the lost spouse 12 months after his or her death occurred in a relatively small minority of subjects.

50. Which of the following statements is *true* regarding panic disorder?

    A. Prognosis is associated with marital status.
    B. About 75% recover completely, 50% have limited impairment, and <20% have major impairment.
    C. Poor prognosis has been associated with less severe initial panic attacks because panic attacks precipitously worsen thereafter.

    D. Panic disorder has a consistent and gradually worsening, then remitting, course, with fairly predictable periods of exacerbations and remissions.
    E. Prognosis is not associated with depression.

51. A number of different brain regions are involved in attentional processes. Which brain region plays a pivotal role in attention by contributing important energetic components of drive and motivation?

    A. Dorsolateral prefrontal cortex.
    B. Reticular activating system (RAS).
    C. Hypothalamus.
    D. Anterior cingulate gyrus.
    E. Orbitomedial prefrontal circuit.

52. Quantitative electroencephalography (QEEG) may have utility in the understanding of neuropsychiatric disorders and may even have prognostic significance. All of the following statements are true *except*

    A. Patients with schizophrenia have more delta activity compared with control subjects.
    B. Delta activity is more pronounced in patients with schizophrenia treated with antipsychotics.
    C. Increased delta activity is present in children with high genetic loading for schizophrenia.
    D. Alpha and beta power during photic stimulation is decreased in patients with presenile dementia.
    E. Intoxication, delirium, and dementia are associated with increased delta activity.

53. Which of the following statements regarding the use of antidepressants in bipolar disorder is *true?*

    A. Antidepressants should never be used in bipolar disorder.
    B. Newer antidepressants should be considered over tricyclic antidepressants (TCAs) because of lower switch rates.
    C. Lamotrigine may have effectiveness as an antidepressant and antimanic agent.
    D. Olanzapine does not have antidepressant activity in acute bipolar depression.
    E. None of the above.

54. Some physical anomalies are stable through childhood and give clues to abnormal neurodevelopment in adulthood. A scale that is in common use to note these anomalies is called the *Waldrop scale*. Which of the following minor physical anomalies is *not* included in this scale?

    A. Small nails.
    B. Wide-spaced eyes.
    C. Adherent ear lobes.
    D. Furrowed tongue.
    E. Abnormal palm crease.

55. In the clinical classification of substance dependence, DSM-IV-TR provides several course specifiers by which the clinician may represent the course of illness. Which of the following is *not* a valid DSM-IV-TR course specifier for substance dependence?

    A. Early full remission.
    B. Sustained partial remission.
    C. On agonist therapy.
    D. On aversive therapy.
    E. In a controlled environment.

56. Which of the following is *true* regarding electroencephalograph (EEG) findings in various conditions?

    A. The EEG of a healthy, awake individual is dominated by frequencies in the alpha range. This pattern shows a gradual, but significant decline in the mean alpha frequency in normal aging.
    B. EEG findings in delirium include slowing.
    C. EEG findings in dementia are characterized by a decrease in low-frequency (delta and theta) activity and a slowing of alpha frequencies.
    D. Quantitative EEG signals tend not to correlate with the severity and duration of delirium.
    E. Normal aging is generally associated with significant increases in delta activity.

57. All of the following are *true* regarding the issue of driving among patients with dementia *except*

    A. Local offices of the departments of motor vehicles (DMVs) rarely provide independent driving evaluations when requested by family members or patients' physicians.

    B. Psychiatrists are bound by ethical principles such as confidentiality to notify local DMVs about an individual's impaired driving skills without the express written consent of the individual.
    C. Some state DMVs automatically revoke the driver's licenses of individuals diagnosed with moderate or severe dementia.
    D. Because symptoms of dementia are likely to worsen over time, individuals who pass a driving evaluation should continue to be reevaluated yearly.
    E. Psychiatrists should recommend against caregivers mechanically disabling the car of an individual with dementia because this could further exacerbate familial relationships as well as erode the patient-physician relationship.

58. Dysfunction in _____ is more common in depressed patients with psychotic features than in depressed patients without psychotic features.

    A. Measures of speed of processing.
    B. Mental flexibility.
    C. Language.
    D. Memory.
    E. Visuospatial abilities.

59. Which of the following antidepressants is an inhibitor of both dopamine and norepinephrine transporters?

    A. Bupropion.
    B. Tricyclic antidepressants (TCAs).
    C. Venlafaxine.
    D. Monoamine oxidase inhibitors (MAOIs).
    E. Mirtazapine.

60. Pharmacoelectroencephalography (pharmaco-EEG) in clinical applications offers an attractive technique to fine-tune drug development and is likely to play an expanded role in the future of applied psychopharmacology. All of the following statements are true *except*

    A. Decreased quantitative electroencephalography (QEEG) theta and alpha activity has been reported in patients with schizophrenia who were being treated with high-potency antipsychotics.
    B. Slow alpha changes identify nonresponders versus responders to antipsychotics.
    C. Medication-associated increases in beta waves correlate with decrease in depression symptoms.

D. QEEG profile after a single dose of an acetyl-cholinesterase inhibitor predicted cognitive modifications in dementia patients.

E. With antipsychotic treatment, increased QEEG alpha activity correlates with a favorable clinical response.

61. A disadvantage of a screening head computed tomography (CT) scan over a magnetic resonance imaging (MRI) scan is that

A. It takes longer.
B. It is more expensive.
C. It is less sensitive.
D. It is not useful for rapid screening.
E. It produces more discomfort.

62. Which of the following is *not* a typical defense encountered in substance abusers?

A. Denial.
B. Minimization.
C. Sublimation.
D. Rationalization.
E. Externalization.

63. Principle-based ethics advocates a technique of balancing four ethical principles in the actions of a particular case. Which of the following is *not* one of the four principles emphasized in this model?

A. Privacy.
B. Nonmaleficence.
C. Beneficence.
D. Respect for autonomy.
E. Justice.

64. In the middle of the night, the general medicine team urgently consults the psychosomatic medicine (PSM) team regarding a 79-year-old man who is threatening to leave the hospital against medical advice. The consulting team requests that an evaluation be made regarding the patient's ability to make this decision. Of the following, which statement reflects accurately an important issue that the PSM team must address?

A. The patient may or may not possess the competency to make medical decisions regarding his health care.

B. By law, only a psychiatrist (and/or a PSM team) can determine whether the patient has necessary insight and judgment to refuse medical care.

C. Competency requires a court decision, not a medical one.

D. Making a will and executing a power of attorney require the same level of competency.

E. The court may request a written report but may not compel the physician to personally testify in competency cases.

65. Which of the following sexual dysfunctions has the *lowest* estimated prevalence in the U.S. population?

A. Male orgasmic disorder.
B. Female orgasmic disorder.
C. Male dyspareunia.
D. Female arousal disorder.
E. Erectile dysfunction.

66. Among the suicide risk factors identified in a 10-year prospective study of patients with affective disorders, which of the following was considered to be a long-term suicide risk factor rather than a short-term one?

A. Severe hopelessness.
B. Panic attacks.
C. Psychic anxiety.
D. Diminished concentration.
E. Global insomnia.

67. Changes of aging that occur in dopamine and dopamine receptors include

A. Decreased numbers of dopamine type 2 ($D_2$) receptors in the striatum with increasing age correlated with decreased cognitive function.

B. Decreased dopamine transporter in caudate/putamen in oldest subjects.

C. Correlation with decreased glucose metabolism of the frontal, temporal, and cingulate cortices.

D. All of the above.

E. None of the above.

68. Personality change due to degenerative frontal lobe disease is associated with difficulties in planning, conformity to social norms, experience of reward and punishment, and management of complex emotions. Clinically, these symptoms may bear strong resemblance to several DSM-IV-TR personality disorders. These specific behaviors may commonly overlap with all of the following personality disorders *except*

    A. Obsessive-compulsive personality disorder.
    B. Narcissistic personality disorder.
    C. Antisocial personality disorder.
    D. Borderline personality disorder.
    E. Paranoid personality disorder.

69. All of the following symptoms seen in psychotic illness have been found to increase violence risk *except*

    A. Delusions characterized by "threat/control override" symptoms.
    B. Hallucinations associated with "negative" emotions.
    C. Command hallucinations to harm others.
    D. Persecutory delusions.
    E. Negative symptoms such as social withdrawal.

70. Medications typically used in the treatment of narcolepsy include all of the following *except*

    A. Dextroamphetamine.
    B. Methylphenidate.
    C. Atomoxetine.
    D. Gamma-aminobutyric acid (GABA)–hydroxybutyrate.
    E. Modafinil.

71. Which of the following is *true* regarding conversion disorder?

    A. Conversion disorder is more common in elderly women than in younger women.
    B. Conversion disorder is seen almost exclusively in women.
    C. Comorbidity in conversion disorder includes substance abuse and head injury.
    D. Although nonepileptic seizures (often referred to as pseudoseizures) are a subtype of conversion disorder, they rarely are seen in patients with a bona fide seizure disorder.

E. Like younger patients, elderly patients with conversion disorder infrequently have an "actual" comorbid neurological disorder.

72. Which particular type of serotonin receptor agonists is known to facilitate strongly cocaine reward?

    A. Serotonin type 1A receptor ($5\text{-HT}_{1A}$).
    B. $5\text{-HT}_{1B}$.
    C. $5\text{-HT}_{1C}$.
    D. $5\text{-HT}_{2A}$.
    E. $5\text{-HT}_3$.

73. A 47-year-old woman with schizoaffective disorder is brought to the emergency department by her caregiver, who reported that the patient has become increasingly disoriented in the past week. The patient has been sick with the "flu" and complained of a sore throat earlier in the week. The caregiver insists that the patient has no history of drug abuse and has "never" been suicidal. After taking an antipsychotic for a year, the patient experienced stabilization of her psychotic symptoms for the first time in 20 years, but she gained 40 lb. during that time. Ten days ago, she was prescribed a low dose of fluvoxamine because of persistently depressed mood and obsessive-compulsive symptoms. On examination, the patient is pale and unresponsive to verbal stimuli. Her blood pressure is 95/60 mmHg, respiratory rate 15 breaths/minute, and heart rate 105 bpm, and her temperature is normal. Of the following, which laboratory test and/or intervention would most assist the treatment team to narrow down the differential diagnosis and develop an appropriate course of action?

    A. A comprehensive urine toxicology screen and blood alcohol level.
    B. Random blood glucose and electrolytes.
    C. Complete blood count with differential.
    D. Electrolytes and lithium level.
    E. Obtain liver function test and ammonia level; provide intravenous glucose and thiamine.

74. Which of the following is considered to be a restoration-oriented rather than a loss-oriented stressor in the dual-process model of bereavement (Stroebe and Schut 1999)?

    A. Emotional symptoms.
    B. Behavioral symptoms.

C. New identity development.
D. Physiological symptoms.
E. Cognitive symptoms.

75. Dysregulation of dopaminergic release in which of the following brain structures is associated with helplessness behaviors and delayed extinction of conditioned fear responses?

   A. Amygdala.
   B. Nucleus accumbens.
   C. Medial prefrontal cortex.
   D. Tuberoinfundibular tract.
   E. Cingulate gyrus.

76. Bipolar disorder in the elderly may have all of the following characteristics *except*

   A. Tendency toward more rapid recurrences late in the illness.
   B. Stressful events more likely to precede early-onset mania than late-onset mania.
   C. Increased cerebral vulnerability playing a stronger role than life events in precipitating late-onset mania.
   D. Association with low rates of familial affective disorder.
   E. Genetic factors weighing heavily in the etiology.

77. Epidemiological findings concerning autism include all of the following *except*

   A. Onset typically occurs before age 3 years.
   B. The overall rate of autism in second-degree relatives of children with autism is 0.2%.
   C. The male-to-female ratio is 1.5 to 1.0.
   D. Rates of autism in siblings of affected individuals are in the range of 2% to 6%.
   E. The concordance rate for monozygotic twins has been estimated to be between 36% and 91%.

78. Which of the following is a feature of progressive supranuclear palsy (PSP)?

   A. Does not include vertical gaze palsy.
   B. Features parkinsonism without prominent tremor.
   C. Has appendicular rigidity that is greater than axial rigidity.
   D. Has good response to levodopa.

E. Is characterized by a bilateral, symmetric parkinsonism that is poorly responsive to levodopa therapy.

79. A number of physicians in the eighteenth and nineteenth centuries made important contributions to the understanding of schizophrenia. Which of the following individuals outlined a set of "first-rank" symptoms in an attempt to establish a discrete criteria set for the diagnosis?

   A. Kahlbaum.
   B. Kraepelin.
   C. Morel.
   D. Pinel.
   E. Schneider.

80. Which of the following is the likely final common neural pathway in delirium?

   A. Low cholinergic/high dopaminergic state.
   B. High cholinergic/high dopaminergic state.
   C. High gamma-aminobutyric acid (GABA)/low dopaminergic state.
   D. Low GABA/high dopaminergic state.
   E. Low serotonin/high GABA state.

81. Which of the following antiepileptic drugs (AEDs) has been shown to be effective in the treatment of agitation and aggression in patients with dementia?

   A. Lamotrigine.
   B. Levetiracetam.
   C. Gabapentin.
   D. Valproate.
   E. Phenytoin.

82. Depression is associated with all of the following neurochemical alterations *except*

   A. Lower levels of cerebrospinal fluid (CSF) serotonin metabolites.
   B. Decreased serotonin transporter binding.
   C. Serotonin receptor abnormalities.
   D. Decreased CSF homovanillic acid.
   E. Increased dopamine transporter activity.

83. The current American Academy of Neurology (2007) practice recommendations for evaluation of reversible causes of dementia include laboratory testing to rule out which of the following medical disorders?

    A. Hypocalcemia.
    B. Hypothyroidism.
    C. Hyponatremia.
    D. Iron deficiency.
    E. Hyperparathyroidism.

84. A psychiatrist is asked to participate in a research project in which residents of a neighborhood that was recently devastated by an earthquake are asked to provide detailed accounts of their experiences during the earthquake. Which is the most relevant ethical principle to consider at this time?

    A. Value.
    B. Scientific validity.
    C. Informed consent.
    D. Favorable risk-benefit ratio.
    E. Independent review.

85. "Drug courts" have been developed as an alternative method to deal with substance abusers who commit crimes. Which of the following statements is *false* regarding drug courts in the United States?

    A. They are a type of "diversion."
    B. They are found in a limited number of jurisdictions.
    C. They have low recidivism rates.
    D. They are used for nonviolent offenders with misdemeanor charges.
    E. None require a comorbid psychiatric illness for participation.

86. Which of the following statements is *true* regarding the DSM-IV-TR (American Psychiatric Association 2000) diagnosis of gender identity disorder?

    A. The diagnosis applies only to adults and not to children or adolescents.
    B. The diagnosis should not be used for transsexualism.
    C. The diagnosis would apply to someone with androgen insensitivity syndrome.
    D. The diagnosis requires a strong and persistent cross-gender identification.

    E. The diagnosis is not given in the absence of discomfort with one's sex.

87. Which of the following does *not* predict greater risk of violence?

    A. Younger age at first arrest for serious crime.
    B. Prior violent acts.
    C. Being employed.
    D. Past use of weapons in assaults.
    E. History of formal military discipline.

88. Regarding neuropsychological deficits from parietal lobe lesions, which of the following is *true?*

    A. Wernicke's aphasia is characterized by fluent paraphasic speech and defective aural comprehension but preserved simple repetition.
    B. Conduction aphasia is associated with profoundly defective verbatim repetition, nonfluent speech, and impaired reading comprehension.
    C. Lesions to the inferior parietal lobule may lead to acalculia, an acquired inability to perform simple mathematical calculations.
    D. Neglect syndromes from right-sided inferior parietal lobule lesions are confined to neglect of intrapersonal space.
    E. Anosognosia refers to the patient's lack of concern with (rather than lack of recognition of) a neurological and/or neuropsychological deficit.

89. Which of the following personality disorders is most commonly associated with violence?

    A. Borderline personality disorder.
    B. Paranoid personality disorder.
    C. Narcissistic personality disorder.
    D. Antisocial personality disorder.
    E. Schizotypal personality disorder.

90. Which of the following is characteristic of violence associated with traumatic brain injury (TBI)?

    A. Episodes of violence with long periods of relative calm.
    B. Violence often motivated by revenge.
    C. Calculated acts of violence.
    D. Violence perpetrated against nonfamily members and involving an altercation with the victim prior to violence.
    E. Lack of remorse.

91. In a long-term follow-up study of patients with schizophrenia (the Vermont Longitudinal Study), the majority of these patients, after 10 years of follow-up and approximately 15–20 years of illness, showed

    A. A marked deterioration in mental functioning.
    B. No psychotic symptoms.
    C. A poor level of overall functioning, especially those over 50 years of age.
    D. A deteriorating long-term course.
    E. Little heterogeneity in outcome.

92. Psychophysiological insomnia is a troubling sleep disorder with specific behavioral characteristics. Which of the following is *not* a feature of this condition?

    A. Excessive worry about not being able to sleep.
    B. Trying too hard to sleep.
    C. Rumination.
    D. Sleeping poorly in a novel environment.
    E. Increased muscle tension when retiring.

93. Which of the following is *false* regarding pain disorders?

    A. Alzheimer's disease may lower the pain threshold and thus alter the pain perception in these patients.
    B. Nearly 50% of elderly individuals have chronic pain; 70% of those in long-term care have chronic pain.
    C. Individuals with chronic back pain have an estimated 80% lifetime prevalence of a psychiatric disorder.
    D. Pain is the most common medical complaint in elderly persons, with pain caused by musculoskeletal disease being the most common type of pain.
    E. Depressive disorder is the most common comorbidity in individuals with pain disorder.

94. Loci influencing the risk for alcohol dependence map close to an alcohol dehydrogenase gene cluster on the long arm of which chromosome?

    A. Chromosome 4.
    B. Chromosome 6.
    C. Chromosome 12.
    D. Chromosome 15.
    E. Chromosome 16.

95. Substance withdrawal states may be associated with periods of autonomic instability. Which of the following substances is *not* associated with actual physiologic withdrawal?

    A. Alcohol.
    B. Benzodiazepines.
    C. Cocaine.
    D. Barbiturates.
    E. Opioids.

96. Treatment of pain states may be an appropriate application of tricyclic antidepressants (TCAs). Unfortunately, a host of cardiac concerns make electrocardiogram (ECG) monitoring necessary with these agents. Which of the following is *not* a characteristic ECG change associated with TCAs?

    A. Flattened T-wave.
    B. Prolonged Q-T interval.
    C. Prolonged QRS interval.
    D. Prolonged PR interval.
    E. Elevated S-T segment.

97. An application of Stroebe and Schut's (1999) dual-process model of grief is to focus on specific tasks required of the survivor. Which of the following is *true* regarding this model?

    A. The tasks can be divided into grief tasks and loss tasks.
    B. The tasks can be divided into grief tasks (such as confronting the loss) and restoration tasks (such as emotionally withdrawing from the deceased person).
    C. Restructuring thoughts and memories about the deceased person are grief tasks.
    D. Emotional withdrawing from the deceased person includes actively attempting to forget the deceased person.
    E. A loss task includes spending time away from grieving.

98. Which of the following augmentation strategies has been found to be effective in treatment-resistant obsessive-compulsive disorder (OCD)?

    A. Addition of venlafaxine to buspirone.
    B. Addition of lithium to risperidone.
    C. Addition of risperidone to a selective serotonin reuptake inhibitor (SSRI).

D. Addition of valproate to clomipramine.

E. Addition of gabapentin to an SSRI.

99. Hyperthyroidism has been associated with a specific range of neuropsychiatric symptoms and syndromes. Which of the following is *true?*

    A. Because of the degree of systemic metabolic disturbances in hyperthyroidism, the majority of patients exhibit psychopathology as a result of hyperthyroidism.
    B. In studies of both selected and unselected hyperthyroidism patients, anxiety disorders are the most common neuropsychiatric illnesses.
    C. Cognitive disturbance in hyperthyroidism is as common as it is in hypothyroidism.
    D. In hyperthyroid patients with depressive symptoms, the physical symptoms of hyperthyroidism precede mood symptoms in the vast majority of cases.
    E. In hyperthyroidism, both mania and psychosis are uncommon.

100. The increasing multiethnicity of Western English-speaking countries has sparked a debate about alternative models of culturally sensitive models of care. One such model acknowledges that following both prescribed medication and ethnic spiritual therapy may be the best hope for securing adherence. This model also encourages a more honest discussion of the other therapies being tried and their interaction, from the reading of sacred texts to the possible infliction of physical harm. This model is called

    A. A cultural consultation model.
    B. A hedge-your-bets approach.
    C. A melting pot approach.
    D. A separate services model.
    E. A cultural recovery model.

101. The emergence of lateralization and hemispheric asymmetry are important to neurobehavioral development. All of the following statements are true *except*

    A. Lateralization is largely established by age 5 years.
    B. Differential development of the two hemispheres in early growth is caused by delayed myelination of the corpus callosum.
    C. In early development, the left hemisphere develops more rapidly than the right because of its usual dominance.

D. Development of the right hemisphere accelerates between ages 3 and 6 years.

E. Gray matter density tends to be greater in the right posterior temporal regions than the left.

102. Delirium in the elderly is characterized by which of the following?

    A. Usually resolves within a week after being discharged from a medical or surgical hospitalization.
    B. Usually results in a full resolution of symptoms once the underlying acute medical problems are resolved.
    C. Is often the initial presentation of an underlying dementia.
    D. Tends to occur abruptly in elderly persons, as with other populations. Thus, gradualness of mental status changes usually rules out delirium in older individuals.
    E. All of the above.

103. Which of the following statements is *true* regarding treatment of behavioral disturbances in dementia?

    A. Benzodiazepines are the treatment of choice to treat behavioral disturbances in patients with dementia.
    B. Clonazepam is preferred over lorazepam when treating agitation in patients with dementia.
    C. Benzodiazepines can be used for short-term treatment of behavioral disturbances associated with disruptions to routines or adjustments to changes.
    D. Diphenhydramine is an appropriate treatment option for most patients with dementia.
    E. Benzodiazepines should be given with antipsychotics whenever possible.

104. Which of the following statements is *true* regarding specific psychiatric illnesses and comorbid substance use disorders?

    A. When comorbid with substance use disorder, conduct disorder usually follows substance use disorder.
    B. Rates of conduct disorder in adolescent substance abusers are between 30% and 50%.
    C. Mood disorders, particularly depression, frequently precede adolescent drug abuse.

D.  Depressive disorders are reported in 15%–20% of adolescent substance abusers.

E.  Social phobia and panic disorder usually follow the onset of substance abuse in adolescents.

105.  Which of the following tests assesses the cognitive domain of executive ability?

A.  Continuous Performance Test.
B.  Trail Making Test.
C.  Wisconsin Card Sorting Test.
D.  Judgment of Line Orientation.
E.  Boston Naming Test.

106.  A patient with schizophrenia asks his outpatient psychiatrist to document a less-stigmatizing diagnosis when completing insurance forms. Of the following, which is the most relevant ethical principle to consider in this case?

A.  Nonmaleficence.
B.  Fiduciary.
C.  Empathy.
D.  Conflict of interest.
E.  Personhood.

107.  Damage to this brain structure frequently produces symptoms of aggression, violence, anorexia, depression, impaired short-term memory, dementia, laughing, seizures, and altered sleep–wake cycle.

A.  Hypothalamus.
B.  Thalamus.
C.  Cerebellum.
D.  Mammillary bodies.
E.  Putamen.

108.  Evoked potentials, particularly the P300 potential, may be useful in the diagnosis and management of neuropsychiatric illness. All of the following statements are true *except*

A.  The most consistent P300 finding in schizophrenia is a reduction in amplitude.
B.  In schizophrenia, P300 abnormalities present in nonmedicated and medicated patients.
C.  P300 abnormalities correlate with the amount of negative symptoms and formal thought disorder in schizophrenia.

D.  In schizophrenia, asymmetrical auditory P300 reduction is frequently reported, with smaller amplitudes over the right temporal region.
E.  P300 abnormalities have been reported in relatives of schizophrenia patients and high-risk subjects for psychosis.

109.  A defendant is charged with involuntary manslaughter because of his involvement in a three-car collision that led to the death of a passenger in another car. The accident occurred after a the windshield of defendant's car was suddenly struck by a broken tree branch, and he swerved to avoid hitting a large group of pedestrians. Police reports say that the defendant immediately called 911 on his cell phone, aided the other victims, and cooperated fully with authorities. A routine blood alcohol level found that the defendant just barely met the legal criterion for alcohol intoxication. The defendant has no prior drug or other criminal record. Which of the following statements is *true* regarding this case?

A.  Because ample evidence demonstrates that alcohol had little role to play in causing the accident, the charges will probably be dropped.
B.  He is unlikely to be convicted of the crime because he barely met the legal limit for alcohol intoxication and clearly demonstrated by his actions that his mental and physical status were largely unimpaired during and immediately after the accident.
C.  Even if strict liability is mandated, the defendant will unlikely be convicted because a "freak accident"—not alcohol—led to the accident.
D.  Under strict liability, the defendant's blood alcohol level may be enough to convict him of the crime.
E.  In such crimes, mandated minimum sentences for deaths resulting from driving while intoxicated apply only if the intoxication plays a substantial role in the death.

110.  Which of the following personality disorders has been found to be common in arsonists?

A.  Narcissistic.
B.  Histrionic.
C.  Schizoid.
D.  Borderline.
E.  Avoidant.

111. Which of the following is *not* true regarding the epidemiology of violence?

    A. In the general population, males perpetrate violence at a rate 10 times that of females.
    B. Among mentally ill patients, men are five times more likely than women to commit violence.
    C. Among violent, mentally ill persons, women are more likely than men to commit violence toward family members.
    D. Among violent, mentally ill persons, men are more likely than women to commit violence resulting in arrest.
    E. Among psychiatric inpatients, men and women have similar rates of physical assault.

112. A patient with traumatic brain injury with eye opening to speech (but not spontaneously), decorticate motor response, and intelligible but incoherent speech would score ____ on the Glasgow Coma Scale.

    A. 8.
    B. 9.
    C. 10.
    D. 11.
    E. 12.

113. Which of the following statements is *false* regarding suicidality in various psychiatric disorders?

    A. Among personality disorders, antisocial and borderline personality disorders have a particularly high rate of suicide.
    B. The lifetime risk of suicide in schizophrenia is approximately 10%.
    C. Suicide is the leading cause of death among schizophrenic individuals younger than age 35 years.
    D. Individuals with schizophrenia are at particular risk of suicide during exacerbations of illness and in early stages of schizophrenia.
    E. Depressed patients with melancholic features have a rate of suicide that is two times that of nonmelancholic depressed patients.

114. Which of the following statements is *true* regarding schizophrenia in women?

    A. Men and women have similar incidence rates for schizophrenia.

    B. The onset of schizophrenia is approximately 5 years later in women than in men.
    C. Approximately 25% of women with schizophrenia develop their illness in the mid to late 40s.
    D. Relatives of men with schizophrenia are more likely to themselves develop schizophrenia than are the relatives of women with schizophrenia.
    E. Neuroanatomical study shows that women with schizophrenia are more likely to have anatomical abnormalities than are men with schizophrenia.

115. Which of the following antidepressive agents increases rapid eye movement (REM) sleep?

    A. Bupropion.
    B. Clomipramine.
    C. Phenelzine.
    D. Venlafaxine.
    E. Sertraline.

116. Which of the following is *true* regarding the etiology of somatoform disorders?

    A. The prevalence of all definitively diagnosed somatoform disorders increases with age.
    B. When somatoform disorders present in the older patient, comorbid neurological illness may be associated with them but neuropsychological (cognitive) impairment is not.
    C. Somatoform disorders are associated with a history of serious illness of a parent, but not in the patient, early in life.
    D. Comorbid panic disorder is common in somatoform disorders, but other anxiety disorders are not.
    E. The personality trait of neuroticism, wherein the subject experiences more negative emotions, is associated with the development of somatoform disorders.

117. Laboratory assessment is invaluable in the clinical care of substance abusers. Which of the following occurrences is *not* characteristic of the effects of alcohol?

    A. Increased glycoprotein carbohydrate–deficient transferrin.
    B. Increased glutamyltranspeptidase.
    C. Increased aspartate aminotransferase.
    D. Increased alanine aminotransferase.
    E. Decreased mean corpuscular hemoglobin.

118. Many chemicals present in blood and tissue are analgesic. Which of the following substances does *not* itself directly excite primary noxious afferents?

    A. Prostaglandins.
    B. Serotonin.
    C. Histamine.
    D. Acetylcholine.
    E. Bradykinin.

119. A 38-year-old woman with a history of treatment-resistant major depressive disorder (not currently receiving any medication) returns for a routine outpatient visit and is now 3 weeks postpartum and plans to continue breastfeeding for at least 1 year. Her baby was full-term and healthy and is developing well. The woman's depressive symptoms are recurring, and she would like to restart nortriptyline, which was, according to her, the "only" medication among several selective serotonin reuptake inhibitors (SSRIs) and other antidepressants that had been effective for her depression. Five years ago, she developed severe depression after the birth of her first child and required emergent inpatient psychiatric treatment. The most prudent treatment recommendation is to

    A. Recommend doxepin, a tricyclic antidepressant (TCA) that is safer for infants than nortriptyline during lactation.
    B. Advise against starting nortriptyline while she is still breastfeeding, and recommend a trial of citalopram or escitalopram.
    C. Start low-dose nortriptyline, and titrate the dose to her previous dose, as tolerated.
    D. Advise against starting any antidepressants until the infant is at least 6 months old.
    E. Recommend imipramine, a TCA that is safer for infants than nortriptyline during lactation.

120. Studies of ethnic and cultural differences in end-of-life and bereavement issues have revealed distinctions of clinical importance. Regarding Block's 1998 study of Latinos, particularly first- and second-generation, which of the following is *not* true?

    A. Patients valued family input into treatment decisions.
    B. Patients had extensive social networks.
    C. Patients placed family interests above those of the self.

    D. Patients resisted accepting death as unavoidable.
    E. Patients preferred a caring rather than a scientific approach by a physician.

121. A patient with panic disorder develops agitation, insomnia, and nausea while taking fluoxetine. Which of the following agents might be useful in reducing these symptoms?

    A. Mirtazapine.
    B. Buspirone.
    C. Lithium.
    D. Venlafaxine.
    E. Valproate.

122. Which of the following statements is *false* regarding the American Psychiatric Association (APA) (2006) guideline for treatment of manic or mixed episodes?

    A. Antidepressants should be tapered and discontinued during acute treatment of a manic or mixed episode.
    B. The first-line pharmacological treatment for severe manic or mixed episodes is either lithium plus an antipsychotic, or valproate plus an antipsychotic.
    C. It is not recommended that benzodiazepines be used in severely ill or agitated patients who are in the midst of a mixed or manic episode.
    D. The first-line pharmacological treatment for serious but less severe manic or mixed episodes is monotherapy with lithium, valproic acid, or an antipsychotic such as olanzapine.
    E. If first-line medication treatment at optimal doses fails to control symptoms, it is recommended that another first-line agent be added.

123. The Swedo (Swedo et al. 1998) criteria for pediatric autoimmune neuropsychiatric disorders associated with streptococcal infection (PANDAS) include all of the following *except*

    A. Presence of obsessive-compulsive disorder (OCD) and/or tic disorder.
    B. Onset before age 7 years.
    C. Episodic course of symptom severity.
    D. Association with group A beta-hemolytic streptococcal (GABHS) infection.
    E. Association with neurological abnormalities.

124. Which of the following statements concerning socio-demographic correlates of mood disorders is *true?*

    A. The mean age at onset of major depressive disorder (MDD) is in the late 30s.
    B. The rates of bipolar disorder among men and women appear to be similar.
    C. Prior to adolescence, depression is twice as common in girls as in boys.
    D. People with bipolar disorder tend to develop symptoms in a unimodal distribution from ages 18–44 years.
    E. In clinical samples, bipolar disorder and MDD appear to be associated with a higher socioeconomic status.

125. All of the following attenuate (decrease) essential tremor *except*

    A. Propranolol.
    B. Primidone.
    C. Alcohol.
    D. Deep brain stimulation of the ventral intermediate nucleus of the contralateral thalamus.
    E. Trihexyphenidyl.

126. Schizophrenia, whether broadly or narrowly defined, is familial. Which of the following is a subclinical phenotype that is elevated in the relatives of patients with schizophrenia?

    A. Positive symptoms measured by the Thought Disorder Index.
    B. Negative symptoms measured by the Scale for the Assessment of Negative Symptoms.
    C. Neuropsychological signs such as deficits in abstraction and in short-term verbal memory.
    D. Eye movement dysfunction on smooth pursuit and visual fixation tasks.
    E. Neurological soft signs.

127. The Minnesota Multiphasic Personality Inventory (MMPI) and its successor, the MMPI-2, employ nine clinical scales. Which of the following is *not* one of the scales?

    A. Hypochondriasis.
    B. Hysteria.
    C. Paranoia.
    D. Schizophrenia.
    E. Anxiety.

128. Standards for determination of competency in decision making include all of the following *except*

    A. Communication of clinical choice.
    B. Understanding of relevant information provided.
    C. Appreciation of available options and consequences.
    D. Rational decision making.
    E. Performance in the "unimpaired" range on formal cognitive testing.

129. Antidepressants may sometimes interfere with sexual functioning. Of the following, which antidepressant medication is *least* likely to produce sexual dysfunction?

    A. Tricyclic antidepressants (TCAs).
    B. Mirtazapine.
    C. Monoamine oxidase inhibitors.
    D. Selective serotonin reuptake inhibitors (SSRIs).
    E. Venlafaxine.

130. The amygdala plays an important role in all of the following *except*

    A. Recognition of emotion.
    B. Classical conditioning of autonomic responses.
    C. Processing of stimuli that communicate emotional significance in social situations.
    D. Decision-making process.
    E. Declarative memory.

131. Since DSM-III (American Psychiatric Association 1980), personality disorders have been grouped into three clusters: A, B, and C. Which of the following disorders fall within cluster C?

    A. Borderline, histrionic, narcissistic, antisocial.
    B. Histrionic, obsessive-compulsive, narcissistic.
    C. Paranoid, borderline, antisocial.
    D. Avoidant, dependent, obsessive-compulsive.
    E. Schizotypal, schizoid, paranoid.

132. Which of the following statements is *false* regarding postpartum psychosis?

    A. Postpartum psychosis occurs in 1–2 of every 1,000 live births.
    B. Postpartum psychosis is considered to be a manifestation of bipolar disorder, not schizophrenia.

C. A history of both bipolar disorder and prior episodes of postpartum psychosis increases the risk of subsequent postpartum psychosis to 80%.

D. Because of risks to the patient and the newborn, postpartum psychosis patients should be hospitalized.

E. Systemic etiologies such as Sheehan's syndrome and postpartum thyroiditis may mimic postpartum psychosis.

133. Which of the following approaches is recommended in the treatment of somatoform disorders?

A. The physician should arrange appointments on an as-needed basis.

B. A focus on obtaining insight into the psychological context of somatoform symptoms should be the first priority for intervention.

C. The physician should not offer to review all prior medical records because this merely reinforces maladaptive somatization behavior.

D. Hypochondriasis has been shown to respond to antidepressants and anxiolytics.

E. Hypnosis should be avoided in conversion disorder as these patients are rarely subject to induction of hypnosis.

134. Which one of the following substances is associated with clearly defined withdrawal symptoms?

A. Cannabis.
B. Hallucinogens.
C. Phencyclidine (PCP).
D. Amphetamines.
E. Inhalants.

135. If valproic acid must be used during pregnancy, what are the recommendations regarding its dosing and folic acid supplementation?

A. No more than 1,000 mg/day of valproic acid, and take 1–2 mg/day of a folic acid supplement.

B. No more than 1,000 mg/day of valproic acid, and take 4–5 mg/day of folic acid during the first trimester and at least 1–2 mg/day for the rest of gestation.

C. No more than 1,000 mg/day of valproic acid, and take 4–5 mg/day of folic acid throughout gestation.

D. For doses of valproic acid greater than 1,000 mg/day, take 40–50 mg/day of folic acid during the first trimester, then 4–5 mg/day thereafter.

E. No more than 1,000 mg/day of valproic acid, and take a daily multivitamin with 1–2 mg of folic acid throughout gestation.

136. Which of the following statements is *true* regarding culture and bereavement?

A. The manifestations, duration, and intensity of grief are universal.

B. The literature describing cross-cultural and ethnic expressions after death indicates that bereavement is most likely communicated and regulated through the same pathway across cultures.

C. The concept of performing grief tasks is equally applicable to all cultures.

D. In contrast to other cultures that focus on rituals, expressions, and meanings that are shared interpersonally and socially, Euro-American culture generally has conceptualized grief as loss oriented, with a focus on individual manifestations of grief.

E. Culturally mainstream Americans tend to view death as an active, ongoing interaction with a deceased individual.

137. Lamotrigine is being evaluated for efficacy in treating depressive, manic, and mixed episodes in bipolar patients as well as for rapid cycling. Which of the following statements is *true* about lamotrigine?

A. It is efficacious for bipolar depression.
B. It is efficacious for bipolar depression with psychosis.
C. It lacks efficacy for bipolar mania.
D. It lacks efficacy for rapid cycling.
E. It lacks efficacy as an adjunct to other treatments.

138. A childhood seizure that features alterations in consciousness; auras of unpleasant odors, tastes, and sensations; and simple, repetitive, and purposeless automatisms is classified as what type of seizure?

A. Simple partial seizure.
B. Partial sensory seizure.
C. Rolandic epilepsy.
D. Complex partial seizure.
E. Frontal lobe epilepsy.

139. Which of the following is *true* regarding mood disorders in nursing home residents?

    A. Dementia is the most common psychiatric illness in nursing home residents (50%–75%), followed by depressive disorder (15%–50%).
    B. The rate of mood disorders in nursing home residents in the United States is substantially higher than in other industrialized nations.
    C. Depression in nursing home residents increases morbidity, but not mortality, rates.
    D. Because of concurrent chronic medical illnesses, the DSM-IV-TR diagnostic criteria for mood disorders are not clinically valid in predicting treatment response in nursing home residents.
    E. A subtype of depression in nursing home residents that includes low serum albumin and high levels of psychosocial disability usually responds promptly to treatment with nortriptyline.

140. Which of the following measures uses a clinical interview for data collection?

    A. Symptom Checklist–90—Revised.
    B. Brief Symptom Inventory.
    C. Brief Psychiatric Rating Scale.
    D. Personality Assessment Inventory.
    E. Millon Clinical Multiaxial Inventory–III.

141. There are a number of different types of paraphilias. Klismaphilia involves which of the following?

    A. Enemas.
    B. Urine.
    C. Animals.
    D. Corpses.
    E. Nonliving objects.

142. Which of the following is *not* considered a perceptual disturbance?

    A. Derealization.
    B. Illusion.
    C. Depersonalization.
    D. Delusion.
    E. Hallucination.

143. Which of the following statements is *true* regarding the neuropsychological correlates of frontal lobe dysfunction?

    A. Akinetic mutism may follow lesions to the superior mesial aspect of the frontal lobe.
    B. The patient with akinetic mutism makes no effort to communicate by any modality and will not track moving targets with smooth pursuit eye movements.
    C. Akinetic mutism is typically more severe with right- as opposed to left-sided lesions.
    D. Acquired sociopathy is associated with memory disturbances.
    E. The dorsolateral frontal cortices have not been linked to verbal regulation of behavior.

144. Patients with this personality disorder are mostly women who spend an excessive amount of time seeking attention and making themselves attractive. They also display an effusive but labile and shallow range of feelings, often being overly impressionistic and given to hyperbolic descriptions of others. Which personality disorder is being described?

    A. Narcissistic personality disorder.
    B. Borderline personality disorder.
    C. Dependent personality disorder.
    D. Histrionic personality disorder.
    E. Avoidant personality disorder.

145. Which of the following mood stabilizers is considered to be a first-line augmenting agent for schizophrenic patients with persistent aggressiveness?

    A. Phenytoin.
    B. Carbamazepine.
    C. Oxcarbazepine.
    D. Lithium.
    E. Valproate.

146. *Ataque de nervios*, which is prevalent in Latin America, is an example of which type of dissociative disorder?

    A. Dissociative amnesia.
    B. Dissociative fugue.
    C. Dissociative identity disorder.
    D. Dissociative trance disorder.
    E. Acute stress disorder.

147. Twin, family, and adoption studies have demonstrated that familial and genetic factors are important for the development of alcohol dependence. The largest twin studies have yielded heritability estimates in which range?

    A. 10%–20%.
    B. 20%–30%.
    C. 30%–40%.
    D. 40%–50%.
    E. 50%–60%.

148. Which of the following statistics is *true* regarding substance abuse and dependence?

    A. The most commonly abused benzodiazepine is lorazepam.
    B. Among the 1%–2% of individuals using benzodiazepines without medical supervision, about 15% meet DSM-IV-TR criteria for sedative abuse or dependence.
    C. Of individuals admitted for addiction treatment, benzodiazepines are the drug of choice in about 5%–10% of these patients.
    D. About a quarter of benzodiazepine abusers in substance abuse treatment programs have a comorbid psychiatric disorder.
    E. Benzodiazepine abuse is uncommon in opioid-dependent patients undergoing methadone maintenance treatment.

149. Lithium has been reported to have a robust effect on which particular type of mania?

    A. Mania associated with human immunodeficiency virus.
    B. Mania associated with traumatic brain injury.
    C. Mania associated with steroid use.
    D. Mania associated with Parkinson's disease.
    E. Mania associated with multiple sclerosis.

150. Psychiatric comorbidity in attention-deficit/hyperactivity disorder (ADHD) often complicates this already difficult-to-manage disorder. Which of the following statements is *true?*

    A. Conduct disorder occurs in 20%–40% of ADHD cases.
    B. Abused children with both posttraumatic stress disorder (PTSD) and ADHD have the same degree of motor hyperactivity as do children with classic ADHD alone.

    C. Thyroid hormone resistance is a common cause of ADHD.
    D. A high incidence of ADHD is found with girls, but not boys, with Tourette's syndrome.
    E. ADHD-type symptoms may indicate genetic risk in schizophrenia pedigrees.

151. All of the following characterize the sleep electroencephalography (EEG) of depressed patients *except*

    A. Decreased rapid eye movement (REM) latency.
    B. Prolonged sleep latency.
    C. Decreased slow-wave sleep.
    D. Increased REM latency.
    E. Decreased time in non-REM sleep.

152. DeCuypere et al. (2005) conducted a follow-up study of 55 transsexual patients (both male-to-female and female-to-male) after sex reassignment surgery. Among their findings was that

    A. Only 20% of patients reported improvement in their sexuality.
    B. Male-to-female patients experienced more general health problems.
    C. Most patients reported that their expectations concerning the surgery had not been met on a social and emotional level.
    D. Major problems were observed in the patients.
    E. Few patients experienced a positive change in orgasmic sensations.

153. Delusions that cannot be understood by other psychological processes are referred to as *primary delusions*. Which of the following is an example of this type of delusion?

    A. Poverty.
    B. Nihilism.
    C. Thought insertion.
    D. Persecution.
    E. Guilt.

154. The abilities involved in formulating goals, planning, effectively carrying out goal-directed plans, monitoring, and self-correcting are collectively called

    A. Executive functions.
    B. Motor functions.
    C. Perception.
    D. Praxis.
    E. Constructional ability.

155. Which of the following medications commonly prescribed for the management of impulsivity may potentially worsen symptoms?

    A. Monoamine oxidase inhibitors.
    B. Serotonin reuptake inhibitors.
    C. Benzodiazepines.
    D. Atypical neuroleptics.
    E. Mood stabilizers.

156. A 22-year-old female patient whom you are treating is concerned that she may develop schizophrenia, given that her mother has been treated for many years for paranoid schizophrenia. The patient is an only child, and her biological father has no psychiatric history. This patient's risk rate is

    A. 6%.
    B. 13%.
    C. 25%.
    D. 46%.
    E. 53%.

157. Which of the following features is descriptive of depersonalization disorder?

    A. Patients frequently have impaired reality testing.
    B. Patients are rarely distressed by the symptoms.
    C. Derealization rarely co-occurs with depersonalization.
    D. Patients are frequently delusional.
    E. The symptoms are usually transient.

158. Which of the following factors was identified as an important predictor of subsequent early alcohol use?

    A. Family history of depression.
    B. Divorced parents.
    C. Maltreatment.
    D. Poor school performance.
    E. Premature birth.

159. Which of the following statements is *true* regarding the National Institute of Mental Health (NIMH) Treatment of Depression Collaborative Research Program?

    A. The treatment outcomes of psychodynamic psychotherapy were comparable to those of pharmacotherapy and clinical management.

    B. The treatment outcomes of psychodynamic psychotherapy were comparable to those of the manually driven therapies, interpersonal therapy (IPT), and cognitive-behavioral therapy (CBT).
    C. There was no evidence of greater effectiveness of the psychotherapies compared with pharmacotherapy and clinical management.
    D. Patients were assigned to one of four 32-week treatment conditions: interpersonal therapy (IPT), cognitive-behavioral therapy, (CBT) imipramine plus clinical management, or placebo plus clinical management.
    E. The psychotherapies were shown to be more effective than pharmacotherapy and clinical management.

160. Family studies of bipolar disorder have demonstrated all of the following findings *except*

    A. A sevenfold increase in lifetime risk for bipolar disorder in families with the disorder compared with family members of control subjects.
    B. Recurrence risks were found to be higher in females, either of the relative or of the bipolar proband.
    C. The age at onset of the first manic or depressive episode has been shown to be earlier in the younger generation of two generations of affected relative pairs.
    D. The risk for bipolar disorder appears to be especially elevated in the relatives of probands with early-onset disorder.
    E. The risk for bipolar disorder increases with the number of psychiatrically ill relatives.

161. Imaging studies have helped to delineate a constellation of brain regions involved in attention-deficit/hyperactivity disorder (ADHD). Which of the following is the most consistent neuroanatomical finding in ADHD subjects relative to non-ADHD control subjects?

    A. Decreased size of the caudate.
    B. Increased size of the frontal cortex.
    C. Increased size of the posterior portion of the corpus callosum.
    D. Decreased size of the cerebellar vermis.
    E. Increased size of the anterior portion of the corpus callosum.

162. The neurobiology of depression involves hypo-activity in the following cortical structures *except*

    A. Dorsolateral prefrontal cortex.
    B. Ventrolateral prefrontal cortex.
    C. Orbitofrontal prefrontal cortex.
    D. Anterior cingulate cortex.
    E. Amygdala.

163. DSM-IV-TR (American Psychiatric Association 2000) includes within the impulse-control disorder category five distinct impulse-control disorders not elsewhere classified. Which of the following is *not* one of these five disorders?

    A. Intermittent explosive disorder.
    B. Kleptomania.
    C. Pyromania.
    D. Trichotillomania.
    E. Binge-eating disorder.

164. When interviewing a depressed or suicidal patient, the psychiatrist is advised to do all of the following *except*

    A. Begin with assessment of physical appearance and motor behavior.
    B. Thoroughly explore neurovegetative signs or symptoms and their effect on patient function.
    C. Be attentive to recent psychosocial stressors (especially losses) and recent anniversaries of significant past losses.
    D. Allow the patient to set the pace of the interview, avoid excessive engagement, and tolerate long silences.
    E. Assess both suicidal cognitions and the patient's ability to control self-destructive impulses.

165. Regarding chemically mediated synapses and their neurotransmitters, which of the following is *true?*

    A. Chemical synapses are faster than electrical synapses.
    B. Chemical synapses are limited in utility because they do not allow for signal amplification.
    C. Chemical synapses can modulate the activity of other cells through activation of second-messenger cascades.
    D. Small molecule transmitters (e.g., glutamate, gamma-aminobutyric acid, and glycine) are stored in large dense-core vesicles.

E. Neuropeptides (e.g., somatostatin, endorphins, and enkephalins) mediate fast synaptic transmission.

166. The primary differential diagnostic issue for antisocial personality disorder involves which of the following diagnoses?

    A. Narcissistic personality disorder.
    B. Paranoid personality disorder.
    C. Obsessive-compulsive personality disorder.
    D. Avoidant personality disorder.
    E. Schizoid personality disorder.

167. Which of the following candidate genes implicated in schizophrenia has also been associated with velo-cardiofacial syndrome?

    A. Dystrobrevin binding protein–1.
    B. Neuregulin-1.
    C. Catechol-*O*-methyltransferase (COMT).
    D. Disrupted-in-schizophrenia–1 and –2.
    E. Metabotropic glutamate receptor–3.

168. Which of the following characteristics is indicative of dissociative amnesia?

    A. The memory loss is wide-ranging rather than limited to a discrete period of time.
    B. There is difficulty learning new information.
    C. The amnesia is typically anterograde.
    D. The memory loss is episodic.
    E. The memory loss is generally not limited to events of a traumatic nature.

169. Which of the following DSM-IV-TR clinical criteria does not apply to a diagnosis of substance abuse?

    A. Withdrawal symptoms or the taking of a substance to avoid withdrawal symptoms.
    B. Recurrent substance use resulting in failure to fulfill major role obligations.
    C. Recurrent substance use in situations in which it is physically hazardous.
    D. Recurrent substance-related legal problems.
    E. Continued substance use despite persistent or recurrent social problems caused by the effects of the substance.

170. All of the following statements describe either benefits of naltrexone treatment for opiate dependence or patient populations who may respond well to naltrexone treatment *except*

A. Patients with a history of recent employment do well while taking naltrexone.
B. Naltrexone may be prescribed by any physician in his or her office.
C. Naltrexone has been shown to be effective in treating opiate dependence even when simply prescribed as a medication in the absence of a structural rehabilitation program.
D. Naltrexone is not a controlled substance.
E. Health care professionals have done well in naltrexone treatment programs as patients.

171. What is the the first-line treatment recommendation of the American Psychiatric Association during the acute phase of rapid cycling?

A. Lithium, valproic acid, or lamotrigine.
B. Lithium or valproic acid but not lamotrigine.
C. Lithium plus valproic acid.
D. Lithium or valproic acid plus an antipsychotic.
E. Lithium but not valproic acid.

172. Psychostimulant medications remain the cornerstone of attention-deficit/hyperactivity disorder (ADHD) treatment. Of the following, which is the least common side effect of psychostimulants?

A. Anorexia.
B. Irritability.
C. Dysphoria.
D. Tics and other stereotypic movements.
E. Insomnia.

173. Which of the following statements is *true* regarding sexual orientation as addressed in DSM-IV-TR?

A. A diagnosis of transvestic fetishism requires the presence of homosexual sexual orientation.
B. Transvestic fetishism may be diagnosed in either homosexual or heterosexual men.
C. Homosexual orientation is an exclusionary criterion for transvestic fetishism.
D. Gender identity disorder is the appropriate diagnosis for "sissy" behavior in young boys.
E. Sexual disorder not otherwise specified (NOS) does not encompass distress about sexual orientation.

174. After fully exploring the patient's personal history, the psychiatrist proceeds to the next history item by asking, "Is there a family history of psychiatric illness, for example, suicidal behavior, mental retardation, or anxiety, mood, psychotic, substance abuse, or personality disorder?" This would be an example of

A. Excessive direct questions.
B. Preemptive topic shift.
C. Run-on questioning.
D. Put down.
E. Checklist questioning.

175. Regarding gamma-aminobutyric acid (GABA) receptors, which of the following is *true?*

A. Excitatory postsynaptic potentials in the brain are mediated primarily by GABA receptors.
B. The GABA$_A$ receptor–channel complex is composed of five subunits.
C. GABA receptors are metabotropic receptors.
D. Clinical actions of benzodiazepines and barbiturates are proportional to their binding potential at GABA$_B$ receptors.
E. Benzodiazepines increase GABA current by increasing the amount of "open" time in receptor channels.

176. The police bring to the emergency department a young adult male who was found talking to himself in public and chuckling and gesturing for no apparent reason. The patient is unkempt; his speech is odd and idiosyncratic, although there is no overt psychosis. A drug screen is negative. There is no information on whether gradual social deterioration has occurred. Of the personality disorders, which of the following is the most likely diagnosis in this patient?

A. Paranoid personality disorder.
B. Schizoid personality disorder.
C. Schizotypal personality disorder.
D. Antisocial personality disorder.
E. Avoidant personality disorder.

177. Magnetic resonance imaging (MRI) studies of the brains of patients with schizophrenia have revealed a volume decrease in all of the following brain structures *except*

A. Hippocampus.
B. Amygdala.

C. Parahippocampal gyrus.

D. Superior temporal gyrus.

E. Caudate nucleus.

178. Repression, as a general model for keeping information out of conscious awareness, differs from dissociation in a number of important ways. Which of the following statements describes repression?

A. The organizational structure of mental contents is horizontal, with subunits of information divided from one another but equally available to consciousness.

B. Motivated forgetting is the underlying mechanism.

C. The information is kept out of awareness for a discrete and sharply delimited time.

D. The information is stored in a discrete and untransformed manner.

E. Retrieval of information can be direct to uncover warded-off memories.

179. Which of the following statements is *true* regarding the Epidemiologic Catchment Area (ECA) study?

A. The study sampled adults and adolescents.

B. It used DSM-IV-TR diagnostic criteria.

C. The study reported a lifetime prevalence of alcohol abuse and dependence of more than 10% of the population for each disorder.

D. Lifetime prevalence of alcohol abuse was highest for subjects ages 30–39 years.

E. Marijuana abuse/dependence was the most common disorder due to illicit drugs.

180. Which of the following statements is *true* regarding opioid antagonists?

A. Naltrexone is poorly absorbed in the gut.

B. Naloxone is poorly absorbed from the gut but is effective when given parenterally.

C. Naltrexone does not block opiate-induced euphoria, respiratory depression, and other opiate effects.

D. Naltrexone must be dosed daily to be effective.

E. In cases of overdose, a one-time dose of naloxone should be given initially.

181. Which of the following symptoms is *not* characteristic of fragile X syndrome?

A. Social withdrawal and reduced caregiver attachment.

B. Gaze avoidance.

C. Hand flapping.

D. Tactile defensiveness.

E. Perseveration.

182. A core feature associated with impulse-control disorders is that at the time of committing the act the person normally experiences

A. Regret.

B. Pleasure or gratification.

C. A heightened sense of tension or arousal.

D. A sense of relief from the urge.

E. Self-reproach or guilt.

183. Which of the following statements about studies of amnesia as it is associated with hippocampal damage is *false*?

A. Neuropsychological findings have demonstrated selective impairments in relational memory.

B. The hippocampal system mediates long-term relational memory.

C. There is a consistent relationship between the side of the hippocampal lesion and the type of learning impairment.

D. The hippocampal system plays a role in the learning of perceptuomotor skills.

E. The hippocampal system is not the principal repository for old memories.

184. An important theoretical issue is whether the personality disorders are best classified as dimensions or categories. Which of the following arguments supports a categorical approach to personality disorder classification?

A. The thresholds for diagnosing personality disorders are arbitrary.

B. Excessive diagnostic co-occurrence between personality disorders has been observed in many studies.

C. The residual category of personality disorder not otherwise specified (NOS) may be the most commonly assigned personality disorder diagnosis in clinical practice.

D. There is considerable heterogeneity of features among patients receiving the same diagnosis.

E. Categorical models better reflect how clinicians think about pathological syndromes.

185. Which of the following psychosocial treatments for schizophrenia has been found *not* to be effective and may increase the risk for decompensation?

A. Assertive community treatment (ACT).
B. Cognitive-behavioral therapy (CBT).
C. Individual psychoanalytically oriented psychotherapy.
D. Family therapy.
E. Personal therapy.

186. Which of the following is more indicative of somatization disorder than of physical illness?

A. Laboratory abnormalities of the suggested physical disorder.
B. Physical signs of structural abnormalities.
C. Involvement of multiple organ systems.
D. Late onset and acute course.
E. Involvement of only one organ system.

187. Which of the following is associated with intravenous use of cocaine?

A. Ischemic necrosis of the nasal septum.
B. Dyspnea.
C. Pneumothorax.
D. Pulmonary infarction.
E. Endocarditis.

188. Which of the following statements is *true* regarding fluctuations of medication levels?

A. Nortriptyline doses are likely to require increases in order to maintain stable maternal blood levels as pregnancy progresses.
B. Neonates are not prone to lithium toxicity as long as their serum concentrations are lower than maternal concentrations.
C. Maternal valproic acid concentrations increase as pregnancy progresses.

D. Lamotrigine clearance decreases as pregnancy progresses.
E. The mean fetal-to-maternal ratio of the plasma concentrations of selective serotonin reuptake inhibitors (SSRIs) is about 20 to 1.

189. All of the following statements are true *except*

A. Obsessive-compulsive disorder (OCD) is seen in approximately 10% of patients with Tourette's syndrome.
B. OCD symptoms usually appear 1–2 years before simple tics in these patients.
C. Tic-related OCD has an earlier onset than does classic OCD.
D. Tic-related OCD features more ritualized touching and tapping than does classic OCD.
E. Tic-related OCD has a less favorable response to selective serotonin reuptake inhibitors (SSRIs) and a more favorable response to antipsychotic augmentation compared with classic OCD.

190. Which of the following disorders has been found to frequently co-occur with pathological gambling?

A. Generalized anxiety disorder.
B. Panic disorder.
C. Attention deficit/hyperactivity disorder (ADHD).
D. Somatization disorder.
E. Dissociative identity disorder.

191. Where is the hippocampus located?

A. Nonmesial portion of the temporal lobe.
B. The mesial temporal lobe.
C. Temporoparietal junction of the parietal lobe.
D. Basal ganglia.
E. Dorsolateral prefrontal region.

192. A number of studies that have compared patients with personality disorders with patients with no personality disorders or with Axis I disorders have found that patients with personality disorders

A. Were more likely to be married.
B. Had less unemployment.
C. Were rarely less well educated.
D. Had fewer periods of disability.
E. Had better social functioning.

193. Which of the following statements is *true* regarding second-generation antipsychotics (SGAs) (or atypical antipsychotics) and first-generation antipsychotics (FGAs)?

    A. SGAs have efficacy comparable to that of FGAs in treating positive symptoms of schizophrenia.
    B. FGAs are superior to SGAs in treating negative symptoms of schizophrenia.
    C. FGAs are superior to SGAs in treating refractory schizophrenia.
    D. The incidence of extrapyramidal symptoms in patients treated with FGAs is comparable to that in patients treated with SGAs.
    E. The frequency of tardive dyskinesia in patients treated with SGAs is comparable with that in patients treated with FGAs.

194. Other psychiatric disorders must be carefully considered in the differential diagnosis of somatization disorder. The most troublesome distinction is between somatization disorder and which of the following psychiatric disorders?

    A. Dissociative disorders.
    B. Anxiety disorders.
    C. Substance use disorders.
    D. Impulse control disorders.
    E. Adjustment disorders.

195. In addition to the substance use disorders characterized by patterns of use, there are several substance-related disorders whose descriptions are based on the pharmacological effects of the substance. Which of the following is *not* true of these illnesses?

    A. This category includes both intoxication and withdrawal syndromes.
    B. Examples of substance-induced syndromes include dementia and amnestic and mood disorders.
    C. All abused substances have a specific intoxication syndrome.
    D. All categories of abused substances produce a withdrawal syndrome.
    E. Not all categories of abused substances produce all of the substance-induced disorders.

196. All of the following are common medical complications of bulimia nervosa *except*

    A. Elevated serum bicarbonate levels.
    B. Parotid gland enlargement.
    C. Cardiomyopathy.
    D. Elevated amylase levels.
    E. Hyperkalemia.

197. Which of the following symptoms is characteristic of temporal, rather than frontal, lobe symptoms?

    A. Heightened interpersonal sensitivity and paranoid ideation.
    B. Social disinhibition.
    C. Reduced attention.
    D. Distractibility.
    E. Impaired judgment.

198. Patients with paranoid personality disorder exhibit which of the following symptoms?

    A. Delusions.
    B. Suspiciousness.
    C. Marginal thinking.
    D. Perceptual distortions.
    E. Odd thinking.

199. Phencyclidine (PCP) and ketamine cause a schizophrenic-like reaction in humans and affect which of the following neurotransmitters?

    A. Dopamine.
    B. Serotonin.
    C. Nicotine.
    D. Glutamine.
    E. Acetylcholine.

200. Which of the following symptoms or characteristics is less consistent with malingering of psychosis than with true psychosis?

    A. Atypical hallucinations or delusions.
    B. Marked discrepancies in interview and noninterview behavior.
    C. Blatant contradictions between reported prior episodes and documented psychiatric history.
    D. Psychotic symptoms with common paranoid, grandiose, or religious themes.
    E. Gross inconsistencies in reported psychotic symptoms.

# Answer Guide to Exam 2

1. Which of the following is not one of Eugen Bleuler's "four As" of schizophrenia?

   A. Affective flattening.
   B. Alogia.
   C. Ambivalence.
   D. Loosening of associations.
   E. Autism.

**The correct response is option B.**

*Alogia*, which describes the significant decrease in the amount of unprompted speech given by a patient, is not one of Bleuler's four As: 1) looseness of **A**ssociations, 2) **A**ffective flattening, 3) **A**utism, and 4) **A**mbivalence. This description is essentially an emphasis on cognition, apparent in the link between the term *schizophrenia* (or "split mind") and the formal thought disorder manifest in disturbed associations.

Minzenberg MJ, Yoon JH, Carter CS: Schizophrenia, in The American Psychiatric Publishing Textbook of Psychiatry, 5th Edition. Edited by Hales RE, Yudofsky SC, Gabbard GO. Washington, DC, American Psychiatric Publishing, 2008, p 409

2. Which of the following physical signs is *not* characteristic of opioid withdrawal?

   A. Dysphoria.
   B. Muscle aches.
   C. Nausea and vomiting.
   D. Miotic ("pinpoint") pupils.
   E. Piloerection (gooseflesh).

**The correct response is option D.**

Opioid withdrawal can be a polysymptomatic and physically uncomfortable condition that may, upon assessment, benefit from inpatient medical detoxification. Signs and symptoms of opioid withdrawal include dysphoric mood, muscle aches, nausea or vomiting, lacrimation or rhinorrhea, yawning, fever, insomnia, as well as pupillary dilation, piloerection, and diaphoresis. Although opioid withdrawal is not associated with severe medical complications, inpatient detoxification may be necessary to ameliorate withdrawal symptoms that if left untreated could result in ongoing opioid use.

Greenfield SF, Hennessy G: Assessment of the patient, in The American Psychiatric Publishing Textbook of Substance Abuse Treatment, 4th Edition. Edited by Galanter M, Kleber HD. Washington, DC, American Psychiatric Publishing, 2008, p 58

3. Which of the following criteria is *not* necessary in order to diagnose factitious disorder?

   A. Intentional production of physical or psychological signs and symptoms.
   B. Unconscious production of signs or symptoms.
   C. Motivation to assume the sick role.
   D. Absence of external incentives beyond assumption of the sick role.
   E. Factitious symptoms of predominantly physical or psychological origin.

**The correct response is option B.**

Unconsciously produced signs or symptoms are not consistent with factitious disorder, in which signs and symptoms are, by definition, consciously produced.

McDermott BE, Leamon MH, Feldman MD, et al: Factitious disorder and malingering, in The American Psychiatric Publishing Textbook of Psychiatry, 5th Edition. Edited by Hales RE, Yudofsky SC, Gabbard GO. Washington, DC, American Psychiatric Publishing, 2008, p 644; see Table 14–1

4. Which of the following is a definition of acculturation?

   A. A diversity of cultural backgrounds, in which people from each background share a common national culture.
   B. Identity with a natural and/or shared language of origin, religious practice, dress, diet, holidays, family rituals, and leisure activities.
   C. The accumulative social learning process in which people assimilate the values of the host culture while retaining the values of the original culture.
   D. The comparison of characteristics across culture groups.
   E. Distinct groupings resulting, for example in the context of addiction, from substance use, abuse, or dependence.

**The correct response is option C.**

*Acculturation* is the accumulative social learning process in which people assimilate the values of the host culture while retaining the values of the original culture. Option A is incorrect because this statement describes *ethnicity*. Option B describes *background*. Option D describes the term *cross-cultural*. Option E describes *subcultures*.

El-Guebaly N: Cross-cultural aspects of addiction, in The American Psychiatric Publishing Textbook of Substance Abuse Treatment, 4th Edition. Edited by Galanter M, Kleber HD. Washington, DC, American Psychiatric Publishing, 2008, p 45

5. A 72-year-old woman lost two brothers to cancer, one 12 months ago and the other 10 months ago. Following each loss, the woman experienced a 3- to 4-week period of mildly depressed mood and sleep disturbance, and had visual hallucinations of her brothers walking around in her home. Eight months ago, she voluntarily retired from running a small business that she thoroughly enjoyed for the previous 20 years in order to spend more time with her grandchildren. Two months later, this formerly physically and socially active woman underwent routine urologic surgery that led to multiple medical complications and has prevented her from participating in a bowling league and other activities. She denies depressed mood, but family members have noticed that in the past 6 months she has been more "weepy" than usual, crying at the slightest provocation; watches television all day, rarely leaving the house; and does not seem to be as talkative as before. Of the following, which is the most likely current diagnosis?

   A. Bereavement and major depressive disorder.
   B. Chronic adjustment disorder with depressed mood.
   C. Acute adjustment disorder with depressed mood.
   D. Bereavement and adjustment disorder with depressed mood.
   E. Major depressive disorder.

**The correct response is option B.**

When a stressor has resulted in impaired function or distress, together with depressed mood, then the diagnosis of adjustment disorder with depressed mood is appropriate. The adjustment disorder is considered chronic, not acute, because her symptoms have lasted longer than 6 months, therefore option C is incorrect.

Option A is incorrect because although the woman underwent a period of bereavement that included sleep disturbance and vivid hallucinations, 2 months of these symptoms are considered "normal" according to DSM-IV-TR criteria. She seems to have undergone a period of bereavement after the death of each brother that lasted for at least 4 weeks. Subsequent stressors, however, led to persistent symptoms of depressed mood. The association between depression and loss is common. However, not all depressive episodes that follow a stressor develop into major depressive episodes, and chronic adjustment disorder with depressed mood is the most precise diagnosis at this time.

American Psychiatric Association: Diagnostic and Statistical Manual of Mental Disorders, 4th Edition, Text Revision. Washington, DC, American Psychiatric Association, 2000

6. Which of the following statements is *true* regarding selective mutism?

   A. Most children with selective mutism do not meet DSM-IV-TR criteria for either social phobia or avoidant disorder.
   B. Social situations are usually difficult to dichotomize into mute versus nonmute situations.
   C. Early trauma has been shown to be a significant risk factor for selective mutism.
   D. Selective mutism is associated with a history of delayed speech and language development and

high incidences of enuresis, encopresis, depression, and separation anxiety.

E. Selective mutism has been associated with oppositional, stubborn, and negative personality traits.

## The correct response is option B.

The severity of mutism tends to vary across a spectrum from situations in which speech is completed avoided, to situations in which speech is completely uninhibited, which is similar to what occurs in social phobia. Option A is incorrect because most children with selective mutism do meet DSM-IV-TR criteria for either social phobia or avoidant disorder. Options C, D, and E are incorrect because studies have not demonstrated an association between selective mutism and histories of delayed speech and language development or early trauma; high incidences of enuresis, encopresis, depression, or separation anxiety; or oppositional, stubborn, and negative personality traits.

Black B, Garcia AM, Freeman JB, et al: Specific phobia, panic disorder, social phobia, and selective mutism, in The American Psychiatric Publishing Textbook of Child and Adolescent Psychiatry, 3rd Edition. Edited by Wiener JM, Dulcan MK. Washington, DC, American Psychiatric Publishing, 2004, p 596

7. A number of tasks place demands on attentional capacity and focus because of the requirement to divide attention or to inhibit interfering stimuli or responses. An example is a test in which the subject is required to name the color of a word while ignoring the actual word. What is the name of this test?

A. Wisconsin Card Sorting Test.
B. Trail Making Test.
C. Controlled Word Association Test.
D. Continuous Performance Test.
E. Stroop Test.

## The correct response is option E.

In the Stroop Test, the subject is required to name the color of a word while ignoring the actual word. Interference is created because the color and the meaning of the word are mismatched. This test places strong demands on inhibitory systems, which must suppress both the other stimulus feature and a strong response tendency.

Option A is incorrect because the Wisconsin Card Sorting Test measures concept formation and hypothesis testing. Subjects are presented with cards containing features for color, shape, and number. The task is to determine the correct category for a response based on feedback provided by the examiner. Subjects sort cards to the appropriate category but must switch to a new category when the response criteria change. Poor performance on the Wisconsin Card Sorting Test is often associated with impairments of conceptual flexibility and switching and perseveration secondary to frontal lobe damage affecting the dorsolateral region.

Option B is incorrect because in the Trail Making Test, subjects are initially required to connect a sequence of numbers by drawing a line between numbers that are placed randomly on a sheet of paper (Trails A). On Trails B, subjects are required to alternate between numbers and letters in ascending order. Errors occur when the patient fails to alternate and connects two letters or numbers or when there is a break in the sequence and a particular item is omitted. Each task is timed.

Option C is incorrect because in the Controlled Word Association Test, subjects are given 60 seconds to produce as many words as possible that start with a particular letter (e.g., F, A, or S) or that belong to a specific semantic category (e.g., animals). The total number of words generated is then scored. Option D is incorrect because the Continuous Performance Test measures signal detection performance over blocks of trials. Visual or auditory stimuli are presented sequentially. Intermixed among distractor stimuli are particular target stimuli, such as the letter A. The task is to respond to the target and not to the distractors.

Cohen RA, Salloway S, Sweet LH: Neuropsychiatric aspects of disorders of attention, in The American Psychiatric Publishing Textbook of Neuropsychiatry and Behavioral Neurosciences, 5th Edition. Edited by Yudofsky SC, Hales RE. Washington, DC, American Psychiatric Publishing, 2008, pp 417, 419, 420

8. Which of the following is *least* likely to be associated with psychosis?

A. Stroke.
B. Complex partial seizures.
C. Huntington's disease.
D. HIV disease.
E. Late-stage Parkinson's disease.

## The correct response is option A.

Psychosis is relatively uncommon in stroke and multiple sclerosis and is less common in traumatic brain injury and early and middle-phase Parkinson's disease. It is more commonly associated with complex partial epilepsy, Huntington's disease and late-stage Parkinson's disease, HIV infection, limbic encephalitis, multi-infarct and Alzheimer's dementias, and tumors involving the temporal lobe and diencephalon. Psychosis complicating neuropsychiatric illness can be seen in a number of syndromes but is generally less common than mood disorders.

Holtzheimer PE III, Snowden M, Roy-Byrne PP: Psychopharmacological treatments for patients with neuropsychiatric disorders, in The American Psychiatric Publishing Textbook of Neuropsychiatry and Behavioral Neurosciences, 5th Edition. Edited by Yudofsky SC, Hales RE. Washington, DC, American Psychiatric Publishing, 2008, p 1157

9.    All of the following medications have been shown to have little to no efficacy in the treatment of acute mania *except*

A.   Gabapentin.
B.   Topiramate.
C.   Clonazepam.
D.   Carbamazepine.
E.   Lamotrigine.

**The correct response is option D.**

Carbamazepine was superior to placebo in one crossover trial and one parallel-group trial, comparable with lithium in two comparison studies, and comparable with chlorpromazine in two other comparison trials. The other drugs listed have not yet shown efficacy in acute mania.

Keck PE Jr, McElroy SL: Treatment of bipolar disorder, in The American Psychiatric Publishing Textbook of Psychopharmacology, 3rd Edition. Edited by Schatzberg AF, Nemeroff CB. Washington, DC, American Psychiatric Publishing, 2004, p 869

10.   Which of the following is *not* considered a risk factor for adolescent suicide?

A.   Prior suicide attempts.
B.   Mood disorder.
C.   Substance abuse.
D.   Female gender.
E.   Age 16 years or older.

**The correct response is option D.**

Female gender is not considered a risk factor for adolescent suicide. Suicide risk in certain clinical populations may not reflect suicide risk in the population at large and thus needs to be considered by the clinician when treating certain patient groups. Risk factors for adolescent suicide include prior attempts, affective disorder, substance abuse, living alone, male gender, age 16 years or older, and a history of physical and/or sexual abuse. Adverse childhood experiences such as emotional, physical, and sexual abuse are associated with an increased risk of attempted suicide throughout the lifespan (Dube et al. 2001).

Dube SR, Anda RF, Felitti VJ, et al: Childhood abuse, household dysfunction and the risk of attempted suicide throughout the lifespan: findings from the Adverse Childhood Experiences Study. JAMA 286:3089–3096, 2001

Simon RI: Suicide, in The American Psychiatric Publishing Textbook of Psychiatry, 5th Edition. Edited by Hales RE, Yudofsky SC, Gabbard GO. Washington, DC, American Psychiatric Publishing, 2008, p 1643

11.   Delirium is frequently mistaken for a depressive disorder. Which of the following statements is *true* regarding delirium compared to depression?

A.   Hypoactive delirium is frequently mistaken for depression in the acute medical setting.
B.   Delirium tends to have a diurnal course, whereas depression has a fluctuating course.
C.   Level of consciousness is usually impaired in both delirium and depression in acutely ill hospitalized patients.
D.   Acutely ill patients with depressed mood usually have auditory, tactile, gustatory, and olfactory hallucinations, if at all. Patients with delirium usually only have auditory hallucinations.
E.   If present, the delusions seen in acutely ill patients with depressed mood tend to be fleeting and fragmented; delusions in delirium tend to be complex and mood congruent.

**The correct answer is option A.**

Hypoactive, as opposed to hyperactive, delirium tends to be mistaken for depression in acutely ill patients. Studies have shown that >50% of patients who were referred to a psychiatric consultation-liaison service for "depression" and had thoughts of death were actually delirious. Option B is incorrect because depression tends to have a diurnal course, whereas delirium has a fluctuating course.

Option C is incorrect because level of consciousness is impaired in delirium but not usually in depression. Option D is incorrect because the hallucinations seen in depression are usually only auditory; hallucinations in delirium are usually visual but can be auditory, tactile, gustatory, and olfactory. Option E is incorrect because the delusions in depressed patients tend to be complex and mood congruent; in delirium, the delusions are fleeting, fragmented, and usually persecutory.

Trzepacz PT, Meagher DJ: Neuropsychiatric aspects of delirium, in The American Psychiatric Publishing Textbook of Neuropsychiatry and Behavioral Neurosciences, 5th Edition. Edited by Yudofsky SC, Hales RE. Washington, DC, American Psychiatric Publishing, 2008, pp 450–451; Table 11–3

12. Which of the following is *true* of essential tremor, also called benign essential tremor and familial tremor?

   A. Essential tremor is defined as a rhythmic oscillation across a joint resulting from voluntary, alternating activation of agonist and antagonist muscles.
   B. The prevalence of essential tremor increases with age and by definition cannot result in severe impairment in activities of daily living.
   C. Early on, a key feature of essential tremor is that the tremor is usually present at rest.
   D. Essential tremor tends to manifest as postural and kinetic tremors of the arms and hands and occasionally of the head and neck.
   E. Essential tremor is similar to the type of tremors that are seen in Parkinson's disease.

**The correct response is option D.**

Essential tremor tends to manifest as postural and kinetic tremors of the arms and hands and occasionally of the head and neck. Essential tremor is the most prevalent movement disorder among adults and elderly persons, affecting up to 2% of the general population. The prevalence of essential tremor increases with age, and in individuals older than 70 years estimates of the prevalence of essential tremor range to more than 10%. A key feature of essential tremor, at least early on, is that the tremor is absent at rest, only occurring during action or when a posture is being held. There is usually a clear family history of tremor, and often the tremor attenuates with alcohol use, a phenomenon that can contribute to development of alcoholism in susceptible individuals.

Option A is incorrect because essential tremor is defined as a rhythmic oscillation across a joint resulting from involuntary (not voluntary), alternating activation of agonist and antagonist muscles. Option B is incorrect because although it is true that the prevalence of essential tremor increases with age, essential tremor may result in severe impairment in activities of daily living. Option C is incorrect because essential tremor is usually absent at rest. Option E is incorrect because the tremor of Parkinson's disease is a resting tremor, which is distinct from both postural and kinetic tremors (see box).

Scott B: Movement disorders, in The American Psychiatric Publishing Textbook of Geriatric Psychiatry, 3rd Edition. Edited by Blazer DG, Steffens DC, Busse EW. Washington, DC, American Psychiatric Publishing, 2004, pp 232, 236

---

*Postural tremor* is tremor that appears when a posture is being held against gravity.

*Kinetic tremor* is tremor that occurs with action, or when approximating a target, such as during finger-to-nose testing. Kinetic tremor interferes with eating and drinking.

*Resting tremor* is tremor that typically attenuates transiently during voluntary movement, such as when an individual picks up an object. This type of tremor is seen in some types of Parkinson's disease.

(From Scott 2004, pp. 232, 236)

---

13. Twin studies of schizophrenia have contributed a great deal to our understanding of the genetic transmission of this illness. Which of the following statements is *true* regarding twin studies of schizophrenia?

   A. The risk of schizophrenia in monozygotic (MZ) cotwins of affected probands is at least three times that of dizygotic (DZ) cotwins.
   B. About 95% of MZ twin pairs are concordant for schizophrenia despite being genetically identified.
   C. The risk of schizophrenia in MZ cotwins of affected probands is about five times that in the general population.
   D. Monochorionic MZ twins are less likely to be concordant than are dichorionic MZ twins.
   E. Most (up to 75%) nonschizophrenic MZ cotwins of affected probands show a variety of psychiatric disorders.

**The correct response is option A.**

The risk of schizophrenia in MZ cotwins of affected probands is at least three times that in DZ cotwins and about 40–60 times that in the general population. Just as noteworthy, however, is that only about half of MZ twin pairs are concordant for schizophrenia despite genetic identity. Monochorionic MZ twins are more likely to be concordant that are dichorionic MZ twins, perhaps because the former share not only identical genes but also a similar in utero environment. Although many nonschizophrenic MZ cotwins of affected probands show a variety of psychiatric disorders, including "neurotic" and character disorders and "schizoid" conditions, up to 43% monoseries appear to harbor no psychiatric disorder.

Choudary PV, Knowles JA: Genetics, in The American Psychiatric Publishing Textbook of Psychiatry, 5th Edition. Edited by Hales RE, Yudofsky SC, Gabbard GO. Washington, DC, American Psychiatric Publishing, 2008, p 209

14. Dementia with Lewy bodies includes all of the following neuropathological correlates *except*

    A. Neurofibrillary tangles.
    B. Neuritic plaques.
    C. More Lewy bodies in the substantia nigra than in idiopathic Parkinson's disease.
    D. Alpha-synuclein expressed in Lewy bodies.
    E. Weight of the brain typically less than the weight of the brain of the patient with Alzheimer's disease.

**The correct response is option E.**

Generally, the weight of the brain of the patient with dementia with Lewy bodies is nearly normal and therefore greater than the weight of the brain of the patient with Alzheimer's disease, which tends to be reduced. Diffuse and neuritic plaques may be frequent, but neurofibrillary change is generally less intense than in "pure" Alzheimer's disease. The frequency of Lewy bodies in the substantia nigra of patients with dementia with Lewy bodies may be greater than in patients dying of idiopathic Parkinson's disease. Alpha-synuclein is a protein that has been found to be mutated in rare families with early onset familial Parkinson's disease.

Byrun CE, Moore SD, Hulette CM: Neuroanatomy, neurophysiology, and neuropathology of aging, in The American Psychiatric Publishing Textbook of Geriatric Psychiatry, 3rd Edition. Edited by Blazer DG, Steffens DC, Busse EW. Washington, DC, American Psychiatric Publishing, 2004, pp 73–74

15. Symptoms of neurological illness may mimic or mask the symptoms of mood disturbance. All of the following symptoms are relatively nonspecific, commonly occurring in neurologic illness but not necessarily a symptom of a primary mood disorder, *except*

    A. Apathy.
    B. Mood disturbance with incongruent affect.
    C. Mood disturbance with congruent affect.
    D. Agitation.
    E. Decreased psychomotor speed.

**The correct response is option C.**

Specific symptoms for a primary mood disorder include mood disturbances with congruent affect, anhedonia, excessive guilt, and suicidality. Option B is incorrect because neurologic illnesses often present with incongruent affects in contrast with primary mood disorders. Options A, D, and E are relatively nonspecific symptoms that tend to be associated with neurologic illnesses regardless of the presence of a mood disorder.

Hales RE, Bourgeois JA, Shahrokh NC: Study Guide to Neuropsychiatry and Behavioral Neurosciences: A Companion to The American Psychiatric Publishing Textbook of Neuropsychiatry and Behavioral Neurosciences, 5th Edition, Washington, DC, American Psychiatric Publishing, 2008, p 175

Holtzheimer PE III, Mayberg HS: Neuropsychiatric aspects of mood disorders, in The American Psychiatric Publishing Textbook of Neuropsychiatry and Behavioral Neurosciences, 5th Edition. Edited by Yudofsky SC, Hales RE. Washington, DC, American Psychiatric Publishing, 2008, pp 1011–1017

16. Based on a variety of studies, it appears that patients with psychiatric complaints alone, without other medical problems or symptoms, would benefit from which of the following screening tests?

    A. Serum glucose.
    B. Serum $B_{12}$.
    C. Serum calcium.
    D. Computed tomography scan.
    E. Serum folate.

**The correct response is option A.**

Results of various studies suggest that patients with psychiatric complaints alone will benefit from a few screening tests such as serum glucose concentration, blood urea nitrogen concentration, creatinine clearance, and urinalysis. More extensive screening panels appear to be unnecessary.

Kim HF, Schulz PE, Wilde EA, et al: Laboratory testing and imaging studies in psychiatry, in The American Psychiatric Publishing Textbook of Psychiatry, 5th Edition. Edited by Hales RE, Yudofsky SC, Gabbard GO. Washington, DC, American Psychiatric Publishing, 2008, p 21

17. Sanctions by the American Psychiatric Association for misconduct include all of the following *except*

    A. Admonishment.
    B. Reprimand.
    C. Suspension of membership.
    D. Expulsion from membership.
    E. Direction for state medical board to suspend medical license.

**The answer is option E.**

The American Psychiatric Association (2001) may impose four possible sanctions for misconduct:

1. Admonishment—an informal warning.
2. Reprimand—a formal censure.
3. Suspension (for a period not to exceed 5 years).
4. Expulsion.

American Psychiatric Association: The Principles of Medical Ethics With Annotations Especially Applicable to Psychiatry, 2001 Edition. Washington, DC, American Psychiatric Association, 2001

18. Which of the following is *not* true regarding federal regulation of nursing homes in the United States?

    A. Regulatory concern in the 1980s focused on the inappropriate use of chemical restraints.
    B. Regulatory concern in the 1980s focused on the inappropriate use of physical restraints.
    C. In the 1980s, there was concern that antidepressants were being prescribed excessively in nursing homes.
    D. The Omnibus Budget Reconciliation Act of 1987, which contained the Nursing Home Reform Act, addressed mental health care issues in nursing homes.
    E. Nursing home applicants must now have a preadmission assessment to establish psychiatric needs and appropriate placement.

**The correct response is option C.**

Regulatory focus on nursing homes was prompted in the 1980s by a combination of factors: 1) concerns about the inappropriate use of physical and chemical restraints, 2) concerns about inadequate treatment of depression (Institute of Medicine 1986), and 3) cautions from the Federal Office of Management and Budget that older adults with chronic mental illness were being discharged from state mental hospitals and admitted to nursing homes, thereby shifting the cost of their care from the states to the federal government. Congress responded by passing the Nursing Home Reform Act as part of OBRA-87. The resultant Health Care Financing Administration regulations required preadmission assessment to identify nursing home applicants with mental illness who required acute psychiatric care and to ensure that they were appropriately placed in residential or treatment settings.

Institute of Medicine, Committee on Nursing Home Regulation: Improving the Quality of Care in Nursing Homes. Washington, DC, National Academy Press, 1986

Reichman WE, Streim JE, Loebel JP: Legal, ethical, and policy issues, in The American Psychiatric Publishing Textbook of Geriatric Psychiatry, 3rd Edition. Edited by Blazer DG, Steffens DC, Busse EW. Washington, DC, American Psychiatric Publishing, 2004, p 517

19. According to DSM-IV-TR (American Psychiatric Association 2000), sexual aversion disorder is an example of which of the following sexual dysfunctions?

    A. Sexual desire disorder.
    B. Sexual arousal disorder.
    C. Orgasmic disorder.
    D. Sexual pain disorder.
    E. Sexual dysfunction due to a general medical condition.

**The correct response is option A.**

Sexual aversion disorder is an example of a sexual desire disorder.

American Psychiatric Association: Diagnostic and Statistical Manual of Mental Disorders, 4th Edition, Text Revision. Washington, DC, American Psychiatric Association, 2000

Becker JV, Stinson JD: Human sexuality and sexual dysfunctions, in The American Psychiatric Publishing Textbook of Psychiatry, 5th Edition. Edited by Hales RE, Yudofsky SC, Gabbard GO. Washington, DC, American Psychiatric Publishing, 2008, p 712; Table 16–1

---

## DSM-IV-TR Classification of Sexual Dysfunctions

Sexual desire disorders (hypoactive sexual desire disorder, sexual aversion disorder)

Sexual arousal disorders (female sexual arousal disorder, male erectile disorder)

Orgasmic disorders (female orgasmic disorder, male orgasmic disorder, premature ejaculation)

Sexual pain disorders (dyspareunia [not due to a general medical condition], vaginismus [not due to a general medical condition])

Others (sexual dysfunction due to a general medical condition, substance-induced sexual dysfunction, sexual dysfunction not otherwise specified)

---

20. Barriers to effective communication between the older patient and clinician can include

    A. Physician perceiving the older adult patient incorrectly because of personal fears of aging and death.
    B. Patient having perceptual problems.
    C. Patient taking longer to respond to inquiries, resisting the physician who attempts to hurry through the interview.
    D. Patient perceiving the physician unrealistically.
    E. All of the above.

## The correct response is option E.

The clinician may perceive the older adult patient incorrectly because of personal fears of aging and death or because of previous negative experiences with his or her own parents. Perceptual problems, such as hearing and visual impairments, may exacerbate disorientation and complicate the communication of problems to the clinician. Elderly persons frequently take longer to respond to inquiries and resist the clinician who attempts to rush through the history-taking interview. The elderly patient may perceive the physician unrealistically on the basis of previous life experiences (i.e., transference may occur).

Blazer DG: The psychiatric interview of older adults, in The American Psychiatric Publishing Textbook of Geriatric Psychiatry, 3rd Edition. Edited by Blazer DG, Steffens DC, Busse EW. Washington, DC, American Psychiatric Publishing, 2004, p 175

21. Which of the following is *true* regarding serotonin (5-hydroxytryptamine [5-HT]) receptors?

    A. To date, three 5-HT receptors have been identified.
    B. 5-HT is synthesized from the essential fatty acid (EFA) tyrosine.
    C. The $5\text{-HT}_{2A}$ receptor is most abundant in the cerebral cortex.
    D. No 5-HT receptors are known to project to the dorsal raphe, median raphe, or subcortical structures.
    E. 5-HT is metabolized to 5-hydroxyindoleacetic acid (5-HIAA) via the enzyme catechol-*O*-methyltransferase (COMT).

## The correct response is option C.

The $5\text{-HT}_{2A}$ receptor, which is the most widely studied of the 5-HT receptors, is most abundant in the cerebral cortex. Option A is incorrect because to date 14 5-HT receptors have been identified. Option B is incorrect because 5-HT is synthesized from the EFA tryptophan. Tyrosine is an EFA that is the precursor for L-dopa in the noradrenergic system. Option D is incorrect because the $5\text{-HT}_{1A}$ and $5\text{-HT}_{1B}$ receptors are present in the cerebral cortex, in the projection sites in dorsal and median raphe, and in subcortical structures such as the caudate, nucleus accumbens, hippocampus, thalamus, and amygdala. Option E is incorrect because serotonin is metabolized to 5-HIAA via monoamine oxidase (MAO).

Melchitzky DS, Austin MC, Lewis DA: Chemical neuroanatomy of the primate brain, in The American Psychiatric Publishing Textbook of Psychopharmacology, 3rd Edition. Edited by Schatzberg AF, Nemeroff CB. Washington, DC, American Psychiatric Publishing, 2004, p 78

22. In the evaluation of personality disorders in the elderly patient, the physician can be assisted by several objective and semistructured instruments. Which of the following clinical assessment instruments is a *semistructured interview* rather than an ancillary self-report measure?

    A. Millon Clinical Multiaxial Inventory–III.
    B. Personality Disorders Examination.
    C. Personality Diagnostic Questionnaire.
    D. Schedule for Nonadaptive and Adaptive Personality.
    E. Wisconsin Personality Disorders Inventory.

## The correct response is option B.

The Personality Disorders Examination is a semistructured interview.

Oxman TE, Ferrell RB: Personality disorders, in The American Psychiatric Publishing Textbook of Geriatric Psychiatry, 3rd Edition. Edited by Blazer DG, Steffens DC, Busse EW. Washington, DC, American Psychiatric Publishing, 2004, p 372

23. When the physician evaluates the older patient with suspicious and/or paranoid complaints, which of the following is *not* recommended?

   A. Determine whether suspicious behavior is warranted; for example, consider the possibility of neglect or abuse.
   B. Challenge the delusion to verify that it is indeed fixed in the patient's mind.
   C. Obtain routine laboratory studies, including chemistry and complete blood count.
   D. Consider use of neuroimaging (e.g., computed tomography or magnetic resonance imaging of the head).
   E. Consider specialty referrals for vision and hearing examination and correction.

## The correct response is option B.

Challenging the delusional patient is usually not recommended. Routine laboratory studies needed in new cases of paranoia include blood chemistry, a complete blood count, and a thyroid profile. Use of neuroimaging and examinations of vision and hearing may be indicated to identify potential areas for intervention.

Gwyther LP, Steffens DC: Agitation and suspiciousness, in The American Psychiatric Publishing Textbook of Geriatric Psychiatry, 3rd Edition. Edited by Blazer DG, Steffens DC, Busse EW. Washington, DC, American Psychiatric Publishing, 2004, p 378

24. Sleep disturbances in major depression include all of the following *except*

   A. Increased sleep latency.
   B. Decrease in slow-wave sleep in the first non–rapid eye movement (NREM)–rapid eye movement (REM) cycle.
   C. Increased latency to REM sleep.
   D. Occurrence of REM sleep earlier in the night.
   E. Increase in REM density.

## The correct response is option C.

REM latency is shortened, not lengthened, in sleep disturbances in depressed patients. Sleep disturbances in major depression include increased sleep latency (time to fall asleep), increased nocturnal awakening and early morning awakenings, decrease in slow-wave (or deep) sleep during the first NREM–REM cycle, occurrence of REM sleep earlier in the night, and increase in REM density. Option C is incorrect because latency to REM sleep is decreased, not increased.

Hirshkowitz M, Sharafkhaneh A: Neuropsychiatric aspects of sleep and sleep disorders, in The American Psychiatric Publishing Textbook of Neuropsychiatry and Behavioral Neurosciences, 5th Edition. Edited by Yudofsky SC, Hales RE. Washington, DC, American Psychiatric Publishing, 2008, p 683

25. Which of the following is *true* regarding somatization disorder in geriatric patients?

   A. Paralleling the relative risk for depressive disorders, the risk for somatization disorder in women is twice that in men.
   B. Somatization disorder is common in patients with irritable bowel disease.
   C. As patients with somatization disorder age, their reported symptoms tend to change and symptoms are reported in a less consistent pattern.
   D. Prominent pain symptoms are the typical "pseudoneurological" presentation.
   E. Another term for somatization disorder is *Munchausen syndrome.*

## The correct response is option B.

Somatization disorder was diagnosed in 42% of a sample of 50 medical outpatients with irritable bowel disease and is seen almost exclusively in women. The majority of individuals with somatization disorder demonstrate consistent symptom patterns as they age. Somatization disorder is characterized by multiple physical complaints that include pain at four or more sites, two gastrointestinal symptoms, one sexual symptom, and one pseudoneurological symptom (other than pain). Another term used to describe somatization disorder is Briquet's syndrome.

Agronin ME: Somatoform disorders, in The American Psychiatric Publishing Textbook of Geriatric Psychiatry, 3rd Edition. Edited by Blazer DG, Steffens DC, Busse EW. Washington, DC, American Psychiatric Publishing, 2004, p 296

26. Several neurobiological substrates have been identified to explain the acute reinforcing effects of abused drugs. These models include both specific neurotransmitters and anatomical foci. Which drug of abuse is associated with the neurotransmitters glutamate, dopamine, gamma-aminobutyric acid (GABA), and opioid peptides and the anatomic loci of the nucleus accumbens, ventral tegmental area, and amygdala?

    A. Alcohol.
    B. Nicotine.
    C. Cocaine.
    D. Amphetamines.
    E. Opioids.

**The correct response is option A.**

Alcohol is associated with glutamate, dopamine, GABA, and opioid peptides at the nucleus accumbens, ventral tegmental area, and amygdala sites (see table below). Option B is incorrect because nicotine is associated with dopamine, GABA, and opioid peptides but not glutamate. Options C and D are incorrect because cocaine and amphetamines are associated with dopamine and GABA but not opioid peptides or glutamate. Option E is incorrect because opioids are associated with opioid peptides, dopamine, and endocannaboids but not glutamate dopamine.

Koob GF: Neurobiology of addiction, in The American Psychiatric Publishing Textbook of Substance Abuse Treatment, 4th Edition. Edited by Galanter M, Kleber HD. Washington, DC, American Psychiatric Publishing, 2008, p 7; Table 1–2

### Neurobiological substrates for the acute reinforcing effects of drugs of abuse

| Drug of abuse | Neurotransmitter | Site |
| --- | --- | --- |
| Cocaine and amphetamines | Dopamine<br>Gamma-aminobutyric acid | Nucleus accumbens<br>Amygdala |
| Opioids | Opioid peptides<br>Dopamine<br>Endocannabinoids | Nucleus accumbens<br>Ventral tegmental area |
| Nicotine | Dopamine<br>Gamma-aminobutyric acid<br>Opioid peptides | Nucleus accumbens<br>Ventral tegmental area<br>Amygdala |
| $\Delta^9$-Tetrahydrocannabinol | Endocannabinoids<br>Opioid peptides<br>Dopamine | Nucleus accumbens<br>Ventral tegmental area |
| Alcohol | Dopamine<br>Opioid peptides<br>Gamma-aminobutyric acid<br>Glutamate<br>Endocannabinoids | Nucleus accumbens<br>Ventral tegmental area<br>Amygdala |

*Source.* Koob GF: "Neurobiology of Addiction," in *The American Psychiatric Publishing Textbook of Substance Abuse Treatment.* Edited by Galanter M, Kleber HD. Washington, DC, American Psychiatric Publishing, 2008, pp. 3–16. Used with permission.

27. All of the following symptoms may be present in neuroleptic malignant syndrome (NMS) *except*

    A. Autonomic instability that may include labile blood pressure, tachycardia, hyperthermia, and diaphoresis.
    B. Altered level of consciousness.
    C. Muscular rigidity.
    D. Elevated creatine phosphokinase level and white blood cell count.
    E. Hyperreflexia and nystagmus.

**The correct response is option E.**

Hyperreflexia often occurs in serotonin syndrome, not NMS. Characterized by muscle rigidity, hyperthermia, altered mental status, autonomic instability, and evidence of muscle injury, NMS is a potentially fatal condition and has been estimated to occur in 0.01%–0.02% of patients treated with antipsychotics (Strawn et al. 2007). Options A, B, C, and D are incorrect because NMS includes these findings. Other symptoms include dysphagia and bowel obstruction. The pathophysiology of NMS was once believed to stem from dopamine blockade, so atypical antipsychotics initially were assumed to have a low risk of NMS because of their relatively weak dopamine blockade compared with typical antipsychotics. However, case reports and retrospective data in recent years now suggest otherwise, and questions have been raised about whether cases of NMS from atypical antipsychotics represent the need for more flexible diagnostic criteria that include an atypical variant (Picard et al. 2008).

Garlow SJ, Purselle D, D'Orio B: Psychiatric emergencies, in The American Psychiatric Publishing Textbook of Psychopharmacology, 3rd Edition. Edited by Schatzberg AF, Nemeroff CB. Washington, DC, American Psychiatric Publishing, 2004, p 1080

Picard LS, Lindsay S, Strawn JR, et al: Atypical neuroleptic malignant syndrome: diagnostic controversies and considerations. Pharmacotherapy 28:530–535, 2008

Strawn JR, Keck PE Jr, Caroff SN: Neuroleptic malignant syndrome. Am J Psychiatry 164:870–876, 2007

28. Which of the following is *true* regarding widowhood and widowerhood in the United States?

    A. The mean age at spousal loss is 3 years older for women than for men.
    B. The mean duration of widowhood for women is twice that of widowerhood for men.
    C. The rates of widowhood among persons older than 65 are much higher for Hispanic and Asian Americans than for Caucasian individuals.
    D. Among those older than 65, women are twice as likely as men (30% vs. 15%) to have lost a spouse.
    E. Following the loss of a spouse, women are at a higher risk for mortality than are men.

**The correct response is option B.**

The mean duration of widowhood or widowerhood is approximately 14 years for women and 7 years for men. The mean age at spousal loss is 69 years for men and 66 years for women. Option C is incorrect because the rates of widowhood among people age 65 or older are similar for whites, Hispanics, and Asian Americans and are slightly higher for African Americans. Option D is incorrect because among people age 65 or older, about 45% of women and 15% of men have lost a spouse. Option E is incorrect because after the loss of a spouse, older men are at higher risk for mortality than are women.

Thompson LW, Kaye JL, Tang PCY, et al: Bereavement and adjustment disorders, in The American Psychiatric Publishing Textbook of Geriatric Psychiatry, 3rd Edition. Edited by Blazer DG, Steffens DC, Busse EW. Washington, DC, American Psychiatric Publishing, 2004, pp 319–320

29. Panic disorder has been associated with all of the following *except*

    A. Hyperreactivity of the locus coeruleus.
    B. Dysregulated serotonergic modulation.
    C. Decreased GABA–benzodiazepine receptor complex binding.
    D. Hypersensitive brainstem carbon dioxide chemoreceptors.
    E. Elevated plasma levels of epinephrine.

**The correct response is option E.**

Plasma levels of epinephrine do not rise consistently in panic disorder. Researchers in the 1930s and 1940s demonstrated that epinephrine infusions caused the physical but not the emotional symptoms of anxiety in human subjects. Options A, B, C, and D are incorrect because all of these answers reflect true statements.

Hollander E, Simeon D: Anxiety disorders, in The American Psychiatric Publishing Textbook of Psychiatry, 5th Edition. Edited by Hales RE, Yudofsky SC, Gabbard GO. Washington, DC, American Psychiatric Publishing, 2008, p 512, Table 12–4

30. Recent studies suggest that the antidepressant-associated switch rate—the proportion of bipolar disorder patients who switch to manic symptoms in response to antidepressant treatment—is lower than the previously believed 70%. Which of the following best represents the current estimate of this rate?

    A. 20%.
    B. 30%.
    C. 5%–15%.
    D. <2%.
    E. 50%.

**The correct response is option C.**

Until recently, some treatment guidelines suggested avoiding or minimizing use of antidepressants for bipolar depression, based on reported antidepressant-associated switch rates, which ranged widely, from 10% to 70%. However, many of these earlier estimates of the incidence of antidepressant-associated switching were based on naturalistic studies that did not control for the switch rate associated with the illness itself. The switch rates reported in recent randomized, controlled trials of lamotrigine monotherapy and combinations of paroxetine and lithium or of lithium and valproate have ranged from 3% to 8%. In addition, Post et al. (2001) reported a switch rate of 14% (8% hypomania, 6% mania) in a 10-week acute treatment trial comparing bupropion, venlafaxine, and sertraline in combination with mood stabilizers.

Keck PE, McElroy SL: Treatment of bipolar disorder, in The American Psychiatric Publishing Textbook of Psychopharmacology, 3rd Edition. Edited by Schatzberg AF, Nemeroff CB. Washington, DC, American Psychiatric Publishing, 2004, pp 871–872

Post RM, Altshuler LL, Frye MA, et al: Rate of switch in bipolar patients prospectively treated with second-generation antidepressants as augmentation to mood-stabilizers. Bipolar Disorders 3:259–265, 2001

31. Although definitive data on birth defects and selective serotonin reuptake inhibitors (SSRIs) are lacking, a range of transient perinatal symptoms (which may require admission to special care nurseries) have been reported. These perinatal symptoms include all of the following *except*

    A. Jitteriness.
    B. Poor muscle tone.
    C. Weak/absent cry.
    D. Hyperglycemia.
    E. Low Apgar scores.

**The correct response is option D.**

Hyperglycemia is not a perinatal symptom of third-trimester exposure to SSRIs. Third-trimester exposure to SSRIs is associated with an increased risk of perinatal symptoms sometimes requiring admission to special care nurseries (including jitteriness, poor muscle tone, weak or absent cry, respiratory distress, hypoglycemia, low Apgar score, and seizures).

Burt VK, Stein K: Treatment of women, in The American Psychiatric Publishing Textbook of Psychiatry, 5th Edition. Edited by Hales RE, Yudofsky SC, Gabbard GO. Washington, DC, American Psychiatric Publishing, 2008, pp 1497–1498

32. In their study examining differences in symptom profile between patients with delirium and patients with dementia, which of the following symptoms or disorders were more common in delirium than in dementia?

    A. Delusions.
    B. Affective lability.
    C. Thought process abnormalities.
    D. Disorders of short-term memory.
    E. Disorders of long-term memory.

**The correct response is option C.**

Significant differences have been found between delirium and dementia for thought process abnormalities, sleep-wake cycle disturbances, motor agitation, attention, and visuospatial ability, which were more impaired in delirium. Options A, B, D, and E are incorrect because no differences were found for the disorders for delusions, affective lability, language, motor retardation, orientation, and short- or long-term memory.

Trzepacz PT, Meagher DJ: Neuropsychiatric aspects of delirium, in The American Psychiatric Publishing Textbook of Neuropsychiatry and Behavioral Neurosciences, 5th Edition. Edited by Yudofsky SC, Hales RE. Washington, DC, American Psychiatric Publishing, 2008, p 450

33. When handling diagnostic/prognostic communications and while recommending additional services to the family of patients with dementia, which of the following is *true*?

A. Some Asian American families regard use of formal supportive services as a moral failure.

B. Families rarely tolerate the demands of terminal care of an immobile and incontinent patient but usually can manage the disruptive sleep and behavior of moderate dementia.

C. Combined interventions, although appealing, have not been shown to decrease caregiver depression.

D. Health care decisions should not be made until the diagnosis of dementia is clear and there have been several months of follow-up to estimate rapidity of progression.

E. Families should be advised that judgment about financial matters is usually unimpaired in early dementia.

**The correct response is option A.**

In some Asian American families, use of any formal services may be viewed as a moral failure of the family. Some families cope well with end-of-life care for an immobile or incontinent older adult but are unable to tolerate the disruptive behaviors or sleep patterns of persons with moderate dementia. Combining individual and family counseling, family education, support group participation, and sustained availability of a care manager is associated with decreased caregiver burden and depression; decreases in the elder's disruptive symptoms; and increased caregiver satisfaction, subjective well-being, and self-efficacy. Handling of money and health care decisions should be addressed soon after diagnosis to ensure time for patients to select a surrogate. Families must be reminded that financial judgment is impaired early in dementia.

Gwyther LP: Working with the family of the older adult, in The American Psychiatric Publishing Textbook of Geriatric Psychiatry, 3rd Edition. Edited by Blazer DG, Steffens DC, Busse EW. Washington, DC, American Psychiatric Publishing, 2004, pp 465–468

34. Compared with control subjects, depressed patients perform relatively poorly in measures of

A. Incidental learning.
B. Automatic cognitive processing.
C. Declarative memory.
D. Nondeclarative memory.
E. Procedural memory.

**The correct response is option C.**

Compared with healthy individuals, those who are depressed perform poorly on cognitive tasks requiring effort and a relatively deep level of processing, which occurs in the *declarative*, or explicit, domain of memory. Effortful processing requires attention, must be initiated intentionally, and benefits from rehearsal (e.g., memorizing DSM-IV-TR diagnostic critiera). Because of impaired attention and executive functions (planning, organizing, short-term declarative memory), depressed individuals have a shallow depth of encoding information when compared with healthy individuals, resulting in impaired learning and retrieval. Options A, B, D, and E are incorrect because they are all associated with *automatic processing*, which requires limited attentional capacity, and can occur without intention or awareness. An example of incidental learning is an individual's capacity to learn and retain what was eaten for breakfast.

Stern Y, Sackeim HA: Neuropsychiatric aspects of memory and amnesia, in The American Psychiatric Publishing Textbook of Neuropsychiatry and Behavioral Neurosciences, 5th Edition. Edited by Yudofsky SC, Hales RE. Washington, DC, American Psychiatric Publishing, 2008, pp 576–577

35. According to DSM-IV-TR (American Psychiatric Association 2000) diagnostic criteria for somatoform disorders, pseudocyesis falls under which specific diagnostic category?

A. Undifferentiated somatoform disorder.
B. Conversion disorder.
C. Somatoform disorder not otherwise specified (NOS).
D. Body dysmorphic disorder.
E. Hypochondriasis.

**The correct response is option C.**

The basic DSM-IV-TR requirement for a diagnosis of somatoform disorder NOS is that a disorder with somatoform symptoms must not meet criteria for a specific somatoform disorder. The first example listed in DSM-IV-TR is *pseudocyesis*. In DSM-III (American Psychiatric Association 1980) and DSM-III-R (American Psychiatric Association 1987), pseudocyesis was included as a conversion disorder under criteria broadened to include an alteration or loss of physical functioning, suggesting a physical disorder that was an expression of psychological conflict or need. After contraction of conversion disorder to voluntary motor and sensory dysfunction in DSM-IV (American Psychiatric Association 1994), pseudocyesis was excluded and relegated to the NOS category.

American Psychiatric Association: Diagnostic and Statistical Manual of Mental Disorders, 3rd Edition. Washington, DC, American Psychiatric Association, 1980

American Psychiatric Association: Diagnostic and Statistical Manual of Mental Disorders, 3rd Edition, Revised. Washington, DC, American Psychiatric Association, 1987

American Psychiatric Association: Diagnostic and Statistical Manual of Mental Disorders, 4th Edition. Washington, DC, American Psychiatric Association, 1994

American Psychiatric Association: Diagnostic and Statistical Manual of Mental Disorders, 4th Edition, Text Revision. Washington, DC, American Psychiatric Association, 2000

Yutzy SH, Parish BS: Somatoform disorders, in The American Psychiatric Publishing Textbook of Psychiatry, 5th Edition. Edited by Hales RE, Yudofsky SC, Gabbard GO. Washington, DC, American Psychiatric Publishing, 2008, p 636

36.  Which of the following statements is *true* regarding sociodemographic variables or migration?

A.  Because Mexican societal attitudes toward women's alcohol consumption are more negative than in other ethnic groups, the rates of alcohol abuse among Mexican women is likely to be less than that of other cultural groups.
B.  The higher proportion of youth within Native American populations should lead to lower substance abuse rates.
C.  Differences in family stability and the occurrence of domestic violence in a given ethnic group are unlikely to influence the prevalence of substance use in that group.
D.  The stronger the ties to Hispanic culture among persons born outside the United States who speak Spanish, the more likely that group is to use drugs, compared with Hispanics born in the United States who speak mostly English.
E.  Hawaiian residents of Chinese and Japanese ancestry have higher levels of alcohol use if born in Asia than if born in Hawaii.

**The correct response is option A.**

Mexican societal attitudes toward women's alcohol consumption are more negative than in other ethnic groups. Therefore, this societal norm is likely to have a protective effect on the prevalence estimates of women's alcohol consumption. Differences in age distribution must be taken into account. For example, the higher proportion of

youth, a high-risk group for substance use among Native Americans, influences the prevalence of substance abuse in that ethnic group. Thus, option B is incorrect. Differences in family stability and the occurrence of domestic violence in a given ethnic group may also be a cause and/or consequence of the prevalence of substance use in that group. The same can be said about differences in socioeconomic status and work history. The extent of recent migration in an ethnic group is viewed as both a risk and a protective factor. For example, first- and second-generation acculturation may create socioeconomic stressors, which increase the vulnerability to addiction. Yet, evidence also shows that the stronger the ties to Hispanic culture among persons born outside the United States who speak mostly Spanish, the less likely that group is to use drugs, compared with Hispanics born in the United States who speak mostly English. Hawaiian residents of Chinese and Japanese ancestry also have lower levels of alcohol use if born in Asia than if born in Hawaii.

El-Guebaly N: Cross-cultural aspects of addiction, in The American Psychiatric Publishing Textbook of Substance Abuse Treatment, 4th Edition. Edited by Galanter M, Kleber HD. Washington, DC, American Psychiatric Publishing, 2008, pp 46–47

37.  When should a screening electrocardiogram (ECG) be ordered for a psychiatric patient?

A.  All psychiatric patients should receive an ECG.
B.  An ECG should be obtained for all psychiatric patients older than 50 years.
C.  An ECG should be obtained for a psychiatric patient prior to receiving a selective serotonin reuptake inhibitor.
D.  An ECG should be obtained for a psychiatric patient prior to initiating treatment with a psychotropic drug such as an atypical antipsychotic, which is known to increase cardiac conduction times.
E.  Medically healthy psychiatric patients without cardiovascular symptoms would benefit from routine screening.

**The correct response is option D.**

Regardless of patient age, an ECG is indicated when the history, review of systems, or findings from the physical examination suggest cardiovascular disease, or if a patient is initiating treatment with a psychotropic drug, such as a tricyclic antidepressant or an antipsychotic, that is known to alter cardiac function or increase cardiac conduction times. Routine ECG screening of young, medically healthy psychiatric patients who do not have cardiovascular symptoms is unnecessary. However, studies differ regarding the importance of electrocardiography in the elderly.

Kim HF, Schulz PE, Wilde EA, et al: Laboratory testing and imaging studies in psychiatry, in The American Psychiatric Publishing Textbook of Psychiatry, 5th Edition. Edited by Hales RE, Yudofsky SC, Gabbard GO. Washington, DC, American Psychiatric Publishing, 2008, pp 21, 36

38. Several key principles apply to the exercise of moral behavior and are especially applicable to medical ethics. The movement toward "parity" legislation to ensure that provision of care for mental illness is analogous to care for systemic illness illustrates the ethical principle of

    A. Nonmaleficence.
    B. Beneficence.
    C. Autonomy.
    D. Respect for persons.
    E. Justice.

**The correct response is option E.**

*Justice* is a moral principle that relates to treating people fairly and, in modern society, without prejudice. *Distributive justice* refers to equitable distribution of benefits and burdens among members of society. Parity legislation that seeks to ensure the provision of insurance for mental illness and related conditions that is equal or equivalent to insurance for physical illness illustrates a real-life effort at distributive justice in the United States. *Nonmaleficence* is a modern term for the old, perhaps ancient, rule of *primum non nocere* (first, do no harm). *Beneficence* refers to the belief that individuals should try to do good, to try to seek benefit for others. *Autonomy*, which means "self-rule," suggests a moral principle based on the importance of respecting others' right to personal self-governance. *Respect for persons* is a broad concept that encompasses respect for autonomy plus a deep regard for the worth and dignity of all human beings.

Roberts LW, Hoop JG, Dunn LB: Ethical aspects of psychiatry, in The American Psychiatric Publishing Textbook of Psychiatry, 5th Edition. Edited by Hales RE, Yudofsky SC, Gabbard GO. Washington, DC, American Psychiatric Publishing, 2008, pp 1605, 1607

39. Which of the following is *true* regarding advance directives?

    A. Patients receiving care funded by Medicare or Medicaid are required to execute advance directives.
    B. Notarization is required for a power of attorney for health care in all 50 states.
    C. "Durable power of attorney" is synonymous with "legal guardianship."
    D. A living will confers a wider scope of decision making than a power of attorney for health care.
    E. Compliance with advance directives by medical institutions remains poor.

**The correct response is option E.**

The level of compliance by the health care profession with the preferences of patients, even when these have been explicitly stated, continues to be poor. The Patient Self-Determination Act of 1991 requires hospitals, nursing homes, and organizations receiving Medicare and Medicaid funds from the federal government to notify patients of their right to express their wishes concerning life-sustaining care and of the laws of the relevant state with respect to advance directives. Option A is incorrect because the law does not require patients to sign such a document. Option B is incorrect because not all states require notarization of power of attorney documents. Option C is incorrect because power of attorney is given by a competent individual, but guardianship is obtained on an individual who has been deemed incompetent. The durable power of attorney (DPOA) is one that survives (or comes into existence upon) the disability of the principal. Option D is incorrect because a living will confers a narrower, not wider, scope on the decision making than does the DPOA.

Reichman WE, Streim JE, Loebel JP: Legal, ethical, and policy issues, in The American Psychiatric Publishing Textbook of Geriatric Psychiatry, 3rd Edition. Edited by Blazer DG, Steffens DC, Busse EW. Washington, DC, American Psychiatric Publishing, 2004, p 522

40. Which of the following statements is *false* regarding hypoactive sexual desire disorder?

    A. Hypoactive sexual desire disorder is the most common sexual complaint among females.
    B. Hypoactive sexual desire disorder is the most difficult of all the sexual dysfunctions to treat.

C. There is no consistent evidence to indicate that testosterone increases sexual interest in men.

D. Bupropion has been found to be beneficial for more than 50% of women with hypoactive sexual desire disorder in women.

E. Low-dose testosterone therapy has been found to increase sexual interest and desire in women.

**The correct response is option D.**

Hypoactive sexual desire disorder is perhaps the most common sexual complaint among women, but it has been the most difficult of all the dysfunctions to treat. Results from an empirical study evaluating bupropion's effectiveness in nondepressed women indicated that only 29% of the evaluable participants responded to the treatment. Testosterone has been used for both males and females to treat inhibited sexual desire; however, masculinizing side effects make its use problematic in women. There is no consistent evidence to indicate its success in increasing sexual interest in men, even when initial serum testosterone levels are low. In women, there appears to be some evidence suggestive of improvement in sexual interest and desire after application of low-dose testosterone therapy.

Becker JV, Stinson JD: Human sexuality and sexual dysfunctions, in The American Psychiatric Publishing Textbook of Psychiatry, 5th Edition. Edited by Hales RE, Yudofsky SC, Gabbard GO. Washington, DC, American Psychiatric Publishing, 2008, p 718

41. Which of the following statements is *false* regarding suicide in the United States?

A. The male suicide rate is approximately four times the female rate.

B. The rate of suicide attempts among females is three times the rate of attempts among males.

C. Suicide attempts are far more common than suicide deaths, approximately 25 attempts for each suicide death.

D. The most common method of suicide death is poisoning.

E. The suicide death rate in bipolar disorder is nearly 20 times that of the general population.

**The correct response is option D.**

Suicide statistics help to give the clinician a sense of the extent of this clinical problem and, when put into context, may guide clinical risk assessment and decision making. According to the American Associaton of Suicidology, the most common methods of suicide in 2004 were firearms (51.6%), suffocation/hanging (22.6%), and poisoning (17.9%). The suicide rate was 17.7 per 100,000 for males and 4.6 per 100,000 for females. Women attempt suicide about three times as often as men. In 2004, there were 3.7 male suicides for each female suicide and 3 female attempts for each male attempt. It is estimated that 811,000 suicide attempts occur annually in the United States (25 attempts for every suicide). The suicide rate for individuals with bipolar disorders is estimated at 193 per 100,000 (absolute risk), or 18 times higher (relative risk) compared with the suicide rate for the general population.

Simon RI: Suicide, in The American Psychiatric Publishing Textbook of Psychiatry, 5th Edition. Edited by Hales RE, Yudofsky SC, Gabbard GO. Washington, DC, American Psychiatric Publishing, 2008, pp 1637–1638

42. The inhibitory postsynaptic potentials in the brain are mediated primarily by which of the following receptors?

A. *N*-methyl-D-aspartate (NMDA) receptors.

B. Non-NMDA receptors.

C. Alpha-amino-3-hydroxy-5-methylisoxazole-4-propionic acid (AMPA) receptors.

D. Kainate receptors.

E. Gamma-aminobutyric acid (GABA) receptors.

**The correct response is option E.**

Inhibitory postsynaptic potentials in the brain are mediated primarily by GABA receptors. Several classes of GABA receptors have been identified. Excitatory postsynaptic potentials are mediated by two classes of ionotropic glutamate receptors: NMDA receptors, and non-NMDA or AMPA receptors. The non-NMDA glutamate receptors are further divided into AMPA receptors and kainate receptors on the basis of their affinities for these glutamate analogs.

McAllister AK, Usrey WM, Noctor SC, et al: Cellular and molecular biology of the neuron, in The American Psychiatric Publishing Textbook of Psychiatry, 5th Edition. Edited by Hales RE, Yudofsky SC, Gabbard GO. Washington, DC, American Psychiatric Publishing, 2008, pp 124, 126

43. Vaillant's studies of the hierarchy of psychological defenses have been cited to explain personality function in old age. All of the following defense mechanisms are considered to be mature and thus adaptive *except*

A. Humor.
B. Altruism.
C. Repression.
D. Sublimation.
E. Suppression.

**The correct response is option C.**

Repression is not considered a mature defense mechanism. Mature defense mechanisms include humor, altruism, sublimation, anticipation, and suppression.

Oxman TE, Ferrell RB: Personality disorders, in The American Psychiatric Publishing Textbook of Geriatric Psychiatry, 3rd Edition. Edited by Blazer DG, Steffens DC, Busse EW. Washington, DC, American Psychiatric Publishing, 2004, p 371

44. The clinical evaluation of the suspicious and/or paranoid older patient requires consideration of specific concerns about psychotic disorders in older patients. Which of the following is *true?*

   A. Because of schizophrenia patients' tendency to isolate and have a shorter life expectancy, chronic paranoid schizophrenia is an infrequent cause of suspiciousness in elderly patients.
   B. Elderly schizophrenia patients are best managed with medication alone, rather than comprehensive treatment models.
   C. New-onset delusions in older patients are usually bizarre in nature.
   D. Antipsychotic medication should be used in all cases of sporadic agitation related to delusions.
   E. Agitation may follow family members' challenging of the patient's delusions.

**The correct response is option E.**

Agitation may become an issue in the elderly when they are confronted by family or clinicians about their delusions. Chronic paranoid schizophrenia is a major cause of suspiciousness and agitation in elderly patients. Multimodal treatment is best in elderly schizophrenia patients. New-onset delusions in older patients are usually nonbizarre. Neuroleptic medications and behavioral interventions are best used in cases of sporadic agitation related to delusions.

Gwyther LP, Steffens DC: Agitation and suspiciousness, in The American Psychiatric Publishing Textbook of Geriatric Psychiatry, 3rd Edition. Edited by Blazer DG, Steffens DC, Busse EW. Washington, DC, American Psychiatric Publishing, 2004, pp 377–378

45. Many changes in sleep architecture are seen in aging, and these changes may play a role in late-life insomnia. Which of the following is a typical sleep architecture change affecting the elderly?

   A. Increased total sleep time.
   B. Decreased percentages of Stage 1 and 2 sleep.
   C. Increased percentages of Stage 3 and 4 sleep.
   D. Increased arousal threshold.
   E. Decreased absolute amounts of rapid eye movement (REM) sleep.

**The correct response is option E.**

Aging is associated with decreased absolute amounts of REM sleep, frequent arousals, and a redistribution of sleep across the 24-hour day (e.g., napping during the day).

Option A is incorrect because total sleep time decreases, not increases, with aging. Options B and C are incorrect because with aging, the proportion of Stages 1 and 2 (light sleep) increases, whereas the proportion of Stages 3 and 4 (deep sleep, or slow-wave sleep) decreases. Option D is incorrect because arousal threshold decreases with aging, which is thought to partially explain the increased frequency of arousals.

Hales RE, Bourgeois JA, Shahrokh NC: Study Guide to Psychiatry: A Companion to The American Psychiatric Publishing Textbook of Psychiatry, 5th Edition, Washington, DC, American Psychiatric Publishing, 2008, p 234

Krystal AD, Edinger JD, Wohlgemuth WK, et al: Sleep and circadian rhythm disorders, in The American Psychiatric Publishing Textbook of Geriatric Psychiatry, 3rd Edition. Edited by Blazer DG, Steffens DC, Busse EW. Washington, DC, American Psychiatric Publishing, 2004, pp 342–343

46. Undifferentiated somatoform disorder and hypochondriasis may present in the geriatric psychiatric patient. Which of the following statements is *true?*

   A. Undifferentiated somatoform disorder requires the presence of persistent physical complaints for at least 12 months.
   B. Patients with chronic pain rarely also qualify for a diagnosis of undifferentiated somatoform disorder.
   C. The psychological preoccupation in hypochondriasis relates to the symptoms experienced, rather than the possible disease "represented" by the symptoms.

D. High educational level and high socioeconomic status predispose individuals to hypochondriasis.

E. Comorbid depressive and anxiety disorders are common in hypochondriasis.

**The correct response is option E.**

Comorbid psychiatric disorders, especially major depression, panic disorder, and obsessive-compulsive disorder, are common in hypochondriasis. Undifferentiated somatoform disorder requires the presence of persistent physical pain for at least 6 months. Patients with chronic pain have high rates of undifferentiated somatoform disorder. Hypochondriasis is characterized by a preoccupation with fears of having a serious illness. Option D is incorrect because low education level and low socioeconomic status, not high, seem to increase the risk of hypochondriasis.

Agronin ME: Somatoform disorders, in The American Psychiatric Publishing Textbook of Geriatric Psychiatry, 3rd Edition. Edited by Blazer DG, Steffens DC, Busse EW. Washington, DC, American Psychiatric Publishing, 2004, pp 296–297

47. Many neurotransmitters are involved in the development of drug dependence, both in the acute reinforcing effects of drugs and in the recruitment of the brain stress system. All of the following neurotransmitters have been identified as being involved in the acute reinforcing effects of drugs *except*

A. Norepinephrine.
B. Dopamine.
C. Opioid peptides.
D. Serotonin.
E. Gamma-aminobutyric acid (GABA).

**The correct response is option A.**

During the development of dependence, a change in the function of neurotransmitters associated with the acute reinforcing effects of drugs (dopamine, opioid peptides, serotonin, GABA, and endocannabinoids), recruitment of the brain stress system (corticotropin-releasing factor and norepinephrine), and dysregulation of the neuropeptide Y brain antistress system are evident.

Koob GF: Neurobiology of addiction, in The American Psychiatric Publishing Textbook of Substance Abuse Treatment, 4th Edition. Edited by Galanter M, Kleber HD. Washington, DC, American Psychiatric Publishing, 2008, p 6

48. A 43-year-old man with a long history of treatment-resistant major depressive disorder was precribed and started taking a new antidepressant about 2 months ago. For the first time he has had some improvement in his symptoms after adequate trials of multiple antidepressant agents. Twenty-four hours after undergoing outpatient arthroscopic knee surgery, he goes to the emergency department, saying he "doesn't feel right" after taking an unknown pain medication by mouth. He has barely eaten anything in the past 48 hours. His blood pressure is 210/120 mmHg, heart rate 140 bpm, and temperature 103°F. On exam, the patient is somnolent and disoriented and noted to have nystagmus, myoclonus, hyperreflexia, and muscle rigidity. All of the following treatments may be beneficial *except*

A. Benzodiazepines.
B. Cyproheptadine.
C. Chlorpromazine.
D. Bromocriptine.
E. Propranolol.

**The correct response is option D.**

This case describes the typical features of serotonin syndrome, the symptoms of which improve with benzodiazepines, cyproheptadine, chlorpromazine, propranolol, or methysergide. Bromocriptine, which could be helpful for neuroleptic malignant syndrome, could exacerbate serotonin syndrome. The serotonin syndrome is a delirium characterized by altered level of consciousness, autonomic instability, and neuromuscular abnormalities such as myoclonus, hyperreflexia, nystagmus, akathisia, and muscle rigidity.

Several different drugs, usually administered in combination, can cause this adverse event. Because of the severity of this case, and based on clues in the history, the patient's pain medication may have been meperidine. Meperidine, when taken with monoamine oxidase inhibitors (MAOIs)—especially phenelzine or tranylcypromine—can induce a severe case of serotonin syndrome. Similar reactions have not been reported with opioids such as morphine or codeine. His long history of refractory depression suggests that he had been started on an MAOI, which has similar treatment efficacy with other antidepressant classes, but is considered second-line treatment because of its side effect profile, and the potential for significant drug-drug interactions. Other drugs causing this syndrome include combinations of the following: selective serotonin reuptake inhibitors, venlafaxine, trazodone, nefazodone, lithium, tryptophan, sumatriptan, buspirone, and amphetamines. Discontinuation of the offending agent and general supportive measures are the principal interventions.

Besides serotonin syndrome, lower on the differential diagnosis is an MAOI-induced hypertensive crisis after ingestion of a large amount of tyramine-containing foods. An MAOI-induced hypertensive crisis is unlikely because he has had little food intake in the past 48 hours, and these hypertensive crises usually occur 20–60 minutes after eating the offending food. Tyramine/MAOI-induced hypertensive crises are characterized by hypertension, occipital headache, palpitations, nausea, vomiting, apprehension, occasional chills, sweating, and restlessness. On exam, neck stiffness, pallor, mild pyrexia, dilated pupils, and motor agitation may be seen.

Garlow SJ, Purselle D, D'Orio B: Psychiatric emergencies, in The American Psychiatric Publishing Textbook of Psychopharmacology, 3rd Edition. Edited by Schatzberg AF, Nemeroff CB. Washington, DC, American Psychiatric Publishing, 2004, p 1080

Krishnan KRR: Monoamine oxidase inhibitors, in The American Psychiatric Publishing Textbook of Psychopharmacology, 3rd Edition. Edited by Schatzberg AF, Nemeroff CB. Washington, DC, American Psychiatric Publishing, 2004, pp 308–309

=====

### Tyramine-containing foods that should be avoided when taking MAOIs include:

Cheese, overripe fruit (e.g., banana peel), fava beans, sausage, salami, sherry/liqueurs/red wine, sauerkraut, monosodium glutamate (MSG), pickled fish, Brewer's yeast, beef or chicken liver, fermented foods.

=====

49. Which of the following statements is *true* regarding bereavement and theories of attachment?

   A. Bowlby's (1961) attachment theory holds that separation anxiety and pining serve to facilitate emotional withdrawal from the lost object.
   B. In accordance with theories of adaptation, grief symptoms typically abate in elderly widows and widowers within 6 months of a spouse's death.
   C. Visual, but not auditory, hallucination-like experiences are a common part of grieving.
   D. The survivor who maintains abstract rather then concrete ties with the lost partner is more likely to manifest healthy adaptation to loss.
   E. Bowlby (1980) found that preoccupation with the lost spouse 12 months after his or her death occurred in a relatively small minority of subjects.

### The correct response is option D.

Reports indicate that survivors who comforted themselves with concrete objects, such as possessions of the deceased, experienced more psychological distress and grief-specific symptoms than did those who engaged in less searching behavior and were more inclined to maintain a bond with the deceased spouse through positive memories.

Option A is incorrect because Bowlby's attachment theory emphasizes that bereavement gives rise to many forms of attachment behavior, the functions of which are not withdrawal from the object but reunion with it. Bowlby's attachment theory holds that bereavement gives rise to separation anxiety and pining. He proposed that the desire to reunite with or regain proximity to the deceased person would gradually dissipate through a series of stages, including shock, protest, despair, and finally, breakage of the bond and adjustment to a new self.

Grief symptoms often do not abate in elderly widows and widowers, so options B and E are incorrect. Bowlby found that at least half of his subjects were still preoccupied with their lost spouse more than 12 months after the loss. Option C is incorrect because both visual and auditory hallucination-like and "sense of presence" experiences are a common part of grieving.

Bowlby J: Processes of mourning. Int J Psychoanal 42:317–340, 1961

Bowlby J: Attachment and Loss, Vol 3: Loss: Sadness and Depression. London, Hogarth Press, 1980

Thompson LW, Kaye JL, Tang PCY, et al: Bereavement and adjustment disorders, in The American Psychiatric Publishing Textbook of Geriatric Psychiatry, 3rd Edition. Edited by Blazer DG, Steffens DC, Busse EW. Washington, DC, American Psychiatric Publishing, 2004, pp 320–321

50. Which of the following statements is *true* regarding panic disorder?

   A. Prognosis is associated with marital status.
   B. About 75% recover completely, 50% have limited impairment, and <20% have major impairment.

C. Poor prognosis has been associated with less severe initial panic attacks because panic attacks precipitously worsen thereafter.

D. Panic disorder has a consistent and gradually worsening, then remitting, course, with fairly predictable periods of exacerbations and remissions.

E. Prognosis is not associated with depression.

**The correct response is option A.**

Poor prognosis in panic disorder has been associated with a single marital status. Option B is incorrect because only about 33%, not 75%, recover completely; the rest of the statement is true, with 50% showing limited impairment and <20% showing major impairment. Option C is incorrect because poor prognosis has been associated with more severe initial panic attacks. Option D is incorrect because panic disorder typically has a variable course, with periodic exacerbations and remissions. Option E is incorrect because poorer prognosis is associated with depression.

Hollander E, Simeon D: Anxiety disorders, in The American Psychiatric Publishing Textbook of Psychiatry, 5th Edition. Edited by Hales RE, Yudofsky SC, Gabbard GO. Washington, DC, American Psychiatric Publishing, 2008, p 519; Table 12–5

51. A number of different brain regions are involved in attentional processes. Which brain region plays a pivotal role in attention by contributing important energetic components of drive and motivation?

A. Dorsolateral prefrontal cortex.
B. Reticular activating system (RAS).
C. Hypothalamus.
D. Anterior cingulate gyrus.
E. Orbitomedial prefrontal circuit.

**The correct response is option D.**

The anterior cingulate gyrus plays a pivotal role in attention by contributing important energetic components of drive and motivation. Option A is incorrect because the dorsolateral prefrontal cortex is involved in maintaining response flexibility and generating response alternatives, working memory, and the temporal sequencing of information. Option B is incorrect because the RAS plays a major role in modulating arousal and provides global regulation of attentional tone for the forebrain. Option C is incorrect because the hypothalamus influences the intensity of arousal and the direction of attention. Option E is incorrect because the orbitomedial prefrontal circuit modulates impulses and participates in the regulation of mood and working memory.

Cohen RA, Salloway S, Sweet LH: Neuropsychiatric aspects of disorders of attention, in The American Psychiatric Publishing Textbook of Neuropsychiatry and Behavioral Neurosciences, 5th Edition. Edited by Yudofsky SC, Hales RE. Washington, DC, American Psychiatric Publishing, 2008, pp 410–412

52. Quantitative electroencephalography (QEEG) may have utility in the understanding of neuropsychiatric disorders and may even have prognostic significance. All of the following statements are true *except*

A. Patients with schizophrenia have more delta activity compared with control subjects.
B. Delta activity is more pronounced in patients with schizophrenia treated with antipsychotics.
C. Increased delta activity is present in children with high genetic loading for schizophrenia.
D. Alpha and beta power during photic stimulation is decreased in patients with presenile dementia.
E. Intoxication, delirium, and dementia are associated with increased delta activity.

**The correct response is option B.**

Delta activity is more pronounced in untreated schizophrenic patients. Several studies have shown that schizophrenic patients have more delta activity, particularly over the frontal cortex, compared with control subjects. Increased delta activity is also present in children at genetic risk for schizophrenia and in cases of intoxication, delirium, and dementia. Alpha and beta power during photic stimulations is significantly decreased in patients with presenile dementia compared with age-matched control subjects.

Boutros NN, Thatcher RW, Galderisi S: Electrodiagnostic techniques in neuropsychiatry, in The American Psychiatric Publishing Textbook of Neuropsychiatry and Behavioral Neurosciences, 5th Edition. Edited by Yudofsky SC, Hales RE. Washington, DC, American Psychiatric Publishing, 2008, p 197

53. Which of the following statements regarding the use of antidepressants in bipolar disorder is *true?*

    A. Antidepressants should never be used in bipolar disorder.
    B. Newer antidepressants should be considered over tricyclic antidepressants (TCAs) because of lower switch rates.
    C. Lamotrigine may have effectiveness as an antidepressant and antimanic agent.
    D. Olanzapine does not have antidepressant activity in acute bipolar depression.
    E. None of the above.

**The correct response is option B.**

Among antidepressant options, paroxetine, venlafaxine, bupropion, and fluoxetine are the most studied in randomized controlled trials and appear to have a lower switch risk in comparison with TCAs. Combination therapy with an antidepressant can be done in patients who do not respond to mood stabilizers alone or for patients with moderate to severe bipolar depression. Lamotrigine does not appear to have antimanic activity, and both olanzapine and quetiapine do have some efficacy as monotherapy in cases of acute bipolar depression.

Keck PE, McElroy SL: Treatment of bipolar disorder, in The American Psychiatric Publishing Textbook of Psychopharmacology, 3rd Edition. Edited by Schatzberg AF, Nemeroff CB. Washington, DC, American Psychiatric Publishing, 2004, pp 872–873

54. Some physical anomalies are stable through childhood and give clues to abnormal neurodevelopment in adulthood. A scale that is in common use to note these anomalies is called the *Waldrop scale*. Which of the following minor physical anomalies is *not* included in this scale?

    A. Small nails.
    B. Wide-spaced eyes.
    C. Adherent ear lobes.
    D. Furrowed tongue.
    E. Abnormal palm crease.

**The correct response is option A.**

Small nails are not included in the Waldrop scale. Minor physical anomalies included in the Waldrop scale are head circumference; two or more hair whorls; fine, "electric" hair that will not comb down; wide-spaced eyes; epicanthus; adherent ear lobes; malformation or asymmetry of ears; low-seated or soft and pliable ears; high arch of palate; furrowed tongue; geographic tongue; clinodactyly; abnormal palm crease; third toe longer than second toe; partial syndactyly; and a gap between first and second toes.

Ovsiew F: Bedside neuropsychiatry, in The American Psychiatric Publishing Textbook of Neuropsychiatry and Behavioral Neurosciences, 5th Edition. Edited by Yudofsky SC, Hales RE. Washington, DC, American Psychiatric Publishing, 2008, pp 141–142; Table 4–1

55. In the clinical classification of substance dependence, DSM-IV-TR provides several course specifiers by which the clinician may represent the course of illness. Which of the following is *not* a valid DSM-IV-TR course specifier for substance dependence?

    A. Early full remission.
    B. Sustained partial remission.
    C. On agonist therapy.
    D. On aversive therapy.
    E. In a controlled environment.

**The correct response is option D.**

Being on aversive therapy is not a course specifier for substance dependence, according to DSM-IV-TR diagnostic criteria.

Greenfield SF, Hennessy G: Assessment of the patient, in The American Psychiatric Publishing Textbook of Substance Abuse Treatment, 4th Edition. Edited by Galanter M, Kleber HD. Washington, DC, American Psychiatric Publishing, 2008, pp 59–60; Table 5–1

56. Which of the following is *true* regarding electroencephalograph (EEG) findings in various conditions?

    A. The EEG of a healthy, awake individual is dominated by frequencies in the alpha range. This pattern shows a gradual, but significant decline in the mean alpha frequency in normal aging.
    B. EEG findings in delirium include slowing.
    C. EEG findings in dementia are characterized by a decrease in low-frequency (delta and theta) activity and a slowing of alpha frequencies.

D. Quantitative EEG signals tend not to correlate with the severity and duration of delirium.

E. Normal aging is generally associated with significant increases in delta activity.

**The correct response is option B.**

EEG recordings reflect brain activity essentially on the same time scale as the activity of cortical neurons. The spectra of EEG frequencies conventionally are divided into bands defined as delta (<4 Hz), theta (4–8 Hz), alpha (8–13 Hz), and beta (>13 Hz). Alterations in the frequency spectrum associated with neuropathology may be global (e.g., metabolic, toxic, or anoxic encephalopathy) or localized (e.g., focal lesions such as tumors or strokes).

EEG is a standard tool in the evaluation of delirium. Option B is correct because EEG slowing is an almost universal finding in delirium. Option A is incorrect because the EEG of a healthy, awake individual is dominated by frequencies in the alpha range. However, this pattern shows little change with normal aging. A small decline in the mean alpha frequency may be seen starting in the fifth decade, but a significant drop suggests underlying neuropathology.

Option C is incorrect because EEG findings in dementia are characterized by an increase in low-frequency (delta and theta) activity and a slowing of the dominant alpha frequencies. Option D is incorrect because the quantitative EEG signal tends to correlate with the severity and duration of the delirium. Option E is incorrect because normal aging is generally not associated with significant increases in delta activity.

Byrun CE, Moore SD, Hulette CM: Neuroanatomy, neurophysiology, and neuropathology of aging, in The American Psychiatric Publishing Textbook of Geriatric Psychiatry, 3rd Edition. Edited by Blazer DG, Steffens DC, Busse EW. Washington, DC, American Psychiatric Publishing, 2004, pp 65–66

57. All of the following are *true* regarding the issue of driving among patients with dementia *except*

A. Local offices of the departments of motor vehicles (DMVs) rarely provide independent driving evaluations when requested by family members or patients' physicians.

B. Psychiatrists are bound by ethical principles such as confidentiality to notify local DMVs about an individual's impaired driving skills without the express written consent of the individual.

C. Some state DMVs automatically revoke the driver's licenses of individuals diagnosed with moderate or severe dementia.

D. Because symptoms of dementia are likely to worsen over time, individuals who pass a driving evaluation should continue to be reevaluated yearly.

E. Psychiatrists should recommend against caregivers mechanically disabling the car of an individual with dementia because this could further exacerbate familial relationships as well as erode the patient-physician relationship.

**The correct response is option C.**

In the United States, the laws regarding licensure and driving capacity vary from state to state. Anonymous reports to the department of motor vehicles may lead to required testing or removal of the patient's license, but the absence of a license rarely stops a determined older adult with dementia. Families can be encouraged to assess driving capacity based on observations of current driving, with reminders that dementia affects judgment, reaction time, and problem solving. Shaving the patient's keys, substituting another key, removing a distributor cap, or otherwise disabling a car can sometimes reduce the need to confront the patient with lost skills. The family can also work on solutions that limit the need for driving—delivery services, senior vans, or offers of regular rides to church or for visits.

A systematic review of literature (Stav 2008) related to the effects of drivers' license policies and community mobility programs revealed that states can reduce traffic crashes, traffic violations, and traffic-related fatalities through relicensing policies requiring in-person renewal and vision testing as well as driving restrictions.

Gwyther LP: Working with the family of the older adult, in The American Psychiatric Publishing Textbook of Geriatric Psychiatry, 3rd Edition. Edited by Blazer DG, Steffens DC, Busse EW. Washington, DC, American Psychiatric Publishing, 2004, pp 468–469

Stav WB: Review of the evidence related to older adult community mobility and driver licensure policies. Am J Occup Ther 62:149–158, 2008

58. Dysfunction in _____ is more common in depressed patients with psychotic features than in depressed patients without psychotic features.

    A. Measures of speed of processing.
    B. Mental flexibility.
    C. Language.
    D. Memory.
    E. Visuospatial abilities.

**The correct response is option D.**

Cognitive deficits, including deficits in memory, are more common in depressed patients with psychotic features than in depressed patients without psychotic features. The degree of cognitive impairment appears to be related to the number of prior depressive episodes. Depressed patients with or without psychosis often underperform on measures of speed of processing, mental flexibility, and executive function compared with control subjects, but memory in particular is more impaired in psychotically depressed patients. Options C and E are incorrect because these functions usually are not impaired with depression. Note that memory performance may be intact even when memory complaints are present.

Hales RE, Bourgeois JA, Shahrokh NC: Study Guide to Neuropsychiatry and Behavioral Neurosciences: A Companion to The American Psychiatric Publishing Textbook of Neuropsychiatry and Behavioral Neurosciences, 5th Edition, Washington, DC, American Psychiatric Publishing, 2008, p 97

Howieson DB, Lezak MD: The neuropsychological evaluation, in The American Psychiatric Publishing Textbook of Neuropsychiatry and Behavioral Neurosciences, 5th Edition. Edited by Yudofsky SC, Hales RE. Washington, DC, American Psychiatric Publishing, 2008, pp 218–219

59. Which of the following antidepressants is an inhibitor of both dopamine and norepinephrine transporters?

    A. Bupropion.
    B. Tricyclic antidepressants (TCAs).
    C. Venlafaxine.
    D. Monoamine oxidase inhibitors (MAOIs).
    E. Mirtazapine.

**The correct response is option A.**

Bupropion is an inhibitor of both norepinephrine and dopamine reuptake. It may also facilitate presynaptic re-

lease of these monoamines. Option B is incorrect because TCAs act by reuptake inhibition at both the norepinephrine and serotonin transporters. This combined effect is probably mediated by active metabolites of TCAs as much as by primary drug. Option C is incorrect because venlafaxine is an inhibitor of serotonin (5-HT) and norepinephrine transporters. Option D is incorrect because MAOIs act by the inhibition of the presynaptic enzyme, monoamine oxidase, which produces an increase in synaptic concentrations of all monoamines. Option E is incorrect because mirtazapine is a tetracyclic that antagonizes the norepinephrine receptor as well as the 5-HT$_{2A}$ receptor (noradrenergic- and serotonin-specific antidepressant [NASSA]).

Joska JA, Stein DJ: Mood disorders, in The American Psychiatric Publishing Textbook of Psychiatry, 5th Edition. Edited by Hales RE, Yudofsky SC, Gabbard GO. Washington, DC, American Psychiatric Publishing, 2008, p 482

60. Pharmacoelectroencephalography (pharmaco-EEG) in clinical applications offers an attractive technique to fine-tune drug development and is likely to play an expanded role in the future of applied psychopharmacology. All of the following statements are true *except*

    A. Decreased quantitative electroencephalography (QEEG) theta and alpha activity has been reported in patients with schizophrenia who were being treated with high-potency antipsychotics.
    B. Slow alpha changes identify nonresponders versus responders to antipsychotics.
    C. Medication-associated increases in beta waves correlate with decrease in depression symptoms.
    D. QEEG profile after a single dose of an acetylcholinesterase inhibitor predicted cognitive modifications in dementia patients.
    E. With antipsychotic treatment, increased QEEG alpha activity correlates with a favorable clinical response.

**The correct response is option A.**

An increase of QEEG theta and alpha activity, more often in the slow alpha range (7.5–9.5 Hz), has been reported in patients with schizophrenia treated with high-potency neuroleptics. It has been found that slow alpha changes enable the identification of responders and nonresponders to antipsychotics with an overall accuracy ranging from 89.3% to 91.3%. Drug-induced increase of beta waves was found to correlate with the decrease of depression psychopathological ratings. QEEG profile after a single dose of an acetylcholinesterase inhibitor was found to be a good predictor of cognitive modifications in patients with Alzheimer's disease. Increased QEEG alpha activity correlates with a favorable clinical response to antipsychotic treatment.

Boutros NN, Thatcher RW, Galderisi S: Electrodiagnostic techniques in neuropsychiatry, in The American Psychiatric Publishing Textbook of Neuropsychiatry and Behavioral Neurosciences, 5th Edition. Edited by Yudofsky SC, Hales RE. Washington, DC, American Psychiatric Publishing, 2008, p 201

61.    A disadvantage of a screening head computed tomography (CT) scan over a magnetic resonance imaging (MRI) scan is that

A. It takes longer.
B. It is more expensive.
C. It is less sensitive.
D. It is not useful for rapid screening.
E. It produces more discomfort.

### The correct response is option C.

An MRI scan is more sensitive than a screening head CT scan. A screening head CT scan is very easy to perform, takes only a few minutes, produces little discomfort, and has fairly high resolution and sensitivity. Thus it can be easily performed in any psychiatric patient admitted with clinical features that do not appear to be classic for the disorder diagnosed. MRI is much more likely to detect vascular disease and demyelinating disease. It is also useful for detecting mild neurodegenerative changes that might point to degenerative dementias. MRIs take longer (about 45 minutes) than CT scans and are at least twice as expensive.

Kim HF, Schulz PE, Wilde EA, et al: Laboratory testing and imaging studies in psychiatry, in The American Psychiatric Publishing Textbook of Psychiatry, 5th Edition. Edited by Hales RE, Yudofsky SC, Gabbard GO. Washington, DC, American Psychiatric Publishing, 2008, p 36

62.    Which of the following is *not* a typical defense encountered in substance abusers?

A. Denial.
B. Minimization.
C. Sublimation.
D. Rationalization.
E. Externalization.

### The correct response is option C.

In the assessment of substance abuse patients, it is most helpful to evaluate the usual mechanisms of psychological defense. Patients with substance use disorders often report that they do not discuss their substance use openly with physicians because of their feelings of shame, discomfort, fear, distrust, and hopelessness. They often exhibit certain typical defenses, including denial, minimization, rationalization, projection, and externalization.

Greenfield SF, Hennessy G: Assessment of the patient, in The American Psychiatric Publishing Textbook of Substance Abuse Treatment, 4th Edition. Edited by Galanter M, Kleber HD. Washington, DC, American Psychiatric Publishing, 2008, p 56

63.    Principle-based ethics advocates a technique of balancing four ethical principles in the actions of a particular case. Which of the following is *not* one of the four principles emphasized in this model?

A. Privacy.
B. Nonmaleficence.
C. Beneficence.
D. Respect for autonomy.
E. Justice.

### The correct response is option A.

Principle-based ethics, as described by contemporary theorists James Childress and Thomas Beauchamp, suggests that ethical dilemmas should be resolved through the specification and balancing of the principles of nonmaleficence, beneficence, respect for autonomy, and justice.

Beauchamp TL, Childress JF: Principles of Biomedical Ethics, 5th Edition. New York, Oxford University Press, 2001

Roberts LW, Hoop JG, Dunn LB: Ethical aspects of psychiatry, in The American Psychiatric Publishing Textbook of Psychiatry, 5th Edition. Edited by Hales RE, Yudofsky SC, Gabbard GO. Washington, DC, American Psychiatric Publishing, 2008, p 1608

64. In the middle of the night, the general medicine team urgently consults the psychosomatic medicine (PSM) team regarding a 79-year-old man who is threatening to leave the hospital against medical advice. The consulting team requests that an evaluation be made regarding the patient's ability to make this decision. Of the following, which statement reflects accurately an important issue that the PSM team must address?

    A. The patient may or may not possess the competency to make medical decisions regarding his health care.
    B. By law, only a psychiatrist (and/or a PSM team) can determine whether the patient has necessary insight and judgment to refuse medical care.
    C. Competency requires a court decision, not a medical one.
    D. Making a will and executing a power of attorney require the same level of competency.
    E. The court may request a written report but may not compel the physician to personally testify in competency cases.

### The correct response is option C.

*Competency* is a legal term defined as the ability to understand relevant information and to appreciate the situation and circumstances. A health care team can evaluate clinically an individual's capacity to comprehend the risks and benefits of following or not following recommended treatments but technically cannot determine an individual's legal competency, which is determined by a court of law. Thus, option A is incorrect. Option B is incorrect because a psychiatrist and/or psychosomatic medicine team are not necessary to evaluate a patient's capacity to make a medical decision. Option D is incorrect because making a will requires the lowest level of competency, whereas higher levels are required for executing a power of attorney. Option E is incorrect because a court may require a psychiatrist to testify in person.

Reichman WE, Streim JE, Loebel JP: Legal, ethical, and policy issues, in The American Psychiatric Publishing Textbook of Geriatric Psychiatry, 3rd Edition. Edited by Blazer DG, Steffens DC, Busse EW. Washington, DC, American Psychiatric Publishing, 2004, p 524

Slovenko R: Civil competency, in The American Psychiatric Publishing Textbook of Forensic Psychiatry. Edited by Simon RI, Gold LH. Washington, DC, American Psychiatric Publishing, 2004, p 206

65. Which of the following sexual dysfunctions has the *lowest* estimated prevalence in the U.S. population?

    A. Male orgasmic disorder.
    B. Female orgasmic disorder.
    C. Male dyspareunia.
    D. Female arousal disorder.
    E. Erectile dysfunction.

### The correct response is option C.

Dyspareunia has a 3% prevalence in males and a 15% prevalence in females. A comprehensive survey conducted on a representative sample of the U.S. population between 19 and 59 years of age suggested the following prevalence estimates: 3% for male dyspareunia, 15% for female dyspareunia, 10% for male orgasm problems, 25% for female orgasm problems, 33% for female hypoactive sexual desire, 27% for premature ejaculation, 20% for female arousal problems, and 10% for male erectile difficulties.

Becker JV, Stinson JD: Human sexuality and sexual dysfunctions, in The American Psychiatric Publishing Textbook of Psychiatry, 5th Edition. Edited by Hales RE, Yudofsky SC, Gabbard GO. Washington, DC, American Psychiatric Publishing, 2008, pp 713, 715–716; Table 16–4

66. Among the suicide risk factors identified in a 10-year prospective study of patients with affective disorders, which of the following was considered to be a long-term suicide risk factor rather than a short-term one?

    A. Severe hopelessness.
    B. Panic attacks.
    C. Psychic anxiety.
    D. Diminished concentration.
    E. Global insomnia.

### The correct response is option A.

Differentiating short-term from long-term risk factors for suicide may be important because modifying just a few short-term risk factors may significantly reduce a patient's risk for suicide. Long-term risk factors included suicidal ideation, suicide intent, severe hopelessness, and prior suicide attempts. Long-term suicide risk factors in patients with major affective disorders were associated with suicides completed 2–10 years after assessment. The short-term risk factors were panic attacks, psychic anxiety, loss of pleasure and interest, moderate alcohol abuse, depressive turmoil, diminished concentration, and global insomnia. Short-term risk factors were predominantly severe, anxiety driven, and treatable by a variety of drugs.

Simon RI: Suicide, in The American Psychiatric Publishing Textbook of Psychiatry, 5th Edition. Edited by Hales RE, Yudofsky SC, Gabbard GO. Washington, DC, American Psychiatric Publishing, 2008, p 1640

67. Changes of aging that occur in dopamine and dopamine receptors include

    A. Decreased numbers of dopamine type 2 ($D_2$) receptors in the striatum with increasing age correlated with decreased cognitive function.
    B. Decreased dopamine transporter in caudate/putamen in oldest subjects.
    C. Correlation with decreased glucose metabolism of the frontal, temporal, and cingulate cortices.
    D. All of the above.
    E. None of the above.

**The correct response is option D.**

Decreased numbers of $D_2$ receptors in the striatum with increasing age have been correlated with decreasing cognitive function. The dopamine transporter declines slowly over the entire course of aging, not just at the end stages of life. A loss of dopamine $D_2$ receptor binding of $[^{11}C]$-raclopride in the frontal, temporal, and cingulate cortices is significantly correlated with age-related decline in neuronal glucose metabolism in these regions.

Bissette G: Chemical messengers, in The American Psychiatric Publishing Textbook of Geriatric Psychiatry, 3rd Edition. Edited by Blazer DG, Steffens DC, Busse EW. Washington, DC, American Psychiatric Publishing, 2004, pp 90–92

68. Personality change due to degenerative frontal lobe disease is associated with difficulties in planning, conformity to social norms, experience of reward and punishment, and management of complex emotions. Clinically, these symptoms may bear strong resemblance to several DSM-IV-TR personality disorders. These specific behaviors may commonly overlap with all of the following personality disorders *except*

    A. Obsessive-compulsive personality disorder.
    B. Narcissistic personality disorder.

    C. Antisocial personality disorder.
    D. Borderline personality disorder.
    E. Paranoid personality disorder.

**The correct response is option A.**

Personality changes caused by degenerative frontal lobe disease do not commonly overlap with obsessive-compulsive personality disorder and are more similar to those of the other listed personality disorders.

Oxman TE, Ferrell RB: Personality disorders, in The American Psychiatric Publishing Textbook of Geriatric Psychiatry, 3rd Edition. Edited by Blazer DG, Steffens DC, Busse EW. Washington, DC, American Psychiatric Publishing, 2004, pp 372–373

69. All of the following symptoms seen in psychotic illness have been found to increase violence risk *except*

    A. Delusions characterized by "threat/control override" symptoms.
    B. Hallucinations associated with "negative" emotions.
    C. Command hallucinations to harm others.
    D. Persecutory delusions.
    E. Negative symptoms such as social withdrawal.

**The correct response is option E.**

Negative symptoms such as social withdrawal seem to lower, not increase, the risk of serious violence. Studies indicate that all the other factors listed above tend to increase the risk of violence.

Scott CL, Quanbeck CD, Resnick PJ: Assessment of dangerousness, in The American Psychiatric Publishing Textbook of Psychiatry, 5th Edition. Edited by Hales RE, Yudofsky SC, Gabbard GO. Washington, DC, American Psychiatric Publishing, 2008, pp 1657–1659

70. Medications typically used in the treatment of narcolepsy include all of the following *except*

    A. Dextroamphetamine.
    B. Methylphenidate.
    C. Atomoxetine.
    D. Gamma-aminobutyric acid (GABA)–hydroxybutyrate.
    E. Modafinil.

**The answer is option C.**

Atomoxetine, a selective norepinephrine reuptake inhibitor, is FDA-approved for the treatment of attention-deficit/hyperactivity disorder in children, adolescents, and adults. Although a common side effect of atomoxetine is sleeplessness, no evidence has demonstrated its usefulness in treating narcolepsy. Dopamimetic stimulants such as dextroamphetamine, methylphenidate, or pemoline release presynaptic pools of monoamines, block reuptake of depamine, or inhibit monoamine oxidase metabolism of norepinephrine and dopamine. Additional agents used to treat narcolepsy include GABA-hydroxybutyrate and modafinil. Modafinil, an atypical psychostimulant that affects postsynaptic GABA$_1$-adrenergic receptors, promotes wakefulness and is rarely associated with substance dependence. Modafinil is less effective than amphetamine in controlling cataplexy. Rapid eye movement–suppressing agents such as tricyclic antidepressants and GABA-hydroxybutyrate have been found to control cataplexy.

An important nonpharmacological approach is the use of scheduled naps throughout the wake period.

Buysse DJ, Strollo PJ, Black JE, et al: Sleep disorders, in The American Psychiatric Publishing Textbook of Psychiatry, 5th Edition. Edited by Hales RE, Yudofsky SC, Gabbard GO. Washington, DC, American Psychiatric Publishing, 2008, p 945

71. Which of the following is *true* regarding conversion disorder?

    A. Conversion disorder is more common in elderly women than in younger women.
    B. Conversion disorder is seen almost exclusively in women.
    C. Comorbidity in conversion disorder includes substance abuse and head injury.
    D. Although nonepileptic seizures (often referred to as pseudoseizures) are a subtype of conversion disorder, they rarely are seen in patients with a bona fide seizure disorder.
    E. Like younger patients, elderly patients with conversion disorder infrequently have an "actual" comorbid neurological disorder.

**The correct response is option C.**

Conversion disorder is characterized by motor and/or sensory deficits that suggest neurological illness(es) that cannot be elucidated by the appropriate neurological and neuroimaging evaluations. Comorbidity in conversion disorder includes substance abuse, chronic illness, head trauma, and previous conversion symptoms. Option A is incorrect because conversion disorder is more common in young, not elderly, women. Option B is incorrect because conversion disorder is seen in men, though it predominately occurs in women. Option D is incorrect because nonepileptic seizures are relatively common (5%–20%) in individuals with epilepsy. Option E is incorrect because conversion disorder in late life is likely to be associated with comorbid neurological disorders.

Agronin ME: Somatoform disorders, in The American Psychiatric Publishing Textbook of Geriatric Psychiatry, 3rd Edition. Edited by Blazer DG, Steffens DC, Busse EW. Washington, DC, American Psychiatric Publishing, 2004, p 297

72. Which particular type of serotonin receptor agonists is known to facilitate strongly cocaine reward?

    A. Serotonin type 1A receptor (5-HT$_{1A}$).
    B. 5-HT$_{1B}$.
    C. 5-HT$_{1C}$.
    D. 5-HT$_{2A}$.
    E. 5-HT$_3$.

**The correct response is option B.**

5-HT$_{1B}$ agonists facilitate cocaine reward and decrease alcohol reward.

Koob GF: Neurobiology of addiction, in The American Psychiatric Publishing Textbook of Substance Abuse Treatment, 4th Edition. Edited by Galanter M, Kleber HD. Washington, DC, American Psychiatric Publishing, 2008, p 5

73. A 47-year-old woman with schizoaffective disorder is brought to the emergency department by her caregiver, who reported that the patient has become increasingly disoriented in the past week. The patient has been sick with the "flu" and complained of a sore throat earlier in the week. The caregiver insists that the patient has no history of drug abuse and has "never" been suicidal. After taking an antipsychotic for a year, the patient experienced stabilization of her psychotic symptoms for the first time in 20 years, but she gained 40 lb. during that time. Ten days ago, she was prescribed a low dose of fluvoxamine because of persistently depressed mood and obsessive-compulsive symptoms. On examination, the patient is pale and unresponsive to verbal stimuli. Her blood pressure is 95/60 mmHg, respiratory rate 15 breaths/minute, and heart rate 105 bpm, and her temperature is normal. Of the following,

which laboratory test and/or intervention would most assist the treatment team to narrow down the differential diagnosis and develop an appropriate course of action?

    A.  A comprehensive urine toxicology screen and blood alcohol level.
    B.  Random blood glucose and electrolytes.
    C.  Complete blood count with differential.
    D.  Electrolytes and lithium level.
    E.  Obtain liver function test and ammonia level; provide intravenous glucose and thiamine.

## The correct response is option C.

The patient's history and physical examination findings strongly suggest that she is in the midst of a clozapine-induced agranulocytosis, which is an absolute neutrophil count (ANC) of <500 mm$^3$. Although rare (<1% prevalence), agranulocytosis is a potentially fatal side effect of clozapine and promptly must be ruled out. A clinical clue for agranulocytosis caused by clozapine is that the patient had recently started taking fluvoxamine, which is a potent cytochrome P450 1A2 inhibitor that can substantially elevate blood clozapine levels. Fluoxetine has also been associated with agranulocytosis in patients taking clozapine. The patient's recent history of flulike symptoms and sore throat, hypotension, tachycardia, and abrupt changes in mental status are very concerning for a severe, life-threatening infection that resulted from her impaired immune function.

Clozapine has several other side effects that should be taken into account while considering the differential diagnosis. Clozapine is associated with significant weight gain, hyperlipidemia, hyperglycemia, seizures, respiratory depression, tachycardia, and orthostatic hypotension.

Option A is incorrect because there was little evidence from the patient's history that she is currently intoxicated, and the tests would likely be negative and therefore yield minimal useful information regarding the patient's immediate treatment course. Even though intoxication from substances is low on the differential, her initial evaluation should include these screenings because substance abuse, especially among patients with schizophrenia, is so common.

Electrolyte abnormalities and hyper- and hypoglycemia should be ruled out in this patient, especially because clozapine can cause elevations in blood glucose, which when severe theoretically can lead to electrolyte abnormalities. However, option B is incorrect because the patient's history and exam findings are so indicative of agranulocytosis that these laboratory values will not be as useful in terms of etiology and treatment as a complete blood count with differential would be.

Option D is incorrect because her presentation is more consistent with that of agranulocytosis because of clozapine and fluoxetine than with lithium toxicity. Option E is incorrect because her history and physical exam are more consistent with agranulocytosis than with an alcohol-associated hepatic encephalopathy or Wernicke's encephalopathy because of chronic thiamine deficiency.

Garlow SJ, Purselle D, D'Orio B: Psychiatric emergencies, in The American Psychiatric Publishing Textbook of Psychopharmacology, 3rd Edition. Edited by Schatzberg AF, Nemeroff CB. Washington, DC, American Psychiatric Publishing, 2004, p 1080

Krishnan KRR: Monoamine oxidase inhibitors, in The American Psychiatric Publishing Textbook of Psychopharmacology, 3rd Edition. Edited by Schatzberg AF, Nemeroff CB. Washington, DC, American Psychiatric Publishing, 2004, pp 308–309

Marder SR, Wirshing DA: Clozapine, in The American Psychiatric Publishing Textbook of Psychopharmacology, 3rd Edition. Edited by Schatzberg AF, Nemeroff CB. Washington, DC, American Psychiatric Publishing, 2004, pp 448–453

74.  Which of the following is considered to be a restoration-oriented rather than a loss-oriented stressor in the dual-process model of bereavement (Stroebe and Schut 1999)?

    A.  Emotional symptoms.
    B.  Behavioral symptoms.
    C.  New identity development.
    D.  Physiological symptoms.
    E.  Cognitive symptoms.

## The correct response is option C.

Stroebe and Schut's dual-process model of bereavement synthesizes previously existing conceptualizations of the bereavement process and has been empirically validated (Richardson and Balaswamy 2001). In this model, two types of bereavement-related stressors are distinguished: *loss-oriented stressors*, which focus on the nature of the loss itself, and *restoration-oriented stressors*, which refer to what an individual needs to adapt to the larger, objective environment. Loss-oriented stressors are manifested as emotional, behavioral, physiological, and cognitive symptoms (options A, B, D, and E). Restoration-oriented stressors include developing new identities and learning new skills to perform tasks previously done by the deceased.

Richardson VE, Balaswamy S: Coping with bereavement among elderly widowers. Omega (Westport) 43:129–144, 2001

Stroebe M, Schut H: The dual process model of coping with bereavement: rationale and description. Death Stud 23:197–224, 1999

Thompson LW, Kaye JL, Tang PCY, et al: Bereavement and adjustment disorders, in The American Psychiatric Publishing Textbook of Geriatric Psychiatry, 3rd Edition. Edited by Blazer DG, Steffens DC, Busse EW. Washington, DC, American Psychiatric Publishing, 2004, p 322

75.  Dysregulation of dopaminergic release in which of the following brain structures is associated with helplessness behaviors and delayed extinction of conditioned fear responses?

A.  Amygdala.
B.  Nucleus accumbens.
C.  Medial prefrontal cortex.
D.  Tuberoinfundibular tract.
E.  Cingulate gyrus.

## The correct response is option C.

Dopamine innervation of the medial prefrontal cortex appears to be particularly susceptible to stress. Increasing intensity and/or duration of stress can enhance dopamine release and metabolism in other areas receiving dopamine innervation (e.g., the mesolimbic and nigrostriatal systems). Uncontrollable stress activates dopamine release in the medial prefrontal cortex (Ventura et al. 2002) and inhibits it in the nucleus accumbens. Lesions of medial prefrontal cortex dopamine neurons or reduced medial prefrontal cortex dopamine release delays extinction of the conditioned fear stress response, a situation hypothesized to occur in posttraumatic stress disorder. Increased medial prefrontal cortex dopamine release thus enhances extinction while contributing to helplessness behavior. There may be an optimal range of medial prefrontal cortex dopamine release that facilitates adaptive behavioral responses and extinction of conditioned emotional memories without features of learned helplessness. Too much dopamine release (as in uncontrollable stress) could produce learned helplessness behavior, whereas insufficient medial prefrontal cortex dopamine release could prolong conditioned fear responses.

Bonne O, Drevets WC, Neueister A, et al: Neurobiology of anxiety disorders, in The American Psychiatric Publishing Textbook of Psychopharmacology, 3rd Edition. Edited by Schatzberg AF, Nemeroff CB. Washington, DC, American Psychiatric Publishing, 2004, p 785

Ventura R, Cabib S, Puglisi-Allegra S: Genetic susceptibility of mesocortical dopamine to stress determines liability to inhibition of mesoaccumbens dopamine and to behavioral 'despair' in a mouse model of depression. Neuroscience 999–1007, 2002

76.  Bipolar disorder in the elderly may have all of the following characteristics *except*

A.  Tendency toward more rapid recurrences late in the illness.
B.  Stressful events more likely to precede early-onset mania than late-onset mania.
C.  Increased cerebral vulnerability playing a stronger role than life events in precipitating late-onset mania.
D.  Association with low rates of familial affective disorder.
E.  Genetic factors weighing heavily in the etiology.

## The correct response is option E.

Evidence that genetic factors weigh heavily in the etiology of bipolar disorders in late life is virtually nonexistent, although the biological nature of this disorder would suggest some genetic contribution.

In a review of records of a small number of untreated patients with severe and prolonged bipolar disorder, Cutler and Post (1982) found a tendency toward more rapid recurrences late in the illness, with decreasing periods of normality. Ameblas (1987) emphasized a relationship between life events and onset of mania, noting that stressful events were more likely to precede early-onset mania than late-onset mania. Likewise, Shulman (1989) stressed that increased cerebral vulnerability caused by organic insults (stroke, head trauma, other brain insults) played a stronger role than life events in precipitating late-onset mania (a factor that may also play a role in treatment resistance). Young and Klerman (1992) emphasized the low rates of familial affective disorder.

Ameblas A: Life events and mania. Br J Psychiatry 150:235–240, 1987

Cutler NR, Post RM: Life course of illness in untreated manic-depressive patients. Compr Psychiatry 23:101–115, 1982

Koenig HG, Blazer DG: Mood disorders, in The American Psychiatric Publishing Textbook of Geriatric Psychiatry, 3rd Edition. Edited by Blazer DG, Steffens DC, Busse EW. Washington, DC, American Psychiatric Publishing, 2004, pp 245–246

Shulman KI: The influence of age and aging on manic disorder. Int J Geriatr Psychiatry 4:63–65, 1989

Young RC, Klerman GL: Mania in late life: focus on age at onset. Am J Psychiatry 149:867–876, 1992

77. Epidemiological findings concerning autism include all of the following *except*

 A. Onset typically occurs before age 3 years.
 B. The overall rate of autism in second-degree relatives of children with autism is 0.2%.
 C. The male-to-female ratio is 1.5 to 1.0.
 D. Rates of autism in siblings of affected individuals are in the range of 2% to 6%.
 E. The concordance rate for monozygotic twins has been estimated to be between 36% and 91%.

**The correct response is option C.**

A consistently observed male-to-female ratio of 3–4 to 1 has been noted, with females often having more severe impairment, particularly in IQ. Onset of autism typically occurs before age 3 years. Several studies have suggested an overall rate of autism of 0.2% in second-degree relatives, 0.1% in 3rd-degree relatives, and 2%–6% in siblings of affected individuals. The concordance rate has been estimated to be between 36% and 91% for monozygotic twins and between 0 and 24% for dizygotic twins.

Malaspina D, Corcoran C, Schobel S, et al: Epidemiological and genetic aspects of neuropsychiatric disorders, in The American Psychiatric Publishing Textbook of Neuropsychiatry and Behavioral Neurosciences, 5th Edition. Edited by Yudofsky SC, Hales RE. Washington, DC, American Psychiatric Publishing, 2008, p 318

78. Which of the following is a feature of progressive supranuclear palsy (PSP)?

 A. Does not include vertical gaze palsy.
 B. Features parkinsonism without prominent tremor.
 C. Has appendicular rigidity that is greater than axial rigidity.
 D. Has good response to levodopa.

 E. Is characterized by a bilateral, symmetric parkinsonism that is poorly responsive to levodopa therapy.

**The correct response is option B.**

Progressive supranuclear palsy, or Steele-Richardson-Olszewski syndrome, features parkinsonism without prominent tremor, vertical gaze palsy, axial (midline) more than appendicular (arm and leg) rigidity, early postural instability, and poor response to levodopa. PSP is often associated with frequent falling, lack of eye contact, monotonous speech, sloppy eating, and slowed mentation. Patients may have a surprised or worried facial expression, with raised eyebrows resulting from bradykinesia and increased tone in facial musculature. They may also have difficulty opening their eyes because of eyelid apraxia. Unlike in Parkinson's disease, there is little or no response to levodopa therapy because of degeneration of secondary neurons downstream from the dopaminergic substantia nigra pars compacta neurons.

Option A is incorrect because a characteristic feature of PSP is vertical gaze palsy. Option C is incorrect because axial (midline) is more common than appendicular (arm and leg) rigidity. Option D is incorrect because PSP does not improve with levodopa. Option E is incorrect because this is a description of multiple system atrophy (MSA), not PSP. MSA can be conceived as a "Parkinson's plus" condition characterized by bilateral, symmetric parkinsonism, and absence or virtual absence of tremor.

Scott B: Movement disorders, in The American Psychiatric Publishing Textbook of Geriatric Psychiatry, 3rd Edition. Edited by Blazer DG, Steffens DC, Busse EW. Washington, DC, American Psychiatric Publishing, 2004, pp 234–235

*Apraxia* is the loss of a previously possessed ability to carry out motor activities despite intact comprehension and motor function. May be seen in dementias.

79. A number of physicians in the eighteenth and nineteenth centuries made important contributions to the understanding of schizophrenia. Which of the following individuals outlined a set of "first-rank" symptoms in an attempt to establish a discrete criteria set for the diagnosis?

A. Kahlbaum.
B. Kraepelin.
C. Morel.
D. Pinel.
E. Schneider.

**The correct response is option E.**

Kurt Schneider (1887–1967) outlined a set of "first-rank" symptoms , which represented one of the first attempts at establishing discrete criteria for the diagnosis. Karl Ludwig Kahlbaum (1828–1899), who is known for developing descriptive psychopathology, derived subtypes of schizophrenia such as catatonia and hebetic paraphrenia. Emil Kraepelin (1856–1926), considered to have exerted the single greatest influence in the study of schizophrenia, aimed to classify schizophrenia on the basis of a physical etiology and in general to establish the basis for mental illness in the natural sciences. Bénédict Augustin Morel (1809–1873) first used the term *dementia praecox* to describe schizophrenia as a premature dementia, emphasizing the early onset and progressive clinical decline. The eighteenth century was notable for the emergence of an emphasis on "humane and moral" treatment of the mentally ill. William Tuke (1732–1822) in England and Philippe Pinel (1745–1826) in France led this movement by attempting to treat patients in the least restrictive and most socially supportive environment possible, and they used a scientific perspective to support their arguments.

Minzenberg MJ, Yoon JH, Carter CS: Schizophrenia, in The American Psychiatric Publishing Textbook of Psychiatry, 5th Edition. Edited by Hales RE, Yudofsky SC, Gabbard GO. Washington, DC, American Psychiatric Publishing, 2008, pp 408–410

80. Which of the following is the likely final common neural pathway in delirium?

    A. Low cholinergic/high dopaminergic state.
    B. High cholinergic/high dopaminergic state.
    C. High gamma-aminobutyric acid (GABA)/low dopaminergic state.
    D. Low GABA/high dopaminergic state.
    E. Low serotonin/high GABA state.

**The correct response is option A.**

A low cholinergic/high dopaminergic state is the proposed final common neural pathway for delirium. Option B is incorrect because delirium is associated with a low,

not high, cholinergic state. The activity of cholinergic and dopaminergic pathways can be regulated and affected by other neurotransmitters, including serotonergic, opiatergic, GABAergic, noradrenergic, and glutamatergic systems. However, the strongest evidence points specifically to a low cholinergic state and high dopaminergic state and not other neurotransmitters. Thus, options C, D, and E are incorrect. Other factors that affect the final common pathway and induce delirium include altered metabolic states, physiological changes of inflammatory and stress responses, and glial activity.

A wide variety of medications and medical conditions have anticholinergic effects, increasing the risk of delirium. Many medications that are commonly not recognized as "anticholinergic" have significant anticholinergic action, including digoxin, nifedipine, cimetidine, and codeine. Medical conditions with anticholinergic effects include thiamine deficiency, hypoxia, and hypoglycemia, all of which may reduce acetylcholine by affecting the oxidative metabolism of glucose and the production of acetyl coenzyme A, which is the rate-limiting step for acetylcholine synthesis. The dopamine excess that is associated with delirium has been conceptualized as an imbalance of the activities of dopamine and acetylcholine relative to each other because decreased cholinergic activity tends to result in increased dopaminergic activity. Hypoxia, which is an important risk factor for delirium, is associated with the increased release of dopamine and decreased release of acetylcholine.

Trzepacz PT, Meagher DJ: Neuropsychiatric aspects of delirium, in The American Psychiatric Publishing Textbook of Neuropsychiatry and Behavioral Neurosciences, 5th Edition. Edited by Yudofsky SC, Hales RE. Washington, DC, American Psychiatric Publishing, 2008, pp 495–498

81. Which of the following antiepileptic drugs (AEDs) has been shown to be effective in the treatment of agitation and aggression in patients with dementia?

    A. Lamotrigine.
    B. Levetiracetam.
    C. Gabapentin.
    D. Valproate.
    E. Phenytoin.

**The correct response is option D.**

Of the AEDs, carbamazepine and valproic acid have been found in placebo-controlled trials to lessen agitation and aggression in patients with dementia.

Tune LE: Management of noncognitive symptoms of dementia, in The American Psychiatric Publishing Textbook of Psychopharmacology, 3rd Edition. Edited by Schatzberg AF, Nemeroff CB. Washington, DC, American Psychiatric Publishing, 2004, p 942

82. Depression is associated with all of the following neurochemical alterations *except*

    A. Lower levels of cerebrospinal fluid (CSF) serotonin metabolites.
    B. Decreased serotonin transporter binding.
    C. Serotonin receptor abnormalities.
    D. Decreased CSF homovanillic acid.
    E. Increased dopamine transporter activity.

**The correct response is option E.**

Dopamine transporter activity is often reduced, not increased, in patients with depression. Depressed patients show lower CSF levels of serotonin metabolites, decreased serotonin transporter binding, and abnormalities in serotonin receptors. CSF concentrations of homovanillic acid are also reduced in depression.

Hales RE, Bourgeois JA, Shahrokh NC: Study Guide to Neuropsychiatry and Behavioral Neurosciences: A Companion to The American Psychiatric Publishing Textbook of Neuropsychiatry and Behavioral Neurosciences, 5th Edition, Washington, DC, American Psychiatric Publishing, 2008, p 62

Holtzheimer PE III, Mayberg HS: Neuropsychiatric aspects of mood disorders, in The American Psychiatric Publishing Textbook of Neuropsychiatry and Behavioral Neurosciences, 5th Edition. Edited by Yudofsky SC, Hales RE. Washington, DC, American Psychiatric Publishing, 2008, pp 1007–1008

83. The current American Academy of Neurology (2007) practice recommendations for evaluation of reversible causes of dementia include laboratory testing to rule out which of the following medical disorders?

    A. Hypocalcemia.
    B. Hypothyroidism.
    C. Hyponatremia.
    D. Iron deficiency.
    E. Hyperparathyroidism.

**The correct response is option B.**

Laboratory testing is a major component of the comprehensive evaluation of cognitive decline. The current American Academy of Neurology (2007) practice recommendations for evaluation of reversible causes of dementia include testing for vitamin $B_{12}$ deficiency and hypothyroidism. These laboratory tests are recommended in addition to structural imaging (noncontrast head computed tomography and magnetic resonance imaging studies) and evaluation of depression to rule out so-called pseudodementia or dementia-like symptoms that stem from depression.

American Academy of Neurology: American Academy of Neurology practice guidelines for dementia. Continuum 13(2):Appendix A, 2007

Kim HF, Schulz PE, Wilde EA, et al: Laboratory testing and imaging studies in psychiatry, in The American Psychiatric Publishing Textbook of Psychiatry, 5th Edition. Edited by Hales RE, Yudofsky SC, Gabbard GO. Washington, DC, American Psychiatric Publishing, 2008, p 39

84. A psychiatrist is asked to participate in a research project in which residents of a neighborhood that was recently devastated by an earthquake are asked to provide detailed accounts of their experiences during the earthquake. Which is the most relevant ethical principle to consider at this time?

    A. Value.
    B. Scientific validity.
    C. Informed consent.
    D. Favorable risk-benefit ratio.
    E. Independent review.

**The correct answer is option D.**

The psychiatrist must ensure that there is a favorable risk-benefit ratio for the subjects' prior involvement in this project. The risks of research should be minimized for subjects. The individuals in this devastated community are vulnerable of being exploited as subjects for a research project that ultimately may harm them by forcing them to quickly reexperience their traumas. The potential benefits to the subjects and population in general should be enhanced and exceed the risks associated with intervening at this time. Another required ethical concept, fair subject selection, is also relevant in this case. *Fair subject selection* refers to the principle that communities and people should not be exploited for research purposes; inclusion criteria and study sites should be determined with these principles in mind. The burdens and benefits of research participation should be equally distributed.

Other requirements for ethical clinical research include the principles of value, scientific validity, independent review, informed consent, and respect for enrolled subjects. Options A, B, C, and E are important principles to consider when conducting clinical research but are less potentially damaging. *Value* refers to the principle that research must have the potential to lead to improved knowledge or health; it must answer a nontrivial question.

Roberts LW, Hoop JG, Dunn LB: Ethical aspects of psychiatry, in The American Psychiatric Publishing Textbook of Psychiatry, 5th Edition. Edited by Hales RE, Yudofsky SC, Gabbard GO. Washington, DC, American Psychiatric Publishing, 2008, p 1629

85. "Drug courts" have been developed as an alternative method to deal with substance abusers who commit crimes. Which of the following statements is *false* regarding drug courts in the United States?

    A. They are a type of "diversion."
    B. They are found in a limited number of jurisdictions.
    C. They have low recidivism rates.
    D. They are used for nonviolent offenders with misdemeanor charges.
    E. None require a comorbid psychiatric illness for participation.

**The correct response is option E.**

This statement is false because some states require the presence of an additional mental disorder for a defendant's case to be heard in a drug court. The statements in options A, B, C, and D are all true. A drug court is a type of diversion that is available in a limited number of jurisdictions. These programs are generally for nonviolent offenders with less serious charges.

Mack AH, Barros M: Forensic addiction psychiatry, in The American Psychiatric Publishing Textbook of Substance Abuse Treatment, 4th Edition. Edited by Galanter M, Kleber HD. Washington, DC, American Psychiatric Publishing, 2008, pp 696–697

86. Which of the following statements is *true* regarding the DSM-IV-TR (American Psychiatric Association 2000) diagnosis of gender identity disorder?

    A. The diagnosis applies only to adults and not to children or adolescents.
    B. The diagnosis should not be used for transsexualism.
    C. The diagnosis would apply to someone with androgen insensitivity syndrome.
    D. The diagnosis requires a strong and persistent cross-gender identification.
    E. The diagnosis is not given in the absence of discomfort with one's sex.

**The correct response is option D.**

Currently, it is accepted that there are two necessary components of gender identity disorder: a strong and persistent cross-gender identification and a persistent discomfort with one's sex or a sense of inappropriateness in the gender role of that sex. The diagnosis is not given if the person has a concurrent physical condition such as partial androgen insensitivity syndrome or congenital adrenal hyperplasia, and as with many other diagnoses in DSM-IV-TR, there must be evidence of clinically significant distress or impairment (American Psychiatric Association 2000). The term *transsexualism* was eliminated in DSM-IV (American Psychiatric Association 1994) and was replaced by a single diagnostic term, *gender identity disorder*. The disorder was also placed in the "Sexual and Gender Identity Disorders" section. The term remained the same in the current DSM-IV-TR edition. The elimination of transsexualism alters the sense that it exists as a single disorder and presents it conceptually as a spectrum of disorders. However, the term still appears to describe appropriately what is now referred to as *gender identity disorder of adulthood*.

American Psychiatric Association: Diagnostic and Statistical Manual of Mental Disorders, 4th Edition. Washington, DC, American Psychiatric Association, 1994

American Psychiatric Association: Diagnostic and Statistical Manual of Mental Disorders, 4th Edition, Text Revision. Washington, DC, American Psychiatric Association, 2000

Becker JV, Johnson BR: Gender identity disorders and paraphilias, in The American Psychiatric Publishing Textbook of Psychiatry, 5th Edition. Edited by Hales RE, Yudofsky SC, Gabbard GO. Washington, DC, American Psychiatric Publishing, 2008, pp 730–732, Table 17–1

87. Which of the following does *not* predict greater risk of violence?

    A. Younger age at first arrest for serious crime.
    B. Prior violent acts.
    C. Being employed.
    D. Past use of weapons in assaults.
    E. History of formal military discipline.

**The correct response is option C.**

The clinician is advised to consider the history of past violence in assessing current violence risk. Persons who are laid off from work are six times more likely to be violent than their employed peers. The age at first arrest for a serious offense is highly correlated with persistence of criminal offending. Each prior episode of violence increases the risk of a future violent act. Given four previous arrests, the probability of a fifth is 80%. A person who has used weapons against others in the past may pose a serious risk of future violence. For those individuals who have served in the military, the clinician should review any history of fights, absences without leave, disciplinary measures (Article XV in the Uniform Code of Military Justice), as well as the type of discharge.

Scott CL, Quanbeck CD, Resnick PJ: Assessment of dangerousness, in The American Psychiatric Publishing Textbook of Psychiatry, 5th Edition. Edited by Hales RE, Yudofsky SC, Gabbard GO. Washington, DC, American Psychiatric Publishing, 2008, pp 1656–1657

88. Regarding neuropsychological deficits from parietal lobe lesions, which of the following is *true*?

    A. Wernicke's aphasia is characterized by fluent paraphasic speech and defective aural comprehension but preserved simple repetition.
    B. Conduction aphasia is associated with profoundly defective verbatim repetition, nonfluent speech, and impaired reading comprehension.
    C. Lesions to the inferior parietal lobule may lead to acalculia, an acquired inability to perform simple mathematical calculations.
    D. Neglect syndromes from right-sided inferior parietal lobule lesions are confined to neglect of intrapersonal space.
    E. Anosognosia refers to the patient's lack of concern with (rather than lack of recognition of) a neurological and/or neuropsychological deficit.

**The answer is option C.**

The parietal lobes are crucial for language, mathematical, and recognition functions. Left-sided lesions in the inferior parietal lobule may lead to *acalculia*, wherein patients lose the ability to perform simple mathematical calculations and may even be unable to read or write numbers. *Wernicke's aphasia* is characterized by fluent, paraphasic speech, impaired repetition, and defective aural comprehension. *Conduction aphasia* is associated with marked defects in verbatim repetition, fluent speech, and mildly compromised comprehension. Neglect can involve intrapersonal as well as extrapersonal space. *Neglect of intrapersonal space* is illustrated by the patient failing to use or denying the existence of the contralateral extremity, even when there is no motor impairment. *Neglect of extrapersonal space* is illustrated by the patient failing to attend to "external" stimuli (e.g., external objects in the left visual field). *Anosognosia* is a true recognition defect in which the patient is unaware of acquired motor, sensory, or cognitive deficits.

Taber KH, Hurley RA: Neuroanatomy for the psychiatrist, in The American Psychiatric Publishing Textbook of Psychiatry, 5th Edition. Edited by Hales RE, Yudofsky SC, Gabbard GO. Washington, DC, American Psychiatric Publishing, 2008, pp 181–187; Table 5–1

89. Which of the following personality disorders is most commonly associated with violence?

    A. Borderline personality disorder.
    B. Paranoid personality disorder.
    C. Narcissistic personality disorder.
    D. Antisocial personality disorder.
    E. Schizotypal personality disorder.

**The correct response is option D.**

Although borderline personality disorder and sadistic personality traits are associated with increased violence, the most common personality disorder associated with violence is antisocial personality disorder. The violence by those with antisocial personality disorder is often motivated by revenge or occurs during a period of heavy drinking. Violence among these persons is frequently cold and calculated and lacks emotionality. Low IQ and antisocial personality disorder are a particularly ominous combination for increasing the risk of future violence.

Scott CL, Quanbeck CD, Resnick PJ: Assessment of dangerousness, in The American Psychiatric Publishing Textbook of Psychiatry, 5th Edition. Edited by Hales RE, Yudofsky SC, Gabbard GO. Washington, DC, American Psychiatric Publishing, 2008, p 1659

90.  Which of the following is characteristic of violence associated with traumatic brain injury (TBI)?

 A.  Episodes of violence with long periods of relative calm.
 B.  Violence often motivated by revenge.
 C.  Calculated acts of violence.
 D.  Violence perpetrated against nonfamily members and involving an altercation with the victim prior to violence.
 E.  Lack of remorse.

**The correct response is option A.**

Violent behaviors associated with patients with TBI tend to be episodic in nature, with long periods of relative calm in between. Aggression resulting from TBI often involves reactive behavior triggered by trivial stimuli, nonpurposeful actions with no clear aims or goals, or explosive outbursts without a gradual buildup.

Option B is incorrect because revenge is usually not the motivation behind the violence of patients with TBI. Revenge and heavy drinking are characteristic of the violence seen in individuals with antisocial personality disorder. Option C is incorrect because violent acts by individuals with TBI are usually unpredictable and impulsive, not calculated, which more typifies the violent behaviors of individuals with antisocial personality disorder. Option D is incorrect because the violence described in this option typifies individuals with comorbid schizophrenia and antisocial personality disorder. Option E is incorrect because brain-injured patients typically have feelings of concern and remorse following a violent episode.

Scott CL, Quanbeck CD, Resnick PJ: Assessment of dangerousness, in The American Psychiatric Publishing Textbook of Psychiatry, 5th Edition. Edited by Hales RE, Yudofsky SC, Gabbard GO. Washington, DC, American Psychiatric Publishing, 2008, pp 1659–1660, Table 44–6

91.  In a long-term follow-up study of patients with schizophrenia (the Vermont Longitudinal Study), the majority of these patients, after 10 years of follow-up and approximately 15–20 years of illness, showed

 A.  A marked deterioration in mental functioning.
 B.  No psychotic symptoms.
 C.  A poor level of overall functioning, especially those over 50 years of age.
 D.  A deteriorating long-term course.
 E.  Little heterogeneity in outcome.

**The correct response is option B.**

More than half of the individuals in the Vermont study (Harding et al. 1987a, 1987b) had no psychotic symptoms after 10 years of follow-up, and they were found to have considerable heterogeneity in outcome in later life. After the initial deteriorating years, the later course of the illness settles at a low, but flat, plateau. Surprisingly, symptoms often improve after age 50 years, and most individuals with schizophrenia have a "good" level of functioning in their later lives.

Harding CM, Brooks GW, Ashikga T, et al: The Vermont longitudinal study of persons with severe mental illness, I: methodology, study sample, and overall status 32 years later. Am J Psychiatry 144:718–726, 1987a

Harding CM, Brooks GW, Ashikga T, et al: The Vermont longitudinal study of persons with severe mental illness, II: long-term outcome of subjects who retrospectively met DSM-III criteria for schizophrenia. Am J Psychiatry 144:727–735, 1987b

Tamminga CA, Shad MJ, Ghose S: Neuropsychiatric aspects of schizophrenia, in The American Psychiatric Publishing Textbook of Neuropsychiatry and Behavioral Neurosciences, 5th Edition. Edited by Yudofsky SC, Hales RE. Washington, DC, American Psychiatric Publishing, 2008, p 972

92.  Psychophysiological insomnia is a troubling sleep disorder with specific behavioral characteristics. Which of the following is *not* a feature of this condition?

 A.  Excessive worry about not being able to sleep.
 B.  Trying too hard to sleep.
 C.  Rumination.
 D.  Sleeping poorly in a novel environment.
 E.  Increased muscle tension when retiring.

**The correct response is option D.**

Psychophysiological insomnia is a conditioned inability to sleep. Features of psychophysiological insomnia include excessive worry about not being able to sleep, trying too hard to sleep, rumination, inability to clear one's mind while trying to sleep, increased muscle tension when getting into bed, and other somatic manifestations of anxiety. Persons with psychophysiologic insomnia often report improved sleep in environments other than their own bed and usually do not have problems unintentionally falling asleep (e.g., when watching television). Psychophysiological insomnia may be categorized as dyssomnia not otherwise specified or sleep disorder related to another mental disorder.

American Academy of Sleep Medicine: The International Classification of Sleep Disorders, Second Edition (ICSD-2): Diagnostic and Coding Manual. Westchester, IL, American Academy of Sleep Medicine, 2005

Hirshkowitz M, Sharafkhaneh A: Neuropsychiatric aspects of sleep and sleep disorders, in The American Psychiatric Publishing Textbook of Neuropsychiatry and Behavioral Neurosciences, 5th Edition. Edited by Yudofsky SC, Hales RE. Washington, DC, American Psychiatric Publishing, 2008, p 686

93. Which of the following is *false* regarding pain disorders?

    A. Alzheimer's disease may lower the pain threshold and thus alter the pain perception in these patients.
    B. Nearly 50% of elderly individuals have chronic pain; 70% of those in long-term care have chronic pain.
    C. Individuals with chronic back pain have an estimated 80% lifetime prevalence of a psychiatric disorder.
    D. Pain is the most common medical complaint in elderly persons, with pain caused by musculoskeletal disease being the most common type of pain.
    E. Depressive disorder is the most common comorbidity in individuals with pain disorder.

**The correct response is option A.**

Alzheimer's disease may alter pain perception by increasing the pain threshold, so the statement in option A is incorrect. The statements in options B, C, D, and E are true.

Agronin ME: Somatoform disorders, in The American Psychiatric Publishing Textbook of Geriatric Psychiatry, 3rd Edition. Edited by Blazer DG, Steffens DC, Busse EW. Washington, DC, American Psychiatric Publishing, 2004, pp 297–298

94. Loci influencing the risk for alcohol dependence map close to an alcohol dehydrogenase gene cluster on the long arm of which chromosome?

    A. Chromosome 4.
    B. Chromosome 6.
    C. Chromosome 12.
    D. Chromosome 15.
    E. Chromosome 16.

**The correct response is option A.**

Linkage studies of alcohol dependence by investigators in the Collaborative Studies on the Genetics of Alcoholism and in the intramural program of the National Institute on Alcohol Abuse and Alcoholism have identified promising chromosomal locations for alcohol dependence susceptibility loci, which in some cases have led to discovery of disease-influencing loci. Loci influencing risk for alcohol dependence map close to an alcohol dehydrogenase gene cluster on the long arm of chromosome 4.

Gelernter J, Kranzler HR: Genetics of addiction, in The American Psychiatric Publishing Textbook of Substance Abuse Treatment, 4th Edition. Edited by Galanter M, Kleber HD. Washington, DC, American Psychiatric Publishing, 2008, p 19

95. Substance withdrawal states may be associated with periods of autonomic instability. Which of the following substances is *not* associated with actual physiologic withdrawal?

    A. Alcohol.
    B. Benzodiazepines.
    C. Cocaine.
    D. Barbiturates.
    E. Opioids.

**The correct response is option C.**

Although not considered true physiological withdrawal, the emotional and physiological symptoms associated with amphetamine, cocaine, as well as marijuana, are often substantial and require a period of stabilizing treatment. Options A, B, D, and E are incorrect because these substances are associated with true physiologic withdrawal. Substance-dependent individuals usually experience characteristic rebound "true" physiological withdrawal syndromes about 8–30 hours after the last dose of the drug, depending upon the drug, dosage, and period of use.

McLellan AT: Evolution in addiction treatment concepts and methods, in The American Psychiatric Publishing Textbook of Substance Abuse Treatment, 4th Edition. Edited by Galanter M, Kleber HD. Washington, DC, American Psychiatric Publishing, 2008, p 96

96. Treatment of pain states may be an appropriate application of tricyclic antidepressants (TCAs). Unfortunately, a host of cardiac concerns make electrocardiogram (ECG) monitoring necessary with these agents. Which of the following is *not* a characteristic ECG change associated with TCAs?

    A. Flattened T-wave.
    B. Prolonged Q-T interval.
    C. Prolonged QRS interval.
    D. Prolonged PR interval.
    E. Elevated S-T segment.

## The correct response is option E.

Elevated S-T segments are not an ECG change associated with TCAs. ECG changes observed with TCA use include flattened T-waves; prolonged Q-T, QRS, and PR intervals; and depressed S-T segments.

> Golianu, B, Bhandari R, Shaw RJ, et al: Neuropsychiatric aspects of pain management, in The American Psychiatric Publishing Textbook of Neuropsychiatry and Behavioral Neurosciences, 5th Edition. Edited by Yudofsky SC, Hales RE. Washington, DC, American Psychiatric Publishing, 2008, p 384

97. An application of Stroebe and Schut's (1999) dual-process model of grief is to focus on specific tasks required of the survivor. Which of the following is *true* regarding this model?

    A. The tasks can be divided into grief tasks and loss tasks.
    B. The tasks can be divided into grief tasks (such as confronting the loss) and restoration tasks (such as emotionally withdrawing from the deceased person).
    C. Restructuring thoughts and memories about the deceased person are grief tasks.
    D. Emotional withdrawing from the deceased person includes actively attempting to forget the deceased person.
    E. A loss task includes spending time away from grieving.

## The correct response is option C.

The two categories of tasks have been divided into grief tasks and restoration tasks. Grief tasks include confront-

ing the loss, restructuring of thoughts and memories of the deceased person, and emotionally withdrawing from (but not forgetting) the deceased person. Restoration tasks include accepting the changed world, spending time away from grieving, and developing new relationships and identities.

Option A is incorrect because the tasks are categorized into grief tasks and restoration tasks. Option B is incorrect because emotional withdrawal from the deceased person is a grief, not a restoration, task. Option D is incorrect because forgetting the deceased person is not necessary for emotional withdrawal, which is a grief task.

> Stroebe M, Schat H: The dual process model of copying with bereavement: rationale and description. Death Stud 23:197–224, 1999

> Thompson LW, Kaye JL, Tang PCY, et al: Bereavement and adjustment disorders, in The American Psychiatric Publishing Textbook of Geriatric Psychiatry, 3rd Edition. Edited by Blazer DG, Steffens DC, Busse EW. Washington, DC, American Psychiatric Publishing, 2004, p 322

98. Which of the following augmentation strategies has been found to be effective in treatment-resistant obsessive-compulsive disorder (OCD)?

    A. Addition of venlafaxine to buspirone.
    B. Addition of lithium to risperidone.
    C. Addition of risperidone to a selective serotonin reuptake inhibitor (SSRI).
    D. Addition of valproate to clomipramine.
    E. Addition of gabapentin to an SSRI.

## The correct response is option C.

The following augmentation and/or combination strategies have been reported as offering benefit. Combining fluvoxamine with clomipramine is an approach to consider in individuals who have shown a partial response to clomipramine. Patients with OCD and comorbid tic disorders respond better to haloperidol than to placebo as an addition to fluvoxamine. Olanzapine and risperidone have been added successfully in cases of partial SSRI response.

> Davidson JRT, Connor KM: Treatment of anxiety disorders, in The American Psychiatric Publishing Textbook of Psychopharmacology, 3rd Edition. Edited by Schatzberg AF, Nemeroff CB. Washington, DC, American Psychiatric Publishing, 2004, p 914

99. Hyperthyroidism has been associated with a specific range of neuropsychiatric symptoms and syndromes. Which of the following is *true?*

    A. Because of the degree of systemic metabolic disturbances in hyperthyroidism, the majority of patients exhibit psychopathology as a result of hyperthyroidism.

    B. In studies of both selected and unselected hyperthyroidism patients, anxiety disorders are the most common neuropsychiatric illnesses.

    C. Cognitive disturbance in hyperthyroidism is as common as it is in hypothyroidism.

    D. In hyperthyroid patients with depressive symptoms, the physical symptoms of hyperthyroidism precede mood symptoms in the vast majority of cases.

    E. In hyperthyroidism, both mania and psychosis are uncommon.

## The answer is option E.

Mania or hypomania and psychosis are uncommon in patients with hyperthyroidism, occurring in only about 2.1% of unselected cases. Serious psychopathology occurs in only a minority of patients. Major depression is the most common psychiatric manifestation; however, the mood symptoms may precede the development of physical signs and symptoms of hyperthyroidism in some patients. The prevalence of cognitive disturbance in hyperthyroidism is considerably less than that in hypothyroidism.

Joska JA, Stein DJ: Mood disorders, in The American Psychiatric Publishing Textbook of Psychiatry, 5th Edition. Edited by Hales RE, Yudofsky SC, Gabbard GO. Washington, DC, American Psychiatric Publishing, 2008, pp 464–466

100. The increasing multiethnicity of Western English-speaking countries has sparked a debate about alternative models of culturally sensitive models of care. One such model acknowledges that following both prescribed medication and ethnic spiritual therapy may be the best hope for securing adherence. This model also encourages a more honest discussion of the other therapies being tried and their interaction, from the reading of sacred texts to the possible infliction of physical harm. This model is called

    A. A cultural consultation model.

    B. A hedge-your-bets approach.

    C. A melting pot approach.

    D. A separate services model.

    E. A cultural recovery model.

## The correct response is option B.

Advocates of a hedge-your-bets strategy acknowledge that following both prescribed medication and ethnic spiritual therapy may be the best hope for securing adherence. This model also encourages a more honest discussion of the other therapies being tried and their interaction from the reading of sacred texts to the possible infliction of physical harm. Under a cultural consultation model, a specialized multidisciplinary team brings together clinical experience with cultural knowledge and linguistic skills. It provides consultations to other clinicians rather than taking on patients for continuing care over two to three interviews, which would include the family as well. Team members are involved in the training of interpreters and other culture-link workers.

In the melting pot approach, institutional factors promoting ethnic inequalities are addressed. Culturally influenced or capable services are important to the mainstream delivery of services and not only to minority ethnic groups. Mainstream services are commonly enriched by responding to the needs of all cultural groups, guaranteeing equality of access, and ensuring rights for all individuals.

In the United States, separate public and voluntary sector services for African Americans, Hispanic Americans, and Native Americans are commonplace. Religious denominations sponsor certain hospitals and social services. Lending credibility to the argument for allowing creation of separate services are consistent research findings that show that members of ethnic minorities may experience increased coercive treatment and social encounters that promote their distrust in secular hospitals. Cultural recovery may involve regaining a viable ethnic identity and developing a healthy affiliation with an individual's ethnic group as well as reacquiring a functional social network, a religious or spiritual commitment, a rebuilt social status in the recovering as well as the cultural community, and reestablished vocational and recreational activities.

El-Guebaly N: Cross-cultural aspects of addiction, in The American Psychiatric Publishing Textbook of Substance Abuse Treatment, 4th Edition. Edited by Galanter M, Kleber HD. Washington, DC, American Psychiatric Publishing, 2008, pp 49–50

101. The emergence of lateralization and hemispheric asymmetry are important to neurobehavioral development. All of the following statements are true *except*

    A. Lateralization is largely established by age 5 years.
    B. Differential development of the two hemispheres in early growth is caused by delayed myelination of the corpus callosum.
    C. In early development, the left hemisphere develops more rapidly than the right because of its usual dominance.
    D. Development of the right hemisphere accelerates between ages 3 and 6 years.
    E. Gray matter density tends to be greater in the right posterior temporal regions than the left.

**The correct response is option C.**

During the first few months of development, the right hemisphere develops more rapidly than the left. However, by age 5–6 months, dendritic growth in the left hemisphere surpasses that in the right hemisphere and continues at a rapid pace for the next 2 years. Between ages 3 and 6 years, the right hemisphere accelerates in its development and helps provide the prosodic components of language that flower between ages 5 and 6. Lateralization of the brain is largely established before 5 years of age and emerges through a multistage process that begins in utero.

Teicher MYH, Andersen SL, Navalta CP, et al: Neuropsychiatric disorders of childhood and adolescence, in The American Psychiatric Publishing Textbook of Neuropsychiatry and Behavioral Neurosciences, 5th Edition. Edited by Yudofsky SC, Hales RE. Washington, DC, American Psychiatric Publishing, 2008, p 1048

102. Delirium in the elderly is characterized by which of the following?

    A. Usually resolves within a week after being discharged from a medical or surgical hospitalization.
    B. Usually results in a full resolution of symptoms once the underlying acute medical problems are resolved.
    C. Is often the initial presentation of an underlying dementia.
    D. Tends to occur abruptly in elderly persons, as with other populations. Thus, gradualness of

mental status changes usually rules out delirium in older individuals.
    E. All of the above.

**The correct response is option C.**

Option C is correct because an episode of delirium often is the initial presentation of an underlying dementia. Option A is incorrect because delirium in the elderly usually persists for months, not just days, in elderly patients hospitalized for medical or surgical reasons. Option B is incorrect because full resolution of symptoms of delirium in elderly persons within a short period of time is the exception rather than the rule. Option D is incorrect because in elderly individuals, a delirium secondary to drugs or to illnesses such as renal failure may have an insidious onset.

Raskind MA, Bonner LT, Peskind ER: Cognitive disorders, in The American Psychiatric Publishing Textbook of Geriatric Psychiatry, 3rd Edition. Edited by Blazer DG, Steffens DC, Busse EW. Washington, DC, American Psychiatric Publishing, 2004, p 222

103. Which of the following statements is *true* regarding treatment of behavioral disturbances in dementia?

    A. Benzodiazepines are the treatment of choice to treat behavioral disturbances in patients with dementia.
    B. Clonazepam is preferred over lorazepam when treating agitation in patients with dementia.
    C. Benzodiazepines can be used for short-term treatment of behavioral disturbances associated with disruptions to routines or adjustments to changes.
    D. Diphenhydramine is an appropriate treatment option for most patients with dementia.
    E. Benzodiazepines should be given with antipsychotics whenever possible.

**The correct response is option C.**

The short-term use of short-acting benzodiazepines with few active metabolites, such as lorazepam, may be safely used to manage patients experiencing a difficult adjustment to a change in residence or other disruptions in their normal routine. Option A is incorrect because of the increased risk of delirium, falls, and other side effects in patients with dementia. Option B is incorrect because clonazepam's long half-life and long clearance rate would be problematic in patients with dementia who develop serious side effects such as delirium caused by a benzodiaz-epine. Option D is incorrect because diphenhydramine, an anticholinergic, would increase the risk of delirium in a patient with dementia. Option E is incorrect because benzodiazepines should be used on an as-needed basis for acute symptom management, and routinely administering antipsychotics with benzodiazepines unnecessarily pro-motes polypharmacy, which should be minimized in pa-tients with dementia.

Tune LE: Management of noncognitive symptoms of de-mentia: behavioral and psychological symptoms of demen-tia, in The American Psychiatric Publishing Textbook of Psychopharmacology, 3rd Edition. Edited by Schatzberg AF, Nemeroff CB. Washington, DC, American Psychiatric Publishing, 2004, p 942

104. Which of the following statements is *true* regarding specific psychiatric illnesses and comorbid sub-stance use disorders?

A. When comorbid with substance use disorder, conduct disorder usually follows substance use disorder.
B. Rates of conduct disorder in adolescent sub-stance abusers are between 30% and 50%.
C. Mood disorders, particularly depression, fre-quently precede adolescent drug abuse.
D. Depressive disorders are reported in 15%–20% of adolescent substance abusers.
E. Social phobia and panic disorder usually follow the onset of substance abuse in adolescents.

**The correct response is option C.**

Mood disorders, especially depression, frequently pre-cede substance use and substance use disorders in adoles-cents. Option A is incorrect because conduct disorder usually precedes, not follows, substance use disorders. Option B is incorrect because conduct disorder occurs in 50%–80% of adolescent patients with substance use dis-orders. Option D is incorrect because the prevalence of depressive disorders is higher (24%–50%) among adoles-cent substance abusers. Option E is incorrect because so-cial phobia usually precedes, not follows, substance use disorder. Panic disorder and generalized anxiety disorder usually follow the onset of substance use disorders. To summarize, disorders that usually precede substance use disorders include: conduct disorder, social phobia, mood disorders, follow substance use disorders: panic disorder and generalized anxiety disorder. Attention-deficit/hyper-activity disorder (ADHD) is also frequently observed in

substance-abusing youth; such an association is likely be-cause of the high level of comorbidity between conduct disorder and ADHD as well as a direct causation. The or-der of appearance of anxiety and substance use disorders is variable depending on the specific anxiety disorder.

Kaminer Y: Adolescent substance abuse, in The American Psychiatric Publishing Textbook of Substance Abuse Treat-ment, 4th Edition. Edited by Galanter M, Kleber HD. Washington, DC, American Psychiatric Publishing, 2008, p 527

Hales RE, Bourgeois JA, Shahrokh NC, et al: Study Guide to the American Psychiatric Publishing Textbook of Sub-stance Abuse Treatment, 4th Edition. Washington, DC, American Psychiatric Publishing, 2008, p 214

105. Which of the following tests assesses the cognitive domain of executive ability?

A. Continuous Performance Test.
B. Trail Making Test.
C. Wisconsin Card Sorting Test.
D. Judgment of Line Orientation.
E. Boston Naming Test.

**The correct response is option B.**

The Trail Making Test assesses executive ability by set switching using a visuographic sequence test. The Con-tinuous Performance Test assesses attention through the use of a computerized sustained-attention test. The Wis-consin Card Sorting Test assesses reasoning through con-cept formation and cognitive flexibility. The Judgment of Line Orientation assesses visual perception by matching orientation of straight lines. The Boston Naming Test as-sesses language by having the person name familiar items.

Clarkin JF, Howieson DB, McClough J: The role of psy-chiatric measures in assessment and treatment, in The American Psychiatric Publishing Textbook of Psychiatry, 5th Edition. Edited by Hales RE, Yudofsky SC, Gabbard GO. Washington, DC, American Psychiatric Publishing, 2008, p 90; Table 3–8

106. A patient with schizophrenia asks his outpatient psychiatrist to document a less-stigmatizing diag-nosis when completing insurance forms. Of the fol-lowing, which is the most relevant ethical principle to consider in this case?

A. Nonmaleficence.
B. Fiduciary.

C. Empathy.

D. Conflict of interest.

E. Personhood.

**The correct response is option A.**

*Nonmaleficence* is the duty to avoid doing harm. The psychiatrist's obligation to document the truth is in tension with the desire to avoid the harm that may occur if the insurance company learns of the diagnosis. Options B, C, D, and E are incorrect because these principles are less relevant in this case. *Fiduciary* is an entity in a position of trust with a duty to act on behalf of another for the other's good. Physicians are fiduciaries with respect to their patients. *Empathy* is the act of entering into someone else's frame of reference in terms of thoughts, feelings, and experiences to gain an authentic understanding of the other person's experiences imaginatively as one's own. *Conflict of interest* refers to a situation in which a physician has competing roles, relationships, or interests that could potentially interfere with the ability to care for patients. *Personhood* is the principle of an individual's having full moral status as a human being.

Roberts LW, Hoop JG, Dunn LB: Ethical aspects of psychiatry, in The American Psychiatric Publishing Textbook of Psychiatry, 5th Edition. Edited by Hales RE, Yudofsky SC, Gabbard GO. Washington, DC, American Psychiatric Publishing, 2008, pp 1604, 1606–1607; Tables 42–3, 42–5

107. Damage to this brain structure frequently produces symptoms of aggression, violence, anorexia, depression, impaired short-term memory, dementia, laughing, seizures, and altered sleep–wake cycle.

    A. Hypothalamus.

    B. Thalamus.

    C. Cerebellum.

    D. Mammillary bodies.

    E. Putamen.

**The correct response is option A.**

Behavioral, emotional, and memory symptoms, as well as other deficits, are associated with lesions to the hypothalamus. Examples of commonly reported symptoms are aggression, violence, anorexia, depression, impaired short-term memory, dementia, gelastic (laughing) seizures, and altered sleep–wake cycle. Thalamic injuries are associated with severe memory impairment (thalamic amnesia) and dementia (bilateral damage); deficits in language, verbal intellect, and verbal memory (medial portion of left thal-

amus); and deficits in visuospatial and nonverbal intellect and visual memory (right thalamus). Recent work indicates that cerebellar lesions, particularly to the posterior cerebellum and vermis, can result in a range of cognitive and emotional deficits including executive dysfunction, visuospatial deficits, personality changes, and linguistic abnormalities. Damage to the mammillary bodies or the mammillothalamic tract primarily involves memory deficits and psychosis. Damage to the putamen includes primarily language and behavioral deficits (i.e., atypical aphasia, obsessive-compulsive traits, executive dysfunctions). (See table on next page.)

Taber KH, Hurley RA: Neuroanatomy for the psychiatrist, in The American Psychiatric Publishing Textbook of Psychiatry, 5th Edition. Edited by Hales RE, Yudofsky SC, Gabbard GO. Washington, DC, American Psychiatric Publishing, 2008, pp 168, 178

108. Evoked potentials, particularly the P300 potential, may be useful in the diagnosis and management of neuropsychiatric illness. All of the following statements are true *except*

    A. The most consistent P300 finding in schizophrenia is a reduction in amplitude.

    B. In schizophrenia, P300 abnormalities present in nonmedicated and medicated patients.

    C. P300 abnormalities correlate with the amount of negative symptoms and formal thought disorder in schizophrenia.

    D. In schizophrenia, asymmetrical auditory P300 reduction is frequently reported, with smaller amplitudes over the right temporal region.

    E. P300 abnormalities have been reported in relatives of schizophrenia patients and high-risk subjects for psychosis.

**The correct response is option D.**

Asymmetrical auditory P300 reduction in schizophrenia has been often reported with smaller amplitudes over the left temporal regions. Several studies have found that patients with schizophrenia have abnormal P300 potentials. P300 abnormalities are evident in both medicated and drug-free patients and are associated with several clinical features of schizophrenia, including negative symptoms, thought disorder, illness duration, and age at onset. P300 amplitude reduction or left-lateralized deficit has also been reported in first-degree relatives of schizophrenia patients, in high-risk subjects, and in psychosis-prone groups.

| Brain region | Specific regions included | Functions |
|---|---|---|
| Cortical areas | | |
| Frontal lobe | Broca's area (left), superior mesial, dorsolateral prefrontal regions. | Executive functions, personality, intellect, speech, motor functions, memory. |
| Temporal lobe | Lateral inferior, lateral anterior, dorsolateral, mesial temporal regions (hippocampus, amygdala). | Hearing, naming of objects, memory, emotion, visual recognition. |
| Occipital lobe | Primary visual cortex, visual association cortex. | Vision, visual association (support) areas. |
| Parietal lobe | Wernicke's area (left), inferior parietal lobule, optic tracts, superior parietal lobule. | Sensation, speech, understanding, academics. |
| Insula | | Smell. |
| Basal forebrain | (Common site of lesions for Alzheimer's disease, anterior communicating artery aneurysms) | Memory formation, storage, and retrieval. |
| Subcortical areas | | |
| Basal ganglia | Caudate, globus pallidus, putamen, substantia nigra, subthalamic nucleus. | Movement, emotion. |
| Thalamus | Limbic nuclei, motor nuclei, sensory nuclei, pulvinar. | "Relay station" for the entire basal ganglia and cerebral cortex. |
| Hypothalamus | | Temperature control, sleep, water metabolism, hormone secretion, blood pressure control, satiety, maintenance of balance, circadian rhythms. Modulates physiological reaction to emotional stimuli. |
| Pineal body/gland | | Contains no nerve tracts. Secretes hormones directly into bloodstream, inhibits endocrine gland production, circadian rhythm functions. |
| Reticular activating system | Nuclei and tracts are in the medulla, pons, and midbrain. It receives stimuli from the hypothalamus, basal ganglia, vestibular system, and sensory input from the body. It projects to the thalamus and cerebral cortex. | Consciousness |
| Midbrain | Tectum, tegmentum, red nucleus, cranial nerves 3 and 4 and nuclei. | Consciousness, fiber tracts, cranial nerves. |
| Pons | Locus coeruleus, raphe nucleus, central pons, cranial nerves 4,5,6 and nuclei. | Mood, motor and sensory tracts, wakefulness. |
| Cerebellum | Flocculonodular, anterior, and posterior lobes (anterior/posterior lobes include vermis). | Equilibrium, muscle tone. |
| Brain stem (medulla oblongata) | Cranial nerves 8–12 and nuclei, respiratory and cardiac centers. | Ascending and descending fiber tracts, respiratory centers. |

*Source.* Taber KH, Hurley RA: "Neuroanatomy for the Psychiatrist," in *The American Psychiatric Publishing Textbook of Psychiatry*, 5th Edition. Edited by Hales RE, Yudofsky SC, Gabbard GO. Washington, DC, American Psychiatric Publishing, 2008, pp. 181–187.

Boutros NN, Thatcher RW, Galderisi S: Electrodiagnostic techniques in neuropsychiatry, in The American Psychiatric Publishing Textbook of Neuropsychiatry and Behavioral Neurosciences, 5th Edition. Edited by Yudofsky SC, Hales RE. Washington, DC, American Psychiatric Publishing, 2008, pp 202–203

109. A defendant is charged with involuntary manslaughter because of his involvement in a three-car collision that led to the death of a passenger in another car. The accident occurred after a the windshield of defendant's car was suddenly struck by a broken tree branch, and he swerved to avoid hitting a large group of pedestrians. Police reports say that the defendant immediately called 911 on his cell phone, aided the other victims, and cooperated fully with authorities. A routine blood alcohol level found that the defendant just barely met the legal criterion for alcohol intoxication. The defendant has no prior drug or other criminal record. Which of the following statements is *true* regarding this case?

    A. Because ample evidence demonstrates that alcohol had little role to play in causing the accident, the charges will probably be dropped.
    B. He is unlikely to be convicted of the crime because he barely met the legal limit for alcohol intoxication and clearly demonstrated by his actions that his mental and physical status were largely unimpaired during and immediately after the accident.
    C. Even if strict liability is mandated, the defendant will unlikely be convicted because a "freak accident"—not alcohol—led to the accident.
    D. Under strict liability, the defendant's blood alcohol level may be enough to convict him of the crime.
    E. In such crimes, mandated minimum sentences for deaths resulting from driving while intoxicated apply only if the intoxication plays a substantial role in the death.

## The correct response is option D.

Some states have mandated maximum sentences in cases in which death resulted from a driver who was driving while intoxicated or driving under the influence. These sentences are applied even if the influence of the substance is shown to have played a minimal role in the events leading to the death. In some situations, intoxication alone may directly establish a defendant as guilty. Crimes such as driving while intoxicated or driving under the influence are called *strict liability crimes.* All that is required is evidence that the legal standard for intoxication was met.

Mack AH, Barros M: Forensic addiction psychiatry, in The American Psychiatric Publishing Textbook of Substance Abuse Treatment, 4th Edition. Edited by Galanter M, Kleber HD. Washington, DC, American Psychiatric Publishing, 2008, pp 696–697

110. Which of the following personality disorders has been found to be common in arsonists?

    A. Narcissistic.
    B. Histrionic.
    C. Schizoid.
    D. Borderline.
    E. Avoidant.

## The correct response is option D.

In a study by Virkkunen et al. (1987), all of the arsonists met DSM-III (American Psychiatric Association 1980) criteria for borderline personality disorder.

American Psychiatric Association: Diagnostic and Statistical Manual of Mental Disorders, 3rd Edition. Washington, DC, American Psychiatric Association, 1980

Hollander E, Berlin HA: Neuropsychiatric aspects of aggression and impulse-control disorders, in The American Psychiatric Publishing Textbook of Neuropsychiatry and Behavioral Neurosciences, 5th Edition. Edited by Yudofsky SC, Hales RE. Washington, DC, American Psychiatric Publishing, 2008, p 552

Virkkunen M, Nuutila A, Goodwin FK, et al: Cerebrospinal fluid monoamine metabolite levels in male arsonists. Arch Gen Psychiatry 44:241–247, 1987

111. Which of the following is *not* true regarding the epidemiology of violence?

    A. In the general population, males perpetrate violence at a rate 10 times that of females.
    B. Among mentally ill patients, men are five times more likely than women to commit violence.
    C. Among violent, mentally ill persons, women are more likely than men to commit violence toward family members.
    D. Among violent, mentally ill persons, men are more likely than women to commit violence resulting in arrest.
    E. Among psychiatric inpatients, men and women have similar rates of physical assault.

## The correct response is option B.

Although males in the general population perpetrate violent acts approximately 10 times more often than females, among people with mental disorders, men and women do not significantly differ in their base rates of violent behavior. In fact, rates are remarkably similar and in some cases slightly higher in women. Women were more likely than men to target their aggression toward family members in the home environment. Violent acts by men were more likely to result in an arrest or need for medical treatment.

> Scott CL, Quanbeck CD, Resnick PJ: Assessment of dangerousness, in The American Psychiatric Publishing Textbook of Psychiatry, 5th Edition. Edited by Hales RE, Yudofsky SC, Gabbard GO. Washington, DC, American Psychiatric Publishing, 2008, p 1656

112. A patient with traumatic brain injury with eye opening to speech (but not spontaneously), decorticate motor response, and intelligible but incoherent speech would score ____ on the Glasgow Coma Scale.

A. 8.
B. 9.
C. 10.
D. 11.
E. 12.

## The correct response is option B.

That patient would score 9 on the Glasgow Coma Scale.

> Silver JM, Hales E, Yudofsky SC: Neuropsychiatric aspects of traumatic brain injury, in The American Psychiatric Publishing Textbook of Neuropsychiatry and Behavioral Neurosciences, 5th Edition. Edited by Yudofsky SC, Hales RE. Washington, DC, American Psychiatric Publishing, 2008, p 600; Table 15–3

113. Which of the following statements is *false* regarding suicidality in various psychiatric disorders?

A. Among personality disorders, antisocial and borderline personality disorders have a particularly high rate of suicide.
B. The lifetime risk of suicide in schizophrenia is approximately 10%.
C. Suicide is the leading cause of death among schizophrenic individuals younger than age 35 years.

---

**Glasgow Coma Scale**

**Eye opening**

| None | 1. Not attributable to ocular swelling |
| To pain | 2. Pain stimulus is applied to chest or limbs |
| To speech | 3. Nonspecific response to speech or shout, does not imply the patient obeys command to open eyes |
| Spontaneous | 4. Eyes are open, but this does not imply intact awareness |

**Motor response**

| No response | 1. Flaccid |
| Extension | 2. "Decerebrate." Adduction, internal rotation of shoulder, and pronation of the forearm |
| Abnormal flexion | 3. "Decorticate." Abnormal flexion, adduction of the shoulder |
| Withdrawal | 4. Normal flexor response; withdraws from pain stimulus with adduction of the shoulder |
| Localizes pain | 5. Pain stimulus applied to supraocular region or fingertip causes limb to move so as to attempt to remove it |
| Obeys commands | 6. Follows simple commands |

**Verbal response**

| No response | 1. (Self-explanatory) |
| Incomprehensible | 2. Moaning and groaning, but no recognizable words |
| Inappropriate | 3. Intelligible speech (e.g., shouting or swearing), but no sustained or coherent conversation |
| Confused | 4. Patient responds to questions in a conversational manner, but the responses indicate varying degrees of disorientation and confusion |
| Oriented | 5. Normal orientation to time, place, and person |

*Source.* Silver JM, Hales E, Yudofsky SC: "Neuropsychiatric Aspects of Traumatic Brain Injury," in *The American Psychiatric Publishing Textbook of Neuropsychiatry and Behavioral Neurosciences,* 5th Edition. Edited by Yudofsky SC, Hales RE. Washington, DC, American Psychiatric Publishing, 2008, p. 600; Table 15–3.

D. Individuals with schizophrenia are at particular risk of suicide during exacerbations of illness and in early stages of schizophrenia.

E. Depressed patients with melancholic features have a rate of suicide that is two times that of nonmelancholic depressed patients.

**The correct response is option E.**

No differences exist in rates of suicide between depressed patients with and without melancholic features.

Cluster B personality disorders, especially borderline and antisocial personality disorders, place patients at increased risk for suicide. The lifetime suicide rate for schizophrenia is 9%–13%. Suicide is the leading cause of death among persons with schizophrenia who are younger than 35 years. Suicide tends to occur in the early stages of schizophrenic illness and during acute exacerbations.

Simon RI: Suicide, in The American Psychiatric Publishing Textbook of Psychiatry, 5th Edition. Edited by Hales RE, Yudofsky SC, Gabbard GO. Washington, DC, American Psychiatric Publishing, 2008, pp 1640–1641

114. Which of the following statements is *true* regarding schizophrenia in women?

A. Men and women have similar incidence rates for schizophrenia.
B. The onset of schizophrenia is approximately 5 years later in women than in men.
C. Approximately 25% of women with schizophrenia develop their illness in the mid to late 40s.
D. Relatives of men with schizophrenia are more likely to themselves develop schizophrenia than are the relatives of women with schizophrenia.
E. Neuroanatomical study shows that women with schizophrenia are more likely to have anatomical abnormalities than are men with schizophrenia.

**The correct response is option B.**

The onset of schizophrenia tends to occur approximately 5 years later in women (ages 20–29 years in women vs. ages 15–24 years in men). Although the incidence of schizophrenia has long been thought to be equal between the sexes, a recent meta-analysis has found that the incidence ratio for men relative to women is between 1.31% and 1.42%. Approximately 15% of women develop new-onset symptoms of schizophrenia in their mid to late 40s. More relatives of women with schizophrenia than those

of schizophrenic men are likely to develop the disorder. Neuroanatomical studies suggest that structural brain abnormalities are more likely to be found in men than in women.

Burt VK, Stein K: Treatment of women, in The American Psychiatric Publishing Textbook of Psychiatry, 5th Edition. Edited by Hales RE, Yudofsky SC, Gabbard GO. Washington, DC, American Psychiatric Publishing, 2008, pp 1513, 1515

115. Which of the following antidepressive agents increases rapid eye movement (REM) sleep?

A. Bupropion.
B. Clomipramine.
C. Phenelzine.
D. Venlafaxine.
E. Sertraline.

**The correct response is option A.**

Antidepressants that increase REM sleep include bupropion and nefazodone. However, bupropion tends to cause insomnia ("activating"), whereas nefazodone causes sedation. Tricyclic antidepressants (clomipramine), monoamine oxidase inhibitors (phenelzine), selective serotonin reuptake inhibitors (sertraline), and the serotonin-norepinephrine reuptake inhibitor venlafaxine are associated with an increase in arousals and awakenings and decreased REM sleep. Although bupropion increases REM sleep, it tends to decrease sleep continuity. Antidepressants that block serotonin-2 (5-HT$_2$) receptors (trazodone and nefazodone) and 5-HT$_3$ receptors (mirtazapine) are associated with improved sleep continuity.

Buysse DJ, Strollo PJ, Black JE, et al: Sleep disorders, in The American Psychiatric Publishing Textbook of Psychiatry, 5th Edition. Edited by Hales RE, Yudofsky SC, Gabbard GO. Washington, DC, American Psychiatric Publishing, 2008, p 937

**Insomnia-inducing antidepressants:** bupropion, selective serotonin reuptake inhibitors, venlafaxine, and monoamine oxidase inhibitors.

**Sedating antidepressants:** tricyclic antidepressants (especially amitriptyline and doxepin), trazodone, nefazodone, and mirtazapine.

116. Which of the following is *true* regarding the etiology of somatoform disorders?

    A. The prevalence of all definitively diagnosed somatoform disorders increases with age.
    B. When somatoform disorders present in the older patient, comorbid neurological illness may be associated with them but neuropsychological (cognitive) impairment is not.
    C. Somatoform disorders are associated with a history of serious illness of a parent, but not in the patient, early in life.
    D. Comorbid panic disorder is common in somatoform disorders, but other anxiety disorders are not.
    E. The personality trait of neuroticism, wherein the subject experiences more negative emotions, is associated with the development of somatoform disorders.

**The correct response is option E.**

Neuroticism is associated with the development of somatoform disorders. With the exception of hypochondriasis, the prevalence of somatoform disorders does not increase with age, so option A is incorrect. Option B is incorrect because when present in late life, somatoform disorders may be associated with neuropsychological impairment and/or comorbid neurological illness. Option C is incorrect because somatoform disorders have been associated with serious illness in the patient early in life, childhood abuse, and significant psychological stress. Comorbid depression, anxiety and panic disorders, substance abuse, and personality disorders are common in somatoform disorders.

Agronin ME: Somatoform disorders, in The American Psychiatric Publishing Textbook of Geriatric Psychiatry, 3rd Edition. Edited by Blazer DG, Steffens DC, Busse EW. Washington, DC, American Psychiatric Publishing, 2004, pp 298–299

117. Laboratory assessment is invaluable in the clinical care of substance abusers. Which of the following occurrences is *not* characteristic of the effects of alcohol?

    A. Increased glycoprotein carbohydrate–deficient transferrin.
    B. Increased glutamyltranspeptidase.
    C. Increased aspartate aminotransferase.
    D. Increased alanine aminotransferase.
    E. Decreased mean corpuscular hemoglobin.

**The correct response is option E.**

The mean corpuscular volume of red blood cells may also be increased with heavy alcohol use, demonstrating hepatic damage as well as hematological problems, such as deficiencies in vitamin $B_{12}$ and folate. Alcohol exerts a direct toxic effect on hepatocytes, leading to increased levels of glycoprotein carbohydrate–deficient transferrin, glutamyltranspeptidase, serum glutamic oxaloacetic transaminase (also known as aspartate aminotransferase, or AST) and serum glutamic pyruvic transaminase (also known as alanine aminotransferase, or ALT).

Greenfield SF, Hennessy G: Assessment of the patient, in The American Psychiatric Publishing Textbook of Substance Abuse Treatment, 4th Edition. Edited by Galanter M, Kleber HD. Washington, DC, American Psychiatric Publishing, 2008, p 67

118. Many chemicals present in blood and tissue are analgesic. Which of the following substances does *not* itself directly excite primary noxious afferents?

    A. Prostaglandins.
    B. Serotonin.
    C. Histamine.
    D. Acetylcholine.
    E. Bradykinin.

**The correct response is option A.**

Prostaglandins do not excite pain fibers; however, they appear to sensitize primary afferents to painful substances. Serotonin, histamine, acetylcholine, bradykinin, slow-reacting substance of anaphylaxis (SRS-A), calcitonin gene–related peptide (CGRP), and potassium all excite primary noxious afferents.

Golianu, B, Bhandari R, Shaw RJ, et al: Neuropsychiatric aspects of pain management, in The American Psychiatric Publishing Textbook of Neuropsychiatry and Behavioral Neurosciences, 5th Edition. Edited by Yudofsky SC, Hales RE. Washington, DC, American Psychiatric Publishing, 2008, p 370

119. A 38-year-old woman with a history of treatment-resistant major depressive disorder (not currently receiving any medication) returns for a routine outpatient visit and is now 3 weeks postpartum and plans to continue breastfeeding for at least 1 year. Her baby was full-term and healthy and is developing well. The woman's depressive symptoms are recurring, and she would like to restart nortriptyline, which was, according to her, the "only" medication among several selective serotonin reuptake inhibitors (SSRIs) and other antidepressants that had been effective for her depression. Five years ago, she developed severe depression after the birth of her first child and required emergent inpatient psychiatric treatment. The most prudent treatment recommendation is to

A. Recommend doxepin, a tricyclic antidepressant (TCA) that is safer for infants than nortriptyline during lactation.
B. Advise against starting nortriptyline while she is still breastfeeding, and recommend a trial of citalopram or escitalopram.
C. Start low-dose nortriptyline, and titrate the dose to her previous dose, as tolerated.
D. Advise against starting any antidepressants until the infant is at least 6 months old.
E. Recommend imipramine, a TCA that is safer for infants than nortriptyline during lactation.

**The correct response is option C.**

All TCAs are present in breast milk, but nortriptyline and most other TCAs are considered safe for lactating infants. Her history increases the risk of a recurrence of severe depressive symptoms, especially during the first postpartum year, so prompt treatment with a previously effective antidepressant is important in this patient who has apparently not responded to alternative antidepressants. Up to 13% of psychiatric admissions for women occur during the first postpartum year, which further emphasizes the need to adequately treat her depression at this time. Option A is incorrect because of all the TCAs, doxepin, when used by nursing mothers, leads to the highest blood levels of the drug in lactating infants. Doxepin has been associated with respiratory depression in nursing infants and is contraindicated in lactating women.

Option B is incorrect because the patient's history of a severe depressive episode during the postpartum year necessitates prompt treatment with a previously effective

antidepressant. The patient's report of poor response to several SSRIs suggests that neither of these SSRIs would be of much benefit to the patient. The safety data regarding SSRIs during lactation are unclear and composed of a confusing array of investigations that have used varying assay sensitivities and inconsistent collection methods that have complicated efforts to meaningfully compare rates of breast milk excretion between compounds. The greatest amount of data for SSRIs have been collected for sertraline, paroxetine, and fluoxetine. These data indicate that quantitative infant SSRI exposure during lactation is considerably lower than transplacental exposure to these medications during gestation, suggesting that SSRIs may be safe for lactating infants.

Option D is incorrect because most TCAs, including nortriptyline, are safe for use during lactation, and no data support completely avoiding TCAs other than doxepin. In addition, the risk of this patient developing a recurrent severe depression exceeds the relatively minor risk of this agent for the infant. Option E is incorrect because the only TCA that is contraindicated currently is doxepin, and there is no clinical reason to favor imipramine over nortriptyline at this time.

Newport DJ, Fisher A, Graybeal S, et al: Psychopharmacology during pregnancy and lactation, in The American Psychiatric Publishing Textbook of Psychopharmacology, 3rd Edition. Edited by Schatzberg AF, Nemeroff CB. Washington, DC, American Psychiatric Publishing, 2004, pp 1112, 1120–1121

120. Studies of ethnic and cultural differences in end-of-life and bereavement issues have revealed distinctions of clinical importance. Regarding Block's 1998 study of Latinos, particularly first- and second-generation, which of the following is *not* true?

A. Patients valued family input into treatment decisions.
B. Patients had extensive social networks.
C. Patients placed family interests above those of the self.
D. Patients resisted accepting death as unavoidable.
E. Patients preferred a caring rather than a scientific approach by a physician.

**The correct response is option D.**

First- and second-generation Latinos tended to accept death as unavoidable, value familial input when making treatment decisions, possess extensive social networks, place family interests before self-interest, and prefer a caring, personal approach to a scientific one in the treatment process.

Block JB: The meaning of death, in Healing Latinos: The Art of Cultural Competence in Medicine. Edited by Hayes-Bautista D, Chiprut R. Los Angeles, CA, Cedars-Sinai Health System, 1998, pp 79–85

Thompson LW, Kaye JL, Tang PCY, et al: Bereavement and adjustment disorders, in The American Psychiatric Publishing Textbook of Geriatric Psychiatry, 3rd Edition. Edited by Blazer DG, Steffens DC, Busse EW. Washington, DC, American Psychiatric Publishing, 2004, p 323

121. A patient with panic disorder develops agitation, insomnia, and nausea while taking fluoxetine. Which of the following agents might be useful in reducing these symptoms?

    A. Mirtazapine.
    B. Buspirone.
    C. Lithium.
    D. Venlafaxine.
    E. Valproate.

## The correct response is option A.

Use of serotonin type-2 (5-HT$_2$) or type-3 (5-HT$_3$) antagonists such as mirtazapine, nefazodone, and ondansetron might be considered to limit some of the symptoms that are mediated through these pathways (e.g., insomnia, agitation, gastrointestinal distress).

Davidson JRT, Connor KM: Treatment of anxiety disorders, in The American Psychiatric Publishing Textbook of Psychopharmacology, 3rd Edition. Edited by Schatzberg AF, Nemeroff CB. Washington, DC, American Psychiatric Publishing, 2004, p 915

122. Which of the following statements is *false* regarding the American Psychiatric Association (APA) (2006) guideline for treatment of manic or mixed episodes?

    A. Antidepressants should be tapered and discontinued during acute treatment of a manic or mixed episode.
    B. The first-line pharmacological treatment for severe manic or mixed episodes is either lithium plus an antipsychotic, or valproate plus an antipsychotic.
    C. It is not recommended that benzodiazepines be used in severely ill or agitated patients who are in the midst of a mixed or manic episode.
    D. The first-line pharmacological treatment for serious but less severe manic or mixed episodes is monotherapy with lithium, valproic acid, or an antipsychotic such as olanzapine.
    E. If first-line medication treatment at optimal doses fails to control symptoms, it is recommended that another first-line agent be added.

## The correct response is option C.

The APA recommends with relatively substantial clinical confidence the use of benzodiazepines in severely ill or agitated patients who are in the midst of a mixed or manic episode.

American Psychiatric Association: Practice Guidelines for the Treatment of Psychiatric Disorders: Compendium 2006, Arlington, VA, American Psychiatric Association, 2006, pp 859–861

123. The Swedo (Swedo et al. 1998) criteria for pediatric autoimmune neuropsychiatric disorders associated with streptococcal infection (PANDAS) include all of the following *except*

    A. Presence of obsessive-compulsive disorder (OCD) and/or tic disorder.
    B. Onset before age 7 years.
    C. Episodic course of symptom severity.
    D. Association with group A beta-hemolytic streptococcal (GABHS) infection.
    E. Association with neurological abnormalities.

## The correct response is option B.

Onset of PANDAS occurs before puberty, not necessarily before age 7 years. PANDAS presents a fascinating model of infectious disease–associated neuropsychiatric illness. Swedo et al. (1998), who provided the first characterization of PANDAS, proposed that patients with the syndrome could be identified by the following five criteria: 1) presence of OCD and/or a tic disorder, 2) age at onset before puberty, 3) episodic course of symptom severity, 4) association with GABHS infection, and 5) association with neurological abnormalities.

Swedo SE, Leonard HL, Garvey M, et al: Pediatric autoimmune neuropsychiatric disorders associated with streptococcal infections: clinical description of the first 50 cases. Am J Psychiatry 155:264–271, 1998

Teicher MH, Andersen SL, Navalta CP, et al: Neuropsychiatric disorders of childhood and adolescence, in The American Psychiatric Publishing Textbook of Neuropsychiatry and Behavioral Neurosciences, 5th Edition. Edited by Yudofsky SC, Hales RE. Washington, DC, American Psychiatric Publishing, 2008, p 1083

124. Which of the following statements concerning sociodemographic correlates of mood disorders is *true?*

    A. The mean age at onset of major depressive disorder (MDD) is in the late 30s.
    B. The rates of bipolar disorder among men and women appear to be similar.
    C. Prior to adolescence, depression is twice as common in girls as in boys.
    D. People with bipolar disorder tend to develop symptoms in a unimodal distribution from ages 18–44 years.
    E. In clinical samples, bipolar disorder and MDD appear to be associated with a higher socioeconomic status.

**The correct response is option B.**

Depression is twice as common in women as in men. Option C is incorrect because prior to adolescence rates of MDD among girls and boys are similar. Reasons for the gender difference after, but not before, puberty may include hormonal differences, social factors, or an unequal exposure to abuse and stressful life events. Option A is incorrect because the average age at onset of MDD is earlier, in the late 20s. Option D is incorrect because bipolar disorder symptoms tend to develop in a bimodal distribution from ages 18–44 years. Option E is incorrect because although low socioeconomic status is associated with an increased rate of depression, bipolar disorder is associated with a higher socioeconomic status.

Joska JA, Stein DJ: Mood disorders, in The American Psychiatric Publishing Textbook of Psychiatry, 5th Edition. Edited by Hales RE, Yudofsky SC, Gabbard GO. Washington, DC, American Psychiatric Publishing, 2008, pp 457–503

125. All of the following attenuate (decrease) essential tremor *except*

    A. Propranolol.
    B. Primidone.
    C. Alcohol.
    D. Deep brain stimulation of the ventral intermediate nucleus of the contralateral thalamus.
    E. Trihexyphenidyl.

**The correct response is option E.**

The mainstays of medical treatment for essential tremor are propranolol therapy and primidone therapy. Often the tremor attenuates with alcohol use. Deep brain stimulation targeting the ventral intermediate nucleus of the contralateral thalamus is sometimes helpful in medically refractory cases. Option E is incorrect because trihexyphenidyl, an anticholinergic agent, may be useful in treating dystonia but is not known to attenuate essential tremor.

Scott B: Movement disorders, in The American Psychiatric Publishing Textbook of Geriatric Psychiatry, 3rd Edition. Edited by Blazer DG, Steffens DC, Busse EW. Washington, DC, American Psychiatric Publishing, 2004, p 236

126. Schizophrenia, whether broadly or narrowly defined, is familial. Which of the following is a subclinical phenotype that is elevated in the relatives of patients with schizophrenia?

    A. Positive symptoms measured by the Thought Disorder Index.
    B. Negative symptoms measured by the Scale for the Assessment of Negative Symptoms.
    C. Neuropsychological signs such as deficits in abstraction and in short-term verbal memory.
    D. Eye movement dysfunction on smooth pursuit and visual fixation tasks.
    E. Neurological soft signs.

**The correct response is option D.**

Subclinical phenotypes that are elevated in the relatives of probands with schizophrenia include 1) disturbances in thinking, social relatedness, volition, and affective expressivity as measured by a psychometric index derived from the Minnesota Multiphasic Personality Inventory (Moldin et al. 1990); 2) eye movement dysfunction on smooth pursuit (Trillenberg et al. 2004) and visual fixation tasks (Amador et al. 1995); 3) impairments in suppression of the 50 msec preattentional component (P50) of the auditory evoked potential in a conditioning testing paradigm (Clementz et al. 1998); and 4) attentional disturbances as measured by the Continuous Performance Test (Keefe et al. 1997), Forced-Choice Span of Apprehension Task, and Digit Symbol Substitution Test (Laurent et al. 2000).

Elevated quantitative phenotypes that are clinically apparent in the relatives of schizophrenia probands include 1) positive symptoms (as measured by the Thought Disorder Index; Shenton et al. 1989), 2) negative symptoms (as measured by the Scale for the Assessment of Negative Symptoms; Tsuang et al. 1991), 3) neuropsychological signs such as deficits in abstraction (as measured by the Wisconsin Card Sorting Test) and in short-term verbal memory (Franke et al. 1992), and 4) neurological soft signs (Kinney et al. 1991) (for references, see Choudary and Knowles 2008).

Choudary PV, Knowles JA: Genetics, in The American Psychiatric Publishing Textbook of Psychiatry, 5th Edition. Edited by Hales RE, Yudofsky SC, Gabbard GO. Washington, DC, American Psychiatric Publishing, 2008, p 208

127. The Minnesota Multiphasic Personality Inventory (MMPI) and its successor, the MMPI-2, employ nine clinical scales. Which of the following is *not* one of the scales?

    A. Hypochondriasis.
    B. Hysteria.
    C. Paranoia.
    D. Schizophrenia.
    E. Anxiety.

**The correct response is option E.**

Anxiety is not one of the nine MMPI clinical scales. The MMPI used the method of contrasting criterion groups to construct the following nine clinical scales: Hypochondriasis (Scale 1), Depression (Scale 2), Hysteria (Scale 3), Psychopathic Deviance (Scale 4), Masculinity–Femininity (Scale 5), Paranoia (Scale 6), Psychasthenia (Scale 7), Schizophrenia (Scale 8), and Mania (Scale 9).

Clarkin JF, Howieson DB, McClough J: The role of psychiatric measures in assessment and treatment, in The American Psychiatric Publishing Textbook of Psychiatry, 5th Edition. Edited by Hales RE, Yudofsky SC, Gabbard GO. Washington, DC, American Psychiatric Publishing, 2008, p 80

128. Standards for determination of competency in decision making include all of the following *except*

    A. Communication of clinical choice.
    B. Understanding of relevant information provided.
    C. Appreciation of available options and consequences.
    D. Rational decision making.
    E. Performance in the "unimpaired" range on formal cognitive testing.

**The correct response is option E.**

Performance in the unimpaired range on formal cognitive testing is not used for determination of competency in decision making. A review of case law and scholarly literature reveals four standards for determining incompetency in decision making. In order of increasing levels of mental capacity required, these standards are 1) communication of choice, 2) understanding of relevant information provided, 3) appreciation of available options and consequences, and 4) rational decision making.

Simon RI, Shuman DW: Psychiatry and the law, in The American Psychiatric Publishing Textbook of Psychiatry, 5th Edition. Edited by Hales RE, Yudofsky SC, Gabbard GO. Washington, DC, American Psychiatric Publishing, 2008, p 1558

129. Antidepressants may sometimes interfere with sexual functioning. Of the following, which antidepressant medication is *least* likely to produce sexual dysfunction?

    A. Tricyclic antidepressants (TCAs).
    B. Mirtazapine.
    C. Monoamine oxidase inhibitors.
    D. Selective serotonin reuptake inhibitors (SSRIs).
    E. Venlafaxine.

**The correct response is option B.**

Mirtazapine rarely interferes with sexual functioning. Commonly used antidepressants that may interfere with sexual functioning include TCAs, SSRIs (especially paroxetine and fluoxetine), trazodone, and mirtazapine (albeit rare). Antidepressants that are least likely to cause sexual side effects include bupropion and nefazodone.

Becker JV, Stinson JD: Human sexuality and sexual dysfunctions, in The American Psychiatric Publishing Textbook of Psychiatry, 5th Edition. Edited by Hales RE, Yudofsky SC, Gabbard GO. Washington, DC, American Psychiatric Publishing, 2008, p 715; Table 16–2

130. The amygdala plays an important role in all of the following *except*

    A. Recognition of emotion.
    B. Classical conditioning of autonomic responses.
    C. Processing of stimuli that communicate emotional significance in social situations.
    D. Decision-making process.
    E. Declarative memory.

**The correct response is option E.**

The amygdala does not appear to play a crucial role in declarative memory. Thus, patients with bilateral amygdala damage can acquire declarative knowledge normally but have impairment in their conditioned autonomic responses. Options A, B, C, and D are incorrect because these statements are true regarding the amygdala.

The amygdala is important for the recognition of emotion, especially fear. It is also important for classical conditioning of autonomic responses, for processing stimuli that communicate emotional significance in social situations, and in decision making.

Harel BT, Tranel D: Functional neuroanatomy, in The American Psychiatric Publishing Textbook of Neuropsychiatry and Behavioral Neurosciences, 5th Edition. Edited by Yudofsky SC, Hales RE. Washington, DC, American Psychiatric Publishing, 2008, p 53

131. Since DSM-III (American Psychiatric Association 1980), personality disorders have been grouped into three clusters: A, B, and C. Which of the following disorders fall within cluster C?

    A. Borderline, histrionic, narcissistic, antisocial.
    B. Histrionic, obsessive-compulsive, narcissistic.
    C. Paranoid, borderline, antisocial.
    D. Avoidant, dependent, obsessive-compulsive.
    E. Schizotypal, schizoid, paranoid.

**The correct response is option D.**

Since DSM-III, the personality disorders have been grouped into three clusters: the odd or eccentric cluster A (schizotypal, schizoid, and paranoid); the dramatic, emotional, or erratic cluster B (borderline, histrionic, narcissistic, and antisocial); and the anxious or fearful cluster C (avoidant, dependent, and obsessive-compulsive).

American Psychiatric Association: Diagnostic and Statistical Manual of Mental Disorders, 3rd Edition. Washington, DC, American Psychiatric Association, 1980

Skodol AE, Gunderson JG: Personality disorders, in The American Psychiatric Publishing Textbook of Psychiatry, 5th Edition. Edited by Hales RE, Yudofsky SC, Gabbard GO. Washington, DC, American Psychiatric Publishing, 2008, pp 823, 825; Table 20–1

132. Which of the following statements is *false* regarding postpartum psychosis?

    A. Postpartum psychosis occurs in 1–2 of every 1,000 live births.
    B. Postpartum psychosis is considered to be a manifestation of bipolar disorder, not schizophrenia.
    C. A history of both bipolar disorder and prior episodes of postpartum psychosis increases the risk of subsequent postpartum psychosis to 80%.
    D. Because of risks to the patient and the newborn, postpartum psychosis patients should be hospitalized.
    E. Systemic etiologies such as Sheehan's syndrome and postpartum thyroiditis may mimic postpartum psychosis.

**The correct response is option C.**

Having both bipolar disorder and a prior postpartum psychotic episode increases the risk of subsequent postpartum psychosis to 50%. The most serious postpartum illness, postpartum psychosis, occurs in 1–2 of every 1,000 births. Postpartum psychosis is thought to be a manifestation of bipolar disorder. Women who have had an episode of postpartum psychosis are at risk for subsequent bipolar disorder, suggesting that postpartum psychosis may be a subcategory of bipolar disorder. Because postpartum psychosis carries with it the risk of suicide, infant neglect, and infanticide, patients should be hospitalized. The initial evaluation includes a medical assessment to rule out organic etiologies such as postpartum thyroiditis, Sheehan's syndrome, pregnancy-related autoimmune disorders, HIV-related infection, and intoxication/withdrawal states.

Burt VK, Stein K: Treatment of women, in The American Psychiatric Publishing Textbook of Psychiatry, 5th Edition. Edited by Hales RE, Yudofsky SC, Gabbard GO. Washington, DC, American Psychiatric Publishing, 2008, p 1508

133. Which of the following approaches is recommended in the treatment of somatoform disorders?

    A. The physician should arrange appointments on an as-needed basis.
    B. A focus on obtaining insight into the psychological context of somatoform symptoms should be the first priority for intervention.
    C. The physician should not offer to review all prior medical records because this merely reinforces maladaptive somatization behavior.
    D. Hypochondriasis has been shown to respond to antidepressants and anxiolytics.
    E. Hypnosis should be avoided in conversion disorder as these patients are rarely subject to induction of hypnosis.

**The correct response is option D.**

Treatment of somatoform disorders calls for an integrative biopsychosocial approach. Hypochondriacal symptoms have responded to selective serotonin reuptake inhibitors and anxiolytics. The physician should arrange periodic but regularly scheduled appointments and should focus on symptom reduction and rehabilitation. Offering to review all available medical records can be a tangible way for the physician to convey the seriousness given to the patient's symptoms. In conversion disorders, hypnosis is sometimes used as both a diagnostic and a therapeutic tool.

Agronin ME: Somatoform disorders, in The American Psychiatric Publishing Textbook of Geriatric Psychiatry, 3rd Edition. Edited by Blazer DG, Steffens DC, Busse EW. Washington, DC, American Psychiatric Publishing, 2004, pp 299–300

134. Which one of the following substances is associated with clearly defined withdrawal symptoms?

    A. Cannabis.
    B. Hallucinogens.
    C. Phencyclidine (PCP).
    D. Amphetamines.
    E. Inhalants.

**The correct response is option D.**

Patients withdrawing from either amphetamines or cocaine may present with dysphoria, psychomotor agitation or retardation, and signs of fatigue; they may complain of increased appetite, vivid and unpleasant dreams, insomnia, or hypersomnia. Cannabis, hallucinogens, PCP, and inhalants do not have defined withdrawal syndromes.

Greenfield SF, Hennessy G: Assessment of the patient, in The American Psychiatric Publishing Textbook of Substance Abuse Treatment, 4th Edition. Edited by Galanter M, Kleber HD. Washington, DC, American Psychiatric Publishing, 2008, pp 66–67

135. If valproic acid must be used during pregnancy, what are the recommendations regarding its dosing and folic acid supplementation?

    A. No more than 1,000 mg/day of valproic acid, and take 1–2 mg/day of a folic acid supplement.
    B. No more than 1,000 mg/day of valproic acid, and take 4–5 mg/day of folic acid during the first trimester and at least 1–2 mg/day for the rest of gestation.
    C. No more than 1,000 mg/day of valproic acid, and take 4–5 mg/day of folic acid throughout gestation.
    D. For doses of valproic acid greater than 1,000 mg/day, take 40–50 mg/day of folic acid during the first trimester, then 4–5 mg/day thereafter.
    E. No more than 1,000 mg/day of valproic acid, and take a daily multivitamin with 1–2 mg of folic acid throughout gestation.

**The correct response is option C.**

If valproic acid must be used during pregnancy, its risk may be reduced by limiting the dose to 1,000 mg/day or maintaining a serum concentration of 70 μg/mL. Folic acid supplementation with 4–5 mg/day of folic acid throughout pregnancy is also recommended, although no evidence shows that this reduces the risk of valproic acid–associated anomalies. Because nearly half of the pregnancies in the United States are unplanned, and women with unplanned pregnancies typically recognize that they are pregnant during the sixth week of gestation or even later (2 full weeks after neural tube closure), all women of childbearing potential who are taking valproic acid should receive concomitant folic acid supplementation, regardless of whether they plan to conceive. The preliminary evidence that aspects of fetal valproic acid syndrome other than neural tube defects may be associated with valproic acid's antagonism of folic acid metabolism suggests that folic acid supplementation should be administered not only in the first trimester but also throughout gestation.

Option A is incorrect because the recommendation is for 4–5 mg/day, not 1–2 mg/day. Option B is incorrect because the valproic acid syndrome may affect fetal development in all trimesters, not only during the first trimester, which is the high-risk period for neural tube defects in general. Because the time beyond the first trimester is not necessarily protective for women on valproic acid, the recommendation is to take 4–5 mg/day of folic acid throughout pregnancy. Option D is incorrect because the current recommendation for valproic acid is to not exceed doses of 1,000 mg/day during pregnancy; megadoses (10 times the recommended dose) of folic acid may not necessarily be protective. Option E is incorrect because even though a multivitamin is recommended for pregnant women in general, 1–2 mg of folic acid is an inadequate dose.

Newport DJ, Fisher A, Graybeal S, et al: Psychopharmacology during pregnancy and lactation, in The American Psychiatric Publishing Textbook of Psychopharmacology, 3rd Edition. Edited by Schatzberg AF, Nemeroff CB. Washington, DC, American Psychiatric Publishing, 2004, p 1125

136. Which of the following statements is *true* regarding culture and bereavement?

    A. The manifestations, duration, and intensity of grief are universal.
    B. The literature describing cross-cultural and ethnic expressions after death indicates that bereavement is most likely communicated and regulated through the same pathway across cultures.
    C. The concept of performing grief tasks is equally applicable to all cultures.
    D. In contrast to other cultures that focus on rituals, expressions, and meanings that are shared interpersonally and socially, Euro-American culture generally has conceptualized grief as loss oriented, with a focus on individual manifestations of grief.
    E. Culturally mainstream Americans tend to view death as an active, ongoing interaction with a deceased individual.

**The correct response is option D.**

Option A is incorrect because the manifestations, duration, and intensity of grief are likely to be culturally specific, not universal. Option B is incorrect because the literature describing cross-cultural and ethnic expressions

after death indicates that bereavement can be communicated and regulated through the various pathways across cultures. Option C is incorrect because the performance of grief tasks may not be applicable to all cultures. Option E is incorrect because the culturally mainstream American view of death is of death being the end of the relationship with the person. In contrast, traditional Asian cultures may consider death as merely a change in an ongoing relationship with an individual.

Thompson LW, Kaye JL, Tang PCY, et al: Bereavement and adjustment disorders, in The American Psychiatric Publishing Textbook of Geriatric Psychiatry, 3rd Edition. Edited by Blazer DG, Steffens DC, Busse EW. Washington, DC, American Psychiatric Publishing, 2004, p 323

137. Lamotrigine is being evaluated for efficacy in treating depressive, manic, and mixed episodes in bipolar patients as well as for rapid cycling. Which of the following statements is *true* about lamotrigine?

    A. It is efficacious for bipolar depression.
    B. It is efficacious for bipolar depression with psychosis.
    C. It lacks efficacy for bipolar mania.
    D. It lacks efficacy for rapid cycling.
    E. It lacks efficacy as an adjunct to other treatments.

**The answer is option A.**

Lamotrigine was found in controlled trials to be useful in bipolar depression.

Shelton MD, Calabrese JR: Lamotrigine, in The American Psychiatric Publishing Textbook of Psychopharmacology, 3rd Edition. Edited by Schatzberg AF, Nemeroff CB. Washington, DC, American Psychiatric Publishing, 2004, p 618

138. A childhood seizure that features alterations in consciousness; auras of unpleasant odors, tastes, and sensations; and simple, repetitive, and purposeless automatisms is classified as what type of seizure?

    A. Simple partial seizure.
    B. Partial sensory seizure.
    C. Rolandic epilepsy.
    D. Complex partial seizure.
    E. Frontal lobe epilepsy.

**The correct response is option D.**

*Complex partial seizures*, also known as *psychomotor* or *temporal lobe seizures*, are the most frequent form of focal epilepsy in children and are distinguished from other partial seizures by alterations in consciousness. *Frontal lobe epilepsy* is the second most frequent localized form of epilepsy. Initial manifestations of frontal lobe seizures depend on the location of the epileptogenic zone. *Simple partial seizures* may be motor or sensory. A simple partial motor seizure consists of recurrent clonic movements of one part of the body without loss of consciousness. *Partial sensory seizures* consist of paresthesias or pain referred to a single part of the body. They also can spread. In general, partial seizures last 1–2 minutes and are not associated with loss of consciousness. *Rolandic epilepsy* is a benign, inherited focal epileptic disorder of childhood that is the most common form of focal seizure seen in children younger than 15 years.

Teicher MYH, Andersen SL, Navalta CP, et al: Neuropsychiatric disorders of childhood and adolescence, in The American Psychiatric Publishing Textbook of Neuropsychiatry and Behavioral Neurosciences, 5th Edition. Edited by Yudofsky SC, Hales RE. Washington, DC, American Psychiatric Publishing, 2008, pp 1077–1078

139. Which of the following is *true* regarding mood disorders in nursing home residents?

    A. Dementia is the most common psychiatric illness in nursing home residents (50%–75%), followed by depressive disorder (15%–50%).
    B. The rate of mood disorders in nursing home residents in the United States is substantially higher than in other industrialized nations.
    C. Depression in nursing home residents increases morbidity, but not mortality, rates.
    D. Because of concurrent chronic medical illnesses, the DSM-IV-TR diagnostic criteria for mood disorders are not clinically valid in predicting treatment response in nursing home residents.
    E. A subtype of depression in nursing home residents that includes low serum albumin and high levels of psychosocial disability usually responds promptly to treatment with nortriptyline.

**The correct response is option A.**

Dementia is the most common psychiatric illness in nursing home residents (50%–75%), followed by depressive disorder (estimates of 15%–50%). Option B is incorrect because rates of mood disorders among nursing home residents are similar in the United States and other industrialized nations. Option C is incorrect because depres-

sion in nursing homes increases both morbidity and mortality rates. Option D is incorrect because DSM criteria have been shown to remain valid as predictors of treatment response in this population. Option E is incorrect because this subtype is typically not responsive to treatment with nortriptyline.

Benjamin L, Bourgeois JA, Shahrokh NC, et al: Study Guide to Geriatric Psychiatry: A Companion to The American Psychiatric Publishing Textbook of Geriatric Psychiatry, 3rd Edition, Washington, DC, 2006, p 160

Streim JE, Katz IR: Clinical psychiatry in the nursing home, in The American Psychiatric Publishing Textbook of Geriatric Psychiatry, 3rd Edition. Edited by Blazer DG, Steffens DC, Busse EW. Washington, DC, American Psychiatric Publishing, 2004, pp 475–476

140. Which of the following measures uses a clinical interview for data collection?

    A. Symptom Checklist–90—Revised.
    B. Brief Symptom Inventory.
    C. Brief Psychiatric Rating Scale.
    D. Personality Assessment Inventory.
    E. Millon Clinical Multiaxial Inventory–III.

**The correct response is option C.**

The Brief Psychiatric Rating Scale is administered by a physician. The other tests listed above are self-report instruments.

Clarkin JF, Howieson DB, McClough J: The role of psychiatric measures in assessment and treatment, in The American Psychiatric Publishing Textbook of Psychiatry, 5th Edition. Edited by Hales RE, Yudofsky SC, Gabbard GO. Washington, DC, American Psychiatric Publishing, 2008, pp 79–80; Table 3–5

141. There are a number of different types of paraphilias. Klismaphilia involves which of the following?

    A. Enemas.
    B. Urine.
    C. Animals.
    D. Corpses.
    E. Nonliving objects.

**The correct response is option A.**

*Klismaphilia* is defined as sexually deviant behavior involving enemas. Sexually deviant behavior involving urine is termed *urophilia*, that involving animals is termed *zoophilia*, and that involving corpses is termed *necrophilia*. Arousal to nonliving objects is termed *fetishism*.

Becker JV, Johnson BR: Gender identity disorders and paraphilias, in The American Psychiatric Publishing Textbook of Psychiatry, 5th Edition. Edited by Hales RE, Yudofsky SC, Gabbard GO. Washington, DC, American Psychiatric Publishing, 2008, p 737; Table 17–2

142. Which of the following is *not* considered a perceptual disturbance?

    A. Derealization.
    B. Illusion.
    C. Depersonalization.
    D. Delusion.
    E. Hallucination.

**The answer is option D.**

Perceptual disturbances encompass hallucinations, illusions, depersonalization, and derealization.

143. Which of the following statements is *true* regarding the neuropsychological correlates of frontal lobe dysfunction?

    A. Akinetic mutism may follow lesions to the superior mesial aspect of the frontal lobe.
    B. The patient with akinetic mutism makes no effort to communicate by any modality and will not track moving targets with smooth pursuit eye movements.
    C. Akinetic mutism is typically more severe with right- as opposed to left-sided lesions.
    D. Acquired sociopathy is associated with memory disturbances.
    E. The dorsolateral frontal cortices have not been linked to verbal regulation of behavior.

**The answer is option A.**

The frontal lobes are responsible for a wide array of behaviors, ranging from simple interpersonal communication to memory to interpersonal conduct. The superior mesial aspect of the frontal lobes is crucial in the initiation of movement and emotional expression. Lesions in this region cause akinetic mutism, a syndrome in which the patient does not communicate, either verbally or by gesture, and maintains a noncommunicative facial expression. Movements are limited to tracking of moving targets. There does not appear to be a significant difference in the profile of akinetic mutism as a function of the side of the lesion. Patients with ventromedial frontal lobe damage develop a severe disruption of social conduct, a condition termed *acquired sociopathy*. This condition does not provoke memory disturbances, and the patients are free of conventional neuropsychological defects. The dorsolateral frontal cortices have been linked to the verbal regulation of behavior and verbal fluency.

Luria AR: Higher Cortical Functions in Man, 2nd Edition. New York, Basic Books, 1980

Taber KH, Hurley RA: Neuroanatomy for the psychiatrist, in The American Psychiatric Publishing Textbook of Psychiatry, 5th Edition. Edited by Hales RE, Yudofsky SC, Gabbard GO. Washington, DC, American Psychiatric Publishing, 2008, pp 181–187; Table 5–1

144. Patients with this personality disorder are mostly women who spend an excessive amount of time seeking attention and making themselves attractive. They also display an effusive but labile and shallow range of feelings, often being overly impressionistic and given to hyperbolic descriptions of others. Which personality disorder is being described?

    A. Narcissistic personality disorder.
    B. Borderline personality disorder.
    C. Dependent personality disorder.
    D. Histrionic personality disorder.
    E. Avoidant personality disorder.

**The correct response is option D.**

In addition to the traits listed above, histrionic individuals are often willing to have others make decisions and organize their activities for them. In contrast to persons with dependent personality disorder, histrionic persons are uninhibited and lively companions who willfully forgo appearing autonomous because they believe that by doing so, they can attract others. Unlike persons with borderline personality disorder, they do not perceive themselves as bad, and they lack ongoing problems with rage or willful self-destructiveness. Persons with narcissistic personality disorder also seek attention to sustain their self-esteem but differ in that their self-esteem is characterized by grandiosity and the attention they crave must be admiring.

Skodol AE, Gunderson JG: Personality disorders, in The American Psychiatric Publishing Textbook of Psychiatry, 5th Edition. Edited by Hales RE, Yudofsky SC, Gabbard GO. Washington, DC, American Psychiatric Publishing, 2008, pp 843–844

145. Which of the following mood stabilizers is considered to be a first-line augmenting agent for schizophrenic patients with persistent aggressiveness?

    A. Phenytoin.
    B. Carbamazepine.
    C. Oxcarbazepine.
    D. Lithium.
    E. Valproate.

**The correct response is option E.**

Phenytoin, oxcarbazepine, carbamazepine, and lithium have shown some efficacy in decreasing impulsive aggression behaviors among nonschizophrenic individuals. But valproic acid is the only mood stabilizer considered to be a first-line augmenting agent for patients with schizophrenia who are persistently aggressive.

Scott CL, Quanbeck CD, Resnick PJ: Assessment of dangerousness, in The American Psychiatric Publishing Textbook of Psychiatry, 5th Edition. Edited by Hales RE, Yudofsky SC, Gabbard GO. Washington, DC, American Psychiatric Publishing, 2008, pp 1664–1665

146. *Ataque de nervios*, which is prevalent in Latin America, is an example of which type of dissociative disorder?

    A. Dissociative amnesia.
    B. Dissociative fugue.
    C. Dissociative identity disorder.
    D. Dissociative trance disorder.
    E. Acute stress disorder.

**The correct response is option D.**

*Ataque de nervios* is a dissociative trance phenomenon that frequently involves sudden, extreme changes in sensory and motor control. Typically, the individual suddenly starts to shake convulsively, hyperventilate, scream, and show agitation and aggressive movements. These behaviors may be followed by collapse and loss of consciousness. Afterward, such individuals report being exhausted and may have some amnesia for the event.

Maldonado JR, Spiegel D: Dissociative disorders, in The American Psychiatric Publishing Textbook of Psychiatry, 5th Edition. Edited by Hales RE, Yudofsky SC, Gabbard GO. Washington, DC, American Psychiatric Publishing, 2008, p 696

147. Twin, family, and adoption studies have demonstrated that familial and genetic factors are important for the development of alcohol dependence. The largest twin studies have yielded heritability estimates in which range?

    A. 10%–20%.
    B. 20%–30%.
    C. 30%–40%.
    D. 40%–50%.
    E. 50%–60%.

**The correct response is option E.**

Gelernter J, Kranzler HR: Genetics of addiction, in The American Psychiatric Publishing Textbook of Substance Abuse Treatment, 4th Edition. Edited by Galanter M, Kleber HD. Washington, DC, American Psychiatric Publishing, 2008, p 18

148. Which of the following statistics is *true* regarding substance abuse and dependence?

    A. The most commonly abused benzodiazepine is lorazepam.
    B. Among the 1%–2% of individuals using benzodiazepines without medical supervision, about 15% meet DSM-IV-TR criteria for sedative abuse or dependence.
    C. Of individuals admitted for addiction treatment, benzodiazepines are the drug of choice in about 5%–10% of these patients.
    D. About a quarter of benzodiazepine abusers in substance abuse treatment programs have a comorbid psychiatric disorder.
    E. Benzodiazepine abuse is uncommon in opioid-dependent patients undergoing methadone maintenance treatment.

**The correct response is option B.**

Despite the widespread perception that a high proportion of patients taking benzodiazepines are doing so without medical supervision, only 1%–2% of patients have taken these medications without supervision. As stated in the answer, 15% of these patients meet criteria for sedative abuse or dependence. Option A is incorrect because the most commonly abused benzodiazepine is alprazolam, not lorazepam. Option C is incorrect because benzodiazepines rarely are a primary substance of abuse in individuals admitted for addiction treatment, comprising less than 1% of all admissions. The most commonly misused benzodiazepine is alprazolam, which is also the most often prescribed sedative-hypnotic medication. Option D is incorrect because nearly half of individuals in substance abuse treatment programs who abuse benzodiazepines have another psychiatric disorder—a rate that is twice that seen with patients admitted for other drugs of abuse. This suggests that benzodiazepine use, abuse, or dependence is a useful clinical sign indicating that other co-occurring psychiatric disorders (mood, anxiety, personality, etc.) may be present. Option E is incorrect because benzodiazepine abuse is particularly common among persons receiving methadone maintenance, 40%–50% of whom abuse benzodiazepines at any one time.

> Bisaga A: Benzodiazepines and other sedatives and hypnotics, in The American Psychiatric Publishing Textbook of Substance Abuse Treatment, 4th Edition. Edited by Galanter M, Kleber HD. Washington, DC, American Psychiatric Publishing, 2008, p 222

149. Lithium has been reported to have a robust effect on which particular type of mania?

    A. Mania associated with human immunodeficiency virus.
    B. Mania associated with traumatic brain injury.
    C. Mania associated with steroid use.
    D. Mania associated with Parkinson's disease.
    E. Mania associated with multiple sclerosis.

## The correct response is option C.

Lithium appears to have a robust effect on steroid-induced mania and agitation. However, because of its proconvulsant effects and its ability to cause or aggravate extrapyramidal side effects, it is not considered a first-line choice for most neuropsychiatric patients.

> Holtzheimer PE III, Snowden M, Roy-Byrne PP: Psychopharmacological treatments for patients with neuropsychiatric disorders, in The American Psychiatric Publishing Textbook of Neuropsychiatry and Behavioral Neurosciences, 5th Edition. Edited by Yudofsky SC, Hales RE. Washington, DC, American Psychiatric Publishing, 2008, p 1167

150. Psychiatric comorbidity in attention-deficit/hyperactivity disorder (ADHD) often complicates this already difficult-to-manage disorder. Which of the following statements is *true*?

    A. Conduct disorder occurs in 20%–40% of ADHD cases.

    B. Abused children with both posttraumatic stress disorder (PTSD) and ADHD have the same degree of motor hyperactivity as do children with classic ADHD alone.
    C. Thyroid hormone resistance is a common cause of ADHD.
    D. A high incidence of ADHD is found with girls, but not boys, with Tourette's syndrome.
    E. ADHD-type symptoms may indicate genetic risk in schizophrenia pedigrees.

## The correct response is option E.

ADHD-type symptoms may indicate genetic risk in children with a family history of schizophrenia. Conduct disorder is found in 40%–70% of subjects with ADHD. Abused children with PTSD and ADHD are more active than normal children but substantially less active than children with classic ADHD. Thyroid hormone resistance is very rare and almost never found in children with ADHD. A high incidence of ADHD is also found in boys with Tourette's syndrome.

> Teicher MYH, Andersen SL, Navalta CP, et al: Neuropsychiatric disorders of childhood and adolescence, in The American Psychiatric Publishing Textbook of Neuropsychiatry and Behavioral Neurosciences, 5th Edition. Edited by Yudofsky SC, Hales RE. Washington, DC, American Psychiatric Publishing, 2008, p 1050

151. All of the following characterize the sleep electroencephalography (EEG) of depressed patients *except*

    A. Decreased rapid eye movement (REM) latency.
    B. Prolonged sleep latency.
    C. Decreased slow-wave sleep.
    D. Increased REM latency.
    E. Decreased time in non-REM sleep.

## The correct response is option D.

Reduced REM latency is the best-studied and most reproducible sleep-related EEG finding in depressed patients, and this abnormality is reversed by most antidepressants. *REM latency* refers to the time it takes to enter REM sleep. Normal sleep architecture consists of two major stages: non-REM and REM.

The sleep EEG of depressed patients coincides with depressed patients' complaints of taking "forever" to fall asleep, frequent awakenings, early morning awakenings, and nonrestorative sleep. Three common EEG patterns among depressed patients are 1) REM sleep abnormalities such as reduced REM latency and increased REM sleep percentage (which, by default, decreases time in non-REM sleep); 2) sleep continuity disturbances characterized by prolonged sleep latency (time to fall asleep), increased wake time during sleep, and decreased total sleep time; and 3) decreased proportion and length of slow-wave (or deep) sleep (Peterson and Benca 2006).

Hales RE, Bourgeois JA, Shahrokh NC: Study Guide to Neuropsychiatry and Behavioral Neurosciences: A Companion to The American Psychiatric Publishing Textbook of Neuropsychiatry and Behavioral Neurosciences, 5th Edition. Washington, DC, American Psychiatric Publishing, 2008, p 174

Holtzheimer PE III, Mayberg HS: Neuropsychiatric aspects of mood disorders, in The American Psychiatric Publishing Textbook of Neuropsychiatry and Behavioral Neurosciences, 5th Edition. Edited by Yudofsky SC, Hales RE. Washington, DC, American Psychiatric Publishing, 2008, p 1014

Peterson MJ, Benca RM: Sleep in mood disorders. Psychiatr Clin North Am 29:1009–1032, 2006

### Non-REM Sleep
75%–80% of total sleep time.
Relatively inactive EEG pattern. No muscle atonia or paralysis.
Includes four stages (S1–S4), with each stage leading to a progressively deeper sleep. S3 and S4 are considered to be slow-wave sleep, or deep sleep, which increases over the night. Slow-wave sleep is necessary for physiologic restoration.

### REM Sleep
20%–25% of total sleep time.
Activated EEG pattern, muscle atonia, and episodic bursts of rapid eye movements.
REM sleep is associated with dreaming and is essential for maintaining emotional and cognitive well-being.

152. DeCuypere et al. (2005) conducted a follow-up study of 55 transsexual patients (both male-to-female and female-to-male) after sex reassignment surgery. Among their findings was that

   A. Only 20% of patients reported improvement in their sexuality.
   B. Male-to-female patients experienced more general health problems.

   C. Most patients reported that their expectations concerning the surgery had not been met on a social and emotional level.
   D. Major problems were observed in the patients.
   E. Few patients experienced a positive change in orgasmic sensations.

### The correct response is option B.

Male-to-female patients experienced more general health problems. The researchers stated that this might have been explained by smoking habits or older age (DeCuypere et al. 2005). Eighty percent reported improvement in their sexuality. One specific sexual change noted was that the female-to-male patients reported an increase in masturbation and a trend toward more sexual excitement, satisfaction, and orgasm. The patients reported that their expectations regarding the surgery were met on a social and emotional level but not so much on a physical and sexual level. Researchers found that few and minor problems were observed in the patients and most were reversible with appropriate treatment. The majority of patients reported a more powerful change in orgasmic feeling.

Becker JV, Johnson BR: Gender identity disorders and paraphilias, in The American Psychiatric Publishing Textbook of Psychiatry, 5th Edition. Edited by Hales RE, Yudofsky SC, Gabbard GO. Washington, DC, American Psychiatric Publishing, 2008, pp 734–735

DeCuypere G, T-Sjoen G, Beerten R, et al: Sexual and physical health after sex reassignment surgery. Arch Sex Behav 34:679–690, 2005

153. Delusions that cannot be understood by other psychological processes are referred to as *primary delusions*. Which of the following is an example of this type of delusion?

   A. Poverty.
   B. Nihilism.
   C. Thought insertion.
   D. Persecution.
   E. Guilt.

### The answer is option C.

Examples of primary delusions include thought insertion, thought broadcasting, and beliefs about world destruction.

154. The abilities involved in formulating goals, planning, effectively carrying out goal-directed plans, monitoring, and self-correcting are collectively called

    A. Executive functions.
    B. Motor functions.
    C. Perception.
    D. Praxis.
    E. Constructional ability.

**The answer is option A.**

Executive functions include abilities to formulate a goal, to plan, to carry out goal-directed plans effectively, and to monitor and self-correct spontaneously and reliably. Executive function tasks are difficult for patients with frontal lobe or diffuse brain injuries.

Luria AR: Higher Cortical Functions in Man, 2nd Edition. New York, Basic Books, 1980

155. Which of the following medications commonly prescribed for the management of impulsivity may potentially worsen symptoms?

    A. Monoamine oxidase inhibitors.
    B. Serotonin reuptake inhibitors.
    C. Benzodiazepines.
    D. Atypical neuroleptics.
    E. Mood stabilizers.

**The correct response is option C.**

Benzodiazepines may worsen symptoms of borderline personality disorder, in particular impulsivity.

Skodol AE, Gunderson JG: Personality disorders, in The American Psychiatric Publishing Textbook of Psychiatry, 5th Edition. Edited by Hales RE, Yudofsky SC, Gabbard GO. Washington, DC, American Psychiatric Publishing, 2008, p 843; Table 20–16

156. A 22-year-old female patient whom you are treating is concerned that she may develop schizophrenia, given that her mother has been treated for many years for paranoid schizophrenia. The patient is an only child, and her biological father has no psychiatric history. This patient's risk rate is

    A. 6%.
    B. 13%.
    C. 25%.
    D. 46%.
    E. 53%.

**The correct response is option B.**

First-degree relatives of probands with schizophrenia have a risk rate of 13% when one parent is affected, 46% when both are.

Malaspina D, Corcoran C, Schobel S, et al: Epidemiological and genetic aspects of neuropsychiatric disorders, in The American Psychiatric Publishing Textbook of Neuropsychiatry and Behavioral Neurosciences, 5th Edition. Edited by Yudofsky SC, Hales RE. Washington, DC, American Psychiatric Publishing, 2008, p 338

157. Which of the following features is descriptive of depersonalization disorder?

    A. Patients frequently have impaired reality testing.
    B. Patients are rarely distressed by the symptoms.
    C. Derealization rarely co-occurs with depersonalization.
    D. Patients are frequently delusional.
    E. The symptoms are usually transient.

**The correct response is option E.**

Patients with depersonalization disorder have intact reality testing, unlike patients with delusional disorder and other psychotic processes. Individuals who have depersonalization disorder are distressed by it. Derealization frequently co-occurs with depersonalization disorder. Patients are aware of some distortion in their perceptual experience and therefore are not delusional. Symptoms are often transient and may co-occur with a variety of other symptoms.

Maldonado JR, Spiegel D: Dissociative disorders, in The American Psychiatric Publishing Textbook of Psychiatry, 5th Edition. Edited by Hales RE, Yudofsky SC, Gabbard GO. Washington, DC, American Psychiatric Publishing, 2008, p 680

158. Which of the following factors was identified as an important predictor of subsequent early alcohol use?

    A. Family history of depression.
    B. Divorced parents.
    C. Maltreatment.
    D. Poor school performance.
    E. Premature birth.

**The correct response is option C.**

A 2007 case-controlled study of adolescents found that predictors of early alcohol use included maltreatment, substance dependence family loading, and the serotonin transporter genotype (the 5-HTTLPR polymorphism) (Kaufman et al. 2007). The rate of alcohol use among the maltreated children was more than seven times the rate observed in control subjects, and maltreated children also initiated drinking, on average, more than 2 years earlier than control subjects.

Gelernter J, Kranzler HR: Genetics of addiction, in The American Psychiatric Publishing Textbook of Substance Abuse Treatment, 4th Edition. Edited by Galanter M, Kleber HD. Washington, DC, American Psychiatric Publishing, 2008, p 23

Kaufman J, Yang BZ, Douglas-Palumberi H, et al: Genetic and environmental predictors of early alcohol use. Biol Psychiatry 61:1228–1234, 2007

159. Which of the following statements is *true* regarding the National Institute of Mental Health (NIMH) Treatment of Depression Collaborative Research Program?

   A. The treatment outcomes of psychodynamic psychotherapy were comparable to those of pharmacotherapy and clinical management.
   B. The treatment outcomes of psychodynamic psychotherapy were comparable to those of the manually driven therapies, interpersonal therapy (IPT), and cognitive-behavioral therapy (CBT).
   C. There was no evidence of greater effectiveness of the psychotherapies compared with pharmacotherapy and clinical management.
   D. Patients were assigned to one of four 32-week treatment conditions: interpersonal therapy (IPT), cognitive-behavioral therapy, (CBT) imipramine plus clinical management, or placebo plus clinical management.
   E. The psychotherapies were shown to be more effective than pharmacotherapy and clinical management.

**The correct response is option C.**

The NIMH Treatment of Depression Collaborative Research Program compared two manually driven therapies, IPT and CBT, with treatment with imipramine plus clinical management and with placebo plus clinical management. Options A and B are incorrect because this study did not as-

sess psychodynamic therapy. Option C is correct because because imipramine plus clinical management was generally superior to psychotherapy (both models). Option E is incorrect because the opposite it true. Option D is incorrect because the design was for 16-week treatment conditions.

Elkin I, Shea MT, Watkins JT, et al: National Institute of Mental Health Treatment of Depression Collaborative Research Program: general effectiveness of treatments. Arch Gen Psychiatry 46:971–982, 1989

Gabbard GO: The evolving role of the psychiatrist from the perspective of psychotherapy, in American Psychiatry After World War II: 1944–1994. Edited by Menninger RW, Nemiah JC. Washington, DC, American Psychiatric Publishing, 2000, pp 109–110

160. Family studies of bipolar disorder have demonstrated all of the following findings *except*

   A. A sevenfold increase in lifetime risk for bipolar disorder in families with the disorder compared with family members of control subjects.
   B. Recurrence risks were found to be higher in females, either of the relative or of the bipolar proband.
   C. The age at onset of the first manic or depressive episode has been shown to be earlier in the younger generation of two generations of affected relative pairs.
   D. The risk for bipolar disorder appears to be especially elevated in the relatives of probands with early-onset disorder.
   E. The risk for bipolar disorder increases with the number of psychiatrically ill relatives.

**The correct response is option B.**

Recurrence risks do not vary by gender, either of the relative or of the bipolar proband. A sevenfold increase in lifetime risk for bipolar disorder has been found in families of individuals with the disorder compared with families of control subjects. The age at onset of the first manic or depressive episode has been shown to be earlier, and the frequency of episodes greater, in the younger generation of two generations of affected relative pairs.

Malaspina D, Corcoran C, Schobel S, et al: Epidemiological and genetic aspects of neuropsychiatric disorders, in The American Psychiatric Publishing Textbook of Neuropsychiatry and Behavioral Neurosciences, 5th Edition. Edited by Yudofsky SC, Hales RE. Washington, DC, American Psychiatric Publishing, 2008, p 327

161. Imaging studies have helped to delineate a constellation of brain regions involved in attention-deficit/hyperactivity disorder (ADHD). Which of the following is the most consistent neuroanatomical finding in ADHD subjects relative to non-ADHD control subjects?

    A. Decreased size of the caudate.
    B. Increased size of the frontal cortex.
    C. Increased size of the posterior portion of the corpus callosum.
    D. Decreased size of the cerebellar vermis.
    E. Increased size of the anterior portion of the corpus callosum.

## The correct response is option D.

The most consistently documented morphometric difference between ADHD subjects and control subjects is a reduction in the size of the cerebellar vermis, a midline gray and white matter region that connects left and right cerebellar hemispheres. Interestingly, this is the brain region that shows the greatest degree of growth during the postnatal period. The caudate volume appears to decrease with age in boys without ADHD, presumably as a consequence of pruning, but does not appear to change with age in boys with ADHD. Some studies have documented a decrease in the size of the posterior corpus callosum, whereas others have reported that the anterior portion of the corpus callosum is reduced in size in boys with ADHD.

Teicher MYH, Andersen SL, Navalta CP, et al: Neuropsychiatric disorders of childhood and adolescence, in The American Psychiatric Publishing Textbook of Neuropsychiatry and Behavioral Neurosciences, 5th Edition. Edited by Yudofsky SC, Hales RE. Washington, DC, American Psychiatric Publishing, 2008, pp 1051–1052

162. The neurobiology of depression involves hypoactivity in the following cortical structures *except*

    A. Dorsolateral prefrontal cortex.
    B. Ventrolateral prefrontal cortex.
    C. Orbitofrontal prefrontal cortex.
    D. Anterior cingulate cortex.
    E. Amygdala.

## The correct response is option E.

The most common functional neuroanatomical abnormality associated with depression is resting state hypometabolism or decreased flow in the prefrontal cortex, including the dorsolateral, ventrolateral, and orbitofrontal prefrontal cortex. Hypoactivity has also been found in dorsal parts of the anterior cingulate cortex. Depression appears to be associated with increased activity in subcortical regions such as the amygdala, anterior temporal, insula, basal ganglia, and thalamus.

Holtzheimer PE III, Mayberg HS: Neuropsychiatric aspects of mood disorders, in The American Psychiatric Publishing Textbook of Neuropsychiatry and Behavioral Neurosciences, 5th Edition. Edited by Yudofsky SC, Hales RE. Washington, DC, American Psychiatric Publishing, 2008, p 1011

163. DSM-IV-TR (American Psychiatric Association 2000) includes within the impulse-control disorder category five distinct impulse-control disorders not elsewhere classified. Which of the following is *not* one of these five disorders?

    A. Intermittent explosive disorder.
    B. Kleptomania.
    C. Pyromania.
    D. Trichotillomania.
    E. Binge-eating disorder.

## The correct response is option E.

Binge-eating disorder is not classified as an impulse-control disorder but rather as an eating disorder. The impulse-control disorders not elsewhere classified include intermittent explosive disorder (failure to resist aggressive impulses), kleptomania (failure to resist urges to steal items), pyromania (failure to resist urges to set fires), pathological gambling (failure to resist urges to gamble), and trichotillomania (failure to resist urges to pull one's hair).

American Psychiatric Association: Diagnostic and Statistical Manual of Mental Disorders, 4th Edition, Text Revision. Washington, DC, American Psychiatric Association, 2000

Hollander E, Berlin HA, Stein DJ: Impulse control disorders not elsewhere classified, in The American Psychiatric Publishing Textbook of Psychiatry, 5th Edition. Edited by Hales RE, Yudofsky SC, Gabbard GO. Washington, DC, American Psychiatric Publishing, 2008, pp 777–778; Table 19–1

164. When interviewing a depressed or suicidal patient, the psychiatrist is advised to do all of the following *except*

    A. Begin with assessment of physical appearance and motor behavior.
    B. Thoroughly explore neurovegetative signs or symptoms and their effect on patient function.
    C. Be attentive to recent psychosocial stressors (especially losses) and recent anniversaries of significant past losses.
    D. Allow the patient to set the pace of the interview, avoid excessive engagement, and tolerate long silences.
    E. Assess both suicidal cognitions and the patient's ability to control self-destructive impulses.

**The answer is option D.**

The psychiatrist takes an active role when interviewing the depressed patient. The patient is encouraged to verbalize what he or she is experiencing. The psychiatrist empathizes with the patient's pain and mental anguish. Prolonged silences on the part of the psychiatrist are rarely helpful with these patients and should be discouraged.

Simon RI: Suicide, in The American Psychiatric Publishing Textbook of Psychiatry, 5th Edition. Edited by Hales RE, Yudofsky SC, Gabbard GO. Washington, DC, American Psychiatric Publishing, 2008, pp 1637–1654

165. Regarding chemically mediated synapses and their neurotransmitters, which of the following is *true*?

    A. Chemical synapses are faster than electrical synapses.
    B. Chemical synapses are limited in utility because they do not allow for signal amplification.
    C. Chemical synapses can modulate the activity of other cells through activation of second-messenger cascades.
    D. Small molecule transmitters (e.g., glutamate, gamma-aminobutyric acid, and glycine) are stored in large dense-core vesicles.
    E. Neuropeptides (e.g., somatostatin, endorphins, and enkephalins) mediate fast synaptic transmission.

**The answer is option C.**

In the central nervous system (CNS), both chemical and electrical synapses are critical for neural activity. Most CNS synaptic connections are mediated by chemical neurotransmitters.

Although chemical synapses are slower than electrical ones, they allow for signal amplification, may be inhibitory as well as excitatory, are susceptible to a wide range of modulation, and can modulate the activities of other cells through the release of transmitters activating second-messenger cascades.

McAllister AK, Usrey WM, Noctor SC, et al: Cellular and molecular biology of the neuron, in The American Psychiatric Publishing Textbook of Psychiatry, 5th Edition. Edited by Hales RE, Yudofsky SC, Gabbard GO. Washington, DC, American Psychiatric Publishing, 2008, pp 114–120

166. The primary differential diagnostic issue for antisocial personality disorder involves which of the following diagnoses?

    A. Narcissistic personality disorder.
    B. Paranoid personality disorder.
    C. Obsessive-compulsive personality disorder.
    D. Avoidant personality disorder.
    E. Schizoid personality disorder.

**The correct response is option A.**

Antisocial personality disorder and narcissistic personality disorder may be variants of the same basic type of psychopathology. Unlike the narcissistic person, the antisocial person is likely to be reckless and impulsive. In addition, narcissistic individuals' exploitiveness and disregard for others are attributable to their sense of uniqueness and superiority rather than to a desire for materialistic gains.

Skodol AE, Gunderson JG: Personality disorders, in The American Psychiatric Publishing Textbook of Psychiatry, 5th Edition. Edited by Hales RE, Yudofsky SC, Gabbard GO. Washington, DC, American Psychiatric Publishing, 2008, p 839

167. Which of the following candidate genes implicated in schizophrenia has also been associated with velocardiofacial syndrome?

    A. Dystrobrevin binding protein–1.
    B. Neuregulin-1.
    C. Catechol-*O*-methyltransferase (COMT).
    D. Disrupted-in-schizophrenia–1 and –2.
    E. Metabotropic glutamate receptor–3.

**The correct response is option C.**

COMT maps to 22q11, the deletion of which produces velocardiofacial syndrome, a disease associated with a high incidence of psychosis.

Tamminga CA, Shad MJ, Ghose S: Neuropsychiatric aspects of schizophrenia, in The American Psychiatric Publishing Textbook of Neuropsychiatry and Behavioral Neurosciences, 5th Edition. Edited by Yudofsky SC, Hales RE. Washington, DC, American Psychiatric Publishing, 2008, p 974

168. Which of the following characteristics is indicative of dissociative amnesia?

    A. The memory loss is wide-ranging rather than limited to a discrete period of time.
    B. There is difficulty learning new information.
    C. The amnesia is typically anterograde.
    D. The memory loss is episodic.
    E. The memory loss is generally not limited to events of a traumatic nature.

## The correct response is option D.

The memory loss in dissociative amnesia is episodic. Dissociative amnesia has three primary characteristics:

1. The memory loss is episodic. The first-person recollection of certain events is lost, rather than knowledge of procedures.
2. The memory loss encompasses a discrete period of time, ranging from minutes to years. It is not vagueness or inefficient retrieval of memories but rather a dense unavailability of memories that previously had been clearly accessible. There is usually no difficulty in learning new episodic information. Thus, the amnesia is typically retrograde rather than anterograde.
3. The memory loss is generally for events of a traumatic or stressful nature.

Maldonado JR, Spiegel D: Dissociative disorders, in The American Psychiatric Publishing Textbook of Psychiatry, 5th Edition. Edited by Hales RE, Yudofsky SC, Gabbard GO. Washington, DC, American Psychiatric Publishing, 2008, pp 675–676

169. Which of the following DSM-IV-TR clinical criteria does not apply to a diagnosis of substance abuse?

    A. Withdrawal symptoms or the taking of a substance to avoid withdrawal symptoms.
    B. Recurrent substance use resulting in failure to fulfill major role obligations.

    C. Recurrent substance use in situations in which it is physically hazardous.
    D. Recurrent substance-related legal problems.
    E. Continued substance use despite persistent or recurrent social problems caused by the effects of the substance.

## The correct response is option A.

Withdrawal symptoms are a characteristic of substance dependence, not substance abuse. Substance abuse is assessed using the following four criteria: 1) recurrent substance use resulting in failure to fulfill major role obligations at work, school, or home; 2) recurrent substance use in situations in which it is physically hazardous; 3) recurrent substance-related legal problems; and 4) continued substance use despite persistent or recurrent social or interpersonal problems caused or exacerbated by the effects of the substance.

Brook JS, Pahl K, Rubenstone E: Epidemiology of addiction, in The American Psychiatric Publishing Textbook of Substance Abuse Treatment, 4th Edition. Edited by Galanter M, Kleber HD. Washington, DC, American Psychiatric Publishing, 2008, p 29

170. All of the following statements describe either benefits of naltrexone treatment for opiate dependence or patient populations who may respond well to naltrexone treatment *except*

    A. Patients with a history of recent employment do well while taking naltrexone.
    B. Naltrexone may be prescribed by any physician in his or her office.
    C. Naltrexone has been shown to be effective in treating opiate dependence even when simply prescribed as a medication in the absence of a structural rehabilitation program.
    D. Naltrexone is not a controlled substance.
    E. Health care professionals have done well in naltrexone treatment programs as patients.

## The correct response is option C.

Naltrexone is not effective when simply prescribed as a medication for street heroin–addicted patients in the absence of a structured rehabilitation program. Options A and E are correct because within a structured program naltrexone appears to be effective, particularly with specific motivated populations such as health care professionals and individuals with a history of recent employment and strong educational backgrounds. Unlike methadone, naltrexone is not a controlled substance and can be prescribed by any physician in his or her office. Methadone maintenance often requires daily clinic visits, and practitioners who prescribe and dispense controlled substances for narcotic addiction must be registered with the U.S. Drug Enforcement Agency. Thus, options B and C reflect true statements and are therefore incorrect. Although high-functioning patients may be strongly motivated to be drug free, they remain susceptible to impulsive drug use. Using naltrexone as a kind of "insurance" is often a very appealing idea.

O'Brien C, Kampman KM: Antagonists of opioids, in The American Psychiatric Publishing Textbook of Substance Abuse Treatment, 4th Edition. Edited by Galanter M, Kleber HD. Washington, DC, American Psychiatric Publishing, 2008, p 326

U.S. Department of Health and Human Services, Substance Abuse and Mental Health Services Administration, Center for Substance Abuse Treatment: What Every Individual Needs to Know About Methadone Maintenance Treatment (DHHS Publ No SMA-06-4123; NCADI Publ No PHD1124). Washington, DC, U.S. Department of Health and Human Services, 2005

171. What is the the first-line treatment recommendation of the American Psychiatric Association during the acute phase of rapid cycling?

    A. Lithium, valproic acid, or lamotrigine.
    B. Lithium or valproic acid but not lamotrigine.
    C. Lithium plus valproic acid.
    D. Lithium or valproic acid plus an antipsychotic.
    E. Lithium but not valproic acid.

### The correct response is option A.

Some patients may require combinations of medications, but the initial treatment recommendation is to attempt monotherapy with lithium, valproic acid, or lamotrigine. Thus, options B, C, and E are incorrect. Lithium or valproic acid plus an antipsychotic is the first-line treatment recommendation for severe manic or mixed episodes during the acute phase of treatment, not rapid cycling.

American Psychiatric Association: Practice Guidelines for the Treatment of Psychiatric Disorders, Compendium 2006. Arlington, VA, American Psychiatric Association, 2006, pp 859–861

172. Psychostimulant medications remain the cornerstone of attention-deficit/hyperactivity disorder (ADHD) treatment. Of the following, which is the least common side effect of psychostimulants?

    A. Anorexia.
    B. Irritability.
    C. Dysphoria.
    D. Tics and other stereotypic movements.
    E. Insomnia.

### The correct response is option D.

The side effects most commonly reported with psychostimulant medications are anorexia, stomachaches, insomnia, and mood changes (irritability, mood lability, dysphoria). Tics and other stereotypic movements are uncommon side effects of psychostimulants.

Teicher MYH, Andersen SL, Navalta CP, et al: Neuropsychiatric disorders of childhood and adolescence, in The American Psychiatric Publishing Textbook of Neuropsychiatry and Behavioral Neurosciences, 5th Edition. Edited by Yudofsky SC, Hales RE. Washington, DC, American Psychiatric Publishing, 2008, p 1056

173. Which of the following statements is *true* regarding sexual orientation as addressed in DSM-IV-TR?

    A. A diagnosis of transvestic fetishism requires the presence of homosexual sexual orientation.
    B. Transvestic fetishism may be diagnosed in either homosexual or heterosexual men.
    C. Homosexual orientation is an exclusionary criterion for transvestic fetishism.
    D. Gender identity disorder is the appropriate diagnosis for "sissy" behavior in young boys.
    E. Sexual disorder not otherwise specified (NOS) does not encompass distress about sexual orientation.

### The correct response is option C.

DSM-IV-TR (American Psychiatric Association 2000) contains few specific mentions of sexual orientation. Homosexual sexual orientation is an exclusionary criterion for transvestic fetishism. Gender identity disorder in childhood is not to be diagnosed simply for "tomboyish" behavior in girls or "sissyish" behavior in boys; this exclusion reflects an effort to focus on distress about gender rather than stereotypes about sexual orientation. In one study, 75% of children with this diagnosis became homosexual or bisexual as adults (Green 1987). Sexual disorder NOS includes a category of "persistent and marked distress about sexual orientation."

American Psychiatric Association: Diagnostic and Statistical Manual of Mental Health Disorders, 4th Edition, Text Revision. Washington, DC, American Psychiatric Association, 2000

Drescher J, McCommon BH, Jones BE: Treatment of lesbian, gay, bisexual, and transgender patients, in The American Psychiatric Publishing Textbook of Psychiatry, 5th Edition. Edited by Hales RE, Yudofsky SC, Gabbard GO. Washington, DC, American Psychiatric Publishing, 2008, p 1478

Green R: The "Sissy Boy Syndrome" and the Development of Homosexuality. New Haven, CT, Yale University Press, 1987

174. After fully exploring the patient's personal history, the psychiatrist proceeds to the next history item by asking, "Is there a family history of psychiatric illness, for example, suicidal behavior, mental retardation, or anxiety, mood, psychotic, substance abuse, or personality disorder?" This would be an example of

   A. Excessive direct questions.
   B. Preemptive topic shift.
   C. Run-on questioning.
   D. Put down.
   E. Checklist questioning.

## The answer is option C.

By lumping several questions into a single sentence, the psychiatrist overwhelms the patient and demonstrates a lack of regard for the importance of the patient's answers to the individual questions.

175. Regarding gamma-aminobutyric acid (GABA) receptors, which of the following is *true?*

   A. Excitatory postsynaptic potentials in the brain are mediated primarily by GABA receptors.
   B. The $GABA_A$ receptor–channel complex is composed of five subunits.
   C. GABA receptors are metabotropic receptors.
   D. Clinical actions of benzodiazepines and barbiturates are proportional to their binding potential at $GABA_B$ receptors.
   E. Benzodiazepines increase GABA current by increasing the amount of "open" time in receptor channels.

## The answer is option B.

GABA receptors are ubiquitous in the central nervous system (CNS) and have different conformational and neurophysiological properties. Inhibitory, not excitatory, postsynaptic potentials in the brain are mediated primarily by GABA receptors, so option A is incorrect.

$GABA_A$ receptors are members of the nicotinic acetylcholine receptor superfamily and are ionotropic receptors, so option C is incorrect. The $GABA_A$ receptor–channel complex is composed of five subunits. This gives rise to receptors with varying properties. Because most of the subunits have multiple subtypes, there is a potential for an extraordinary diversity of $GABA_A$-receptor function.

The clinical actions of benzodiazepines, along with two other classes of CNS-depressant drugs (barbiturates and anesthetic steroids), seem to be related to their ability to bind to $GABA_A$ receptors and to enhance $GABA_A$ receptor currents, not $GABA_B$, so option D is incorrect. Individual $GABA_A$ channels do not open continuously in the presence of GABA but rather flicker open and closed, often in bursts. Benzodiazepines increase GABA current by increasing the frequency of channel openings without altering open time or conductance.

McAllister AK, Usrey WM, Noctor SC, et al: Cellular and molecular biology of the neuron, in The American Psychiatric Publishing Textbook of Psychiatry, 5th Edition. Edited by Hales RE, Yudofsky SC, Gabbard GO. Washington, DC, American Psychiatric Publishing, 2008, p 126

176. The police bring to the emergency department a young adult male who was found talking to himself in public and chuckling and gesturing for no apparent reason. The patient is unkempt; his speech is odd and idiosyncratic, although there is no overt psychosis. A drug screen is negative. There is no information on whether gradual social deterioration has occurred. Of the personality disorders, which of the following is the most likely diagnosis in this patient?

   A. Paranoid personality disorder.
   B. Schizoid personality disorder.
   C. Schizotypal personality disorder.
   D. Antisocial personality disorder.
   E. Avoidant personality disorder.

## The correct response is option C.

Individuals with schizotypal personality disorder may, for example, talk to themselves in public, gesture for no apparent reason, or dress in a peculiar or unkempt fashion. Their speech is often odd and idiosyncratic—unusually circumstantial, metaphorical, or vague, for instance—and their affect is constricted or inappropriate. Such a person may, for example, laugh inappropriately when discussing his or her problems. Schizotypal personality disorder shares the feature of suspiciousness with paranoid personality disorder and that of social isolation with schizoid personality disorder, but the latter two disorders lack the markedly peculiar behavior and significant cognitive and perceptual distortions typical of schizotypal personality disorder. The symptoms of schizotypal personality disorder appear to be attenuated versions of the symptoms of schizophrenia, but enduring periods of overt psychosis and social deterioration over time are not characteristic.

Skodol AE, Gunderson JG: Personality disorders, in The American Psychiatric Publishing Textbook of Psychiatry, 5th Edition. Edited by Hales RE, Yudofsky SC, Gabbard GO. Washington, DC, American Psychiatric Publishing, 2008, p 837

177. Magnetic resonance imaging (MRI) studies of the brains of patients with schizophrenia have revealed a volume decrease in all of the following brain structures *except*

A. Hippocampus.
B. Amygdala.
C. Parahippocampal gyrus.
D. Superior temporal gyrus.
E. Caudate nucleus.

## The correct response is option E.

A volume decrease of the caudate nucleus has not been revealed in MRI studies of patients with schizophrenia. MRI studies have consistently revealed a volume decrease in the medial temporal cortical structures, hippocampus, amygdala, and parahippocampal gyrus. The volume of the superior temporal gyrus has also been reported as being reduced in schizophrenia, and the magnitude of the reduction has been correlated with the presence of hallucinations and with electrophysiological changes in the patients.

Tamminga CA, Shad MJ, Ghose S: Neuropsychiatric aspects of schizophrenia, in The American Psychiatric Publishing Textbook of Neuropsychiatry and Behavioral Neurosciences, 5th Edition. Edited by Yudofsky SC, Hales RE. Washington, DC, American Psychiatric Publishing, 2008, p 977

178. Repression, as a general model for keeping information out of conscious awareness, differs from dissociation in a number of important ways. Which of the following statements describes repression?

A. The organizational structure of mental contents is horizontal, with subunits of information divided from one another but equally available to consciousness.
B. Motivated forgetting is the underlying mechanism.
C. The information is kept out of awareness for a discrete and sharply delimited time.
D. The information is stored in a discrete and untransformed manner.
E. Retrieval of information can be direct to uncover warded-off memories.

## The correct response is option B.

Dynamic conflict, or motivated forgetting, is the mechanism underlying repression. Repression, as a general model for keeping information out of conscious awareness, differs from dissociation in several important ways:

1. The organization structure of mental contents in dissociation is thought of as horizontal, with subunits of information divided from one another but equally available to consciousness. Repressed information, on the other hand, is presumed to be stored in an archeological manner, at various depths, and therefore different components are not equally accessible.
2. Subunits of information are presumed to be divided by amnesic barriers in dissociation, whereas dynamic conflict, or motivated forgetting, is the mechanism underlying repression.
3. The information kept out of awareness in dissociation is often for a discrete and sharply delimited time, usually for a traumatic experience, whereas repressed information may be for a variety of experiences, fears, or wishes scattered across time.
4. Dissociation is often elicited as a defense, especially after episodes of physical trauma, whereas repression is a response to warded-off fears and wishes or in response to other dynamic conflicts.
5. Dissociated information is stored in a discrete and untransformed manner, whereas repressed information is usually disguised and fragmented. Even when repressed information becomes available to consciousness, its meaning is hidden (e.g., in dreams, slips of the tongue).

6. Retrieval of dissociated information often can be direct. Techniques such as hypnosis can be used to access warded-off memories. In contrast, uncovering of repressed information often requires repeated recall trials through intense questioning, psychotherapy, or psychoanalysis with subsequent interpretation (i.e., of dreams).

7. The focus of psychotherapy for dissociation is integration via control of access to dissociated states and working through of traumatic memories. The classical psychotherapy for repression involves interpretation, including working through of the transference.

Maldonado JR, Spiegel D: Dissociative disorders, in The American Psychiatric Publishing Textbook of Psychiatry, 5th Edition. Edited by Hales RE, Yudofsky SC, Gabbard GO. Washington, DC, American Psychiatric Publishing, 2008, p 667, Table 15–2

179. Which of the following statements is *true* regarding the Epidemiologic Catchment Area (ECA) study?

    A. The study sampled adults and adolescents.
    B. It used DSM-IV-TR diagnostic criteria.
    C. The study reported a lifetime prevalence of alcohol abuse and dependence of more than 10% of the population for each disorder.
    D. Lifetime prevalence of alcohol abuse was highest for subjects ages 30–39 years.
    E. Marijuana abuse/dependence was the most common disorder due to illicit drugs.

### The correct response is option E.

The ECA study was carried out in the early 1980s in five large metropolitan areas and sampled approximately 20,000 people. Option A is incorrect because the ECA sample included only adults (>18 years). Option B is incorrect because DSM-III criteria, not DSM-IV-TR, were used. Option C is incorrect because the results showed a <10% lifetime prevalence of these disorders (7.9% of alcohol dependence and 5.8% of alcohol abuse). Option D is incorrect because alcohol abuse was highest in people between ages 18 and 29 years, not people in their 30s. Findings from the ECA study revealed that marijuana abuse and dependence had the highest lifetime prevalence rate (4.4%) when compared with cocaine, amphetamines, sedatives, opioids, and hallucinogens.

Brook JS, Pahl K, Rubenstone E: Epidemiology of addiction, in The APP Textbook of Substance Abuse Treatment, 4th Edition. Edited by Galanter M, Kleber HD. Washington, DC, American Psychiatric Publishing, 2008, p 30

180. Which of the following statements is *true* regarding opioid antagonists?

    A. Naltrexone is poorly absorbed in the gut.
    B. Naloxone is poorly absorbed from the gut but is effective when given parenterally.
    C. Naltrexone does not block opiate-induced euphoria, respiratory depression, and other opiate effects.
    D. Naltrexone must be dosed daily to be effective.
    E. In cases of overdose, a one-time dose of naloxone should be given initially.

### The correct response is option B.

Naloxone is poorly absorbed from the gut but is effective when given parenterally. However, naloxone delivered parenterally is metabolized rapidly. Option A is incorrect because naltrexone, in contrast with naloxone, is well absorbed in the gut. Available in oral form, naltrexone is long acting and is ideal for use in preventing opioid relapse. Naltrexone is a relatively pure antagonist in that it produces little or no agonist activity at usual doses and prevents opiate agonists from binding to the receptor and producing opiate effects.

Option C is incorrect because its high receptor affinity blocks virtually all the effects of the usual doses of opioids and opiates such as heroin. Option D is incorrect because although a daily dose of oral naltrexone would presumably be most protective against relapse, its long duration of action allows for dosing as infrequently as 2–3 times a week. Option E is incorrect because naloxone has a short duration of action. With its effects disappearing in 20–30 minutes of administration, naloxone would need to be given repeatedly in cases of an overdose.

O'Brien C, Kampman KM: Antagonists of opioids, in The American Psychiatric Publishing Textbook of Substance Abuse Treatment, 4th Edition. Edited by Galanter M, Kleber HD. Washington, DC, American Psychiatric Publishing, 2008, pp 325–326

| Naloxone | Naltrexone |
| --- | --- |
| Short duration of action | Long duration of action |
| Parenteral (poor gut absorption) | Oral (good gut absorption) |

181. Which of the following symptoms is *not* characteristic of fragile X syndrome?

     A. Social withdrawal and reduced caregiver attachment.
     B. Gaze avoidance.
     C. Hand flapping.
     D. Tactile defensiveness.
     E. Perseveration.

## The correct response is option A.

Fragile X syndrome, the most common known inherited cause of mental retardation, is often associated with autism spectrum behaviors. Social withdrawal and reduced attachment to caregivers are not characteristic of fragile X syndrome. Many patients affected by fragile X syndrome show autistic features such as gaze avoidance, hand flapping, tactile defensiveness, and perseveration.

Teicher MYH, Andersen SL, Navalta CP, et al: Neuropsychiatric disorders of childhood and adolescence, in The American Psychiatric Publishing Textbook of Neuropsychiatry and Behavioral Neurosciences, 5th Edition. Edited by Yudofsky SC, Hales RE. Washington, DC, American Psychiatric Publishing, 2008, p 1064

182. A core feature associated with impulse-control disorders is that at the time of committing the act the person normally experiences

     A. Regret.
     B. Pleasure or gratification.
     C. A heightened sense of tension or arousal.
     D. A sense of relief from the urge.
     E. Self-reproach or guilt.

## The correct response is option B.

At the time of committing the act, the individual experiences pleasure, gratification, or relief. DSM-IV-TR impulse-control disorders are characterized by a sequence of symptomatic feelings and behaviors. Before committing the act, the individual experiences an increased sense of tension or arousal. At the time of committing the act, the individual experiences pleasure, gratification, or relief. After committing the act, the person experiences a sense of relief from the urge that may be accompanied by regret, self-reproach, or guilt.

Hollander E, Berlin HA, Stein DJ: Impulse-control disorders not elsewhere classified, in The American Psychiatric Publishing Textbook of Psychiatry, 5th Edition. Edited by Hales RE, Yudofsky SC, Gabbard GO. Washington, DC, American Psychiatric Publishing, 2008, pp 777–778, Table 19–2

183. Which of the following statements about studies of amnesia as it is associated with hippocampal damage is *false?*

     A. Neuropsychological findings have demonstrated selective impairments in relational memory.
     B. The hippocampal system mediates long-term relational memory.
     C. There is a consistent relationship between the side of the hippocampal lesion and the type of learning impairment.
     D. The hippocampal system plays a role in the learning of perceptuomotor skills.
     E. The hippocampal system is not the principal repository for old memories.

## The correct response is option D.

The hippocampal system does not appear to play a role in the learning of perceptuomotor skills and other knowledge (referred to as *nondeclarative memory*). Neuropsychological findings have demonstrated selected impairments in relational memory, and this has been supported by functional neuroimaging research as well. More recent work has suggested that the hippocampal system specifically mediates long-term relational memory. There is a consistent relationship between the side of the lesion and the type of learning impairment. Specifically, damage to the left hippocampal system produces an amnesic syndrome that affects verbal material but spares nonverbal material; conversely, damage to the right hippocampal system affects nonverbal material but spares verbal material. The hippocampal system is not the principal repository for old memories.

Harel BT, Tranel D: Functional neuroanatomy, in The American Psychiatric Publishing Textbook of Neuropsychiatry and Behavioral Neurosciences, 5th Edition. Edited by Yudofsky SC, Hales RE. Washington, DC, American Psychiatric Publishing, 2008, pp 51–52

184. An important theoretical issue is whether the personality disorders are best classified as dimensions or categories. Which of the following arguments supports a categorical approach to personality disorder classification?

    A. The thresholds for diagnosing personality disorders are arbitrary.
    B. Excessive diagnostic co-occurrence between personality disorders has been observed in many studies.
    C. The residual category of personality disorder not otherwise specified (NOS) may be the most commonly assigned personality disorder diagnosis in clinical practice.
    D. There is considerable heterogeneity of features among patients receiving the same diagnosis.
    E. Categorical models better reflect how clinicians think about pathological syndromes.

## The correct response is option E.

An argument in favor of categorical models is that they better reflect how clinicians think—that is, in terms of pathological syndromes that a person either has or does not have. The use of categories also makes it possible for clinicians to summarize patients' difficulties succinctly and facilitates communication about them. Categorical diagnoses of personality disorders have been criticized for a number of reasons. First, excessive diagnostic co-occurrence between personality disorders has been observed in many studies: most patients with personality disorders meet criteria for more than one disorder. Second, there is considerable heterogeneity of features among patients receiving the same diagnosis. Third, the thresholds for making personality disorder diagnoses are arbitrary in that they were decided on the basis of expert consensus and not on the basis of empirical research. Finally, despite the inclusion of 10 specific personality disorder types in DSM-IV-TR (American Psychiatric Association 2000), the residual category of personality disorder NOS may be the most commonly applied personality disorder diagnosis in clinical practice, suggesting inadequate coverage of personality psychopathology by the DSM.

American Psychiatric Association: Diagnostic and Statistical Manual of Mental Disorders, 4th Edition, Text Revision. Washington, DC, American Psychiatric Association, 2000

Skodol AE, Gunderson JG: Personality disorders, in The American Psychiatric Publishing Textbook of Psychiatry, 5th Edition. Edited by Hales RE, Yudofsky SC, Gabbard GO. Washington, DC, American Psychiatric Publishing, 2008, pp 823–827

185. Which of the following psychosocial treatments for schizophrenia has been found *not* to be effective and may increase the risk for decompensation?

    A. Assertive community treatment (ACT).
    B. Cognitive-behavioral therapy (CBT).
    C. Individual psychoanalytically oriented psychotherapy.
    D. Family therapy.
    E. Personal therapy.

## The correct response is option C.

After landmark studies in the early 1980s demonstrated its ineffectiveness for schizophrenia, individual psychoanalytically oriented psychotherapy was largely abandoned in the treatment of schizophrenia patients. Psychoanalytic psychotherapy is now generally considered to elevate the risk for psychotic decompensation, probably because of the unstructured and anxiety-provoking nature of this treatment.

One particularly successful form of case management used in the United States is ACT. Candidates for this care are typically identified in community mental health settings as those with the highest service needs and are referred to a multidisciplinary team comprising a psychiatric nurse, a psychiatrist, and other psychiatric support staff. ACTs appear to reduce the time spent in the hospital and improve the stability of housing maintenance.

CBT is used in the United Kingdom for the treatment of schizophrenia. Randomized, controlled studies show that CBT decreases symptom severity in comparison with supportive therapy and treatment as usual. Family therapy seems to reduce relapse rates in schizophrenia.

Supportive therapy encompasses a diverse set of approaches with a common goal of providing reassurance, guidance, and an interpersonal environment that is stable, predictable, and tolerant of the patient's expression, symptoms, and problems in living.

Personal therapy, a supportive approach, utilizes techniques that are individualized for the patient, with progressive focus first on stress reduction, followed by cognitive reframing and later vocational rehabilitation, as the emphasis follows the patient's stage of recovery.

Minzenberg MJ, Yoon JH, Carter CS: Schizophrenia, in The American Psychiatric Publishing Textbook of Psychiatry, 5th Edition. Edited by Hales RE, Yudofsky SC, Gabbard GO. Washington, DC, American Psychiatric Publishing, 2008, pp 444–446

186. Which of the following is more indicative of somatization disorder than of physical illness?

    A. Laboratory abnormalities of the suggested physical disorder.
    B. Physical signs of structural abnormalities.
    C. Involvement of multiple organ systems.
    D. Late onset and acute course.
    E. Involvement of only one organ system.

**The correct response is option C.**

The symptoms in somatization disorder are frequently nonspecific and can overlap with a multitude of medical disorders. Three features are useful in discriminating between somatization disorder and physical illness: 1) involvement of multiple organ systems, 2) early onset and chronic course without development of physical signs of structural abnormalities, and 3) absence of characteristic laboratory abnormalities of the suggested physical disorder.

Yutzy SH, Parish BS: Somatoform disorders, in The American Psychiatric Publishing Textbook of Psychiatry, 5th Edition. Edited by Hales RE, Yudofsky SC, Gabbard GO. Washington, DC, American Psychiatric Publishing, 2008, pp 617–618; Table 13–5

187. Which of the following is associated with intravenous use of cocaine?

    A. Ischemic necrosis of the nasal septum.
    B. Dyspnea.
    C. Pneumothorax.
    D. Pulmonary infarction.
    E. Endocarditis.

**The correct response is option E.**

Intravenous cocaine use may cause cellulitis or endocarditis. Ischemic necrosis of the nasal septum is associated with insufflating or snorting powder cocaine; smoking crack cocaine may lead to dyspnea, pneumothorax, pneumomediastinum, and pulmonary infarction.

Greenfield SF, Hennessy G: Assessment of the patient, in The American Psychiatric Publishing Textbook of Substance Abuse Treatment, 4th Edition. Edited by Galanter M, Kleber HD. Washington, DC, American Psychiatric Publishing, 2008, p 64

188. Which of the following statements is *true* regarding fluctuations of medication levels?

    A. Nortriptyline doses are likely to require increases in order to maintain stable maternal blood levels as pregnancy progresses.
    B. Neonates are not prone to lithium toxicity as long as their serum concentrations are lower than maternal concentrations.
    C. Maternal valproic acid concentrations increase as pregnancy progresses.
    D. Lamotrigine clearance decreases as pregnancy progresses.
    E. The mean fetal-to-maternal ratio of the plasma concentrations of selective serotonin reuptake inhibitors (SSRIs) is about 20 to 1.

**The correct response is option A.**

Doses of up to 1.6 times the usual dose of nortriptyline may be required in late pregnancy to maintain therapeutic serum concentrations.

Option B is incorrect because neonates may show signs of lithium toxicity at serum concentrations that are lower than maternal levels. Neonatal symptoms of lithium toxicity—flaccidity, lethargy, and poor suck reflexes—may persist for more than 7 days postpartum. Option C is incorrect because maternal valproic acid concentrations appear to steadily decline during pregnancy, reaching levels as much as 50% lower than preconception concentrations. Option D is incorrect because lamotrigine clearance steadily increases during gestation. Option E is incorrect because the mean fetal-to-maternal ratio of SSRIs is uniformly <1.

Newport DJ, Fisher A, Graybeal S, et al: Psychopharmacology during pregnancy and lactation, in The American Psychiatric Publishing Textbook of Psychopharmacology, 3rd Edition. Edited by Schatzberg AF, Nemeroff CB. Washington, DC, American Psychiatric Publishing, 2004, pp 1118, 1121, 1123–1124, 1126–1127

189. All of the following statements are true *except*

    A. Obsessive-compulsive disorder (OCD) is seen in approximately 10% of patients with Tourette's syndrome.
    B. OCD symptoms usually appear 1–2 years before simple tics in these patients.
    C. Tic-related OCD has an earlier onset than does classic OCD.
    D. Tic-related OCD features more ritualized touching and tapping than does classic OCD.

E. Tic-related OCD has a less favorable response to selective serotonin reuptake inhibitors (SSRIs) and a more favorable response to antipsychotic augmentation compared with classic OCD.

**The correct response is option B.**

Tic disorders are often comorbid with OCD. However, the OCD symptoms in tic disorder patients often differ from the symptoms in patients with classic OCD. In patients with Tourette's syndrome who develop OCD, the symptoms usually appear 5–10 years after the first appearance of simple tics. Tic-related OCD may differ from classic OCD, with an earlier onset; more prominent symptoms of ritualized touching, tapping, and rubbing; a less satisfactory response to SSRIs; and an enhanced response to neuroleptic augmentation.

Teicher MYH, Andersen SL, Navalta CP, et al: Neuropsychiatric disorders of childhood and adolescence, in The American Psychiatric Publishing Textbook of Neuropsychiatry and Behavioral Neurosciences, 5th Edition. Edited by Yudofsky SC, Hales RE. Washington, DC, American Psychiatric Publishing, 2008, p 1059

190. Which of the following disorders has been found to frequently co-occur with pathological gambling?

    A. Generalized anxiety disorder.
    B. Panic disorder.
    C. Attention deficit/hyperactivity disorder (ADHD).
    D. Somatization disorder.
    E. Dissociative identity disorder.

**The correct response is option C.**

Pathological gambling has been associated with ADHD. Because an association between alcoholism and childhood ADHD has been found, as well as high co-occurrence between pathological gambling and alcohol abuse, inadequate impulse control may be a key factor that links these three disorders dimensionally.

There also appears to be a strong relationship between pathological gambling and substance abuse, and these are also highly comorbid with affective disorders among inpatient and outpatient samples.

Hollander E, Berlin HA, Stein DJ: Impulse control disorders not elsewhere classified, in The American Psychiatric Publishing Textbook of Psychiatry, 5th Edition. Edited by Hales RE, Yudofsky SC, Gabbard GO. Washington, DC, American Psychiatric Publishing, 2008, p 796

191. Where is the hippocampus located?

    A. Nonmesial portion of the temporal lobe.
    B. The mesial temporal lobe.
    C. Temporoparietal junction of the parietal lobe.
    D. Basal ganglia.
    E. Dorsolateral prefrontal region.

**The correct response is option B.**

The hippocampus is in a region of temporal lobe called the *mesial temporal lobe*, which also includes the amygdala, the entorhinal and perirhinal cortices, and a portion of the anterior parahippocampal gyrus. In addition to the mesial temporal lobe, other subdivisions of the temporal lobe include the temporal pole, inferotemporal lobe, and occipitotemporal junction. Option A is incorrect because the hippocampus is part of the mesial, not nonmesial, portion of the temporal lobe. Option C is incorrect because the hippocampus is part of the temporal, not parietal, lobe. A lesion of the temporoparietial junction of the left parietal lobe may lead to Wernicke's aphasia. Options D and E are incorrect because the hippocampus is part of the cortical, not subcortical, region of the brain that includes the basal ganglia and the thalamus. (See table on next two pages.)

Harel BT, Tranel D: Functional neuroanatomy, in The American Psychiatric Publishing Textbook of Neuropsychiatry and Behavioral Neurosciences, 5th Edition. Edited by Yudofsky SC, Hales RE. Washington, DC, American Psychiatric Publishing, 2008, p 48

192. A number of studies that have compared patients with personality disorders with patients with no personality disorders or with Axis I disorders have found that patients with personality disorders

    A. Were more likely to be married.
    B. Had less unemployment.
    C. Were rarely less well educated.
    D. Had fewer periods of disability.
    E. Had better social functioning.

**The correct response is option C.**

Patients with personality disorders only rarely have been found to be less well educated. A number of studies have found that patients with personality disorders were more likely to be separated, divorced, or never married and to have had more unemployment, frequent job changes, or

## Neuropsychological manifestations of brain lesions

| Structures and major subdivisions | Hemispheric side of lesion | | |
|---|---|---|---|
| | **Left** | **Right** | **Bilateral** |
| **Temporal lobes** | | | |
| Mesial | Anterograde amnesia for verbal material | Anterograde amnesia for nonverbal material | Severe anterograde amnesia for verbal and nonverbal material |
| Temporal pole | Impaired retrieval of proper nouns | Impaired retrieval of concepts for unique entities | Impaired retrieval of concepts and names for unique entities |
| | | Impaired memory for episodic and declarative knowledge | Impaired episodic memory |
| Inferotemporal | Impaired retrieval of common nouns | Impaired retrieval of concepts for some nonunique entities | Impaired retrieval of concepts and names for some nonunique entities |
| Occipito-temporal junction | "Deep" prosopagnosia Impaired retrieval of concepts for some nonunique entities | Transient or mild prosopagnosia Impaired retrieval of concepts for some nonunique entities | Severe, permanent prosopagnosia Visual object agnosia |
| **Occipital lobes** | | | |
| Dorsal | Partial or mild Balint's syndrome | Partial or mild Balint's syndrome | Balint's syndrome (visual disorientation, ocular apraxia, optic ataxia) Defective motion perception Astereopsis |
| Ventral | Right hemiachromatopsia "Pure" alexia Impaired mental imagery | Left hemiachromatopsia Apperceptive visual agnosia Defective facial imagery | Full-field achromatopsia Visual object agnosia Impaired mental imagery Prosopagnosia |
| **Parietal lobes** | | | |
| Temporoparietal junction | Wernicke's aphasia | Amusia Defective music recognition "Phonagnosia" | Auditory agnosia |
| Inferior parietal lobule | Conduction aphasia Tactile object agnosia Acalculia | Neglect Anosognosia Anosodiaphoria Tactile object agnosia | Body schema disturbances Anosognosia Anosodiaphoria |
| **Frontal lobes** | | | |
| Frontal operculum | Broca's aphasia Defective retrieval of words for actions (verbs) | "Expressive" aprosody | Broca's aphasia Defective retrieval of words for actions (verbs) |
| Superior mesial region | Akinetic mutism | Akinetic mutism | Severe akinetic mutism |

## Neuropsychological manifestations of brain lesions *(continued)*

| Structures and major subdivisions | Hemispheric side of lesion | | |
| --- | --- | --- | --- |
| | **Left** | **Right** | **Bilateral** |
| **Frontal lobes (continued)** | | | |
| Basal forebrain (inferior mesial region) | Anterograde and retrograde amnesia with confabulation (worse for verbal stimuli) | Anterograde and retrograde amnesia with confabulation (worse for nonverbal stimuli) | Anterograde and retrograde amnesia with confabulation for verbal and nonverbal stimuli |
| Orbital (inferior mesial region) | Defective social conduct "Acquired" sociopathy Prospective memory defects | Defective social conduct "Acquired" sociopathy Prospective memory defects | Defective social conduct "Acquired" sociopathy Prospective memory defects |
| Dorsolateral prefrontal region | Impaired working memory for verbal material Impaired verbal intellect Defective recency and frequency judgments for verbal material Defective verbal fluency Impaired "executive functions" | Impaired working memory for nonverbal spatial material Impaired nonverbal intellect Defective recency and frequency judgments for nonverbal material Defective design fluency Impaired "executive functions" | Impaired working memory for verbal and nonverbal spatial material Impaired verbal and nonverbal intellect Defective recency and frequency judgments for verbal and nonverbal material Defective verbal and design fluency Impaired "executive functions" |
| **Subcortical structures** | | | |
| Basal ganglia | Atypical aphasia Dysarthria Aprosody Impaired nondeclarative memory Defective motor skill learning | Dysarthria Aprosody Impaired nondeclarative memory Defective motor skill learning | Atypical aphasia Dysarthria Aprosody Impaired nondeclarative memory Defective motor skill learning |
| Thalamus | Thalamic aphasia Anterograde amnesia with confabulation Retrograde amnesia with temporal gradient Impairments in "executive functions" Attention or concentration defects | Anterograde amnesia with confabulation Retrograde amnesia with temporal gradient Impairments in "executive functions" Attention or concentration defects | Thalamic aphasia Anterograde amnesia with confabulation Retrograde amnesia with temporal gradient Impairments in "executive functions" Attention or concentration defects |

periods of disability. Studies that have examined quality of functioning have found poorer social functioning or interpersonal relationships and poorer work functioning or occupational achievement and satisfaction in patients with personality disorders.

Skodol AE, Gunderson JG: Personality disorders, in The American Psychiatric Publishing Textbook of Psychiatry, 5th Edition. Edited by Hales RE, Yudofsky SC, Gabbard GO. Washington, DC, American Psychiatric Publishing, 2008, p 830

193. Which of the following statements is *true* regarding second-generation antipsychotics (SGAs) (or atypical antipsychotics) and first-generation antipsychotics (FGAs)?

A. SGAs have efficacy comparable to that of FGAs in treating positive symptoms of schizophrenia.
B. FGAs are superior to SGAs in treating negative symptoms of schizophrenia.
C. FGAs are superior to SGAs in treating refractory schizophrenia.
D. The incidence of extrapyramidal symptoms in patients treated with FGAs is comparable to that in patients treated with SGAs.
E. The frequency of tardive dyskinesia in patients treated with SGAs is comparable with that in patients treated with FGAs.

## The correct response is option A.

SGAs appear to have efficacy in treatment of positive symptoms that is comparable to that of FGAs. However, SGAs are consistently superior to FGAs (and placebo) in the treatment of negative symptoms. There is some evidence that SGAs (clozapine in particular) exhibit greater efficacy in treatment-refractory schizophrenia. The empirical literature strongly indicates that SGAs are superior to FGAs in terms of the lower incidence of extrapyramidal symptoms resulting from their use. It appears likely that tardive dyskinesia, an important cause of nonadherence, will also emerge as a less frequent effect of SGAs.

Minzenberg MJ, Yoon JH, Carter CS: Schizophrenia, in The American Psychiatric Publishing Textbook of Psychiatry, 5th Edition. Edited by Hales RE, Yudofsky SC, Gabbard GO. Washington, DC, American Psychiatric Publishing, 2008, pp 438–440

194. Other psychiatric disorders must be carefully considered in the differential diagnosis of somatization disorder. The most troublesome distinction is between somatization disorder and which of the following psychiatric disorders?

A. Dissociative disorders.
B. Anxiety disorders.
C. Substance use disorders.
D. Impulse control disorders.
E. Adjustment disorders.

## The correct response is option B.

The following three psychiatric disorders must be carefully considered in the differential diagnosis of somatization disorder: anxiety disorders, mood disorders, and schizophrenia. The most troublesome distinction is between anxiety disorders and somatization disorder. Individuals with anxiety disorders also may have disease concerns and hypochondriacal complaints common to somatization disorder. Similarly, patients with somatization disorder often report panic (anxiety) attacks. Although the usual parameters of age at onset and course may be helpful in differentiating between an anxiety disorder and somatization disorder, the presence of certain traits, symptoms, and social factors can be of assistance. In particular, the presence of histrionic personality traits, conversion and dissociative symptoms, sexual and menstrual problems, and social impairment supports a diagnosis of somatization disorder.

Yutzy SH, Parish BS: Somatoform disorders, in The American Psychiatric Publishing Textbook of Psychiatry, 5th Edition. Edited by Hales RE, Yudofsky SC, Gabbard GO. Washington, DC, American Psychiatric Publishing, 2008, p 617

195. In addition to the substance use disorders characterized by patterns of use, there are several substance-related disorders whose descriptions are based on the pharmacological effects of the substance. Which of the following is *not* true of these illnesses?

A. This category includes both intoxication and withdrawal syndromes.
B. Examples of substance-induced syndromes include dementia and amnestic and mood disorders.
C. All abused substances have a specific intoxication syndrome.
D. All categories of abused substances produce a withdrawal syndrome.

E. Not all categories of abused substances produce all of the substance-induced disorders.

## The correct response is option D.

According to DSM-IV-TR, not all categories of substances produce a withdrawal syndrome or all of the other substance-induced disorders. Disorders produced by the direct pharmacological effects of the substance, referred to as *substance-induced disorders*, include the intoxication and withdrawal syndromes as well as syndromes such as substance-induced dementia and amnestic, psychotic, mood, anxiety, sleep, and sexual dysfunction disorders. Although all categories of substances produce an intoxication syndrome, the symptoms, signs, and durations of the syndromes vary by substance category.

Greenfield SF, Hennessy G: Assessment of the patient, in The American Psychiatric Publishing Textbook of Substance Abuse Treatment, 4th Edition. Edited by Galanter M, Kleber HD. Washington, DC, American Psychiatric Publishing, 2008, p 61

196. All of the following are common medical complications of bulimia nervosa *except*

    A. Elevated serum bicarbonate levels.
    B. Parotid gland enlargement.
    C. Cardiomyopathy.
    D. Elevated amylase levels.
    E. Hyperkalemia.

## The correct response is option E.

Patients with bulimia nervosa who engage in self-induced vomiting and abuse purgatives or diuretics are susceptible to hypokalemic alkalosis. These patients have electrolyte abnormalities, including elevated serum bicarbonate levels, hypochloremia, hypokalemia, and in a few cases low serum bicarbonate levels indicating a metabolic acidosis. Cardiac failure caused by cardiomyopathy from ipecac intoxication is a medical emergency that is being reported more frequently and that usually results in death. Laboratory findings may include elevated liver enzymes and an increased erythrocyte sedimentation rate. Parotid gland enlargement associated with elevated serum amylase levels is commonly observed in patients who binge and vomit. In fact, the serum amylase level is an excellent way to follow reduction of vomiting in patients with eating disorders who deny purging episodes. Esophageal tears also can occur throughout the process.

Halmi KA: Eating disorders, in The American Psychiatric Publishing Textbook of Psychiatry, 5th Edition. Edited by Hales RE, Yudofsky SC, Gabbard GO. Washington, DC, American Psychiatric Publishing, 2008, pp 983–985; Table 23–10

197. Which of the following symptoms is characteristic of temporal, rather than frontal, lobe symptoms?

    A. Heightened interpersonal sensitivity and paranoid ideation.
    B. Social disinhibition.
    C. Reduced attention.
    D. Distractibility.
    E. Impaired judgment.

## The correct response is option A.

Patients with frontal lobe impairments often have different rehabilitative needs than those with temporal lobe deficits. Individuals with temporal lobe dysfunction can show heightened interpersonal sensitivity, which can evolve into frank paranoid ideation. In contrast, individuals with frontal lobe dysfunction caused by stroke, tumor, or other disease processes often show a cluster of symptoms that includes social disinhibition. Other symptoms of frontal lobe dysfunction include reduced attention, distractibility, impaired judgment, affective lability, and more pervasive mood disorders, therefore options B, C, D, and E are incorrect.

Franzen MD, Lovell MR: Cognitive rehabilitation and behavior therapy for patients with neuropsychiatric disorders, in The American Psychiatric Publishing Textbook of Neuropsychiatry and Behavioral Neurosciences, 5th Edition. Edited by Yudofsky SC, Hales RE. Washington, DC, American Psychiatric Publishing, 2008, p 1253

198. Patients with *paranoid personality disorder* exhibit which of the following symptoms?

    A. Delusions.
    B. Suspiciousness.
    C. Marginal thinking.
    D. Perceptual distortions.
    E. Odd thinking.

## The correct response is option B.

Persons with paranoid personality disorder have a pervasive, persistent, and inappropriate mistrust of others. They are suspicious of others' motives and assume that others intend to exploit, harm, or deceive them. Unlike paranoid personality disorder, the Axis I disorders paranoid schizophrenia and delusional disorder, persecutory type, are both characterized by prominent and persistent paranoid delusions of psychotic proportions; paranoid schizophrenia is also accompanied by hallucinations and other core symptoms of schizophrenia. Although paranoid and schizotypal personality disorders both involve suspiciousness, paranoid personality disorder does not include magical thinking, perceptual distortions, or odd thinking or speech.

Skodol AE, Gunderson JG: Personality disorders, in The American Psychiatric Publishing Textbook of Psychiatry, 5th Edition. Edited by Hales RE, Yudofsky SC, Gabbard GO. Washington, DC, American Psychiatric Publishing, 2008, p 833

199. Phencyclidine (PCP) and ketamine cause a schizophrenic-like reaction in humans and affect which of the following neurotransmitters?

    A. Dopamine.
    B. Serotonin.
    C. Nicotine.
    D. Glutamine.
    E. Acetylcholine.

**The correct response is option D.**

The glutamatergic system has become a focus of study in schizophrenia because of its ubiquitous and prominent location in the central nervous system and because the antiglutamatergic drugs PCP and ketamine cause a schizophrenic-like reaction in humans.

Tamminga CA, Shad MJ, Ghose S: Neuropsychiatric aspects of schizophrenia, in The American Psychiatric Publishing Textbook of Neuropsychiatry and Behavioral Neurosciences, 5th Edition. Edited by Yudofsky SC, Hales RE. Washington, DC, American Psychiatric Publishing, 2008, p 980

200. Which of the following symptoms or characteristics is less consistent with malingering of psychosis than with true psychosis?

    A. Atypical hallucinations or delusions.
    B. Marked discrepancies in interview and noninterview behavior.
    C. Blatant contradictions between reported prior episodes and documented psychiatric history.
    D. Psychotic symptoms with common paranoid, grandiose, or religious themes.
    E. Gross inconsistencies in reported psychotic symptoms.

**The correct response is option D.**

Psychotic symptoms associated with common paranoid, grandiose, or religious themes are not consistent with malingering of psychosis.

McDermott BE, Leamon MH, Feldman MD, et al: Factitious disorder and malingering, in The American Psychiatric Publishing Textbook of Psychiatry, 5th Edition. Edited by Hales RE, Yudofsky SC, Gabbard GO. Washington, DC, American Psychiatric Publishing, 2008, p 655; Table 14–6

# References

American Academy of Sleep Medicine: The International Classification of Sleep Disorders, Second Edition (ICSD-2): Diagnostic and Coding Manual. Westchester, IL, American Academy of Sleep Medicine, 2005

American Psychiatric Association: Practice Guidelines for the Treatment of Psychiatric Disorders: Compendium 2006. Arlington, VA, American Psychiatric Association, 2006

American Psychiatric Association: Diagnostic and Statistical Manual of Mental Disorders, 4th Edition, Text Revision. Washington, DC, American Psychiatric Association, 2000

American Psychiatric Association: The Principles of Medical Ethics With Annotations Especially Applicable to Psychiatry, 2001 Edition. Washington, DC, American Psychiatric Association, 2001

Beauchamp TL, Childress JF: Principles of Biomedical Ethics, 5th Edition. New York, Oxford University Press, 2001

Benjamin L, Bourgeois JA, Shahrokh NC, et al: Study Guide to Geriatric Psychiatry: A Companion to The American Psychiatric Publishing Textbook of Geriatric Psychiatry, Third Edition. Washington, DC, American Psychiatric Publishing, 2006

Blazer DG, Steffens DC, Busse EW: The American Psychiatric Publishing Textbook of Geriatric Psychiatry, 3rd Edition. Washington, DC, American Psychiatric Publishing, 2004

Blazer DG, Steffens DC, Busse EW (eds): Essentials of Geriatric Psychiatry. Washington, DC, American Psychiatric Publishing, 2007, pp 242–243

Bourgeois JA, Hales RE, Yudofsky SC: The American Psychiatric Publishing Board Prep and Review Guide for Psychiatry. Washington, DC, American Psychiatric Publishing, 2007

Cozza KL, Armstrong SC, Oesterheld JR, et al: Study Guide to Clinical Psychopharmacology: A Companion to The American Psychiatric Publishing Textbook of Psychopharmacology, Third Edition. Washington, DC, American Psychiatric Publishing, 2004

Fuller MA, Sajatovic M. Drug Information Handbook for Psychiatry, 6th Edition. Hudson, OH, Lexi-Comp, 2007

Galanter M, Kleber HD (eds): The American Psychiatric Publishing Textbook of Substance Abuse Treatment, 4th Edition. Washington, DC, American Psychiatric Publishing, 2008

Grant JE, Potenza MN (eds): Textbook of Men's Mental Health. Washington, DC, American Psychiatric Publishing, 2007, pp 179–180

Hales RE, Bourgeois JA, Shahrokh NC: Study Guide to Neuropsychiatry and Behavioral Neurosciences: A Companion to The American Psychiatric Publishing Textbook of Neuropsychiatry and Behavioral Neurosciences, Fifth Edition. Washington, DC, American Psychiatric Publishing, 2008

Hales RE, Bourgeois JA, Shahrokh NC: Study Guide to Psychiatry: A Companion to The American Psychiatric Publishing Textbook of Psychiatry, Fifth Edition. Washington, DC, American Psychiatric Publishing, 2008

Hales RE, Bourgeois JA, Shahrokh NC, et al: Study Guide to The American Psychiatric Publishing Textbook of Substance Abuse Treatment, Fourth Edition. Washington, DC, American Psychiatric Publishing, 2008

Hales RE, Yudofsky SC, Gabbard GO (eds): The American Psychiatric Publishing Textbook of Psychiatry, 5th Edition. Washington, DC, American Psychiatric Publishing, 2008

Kaufman DM: Clinical Neurology for Psychiatrists, 6th Edition. Philadelphia, PA, Saunders Elsevier, 2008

Leo RJ. Clinical Manual of Pain Management in Psychiatry. Washington, DC, American Psychiatric Publishing, 2007

Levenson JL (ed). The American Psychiatric Publishing Textbook of Psychosomatic Medicine. Washington, DC, American Psychiatric Publishing, 2005

Luria AR: Higher Cortical Functions in Man, 2nd Edition. New York, Basic Books, 1980

MacKinnon RA, Michels R, Buckley PJ: The Psychiatric Interview in Clinical Practice, 2nd Edition. Washington, DC, American Psychiatric Publishing, 2006

McGee S. Evidence-Based Physical Diagnosis. Philadelphia, PA, Saunders Elsevier, 2001

Menninger RW, Nemiah JC (eds): American Psychiatry After World War II, 1944–1994. Washington, DC, American Psychiatric Press, 2000

Moore DP, Jefferson JW: Handbook of Medical Psychiatry, 2nd Edition. Philadelphia, PA, Elsevier Mosby, 2004

Narrow WE, First MB, Sirovatka PJ, et al (eds): Age and Gender Considerations in Psychiatric Diagnosis: A Research Agenda for DSM-V. Arlington, VA, American Psychiatric Association, 2007

Powell AD: Grief, bereavement, and adjustment disorders, in Massachusetts General Hospital Comprehensive Clinical Psychiatry. Edited by Stern TA, Rosenbaum JF, Fava M, et al. Philadelphia, PA, Mosby Elsevier, 2008, p 522

Roberts LW, Hoop JG: Professionalism and Ethics: Q&A Self-Study Guide for Mental Health Professionals. Washington, DC, American Psychiatric Publishing, 2008

Sandson NB: Drug–Drug Interaction Primer: A Compendium of Case Vignettes for the Practicing Clinician. Washington, DC, American Psychiatric Publishing, 2007

Schatzberg AF, Nemeroff CB (eds): The American Psychiatric Publishing Textbook of Psychopharmacology, 3rd Edition. Washington, DC, American Psychiatric Publishing, 2004

Shahrokh NC, Hales RE: American Psychiatric Glossary, 8th Edition. Washington, DC, American Psychiatric Publishing, 2003

Simon RI, Tardiff K: Textbook of Violence Assessment and Management. Washington, DC, American Psychiatric Publishing, 2008

Simon RI, Gold LH (eds): The American Psychiatric Publishing Textbook of Forensic Psychiatry. Washington, DC, American Psychiatric Publishing, 2004

Stewart DE: Menopause: A Mental Health Practitioner's Guide. Washington, DC, American Psychiatric Publishing, 2005

Wiener JM, Dulcan MK (eds): The American Psychiatric Publishing Textbook of Child and Adolescent Psychiatry, 3rd Edition. Washington, DC, American Psychiatric Publishing, 2004

Yudofsky SC, Hales RE (eds): The American Psychiatric Publishing Textbook of Neuropsychiatry and Behavioral Neurosciences, 5th Edition. Washington, DC, American Psychiatric Publishing, 2008

# Index

Page numbers printed in **boldface** type refer to tables or figures.

Hyperinsulinemia, Alzheimer's disease
and, 134
Hyperkinetic movement disorders, tic
disorders, 210–213
Hyperparathyroidism, lithium-induced,
558
Hyperphagia, in depression, 301
Hyperpolarization, 54
Hyperprolactinemia, antipsychotic-
induced, 540, 544, 551, 553
Hyperreflexia, lithium-induced, 317
Hypersalivation, clozapine-induced, 549
Hypersomnia. *See also* Narcolepsy
in depression, 301
Hypertension
Alzheimer's disease and, 134
drug-induced
mirtazapine, **521**
phencyclidine, 271
venlafaxine, 238, **521,** 523
in metabolic syndrome, 544
obstructive sleep apnea and, 458
Hypertensive crisis, monoamine oxidase
inhibitor–induced, 207, 316,
529–531
Hyperthermia
malignant, 543
in neuroleptic malignant syndrome,
543
Hyperthyroidism
anxiety and, 337
mood disorders and, 313
Hypertonus, 150
Hypnotherapy
for depersonalization disorder, 401
for dissociative amnesia, 399–400
for dissociative fugue, 400
for dissociative identity disorder,
404–405
Freud's use of, 582
for male erectile disorder, 417
in pain disorder, 616, **616**
Hypoactive delirium, 221
Hypoactive sexual desire disorder, **413,**
**415,** 415–416
Hypochondriasis, 381–382, 384
clinical features of, 381
diagnostic criteria for, **381**
differential diagnosis of, 381
epidemiology of, 381
etiology of, 381
natural history of, 381
treatment of, 381–382
Hypocretin/orexin, in narcolepsy, 460

Hypoglycemia
monoamine oxidase inhibitor–
induced, 316
Hypogonadism, opioid-induced, **618**
Hypomania, **300,** 302
in bipolar II disorder, 304
in cyclothymic disorder, 305
recurrent brief, **300**
Hyponatremia, oxcarbazepine-induced,
563
Hypopnea, 458
Hypotension, drug-induced
alpha-agonists, 206
antipsychotics, 544
clozapine, 548
mirtazapine, **521**
monoamine oxidase inhibitors, **521,**
529, 531
risperidone, 551
trazodone, **521,** 525
tricyclic antidepressants, 314, **521,**
526, 527
Hypothalamic-pituitary-adrenal (HPA)
axis
in depression, 313
in multiple sclerosis, 73
in panic disorder, 335
in posttraumatic stress disorder, 362
Hypothalamic-pituitary-gonadal (HPG)
axis, in mood disorders, 313–314
Hypothalamic-pituitary-thyroid (HPT)
axis, in mood disorders, 313
Hypothalamic-releasing hormones, 53
Hypothetical thinking, 19
Hypothyroidism
anxiety and, 337
congenital, 199
lithium-induced, **557,** 558
mood disorders and, 313
Hypoxyphilia, 429

Ibuprofen, for HIV dementia, 239
ICD-10. *See International Classification of
Diseases*
ICDs. *See* Impulse-control disorders
"Ice." *See* Methamphetamine, abuse of
Id, 4
Id anxiety, 335
Ideas of reference, 278
Identification, 11, **590**
Identification with the aggressor, **590, 591**
Identity
emancipated, 19–20, **20**
false, 20

gender, 8, 10, 12, 18
peer, 12, 15
sexual, 12, 14, 18
social, 15
Identity confusion, 20
IED. *See* Intermittent explosive disorder
*Ikota,* 109
Imagery, in cognitive therapy, 601, 604
Imagery rehearsal, for nightmare
disorder, 465
Imaginal desensitization, for
kleptomania, 474
Imipramine, 526
dosage and half-life of, **519, 527**
indications for
bulimia nervosa, 446, **446,** 447
generalized anxiety disorder, **344,**
345
kleptomania, 474
panic disorder, 338, **339**
posttraumatic stress disorder, 365
therapeutic plasma levels of, 173,
**175,** 527
Imitation, deferred, 9
Immune deficiencies, 71–72. *See also*
Human immunodeficiency virus
disease
Immune system, 71–75
cytokines, 71, 75
diseases due to dysfunction of, 71–72
primary and secondary immune
tissues, 71
psychiatric illness and, 74–75
bipolar disorder, 75
depression, 74–75
schizophrenia, 75
stress, depression and, 72–74
in AIDS, 73
in cancer, 72–73
in Graves' disease, 74
in multiple sclerosis, 73
in systemic lupus erythematosus,
74
types of cells in, 71
Immunocompromised patients,
clozapine in, 549
Immunoglobulin G, **167**
Impulse anxiety, 335
Impulse-control disorders (ICDs),
469–478
assessment instruments for, 478
classification of, 469, **470**
intermittent explosive disorder,
469–472, **470**

Multiple personality disorder. *See* Dissociative identity disorder

Multiple sclerosis (MS), 73
   dementia due to, 232
   magnetic resonance imaging in, **186**

Multiple sleep latency test (MSLT), 460, 461

Multisystemic therapy, for conduct disorder, 207

Munchausen syndrome, 387, 391. *See also* Factitious disorder
   by proxy, 389–390

Muscarinic receptors, drug affinity for
   antipsychotics, 290, **290**
      clozapine, 548
      olanzapine, 549
   mirtazapine, 526
   tricyclic antidepressants, 526

Muscle cramps, drug-induced
   acetylcholinesterase inhibitors, 236
   monoamine oxidase inhibitors, 316

Muscle relaxants
   interaction with lithium, 558
   for pain disorders, **617,** 621

Mutism
   akinetic, 38, **41, 46,** 149
   definition of, 148
   examination for, 148–149
   selective, cultural factors and, 106

Myelin basic protein, **167**

Myelination, 53

Myeloid immune cells, 71

Myocardial infarction, drug-related. *See also* Cardiovascular effects of drugs
   alcohol, 258
   cocaine, 264

Myoclonus
   lithium-induced, 317
   monoamine oxidase inhibitor–induced, 316
   in serotonin syndrome, 522, 531

Myoglobin, urine, **168**

*Myriachit,* 109

Nadolol, for aggression in patients with traumatic brain injury, 674

Naloxone, for opioid overdose, 264, **265**

Naltrexone
   for alcoholism, **262,** 273
   for kleptomania, 474

Naming, 149
   defects in
      in Broca's aphasia, 37
      due to parietal lobe lesion, 34, **37**

role of temporal lobe structures in, 30
   testing of, 149

Narcissism, 12–13

Narcissistic personality disorder, 489, 502–504
   clinical features of, **490,** 502–503
   diagnostic criteria for, **503**
   differential diagnosis of, 503
      antisocial personality disorder, 498
   epidemiology of, 502
   etiology of, 503
   gender identity disorder and, 425
   treatment of, **493,** 503–504

Narcolepsy, 459–460, 466
   assessment and diagnosis of, 460
   with cataplexy, 459
   clinical features of, 459
   epidemiology of, **132,** 460
   pathophysiology of, 460
   relative risk for, **132**
   treatment of, 460, **461**

Narcotics Anonymous, **258,** 477

Nardil. *See* Phenelzine

NASSA (norepinephrine and serotonin specific antidepressant), **315, 520.** *See also* Mirtazapine

National Comorbidity Survey (NCS), 137, 272, 307, 308, **312,** 336, 346, 359, 628

National Comorbidity Survey Replication (NCS-R), 307, **312**

National Epidemiologic Survey on Alcohol and Related Conditions (NESARC), 333, 342, 346

National Institute of Clinical Excellence, 320

National Institute of Mental Health (NIMH)
   Clinical Antipsychotic Trials of Intervention Effectiveness (CATIE), 291, 544, 545, 547, 550, 553, 637
   Collaborative Study of Affective Disorders, 64, **64**
   Epidemiologic Catchment Area study, 110, 137, 256, 272, 307, **312,** 333, 336, 377, 381

National Practitioner Data Bank, 119

National Survey on Drug Use and Health, 255, 259, 263, 264

Natural killer (NK) cells, 71, 73, 74

Nausea/vomiting
   antipsychotics for treatment of, 538
   drug-induced
      acetylcholinesterase inhibitors, 236
      aripiprazole, 553
      bupropion, **521**
      buspirone, 536
      carbamazepine, 317
      clomipramine, 357
      duloxetine, **521,** 524
      lamotrigine, 318
      lithium, 317
      monoamine oxidase inhibitors, 316
      opioids, 264, **618**
      selective serotonin reuptake inhibitors, 521, **521**
      valproate, 317, 559, 560
      venlafaxine, 345
      ziprasidone, 553
   self-induced vomiting
      in anorexia nervosa, 438
      in bulimia nervosa, 443, 444

Navane. *See* Thiothixene

NBRS (Neurobehavioral Rating Scale), **664**

NCS (National Comorbidity Survey), 137, 272, 307, 308, **312,** 336, 346, 359, 628

NCS-R (National Comorbidity Survey Replication), 307, **312**

NDI (nephrogenic diabetes insipidus), lithium-induced, 555, **556**

NDRIs (norepinephrine and dopamine reuptake inhibitors), **315, 520.** *See also* Bupropion

NE. *See* Norepinephrine

Necrophilia, **429,** 430

Nefazodone, **315, 321**
   dosage and half-life of, **520**
   interaction with eszopiclone, 537

Neglect, 34, **38**
   testing for, 98

Negligence, 117–119, **650**
   related to electroconvulsive therapy, 119
   related to psychopharmacotherapy, 117–119, **118**

Nembutal. *See* Pentobarbital

NEMESIS (Netherlands Mental Health Survey and Incidence Study), 307, 308, **312**